# Psychiatric Nursing

**Norman L. Keltner, EdD, RN, APRN**
Professor
School of Nursing
University of Alabama at Birmingham
Birmingham, Alabama

**Lee Hilyard Schwecke, RN, MSN, EdD**
Associate Professor
School of Nursing
Indiana University
Indianapolis, Indiana

**Carol E. Bostrom, MSN, APRN, BC**
Clinical Assistant Professor
School of Nursing
Indiana University
Indianapolis, Indiana

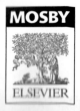

MOSBY
ELSEVIER

203.

(ENSYD)

# MOSBY
### ELSEVIER

11830 Westline Industrial Drive
St. Louis, MO 63146

PSYCHIATRIC NURSING

ISBN-13: 978-0-323-03906-2
ISBN-10: 0-323-03906-5

Copyright © 2007, 1995, 1991 by Mosby, Inc., an affiliate of Elsevier Inc.

---

### Notice

Knowledge and best practice in this field are constantly changing. As new research and experience broaden our knowledge, changes in practice, treatment and drug therapy may become necessary or appropriate. Readers are advised to check the most current information provided (i) on procedures featured or (ii) by the manufacturer of each product to be administered, to verify the recommended dose or formula, the method and duration of administration, and contraindications. It is the responsibility of the practitioner, relying on their own experience and knowledge of the patient, to make diagnoses, to determine dosages and the best treatment for each individual patient, and to take all appropriate safety precautions. To the fullest extent of the law, neither the Publisher nor the Authors assume any liability for any injury and/or damage to persons or property arising out or related to any use of the material contained in this book.

---

ISBN-13: 978-0-323-03906-2
ISBN-10: 0-323-03906-5

Executive Editor: Tom Wilhelm
Developmental Editor: Allison M. Brock
Publishing Services Manager: John Rogers
Project Manager: Doug Turner
Cover Design Direction: Paula Ruckenbrod
Text Design: Paula Ruckenbrod

Printed in the United States of America

Last digit is the print number: 9 8 7 6 5 4 3 2 1

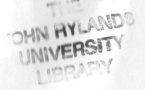

# Contributors

**Beverly K. Hogan, BSN, MSN, APRN, BC**
School of Nursing
University of Alabama at Birmingham
Birmingham, Alabama

**Maryellen Pachler, MSN**
Child Psychiatric Nurse Practitioner
Yale Child Study Center
Yale University
New Haven, Connecticut

**Gordon Pugh, M Div, M Phil, BCC, MLAP, ICADC**
Chaplain
Children's Health System
Birmingham, Alabama

**Lawrence Scahill, MSN, PhD**
Professor
Yale Child Study Center
Yale University School of Nursing
New Haven, Connecticut

**Mona Shattell, PhD, RN**
Assistant Professor
School of Nursing
University of North Carolina at Greensboro
Greensboro, North Carolina

**Richard A. Sugerman, PhD**
Professor of Anatomy
Executive Assistant Dean for Basic Sciences
    and Research
College of Osteopathic Medicine of the Pacific
Western University of Health Sciences
Pomona, California

**Barbara Jones Warren, PhD, APRN, BC**
Associate Clinical Professor
College of Nursing
Ohio State University
Columbus, Ohio
Executive Nurse
The Ohio Department of Mental Health
Columbus, Ohio

**Judith A. Wilson, APRN, BC**
Clinical Nurse Specialist
Geriatric Psychiatry
Center for Psychiatric Medicine
UAB Hospital
University of Alabama at Birmingham
Birmingham, Alabama

**Sandra Jean Wood, MSN, APRN, BC**
Clinical Assistant Professor
School of Nursing
Indiana University
Indianapolis, Indiana

# Reviewers

**Kim Abel, MSN**
Nursing Instructor
Health Professions
Illinois Valley Community College
Oglesby, Illinois

**Catherine L. Batscha, APRN, BC**
Instructor
College of Nursing
University of Illinois at Chicago
Chicago, Illinois

**Linnea Carlson-Sabelli, PhD, APRN-BC, TEP**
Associate Professor
Community Mental Health Nursing
Rush University College of Nursing
Chicago, Illinois

**Joan C. Masters, MA, MBA, RN**
Assistant Professor of Nursing
Lansing School of Nursing and Health Sciences
Bellarmine University
Louisville, Kentucky

**Deborah L. Schiavone, DNSc, APRN, BC**
Assistant Professor
Division of Nursing
Howard University
Washington, D.C.

**April Lynne Shapiro, RN, BSN, MSN, MS**
Nursing Instructor
Mineral County School of Practical Nursing
Keyser, West Virginia

**Betty L. Sherrard, RN, MSN, DCC**
RN Admission Coordinator
Call Center
Sutter Center for Psychiatry
Sacramento, California

**Donna R. Talty, RN, MSN, FNP**
Associate Professor, Nursing
Oakton Community College
Des Plaines, Illinois

**Judy Walker, BSN, MSN**
Assistant Professor
Associate Degree Nursing Program
Western Kentucky University
Bowling Green, Kentucky

# Preface

The first edition of *Psychiatric Nursing,* published in 1991, coincided with the dawning of the Decade of the Brain. When we wrote the prospectus for the book in late 1987, we had not heard of the Decade of the Brain—but we anticipated it. From the beginning we emphasized the psychobiologic nature of some mental disorders and the need for psychiatric nurses to grapple with these concepts without letting go of their traditional emphasis on the nurse-patient relationship. These ideas were first presented in an article that was featured in *Perspectives in Psychiatric Care* and entitled "Psychotherapeutic Management: A Model for Nursing Practice." Alice R. Clarke, the editor of *Perspectives* at the time, enthusiastically embraced the idea of this "new" but old approach to psychiatric nursing. She leapfrogged this manuscript past others and published these ideas in the next edition. Alice understood the need for a change in thinking in psychiatric nursing practice.

The psychotherapeutic management model simply states that psychiatric nurses have three primary tools:

- Themselves
- Medications
- Environment

This simple paradigm is informed by an in-depth understanding of psychopathology. Based on this model therapeutic language, psychotropic medications, and environmental considerations change depending on the patient's diagnosis. In other words, one size does not fit all. For example, an understanding of the psychopathology of schizophrenia leads a nurse to recognize that nursing interactions, medications, and environmental concerns for a schizophrenic patient differ from those of a patient with a substance abuse disorder.

Though the psychotherapeutic management model is simple, implementation requires diligent study and practice. Thus, to use the model, the nurse must understand the psychobiologic basis for mental disorders. However, for many students and for some faculty members, developing this understanding is a daunting task. Nonetheless, a solid grounding in psychobiologic concepts will elevate the nurse's level of practice. The same is true for psychopharmacology. This field is changing so rapidly that without an appreciation of basic concepts, the nurse is left bewildered and even unsafe.

We believe the straightforward approach to psychiatric care presented in *Psychiatric Nursing* is an effective method of care and is readily learned by students. New students can use the model almost immediately. The model directs students' attention toward important parameters of care. More experienced students and seasoned nurses can examine each intervention approach and the related psychopathologic factors to gain a deeper understanding and to refine their nursing care practice. The original article published in the 1980s captured the potential of this approach:

*Psychotherapeutic management is "real world" nursing. Mastery of the components—psychopharmacology, therapeutic nurse-patient communication, and milieu management—grounded in psychopathological concepts is a challenging but achievable undertaking: one that will provide a model for productive psychiatric nursing and a distinct sense of professional achievement and role clarity for the psychiatric nurse (Keltner, 1985).*

## ORGANIZATION

The book is organized into six units:

Unit I: Introduction to Psychiatric Nursing
Unit II: Therapeutic Nurse-Patient Relationship
Unit III: Psychopharmacology
Unit IV: Milieu Management
Unit V: Psychopathology

Unit VI: Special Populations and Therapies in Psychiatric Nursing

The crucial units are those that flesh out the three psychotherapeutic interventions (Units II, III, and IV) and the unit on psychopathology (Unit V). The material in the other units (e.g., electroconvulsive therapy in Unit VI) support the model or touch on issues not expressly addressed by the model.

## WHAT'S NEW

- Chapter 22, **Antidementia Drugs**, introduces what nurses need to know about up-to-date psychopharmacology for antidementia disorders.
- Updated *DSM-IV-TR* **content** based on the latest Text Revision is provided throughout the text.
- **Putting It All Together** headings identify end-of-chapter psychopathology summary in each of the clinical chapters.
- **Norm's Notes,** direct author-to-student communications in the form of a Post-it Note, communicate helpful tips for understanding difficult topics.
- **Highlighting the Evidence** boxes, found in the Psychopathology and Milieu Management units, summarize research articles that demonstrate the effects of research on today's practice.

## FEATURES

- **Patient and Family Education** boxes in selected disorders chapters highlight information that nurses need to provide to patients and families.
- **Critical Thinking Questions** are interspersed throughout the narrative to expand students' clinical reasoning skills.
- **Family Issues** boxes in selected chapters discuss issues that families confront when a family member experiences mental illness.
- **Clinical Examples,** concise vignettes drawn from the authors' experiences, provide realistic illustrations of specific content.
- **Case Studies,** detailed depictions of psychiatric disorders, are used in selected chapters to help the student conceptualize the development of effective nursing care strategies.
- **Nursing Care Plans,** based on the six steps of the nursing process, are carefully developed from the case studies.

- *DSM-IV-TR* and **NANDA International** diagnoses are compared to help students understand their interrelationship.
- Boxes and tables with **pharmacologic content** are highlighted with a special symbol ⊘.
- **Study Notes** are placed at the end of each chapter to summarize important content.
- A **Glossary** with up-to-date definitions for key psychiatric terms provides a quick reference.

## RESOURCES FOR THE STUDENT AND INSTRUCTOR

- New **Student Study CD-ROM** contains review questions for the NCLEX examination, animations (including a neurology review), interactive exercises, and an audio glossary.
- Updated **Evolve web site for Students** includes open-book quizzes, answers to Critical Thinking Questions found in the textbook, and supplemental appendixes.
- Updated **Evolve web site for Instructors** includes:
  - All elements from Evolve web site for Students
  - An **instructor's manual** with chapter focus, key terms, learning objectives, chapter outlines, and teaching strategies for each chapter
  - Completely revised computerized **test bank** with approximately 900 questions with correct answers, rationale for the correct answers, objectives, stages of the nursing process, and cognitive level
  - More than 400 **PowerPoint slides** containing full-color figures from this textbook, as well as unique psychobiology slides from additional resources

As is true of all nursing text authors, our goal is to present accurate and meaningful information to the student without the distraction of sexist language. Where possible, we have made every attempt to avoid the use of sexist pronouns by using plural nouns and pronouns or "his or her" rather than risk stigmatizing by gender. To avoid awkwardness of style, we have sometimes referred to the nurse as "she" and the patient as "he."

**Norman L. Keltner**
**Lee Hilyard Schwecke**
**Carol E. Bostrom**

# Acknowledgments

The fact that *Psychiatric Nursing* warrants a fifth edition humbles me. Past editions mention those who guided my thinking, encouraged me at the right time, or pushed me to develop my philosophy of and approach to psychiatric nursing care. I remember these individuals and their contributions to my life and others who mean so much. So, if my list grows long, it is because my debt runs high.

1963: Jeanne Lough, Stockton State Hospital: My first "psychiatric" teacher

1964: Vi Torres Lawrence, Delta College: Told me to shape up or ship out—old-fashioned motivation; Willie Smith, Mitch Patterson, and Dan Ramsey: fellow students at Delta College

1967: Army Nurse Corp: Where I learned the importance of an education

1971: John Bergey and Cleo Metcalf, Fresno State College: Encouraged me to pursue a Master's in psychiatry

1972: Jo Bacci, Stockton State Hospital: Gave me my first job as a teacher

1973: Sarah

1977: Amanda

1982: Alex

1987: Alice Clarke, editor of *Perspectives in Psychiatric Care*: Really liked my concept of "Psychotherapeutic Management," which led to this and other textbooks

1988: Linda Duncan and Jeff Burnham, Mosby

1989: Lee Schwecke and Carol Bostrom: Agreed to help me birth this book

1990: Rachel Booth, University of Alabama School of Nursing (UASON)

1991: David Folks: Helped me write *Psychotropic Drugs*

1994: Elizabeth Morrison and Arthur Ree Campbell, UASON: Real encouragers

1998: Jeanne Allison and Jeff Downing, Mosby

1999: Mary Paquette, editor of *Perspectives in Psychiatric Care*: She continues to be a wonderful sounding board and friend

2000: Beverly Hogan, psychiatric nursing faculty, UASON: Helped me think through many thorny issues concerning psychiatric nursing

2001: The Elsevier folks—Terri Wood, Cathy Ott, Jeanne Allison, and Dana Peick

2002: Barbara Woodring: Has helped me clarify my thinking on all kinds of stuff and still does

2005: Tom Wilhelm, Allison Brock, and Doug Turner at Elsevier: Continue to help me drain the swamp

2006: Doreen Harper: Kept me honest by encouraging me to resharpen my clinical skills

I also want to thank my students over the years. Many have given ideas on how to improve the book; others have indicated what we are doing right. I particularly want to thank those students who have taken the time to let me know that they actually have read the book. From the beginning I wanted a textbook that students would read. I keep hearing from students that they do.

Finally, I dedicate this book to my three grandsons: Sam, Asher, and Izzy.

**NLK**

This book would not have been possible without the hundreds of patients, victims, and survivors who were willing to share their pain, experiences, and successes. I also appreciate the students, faculty, and colleagues who questioned and challenged the content in the earlier editions and offered input for this edition. Norm Keltner, Carol Bostrom, and Sandy Wood deserve special mention for their insights and support. Over time, the staff of Community Hospital North Psychiatric Pavilion have helped me expand my knowledge and develop more effective intervention strategies. A sincere thank you to all who have touched my life and thereby influenced this book.

**LHS**

I want to thank Norman Keltner, Lee Schwecke, and our contributors for their dedication toward making this fifth edition possible. Most of all, I want to thank the faculty and students who have shared their thoughts and given us valuable feedback about this textbook.

**CEB**

# Contents

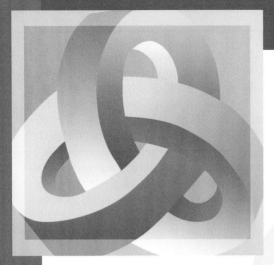

# Chapter 1

# Introduction to Psychiatric Nursing

*Norman L. Keltner*

## Learning Objectives

*After reading this chapter, you should be able to:*
- Describe the enormity of mental health concerns in both human and financial contexts.
- Explain the history of psychiatry as a foundation for current psychiatric nursing practice.
- Identify the significant changes that occurred during the period of the Enlightenment.
- Relate the contributions of early scientists to the current understanding of mental illness.
- Explain the impact of psychotropic drugs on psychiatric care.
- Analyze the immediate and long-term effects of the community mental health movement.
- Describe the impact of the Decade of the Brain on psychiatric care.
- Identify the specific strengths that enable psychiatric nurses to become effective in the new continuum of care.

*Some people's illnesses are so severe that they will always need asylum. A continuum of care is needed: from total freedom to total hospitalization, reflecting the diverse needs of mentally ill people.*

*Mona Wasow (professional social worker [MSW] and mother of a mentally ill adult; 1993)*

**Note to students:** *It is an interesting time to be studying psychiatric nursing. In June of 2001, we were all stunned by the news of a mother of five young children who killed her four boys: Luke, 2; Paul, 3; John, 5; Noah, 7; and her only daughter, Mary, 6 months. Andrea Yeats, 36 at the time, was said to suffer from postpartum depression (Jones, 2001). In March of 2005, Jeff Weise (Lee, 2006), a 16-year-old student from Red Lake, Minnesota, opened fire on faculty and students at his high school, killing nine and wounding seven. Weise, who died also, was being treated for a mental disorder and had been prescribed Prozac. His family wondered whether his medication might have contributed to his loss of control. A long list of similar tragic events can be generated. Whether or not you are sympathetic to these individuals, you have to admit that they provoke interest. Such issues are complex and fall considerably outside the mainstream of psychiatric nursing care; nonetheless, they are related to what you will be studying in this text. Therefore, although most of you will not work full time in psychiatric nursing, you can learn a lot about mental illness, mental health, and yourself, and be better able to understand headlines in your morning papers, by reading this text.*

Epidemiologic evidence has indicated that almost 10% of American adults older than 18 years have a serious mental disorder in any 12-month period (Substance Abuse and Mental Health Services Administration [SAMSHA], 2005)

**Norm's Notes**

Well, here we are—just the two of us alone with the first chapter of your textbook for your new psych course. This chapter discusses history, and when you understand history, you understand context. Without an understanding of history, many things do not and cannot make sense. But more than that, this chapter describes where we have been and how we got here. It can help you understand things better, like the homeless guy sitting on the sidewalk who is acting strangely, or the incessant ads for antidepressants in the media. It is an introduction and, as such, provides a foundation for the rest of the book.

and twice that many suffer when less severe forms are included (U.S. Surgeon General, 1999). When addictive disorders are added, studies reveal that approximately 25%, or 44 million Americans, are affected each year (National Institute of Mental Health [NIMH], 2005; U.S. Surgeon General, 1999). Table 1-1 provides a breakdown by diagnosis of the disorders prevalent at any time in American society. The pervasiveness of these maladies and the tremendous costs that they incur indicate a great need for psychiatric professionals, including nurses, today and in the foreseeable future.

## BENCHMARKS IN PSYCHIATRIC HISTORY

*And a certain woman . . . had suffered many things of many physicians, and had spent all that she had, and was nothing bettered, but rather grew worse.*

Mark 5:25-26, King James Version (1611)

| **Table 1-1** | **12-Month Prevalence Rate of Mental Disorders in the United States*** |

| Disorders | Approximate Number Older Than 17 Years (%) | Approximate Number of Persons | Gender Overrepresentation |
|---|---|---|---|
| **Anxiety Disorders** | 18.0 overall | 36,000,000 | |
| Panic disorder | 3.5 | 7,000,000 | Women |
| Social phobia | 7.0 | 14,000,000 | Women |
| Specific phobia | 8.7 | 17,000,000 | Women |
| Generalized anxiety disorder | 3.0 | 6,000,000 | Women |
| Posttraumatic stress disorder | 3.5 | 7,000,000 | Women |
| Obsessive compulsive disorder | 1.0 | 2,000,000 | Equal |
| **Mood Disorders** | 9.5 overall | 19,000,000 | |
| Major depression | 6.7 | | Women |
| Dysthymia | 1.5 | | Women |
| Bipolar I and II | 2.6 | | BD I: Equal BD II: Women (?) |
| **Impulse Control Disorders** | 9.0 overall | 18,000,000 | |
| Conduct disorders | 1.0 | 2,000,000 | Men |
| Attention-deficit/hyperactivity disorder | 4.0 | 8,000,000 | Men |
| **Substance Abuse Disorders** | 3.8 overall | 7,600,000 | |
| Alcohol abuse and dependence | 3.1 | 6,200,000 | Men |
| Drug abuse and dependence | 1.4 | 2,800,000 | Men |
| **Schizophrenia** | 1.1 | 2,100,000 | Equal |

*Extrapolated from several sources based on current census data.
From Kessler RC, Chiu WT, Demler O, Walters EE: Prevalance, severity, and comorbidity of 12-month DSM-IV disorders in the national comorbidity survey replication. *Arch Gen Psychiatry* 62:617-627, 2005; U.S. Surgeon General: *Mental health: a report from the Surgeon General*, Washington, DC, 1999, Department of Health and Human Services; National Institute of Mental Health: Available at http://www.nimh.nih.gov/; accessed April 18, 2005.

The modern era of psychiatric care can be traced from events that occurred in England and France near the end of the eighteenth century, a time referred to as the Enlightenment. Before this time, the mentally ill were often regarded as no better than wild animals. Rosenblatt (1984) has written of the ABC's of community response during this time: assistance, banishment, and confinement. Assistance, the least restrictive approach, provided food and money and often enabled the family to maintain its integrity as a unit. Banishment occurred in some communities, particularly when the deranged were strangers. Banishment led to wandering bands of "lunatics . . . living no one cared how, and dying no one cared where" (Rosenblatt, 1984). The infamous "Ship of Fools"—boatloads of the mentally disordered cast out to sea to find their "right minds"—occurred during this period.

Confinement was the most restrictive method of coping with the mentally ill, who were often chained. The old and the young, men and women, the insane, criminals, and paupers were indiscriminately mixed. The mentally ill were thought to be immune to normal biologic stressors such as cold, heat, and hunger. Patients were placed on display for the amusement of their caretakers and the paying public. For example, until 1770, a small fee was charged to visitors of St. Mary of Bethlem Hospital (Bedlam) in England. At Bedlam, treatments such as bleeding, bathing, vomiting and purging, and forced feedings were common therapeutic interventions (McMillan, 1997). At Bicêtre in France, the attendants served as "ringmasters," using whips to "encourage" their patients to perform (Rosenblatt, 1984). These warehouses for the tormented discouraged outside intrusion and attracted employees who were at the bottom levels of society, both socially and morally.

As the late 1700s approached, a day of enlightenment dawned, the establishment of the asylum. Five periods stand out as benchmarks in the evolution of modern psychiatric care (Table 1-2):

Benchmark I: ~1790s
Benchmark II: ~late 1800s
Benchmark III: ~1950s
Benchmark IV: 1960s
Benchmark V: 1990s

During each of these five periods, the way of thinking about the mentally ill underwent signifi-

cant changes. After each one, events occurred that were important in their own right, but the inspirational sources of these events can be traced to the aforementioned benchmarks.

## BENCHMARK I: PERIOD OF ENLIGHTENMENT

*To consider madness incurable . . . is constantly refuted by the most authentic facts.*
                    *Philippe Pinel, December 11, 1794*
                            *(cited in Weiner, 1992)*

The modern era of psychiatric care began with the involvement of two men, Philippe Pinel in France and William Tuke in England. In 1793, Pinel became the superintendent of the French institution, Bicêtre (for men) and, later, the Salpêtrière (for women). Pinel was dismayed by the conditions he found and wrote of the patients, "They were abandoned to the incompetence of a callous director and to the cold brutality of servants . . ." (Weiner, 1992). Soon after assuming leadership, Pinel unchained the shackled, clothed the naked, fed the hungry, and abolished the whips and other instruments of abuse. Simultaneously, in England, William Tuke was planning a private facility that would ensure moral treatment for the mentally ill after he witnessed the deplorable conditions in public facilities. In 1796, based on Quaker teachings, the York Retreat opened for patients, providing "a place in which the unhappy might obtain refuge—a quiet haven in which the shattered bark might find a means of reparation or safety" (Gollaher, 1995). Pinel and Tuke were responsible for this first benchmark of modern psychiatric care.

### Asylum

The concept of the asylum developed from the humane efforts of Pinel and Tuke. The term *asylum* can mean protection, social support, or sanctuary from the stresses of life. A touring Chinese gymnast pleading for asylum is a good example of this definition. Currently, however, asylum most often provokes an image of mistreatment and neglect. It was the first definition that motivated Pinel, Tuke, and other similarly minded individuals. Understanding that mental illness worsened with stress, these individuals sought to provide an environment relatively free from stressors. Their language is inappropriate

| Table 1-2 | **Benchmark Periods in Psychiatric History** | | |

| Period | Key People or Developments | Significant Change in Thinking | Result(s) |
| --- | --- | --- | --- |
| Enlightenment, ~1790s | Pinel (1745-1826): Unchained the mentally ill (1793)<br>Tuke (1732-1822): Established the York Retreat | Insane no longer treated as less than human<br>Human dignity upheld | Asylum movement developed |
| Scientific Study, ~1870s | Freud (1856-1939): Emphasized the importance of early life experiences in shaping mental health<br>Kraepelin (1856-1926): Developed classification of mental illness<br>Bleuler (1857-1939): Was optimistic about treatment | Humans could be studied; study held promise for treating and curing mental health problems | Study of the mind and treatment approaches to psychiatric conditions flourished<br>Decade of the Brain can be traced back to Kraepelin's thinking |
| Psychotropic drugs, ~1950s | 1949: Lithium<br>1950: First antipsychotic<br>1952: Monoamine oxidase inhibitors (MAOIs)<br>1957: Haloperidol<br>1958: Tricyclic antidepressants (TCAs)<br>1960: Benzodiazepines | Some mental disorders caused by chemical imbalances; if chemical problem could be found through research, chemical cure could also be found; people would no longer need to be confined | A destigmatization of mental illness occurred; parents and others not to blame; term *least restrictive environment* evolved from this discovery |
| Community Mental Health, ~1960s | Community Mental Health Centers Act (1963) | Individuals do not need to be hospitalized away from family and community; people have the right to be treated in their own community | *Advantage:* Intervention in familiar surroundings has helped many people, is less expensive<br>*Disadvantage:* Homelessness linked to deinstitutionalization; many people "slip through the cracks" of the system |
| Decade of the Brain, 1990s | Congressional mandate | If we can understand the brain, we can help millions of people suffering from mental disorders | An increase in funding for brain research, leading to new treatment strategies; has increased our understanding of mental disorders |

today—"madness, lunacy, insanity, idiocy, feeble-mindedness"—but these were the accepted terms of their day. These early reformers were driven by a desire to improve the lot of abandoned, mentally ill persons and to provide asylum or sanctuary.

Dorothea Dix (1802-1887), one of the first major reformers in the United States, was instrumental in developing the concept of asylum; she played a direct role in opening 32 state hospitals.

Her efforts invariably have been described as a crusade. Several years before launching her crusade, she visited Tuke's York Retreat. Undoubtedly, Tuke's moral treatment influenced her to confront the pain and suffering she had witnessed in her native land. Dix came to believe that the people of the United States had an obligation to their mentally ill brothers and sisters. She proposed to alleviate suffering with adequate shelter, nutritious food, and warm clothing. In Gollaher's biography of Dix (1995), he quotes from one of her Memorials, the documents she wrote to expose the terrible plight of the insane. From her Massachusetts Memorial, he notes:

*Concord:* A woman from the [Worcester] hospital in a cage in the almshouse. In the jail several, decently cared for in general but not properly placed in a prison. Violent, noisy, unmanageable most of the time.
*Lincoln:* A woman in a cage.
*Medford:* One idiotic subject chained, and one in a close [or narrow] stall for 17 years . . .
*Granville:* One often closely confined . . . now losing the use of his limbs from want of exercise.

Although Dix is rightfully credited with being the first reformer to have a nationwide perspective, other more regional sanctuaries had been established before she began her crusade. The first asylum in the United States was the Eastern Lunatic Asylum in Williamsburg, Virginia, founded in 1773. Other institutions followed, such as the Frankford Asylum near Philadelphia (1813), the Bloomingdale Asylum in New York (1818), and the Hartford Retreat in Connecticut (1824). The Philadelphia and New York asylums were established under Quaker influence and thus can be traced to Tuke.

The period of Enlightenment was short-lived. Within 100 years of the establishment of the first asylum, the reformers were being charged with misuse and abuse of their charges. State hospitals were beset with problems. The first definition of asylum *(sanctuary)* had materialized in the form of hospitals built in rural settings. Patients were isolated geographically, socially and, after release, from follow-up care. Patients were also isolated from public scrutiny, which enabled many large institutions to become closed systems. As might be guessed, the beneficence of the reformers was not shared by the many caretakers who followed. Within a relatively brief period, the meaning of asylum changed; it evolved from a place of refuge to a place of torment.

Today, a renewed interest in asylum as a place of rest and restoration exists. This concept can be considered in terms of the four P's: parents, professionals, patients, and public, each of which has a stake in the discussion of asylum. Wasow (1993) has written persuasively of the need for asylum: "Some people's illnesses are so severe that they will always need asylum. A continuum of care is needed: from total freedom to total hospitalization, reflecting the diverse needs of mentally ill people."

| CRITICAL THINKING QUESTION | 1 |
|---|---|

1. Which of the two definitions of "asylum" do you believe is more prevalent in psychiatric nursing today?
2. What are some negative outcomes of deinstitutionalization that you have witnessed or with which you have been personally involved?

## BENCHMARK II: PERIOD OF SCIENTIFIC STUDY

The shift in focus from sanctuary to treatment is linked to the second benchmark in psychiatric care, personified by Sigmund Freud (1856-1939). Toward the last third of the nineteenth century, several scientists devoted themselves to understanding the mind and mental illness. The fruits of their labor held great promise, some of which is still unfulfilled. Nonetheless, the efforts forever changed the world's view: mental illness need not be suffered (however humanely patients were treated) but might be alleviated. In a sense, psychiatric care was popularized.

### *Early Scientists*

Although Freud had the greatest impact on the world's view of mental illness, he neither thought nor worked in a vacuum. Other men and women had tremendous influence on this newly enthusiastic and optimistic approach to mental illness. Emil Kraepelin (1856-1926) made tremendous contributions to the classification of mental disorders. He was a true scientist whose classic descriptions of schizophrenia are valuable reading. Eugene Bleuler (1857-1939) coined the term *schizophrenia* and added a note of optimism to its treatment. Still others, many of whom were colleagues or disciples of Freud, made significant contributions to the emerging field of psychiatry.

Freud's contributions still influence psychiatrical care although, for a number of years, belittling his thinking was popular. Paraphrasing a statement made by Sir Isaac Newton (1642-1727): "If we see far today, it is because we stand on the shoulders of giants."

Freud described human behavior in psychological terms. He developed a theory of motivation, established the usefulness of talking (catharsis), explained the importance of dreams, and proposed to unlock the hidden parts of the mind. He introduced terms that have become part of our language—*psychoanalysis, id, ego, superego,* and *free association.* He felt free to study human beings as he would any other animal because of Charles Darwin's work. The work of others evolved from Freud's studies. Alfred Adler, Carl Jung, Ernest Jones, Otto Rank, Helene Deutsch, Karen Horney, and Anna Freud (Freud's daughter) all made significant and, in most cases, lasting contributions to the field of dynamic psychiatry.

Freud's inspiration, however, reached far beyond those with whom he worked personally. Society in general is indebted to him, even though conflicting opinions about his ideas have emerged. Freud challenged society to look at human beings objectively and fostered a milieu of thinking about the mind and mental disorders. Unit II (Therapeutic Nurse-Patient Relationship) builds on these concepts and is devoted to the implementation of strategies for working with psychiatric patients.

## BENCHMARK III: PERIOD OF PSYCHOTROPIC DRUGS

From this milieu of theory and scientific thought came the third benchmark, which began around 1950 with the discovery of psychotropic drugs. Chlorpromazine (Thorazine), an antipsychotic drug, and lithium, an antimanic agent, were introduced first, and imipramine (Tofranil), an antidepressant, was introduced a few years later. The impact of these drugs has been powerful. Patients who appeared beyond reach became less agitated and experienced a reduction in psychotic thinking. Depressed patients regained normal feelings. Hospital stays were shortened, and hospital environments improved. However, although psychotropic drugs have allowed many patients to be treated in less restrictive environments, ethical, moral, and legal questions have arisen with this treatment modality. Unit III (Psychopharmacology) is devoted to an understanding of the role of psychotropic drugs in the treatment of mental disorders.

## BENCHMARK IV: PERIOD OF COMMUNITY MENTAL HEALTH

The notion that one benchmark period ended entirely before the next one began is inaccurate. Trends overlap as advocates of one view have struggled to defend existing strategies while more dynamic forces have emerged elsewhere. As the various treatment approaches were being developed in the milieu derived from Freud's theories, criticism grew, and the state hospital system continued its plunge into "psychiatric Siberia." The popular movie *The Snake Pit* (1948) portrayed a mindless, ineffective and, at times, cruel system of care. In an even more devastating exposé, the book *The Shame of the States,* by Albert Deutsch (1948), vividly revealed with words and photographs the deplorable conditions in several large state hospitals in the United States.

Legislators were watching, reading, and listening; legislation was passed that would change the approach to psychiatric care. In 1946, President Truman signed the National Mental Health Act, enabling the establishment of the National Institute of Mental Health a few years later (in 1949). In 1947, the Hill-Burton Act legislated funds to build general hospitals that included psychiatric units (Table 1-3). This initiative began the effort for early intervention and helped shorten the length of hospitalization for psychiatric patients.

In 1961, the Joint Commission on Mental Illness and Health, appointed by President Kennedy, published a report entitled *Action for Mental Health.* It urged increased support for the state hospital system in recognition of the need for improved treatment of the mentally ill population. Opponents of the state hospital system overwhelmed

| Table 1-3 | Legislative Events that Changed Psychiatric Care in America |
|---|---|

| Year | Legislative Act |
|---|---|
| 1946 | President Truman signs the National Mental Health Act |
| 1947 | Hill-Burton Act: Allocated funds for general hospitals to develop psychiatric units |
| 1949 | National Institute of Mental Health established |
| 1961 | President Kennedy: Joint Commission on Mental Illness and Health established |
| 1963 | Community Mental Health Centers Act |

supporters of this report. In fact, the more out-spoken critics of state hospitals declared that these hospitals were actually the cause of mental illness. The era of the large state hospitals was over.

Rather than increasing monetary support for the state hospital system, a convergence of forces set the stage for this fourth benchmark period in psychiatric history:

1. The public's declining confidence in the state hospital system
2. The failure of various treatment approaches to eradicate mental illness
3. The legislative climate that had begun in the 1940s, emphasizing the civil rights of the mentally ill
4. The newfound faith in psychotropic drugs

These factors led to the enactment of the Community Mental Health Centers (CMHC) Act in 1963, which virtually destroyed the state hospital system. A deliberate shift was made from institutional to extrainstitutional care; the goal was deinstitutionalization of the state hospital system population. The problem of geographic isolation (see earlier) was addressed with the establishment of community treatment centers and community living arrangements (e.g., halfway houses). Keeping the mentally disordered individual closer to the family addressed the issue of isolation from family members. Isolation from follow-up care was remedied because various levels of care were available locally.

Eventually, community mental health programs were developed to meet the needs of all those living within the boundaries of a designated (e.g., catchment) area. These programs had the following goals:

- Emergency care
- 24-hour inpatient care
- Partial hospitalization care
- Outpatient care
- Consultation and education for the population served by the center
- Screening services

## Deinstitutionalization

*The practice, over the past four decades, of releasing people with severe mental illnesses from institutions has been one of the largest social experiments in twentieth century America.*

*E. Fuller Torrey (1997)*

Deinstitutionalization refers to the depopulating of state mental hospitals. State hospitals reached their peak population in 1955 and then slowly began the process of trimming their census rolls. This process began with the growing concerns about asylum and were nurtured by some of the events previously discussed. A more subtle influence was psychiatry's and psychiatric nursing's growing disillusionment with the chronically mentally ill and a turning to the worried well.

These factors clearly laid the groundwork for deinstitutionalization; however, federal actions fully supported the process. First was the CMHC Act of 1963. The second federal action was legislation that provided mentally disabled persons with an income while living in the community. This legislation was named Aid to the Disabled (ATD), now called Supplemental Security Income (SSI) and Social Security Disability Insurance (SSDI). The number of individuals with mental disorders receiving these benefits increased dramatically.

### Shifting the Cost of Mental Illness

State governments soon found that ATD, even when supplemented by the state, was less expensive than public hospitalization because the federal government paid most of the costs. The federal share grew by 3100% between 1963 and 1994 (Torrey, 1997). Naturally, state financial incentives declined as the involvement of the federal government increased.

Perhaps the final event in the deinstitutionalization movement was the change in commitment laws. Out of concern for the civil rights of mental patients, involuntary commitment of individuals to a state hospital became difficult (Rosenheck, 1997). The state had to demonstrate that those accused were a clear danger to themselves or to others. These sweeping changes were reactions to years of injustice during which persons said to be mentally ill could be detained and involuntarily committed, with little recourse, for long periods. (Rosenhan's classic study [1973] illustrates how difficult it was for a sane person to be discharged from a mental hospital [Box 1-1].) The stage was set for the rapid depopulation of state hospitals.

### Depopulation of State Hospitals

The state hospital population reached its peak in 1955, with 558,922 patients. Today, the state hospital population is about 70,000 patients, a decline

## Box 1-1   On Being Sane in Insane Places

Rosenhan wondered whether the "sane" could be distinguished from the "insane." He selected eight pseudopatients (people who pretended to be mentally ill) and instructed them to attempt to gain admission to public mental hospitals. The task was much easier than anyone had anticipated. Twelve hospitals in five states were used. The pseudopatient group consisted of a graduate student in psychology, three psychologists (including Rosenhan himself), a pediatrician, a psychiatrist, a painter, and a housewife; three were women and five were men. No one in the hospital knew of the deception. The pseudopatients were trained to do the following:

1. Call the hospital and make an appointment.
2. On arriving at the hospital, tell the psychiatrist that they had been hearing voices.
3. On being asked to describe the voices, say that they were not sure but remembered the words "empty," "hollow," and "thud."
4. Other than giving this false information and false information about their names, occupations, and employers, they were to be be truthful and "normal" from that point forward.
5. Immediately on admission, they were to cease simulating abnormal behavior and behave "normally."
6. When asked how they were doing, they were told to respond "fine" and to inform the staff that they were no longer experiencing problems.

Despite behaving normally, none of the pseudopatients were discovered by the staff. However, approximately 25% of the other patients made comments about the pseudopatients' "sanity," and a few even guessed that the pseudopatients were doing some type of undercover work. Rosenhan noted reluctance by the staff to see mental health in their patients. He stated, "Having once been labeled schizophrenic, there is nothing the pseudopatients can do to overcome the tag." Pseudopatient histories were written to support their diagnoses. In other words, psychiatrists saw problems that had never existed.

The pseudopatients were also asked to write down their observations. At first, they followed elaborate precautions to avoid detection; however, they were soon jotting down observations in front of the staff. The pseudopatients discovered that no one was paying any attention to them.

Another part of the experiment was to determine the amount of time spent with patients. This amount was difficult to measure; thus, a proxy behavior was substituted—time the nurses spent outside the nurses' station. Nursing attendants had the highest percentage of time spent outside the station (11.3%). Rosenhan found that measuring registered nurse time outside the nurses' station was impossible, because it occurred so infrequently. Psychiatrists were even worse, because they hid behind their closed office doors; at least the patients were able to see the nurses. Rosenhan concluded, "Those with the most power have least to do with patients, and those with the least power are most involved with them."

Rosenhan decried the powerlessness and the depersonalization experienced by the pseudopatients. He remembered how he was frequently awakened in the hospital to which he had been admitted: "Come on you m----f----s, out of bed."

The pseudopatients were hospitalized on average for 19 days before they were deemed well enough for discharge. The range of stay was from 7 to 52 days.

From Rosenhan DL: On being sane in insane places, *Science* 179:250, 1973.

of over 85%. Almost 1,000,000 people would be in state hospitals today if the same proportions were in effect. Thus, over 900,000 individuals who might have been hospitalized years ago are currently living outside such institutions. This decline has resulted in the closing of many state hospitals. Patients hospitalized today require a high level of care, have few social relationships, are psychotic, and are typically acutely ill young men. Table 1-4 provides insights into where these people might be living.

### Community Effects

The effects of deinstitutionalization are also evident in community agencies. For example, emergency department use by acutely disturbed

### Table 1-4   Where Individuals with Severe Mental Illness Live

**Location**

Nursing homes
Prison
State hospitals
Homeless
Home with families, group or board-and-care homes, or on their own

From Torrey EF: The release of the mentally ill from institutions: a well-intentioned disaster, *Chron High Educ* 43:B4, 1997.

individuals has increased dramatically in the absence of the previous system. Emergency psychiatric services are sagging from the load they now carry. Some general hospital psychiatric units are overwhelmed at times with a continuous flow of patients being admitted and discharged. Many professionals believe that the typical patient is also different. Compared with the patients of the 1960s and 1970s, today's patients are more aggressive and many are armed when first seen in the emergency department (Ries, 1997). Furthermore, approximately 1000 homicides are committed each year by severely mentally ill (SMI) individuals who are not receiving adequate care (Torrey, 1997). Lastly, 10% to 15% of those in state prisons are SMI (Lamb and Weinberger, 1998).

---

### CRITICAL THINKING QUESTION  2

It has been stated that the fields of psychiatry and psychiatric nursing lost interest in the SMI and became more interested in working with the worried well. Do you believe that this is still true in psychiatric nursing? Support your answer.

---

## BENCHMARK V:
## DECADE OF THE BRAIN

The 1990s were declared the Decade of the Brain by Congress. During this decade, a steep increase in brain research occurred that coincided with an increased interest in biologic explanations for mental disorders. The immediate impetus for this benchmark was the significant changes in the diagnostic manual published in 1980 (see subsequent discussions in this chapter). However, in many ways, the emphasis on brain biology represented a completion of the circle started by Kraepelin 100 years before. Kraepelin believed that brain pathology was at the root of serious mental disorders.

Significant changes in public awareness occurred because of the Decade of the Brain, which enabled clinicians to address relatively complex topics with patients and families. Nursing responded to this challenge with a significant augmentation of psychobiologic content in academic nursing programs and a torrent of continuing education programs. In fact, pre-1990 psychiatric nursing textbooks provided very little, if any, information about psychobiology and psychopharmacology, leaving many nursing graduates of that period inadequately prepared. All textbooks now provide this information. Nurses educated in previous decades felt the pressure to upgrade their knowledge to remain viable in the workplace. Most have done so, and

those who did not or could not have, for the most part, moved on.

The Decade of the Brain brought many challenges, but the benefits have been tremendous in terms of making psychiatric nursing a more viable specialty. It crystallized the fact that some behaviors are caused by biologic irregularities and not willful contrariness, or worse. It also enabled individuals to move beyond blaming toward a focus on what could be done. The Decade of the Brain brought nursing back into the mainstream of psychiatric care.

---

### ISSUES THAT AFFECT THE
### DELIVERY OF PSYCHIATRIC CARE

Several important issues affecting the delivery of psychiatric care remain for discussion. Although briefly discussed earlier in this chapter, the paradigm shift that has occurred in the way we think about and treat mental disorders is very important. The way we conceptualize a disorder informs all decisions about that disorder. Homelessness is a problem that also influences psychiatric care. Vast numbers of individuals are standing on street corners with signs pleading for money, and studies have indicated that many of these people have a serious mental disorder. The need for and the reality of community-based care is another issue. What mechanisms are in place to fortify the continuum of care? Finally, we have developed a system of care that is driven by carefully described signs and symptoms. This "bible" of diagnoses is indispensable in our psychiatric care delivery system.

## PARADIGM SHIFT IN PSYCHIATRIC
## CARE

Psychiatry in general lost interest in the SMI as a result of the influx of psychoanalysts in the 1930s and 1940s (Miller, 1984). As Freud himself had discovered, his analytic approach was most helpful to persons with less severe problems and was not particularly helpful to psychotic patients. Thus, as freudian thinking influenced more psychiatrists and psychiatric nurses, a natural withdrawal from the SMI and a refocusing on individuals more amenable to treatment occurred. "Asylum psychiatry, and the Kraepelinian model on which it was based, fell into relative decline" (Wilson, 1993).

Public mental hospitals lost prestige, as did the physicians and nurses working in them. Within the psychiatric nursing fraternity, staff nurses were not as highly valued as were those working in the role of therapist. In many cases, as participants in a self-fulfilling prophecy, the devalued inpatient psychiatric nurses in public hospitals became what they were perceived to be. They were often derisively referred to as either crazy or lazy.

The mainstream of psychiatry and psychiatric nursing turned from chronically disturbed patients to individuals with lowered self-esteem, those who were striving to reach their potential, and those who were existentially unhappy (Detre, 1987). Psychiatry changed its focus from one extreme of the psychiatric care continuum (the SMI) to the other (the worried well) over a few decades. Social issues started to emerge as legitimate professional concerns. Psychiatry and psychiatric nursing became interested in issues such as poverty, racism, alternate lifestyles, and sexism at the professional level. Some clinicians believe that this process of enlightenment and social relevance further distanced the mainstream of psychiatric care from persons most in need of that care.

Psychiatry returned to its roots with the publishing of the *Diagnostic and Statistical Manual-III* in 1980. That edition has been described by Wilson (1993) as the "remedicalization of psychiatry." Psychiatric nursing was much slower to embrace research (i.e., evidence-based diagnosis) and the biologic underpinnings of the more severely mentally ill. But, as the Decade of the Brain (the 1990s) progressed, psychiatric nursing and psychiatric nursing textbooks reflected the "new" understanding.

## HOMELESSNESS

Many psychiatric professionals believe that homelessness can be directly linked to benchmark IV. About 800,000 people are homeless each night (SAMSHA, 2005). Thirty years ago, the most popular view was that homeless people (mostly Caucasian men) were skid row bums, alcoholics, and hobos who chose to be homeless. Current studies have altered that perception considerably. The current belief is that the homeless are people (including entire families) who have been displaced by social policies over which they have no control. Perhaps 25% of the homeless are children, and another 25% are employed in low-paying jobs.

Estimates concerning the prevalence of mental illness among this population also vary. The consensus of opinion, however, is that between 20% and 25% of the adult homeless population has a severe mental illness, and that approximately 50% to 70% suffer from alcohol or drug abuse (SAMSHA, 2005). Many suffer from both.

People who are homeless and mentally ill present a challenge to the mental health and political systems in the United States; these individuals are usually single or divorced, and have a weak social support system. The homeless SMI are found in parks, airport terminals, soup kitchens, jails, and general hospitals, and often present a troubling appearance. Furthermore, the economic windfall experienced by some Americans in recent years has not filtered down to the streets. Many homeless mentally ill persons have become bold in their efforts to survive, assaulting the sensitivities of passersby. From aggressive panhandling to embarrassing public elimination of bodily wastes, societal standards are being affronted. Although much of this alienating behavior is required for survival on the mean streets, it is behavior that offends mainstream America. The dilemma is real, and mental health professionals are searching for answers.

As mentioned, homeless people may live exclusively on the streets (the so-called street people), or they may live in community shelters, halfway houses, or board-and-care homes. A possible third group includes individuals who are able to stay for short periods in cheap hotels, alternating between this and nights in less accommodating surroundings. Still another significant group moves among homeless shelters, rehabilitation programs, jails, and prisons (Haugland et al, 1997).

Homelessness is an end product of chronic mental illness and probably exacerbates it as well. Stated another way, many chronically ill persons end up on the streets because of their inability to succeed in a competitive society and, once they are on the streets, the stresses of the homeless life compound their mental health problems; they are in a no-win situation. As with many societal problems, some groups appear to fare worse than others. Racial and ethnic minorities are overrepresented among the homeless.

Proponents of deinstitutionalization argue that these particular problems are not inherently a part of depopulating state hospitals, but have resulted instead because money has not followed patients into the community. They attempt to make the case that community mental health has never been allocated the resources necessary to realize its promise. Traditionalists, on the other hand, point to the homeless and the disproportionate effect experienced by some minority groups as evidence of the need for change. Homelessness is more than a lack of shelter, these critics maintain—it is a lack of support systems available in the public mental hospital system.

## COMMUNITY-BASED CARE

The future of psychiatric care and psychiatric nursing will be linked to continuing efforts to prevent mental health problems and to treat existing disorders more effectively. Because of economic realities, much of that will be a community-based effort as part of a continuum of care. Nurses will need to continue to train for roles in the community while reestablishing a leadership role in inpatient services. An agenda for mental health has been established in the document *Healthy People 2010* (2000), developed by the U.S. Department of Health and Human Services.

### Developing a Continuum of Care

In the early 1960s, mental health activists were successful in passing federal legislation that dramatically reshaped the way mental health services were delivered in the United States. Converging forces related to these changes have been previously discussed.

Specific problems associated with community mental health (CMH) were the liberalization of commitment laws, which allowed SMI patients to go untreated, and restrictive confidentiality rulings, which made discussing the difficult issues of treatment with family members a legal concern. As newspaper editorials, grassroots mental health organizations, and families have clamored about the obvious unmet needs of the SMI, the mental health and legal communities have rallied to respond. This insistence has culminated in thoughtful and deliberate dialogue among mental health professionals, with the objective of making the mental health system work.

To make the system work, a seamless continuum of care must be developed that coordinates the activities of diverse treatment sources and facilitates movement between and among its enti-

---

**Box 1-2  Systemic Changes**

In the new health care reality, CMH must move rapidly away from some practices and toward new ways of conceptualizing the system:

- Away from symptom stabilization toward recovery and reintegration
- Away from the view that professionals have all the answers, moving toward more involvement of consumers and family members
- Away from medication management toward holistic thinking (e.g., stabilizing housing, medical health, finances)

---

**Box 1-3  Example of a Continuum of Care***

1. Commitment to a state hospital
2. Day treatment (5× week) in a community mental health center; living at a state or county licensed residential facility
3. Day treatment 1 to 3 days per week; seeking or beginning gainful employment
4. Scheduled follow-up with therapist and prescribing clinician; living in the community

*From most restrictive to least restrictive for a patient with a severe mental illness.

---

ties. Until this seamless continuum is developed, many patients will slip through the cracks of the system as both bureaucratic dysfunction and corporate self-interest drain energy away from programs. Box 1-2 suggests how the system is changing to develop this seamless continuum of care. Box 1-3 presents typical individual movement through the continuum of care, from the most restrictive to a less restrictive environment.

### Role for Nursing in the Continuum of Care

CMH nursing has been in existence for many years. In 1982, the American Nurses Association (ANA) defined the CMH nurse's role in the continuum of care as follows: "The nurse participates with other members of the community in assessing, planning, implementing, and evaluating mental health services and community services that include the promotion of the continuum of primary, secondary, and tertiary prevention of mental illness."

Nursing has a natural fit with today's health care realities, because many values traditionally emphasized by psychiatric nursing fit with the concept of a continuum of care. These include the following:

- Viewing the patient as a whole person
- Working with families
- Treating patients in their own homes
- Developing a relationship over time
- Educating patients about medications
- Assessing the environment for safety, hygiene, and support

All these traditional nursing activities position nurses to excel in the world of psychiatric care.

## THE DIAGNOSTIC "BIBLE" OF PSYCHIATRY

*Labels provide an usually false yet comforting sense of being able to control the uncontrollable.*
    *Allen J. Frances and Helen Link Egger (1999)*

The *Diagnostic and Statistical Manual of Mental Disorders (DSM)* outlines the signs and symptoms required in order for clinicians to assign a specific diagnosis to a patient. Not only are diagnoses based on these criteria, but all third-party payers insist on a *DSM* diagnosis before considering reimbursement payments. The *DSM* has been published in six editions since its inception in 1952:

| | |
|---|---|
| *DSM-I* | 1952 |
| *DSM-II* | 1968 |
| *DSM-III* | 1980 |
| *DSM-IIIR* (Revised) | 1987 |
| *DSM-IV* | 1994 |
| *DSM-IV-TR* (Text Revision) | 2000 |

The first edition described about 100 disorders, was published in a spiral-bound notebook, and cost only a few dollars. It was heavily influenced by freudian or psychoanalytic thinking (Wilson, 1993). As Grob (1987) has noted, the *DSM* relied on and reflected, " . . . an extraordinary broadening of psychiatric boundaries and a rejection of the traditional distinction between mental health and mental abnormality. To move from a concern with illness in institutional populations to the incidence in the general population represented an extraordinary intellectual leap."

The development of the third edition was turned over to a psychiatrist in his mid-40s, Robert Spitzer. Working for 6 years on the new manual, he finally pulled together a document that improved the reliability of psychiatric diag-

nosis (Spiegel, 2005). The *DSM-III* grew to 900 pages while defining and describing about 300 conditions; between *DSM-III* and *DSM-IIIR,* over one million copies were sold (Spiegel, 2005). The current edition, *DSM-IV-TR,* might soon approach that level of usage.

The *DSM* provides five axes for the clinician to use in the assessment of the patient:

Axis I: Clinical disorders (e.g., schizophrenia, major depression, bipolar disorder)
Axis II: Personality or developmental disorders (e.g., paranoid and borderline personality disorders, mental retardation)
Axis III: General medical conditions that relate to axes I or II or have a bearing on treatment (e.g., neoplasms, endocrine disorders)
Axis IV: Severity of psychosocial stressors (e.g., divorce, housing, educational issues)
Axis V: Global assessment of functioning, on a scale of 0 to 100 (e.g., a score of 30 means that the patient's behavior is highly influenced by delusions and hallucinations)

It is important to have a basic understanding of the *DSM,* because this is the language of psychiatry. Although axis I is most often used, a cursory knowledge of the other axes is helpful for the beginning student.

## PSYCHIATRIC NURSING EDUCATION: THREE FIRSTS

### First Psychiatric Nurse

The official history of psychiatric nursing in the United States began approximately 100 years ago. Linda Richards, the first American psychiatric nurse, was a graduate of the New England Hospital for Women. Richards spent much of her professional career developing nursing care in psychiatric hospitals and also directed a school of psychiatric nursing in 1880 at the McLean Psychiatric Asylum in Waverly, Massachusetts. Because of her efforts, more than 30 asylums had developed schools for psychiatric nurses by 1890.

### First Psychiatric Nursing Textbook

In 1920, Harriet Bailey wrote the first psychiatric nursing textbook. The title of the book, *Nursing Mental Diseases,* reflects the appropriate terminology of the day. An important distinction for psychiatric nursing is that it was not brought into the greater nursing fold until the 1940s. Because psychiatric nurses were trained in state hospitals, they were allowed to work only in state hospitals. In 1937, the National League for Nursing (then called the National League for Nursing Education) recommended that psychiatric nursing be made part of the curriculum of general nursing programs.

### First Psychiatric Nursing Theorist

In the 1950s, the views of an important figure in psychiatric nursing shaped and gave direction to psychiatric nursing practice and contributed to the development of a professional climate. Hildegarde Peplau (1952, 1959) developed a model for psychiatric nursing practice. Her book, *Interpersonal Relations in Nursing* (1952), influences practice to this day; her approach, heavily influenced by Harry Stack Sullivan, emphasizes the interpersonal dimension of practice. Peplau also wrote a history of psychiatric nursing that carefully traced the unfolding of the profession. She might be the single most important historic figure in psychiatric nursing.

## SUMMARY

Even if we wanted to, we could not get away from psychiatric concerns. Our daily newspapers jog us from any indifference we might have about accounts of mentally disordered individuals committing crimes. Furthermore, the selective serotonin reuptake inhibitors (also called SSRIs, such as Prozac, Paxil, and Zoloft) are ubiquitous. Tens of millions of Americans are taking these drugs.

Humane psychiatric care started to develop in the late 1700s and has evolved through at least five distinct periods: Enlightenment, Scientific Study, Psychotropic Drugs, Community Mental Health, and Decade of the Brain. Intially, the biologic aspect of mental illness was embraced, but this understanding gave way to a freudian or psychoanalytic view, which directed the clinician to search for what was behind the symptoms. Although this detective approach was intellectually stimulating and made for wonderful conversation, it conceptually missed the point. Many patients were not living out some dark drama

from a childhood long ago but, instead, were suffering from present-day biologic disturbances (e.g., low serotonin levels). Finally, in the 1980s and 1990s, respectively, psychiatry and psychiatric nursing returned to their roots and acknowledged that many mental health problems are caused by biologic abnormalities.

The *DSM,* sometimes referred to as the bible of psychiatric diagnosis, is the *lingua franca* of psychiatry. To fully participate in clinical discussions, nurses need a basic understanding of its concepts.

### CRITICAL THINKING QUESTION    3

If it is the patient that truly counts, why get caught up in *DSM* terminology? Doesn't this serve to distance the nurse from the patient?

## Study Notes

1. Understanding the principles of psychiatric nursing is important, because mental health problems affect approximately 25% of the population.
2. Modern psychiatry can be traced through five benchmark periods: Enlightenment, Scientific Study, Psychotropic Drugs, Community Mental Health, and Decade of the Brain.
3. Historically, the mentally ill were banished and confined, but the period of Enlightenment ushered in an era in which the mentally ill were treated humanely.
4. The asylum movement (providing sanctuary from the hostile world) grew out of the humane emphasis of the period of Enlightenment, and resulted in the development of state hospital systems.
5. During the period of scientific study, men such as Freud, Kraepelin, and Bleuler studied people objectively; this effort resulted in both psychodynamic and biologic understanding of mental disorders.
6. During the period of psychotropic drugs, antipsychotic drugs (the early 1950s), antidepressant drugs (late 1950s), and other drugs were developed and greatly contributed to the treatment of specific mental disorders.
7. The period of CMH began as a result of several converging factors, including:
   - Hostility toward state hospitals
   - Psychotropic drugs

- Civil rights
- Financial incentives

8. Deinstitutionalization, which changed the locus of treatment from large public hospitals to the community, is a product of the CMH movement.

9. In 1955, over a half-million patients were in state hospitals; today, approximately 70,000 are in these hospitals.

10. A large percentage of the nation's homeless has a diagnosable mental disorder. Critics of deinstitutionalization place some of the blame for homelessness on the CMH movement.

11. CMH nurses have a major role in the continuum of care because of their specialized training in patient care, comprehensive services, patient education, and case management.

12. Psychiatric care and psychiatric nursing have evolved during the twentieth century. At one time, psychiatric nursing was closely associated with the care of the SMI but, similar to medicine, those in the field became professionally interested in the worried well. Beginning with the Decade of the Brain, many psychiatric nurses renewed their interest in understanding biologic variables affecting patients with mental disorders.

13. The *DSM* is the bible of psychiatric diagnosis. Nurses who seek to provide the best care and who want to advocate for patients most effectively learn these concepts.

14. In 1920, Harriet Bailey wrote the first psychiatric nursing textbook, but Hildegarde Peplau's book, *Interpersonal Relations in Nursing,* has most influenced psychiatric nursing.

## ◼ References

American Nurses Association: *Standards of psychiatric and mental health nursing practice,* Kansas City, 1982, The Association.

Detre T: The future of psychiatry, *Am J Psychiatry* 144:621, 1987.

Deutsch A: *The shame of the states,* New York, 1948, Harcourt Brace.

Frances AJ, Egger HL: Whither psychiatric diagnosis, *Aust N Z J Psychiatry* 33:161, 1999.

Gollaher D: *Voice for the mad: the life of Dorothea Dix,* New York, 1995, Free Press.

Haugland G, Siegel C, Hopper K, Alexander MJ: Mental illness among homeless individuals in a suburban county, *Psychiatr Serv* 48:504, 1997.

Jones D: (2001, June 22). Kids' dad defends his wife. *USA Today,* p. 1A.

Lamb HR, Weinberger LE: Persons with severe mental illness in jails and prisons: a review, *Psychiatr Serv* 49:483, 1998.

Lee S: *Red Lake shootings: A look inside.* Available at: www.grandforks.com/mld/grandforks/11272191.htm. Accessed January 17, 2006.

McMillan I: Insight into Bedlam: one hospital's history, *J Psychosoc Nurs Ment Health Serv* 35:28, 1997.

Miller RD: Public mental hospital work: pros and cons for psychiatrists, *Hosp Community Psychiatry* 35:928, 1984.

National Institute of Mental Health: *Mental health statistics,* Rockville, MD, 1993, Office of Consumer, Family, and Public Information, Center for Mental Health Services.

National Institute of Mental Health (NIMH): *Statistics.* Available at http://www.nimh.nih.gov/. Accessed April 18, 2005.

Peplau H: *Interpersonal relations in nursing,* New York, 1952, Putnam.

Peplau H: Principles of psychiatric nursing. In Arieti S, editor: *American handbook of psychiatry,* vol 2, New York, 1959, Basic Books, pp 1840-1856.

Ries R: Advantages of separating the triage function from the emergency service, *Psychiatr Serv* 48:755, 1997.

Rosenblatt A: Concepts of the asylum in the care of the mentally ill, *Hosp Community Psychiatry* 35:244, 1984.

Rosenhan DL: On being sane in insane places, *Science* 179:250, 1973.

Rosenheck R: Disability payments and chemical dependence: conflicting values and uncertain effects, *Psychiatr Serv* 48:789, 1997.

Spiegel A: The dictionary of disorder. *New Yorker* 56:56-63, 2005.

Substance Abuse and Mental Health Services Administration (SAMSHA): Available at http://www.samsha.gov/. Accessed April 18, 2005.

Torrey EF: The release of the mentally ill from institutions: a well-intentioned disaster, *Chron High Educ* 43:B4, 1997.

U.S. Department of Health and Human Services: *Healthy people 2010,* Washington, DC, 2000, USDHHS.

U.S. Surgeon General: *Mental health: a report from the Surgeon General,* Washington, DC, 1999, USDHHS.

Wasow M: The need for asylum revisited, *Hosp Community Psychiatry* 44:207, 1993.

Weiner DB: Philippe Pinel's "Memoir on Madness" of December 11, 1794: A fundamental text of modern psychiatry, *Am J Psychiatry* 149:725, 1992.

Wilson M: DSM-III and the transformation of American psychiatry: a history, *Am J Psychiatry* 150:399, 1993.

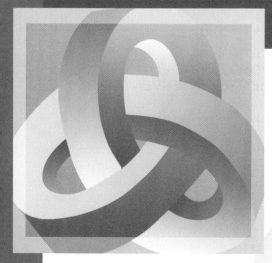

# Chapter 2

# Psychotherapeutic Management in the Continuum of Care

*Norman L. Keltner*

## Learning Objectives

*After reading this chapter, you should be able to:*
- Describe the components of psychotherapeutic management.
- Explain the way in which the balancing of psychotherapeutic management components combine to form a powerful therapeutic model of care.

- Recognize the relationship between the continuum of care and the psychotherapeutic management model.

## PSYCHOTHERAPEUTIC MANAGEMENT

Psychiatric nursing is in search of care delivery models that are not only effective for patient care, but can also capitalize on the uniqueness of the discipline. Psychotherapeutic management proposes a real world approach to psychiatric nursing care that recognizes the interdependence of the mental health professions and exploits the strengths of psychiatric nursing. It answers the question, "What do psychiatric nurses do that is different from that of other mental health professionals, particularly social workers, psychologists, marriage and family counselors, and other therapists?" In 1979, Koldjeski wrote: "Psychiatric nurses must clearly demonstrate the exact nature of their practice and must differentiate their practice from the practice of other nonmedical mental health personnel" (Koldjeski, 1979). After Koldjeski's prescription, psychotherapeutic management was proposed as a model to clarify and

distinguish the role of the psychiatric nurse (Keltner, 1985). Psychiatric treatment can be divided into five basic categories: (1) use of words (which encompass all forms of psychotherapy), (2) drugs, (3) environment, (4) somatic therapies, and (5) behavioral conditioning. Psychotherapeutic management emphasizes three of these categories: (1) the psychotherapeutic nurse-patient relationship (words), (2) psychopharmacology (drugs), and (3) milieu management (environment), all of which must be supported by a sound understanding of psychopathology (Figure 2-1).

Stated another way, the student has three intervention tools:

1. Self (i.e., themselves)
2. Psychotropic drugs
3. Environment (i.e., milieu)

The particular intervention approach depends on the patient's psychopathology. For example, the nurse learns to use different words when he or she speaks with a patient who has been diagnosed

### Norm's Notes

*Take a good look at this chapter. It will make a lot of sense because it gives you a simple approach for conceptualizing what you are doing with patients. When you work with patients, you need to focus on three things: (1) how you will interact with them, (2) the meds they need, and (3) how you can affect their environment. This approach arms you with a strategy. Now, although the framework is simple, the basics of the psychotherapeutic management approach are not simple—far from it. You will spend the entire semester understanding what goes into fleshing out this model.*

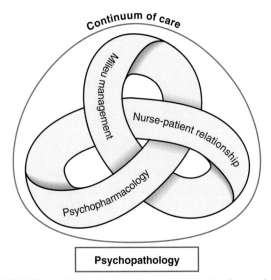

**FIGURE 2-1** Psychotherapeutic management in the continuum of care.

with schizophrenia compared with a patient who has been diagnosed with depression. More than likely, the patient with schizophrenia requires antipsychotic medications, whereas the depressed patient receives antidepressant drugs—hence, drug management is different. Finally, whereas the patient with schizophrenia might need an environment that reduces stressors, a key environmental concern for the depressed patient might be safety (e.g., suicide prevention). In other words, the psychotherapeutic management model recognizes that one size does not fit all.

## APPLICATION OF PSYCHOTHERAPEUTIC MANAGEMENT INTERVENTIONS

The application of psychopathology and the knowledgeable use of psychotherapeutic management skills extend beyond inpatient settings into various care settings, such as outpatient programs, residential services, and home care. The needs of the individual and the setting in which care is delivered influence the degree to which each component of psychotherapeutic management is used within the continuum of care (Figure 2-2).

For example, individuals with schizophrenia in an inpatient setting benefit most when a therapeutic nurse-patient relationship, psychopharmacology, and a well-managed milieu are available. When one component is missing from the equation, treatment is compromised. Ordinarily, when psychotropic drugs and a well-managed milieu are subtracted from this equation, patients decompensate into a pretreatment state. Similarly, when drugs and therapeutic communication are available (perhaps the latter from only a few motivated staff members) but the overall environment is poorly managed, patients are left to fend for themselves and are drained of the internal resources needed for healing. When inpatients receive only drug therapy but are denied therapeutic interaction opportunities in a well-managed milieu, a return to the inadequacies of custodial care takes place. In other words, all components of the psychotherapeutic management equation must be present if patients are to realize the benefits of effective nursing intervention fully. However, one component might take precedence at a given point in time. For example, an individual with schizophrenia has missed his last appointment for an injection of haloperidol decanoate (an antipsychotic drug that lasts for 2 to 4 weeks). The nurse's priority might be to make a home visit to administer the injection. The psychopharmacology component is a priority at this time, but the nurse-patient relationship and milieu aspects are not ignored. In this case, perhaps only the nurse who has developed a relationship with this patient will be allowed to give the injection. Psychotherapeutic management endeavors to bring balance to practice and, with balance, role clarification, thus providing a valuable approach in both inpatient and outpatient settings.

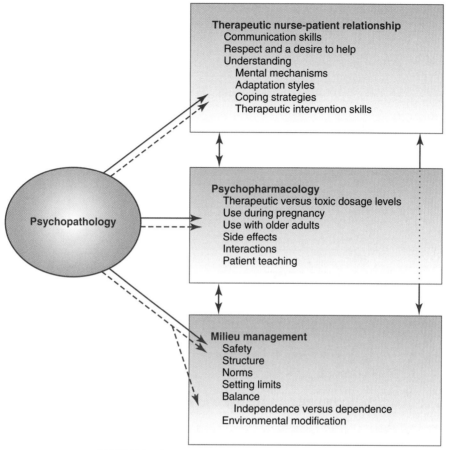

**FIGURE 2-2** Psychotherapeutic management model.

## CONTINUUM OF CARE

Chapter 3 deals with the continuum of care within which the psychotherapeutic management approach is implemented and includes providing services based on the needs of the individual. These services span the continuum from health promotion through prevention, treatment, and rehabilitation, and can be provided in a variety of settings. An important aspect of the continuum of care is that individuals can be guided through treatment or services as their needs change. The individual's initial contact with the mental health system should involve the process of assessment and referral to the least restrictive, most effective, and most cost-conscious source of services. Multiple services might or might not involve the nurse as the primary caregiver; other disciplines or care providers might be responsible for a particular service. The psychotherapeutic management model has relevance in various care settings and can be adapted by the nurse to any level of care.

The way in which the patient is guided to an appropriate level of care is based on a series of decisions (Figure 2-3). Traditionally, the nurse has made these decisions as part of discharge planning before the patient's release from the hospital. Given current trends in mental health care, the decisions might now be made by the nurse or other professionals during the risk assessment phase.

## PSYCHOTHERAPEUTIC MANAGEMENT: THREE INTERVENTIONS

### THERAPEUTIC NURSE-PATIENT RELATIONSHIP

Differentiating therapy from being therapeutic is crucial for the student of psychiatric nursing. Therapy is the focus of graduate-level psychiatric nursing training, and the art of being therapeutic is the domain of undergraduate-level psychiatric

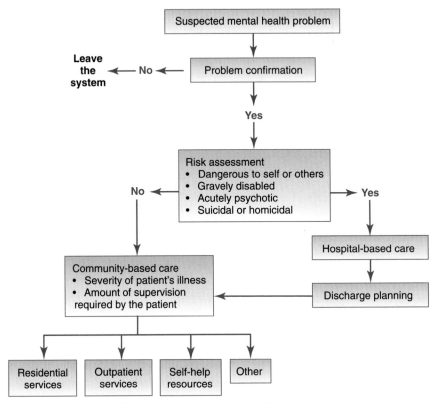

**FIGURE 2-3** Decision tree for continuum of care.

nurses. Therefore, when this course is completed, the student is not a therapist but should be therapeutic.

Unit II is devoted to this first dimension of psychotherapeutic management. The different emphases placed on words and the wide range of styles within the domain of words are discussed, specifically general communication skills (Chapter 7), the nature of the nurse-patient relationship (Chapter 8), the nursing process (Chapter 9), anxiety, coping, and crisis (Chapter 10), working with the aggressive patient (Chapter 11), working with groups of patients (Chapter 12), working with the families of patients (Chapter 13), working with patients from different cultures (Chapter 14), and dealing with the spiritual needs of patients (Chapter 15).

## PSYCHOPHARMACOLOGY

Unit III is devoted to the contribution of psychotropic drugs to psychiatric nursing, the responsibilities of the nurse, and essential information about these drugs. Psychopharmacology is an

important dimension in psychotherapeutic management, because psychotropic drugs have enabled millions of people to live increasingly independent lives. Notably, drug intervention is neither always desirable nor appropriate. However, when drug therapy is indicated, patients usually respond more rapidly than they would without drugs.

The nurse who uses the nursing process model can assess patients' responses to medication, plan to respond to side effects should they occur, implement those plans, and evaluate for desired results. The nurse's pivotal role, particularly in an inpatient setting, allows intervention before serious drug-related problems occur. Additionally, the nurse dispenses medications and makes decisions regarding as needed (prn) medications. For these and other reasons, the nurse must have immediate access to information about psychotropic drugs.

## MILIEU MANAGEMENT

Milieu (or environment) management is a proactive approach to care that forges therapeutic benefits from patients' surroundings, whether in the home, hospital, or outpatient setting. The six environmental elements that nurses must consider in creating a therapeutic milieu include the following:

1. Safety: keeping the patient free from danger or harm
2. Structure: the physical environment, regulations, schedules
3. Norms: specific expectations of behavior e.g., acceptance, nonviolence, privacy
4. Limit setting: clear and enforceable limitations on behaviors
5. Balance: negotiating the line between dependence and independence
6. Environmental modification: changing environment to promote mental health.

These elements might overlap; for example, safety is a component of all the other dimensions of milieu.

Nurses are the consistent force in the milieu. Kyes and Hofling (1974) have stated that "The interpersonal environment in which a patient lives may be therapeutic or nontherapeutic depending almost entirely on the interest and ability of the [nursing] staff." The authors added that the nurse is critical in guiding other staff members toward being therapeutic. Because humans are incapable of *not* interacting with their environment, nurses must make these interactions therapeutic. Various aspects of milieu management are discussed in Unit IV.

## PSYCHOPATHOLOGY

Unit V, which discusses psychopathology, provides the foundation on which the three components of psychotherapeutic management rest; it facilitates therapeutic communication in the nurse-patient relationship and lays the groundwork for an understanding of psychopharmacology and milieu management. Unit V also includes information about the major mental disorders. Schizophrenia, depressive disorders, bipolar disorders, anxiety-related disorders, cognitive disorders, personality disorders, sexual disorders, substance-related disorders, dual diagnosis, and eating disorders are considered in separate chapters of Unit V.

## CRITICAL THINKING QUESTION          1

If you develop a mental health problem, which aspect of psychotherapeutic management would be most important to you?

## SPECIAL THERAPIES

Unit VI discusses special populations and therapies; it contains chapters on behavior therapy, somatic therapies, and alternative and complementary therapies. Although these modalities are important dimensions of psychiatric care and are effective treatments, they do not have the universal clinical applications of the other categories of psychiatric treatment and are not emphasized in this text. Special populations in psychiatric nursing include victims of violence, child and adolescent psychiatric patients, and older mentally ill adults.

## CRITICAL THINKING QUESTION          2

Based on your clinical setting, what is your evaluation of the components of the psychotherapeutic management model that you have observed?

## █ Study Notes

1. Psychotherapeutic management is a model of care that clarifies the nature of psychiatric nursing and differentiates psychiatric nursing practice from the practice of other disciplines.
2. In the continuum of care, the individual is guided to services based on specific needs at a given point in time.
3. The components of psychotherapeutic management include a therapeutic nurse-patient relationship, psychopharmacology, and milieu management, all of which are supported by a basic understanding of psychopathology.
4. The therapeutic nurse-patient relationship emphasizes how important it is for the nurse to understand basic principles of therapeutic communication.
5. Being therapeutic is different from providing therapy in that being therapeutic involves interactions that should occur during every patient contact, whereas therapy indicates a more formal and structured interaction.
6. Psychopharmacologic understanding is important, because nurses administer medication, make decisions about prn medication, and evaluate for therapeutic and adverse responses to medication.
7. Because human beings are incapable of *not* interacting with their environment, milieu

management is an important nursing consideration. Nurses are uniquely responsible for developing the patients' treatment environment.

8. An understanding of psychopathology facilitates the nurse-patient relationship, lays the groundwork for understanding psychopharmacology, and provides a theoretical structure for milieu management.

## References

Keltner NL: Psychotherapeutic management: a model for nursing practice, *Perspect Psychiatr Care* 23:125, 1985.

Koldjeski D: *Mental health and psychiatric nursing and primary health care: issues and prospects,* In Proceedings of the Fourth National Conference in Graduate Education in Psychiatric and Mental Health Nursing, Kansas City, MO, 1979, American Nurses' Association.

Kyes J, Hofling C: *Basic psychiatric concepts in nursing,* ed 3, Philadelphia, 1974, JB Lippincott.

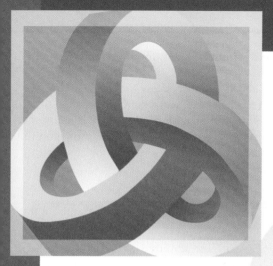

# Chapter 3

# Continuum of Care

*Carol E. Bostrom*

## Learning Objectives

*After reading this chapter, you should be able to:*
- Identify the various levels of care within the continuum of care.
- Understand the types of care that might be available in hospitals and in the community.
- Identify the role of the nurse in implementing the psychotherapeutic management model in hospital and community-based care.
- Apply the nursing process to patients who are receiving care in the community.

The continuum of care provides consumers with a wide range of treatment modalities to help an individual in achieving his or her optimal level of functioning. Continued efforts help integrate all levels of services into a seamless continuum so that an individual can move smoothly among them while receiving quality care. The role of nurses and other professionals is to assess the individual's current level of functioning comprehensively and thus direct the person to appropriate resources to enhance quality of life and decrease fragmentation of care. Coordination of services for the individual necessitates multidisciplinary collaboration. Multidisciplinary care has been expanded to include not only professional staff, but also nonprofessionals, consumers, family, and various nonpsychiatric resources (e.g., representatives from Medicare, Medicaid, nursing homes, group homes, and medical clinics).

The decision tree (see Chapter 2) is used to match the needs of the individual with appropriate services based on safety needs and intensity of supervision needed, severity of symptoms, level of functioning, and type of treatment needed. For example, consider the following:

1. An individual with auditory hallucinations telling her to kill her newborn infant might need inpatient hospitalization with 24-hour nursing care and supervision in a safe environment.
2. An individual with thoughts of suicide but without a plan might be managed effectively by attending a day treatment program 5 days a week for 2 weeks.
3. An individual with a history of medication noncompliance who needs a place to live might be appropriately placed in a group home with 24-hour supervision.
4. An individual with alcoholism who has completed acute detoxification might need referral to outpatient counseling or a self-help group such as Alcoholics Anonymous.

For any individual, additional referrals along the continuum of care can be made if needs change. An individual might be referred to mental health services at the suggestion of a family physician, minister, priest, or rabbi, police, family,

**Norm's Notes**

*The title of this chapter might not grab you like, for instance, a chapter titled "Schizophrenia" or "Working with the Aggressive Patient." However, this concept—the continuum of care—is very important. There must be different options and different levels of care for everyone. Furthermore, people can't be just dropped out of one program with nowhere else to turn. Those with mental disorders should not have to fend for themselves. There needs to be a system in place and, in most places in the United States, there is. The continuum of care provides resources for the neediest among us all the way to those who are almost ready to control all aspects of their lives.*

friends, or staff from the health clinic, emergency room, crisis service, or employee assistance program. Self-referral is also a means whereby individuals can gain entry into the mental health system.

The individual and care provider develop specific problem-oriented goals or outcomes based on objective data and subjective self-reports. Unfortunately, individuals might overestimate their progress toward the outcomes, or they might deny the need for follow-up care and fail to reach the outcomes. Because self-reports can be unreliable, more objective measures of outcomes are needed, such as compliance with medication and treatment, job attendance, and community living skills. Continual monitoring of the achievement of specific outcomes is critical for reimbursement by payers and for determining quality of care.

Managed care has had a major influence on the continuum of care. The mental health system in the United States has been affected by managed care in the public and private service areas. Less money for mental health and addiction services has resulted in the closing of inpatient beds and insufficient community treatment (Appelbaum, 2003). The decreased number of inpatient beds and short length of inpatient stays have influenced the need for intensive community treatment (Benson and Briscoe, 2003). Psychiatric treatment must be cost-effective, occur in the least restrictive setting, and be individualized and outcome-based.

Decreased reimbursement for care and lack of parity for mental health and addiction services have resulted in lack of access to care and lack of needed treatment and services. Other issues that interfere with the provision of care are decreased accessibility to services, especially for those most in need, and stigma that is still associated with how funds are allocated.

## HOSPITAL-BASED CARE

Historically, patients admitted to acute care units often stayed 4 to 6 weeks. Today, length of stay (LOS) in these units is typically 3 to 5 days. As reimbursement has decreased, hospital-based care, including medical, surgical, and other specialties, changed in the following areas: purpose and goals of hospitalization, greater need for risk assessment before admission, implementation of more varied types of care, change in staffing patterns, increased acuity of patients, and increased importance of discharge planning. Hospitals were the point of entry into the health care system, whereas the point of entry now can be anywhere along the continuum of care. As a result, a competent evaluation and triage is required for each individual who requests care (Schreter, 2000).

### PURPOSES OF PSYCHIATRIC HOSPITAL-BASED CARE

The highest priority for admission to hospital-based care is safety for self and others, necessitating 24-hour supervision in a secure environment (Schreter, 2000); this includes recognition of individuals who are actively suicidal, self-mutilating, or threatening others with harm. Individuals who have attempted suicide are often transferred from the emergency room or medical intensive care unit to a psychiatric unit when medically stable.

Other individuals who require hospitalization include those who are at risk for accidental harm—that is, those who are gravely disabled (see Chapter 5). For example, individuals who are acutely psychotic or those who are confused and disoriented might not function well enough to meet their basic needs for food, clothing, shelter, medical care, or physical safety. In addition to safety and protection, hospitalization provides thorough medical and psychiatric evaluation to identify the underlying cause of their symptoms.

Another group that might be admitted includes individuals who are experiencing toxic reactions to medications or other substances and those who need medical intervention when withdrawal from substances might produce life-threatening conditions. Some individuals might be admitted for a medical evaluation or because the medical illness produces or complicates a psychiatric disorder.

The goals of hospital-based care are to assist individuals with attaining initial stabilization and a safe level of functioning and to assess for appropriate referrals for aftercare. Attempts are made to interact with family, support systems, or both to determine the individual's problems and needs, as well as to help the individual after discharge (Kirsch, 2000).

## TYPES OF HOSPITAL-BASED CARE

Inpatient units vary from hospital to hospital and from community to community. For example, a small hospital might have only one closed (i.e., locked) inpatient unit that accepts all patients with all diagnoses. A larger hospital might offer more options for specialized care compared with the smaller hospital. Some common specialty care areas are described in Table 3-1.

An important type of inpatient service is the psychiatric intensive care unit (PICU). The PICU generally has 8 to 10 beds with more safety precautions and more staff than other psychiatric units to handle at-risk behaviors, such as suicide, assault, self-mutilation, sexual acting out, arson, and escape. Seclusion and restraints might be used more often on this type of unit. The purpose of the PICU is initial symptom and behavior control so that individuals can then be transferred to more treatment-oriented units or programs. Group activities might or might not be provided. When group activities occur, the focus is typically reality- or activity-based.

## DISCHARGE PLANNING

Hospital-based care uses multidisciplinary treatment conferences and discharge planning to ensure holistic care. Team members collaborate and coordinate inpatient care and determine aftercare services within the continuum of care based on the individual's needs (Cesta and Falter, 1999). The team might include the psychiatrist, nurse, social worker, dietician, pharmacist, activity therapist, and chaplain. Consultations with other services, such as physical therapy, neurology, internal medicine, and aftercare services, occur as needed. The individual has the opportunity to meet with any or all team members. The multidisciplinary team uses a decision tree in its discharge planning process (Cesta and Falter, 1999). (See Chapter 2 for discussion of the decision tree.)

| Table 3-1 | Types of Programming |
| --- | --- |

| Programming | Examples of Major Target Issues |
| --- | --- |
| **Age-Based** | |
| Child | Family issues, developmental issues, peer relationships, academic issues, behavior management, life stresses, coping strategies |
| Adolescent | Same as above, plus intimate relationships, sexuality, substance abuse |
| Adult | Same as above, plus acceptance of illness and medication compliance; social, occupational, and financial problem solving |
| Older adult | Same as above, plus aging process, death and dying, retirement adjustment, disabilities and chronic illnesses, assistance in living issues |
| **Diagnosis-Based** | |
| Acute or nonpsychotic, or both | Insight into illness and life situations, problem solving, interpersonal relationships |
| Chronic or psychotic, or both | Symptom management, medication compliance, social skills, community living skills, vocational assessment |
| Addictions | Dynamics of addiction, effects of addictions |

## NURSE-PATIENT RELATIONSHIP

Nurses are the only members of the multidisciplinary team who provide 24-hour care during the hospital stay. Individuals admitted to psychiatric units today are more acutely ill than they were in the past and exhibit more severe psychopathology. Within a day or two, with the aforementioned shorter LOS, the nurse must establish a therapeutic relationship, identify immediate needs, and provide holistic quality care. The nurse often begins to intervene while the individual is being admitted to the unit because of behaviors that are dangerous to self or others. Despite the individual's level of illness or the type of behaviors being exhibited, the patient must quickly realize that the nurse is caring, empathetic, supportive, and helpful. The nurse might need to set limits on behaviors but, at the same time, must convey respect and maintain the dignity of the individual.

After the individual acquires a sense of safety and is more able to control behavior, further assessment occurs. The nursing assessment must be direct, specific, and comprehensive. Gathering information from as many sources as possible is important. These sources include family, significant others, old charts and records, and professionals in outpatient services with whom the individual might have had contact.

Discharge planning has always been an important nursing role. With decreased LOS, life after hospitalization has become even more critical. Discharge planning begins at admission and is incorporated into the multidisciplinary treatment plan. For some individuals, discharge planning can be relatively simple, such as "return home with outpatient follow-up." For others, the discharge plan can be complex and involve a number of community services along the continuum of care, such as housing, medicine clinic, dental service, outpatient counseling, and self-help group for the family. Although the nurse might not arrange for these services directly, the nurse coordinates this activity. Including the individual and the family or significant other(s) in multidisciplinary conferences as much as possible is important; thus, they can be involved in the development and implementation of goals, including those after discharge. For more information about the nurse-patient relationship, see Chapter 8.

## PSYCHOPHARMACOLOGY

The nurse is instrumental in obtaining the medication history; this includes information about past and current medications and dosages, medication allergies, the individual's perspective on medication effectiveness, problems with side effects, and present and past compliance. An important role includes monitoring the effectiveness of medication, the presence of side effects, and educating the individual and family about the medication and its side effects. The nurse must carefully assess the need for as-needed (prn) medication so problem behaviors and symptoms can be addressed and alleviated as quickly as possible. The nurse emphasizes the importance of medication compliance in symptom management and control with the individual and family. (For specific information on medications, see Chapters 16 through 22.)

## MILIEU MANAGEMENT

The milieu or inpatient environment is therapeutic and supportive to encourage the individual's return to adequate functioning in the community. The emphasis of milieu activities is on helping the individual cope with immediate needs and with stressors and problems in his or her home or living environment. Because of the current increased incidence of short-term stays, the need exists for structured milieus to include groups that are problem-focused, goal-oriented, and relevant to the needs of the individual. Box 3-1 provides a sample inpatient daily schedule. The nurse assists the individual in applying information obtained in educational groups to his or her own situation. The nurse teaches the individual the best way to solve problems, rather than focusing on resolving all problems before discharge. With these skills, the individual can hopefully continue to solve problems after discharge. Homework assignments, journal writing, and educational handouts provide even more structure in the milieu.

| Box 3-1 | Sample of an Inpatient Daily Schedule* |
|---|---|
| 7:00 AM | Wake-up and morning care |
| 8:00 AM | Breakfast and free time |
| 9:00 AM | Goal-setting group |
| 10:00 AM | Stress management group |
| 11:00 AM | Exercise group |
| 12:00 PM | Lunch and free time |
| 1:00 PM | Medication education group |
| 2:00 PM | Self-esteem group |
| 3:00 PM | Addictions group |
| 4:00 PM | Free time |
| 5:00 PM | Dinner and goal review group |
| 6:00 PM | Family education group |
| 7:00 PM | Visiting or free time, or both |
| 9:00 PM | Relaxation group |
| 10:00 PM | Free time |
| 10:30 PM | Bedtime |

*All group sessions last 40 minutes. Interactions with staff are expected between group sessions, during free time, or both.

## CRITICAL THINKING QUESTION    1

You are admitting a 15-year-old boy to an inpatient unit because of alcohol and marijuana abuse, sexual promiscuity, and failing grades. These behaviors developed over the last 3 months after his father was diagnosed w-[ith terminal cancer. What issues need to be addressed during his hospitalization?

## COMMUNITY-BASED CARE

Nurses have a role in community-based services because of their psychotherapeutic management skills, their knowledge of psychopathology and psychopharmacology, and their ability to adapt the use of the nursing process to any setting. Another valuable asset that the nurse brings to the health care system is knowledge of reimbursement systems and budget restrictions. Using a holistic approach, nurses can deliver direct care to help reintegrate people with mental illness into community living, as well as assist the individual in linking with other community resources. The nurse might need to advocate and negotiate for services such as the following:

- Medical clinics
- Dental services
- Financial services
- Vocational services
- Transportation
- Housing
- Medicare and Medicaid
- Legal or justice system
- Church-related programs
- Employee assistance programs
- Consumer groups
- Telehealth

## TRADITIONAL OUTPATIENT SERVICES

Traditionally, outpatient treatment has occurred in mental health clinics and private offices. The person providing counseling might be a psychiatrist, psychologist, social worker, clinical nurse specialist, nurse, or other professional. The number of visits per week or month varies according to the individual's needs. The typical pattern for an individual with a chronic mental illness might be a visit once a month with a counselor or case manager and periodic appointments with a psychiatrist for medication review. During these counseling visits, an assessment of needs for additional services is made to determine whether the individual needs more intense service or a different type of service.

## CLINICAL EXAMPLE

Larry, a 31-year-old man with the diagnosis of chronic undifferentiated schizophrenia, attends a community support program. He meets with his case manager every other week after he receives his haloperidol decanoate (Haldol Decanoate) injection from the nurse, who assesses for effectiveness of the medication and management of side effects. He also participates in a social club, which offers lunch and social activities twice weekly. The psychiatrist meets with him every 3 months for medication evaluation.

## PARTIAL PROGRAMS AND DAY TREATMENT

Individuals who need some supervision, structured activities, ongoing treatment, and nursing care might benefit from partial programs and day treatment. These programs vary in length from 4 to 8 hours per day and 1 to 5 days per week. Programming can occur during the day, evening, and night. Depending on the community, these programs might provide treatment for specific populations based on age (child, adolescent, adult, or older adult) or type of problem (addiction or chronic mental illness).

### CLINICAL EXAMPLE

John, a 52-year-old man with severe depression resulting from the unexpected death of his wife, is discharged from the hospital but is unable to return to work. He attends a partial program for 2 weeks that meets from 10 AM to 3 PM, Monday through Friday. He attends groups that focus on exercise, spirituality, coping with losses, and self-esteem issues. Lunchtime provides an opportunity for socialization with program members.

## PSYCHIATRIC HOME CARE

Psychiatric home care services are available for the homebound because their illness or disability inhibits their ability to leave home and obtain services elsewhere. Home visits can occur in conjunction with other community-based services. Home care often serves individuals with severe and persistent mental illnesses and those with a combination of psychiatric and medical illnesses. Home care can be provided by traditional public and private home care agencies that have added psychiatric home services. Many psychiatric hospitals and community mental health centers have instituted home care programs.

### CLINICAL EXAMPLE

Joe, an 80-year-old man with Alzheimer's disease, lives at home with his wife. The nurse assesses Joe's mental status and level of functioning. Assistance is given to Joe's wife in implementing safety measures in the home because of Joe's wandering behavior. The nurse assists with arranging respite care so that Joe's wife can go shopping and attend a weekly caregivers' support group.

## COMMUNITY OUTREACH PROGRAMS

Outreach services have been developed to reach individuals in areas in which a lack of traditional medical and social services exists. Programs such as mobile crisis teams are available that attempt to reach particular individuals, such as the homeless or transient groups (e.g., migrant workers and their families), who have had little success with community-based services. Mobile programs that serve the needs of mentally ill individuals on the streets, under bridges, in parks, in missions, and at lunch programs exemplify outreach services. Some programs arrange for physician and nurse volunteers to operate a neighborhood clinic once or twice weekly to serve homeless individuals with medical or psychiatric needs, or both. Outreach services that assess and treat older adults have improved access and outcomes (Van Citters and Bartels, 2004).

## RESIDENTIAL SERVICES

Residential services are available to help individuals who need temporary or long-term housing. Most states have long-term care facilities for individuals needing prolonged 24-hour supervision. The LOS might be 3 to 6 months or longer.

*Extended care facilities* (e.g., nursing homes) are available for people who require 24-hour supervision and medical nursing care. This level of care is often required for individuals with severe developmental disabilities, dementia, or acute and chronic medical illnesses.

*Group homes* might provide temporary or permanent housing for individuals with chronic mental disorders. Depending on the needs of the residents, staff might be present for 24 hours a day or less. Some group homes provide group therapy and structured activities, whereas others might provide only meals, a bed, and laundry facilities.

Traditionally, *halfway houses* were available for individuals with chemical dependency. Residents were expected to seek employment and participate in cooking and cleaning chores. Residents would also attend self-help groups that meet on site, such as Alcoholics Anonymous. Some halfway houses are now open to individuals with other problems.

*Apartment living* programs provide varying degrees of supervision and programming. Staff might be on site on a daily basis, offering group sessions and activities, or they might visit periodically to ensure medication compliance and attendance at various appointments.

*Foster care* and *boarding homes* are generally staffed by nonprofessionals but have professional supervision available on an outpatient basis. *Shelters* provide room and board to the homeless. Some homes might provide services for specific populations, such as victims of violence (e.g., abused women and their families) or those with addictions.

---

### CLINICAL EXAMPLE

Lois, a 63-year-old woman with the diagnosis of bipolar disorder mania, had been living with her son until her behaviors became unmanageable, which resulted from medication noncompliance. Because of her need for more supervision, she was placed in an apartment living program. A nurse visits her three times weekly to monitor medication compliance. The nurse also assists her with keeping outpatient appointments.

---

## SELF-HELP GROUPS

Self-help groups are another source of support on the continuum of care. Self-help group meetings are conducted by members, not professionals, and can take place on a weekly basis. Table 3-2 provides examples of types of self-help groups. See Chapter 12 for additional information.

## INTENSIVE OUTPATIENT PROGRAMS

*Intensive outpatient programs* provide services at a greater level of intensity than traditional outpatient programs (Schreter, 2000). These are designed to stabilize patients in the community by offering a clubhouse model, and are based on a community-based rehabilitation model called Fountain House, which opened in New York City in 1948. This type of program focuses on supporting people with disabilities in their pursuit of recovery. The clubhouse model provides members with opportunities such as (1) daytime work-organized activities focused on the care and maintenance of the housing environment, (2) evening, weekend, and holiday leisure time activities, (3) support for employment, and (4) housing (Aquila et al, 1999).

Many new outpatient programs are based on the concept of recovery, which provides the consumer with control and responsibility for his or her life. Outpatient programs empower the consumer with the ability to maintain and improve in the major domains of life involving work, housing, relationships, and recreation. The recovery model emphasizes consumers' strengths and choices. Power and responsibility are shared in collaboration and involvement with friends, family, supports, and professionals (Jacobson and Curtis, 2000).

Traditional case management is a method used to provide holistic, seamless care by coordinating services and resources needed by an individual to improve quality of life and to live independently in the community. The goal of case management is to prevent rehospitalization by providing comprehensive and cost-effective services. Box 3–2 lists additional goals and purposes. Variations of case management have evolved to correct lack of continuity of care and fragmented services, but have been unsuccessful in achieving

| Table 3-2 | Self-Help Groups | |
| --- | --- |

| Type of Group | Examples |
| --- | --- |
| Addiction-based | Alcoholics Anonymous |
| | Narcotics Anonymous |
| | Overeaters Anonymous |
| Survivor-based | Survivors of Suicide |
| | Incest Survivors Anonymous |
| | Adult Children of Alcoholics |
| Disorder-based | Eating disorders |
| | Bipolar disorder |
| | Family and caregiver support groups |
| | National Alliance for the Mentally Ill |
| Loss-based | Grief, divorce, bereavement support groups |
| Medically based (chronic or terminal illness) | Lupus, cancer, chronic fatigue, AIDS support groups |
| Prevention-based | Parenting, tough love support groups |

| Box 3-2 | Goals and Purposes of Community Treatment |
|---|---|

Hope
Increased quality of life
Participation in treatment
Competency
Empowerment
Decreased readmissions to inpatient units
Increased social, vocational, and emotional
    functioning
Decreased burden on caregivers
Independence and growth
Community involvement
Adaptation to or recovery from mental illness
Satisfaction with environment
Continuous treatment
Cost-effective treatment

their goals fully (Antai-Ontong, 2003). Large caseloads, fragmented care, and the inability of the individual with mental illness to get needs met and achieve positive outcomes are some elements that have contributed to its ineffectiveness.

## ASSERTIVE COMMUNITY TREATMENT

Assertive community treatment (ACT) is a comprehensive, community-based service delivery model in which a team of professionals assumes direct responsibility for providing services needed by the consumer 24 hours a day, 7 days a week. Services are provided in settings in which consumers' problems arise and support or skills are needed (Phillips et al, 2001). Multidisciplinary team members, including a nurse, psychiatrist, social worker, supportive employment person, and substance abuse person, work together and share responsibility for providing comprehensive treatment and support to a specified number of consumers. Small caseloads and provision of direct care rather than making referrals are two differences between ACT and traditional case management (Rapp and Goscha, 2004). Treatment and services include assistance with shopping, laundry, transportation, and housing. Supervising medication, monitoring health care, and responding to emergencies are a few of the many responsibilities that team members share. Members also provide outreach to wherever the consumer lives, such as homeless shelters, the streets, and jails. The ACT program is an evidence-based practice model of community treatment that has reduced hospital admissions and improved social functioning and quality of life for

individuals with severe mental illness (Marshall et al, 2005; Marshall and Lockwood, 2005).

The case manager role in the ACT program is appropriate for the nurse because the nurse has been an important provider of care to consumers, families, and groups along the continuum of care and an active member of the multidisciplinary team (Antai-Ontong, 2003). The nurse uses case management to increase continuity of care, ensure access to care, and provide direct cost-effective care. The nurse might assume multiple roles, such as teacher, counselor, advocate, and coordinator. The nurse must also possess key qualities to be effective, including warmth, sensitivity, creativity, empathy, and patience, which qualities facilitate independent living and enhance the quality of life. Through the nurse-patient relationship, the nurse empowers the individual to pursue positive outcomes and offers hope, support, and guidance. The nurse has been identified as an integral member of the ACT team by other members of the treatment team (McGrew et al, 2003).

## OTHER TYPES OF INTENSIVE SERVICE

### Primary Care

Individuals with mental health–related needs, such as anxiety, depression, and sleep disturbances, sometimes seek help for these problems in primary care offices and clinics. Three reasons for this are (1) the stigma that exists about mental illness, (2) lack of knowledge about who to see and where to get help, and (3) reduced access to care. Psychopharmacologic medications are prescribed at times without a comprehensive history and assessment of the patient. When that happens, the patient's immediate need might be addressed, but other modes of treatment that could benefit the patient might not be recommended or are overlooked. Implementation of other types of interventions related to coping, problem solving, feeling and behavioral management, and substance-related problems could be indicated.

The advanced practice psychiatric nurse or clinical specialist working in primary care areas provides interventions that benefit individuals with mental health–related needs. Short sessions with the patient regarding medication management, methods to decrease anxiety, and relationship issues might be addressed by advanced practice nurses.

## *Integrated Community Treatment*

Individuals with serious mental illnesses have high morbidity and mortality because of physical illness. Diabetes, hypertension, and dyslipidemia are only a few examples. Integrated community treatment is a model of care that provides treatment for physical and mental health care. This model provides increased ease of access to care, completeness of care, support, education, and holistic care in one location or clinic. The focus is on health promotion, illness prevention, and illness care. One such clinic is Old Town Clinic in Oregon, located in the inner city, which provides access to care for the homeless and low-income population in the community (Krautscheid et al, 2004).

Another example of integrated treatment has been described by Kane and Blank (2004). Advanced practice nurses and consumer peer providers were part of an assertive community treatment team. The advanced practice nurse managed the physical and psychiatric care of the patient while the consumer peer provider lended encouragement and support to the patient in the community. Integrated community treatment improves client community functioning, results in moderate-to-high client and staff satisfaction, and makes good use of limited resources.

---

| CRITICAL THINKING QUESTION | 2 |
| --- | --- |

During one of your visits to a homeless shelter, you meet Ann, who is 19 years old. Ann has been homeless for 2 months and, until recently, had been living with friends. Ann was diagnosed with bipolar disorder 5 months ago. She lost her job as a waitress shortly after becoming ill and quickly emptied her small savings account to pay rent and buy food. She has not been taking her medication because of lack of money. Ann is motivated to work but does not know how to go about finding a job and housing. She is feeling overwhelmed and is afraid that she will get sick again. What community resources would be helpful to Ann?

---

## PUTTING IT ALL TOGETHER
### Psychotherapeutic Management

Psychiatric nursing advocates for the inclusion of nurses as members of the multidisciplinary team in any of the settings described in this chapter.

Psychiatric nurses offer valuable contributions to community-based care because of their ability to adapt the nursing process and the psychotherapeutic management model of care to any setting.

## NURSE-PATIENT RELATIONSHIP

Developing a nurse-patient relationship in the community is challenging because of the decreased contact and time spent with the individual. Establishing rapport and trust quickly is critical to implementing the nursing process effectively and efficiently. Individuals are more likely to maintain contact with the nurse over time when they feel valued, respected, and satisfied with their care. The nurse also uses the principles of developing the nurse-patient relationship when working with caregivers and family members. Developing collaborative relationships with other professionals is crucial for maintaining the continuum of care.

## PSYCHOPHARMACOLOGY

In community-based settings, the individual and caregiver or family must have knowledge about medications and about the importance of taking these medications as prescribed. Noncompliance with medication is the major cause of relapse and rehospitalization. The nurse has a major role in teaching about medication effects, side effects, management of side effects, and the relationship between medication and symptom management. The nurse must be astute in recognizing early signs of both side effects and noncompliance so as to be able to intervene quickly. Missing early signs of side effects can result in unnecessary patient discomfort, or worse, and missing noncompliance can lead to poor symptom management.

## MILIEU MANAGEMENT

In community-based care, the principles of milieu management are adapted in assessing agencies, programs, and private homes. After assessing the individual's needs, the nurse is responsible for determining which services in the continuum of care would best meet the individual's needs in the least restrictive setting. The nurse has less direct control and influence over an environment in the community than in an inpatient setting. Furthermore, economic factors affecting the health care system, individuals, and families might put constraints on environmental modifications that can be accomplished and the type of care that can be delivered. This means that the nurse adapts care based on environmental limitations and availability of resources.

## USE OF THE NURSING PROCESS IN THE COMMUNITY

The nursing process is the foundation of case management. Effective use of the nursing process in the areas of psychiatric rehabilitation, crisis intervention, home care, therapy, consultation and liaison, resource linkage, and advocacy provides case management services for psychiatric patients (Figure 3-1). The nurse is skilled in synthesizing these components in an understandable and useful manner for patients.

## ASSESSMENT

The nurse comprehensively assesses the individual's mental and physical health to provide and coordinate holistic and culturally appropriate care. The individual is the center of care and is a key member of the team in identifying needs and outcomes. The following areas are usually assessed:

- Medication compliance and management
- Symptom management
- Social supports
- Family involvement

- Medical needs and limitations
- Skills
- Cognitive functioning
- Vocational skills
- Social skills
- Problem solving
- Spiritual and religious needs and concerns
- Coping abilities

### CLINICAL EXAMPLE

The nurse assesses Jim at his first appointment at the mental health clinic after a recent hospitalization. Jim complains of being bored and tired of watching television. He states that he doesn't have any clean clothes to wear and is uncertain of how to use the washing machine. He is also bothered by increasing hand tremors. Jim discloses that he is worried about not having enough money to buy groceries at the end of the month. The nurse assesses Jim's needs to include hand tremors, ineffective use of leisure time, self-care deficit, and limited finances.

## OUTCOME IDENTIFICATION AND PLANNING

The nurse plans and prioritizes appropriate care based on comprehensive assessment and nursing diagnoses. In the previous clinical example, the nurse prioritizes Jim's needs. The hand tremors must be addressed first, followed by Jim's self-care deficit, ineffective use of leisure time, and financial needs. The nurse's plan includes (1) consulting with the psychiatrist regarding Jim's hand tremors, (2) addressing his self-care, (3) working with Jim in structuring and using his leisure time in a healthful manner, such as walking, (4) connecting Jim with the social worker for further exploration of financial resources and assistance, (5) helping Jim budget his money, and (6) assisting Jim with meal planning and grocery shopping.

## IMPLEMENTATION

Many factors must be considered when prioritizing interventions, and the nurse must take a holistic approach when implementing these interventions. This means recognizing and addressing the interconnectedness of various factors in a patient's life (e.g., physical, mental, emotional,

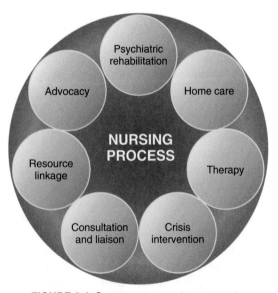

**FIGURE 3-1** Case management components.

spiritual, environmental, financial) to provide culturally appropriate care.

In the previous clinical example, the nurse initiates the plan by building rapport and trust to establish the therapeutic relationship with Jim. The nurse arranges for a psychiatric evaluation before Jim leaves. An adjustment is made in Jim's haloperidol decanoate (Haldol), and he is given a prescription for benztropine mesylate (Cogentin), 1 mg PO daily. The nurse teaches Jim about the purpose and side effects of benztropine. During this discussion, Jim reports that he has insufficient funds to purchase both the benztropine and groceries. The nurse discusses his financial situation with Jim and discovers enough money for a 2-week supply of benztropine. The nurse then consults with the pharmacy to ensure that Jim can purchase a 2-week supply now and fill the remainder of the prescription at the beginning of the following month. The nurse instructs Jim to see the social worker before he leaves the clinic to obtain a bus pass so that he can go to the pharmacy to have his prescription filled. The nurse arranges to visit Jim at his apartment in 2 days to demonstrate how to use the washer and dryer in his apartment building. Jim is sure that he has a small box of laundry detergent in his kitchen. The nurse then proceeds to discuss his food preferences, usual purchases at the grocery store, and budgeting with Jim. Healthy nutrition is also discussed.

Jim states that he enjoys walking and could resume that activity. He asks the nurse about part-time employment because that would help relieve his boredom and he could earn some money. His last job prior to his hospitalization was in janitorial services. He is motivated to work and thinks that he is ready for employment. The nurse refers him to the supportive employment program, which helps individuals with psychiatric disabilities access and retain jobs; an appointment is made with supportive employment in 2 weeks. It is an effective program, and can result in employee and employer satisfaction and employment stability (Dorio, 2004; Perkins et al, 2005).

## EVALUATION

Evaluation is an ongoing process. Each intervention and the overall patient status must be continually evaluated. Patients have changing needs, issues, and concerns. The nurse must be attuned to these changes during all interactions with patients. Responses to medication, including effectiveness and side effects, must be evaluated in an ongoing manner. For example, before Jim leaves the mental health clinic, the nurse evaluates the following:

- Jim's understanding of the medication changes, the desired responses, and the potential side effects
- Jim's plan for purchasing the benztropine
- The purpose, date, and time of the appointment with the nurse
- The purpose, date, and time of the appointment with supportive employment.

## Study Notes

1. The range of services is rapidly evolving to meet the needs of individuals with mental health problems.
2. The goal of managed care is to foster optimal functioning and health by providing the least expensive, least restrictive, and least intensive treatment.
3. Assessment of the individual's needs and level of functioning and the level of supervision that the individual requires determines referral to hospital-based or community-based care.
4. Appropriate and specific outcome-based care is critical to optimizing the individual's level of functioning, as well as reimbursement.
5. Most hospital-based care is now provided on a short-term basis, focusing on crisis intervention and safety.
6. The primary goals of hospital-based care are provision of safety and discharge planning.
7. The type of hospital-based care available to individuals varies according to the size of both the hospital and the community.
8. Discharge planning begins at the time of admission and varies in complexity.
9. The psychotherapeutic management model is the most relevant approach to short-term hospitalization.
10. Community-based services have evolved to meet the needs of individuals and families in the continuum of care.
11. The continuum of care includes inpatient hospitalization, outpatient services, residential care, self-help activities, and other resources.

12. The nursing process and the psychotherapeutic management approach can be adapted in any setting along the continuum of care.

13. The recovery model of care gives the consumer power and responsibility for his or her life.

14. Assertive community treatment provides care 24 hours a day, 7 days a week by a multidisciplinary team.

15. The nurse as case manager provides direct care and links the patient with needed services along the continuum of care.

## References

Antai-Ontong D: Psychosocial rehabilitation, *Nurs Clin North Am* 38:151, 2003.

Appelbaum PS: Presidential address: re-envisioning a mental health system for the United States, *Am J Psychiatry* 160:1758, 2003.

Aquila R, Santos G, Malamud TJ, McCrory D: The rehabilitation alliance in practice: the clubhouse connection, *Psychiatr Rehabil J* 23:19, 1999.

Benson WD, Briscoe L: Jumping the hurdles of health care wearing cement shoes: where does the inpatient psychiatric nurse fit in? *J Am Psychiatr Nurs Assoc* 9:123, 2003.

Cesta TG, Falter EJ: Case management: its value for staff nurses, *Am J Nurs* 99:48, 1999.

Dorio J: Tying it all together—the pass to success: a comprehensive look at promoting job retention for workers with psychiatric disabilities in a supported employment program, *Psychiatr Rehabil J* 28:32, 2004.

Jacobson N, Curtis L: Recovery as policy in mental health services: strategies emerging from the states, *Psychiatr Rehabil J* 23:333, 2000.

Kane CF, Blank MB: NPACT: enhancing programs of assertive community treatment for the seriously mentally ill, *Commun Ment Health J* 40:549, 2004.

Kirsch D: Developing outpatient mental health services for managed care, *Psychiatr Clin North Am* 23:403, 2000.

Krautscheid L, Moos P, Zeller J: Patient and staff satisfaction with integrated services at Old Town Clinic: a descriptive analysis, *Psychosoc Nurs Mental Health Serv* 42:33, 2004.

Marshall M, Gray A, Lockwood A, Green R: Case management for people with severe mental disorders, *Cochrane Database System Reviews* Issue 4, 2005.

Marshall M, Lockwood A: Assertive community treatment for people with severe mental disorders, *Cochrane Database System Rev* Issue 4, 2005.

McGrew JH, Pescosolido B, Wright E: Case managers; perspectives on critical ingredients of assertive community treatment and on its implementation, *Psychiatr Serv* 54:370, 2003.

Perkins DV, Born DL, Raines JA, Galka SW: Program evaluation from an ecological perspective: supported employment services for persons with serious psychiatric disabilities, *Psychiatr Rehabil J* 28:217, 2005.

Phillips SD et al: Moving assertive community treatment into standard practice, *Psychiatr Serv* 52(6):771, 2001.

Rapp CA, Goscha RJ: The principles of effective case management of mental health services, *Psychiatr Rehabil J* 27:319, 2004.

Schreter RK: Alternative treatment programs: the psychiatric continuum of care, *Psychiatr Clin North Am* 23:335, 2000.

Van Citters AD, Bartels SJ: A systematic review of the effectiveness of community-based mental health outreach services for older adults, *Psychiatr Serv* 55:1237, 2004.

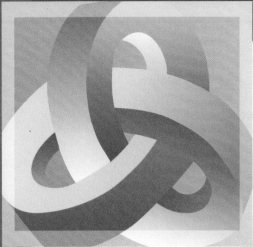

# Models for Working With Psychiatric Patients

*Lee H. Schwecke*

*After reading this chapter, you should be able to:*

- Compare and contrast major therapeutic models that contribute to the understanding of psychiatric patients and their behaviors.

- Identify key concepts of the major therapeutic models.
- Describe the relevance of each therapeutic model to psychiatric nursing practice.

The following models of human behavior have been selected for discussion in this chapter because they provide basic concepts for working with psychiatric patients: psychoanalytic, developmental, interpersonal, cognitive-behavioral, reality therapy, and stress models. These models are summarized in Table 4-1 and throughout the chapter. In addition, behavior therapies are discussed in Chapter 38.

## PSYCHOANALYTIC MODEL

The psychoanalytic model (Freud, 1936; Brill, 1938; Freud and Strachey, 1960) is a theory of the personality that originated with Sigmund Freud and emphasizes unconscious processes or psycho-dynamic factors as the basis for motivation and behavior. Freud believed that the personality is formed during the first 6 years of life. Knowledge of the way in which an individual's drives, instincts, psychic energy or libido, and psycho-sexual attitude are formed is crucial to an understanding of the personality.

## KEY CONCEPTS

### Personality Processes

The personality consists of three processes—the id, the ego, and the superego—that function as a whole to bring about behavior. When these processes function in harmony, the individual experiences stability; when disharmony occurs, the individual is in conflict.

The individual is all *id* at birth, wanting to experience only pleasure. This instinctual drive is known as the pleasure principle; this involves primary process thinking, enabling the individual to strive for pleasure through the use of fantasies and images. The id is compulsive and without morals. The ego controls id impulses and mediates between the id and the reality.

The *ego* focuses on the reality principle and strives to meet the demands of the id while maintaining the well-being of the individual by distinguishing fantasy from environmental reality. Secondary process thinking comprises rational, logical thinking and intelligence. The ego is the

| Table 4-1 | Therapeutic Models | | |
|---|---|---|---|
| **Model** | **Assumptions** | **Goals and Approaches** | **Dialogue** |
| Psychoanalytic (Freud) | Individuals are motivated by unconscious desires and conflicts. Personality is developed by early childhood. | *Insight* into unconscious conflicts and processes Personality reconstruction | Patient: "All women hate me." Immediate response: "Tell me about one woman with whom you are having trouble." |
| | Illness results from childhood conflicts, and ego defenses are inadequate to cope with anxiety. | | |
| | Change is a process of *insight*. | Using free association, dream analysis, and analyses of transference and resistance | *Insight*-oriented response: "Tell me about your relationship with your mother." |
| Developmental (Erikson) | Biologic, psychological, social, and environmental factors influence personality development throughout the life cycle. | Mastering developmental tasks through achievement of insight; continued development through death; analyzing developmental issues, fears, and barriers to *growth* to achieve insight | Patient: "I can't do anything right. Help me." Immediate response: "I hear your doubt in yourself; but I did see you make a positive decision this morning." |
| | *Growth* involves resolution of critical tasks at each of the eight developmental stages. | | |
| | Lack of resolution of tasks causes incomplete development and difficulties in relationships. | | |
| | Change involves reexperiencing and resolving developmental crises. Change is a process of *growth*. | Facilitating mastery of developmental tasks with support and problem solving | *Growth*-oriented response: "I can help you look at ways to develop your self-confidence." |
| Interpersonal (Sullivan, Peplau) | Interpersonal relationships and anxiety facilitate development of the self-system. | Developing satisfactory relationships and maturity; relative freedom from the interference of anxiety; learning effective interpersonal skills | Patient: "I can't sit still. I'm too nervous." Immediate response: "Let's take a walk for a few minutes." |
| | Development occurs in stages with changing types of relationships. | | |
| | Faulty patterns of relating interfere with security and maturity. | | |
| | Security operations protect against anxiety and interfere with learning. | | |
| | Change is a process of *reeducation*. | Examining current interpersonal difficulties; using therapist-patient relationships as a vehicle for analyzing interpersonal processes and testing new skills; consensual validation, validation, reality testing, and reflecting positive appraisals | *Reeducation* response: "Let's talk about what kind of things you get nervous about and what you can do about them." |

| Table 4-1 | Therapeutic Models—cont'd | | |
| --- | --- | --- | --- |
| **Model** | **Assumptions** | **Goals and Approaches** | **Dialogue** |
| Cognitive-behavioral (Beck, Ellis) | An individual has value simply because he or she exists. Individuals have potential *rational* and irrational thinking. Irrational beliefs produce irrational emotions and behaviors. Change involves changing beliefs to change feelings and behaviors. Change is a process of *rational* thinking. | Substituting *rational* beliefs for irrational ones. Eliminating self-defeating behaviors. Increased responsibility for feelings, behaviors, and change. Challenging irrational beliefs; cognitive homework. Role playing and testing out new behaviors | Patient: "My wife makes me so angry." Immediate response: "What did your wife do that you didn't like?" *Cognitive-behavioral* response: "What is self-defeating about the statement you just made?" |
| Reality therapy (Glasser) | An individual's most basic psychological needs are to be loved (to be involved) and to feel worthwhile (to have respect from self and others). Needs must be met responsibly and within the context of reality. Responsibility is fulfilling one's needs without interfering with others who are fulfilling their needs. Illness results from irresponsible behavior. Change is a process of *relearning*. | Facing reality and developing standards for behaving responsibly. Greater maturity, conscientiousness, and responsibility. Being accountable for one's behaviors. Being open, warm, honest, authentic; accepting of the patient as a person. Becoming deeply involved with the patient. Focusing on current behaviors and consequences. Confronting irresponsible behaviors. Assisting with *relearning* of responsible behaviors | Patient: "The stupid doctor revoked my pass for today." Immediate response: "What did you do that showed that you were not ready for a pass?" *Relearning* response: "What behaviors do you think will be necessary before you will be given a pass?" |
| Stress (Selye, Lazarus) | Stress is any positive or negative occurrence or emotion requiring a response. Stress produces physiologic and psychological responses. Inadequate handling of stress can lead to physical or mental illness, or both. Change is a process of *problem solving*. | Developing effective coping mechanisms. Reducing bodily tensions. Increasing resources and social supports. Managing stress. Using biofeedback. Using relaxation training | Patient: "I'm so tense, I can't sleep." Immediate response: "I have a relaxation exercise I can show you." *Problem-solving* approach: "You've said you're worried about seeing your family tomorrow. Let's talk about what you might say to them." |

**Norm's Notes**

*I love this chapter, and I didn't even write it. Dr. Schwecke has done a good job of simplifying some of the great models on which psychiatric care has been based. Although simplified, there is enough information in this chapter to help you really understand the basic premises that guide therapeutic relationships. For example, if you avoid reading this chapter before an exam, but go out with friends instead, then this chapter has a term for that behavior: suppression. You will probably find other ideas to use so you can identify some of your behaviors that might not be beneficial. Remember, the truth always helps.*

part of the personality that experiences anxiety and uses defense mechanisms for protection. Heredity, environmental factors, and maturation influence the formation of the ego.

The *superego* is concerned with right and wrong—that is, the conscience. It provides the ego with an inner control to help cope with the id. The superego is formed from the internalization of what parents teach their children about right and wrong through rewards and punishments. Self-esteem is affected by the perception of a person's actions as good or right. Guilt and inferiority are experienced when the individual cannot live up to parental standards. Inner conflict results when the id, the ego, and the superego are striving for different goals.

### Consciousness

Freud's concepts of the levels of consciousness are central in understanding problems of the personality and behavior. *Consciousness,* or material within an individual's awareness, is only one small part of the mind. The unconscious is a larger area and consists of memories, conflicts, experiences, and material that have been repressed and cannot be recalled at will. Preconscious material refers to memories that can be recalled to consciousness with some effort. Freud believed that uncovering unconscious material generates an understanding of behavior that enables individuals to make choices about behavior and thus improve their

mental health. Insight into the meaning of symptoms facilitates change.

### Defense Mechanisms

The ego usually copes with anxiety through rational means. When anxiety is too painful, the individual copes by using defense mechanisms to protect the ego and diminish anxiety. When these mechanisms are used excessively, individuals are unable to face reality and do not solve their problems. Defense mechanisms are primarily unconscious behaviors; however, some are within voluntary control. Common defense mechanisms are described in Table 4-2.

Painful feelings connected with childhood conflicts are often repressed. Later in life, as similar conflicts are experienced once again, repression fails and these feelings emerge, causing anxiety and discomfort. Freud defined three types of anxiety that form the basis of many mental illnesses: (1) reality anxiety stems from an external real threat; (2) neurotic anxiety deals with the fear that instincts will cause a person to do something to invite punishment, such as being promiscuous; and (3) moral anxiety deals with guilt that is experienced when an individual acts contrary to his or her conscience, such as stealing money from a friend.

## THERAPIST'S ROLE

The goals of freudian psychoanalytic therapy and other psychodynamic therapies are to bring the unconscious into consciousness, enabling individuals to work through the past and understand their past and present behaviors. By overcoming repression and resistance to exploring feelings and thoughts, childhood experiences can be analyzed. Uncovering the causes of current behaviors leads to insight (Miller, 2004a). Only then can individuals decrease their self-defeating behaviors and improve their mental health.

In traditional long-term psychoanalysis, the therapist uses free association (allowing the patient to say everything that comes to mind) so that repressed material can be identified and interpreted for patients. Dream analysis helps patients uncover the meaning of their dreams, which also increases awareness about present behavior. Patients' inconsistencies and resistance to therapy

**Table 4-2    Defense Mechanisms**

| Defense Mechanism | Definition | Patient Example |
|---|---|---|
| Denial | *Unconscious* refusal to admit an unacceptable idea or behavior | Mr. Davis, who is alcohol-dependent, believes that he can control his drinking if he so desires. |
| Repression | *Unconscious* and involuntary forgetting of painful ideas, events, and conflicts | Ms. Young, a victim of incest, no longer remembers the reason she always hated the uncle who molested her. |
| Suppression | *Conscious* exclusion from awareness anxiety-producing feelings, ideas, and situations | Ms. Ames states to the nurse that she is not ready to talk about her recent divorce. |
| Rationalization | *Conscious or unconscious* attempts to make or prove that one's feelings or behaviors are justifiable | Mr. Jones, diagnosed with schizophrenia, states that he cannot go to work because his co-workers are mean, instead of admitting that his illness interferes with working. |
| Intellectualization | *Consciously* or *unconsciously* using only logical explanations without feelings or an affective component | Ms. Mann talks about her son's death from cancer as being merciful and shows no signs of her sadness and anger. |
| Dissociation | The *unconscious* separation of painful feelings and emotions from an unacceptable idea, situation, or object | Ms. Adams recalls that when she was sexually molested as a child, she felt as if she were outside of her body watching what was happening without feeling anything. |
| Identification | *Conscious or unconscious* attempt to model oneself after a respected person | Ms. Kelly states to the nurse, "When I get out of the hospital, I want to be a nurse just like you." |
| Introjection | *Unconsciously* incorporating values and attitudes of others as if they were your own | Without realizing it, Mr. Chad wishes, talks, and acts similarly to his therapist, analyzing other patients. |
| Compensation | *Consciously* covering up for a weakness by overemphasizing or making up a desirable trait | Mr. Hahn, who is depressed and unable to share his feelings with other patients, writes and becomes known for his expressive poetry. |
| Sublimation | *Consciously or unconsciously* channeling instinctual drives into acceptable activities | Mr. Smith, a former perpetrator of incest who fears relapse, forms a local chapter of Sex Addicts Anonymous. |
| Reaction formation | A *conscious* behavior that is the exact opposite of an *unconscious* feeling | Ms. Wren, who unconsciously wishes her mother were dead, continuously tells staff that her mother is wonderful. |
| Undoing | *Consciously* doing something to counteract or make up for a transgression or wrongdoing | After accidentally eating another patient's cookies, Ms. Donnelly apologizes to the patients, cleans the refrigerator, and labels everyone's snack with their names. |
| Displacement | *Unconsciously* discharging pent-up feelings to a less threatening object | A husband comes home after a bad day at work and yells at his wife. |
| Projection | *Unconsciously (or consciously)* blaming someone else for one's difficulties or placing one's unethical desires on someone else | An adolescent comes home late from a dance and states that her date would not bring her home on time. |
| Conversion | The *unconscious* expression of intrapsychic conflict symbolically through physical symptoms | A student awakens with a migraine headache the morning of a final examination and feels too ill to take the test. She does not realize that 2 hours of cramming left her unprepared. |
| Regression | *Unconscious* return to an earlier and more comfortable developmental level | A 6-year-old child has been wetting the bed at night since the birth of his baby sister. |

are confronted. Transference (i.e., the unconscious emotional reaction based on previous experiences) that occurs in the current relationship with the therapist is used to encourage working through feelings that would otherwise remain unconscious. Transference is also discussed in Chapter 8.

Although its roots are in psychoanalytic and psychodynamic therapy, *supportive psychotherapy* was developed for ill patients unable to tolerate the intense probing of intrapsychic conflicts, defenses, and transference issues. It involves interaction with the patient (not silent listening) and emphasizes a focus on the present (not on the past). Questioning is less challenging and critical, and the approach conveys empathy and understanding (Miller, 2004b).

## RELEVANCE TO NURSING PRACTICE

In brief therapeutic encounters, the nurse must recognize and understand maladaptive defense mechanisms that patients use. The nurse carefully points out these mechanisms and works with patients to decrease these behaviors and increase adaptive ones. For example, an individual who denies a problem with alcohol must recognize that an arrest for public intoxication, a pending divorce, and three job losses are, in fact, related to drinking and that abstinence from alcohol is the major adaptive coping mechanism needed. In long-term relationships, patients can be assisted with learning to think, feel, and behave according to their own individual values, beliefs, and needs, not according to someone else's. As an example, a college student who is pursuing an engineering degree at the insistence of a domineering parent can be assisted in deciding his or her career goals, while developing the ego strength to withstand parental pressures. Patients might also need assistance with accepting their desires and drives as normal, for which they need not feel guilt or shame, and with choosing acceptable ways of expressing their desires and drives.

### CLINICAL EXAMPLE

A young divorced woman, who has repressed her memories of childhood sexual abuse, projects blame for her divorce onto her husband, instead of looking at her emotional conflicts about sex. She is beginning a new intimate relationship but has not learned to accept her sexuality and desires as normal. Nursing interventions focus on her feelings about being molested, examining the role of these feelings in fostering the divorce, and accepting her sexual desires as a normal part of being human. The patient might also need guidance in selecting healthy, acceptable outlets for her feelings and desires.

## DEVELOPMENTAL MODEL

Erik Erikson (1963, 1968) built on Freud's psychoanalytic model by including psychosocial and environmental influences along with the freudian psychosexual concepts. Erikson's developmental model spans the total life cycle from birth to death. He believed that each of the eight stages of development afforded opportunities for growth, even up to the acceptance of the person's own death. Table 4-3 delineates adult manifestations of Erikson's eight developmental stages.

## KEY CONCEPTS

Each stage of development is an emotional crisis involving positive and negative experiences. Growth or mastery of critical tasks is the result of having more positive than negative experiences. Nonmastery of tasks inhibits movement to the next stage. Erikson believed that the drive of humans to live and grow is opposed by a drive to return to comfortable earlier states and behaviors; therefore, he saw regression as a possibility. Regression often occurs as a result of trauma, prolonged or severe stress, and physiologic or psychiatric illnesses.

Implied but not clearly described in Erikson's model is the concept of partial mastery of critical tasks in development. The degree of mastery of each stage is related to the degree of maturity that the adult attains. Deficits in development carried from one stage to the next progressively interfere with functioning, until the individual is no longer capable of growing without returning emotionally to an earlier stage to resolve the crisis. For example, a person might develop enough trust in others to engage in superficial relationships but might not be able to develop intimacy with a spouse. Another person might have enough initiative to accept a job but might lack the industry to stay

**Table 4-3    Adult Manifestations of Erikson's Stages of Development**

| Life Stage | Adult Behaviors Reflecting Mastery | Adult Behaviors Reflecting Developmental Problems |
|---|---|---|
| I. Trust versus mistrust (0-18 mo) | Realistic trust of self and others<br>Confidence in others<br>Optimism and hope<br>Sharing openly with others | Suspiciousness or testing of others<br>Fear of criticism and closeness<br>Dissatisfaction and hostility<br>Denial of problems<br>Withdrawal from others<br>*or*<br>Overly trusting of others<br>Naive and gullible<br>Sharing too quickly and easily |
| II. Autonomy versus shame and doubt (18 mo-3 yr) | Self-control and willpower<br>Realistic self-concept and self-esteem<br>Pride and a sense of good will<br>Simple cooperativeness<br>Knowing when to give and take<br>Delayed gratification when necessary | Self-doubt or self-consciousness<br>Dependence on others for approval<br>Feeling of being exposed or attacked<br>Sense of being out of control of self and one's life<br>Ritualistic behaviors<br>Projection of blame and one's feelings<br>*or*<br>Excessive independence or defiance, grandiosity<br>Reckless disregard for safety of self and others<br>Unwillingness to ask for help<br>Impulsiveness or inability to wait |
| III. Initiative versus guilt (3-5 yr) | An adequate conscience<br>Initiative balanced with restraint<br>Appropriate social behaviors<br>Curiosity and exploration<br>Healthy competitiveness<br>Original and purposeful activities | Excessive guilt or embarrassment<br>Passivity and apathy<br>Avoidance of activities or pleasures<br>Rumination and self-pity<br>Assuming a role as victim or self-punishment<br>Reluctance to show emotions<br>Underachievement of potential<br>*or*<br>Multiple incomplete projects<br>Little sense of guilt for actions<br>Excessive expression of emotion<br>Labile emotions<br>Excessive competitiveness or showing off |
| IV. Industry versus inferiority (6-12 yr) | Sense of competence<br>Completion of projects<br>Pleasure in effort and effectiveness<br>Ability to cooperate and compromise<br>Identification with admired others<br>Sense of direction<br>Balance of work and play | Feeling unworthy and inadequate<br>Poor work history (quitting, being fired, lack of promotions, absenteeism, lack of productivity)<br>Inadequate problem-solving and follow through on plans<br>Manipulation of others or violation of others' rights<br>Lack of friends of the same sex<br>*or*<br>Overly high achieving<br>Perfectionistic/obsessive-compulsive<br>Reluctance to try new things for fear of failing<br>Feeling unable to gain love or affection unless totally successful<br>Being a workaholic |

*Continued*

**Table 4-3   Adult Manifestations of Erikson's Stages of Development—cont'd**

| Life Stage | Adult Behaviors Reflecting Mastery | Adult Behaviors Reflecting Developmental Problems |
|---|---|---|
| V. Identity versus role diffusion (12-18 or 20 yr) | Confident sense of self<br>Commitment to peer group values<br>Emotional stability<br>Development of personal values<br>Sense of having a place in society<br>Establishing relationship with the opposite sex<br>Testing out adult roles | Lack of or giving up of goals, beliefs, values, productive roles<br>Feelings of confusion, indecision, and alienation<br>Vacillation between dependence and independence<br>Superficial short-term relationships with opposite sex<br>*or*<br>Dramatic overconfidence<br>Acting out behaviors (including alcohol and drug use)<br>Seductive or "macho" behaviors |
| VI. Intimacy versus isolation (18-25 or 30 yr) | Ability to give and receive love<br>Commitments and mutuality with others<br>Collaboration in work and affiliations<br>Sacrificing for others<br>Responsible sexual behaviors<br>Commitment to career and long-term goals | Persistent aloneness or isolation<br>Emotional distance in all relationships<br>Prejudices against others<br>Lack of established vocation; many career changes<br>Seeking of intimacy through casual sexual encounters<br>*or*<br>Possessiveness, jealousy, abusiveness to loved ones<br>Dependency on parents or partner, or both |
| VII. Generative lifestyle versus stagnation or self-absorption (30-65 yr) | Productive, constructive, creative activity<br>Personal and professional growth<br>Parental and societal responsibilities | Self-centeredness or self-indulgence<br>Exaggerated concern for appearance and possessions<br>Lack of interest in the welfare of others<br>Lack of civic and professional activities or responsibilities<br>Loss of interest in marriage or extramarital affairs, or both<br>*or*<br>Too many professional or community activities to the detriment of the family or self<br>Taking care of others, not oneself |
| VIII. Integrity versus despair (65 yr to death) | Feelings of self-acceptance<br>Sense of dignity, worth, and importance<br>Adaptation to life according to limitations<br>Valuing one's life<br>Sharing of wisdom<br>Exploration of philosophy of life and death | Sense of helplessness, hopelessness, worthlessness, uselessness, meaninglessness, or all of these<br>Withdrawal and loneliness<br>Regression<br>Focusing on past mistakes, failures, and dissatisfactions<br>Feeling too old to start over<br>Giving up on oneself and life<br>*or*<br>Inability to reduce amount of activities when needed<br>Overtaxing strength and abilities<br>Feeling indispensable<br>Acting as if life is forever |

Developed by Schwecke L, Wood S, Indiana University. Revised 2005.

with it. An environmental or social tragedy can shake the early foundations of development, such as when divorce from a spouse threatens the individual's sense of trust in others and results in self-doubt.

An individual can skip a developmental stage because of life circumstances, but might have to return to that stage later to master those critical tasks. For example, a young teenage mother might skip the stages of identity and intimacy as a result of the responsibilities of caring for a child (generativity). However, this new mother will probably be drawn back to the issues of identity and intimacy, often before her child enters school. This creates an inherent conflict in roles, feelings, and behaviors. Mastery of the critical tasks of each stage occurs more easily when it is chronologically appropriate. Overcoming delayed or incomplete development is difficult but possible.

## RELEVANCE TO NURSING PRACTICE

Most psychiatric patients demonstrate developmental delays or only partial mastery of the developmental stages preceding the stage expected for their chronologic age. The nurse conducts an assessment of the patient's level of functioning through the interpretation of verbal and nonverbal behaviors and identifies the degree of mastery of each stage up to the patient's chronologic age. The behavioral manifestations of problems are clues to issues to be addressed in working with the patient. For example, an adolescent is overwhelmed with shame about being sexually abused as a child. Mature intimate relationships will not be achievable until the shame and doubt are resolved through dealing more effectively with the memories and emotions related to the abuse. Patients diagnosed with schizophrenia are often struggling with trust issues because of their suspiciousness and fear of closeness. The nurse must concentrate on trust-building strategies with these patients.

Although Erikson focused on the polarity of each developmental stage (e.g., trust-mistrust) as if the positive pole were the desirable task to be accomplished, it is now recognized that the extremes of either pole produce problems in functioning. For example, being overly trusting can result in being repeatedly taken advantage of by others. Having too much industry might result in working 14 to 16 hours a day, without any time for recreation. Adult manifestations of Erikson's stages are listed in Table 4-3. Nursing interventions involving specific developmental issues are discussed in Chapter 8 and in the chapters on specific disorders.

### CLINICAL EXAMPLE

A patient was admitted because of multiple cuts on the wrists. She is saying that "My boyfriend kicked me out. I just want to die. I knew I shouldn't trust anyone, ever!" She later reveals that she grew up in many foster families, some of whom were abusive to her physically and sexually. She admits to a fear of closeness, anger outbursts, and a sense of being out of control in regard to her emotions and her life in general. She acknowledges her inability to trust anyone and a sense of shame and guilt about being abused as a child. As she begins to trust the nurse, she agrees to work on (1) how to evaluate the trustworthiness of others, (2) sources of anger and ways to express it appropriately, (3) positive ways to get approval from others, (4) a realistic self-concept and self-esteem, (5) taking control of her life with healthy coping strategies, and (6) developing a healthy support system.

## INTERPERSONAL MODEL

Harry Stack Sullivan (1953) developed a comprehensive examination of interpersonal and intergroup relationships called the interpersonal theory of psychiatry, which he believed could be applied to international relations (Brody, 2004). Sullivan considered the healthy person as a social being with the ability to live effectively in relationships with others. Mental illness was viewed as any degree of lack of awareness of or the skills in the processes in interpersonal relationships. Relationships were viewed as the source of anxiety, maladaptive behaviors, and negative personality formation.

### KEY CONCEPTS

Sullivan conceived of the personality as an energy system in which the main goal is to reduce tension. Three types of tension were identified: (1) the *tension of needs* (stemming from the physiochemical requirements of life); (2) the *tension of anxiety* (stemming from interpersonal situations); and (3) the *tension of need for sleep*. Theoretically, a person might vary from a state of complete lack of tension (euphoria) to a state of terror as a result of extreme tension, but Sullivan doubted that the pure extremes existed for very long after birth. The relaxation of the tension of needs is experienced as satisfaction, and the relaxation of the tension of anxiety is experienced as interpersonal security (Sullivan, 1953).

### Self-System

Sullivan labeled the personality a "self-system" that develops relatively enduring patterns for avoiding or minimizing anxiety during interpersonal encounters and the meeting of biologic needs. Sullivan also believed that anxiety might be communicated empathically from one person to another. Anxiety activates behaviors that reduce it and help individuals differentiate among experiences (a process of learning). Severe anxiety and panic fail to convey information and produce confusion, even to the point of amnesia (Sullivan, 1953). Less severe anxiety informs the individual about the different situations and behaviors that cause and relieve tension. As the self-system is developing in infancy, it is initially organized into the "good me" when needs are satisfied, the "bad me" when needs are unmet and anxiety persists, and the "not me" when anxiety is severe and information is not completely integrated into the personality on a conscious level.

As the infant moves to early childhood and develops language, the separate personifications of the self as good and bad begin to fuse into a sense of a whole individual with different behaviors in different situations. However, feedback from others *(reflected appraisals)* continues to shape the child's self-concept in positive and negative ways.

Because infants are unable to avoid poor caregivers or anxiety-producing situations, mechanisms called security operations develop to protect young children from anxiety. In *somnolent detachment,* sleep is used to avoid the anxiety. *Apathy* is an emotional detachment or numbing, even though the experiences are remembered. *Selective inattention* is a process of tuning out details associated with anxiety-producing situations. *Dissociation* prevents situations from integrating into conscious awareness. *Converting anxiety to anger* is another mechanism to reduce anxiety. The powerlessness experienced with anxiety is exchanged for a temporary feeling of power associated with anger directed outwardly.

Although these security operations protect against anxiety, they also interfere with the learning that normally occurs in interpersonal interactions *(socialization processes)*. For example, a child might use selective inattention to tune out a mother's suggestion about a more effective way to express anger. *Focal awareness*—the ability to grasp the details and meanings of situations and the behaviors of others—is necessary for adequate learning. *Consensual validation* is a process of verifying the accuracy of perceptions and meanings of events with others who are involved in those situations.

### Personality Development

Sullivan's model includes a sequence of personality development that focuses on tools or behaviors needed to accomplish developmental tasks. In *infancy* (birth to 1½ years), for example, crying is a tool used to establish contact with others; thus, children can learn to count on others. In *childhood* (1½ to 6 years), language assists with learning to delay the gratification of needs. In the *juvenile period* (6 to 9 years), competition, compromise, and cooperation are tools for developing relationships with peers. In *preadolescence* (9 to 12 years), collaboration and the capacity for love assist in the development of a "chum" relationship with a person of the same gender. These same tools, along with sexual desire, facilitate learning to establish relationships with members of the opposite sex in *early adolescence* (12 to 14 years). The independence developed in early adolescence moves toward interdependence in *later adolescence* (14 to 21 years), and individuals learn to form lasting sexual relationships (Sullivan, 1953). Sullivan's developmental model did not describe changes beyond late adolescence.

## THERAPIST'S ROLE

For Sullivan, the focus of therapy is on a patient's current interpersonal relationships and experiences. The goal of the therapy is to develop mature and satisfactory relationships that are relatively free from anxiety. The therapist-patient relationship is a vehicle for analyzing the patient's interpersonal processes and testing new skills in relating. Although the focus of therapy is on a patient's here-and-now problems, distortions created by past experiences, particularly "not me" experiences, are often revealed. The therapist helps correct these distortions with clear communication, consensual validation, and presentation of reality. In challenging a negative self-image, the therapist presents an appraisal of the patient as a worthwhile, respectable individual with rights, dignity, and valuable abilities. The focus of sessions is often on loneliness, fear of rejection, clarifying emotions and their causes, using anxiety for learning about the self and others, managing interpersonal frustrations, and developing self-respect. An adaptation of the interpersonal model, *interpersonal psychotherapy,* also focuses on resolving grief issues, interpersonal disputes, social role transitions, and interpersonal deficits through the use of the therapeutic relationship (Miller, 2004a).

## RELEVANCE TO NURSING PRACTICE

Hildegard Peplau (1952, 1963) played a significant role in applying Sullivan's concepts to nursing practice. Peplau saw a major goal of nursing as helping patients reduce their anxiety and convert it to constructive action. She elaborated on and applied Sullivan's concept of degrees of anxiety to nursing (pure euphoria, mild anxiety, moderate anxiety, severe anxiety, panic, terror states, and pure anxiety [Peplau, 1963]). Peplau described the effects of mild anxiety through panic levels on perception and learning (see Chapter 10 for a detailed explanation of these processes). She saw the nurse's role as helping patients decrease insecurity and improve functioning through interpersonal relationships that can be seen as microcosms of how patients function in other relationships. For example, a patient says, "My wife always knows when I'm upset and wants to help me, but I just say nothing." The nurse might say, "What are you anxious about when you think about telling her the truth?" Regardless of the current emphasis on psychotropic medications, Peplau's focus on the patients, their issues, and their interpersonal relationships is still relevant. For example, patients with psychosis still have to deal with delusions, hallucinations, and distorted thinking until a medication takes effect or when a medication is not totally effective. Understanding what patients are saying about themselves and their situations

and helping them develop coping skill are always important aspects of patient care (Smoyak, 2004). Specific applications of Sullivan's work as proposed by Peplau are presented in Chapter 8.

### CLINICAL EXAMPLE

The nurse recognizes that a patient experiences increased anxiety whenever he is beginning a relationship with a woman. The patient complains about not knowing what to say or do when he is alone with her (lack of interpersonal skills). "I'm so afraid of acting like an idiot that I get tongue-tied and sweaty (anxiety). It's no wonder that I never see her again." Nursing interventions focus on specific sources of anxiety, overcoming insecurities, rehearsing social conversations with the nurse, and practicing social skills in a small group of patients.

## COGNITIVE-BEHAVIORAL MODELS

Aaron Beck's cognitive therapy (CT) (1967) and Albert Ellis's rational-emotive therapy (RET) (1973) models focus on thinking and behaving rather than on expressing feelings. These models use a cognitive approach based on individuals' abilities to think, analyze, judge, decide, and do. Ellis and Beck view individuals' present perceptions, thoughts, assumptions, beliefs, values, attitudes, and philosophies as needing modification or change (Beck, 1976; Ellis, 1973). Individuals' interpretations of events and expectations of themselves and others (not the actual event or people) are seen as causing the maladaptive responses (Reilly and McDanel, 2005). Even distorted thinking learned from others in childhood can be unlearned. Individuals should value themselves simply because they exist and should not judge themselves by the way they perform or how they are rated by themselves and others.

## KEY CONCEPTS

Beck and Ellis believe that individuals think both rationally and irrationally, and that irrational beliefs or automatic thoughts are responsible for causing problems because self-defeating behaviors are maintained. They also assert that individuals are capable of understanding their limitations and can change their values and beliefs while challenging their self-defeating behaviors. The repetition of irrational thoughts produces emotional disturbances that keep dysfunctional behaviors operant. RET teaches individuals to stop blaming themselves and to accept themselves as they are, with flaws and imperfections. RET attacks problems from a cognitive, emotive, and behavioral standpoint by using the A-B-C theory of personality. A is the activating event, B is the belief about A, and C is the emotional reaction. A (event) does not cause C (emotions); rather, B (irrational beliefs about A) causes C. Intervention, then, is aimed at B (irrational beliefs) and is called D (disputing and changing irrational beliefs) (Ellis, 1973). The outcome is E ("the end result or *profound and effective new philosophies*" or beliefs) (Sacks, 2004). Similarly, Beck (1976) proposed examining the distorted perceptions, erroneous beliefs, self-deceptions, and blind spots that lead to "excessive, inappropriate emotional reactions" to events or stimuli. Reality testing and problem solving are aimed at correcting faulty cognitions and processes; thus, the individual develops "more realistic appraisals of himself and his world" (Beck, 1976).

According to Ellis (1973) and Beck (1976), most individuals subscribe to at least some of the following irrational beliefs and inappropriate rules for living:

- One should feel loved and approved by everyone.
- One must be totally competent to be considered worthwhile.
- Individuals have little ability to change or to control their feelings.
- Influences of the past should determine feelings in the present.
- Rejection or unfair treatment has catastrophic consequences.
- One is disliked when a disagreement exists with another.
- One "should" never make mistakes.
- Individuals who are obnoxious "ought" to be judged as rotten or bad.
- Being passive in life is easier than confronting difficulties and responsibilities.

CT has been adapted for individuals who have experienced traumatic events that often undermine basic assumptions about oneself and life, such as a view of the self as weak, rather than strong, and the world as threatening and fearful, rather than benevolent. The focus of therapy is to challenge these latter assumptions and associated automatic thoughts to help individuals develop more logical assumptions, thoughts, feelings, and behaviors (Robertson et al, 2004).

CT has also been adapted to the use of the computer for patients with depression (Wright et al, 2005):

> The computer program contains a variety of interactive self-help exercises designed to build skills for using the cognitive and behavioral therapy. Video, audio, graphics, and checklists are used extensively . . . Specific content from the program [is] provided at each session: 1) orientation, basic cognitive model; 2) identifying automatic thoughts and cognitive errors using thought records; 3) revising automatic thoughts, finding rational alternatives; 4) behavioral methods, scheduling activities and pleasant events; 5) further behavioral exercises, graded task assignments; 6) identifying and modifying core beliefs; 7) and 8) review and further rehearsal. (pp. 1158-1159)

Cognitive-behavioral therapy (CBT) builds on CT by incorporating techniques based on learning principles (Geffken et al, 2004) and behavior therapy techniques, including exposure (in vitro or imaginal), response prevention, skill training, and reinforcement (see Chapter 38). The goal is to work on directly changing behaviors as well as changing faulty thinking. Especially with very ill patients, such as those with schizophrenia, there is also an emphasis on empathizing with the patient's needs, fostering a *therapeutic alliance,* and using flexibility in approaches as the patient's needs change. Support is essential, especially as the patient begins making better choices and becomes more social (Sudak, 2004).

CBT with seriously ill populations might use a *multicomponent program,* which could include psychoeducation, medication education, and dealing with psychological and practical barriers leading to noncompliance; problem solving about daily realities; social skills training; and cognitive skill practice. Assertive community treatment and family therapy can help with prevention of relapse. Disputing the patient's beliefs, especially those resulting from delusions and perceptual distortions, is done carefully, slowly, and supportively (Sudak, 2004; Turkington et al, 2004). Multicomponent CBT with patients with posttraumatic stress disorder (PTSD) also might add anxiety and anger management, cognitive restructuring, exposure therapy, homework assignments, relaxation training, and breathing retraining to help with the traumatic memories and persistent increased arousal (Frueh et al, 2004; Falsetti and Resnick, 2005). PTSD treatment is discussed in Chapter 31.

Motivational enhancement therapy, a variation of CBT, is more widely used in the treatment of individuals with addictions. The goal is to enhance the patient's readiness and willingness to change habits related to the addictions, using *motivational interviewing*. This nonconfrontational approach includes expressing empathy, pointing out discrepancies between current behaviors and future goals, "rolling with resistance," and promoting self-efficacy (Miller, 2005). Motivational interviewing uses the concepts of "stages of change . . . precontemplation, contemplation, preparation for action, and maintenance" (Miller, 2005).

Rational-emotive behavior therapy (REBT) focuses on behavioral change by integrating "cognitive, emotive, and behavioral techniques" with "a here and now orientation" and "an active directive and re-educative style" (Sacks, 2004). It does acknowledge that there are influences on the individual from social, environmental, and biologic factors, but it still focuses on changing irrational conclusions about these social, environmental, and biologic conditions.

Dialectical behavior therapy (DBT) (Linehan, 1993) was developed for the treatment of borderline personality disorder, which also has been viewed as complex PTSD (Herman, 1992). DBT especially focuses on "parasuicidal" patients who have self-mutilation and suicide attempts in their histories (Oldham, 2004). It concentrates on ways to change these behaviors through concurrent individual therapy and group skills training. It might include contact with the therapist between sessions to intervene with self-harm behaviors. DBT might also include interventions related to dissociation, distress tolerance, affect regulation, and core mindfulness (using meditative practices to focus attention on bodily sensations, feelings, and conscious thoughts) (O'Haver Day and Horton-Deutsch, 2004; Robertson et al, 2004). The combination of cognitive, behavioral, and supportive therapies in DBT typically involves the following goals in a hierarchy (Perseius et al, 2003):

1. Stability and security, aiming toward decreased suicidal behavior and acts of deliberate self-harm, decreased therapy-interfering behaviors, and decreased quality-of-life interfering behaviors
2. Reduction of posttraumatic stress by focusing on traumatic life events
3. Increased self-respect and achievement of individual life goals

## THERAPIST'S ROLE

The patient-therapist relationship is viewed as a collaborative effort to achieve goals for improved self-esteem, coping, relationships, and lifestyles (Beck, 1976). Because patients have many irrational "shoulds," "oughts," and "musts," the therapist actively and directly challenges these beliefs. The therapist demonstrates the degree to which the patient's thinking is illogical. Humor is often used to confront the patient's irrational thinking. The therapist explains ways to replace irrational thinking with rational thinking to reduce dysfunctional feelings and behaviors. The process of therapy focuses on the present. Patients learn to take responsibility for their irrational thoughts, feelings, and behaviors and for eliminating these. The therapist accepts patients as they are and does not allow patients to rate or condemn themselves. Homework assignments are given to promote focusing on positive statements and behaviors and on skill development. New, positive self-statements are encouraged to enable patients to begin to think, feel, and behave differently. Role playing, modeling, and reinforcement are also used.

## RELEVANCE TO NURSING PRACTICE

Nurses help patients change irrational beliefs and reduce stress and anxiety through effective problem solving. Patients have many self-deprecating or negative feelings about themselves that the nurse can dispute by pointing out and reinforcing specific positive behaviors. For example, a nurse, after listening to a patient discuss all of his or her weaknesses, might say, "Let's work on a list of your positive qualities and strengths" to facilitate the patient's beliefs that he or she is worthwhile and has valuable qualities. One message is, "All of us make mistakes at times. Learning from these mistakes helps us grow and become more effective in relating to others." Patients who project blame can be shown that they alone are responsible for their behaviors. For example, patients with alcoholism are skillful at blaming others for their problems when, in fact, they alone are responsible for continuing to drink and for the problems that result from drinking. Other patients who continually function according to "shoulds," "musts," and "oughts" can be taught to act according to their personal wants and beliefs; they need not condemn themselves for being their own person, and their anxiety and hostile feelings toward themselves and others can be eliminated when they can achieve feelings of comfort about themselves.

### CLINICAL EXAMPLE

A depressed young man says to the nurse, "My friends have stopped coming around to see me. They say I'm always bragging about myself, but I feel like I have to prove myself to them and myself (irrational belief)." Nursing interventions focus on the acceptance of himself as a worthwhile person with a few weaknesses but many positive qualities. Interventions also challenge his beliefs that he "must" be totally competent in front of others and never make mistakes.

## REALITY THERAPY MODEL

William Glasser (1965) developed reality therapy because he believed that patients and delinquents share the common characteristic of denying "the reality of the world around them" instead of fulfilling their needs responsibly within the context of reality and society. He defined responsibility as "the ability to fulfill one's needs, and to do so in a way that does not deprive others of the ability to fulfill their needs" (Glasser, 1965). Glasser recognized that he could not change patients' histories or past relationship problems, but that he could help them change current behaviors; thus, their future could improve. He found that an improved sense of responsibility leads to improved mental health.

### KEY CONCEPTS

According to Glasser (1965), all individuals continually strive to meet their needs. The two major psychological needs are (1) to love and be loved (to have relatedness) and (2) to feel worthwhile (to have respect from self and others). Implied in these are the needs for involvement and identity. Children develop a positive identity by being involved with others who teach right, wrong, and responsibility while conveying that the children themselves are worthwhile. Children then learn to be comfortable with and enjoy being around others.

Unfortunately, individuals do not always strive to meet their needs responsibly. An "incapacity or failure at the interpersonal level of functioning" might exist (Glasser, 1965). Glasser believed that illness results from behaving irresponsibly rather than the reverse, and that anger, fear, depression, and anxiety are also the result of irresponsible behavior in relationships. Common forms of irresponsible behavior include violating one's morals, values, or standards; misinforming others about oneself or one's needs (being dishonest); shunning others because of fear of rejection; lying to oneself by rationalizing and excusing one's own behavior; not accepting the consequences of one's behavior; blaming others for problems; and, eventually, losing contact with reality (by denying it). Suicide and denial are major ways of avoiding reality and responsibility. Short-term pleasures such as those derived from alcohol and drugs also interfere with long-term satisfaction and happiness.

### THERAPIST'S ROLE

The goal of reality therapy is to help patients face reality and then to develop responsible behavior patterns; thus, the patient's needs for love and worth can be met more effectively. Directing patients "toward greater maturity, conscientiousness, and responsibility" improves their potential for long-term happiness and pleasure (Glasser, 1965). Glasser emphasized the need for the therapist's authenticity, openness, honesty, responsibility, and deep involvement with patients. Initially, patients need warmth and uncritical acceptance as worthwhile persons who are cared about, even though their irresponsible behaviors, and the excuses for those behaviors, are not accepted, are confronted, and are even disciplined. Their positive behaviors are supported. Patients repeatedly evaluate whether their actions are producing the desired results and whether others are hurt in the process. Patients are asked to choose more effective behaviors and to design specific, realistic plans to try those behaviors. Plans that are unsuccessful are revised until accountability and responsibility have been achieved.

## RELEVANCE TO NURSING PRACTICE

Psychiatric nurses are regularly involved in helping patients identify reality and factors that interfere with meeting their needs effectively (reality testing). An example is helping a patient understand that, if he would like his wife to do something, he must be direct in saying it, instead of hinting about it, as he has been doing. Nurses are routinely responsible for explaining the rules of a program or unit and for outlining expected and appropriate, as well as inappropriate, behaviors. The milieu of a program or unit is normally designed to foster improvement in independence and responsibility, which is rewarded with increases in privileges and freedom. Setting limits on unacceptable (irresponsible) behaviors benefits patients over the long term.

Even without labeling behaviors as irresponsible, nurses are accustomed to helping patients examine the consequences of specific behaviors, particularly in current relationships. For example, with a patient who typically cries instead of getting angry with her husband, the nurse might ask, "How does that solve your anger and your dislike of your husband's behavior?" Supportive confrontation encourages patients to make their own decisions about changes, choose their own solutions, and test new behaviors. This type of relearning process is described in Chapter 8, which discusses the nurse-patient relationship.

---

### CLINICAL EXAMPLE

During a group session with adolescents, they begin complaining about all types of parental and societal rules that they dislike. A common theme among them is the (unrealistic) desire to be totally independent and free from all restrictions (lack of responsibility for behaviors). The nurse asks them to point out the consequences of their recent rebellious behaviors. Begrudgingly, the teens identify continual arguments with parents, loss of friendships, disciplinary actions at school, arrests for alcohol or drug use, sexually transmitted diseases, suicide attempts, and psychiatric hospitalizations. The nurse asks them to describe the benefits of being a mature responsible adult. The teens are then asked to identify their own specific healthy future goals and the positive and responsible behaviors needed to achieve these goals.

---

Stress models provide nurses with a framework for understanding how stress affects individuals and their responses. The ability to adapt to stress leads to conflict resolution, whereas the inability to adapt effectively might result in physical or mental disorders, or even death.

## KEY CONCEPTS: SELYE'S STRESS-ADAPTATION MODEL

Selye (1956) defined stress as wear and tear on the body. He developed his framework to explain the physiologic response to stress. Selye viewed stressors as any positive or negative occurrence or as any emotion requiring a response. Interaction with the environment and others inevitably produces stress, depending on individual perception and definition of the stressor. However, Selye discovered that many individuals demonstrate the same symptoms, regardless of the stressor. These changes became known as the general adaptation syndrome (GAS), and they occur in three stages: (1) alarm, (2) resistance, and (3) exhaustion. Selye did not elaborate on psychosocial changes, but his three stages can be correlated with the levels of anxiety (Chapter 10). The three stages of GAS are summarized in Table 4-4.

### Alarm Reaction

Any type of stressor for individuals activates the preparation for fight or flight. Individuals experience an increase in alertness so as to focus on the immediate task or threat and to mobilize resources and defenses to concentrate on the particular stressor. The levels of anxiety experienced are mild (+1) to moderate (+2). Learning and problem solving can occur. When the stressor continues and is not adaptively or effectively resolved, individuals experience the next stage.

### Stage of Resistance

In this stage, individuals strive to adapt to stress. For adaptation to occur, the use of coping and defense mechanisms is increased. Problem solving and learning are difficult but can be accomplished with assistance. The levels of anxiety experienced are moderate (+2) to severe (+3). When stressors become overwhelming and/or prolonged, individuals experience the next stage.

| Table 4-4 | Stress-Adaptation Syndrome | |
|---|---|---|
| **Stage** | **Physical Changes** | **Psychosocial Changes** |
| **Stage I: Alarm Reaction** Mobilization of the body's defensive forces and activation of the potential for "fight or flight" (+1 to +2 anxiety) | Release of norepinephrine and epinephrine, causing vasoconstriction, increased blood pressure, and increased rate and force of cardiac contraction Increased hormone levels Enlargement of adrenal cortex Marked loss of body weight Shrinkage of the thymus, spleen, and lymph nodes Irritation of the gastric mucosa | Increased level of alertness Increased level of anxiety Task-oriented, defense-oriented, inefficient, or maladaptive behavior might occur |
| **Stage II: Stage of Resistance** Optimal adaptation to stress within the person's capabilities (+2 to +3 anxiety) | Hormone levels readjust Reduction in activity and size of adrenal cortex Lymph nodes return to normal size Weight returns to normal | Increased and intensified use of coping mechanisms Tendency to rely on defense-oriented behavior Psychosomatic symptoms develop |
| **Stage III: Stage of Exhaustion** Loss of ability to resist stress because of depletion of body resources; fight, flight, or immobilization occurs (+3 to +4 anxiety) | Decreased immune response, with suppression of T cells and atrophy of thymus Depletion of adrenal glands and hormone production Weight loss Enlargement of lymph nodes and dysfunction of lymphatic system If exposure to stressor continues, cardiac failure, renal failure, or death might occur | Defense-oriented behaviors become exaggerated Disorganization of thinking Disorganization of personality Sensory stimuli might be misperceived with appearance of illusion Reality contact might be reduced with appearance of delusions or hallucinations If exposure to stressor continues, stupor or violence might occur |

Modified from Kneisl CR, Ames SW: *Adult health nursing: a biopsychosocial approach,* Menlo Park, CA, 1986, Addison-Wesley; ©1986. Reprinted by permission of Pearson Education, Inc., Upper Saddle River, NJ.

### *Stage of Exhaustion*

Exhaustion results from stress that lasts too long, is overwhelming, and/or results from the individual's total inability to cope. Anxiety is experienced at the severe (+3) to panic (+4) levels. Defenses are exaggerated and dysfunctional, and the personality becomes disorganized, thinking becomes illogical, and decision making becomes ineffective. Delusions and hallucinations can occur, with sensory misperception and a greatly reduced orientation to reality. Individuals might become violent, suicidal, or completely immobilized, without even showing the anxiety. Death might occur when exhaustion continues without intervention.

## KEY CONCEPTS: LAZARUS'S INTERACTIONAL MODEL

In contrast to Selye's emphasis on the physiologic effects of stress, Lazarus (1966) focused on the psychological aspects. According to Lazarus, psychological stress is "a relationship between the person and the environment that is appraised by the person as taxing or exceeding his or her resources and endangering his or her well-being" (Lazarus and Folkman, 1984). Lazarus believed that the basis of coping is not a result of anxiety, per se, but of the personal, cognitive appraisal of threat. "Anxiety is the response to threat" (Lazarus, 1966). The significance of the threat or what it means to the individual is of primary importance. For one person, a particular event might be viewed as a challenge; for another, the same event might be viewed as a severe threat or problem.

Three types of cognitive appraisal have been identified. Primary appraisal refers to the judgment that individuals make about a particular event. What does it mean personally? What are its effects? Secondary appraisal is the individual's evaluation of the way to respond to an event. Possible strategies or solutions, as well as resources and supports, are examined. Reappraisal is further appraisal that is made after new or additional information has been received.

Personal and environmental factors influence appraisal—commitments, beliefs, values, feelings, emotions, and views of what is important. A seemingly appropriate solution might not be useful because it conflicts with individual values and beliefs. For example, a passive wife might be unable to be assertive and confrontational with her husband because she was taught and believes that women should be quiet and submissive.

Stressful events often create demands with which individuals cannot effectively cope. Occasionally, personal resources or social supports are inadequate. Preferred methods of coping might be ineffective in resolving the problem and could actually result in more problems. Ineffective coping and the creation of additional problems result in additional stress and can lead to physical illness or mental illness, or both.

## RELEVANCE TO NURSING PRACTICE

Stress theories provide a framework for the nurse to use to assess the effects of stress on patients and their coping processes. To assist patients with developing adaptive or effective coping methods, nurses must help patients identify and evaluate palliative, maladaptive, and dysfunctional behaviors that enable patients to become aware of the consequences of their behavior. Palliative mechanisms decrease the emotions without solving the problems. Maladaptive mechanisms do not manage the emotions sufficiently and do not solve the problems. Dysfunctional mechanisms create new or additional problems. (For further explanation, see Chapter 10 for more on stress, coping, and crisis.)

Patients' appraisal of stressors or problems includes their perception of the stressors, the resources or supports they have to help them cope, and the way in which their beliefs and values influence that coping. For example, an individual who is independent and who has sufficient income and savings, a supportive family, and a belief that divorce is acceptable is likely to cope differently with a partner's affair than an individual who is dependent, unemployed, and without close family and believes that divorce is not an option. In considering patients' perception of stressors, the nurse can facilitate cognitive restructuring or problem solving by helping patients choose adaptive and appropriate coping behaviors. For example, the nurse helps a patient who feels helpless and lonely share these feelings with a group of patients and ask for suggestions for fun (but less threatening) activities with others. Together, the patient and the nurse can then evaluate the effectiveness of strategies used. When patients exhibit behaviors found in Selye's stage of exhaustion or are using primarily dysfunctional coping, the nurse can assess patients' inability to take constructive action; the nurse might be required to make decisions on behalf of patients. After patients gain some control over their situation, they can benefit from classes on stress management, problem solving, relaxation training, and biofeedback.

### CLINICAL EXAMPLE

A male patient is admitted several weeks after his mother has been diagnosed with terminal cancer. He is exhausted and showing symptoms such as misperceptions of reality, delusions, and hallucinations. The patient says, "I can't live without her. I'll lose the house. I can't work if she isn't there to get me up and going in the morning. No one else will help me." The nurse develops a care plan that focuses on (1) protecting the patient from harm and reducing the anxiety level, (2) offering emotional and stress management strategies, (3) engaging the patient in anticipatory grief work, (4) developing a new support system, and (5) designing specific plans for getting up and being ready each morning to be on time for work.

### CRITICAL THINKING QUESTION    1

Which concepts and strategies derived from each of the therapeutic models have you observed being used with patients?

### INTEGRATIVE APPROACH

Most psychiatric nurses adopt an integrative approach with the therapeutic models presented in this chapter. Concepts from various models that best explain a patient's behaviors, problems, and needs are selected. For example, a recently divorced patient states, "I've screwed up my life. All I do is sit at home, cry, and sleep." The nurse might use the psychoanalytic model to identify that the patient is experiencing superego guilt and regression, the developmental model to understand the patient's dissatisfaction with self and withdrawal from others, or the cognitive-behavioral model to identify the irrational belief that one should never make mistakes. In the interpersonal model, the behavior of crying would be seen as a wish for contact with others and sleep as somnolent detachment. In the reality therapy model, the patient would be viewed as feeling unloved, having a loss of self-respect, and being depressed. Using the stress models, the focus is on redefining the meaning of the divorce and using adaptive coping strategies. In addition, psychiatric nurses recognize that the key component in any therapeutic model is the *patient-nurse relationship*. This important component is discussed in depth in Chapter 8. The *therapeutic alliance* is often the best predictor of the outcome of any treatment approach (Bender, 2005).

---

### CRITICAL THINKING QUESTION    2

Using the models presented in this chapter, what goals would you help the patient described below achieve?

Ms. Levy has been admitted after a suicide attempt. During the admission assessment, she says that she recently began having nightmares about her sexual abuse as a child. She reports a lack of trust of men, yet always seeks their approval. Her interpersonal relationships with women are also stormy. Her anxiety interferes with her work performance. She admits to intense anger about the effect of the abuse on her life, but believes that "women shouldn't show their anger." She says that she is afraid to "grow up and be responsible for herself" because she feels overwhelmed by life's stresses.

---

### Study Notes

1. Concepts from various models provide frameworks for understanding patients' behaviors and problems.
2. According to Freud, extensive use of defense mechanisms and maladaptive coping behaviors are assessed and understood by the nurse as inhibitors of healthy or adaptive responses. The nurse helps patients develop adaptive coping responses or behaviors.
3. Unresolved developmental issues (Erikson) interfere with a patient's ability to solve problems and meet his or her own needs. Therefore, these issues must be addressed in the nurse-patient relationship and interventions.
4. Sullivan created the interpersonal model to explain children's and adolescents' skills used in developing healthy adult interpersonal relationships. He also focused on sources of anxiety and coping skills.
5. Peplau used Sullivan's concepts of anxiety as a critical part of her framework in the nurse-patient relationship. Her goal was to help patients manage anxiety and use it for learning interpersonal skills through the nurse-patient relationship.
6. According to the cognitive-behavioral model, replacing irrational beliefs with rational beliefs can reduce stress and anxiety and self-defeating behaviors.
7. Multiple variations of cognitive and cognitive-behavioral therapies have been developed for specific populations.
8. Facing reality and accepting self-responsibility are major goals of reality therapy.
9. Stress models explain many of the physiologic and psychological responses to stress and are a basis for stress reduction strategies.
10. An integrative approach allows the use of concepts from many models so that different aspects of patients' thoughts, feelings, behaviors, problems, and needs can be explained more thoroughly. No one patient "fits" neatly into only one model.

---

### References

Beck AT: *Depression: chemical, experimental and theoretical aspects,* New York, 1967, Noeber Medical Division, Harper & Row.

Beck AT: *Cognitive therapies and the emotional disorders,* New York, 1976, International Universities Press.

Bender DS: The therapeutic alliance in the treatment of personality disorders, *J Psychiatr Pract* 11:73, 2005.

Brill AA, editor: *The basic writings of Sigmund Freud,* New York, 1938, Random House.

Brody EB: Harry Stack Sullivan, Brock Chisholm, Psychiatry, and the World Federation for Mental Health, *Psychiatry* 6:38, 2004.

Ellis A: *Humanistic psychotherapy: the rational-emotive approach,* New York, 1973, Julian Press.

Erikson EH: *Childhood and society,* New York, 1963, Norton.

Erikson EH: *Identity: youth and crisis,* New York, 1968, Norton.

Falsetti SA, Resnick HS, Davis J: Multichannel exposure therapy, *Behav Modif* 29:70, 2005.

Freud S: *The problem of anxiety,* New York, 1936, Norton.

Freud S, Strachey J, editors: *The ego and the id,* New York, 1960, Norton.

Frueh B, et al: Cognitive behavioral treatment of PTSD among people with severe mental illness: a proposed model, *J Psychiatr Pract* 10:26, 2004.

Geffken GR, Storch EA, Gelfand KM, et al: Cognitive behavioral therapy for obsessive-compulsive disorder: review of treatment techniques, *J Psychosoc Nurs Ment Health Serv* 42:44, 2004.

Glasser W: *Reality therapy: a new approach to psychiatry,* New York, 1965, Harper & Row.

Herman J: Complex PTSD: A syndrome in survivors of prolonged and repeated abuse, *J Trauma Stress* 5:377, 1992.

Kneisl CR, Ames SW: *Adult health nursing: a biopsychosocial approach,* Menlo Park, CA, 1986, Addison-Wesley.

Lazarus RS: *Psychological stress and the coping process,* St. Louis, 1966, McGraw-Hill.

Lazarus RS, Folkman S: *Stress, appraisal, and coping,* New York, 1984, Springer.

Linehan MM: *Cognitive behavioral treatment of borderline personality disorder,* New York, 1993, Guilford.

Miller MC, editor: Interpersonal psychotherapy, *Harv Ment Health Lett* 21:1, 2004a.

Miller MC, editor: Supportive psychotherapy, *Harv Ment Health Lett* 20:1, 2004b.

Miller MC, editor: Motivational interviewing, *Harv Ment Health Lett* 21:5, 2005.

O'Haver Day P, Horton-Deutsch S: Using mindfulness-based therapeutic interventions in psychiatric nursing practice—part I: description and empirical support of mindfulness-based interventions, *Arch Psychiatr Nurs* 18:164, 2004.

Oldham JM: Borderline personality disorder: the new treatment dilemma, *J Psychiatr Pract* 10(3):204, 2004.

Peplau HE: *Interpersonal relations in nursing,* New York, 1952, Putnam.

Peplau HE: A working definition of anxiety. In Burd SF, Marshall MA, editors: *Some clinical approaches to psychiatric nursing* (pp. 323-327), Toronto, 1963, Macmillan.

Perseius KI, Ojehagen A, Ekdahl S, et al: Treatment of suicidal and deliberate self-harming patients with borderline personality disorder using dialectical behavioral therapy: the patients' and the therapists' perceptions, *Arch Psychiatr Nurs* 17:218, 2003.

Reilly CE, McDaniel H: Cognitive therapy: A training model for advanced practice nurses, *J Psychosoc Nurs* 43:27, 2005.

Robertson MF, Humphreys L, Ray R: Psychological treatment for posttraumatic stress disorder: recommendations for the clinician based on a review of the literature, *J Psychiatr Pract* 10:106, 2004.

Sacks SB: Rational emotive behavior therapy, *J Psychosoc Nurs* 42:23, 2004.

Selye H: *The stress of life,* St. Louis, 1956, McGraw-Hill.

Smoyak SA: The construction of reality or the deconstruction of the self, *J Psychosoc Nurs* 42:6, 2004.

Sudak DM: Cognitive behavioral therapy for schizophrenia, *J Psychiatric Pract* 10:331, 2004

Sullivan HS: *Interpersonal theory of psychiatry,* New York, 1953, Norton.

Turkington D, Dudley R, Warman D, Beck AT: Cognitive-behavioral therapy for schizophrenia: a review, *J Psychiatr Pract* 10(1):5, 2004.

Wright JH, Wright AS, Albano AM, et al: Computer-assisted cognitive therapy for depression: maintaining efficacy while reducing therapist time, *Am J Psychiatry* 162:1158, 2005.

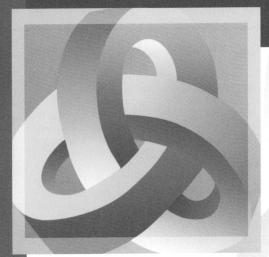

# Chapter 5

# Legal Issues

*Norman L. Keltner*

## Learning Objectives

*After reading this chapter, you should be able to:*
- Define the terms that apply to legal issues in psychiatric care.
- Describe the liability of the nurse in issues such as wrongful commitment, duty to warn, and master-servant rule.
- Identify four landmark court rulings and their impact on psychiatric care.
- Define and discuss involuntary commitment issues and procedures.
- Define and apply the concept of least restrictive alternative.
- Define and apply the concept of confidentiality.
- Define and apply the concept of the right to treatment and the right to refuse treatment.

The evolution of humane treatment of mentally ill persons roughly parallels that of advances made in the jurisprudence system. Historically, movement has been a slow, cautious process from viewing the mentally ill as demonic or weak-willed to viewing them as individuals with legitimate health care problems. Governmental systems and regulatory bodies thoughtfully attempt to achieve balance between the rights of the individuals and the rights of society at large. Although most people are aware of the difficulty in reaching this goal in criminal cases, they are less aware of the struggle for such a balance in psychiatric care.

This chapter begins with a brief review of basic legal principles and sources of law that have influenced mental health delivery and serve as the basis for legally sound psychiatric nursing practice (Box 5-1). The following topics are reviewed:

1. Key legal terms
2. Common law, precedent-setting cases, statutory law, and administrative law
3. Tort law: negligence, assault and battery, and false imprisonment and related nursing liability

Additionally, the nurse's role in these and other legal issues is presented throughout the chapter to help the student understand the applicable legal, regulatory, and compliance issues.

## SOURCES OF LAW

There are three basic sources of law: (1) common law, which is derived from judicial decisions; (2) statutory law, which is created by the federal and state legislatures; and (3) administrative law, developed by administrative agencies. When written laws are not completely clear or are contradictory

## Norm's Notes

*Legal stuff can put most of us to sleep, but there is something to be learned that will help you do something as simple as reading the paper. Almost daily, in any big city newspaper, you read about a mentally ill person who has committed a crime or about a legal defense strategy incorporating the laws mentioned in this chapter. And, what about the rights of the patient? People who have mental problems have important rights. One of the most important things you can do is understand the rights of people with mental health problems, whether it is your patient or a family member.*

### Box 5-1    Sources of Law Affecting Psychiatric Nursing

1. The U.S. Constitution
2. Individual state and federal statutes
3. Precedent-setting legal cases
4. The Joint Commission on Accreditation of Healthcare Organizations (JCAHO)
5. Centers for Medicare and Medicaid Services (CMS)

to other laws, the judicial system is responsible for resolving these disputes. The resulting judicial decisions often influence legislative action to create an appropriate statute.

## COMMON LAW

The term *common law* is applied to the body of legal principles that has evolved and continues to evolve and expand from actual court cases. Many of these legal principles and rules have their origins in English common law.

The judicial system is necessary because having a law that covers every potential event that might occur is impossible. Moreover, the judicial system serves as a mechanism for reviewing legal disputes that arise in the written law; it is an effective review mechanism for those issues in which the written law is silent or confusing, and for situations in which issues involving both written law and common law decisions occur.

Many of these rulings have influenced the current legal view of mental illness. Rules presented here, although they in no way form an exhaustive list of major court decisions, reflect decisions that have shaped the mental health treatment system and have served to improve patient care and protect the public.

1. The M'Naghten rule (1843) states that individuals who do not understand the nature and implications of murderous actions because of insanity cannot be held legally accountable for murder. This ruling was based on the case of Daniel M'Naghten, a Scotsman who felt persecuted by the ruling political party and attempted to kill the Prime Minister. Although he failed to kill the Prime Minister, he did shoot the Prime Minister's secretary. He was ruled not guilty by reason of insanity and was committed to an asylum. This case has provided a basis for legal decisions in American courts since 1851.

   *Comment:* When applied today, the M'Naghten criteria state generally that a person is not criminally responsible at the time of an act if, because of mental "disease or defect," the person did not know the nature and quality of the act, or if the person did know it, he or she did not know that the act was wrong. Because this standard focuses on the knowledge of "right or wrong," it is occasionally referred to as the *cognitive standard*. It is estimated that this defense is successful in only 1% of cases (Moran, 2002).

### CRITICAL THINKING QUESTION    1

"Not guilty by reason of insanity" is a phrase that evokes passion in many people. Jeffrey Dahmer, the cannabilist murderer, did not say that he didn't do it. He said he was not guilty because he did not know what he was doing. His lawyers said he was not guilty by reason of insanity. What do you think about this concept? Do you believe this legal defense is used too often? Is it reasonable to have such protection under the law?

### CLINICAL EXAMPLE

Charles McCoy Jr. dropped building material off overpasses, then began shooting at automobiles on a major highway. He was behind 12 shootings and 200 acts of vandalism in the Columbus, Ohio area in 2003 and 2004. He has pleaded innocence by reason of insanity to murder and 23 other counts. He said voices called him a "wimp." (Highway assailant heard voices.)

2. *Wyatt v. Stickney,* 344 F Supp 373 (MD Ala 1972), confirmed a right to treatment. In this case, the entire mental health system of Alabama was sued for providing an inadequate treatment program. The court ruled that the Alabama mental health system must do the following at each institution:

- Stop using patients for hospital labor needs.
- Ensure a humane environment.
- Develop and maintain minimal staffing standards.
- Establish institutional human rights committees.
- Provide the least restrictive environment for each patient.

*Comment:* After nearly 30 years, this case was settled in 2000 under a consent decree that forced the state of Alabama to implement a wide range of mental health services at the local level.

3. *Rogers v. Okin,* 478 F Supp (D Mass 1979), determined the right to refuse treatment. In this case, the ruling prohibited Boston State Hospital from forcing nonviolent patients to take medications against their will. The court based its decision on the constitutional right to privacy. Furthermore, this decision required patients or their guardians to give informed consent before drug treatment could begin. This case has significant implications for nurses who are tempted to "force" patients to take medications for "their own good."

4. *Tarasoff v. The Regents of the University of California,* (1976) 17 Cal 3rd 425, ruled that mental health professionals have a duty to warn of threats of harm to others. In this case, a patient confided to the therapist that he intended to kill an unnamed but readily identifiable girl when she returned from spending the summer in Brazil. The therapist notified campus police and requested their assistance in confining the man. The officers took the patient into custody but released him because he appeared rational. Shortly after her return from Brazil, the man, Prosenjit Poddar, killed Tatiana Tarasoff on October 27, 1969. Her parents successfully sued the University of California, claiming that the therapist had a duty to warn their daughter of Poddar's threats.

*Comment:* The duty to protect endangered third parties is now a national standard of practice, although some jurisdictions still hold that

---

**Box 5-2    Tips for Monitoring Confidentiality**

1. Keep all patient records secure.
2. Carefully consider the content of all written entries.
3. Release information only with written consent.
4. Disguise clinical material when it is used for educational purposes.
5. Share information only with people who need to know, not with friends or in public areas.
6. Guard written material taken outside the clinical area.
7. Do not access written or electronic information out of curiosity.
8. Fax transmissions to unsecured areas in which a receipt error is a possibility might be prohibited.
9. Know to whom you are talking when relating patient information over the phone; "family" might be a reporter, boss, or insurance attorney.

---

any disclosure of confidential information is a violation of patient rights (Box 5-2).

## STATUTORY LAW

Statutory law is written law developed from a legislative body, such as a state legislature. A statute can abolish any rule of common law by specifically stating the rule. Statutory law follows a chain of command, with the Constitution of the United States being the highest in the hierarchy of enacted written law.

Article VI of the Constitution declares:

> This Constitution, and the Laws of the United States which shall be made in Pursuance thereof; and all Treaties made, or which shall be made, under the Authority of the United States, shall be the supreme Law of the Land; and the Judges in every State shall be bound thereby, any Thing in the Constitution or Laws of any State to the Contrary notwithstanding.

This article means that the U.S. Constitution, federal law, and federal treaties take precedence over the constitutions and laws of states and local jurisdictions, such as state statutes.

## ADMINISTRATIVE LAW

Administrative law is public law issued by administrative agencies authorized by statute to administer the enacted laws of federal and state governments. This branch of law controls the administrative operations of government. One example of these agencies is state boards of nursing. Obviously, monitoring and implementing these laws for federal and state legislative bodies is difficult. For example, states boards of nursing have been created to issue guidelines for nursing practice, licensure, and compliance monitoring in the interest of public safety.

## TORTS (CIVIL LAW)

### NEGLIGENCE

Negligence is a personal wrongdoing that is distinguished from a criminal law violation. Negligence is described as the failure to do or not to do what a reasonably careful person would do under the circumstances. Negligence is a form of conduct that is considered careless and is a departure from the standard of conduct generally imposed on reasonable persons.

The four elements that must be present for a plaintiff to recover damages caused by negligence are:

1. Duty to care
2. An obligation of reasonable care (i.e., standard of care)
3. Breach of duty
4. Injury proximately caused by a breach of duty

All four of these elements should be present for plaintiffs to prevail in suits involving a negligent act. If proof exists of all four elements of negligence, then the plaintiffs are said to have presented a *prima facie* case of negligence, which often enables them to win their case.

### Duty to Care

Duty is defined as a legal obligation of care, performance, or observance imposed on a person who is in a position to safeguard the rights of others. This duty can arise from a special relationship, such as the relationship between a nurse and a patient. The duty to care can arise from a telephone conversation or it can arise out of a voluntary act of assuming the care of a patient. Duty can also be established by statute or contract between the physician and patient.

### Reasonable Care (Standard of Care)

A nurse, for example, who assumes the care of patients has the duty to exercise a standard of care, which is the degree of skill, care, and knowledge ordinarily possessed and exercised by other nurses in the care and treatment of patients. A nurse must be reasonable in the exercise of professional judgment as to the care rendered; however, reasonable judgment must not present a departure from the requirements of accepted nursing practice. In court cases in which nurses are being sued for negligence, the question is always the following: "Did the nurse meet the standard of care?" Typically, expert nursing witnesses provide testimony to answer this question.

### Breach of Duty

Breach of duty is the failure to conform to or the departure from a required duty of care owed to a person. The obligation to perform according to a standard of care might encompass either doing or refraining from doing a particular act.

### CLINICAL EXAMPLE

A patient was admitted to a psychiatric facility late at night from general hospital emergency room $1\frac{1}{2}$ hours away. The patient was known to have overdosed on a long-acting opioid drug. Although pronounced medically stable by the first hospital, the patient was noted to be semi-conscious and incoherent, with an irregular respiration rate of 12 breaths/min. The patient's respiratory irregularity did not improve, but neither the physician on call nor the paramedics were called. The patient died before morning of respiratory arrest. The nurses did not meet their obligation to meet the standard of care.

### Proximate Cause or Causation

The fourth element necessary to establish negligence requires that a reasonable, close, and causal connection or relationship exists between the defendant's negligent conduct and the resulting damages suffered by the plaintiff. In other words, the defendant's negligence must be a substantial factor causing the injury. The mere departure from a proper and recognized procedure is insufficient to enable a patient to recover damages, unless the patient can show that the departure was unreasonable and the proximate cause of the patient's injuries. Foreseeability, as an element of negligence, is the reasonable anticipation that harm or injury is likely to result from an act or an omission to act. The test for foreseeability is whether anyone of ordinary prudence and intelligence should have anticipated the danger to another caused by his or her negligence.

## MALPRACTICE

A form of professional negligence is called malpractice. Malpractice claims can be brought against various professions, including nurses. These claims against nurses are often the result of the nurse's failure to take measures to prevent harm to patients or a failure to maintain the standard of care of nurses in the community.

The psychiatric nurse is responsible for many significant decisions in the care of psychiatric patients. Lapses in attention to specific legal issues related to nursing practice can result in liability and suits against the nurse and the nurse's employer. Areas of concern that can lead to suits include inappropriate dissemination of confidential information, illegal confinement, failure to obtain consent for medication and other treatments, inadequate treatment, medication errors, and the breach of duty to warn of threatened suicide or harm to others.

Understanding the concept of the master-servant rule is vital to both clinical nurses and supervisors. Simply stated, an employer is responsible for the acts of the employee as long as the employee is acting within the scope and authority of employment. A nurse who exceeds clinical boundaries or fails to act as a reasonable and prudent nurse would, in the same or similar circumstances, incurs liability to the employer. Similarly, understanding that unlicensed assistive personnel who exceed their clinical boundaries or authority and are under the direction or supervision of a nurse will cause liability to be incurred on the nurse is critical.

### Nursing Implications

With the push to lower health care costs, the use of unlicensed assistive personnel (UAPs) has increased significantly. More nurses are finding themselves with job responsibilities that include delegating certain tasks to UAPs. When a nurse delegates, the authority to carry out the act on behalf of the nurse is conveyed to the assistant; however, the nurse remains accountable for the consequences of the act and for the adequate supervision of the assistant. When delegating, the nurse at a minimum should:

1. Know and follow the local hospital procedures in order to stay within his or her scope and authority.
2. Ensure that UAPs assigned have been fully trained and are qualified to carry out the tasks they are expected to perform.
3. Know the limitations and responsibilities of nursing practice of his or her state.

### CLINICAL EXAMPLE

Clara Meyers, a 40-year-old woman with a history of recent depression with sleep deprivation and suicidal ideation, is admitted to your unit, sedated, and placed on suicide precautions. The nurse assigns a new nursing assistant to check on the patient every 15 minutes for the entire shift. The nursing assistant, having checked the patient every 15 minutes for 2 hours and finding her asleep, decides that every 30 minutes is sufficient. The nurse who delegated this task was unaware that the new assistant had only general nursing assistant training and had never been oriented on a psychiatric unit. During the 30-minute period when the patient was left alone, she managed to get out of bed and go to the bathroom, where she fell and fractured her pelvis. In the subsequent lawsuit, the nurse was identified as being liable for the UAP's poor decision that resulted in the fall.

## DUTY TO WARN OTHERS

Another area of importance to psychiatric nurses is the "duty to warn of threatened suicide or harm." As noted, this duty is derived in part from the landmark case of *Tarasoff v. The Regents of the University of California.* Before the Tarasoff ruling, mental health professionals had no legal duty to warn of threatened suicide or harm to others. In 1976, the California Supreme Court issued the Tarasoff ruling, which states that failure to warn, coupled with subsequent injury to the threatened person, exposes the mental health professional to civil damages for malpractice. Based on this case and other rulings, the mental health professional must balance a duty to protect confidentiality with a responsibility to warn society of possible danger.

### Nursing Implications

A nurse who is aware of a patient's intention to cause harm to self or others must communicate this information to other professionals and take steps to protect the potential recipient of harm. Not all comments or vague threats should be reported. The Tarasoff ruling specifies that a specific threat to a readily identifiable person or persons must be made. Whenever possible, a decision to communicate confidential patient communications should be discussed with the clinical team before taking action to ensure that patients' rights are balanced with those of third parties. Documentation in the patient's record is crucial for effective communication of this information. The nurse who fails to take prudent action can be held liable. See the following example.

---

### CLINICAL EXAMPLE

Bud Hollman is a 36-year-old man with a history of mental illness that was successfully treated. He has maintained a steady job for the last 12 years. He has a history of abusing his wife over the last 7 years. His wife of 10 years has made a decision to divorce Mr. Hollman and end the abuse; she is currently in a safe house for abused women. Mr. Hollman is obsessed with his wife and with finding her. He goes to the homes of several friends and relatives searching for her. He is unsuccessful in finding her and becomes progressively more agitated. He is delusional, convinced that the only reason she left him is because she is possessed. When he fails to find her at her place of employment, he tells her fellow employees that she is possessed by a demon and that he intends to kill her. The police are called and Mr. Hollman is arrested. He is involuntarily committed for a 72-hour evaluation and is found to have a psychosis manifested by delusions. Mr. Hollman specifically tells the therapist of his wife's demonic possession and his plans to remove the demon. On review, the police and Mrs. Hollman are warned of his threats.

---

## ASSAULT, BATTERY, AND FALSE IMPRISONMENT

### Assault

The distinguishing feature between assault and battery is that assault is the apprehension of physical contact or the person's mental security, and battery is the actual physical contact. An assault is the deliberate threat coupled with the apparent ability to do physical harm to another. No actual contact is necessary. Verbally threatening a patient that you are going to force him or her to take medication against the patient's will constitutes an assault.

### Battery

A battery is an intentional touching of another's person, in a socially impermissible manner, without that person's consent. Battery is intentional conduct that violates the physical security of another. The receiver of the battery does not have to be aware that a battery has occurred. A clinical example of battery would be the force used in unlawful detention of a patient.

### False Imprisonment

False imprisonment is the unlawful **restraint** of an individual's personal liberty or the unlawful restraint or confinement of an individual. The only necessity is that an individual who is physically confined to a given area experiences a reasonable fear that force, which may be implied by words, threats, or gestures, will be used to detain or intimidate him or her without legal justification. Examples include:

1. Excessive force used to restrain a patient: false imprisonment and battery.
2. Preventing a patient from leaving a health care facility: false imprisonment.
3. Wrongfully committing a patient to a psychiatric facility: false imprisonment.

A psychiatric facility should have a policy that defines the parameters of confinement, and the nurse must follow the policy guidelines.

## COMMITMENT ISSUES

The decision to become a patient in a psychiatric facility is important. Patients must admit to themselves and to others that self-management is no longer a viable option for emotional stability. The paradox for individuals who require inpatient care is that the process of becoming a patient can itself cause anxiety and might be depressing. The psychiatric nurse should be aware of this aspect and of the legal status of the patients in his or her charge.

## VOLUNTARY PATIENTS

The vast majority of people with mental health problems are voluntary patients—that is, they seek help voluntarily. Although specific procedures vary from hospital to hospital and from state to state, the basic procedure is that individuals or their therapists request admission and patients sign the appropriate documents, including a consent to treatment. When individuals are ready to leave the treatment setting, they sign themselves out. Most states have a grace period of 48 to 72 hours to allow professional staff the time and opportunity to assess patients before they leave voluntarily. Voluntary patients who want to sign themselves out can be placed on an involuntary commitment status by the court when the staff's assessment indicates a need for further treatment.

## INVOLUNTARY PATIENTS (COMMITMENT)

Mental illness is not equivalent to incompetence. Competence involves the patient's ability to comprehend. Involuntary treatment means that an individual who has the legal capacity to consent to mental health treatment refuses to do so. In every state, individuals who are considered dangerous to self or others because of a mental disorder can be involuntarily treated for that mental disorder. The U.S. Supreme Court has repeatedly held, however, that the civil commitment process is subject to the restraints of the Fourteenth Amendment of the U.S. Constitution. The state must produce clear and convincing evidence to prove that a person is both mentally ill and dangerous. Failure to comply with these guidelines can render a commitment illegal. A third criterion—gravely disabled—is also cause (or required) for involuntary treatment in many states. Involuntary treatment is divided into three common categories:

1. Emergency care
2. Short-term observation and treatment
3. Long-term commitment (3, 6, or 12 months)

Not surprisingly, involuntary treatment is the area of psychiatric care from which most legal issues arise. Although involuntary commitment usually implies inpatient care, it can also be applied to outpatient treatment (e.g., group treatment as a consequence for driving under the influence of alcohol).

### Emergency Care

Individuals who meet any one of these three criteria (i.e., dangerous to self, dangerous to others, or gravely disabled) can be detained involuntarily for evaluation and emergency treatment in most states. An authorized person such as a police officer signs documents to place an individual under involuntary care. The length of the involuntary status varies from state to state; typically, 48 to 72 hours is the average.

### Nursing Implications

Because the law determines the length of this involuntary treatment period, staff must scrupulously adhere to legal time constraints. The nursing staff must be absolutely aware of the point at which the emergency treatment period is over and prepare the patient for discharge at that time. Patients might be asked to remain voluntarily in the facility and, if they refuse, they might then be asked to sign out against medical advice. The following clinical example provides a realistic scenario for involuntary detention.

### CLINICAL EXAMPLE

Bill Wexler is a 52-year-old man who has been informed that his job of 30 years is being eliminated. Although the job loss is part of a larger downsizing effort, Mr. Wexler is deeply and personally affected. Within 1 week, he begins to decompensate. He stops bathing and wears the same suit every day. He shows up for work 2 weeks after being terminated, not having bathed or shaved for a week, and goes to his usual workstation. Another employee occupies the space, and Mr. Wexler demands that the worker move out of his space or he will throw him out. Efforts by other employees who know Mr. Wexler are unsuccessful in trying to calm him. He begins shouting that he is going to kill everyone in human resources and that he has a gun in the car and is going to get it. Security and the police are called and are successful in restraining Mr. Wexler after a brief struggle. Mr. Wexler is taken to the county emergency department and involuntarily committed for 72 hours.

## Short-term Observation and Treatment

Each state has laws that provide for short-term observation and treatment for mental illness. These laws, which differ from state to state, authorize a qualified expert to determine whether a person has a treatable mental disorder. In most states, a qualified expert might be a physician, a psychiatrist, a master's-prepared nurse or social worker, or a psychologist. A treatable mental disorder indicates that the problem is amenable to and can improve with treatment. For example, a person who is hearing voices telling her to kill herself meets this criterion, whereas someone who is simply angry and threatening to kill someone might not.

If, during the emergency evaluation period, it is suspected that further hospitalization is needed, a certification hearing takes place. A complaint or a probable cause statement is written, indicating that the person is a danger to self or others or is gravely disabled. The probable cause statement is required by the Fourth Amendment to the U.S. Constitution, which prohibits "search and seizure of a person without probable cause." In this context, probable cause means that known facts would lead an ordinary person to believe that the person detained is mentally disordered and is a danger to self or others or is gravely disabled. The probable cause hearing is not held to determine whether the person is mentally ill, but whether just cause exists to keep the person for treatment against his or her will.

If probable cause exists, individuals can then be detained for observation and treatment. These individuals must be informed of their rights on being certified for this level of involuntary care. The length of the observation and treatment periods varies from state to state.

## Nursing Implications

Patients must be released when no legal basis exists for continued confinement in the hospital. The hospital staff might suggest voluntary admission and, if it is refused, might require patients to sign out against medical advice. The staff cannot hold someone simply because they believe that the individual needs to be protected from herself or himself.

### CLINICAL EXAMPLE

Mr. Banks, an 82-year-old well-nourished but dirty and malodorous man, has been brought to the hospital by a social worker for psychiatric evaluation. Since his wife's death, 3 years earlier, neighbors report that his house has been taken over by drug dealers and prostitutes. He is often seen outside at night, sleeping on the porch, despite cold weather. Furthermore, Mr. Banks has approached neighbors for food and has told them that the drug dealers have taken his social security check. Mr. Banks insists that he willingly allows others to live in his home, and he enjoys the sex and drugs that come with the arrangement. He is alert and oriented, and no evidence of psychiatric disorder is found during evaluation. He declines offers of assistance to find safe housing, stating that he wants to return to the lifestyle he missed during the years his wife kept him on the straight and narrow.

## Long-term Commitment

Long-term commitment is reserved for persons who need prolonged psychiatric care but refuse to seek such help voluntarily. These hospitalizations can last from about 90 days to much longer. Such individuals are usually brought before a hearing officer, which is a major part of the system of checks and balances that decreases the possibility of someone being railroaded into a mental hospital.

## COMMITMENT OF INCAPACITATED PERSONS

In most states, a procedure is required for establishing a conservator or guardian for a gravely disabled person (the conservatee) because adults are presumed competent before the law. The legal system in the United States maintains that, although a person might be undergoing severe mental and emotional upheaval (as in the clinical example of Mr. Wexler), that person is nonetheless recognized as competent. The person who is identified as being gravely disabled, on the other hand, is viewed by the legal system as incompetent. Once judged incompetent, the individual loses rights such as the right to marry, vote, drive a car, and enter into contracts.

Gravely disabled is defined as the inability to provide food, clothing, and shelter for oneself because of a mental illness. This does not mean that all people living on the streets are gravely disabled, nor that they should be hospitalized for their own good. However, people with money in their pockets who cannot negotiate arrangements for food or shelter are gravely disabled.

---

### CRITICAL THINKING QUESTION    2

Some states have a category of commitment called "gravely disabled," whereas other states do not. Obviously, two firmly held views exist about this type of commitment. Does the state in which you live have this commitment category? Do you find the arguments more compelling for or against this commitment category?

---

### Conservators and Guardians

The appointment of a conservator or guardian is a serious legal matter, and full legal protection is provided for persons being evaluated for conservatee status. The proposed conservatee is entitled to representation by an attorney to challenge conservatorship. An appointed conservator or guardian can be given broad powers, including the right to order the conservatee to receive psychiatric treatment. Technically, although patients might receive treatment against their will, a legal distinction exists between this type of commitment and an involuntary commitment. That distinction is based on the premise that the conservator now speaks for the patient; hence, the treatment is not involuntary. Conservators are legally obligated to act in the best interests of their conservatees.

### Nursing Implications

Because conservators speak for conservatees, the nurse must obtain consent from conservators for decisions that are otherwise made by patients. A nurse who forgets to obtain conservator approval might face legal consequences.

---

### CLINICAL EXAMPLE

Ms. Park, a 73-year-old woman, is found by a social worker to be living in a filthy, roach-infested, older home. A neighbor who has not seen Ms. Park in several months calls the local department of human services. The neighbor explains that no one answers the door when she rings the doorbell. Ms. Park has lived there for years with her husband. Since he died 5 years ago, Ms. Park has lived alone. The stench of cats and cat feces is almost unbearable. Ms. Park is emaciated, incoherent, and paranoid. The social worker decides to initiate involuntary commitment for Ms. Park to evaluate her mental and physical condition and her need for a conservatorship hearing.

---

## PATIENT RIGHTS

In addition to the information discussed in the following section, the *Federal Register*, published by the Centers for Medicare and Medicaid Services (CMS), is a good source of information about patient rights and regulations. Aside from the legal and patient care issues, these rights must be assured for health care providers so they can participate in the Medicare and Medicaid programs.

### RIGHT TO TREATMENT WITH THE LEAST RESTRICTIVE ENVIRONMENT

The concept of the least restrictive alternative or least restrictive environment is central to the ideology of the deinstitutionalization movement. People with mental health problems have the right to treatment of their problems in the least restrictive environment using the least restrictive means (i.e., without restraints and seclusion, unless necessary).

### Nursing Implications

The nurse has treatment responsibilities and can be held liable if the patient does not receive adequate treatment. The following clinical example illustrates the issue of the right to treatment using the least restrictive alternative.

## CLINICAL EXAMPLE

Joe Kelly is a 56-year-old Vietnam veteran who suffers from posttraumatic stress syndrome characterized by periods of flashbacks and depression. After a flashback, Mr. Kelly is often confused and wanders about for days looking for friends he lost in the war. He poses no obvious danger to others or himself. His family is deceased, and he lives alone. When he is picked up by the police for loitering and evaluated by the social worker, Mr. Kelly insists on going home. His case, however, is heard before the court, which rules that he does not need commitment to a psychiatric unit but does need a temporary structured environment. The social worker finds a halfway house with the Veterans Hospital, and Mr. Kelly agrees to temporary placement.

## RIGHT TO CONFIDENTIALITY OF RECORDS

Patient information is privileged material and should be treated confidentially. Both voluntary and involuntary patients are granted this legal consideration. Following this procedure is not always as easy as it might appear hence professional judgment is required. The guidelines in Box 5-2 provide a framework for mandatory confidentiality.

As straightforward as these guidelines are, they do not cover every situation or address exceptions. The rule of confidentiality is not absolute. For example, information about a patient at risk for self-harm must be made available to appropriate individuals. Keeping this type of information confidential constitutes professional malpractice.

### Health Insurance Portability and Accountability Act

The Health Insurance Portability and Accountability Act (HIPAA) took effect in April 2003. Because modern technology is often a two-edged sword, concerns have arisen over its misuse. For example, even though computer technology speeds the transfer and storage of personal medical information, it has also proven to be avenue for invasion of privacy. HIPAA gives patients more control over their medical records. It also creates stiffer penalties for those who handle a patient's medical record in too cavalier a manner. Appelbaum (2002) has outlined the four rights that patients have under HIPAA legislation:

1. Right to be educated about HIPAA privacy regulations
2. Right to access their own medical records
3. Right to correct or add to their medical records
4. Right to demand their authorization before their medical records are disclosed to others

### Nursing Implications

The nurse should document all confidential information that is released in the nursing notes, including the date and circumstances under which disclosure was made, the names of the individuals or agencies receiving the disclosure and their relationship(s) to the patient, and the specific information disclosed.

To release information about patients, a consent form must first be signed. Most states provide legal redress for patients if a nurse willfully discloses confidential information without the proper signature. Confidentiality of the patient's records should not be confused with the doctrine of privileged communication. Under this doctrine, a psychiatrist is not obliged to reveal the contents of sessions with the patient, a privilege that is based on the understanding of the need for trust between physicians and patients. Most states do not include nurses under this provision.

The therapeutic modality of group therapy, which nurses often lead, is particularly vulnerable to violations of confidentiality. The group leader should always address this issue when starting a group or when a new member is introduced to the group. Nurses who lead group sessions must acknowledge the limitations to confidentiality that exist in the group format. After such a proclamation is made, forthrightness by group members concerning their thoughts, feelings, and behaviors might decline. It is absolutely necessary that staff not discuss patients in settings in which those without a clinical need to know can overhear those conversations.

### CRITICAL THINKING QUESTION    3

Confidentiality is stressed in nursing school, but it might be violated. What should you do when one of your classmates is discussing a patient inappropriately? Is it a violation of confidentiality to discuss a patient by name in a clinical conference?

CLINICAL EXAMPLE

Students frequently find themselves in the following situation. After developing a relationship with a patient, the student might hear, "I want to tell you something, but I don't want anyone else to know." What is the proper response? Is it a breach of the patient's right to confidentiality to tell others or to record what is said in the patient's chart? The student must let the patient know that anything said within the context of the nurse-patient relationship will be shared with other team members when appropriate.

## RIGHT TO FREEDOM FROM RESTRAINTS AND SECLUSION

Throughout history, mechanical restraints and segregation have been used to manage the out of control behavior that accompanies some psychiatric disorders. *Restraint* is a broad term used to characterize any form of limiting a person's movement or access to his or her own body. The limits can be the result of physical holds, bed rails, lap trays, restraint devices, or medications. *Seclusion* is defined as the process of isolating a person in a room in which they are physically prevented from leaving. The real value of judiciously used restraint and seclusion to protect severely ill patients and those with whom they come into contact has been overshadowed in recent years by attention to injuries and deaths associated with their use. The U.S. Food and Drug Administration (FDA) has estimated that at least 100 restraint-related deaths occur each year. In some instances, restraints and seclusion have been substituted for more appropriate management interventions. The patient's right to the least restrictive interventions to manage behavioral disturbances has been violated, with resulting disability, injury, and death.

The 1987 Omnibus Reconciliation Act (OBRA) placed stringent limits on the use of physical and chemical restraints (e.g., antipsychotics, benzodiazepines) in nursing homes to ensure that their use is limited to medical necessity, not staff convenience. Many nursing homes have since implemented innovative strategies to preserve the safety of frail older adults, with a goal of becoming restraint free. The Joint Commission on Accreditation of Healthcare Organizations (JCAHO) has developed standards to guide efforts to reduce the use of restraints in both medical and psychiatric facilities. The CMS has also published, within their Patients Rights document, strict rules for restraint and seclusion use in hospitals that receive Medicare and Medicaid funds (Medicare and Medicaid programs, 1999).

CLINICAL EXAMPLE

Mr. Buck Tindal, 75, has been admitted to the geropsychiatric unit of a large teaching hospital for observation and treatment related to recent behaviors suggestive of dementia. Mr. Tindal, although confused at times, is able to feed himself, bathe without assistance, and self-manage toileting needs on admission. As do many men older than 60 years, Mr. Tindal experiences nocturia most nights. Because the staff is concerned about falling and consequent broken bones, Mr. Tindal has been "legally" restrained. Immediately, he begins wetting the bed, something he had not done since childhood. Within 2 weeks, Mr. Tindal is not able to feed and bathe himself, and is described in his chart as incontinent.

### Nursing Implications

Reduction in the use of restraints is difficult to achieve given the rather prevalent belief that a restrained patient is a safe one. Nurses who are aware of the potential negative physical, psychological, and legal consequences associated with restraint and seclusion are more apt to look for alternate strategies. Most valuable are those interventions aimed at preventing a patient's escalation in behavior and loss of control. Attention to the nurse-patient relationship, therapeutic milieu, and principles of pharmacologic management can reduce the need for restrictive measures. Guidelines issued by the CMS for use of restraint and seclusion are substantially different in medically necessary and behavioral control situations. Although laws differ from state to state, general guidelines for use in psychiatry include multiple elements important for the nurse to document:

1. Staff members involved in decisions to restrain or seclude and those who apply or remove restraints must receive special training and demonstrate competency.
2. Alternatives to restraint and seclusion must be considered before their use.

3. Although nurses might be allowed to implement restraint or seclusion in emergent situations, a physician's order is required within 1 hour. Physician assistants and advanced practice nurses can also write restraint and seclusion orders.
4. The least restrictive method or device possible must be chosen.
5. Nurses should carefully document events leading up to the intervention and justification for use.
6. Orders must contain the type of restraint, rationale for use, and time limitations.
7. As needed (prn) orders are not permitted. Each episode must be based on eminent risk.
8. Restraint and seclusion are used for the shortest possible time. The nurse must tell the patients what behaviors are expected before release and reevaluate the patients at least every 2 hours for continued necessity.
9. Patients must be observed constantly during restraint and seclusion, with documentation of safety and comfort interventions at least every 15 minutes.
10. Patients must be debriefed after restrictive interventions.
11. Patients have the right to request notification of a family member or other person in the event that restraints or seclusion are implemented.
12. Death of any patient while in restraints, even when restraints did not contribute to death in the judgment of the health care provider, is required to be reported to the FDA.

## CRITICAL THINKING QUESTION    4

Some psychiatric professionals believe that the courts have gone too far in protecting the rights of patients and have actually set up barriers to effective mental health care. What do you think?

## CLINICAL EXAMPLE

Kim Young is a 28-year-old Korean national married to an American serviceman who is currently assigned overseas. Ms. Young is extremely well versed in the American culture and language, and is exceptionally bright and talented. Ms. Young has performed endless hours of volunteer work in her community and church. She is viewed as a person with boundless energy who never appears to stop. Her volunteer hours continue to increase, and she begins to preach in local bars and taverns. Her language becomes incoherent at times, and English and Korean are often mixed in the same sentence. When the owner of a local tavern calls the police after she refuses to leave, she begins to curse him and tries to hit him with a beer bottle. The police are able to restrain her, and she is involuntarily committed to a psychiatric unit. When approached by the staff, she spits, curses, and tries to strike them. Four-point physical restraint is ordered. Ms. Young requires seclusion and restraint thereafter for her aggressive behavior on several occasions. The nursing progress record (Box 5-3) and the restraint and seclusion nursing notes provide a record of her behavior and the nursing responses to that behavior.

### Box 5-3   Nursing Progress Record

| Time | Format |
|---|---|
| 0210 | Patient continues to pace hallway, dayroom, and room; at 0045, is asking for sleep medications; patient states the best way to get well is walking. |
| 0315 | Patient refuses to go to room and tries to rest, pacing dayroom and at times kneeling as if in prayer. |
| 0430 | Patient is asleep on top of bed, naked; door is open. |
| 0830 | Patient refuses medication; appears very agitated. |
| 0930 | Patient is very agitated, tearing up another patient's magazine and throwing into trash; patient is placed in seclusion. |
| 1030 | Agitation is escalated; when staff goes into room to check on the patient, she swings at staff and attempts to bite the nurse; patient placed in four-point restraint by four female and two male staff members; patient states that she is being "raped" and that "Christ lives in me"; Haldol 5 mg IM and Cogentin 2 mg IM are given. |

## RIGHT TO GIVE OR REFUSE CONSENT TO TREATMENT

The right of voluntary patients to refuse treatment has been recognized for a long time. When voluntary patients believe that the treatment they are receiving is helpful, they can accept it; when they believe that the treatment is not helpful, they can refuse it. Involuntary patients, on the other hand, have not always been understood to have the same right to refuse treatment. Through the years, many involuntary patients have been forced to take medications against their will. Legally, involuntarily admitted patients do not lose their right to give informed consent to the administration of psychotropic drugs. The key issue is whether patients have the capacity to give informed consent to the administration of these drugs. After the court decides that a person is not competent to understand the need for treatment, medications can then be imposed on that person. The way in which this decision is implemented varies from state to state.

In cases of a psychiatric emergency, medications can be given without consent to prevent harm to the patient or to others.

### Nursing Implications

Nurses administer medications to patients. Because it is not uncommon for patients to refuse medications and for nurses to coax those patients into taking medications, nurses must be sure that coaxing does not escalate to the point of forcing medication on a patient. Furthermore, although it might be tempting to hide medications in food or liquid when patients refuse them, these actions are considered forcing. The deception is also counterproductive when trying to establish a therapeutic nurse-patient relationship. Factors that constitute a psychiatric emergency are also not always clear. Nurses might be held liable if their interpretation of a psychiatric emergency differs from that of another professional or a judge.

## SUSPENSION OF PATIENT RIGHTS

Occasionally, suspending rights for the protection of patients or others and for therapeutic purposes is necessary. For example, no units have unlimited telephone privileges, primarily because this policy might be nontherapeutic.

### Nursing Implications

Suspension of a patient's rights requires the nurse to document clearly that allowing the patient to

continue to exercise the specific right might result in harm to the patient or others. For example, a suicidal patient's right to access personal belongings might be suspended because it is believed that such a patient might attempt to harm himself or herself with those objects. The nurse must document the concern and suspension of this right in the nurse's notes.

## ADVANCE DIRECTIVES FOR HEALTH CARE

A majority of states have recognized the rights of individuals to choose the type of medical treatment they receive in case of a life-threatening medical condition, which is accomplished through the use of living wills and health care directives. In the spring of 2005, the Terri Schiavo case brought this matter to the forefront. Ms. Schiavo had not executed a directive, and the world witnessed the drama that became her final days as her husband and the court decided to remove her feeding tube. Many people, inspired by this case, acted swiftly and legally to set forth their wishes in case of their incapacitation.

The U.S. Congress passed the Patient Self-Determination Act in 1990. This requires all health care facilities that serve Medicare or Medicaid patients to provide each of their adult patients with written information regarding their right to make decisions about their medical care. These instructions must be consistent with the laws of each state. Patients are also made aware of the right to execute a living will or durable power of attorney. Both the living will and the health care directive list specific actions that the patient can choose to implement or not under a life-threatening medical condition, such as mechanical ventilator support or artificial nutrition. A durable power of attorney is a written document in which one person (the principal) authorizes another person (the attorney in fact) to act on the principal's behalf in the event the principal becomes unable to act on his or her own behalf secondary to a physical or mental disability. The disability causes this type of power of attorney to take effect.

Advance directives for mental health treatment are similar to medical care advance directives in many ways, but have a number of additional challenges. The issue of ensuring competency when directives are executed is problematic, particularly for patients with fluctuating mental disorders. Nonetheless, in advance of a mental health crisis, individuals can issue directives about treatment in a number of areas, including but not limited to (1) the use of specific medications, including dose and route; (2) the use of specific treatment options, such as electroconvulsive therapy (ECT); (3) the use of behavior management including restraint, seclusion, and sedation; (4) a list of the individuals who are to be notified and allowed to visit; (5) a consent to contact health care providers and obtain treatment records; and (6) a willingness to participate in research studies (Srebnik and LaFond, 1999).

## Nursing Implications

Nurses should be aware of the patient's right to establish advance directives for both physical and mental health care in the form of written statement of preference, or by legal documentation of a durable power of attorney. Nurses should also be familiar with and follow employer procedures and laws that govern how the patient is made aware of this right. The following actions are also important to ensure that the patient's right to self-determination is exercised:

1. Documentation in the medical record of either properly executed forms or a statement or signed waiver must be made indicating that the patient chooses not to exercise his or her right to provide advance directives.
2. The attorney in fact chosen by the patient is consulted before making decisions regarding the patient in areas specified by the document.
3. All members of the health care team are made aware of advance directives and that they are considered in treatment planning.

## ▋ Study Notes

1. The understanding of the rights of mentally ill persons has evolved over the centuries. Today, based on several precedent-setting legal decisions and laws, protection of the mentally ill person's rights has been established.

2. These landmark cases triggered several states to legislate the end of inappropriate, indefinite, and involuntary commitment to mental hospitals.
3. Three categories of commitment include:
   a. Voluntary patient: the person requests hospitalization and voluntarily agrees to be admitted.
   b. Involuntary commitment: a person with the legal capacity to consent refuses to do so and is treated against his or her will.
   c. Commitment of an incapacitated person: treatment of a person who does not have the legal capacity to consent to treatment.
4. Patients under psychiatric care have many rights guaranteed by the U.S. Constitution and the constitutions of individual states.
5. Seclusion and restraint are special procedures for coping with assaultive and dangerous patients; thus, these patients can be isolated or mechanically restrained to prevent injury to the patient, other patients, or staff.
6. Patients, even involuntarily admitted patients, must give informed consent before they are given psychotropic drugs and retain the right to refuse medication. Except for emergency situations, involuntarily admitted patients cannot be given medication against their will without judicial approval.
7. Psychiatric patients have the right to be treated in the least restrictive alternative or least restrictive environment. In other words, if persons can receive appropriate care close to home in a community agency, then they cannot be forced to go to a public mental hospital, far away from family and friends.

## ▋ References

Appelbaum PS: Privacy in psychiatric treatment: threats and responses, *Am J Psychiatry* 159:1809, 2002.

Eskreis TR: Seven common legal pitfalls in nursing, *Am J Nurs* 98:34, 1998.

Highway assailant heard voices. (2005, May 3). *Birmingham News,* p. 3A.

Medicare and Medicaid programs: Hospital conditions of participation: patients' rights; interim final rule, *Fed Reg* 64:36069, 1999 (42 CFR pt 482).

Moran M: Insanity standards may vary, but plea rarely succeeds, *Psychiatr News* 37:24, 2002.

Srebnik D, LaFond J: Advance directives for mental health treatment, *Psychiatr Serv* 50:919, 1999.

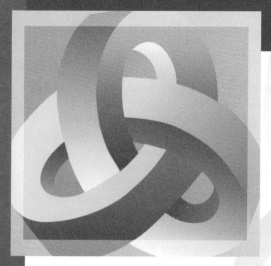

# Chapter 6

# Psychobiologic Bases of Behavior

*Richard A. Sugerman*

## Learning Objectives

*After reading this chapter, you should be able to:*
- Describe the importance of the psychiatric nurse's understanding of brain biology.
- Identify and describe gross neuroanatomic structures.
- Discuss the significance and role of five specific neurotransmitters in normal brain function.
- Identify the role of five specific neurotransmitters in schizophrenia, depression, anxiety, and dementia.
- Differentiate the functions of the sympathetic and parasympathetic nervous systems.
- Describe the function of the basal ganglia system and its significance for movement disorders.
- Discuss key psychobiologic assessment issues for the psychiatric nurse.

The central nervous system (CNS) is composed of the brain and the spinal cord. The brain can be further divided into the cerebrum, the brainstem, and the cerebellum. The brain weighs only approximately 3 to 4 pounds but contains 100 billion neurons, roughly the same as the number of stars in the Milky Way galaxy. The brain is incredibly complex, and a great deal about the brain remains that science does not know. What is known, however, is that many mental disorders that were formerly thought to be caused by psychosocial stressors, traumatic early life experiences, or both are the result of altered or disordered brain biology.

The U.S. Congress declared the 1990s as the Decade of the Brain. Before this time, psychiatric nursing had been influenced primarily by the dominant ideas of the nineteenth century, the ideas of Freud, Bleuler, and Jung, asserting that mental disorders originate from psychodynamic causes. However, psychiatric nursing accepted the congressional mandate, and the 1990s witnessed significant changes in the education and practice of psychiatric nurses. Psychiatric nursing is now fully integrating biologic concepts and, consequently, is now being practiced holistically. The foundation of today's practice includes understanding basic neuroanatomy and neurophysiology.

The objective of this chapter is to present a balanced view of biologic information; thus, the student can be more engaged in the rest of this book, participate in interdisciplinary discussions, and read the psychiatric literature with understanding. Understanding psychobiologic concepts enables the nurse to assess patients' behaviors better and plan appropriate nursing interventions.

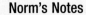

## Norm's Notes

*In Chapter 5, I mentioned that, for some of you, discussing legal parameters of mental illness might cause you to fall asleep. Well, maybe I jumped the gun. There is nothing like a good healthy dose of central nervous system pathways superimposed on a scintillating discussion of presynaptic and postsynaptic receptors to turn the most dedicated student into someone longing for the good old days of fundamentals. Well, it's funny that I should say that, because learning some of the basics of brain biology is crucial to understanding the basics of mental illness. This is fundamental information.*

Specifically, the nurse should have an appreciation for the neuroanatomy of the brain, neurons and neurotransmitters, the autonomic nervous system, and the ventricular system, and should be able to carry out the clinical application of this information to major psychiatric disorders.

## NEUROANATOMY OF THE BRAIN

The nervous system is divided into the CNS and the peripheral nervous system (PNS). The CNS (Figure 6-1) can be further divided into the brain and spinal cord. The brain is composed of the cerebrum, brainstem, and cerebellum.

## CEREBRUM

The cerebrum is divided into two cerebral hemispheres and constitutes the bulk of the nervous system. The hemispheres are composed of a multitude of nervous system pathways, the cerebral cortex, certain limbic structures, the basal ganglia, and the diencephalons (i.e., various thalamic nuclei). These structures are described in the following section.

### Nervous System Pathways

Some specialized neurons in the cerebral cortex transmit information via pathways throughout the CNS. A pathway is a bundle of these communicating neurons. In the CNS, a neuronal pathway (a bundle of neurons) may be called a *tract, fasciculus, peduncle,* or *lemniscus.* (In neuroanatomy, a single anatomic entity can have several names.) In the PNS, a neuronal pathway is called a *nerve.* Hence, cranial nerve III (CN III) is part of the PNS.

A number of large CNS pathways are readily apparent structures within white areas of the brain (white matter). For example, major pathways include the corpus callosum (Figures 6-2 and 6-3), the internal capsule in each hemisphere (Figure 6-4; see also Figure 6-3), and the corona radiata (see Figures 6-3 and 6-4). Although a great deal of interest exists in differences between the right brain (visual-spatial, experiential tasks) and the left brain (language, mathematics, reasoning), many scientists now have a greater appreciation for the interrelatedness of the two hemispheres. The corpus callosum connects the two hemispheres and is the major communication pathway between them. When the corpus callosum is severed, a split-brain syndrome develops. The internal capsule and the corona radiata are pathways through which motor and sensory information passes; for example, motor impulses from the motor cortex (precentral gyrus) to the foot pass through these pathways. In addition to these large pathways, many smaller tracts interconnect the four lobes of the cerebral cortex.

### Cerebral Cortex

The cerebral cortex is the outermost part of the brain and is composed of gray matter. The gray matter, actually taupe (gray-brown) in color, does the work of the brain. Gray matter consists of neuronal cell bodies, dendrites, and synapses and is not myelinated (myelinated axons make up the white matter). The cerebral cortex of the cerebrum is divided into four lobes: the frontal, temporal, parietal, and occipital lobes (see Figures 6-1 and 6-2). Visual examination of the brain reveals the raised areas, or convolutions, and the grooves between these areas. Convoluted gray matter is referred to as a gyrus (plural, *gyri*), and the groove between two gyri is called a sulcus (plural, *sulci*). A deep sulcus is referred to as a *fissure*.

The net effect of this convoluted configuration is that more gray matter can be provided to perform the work of the brain. This principle can be visualized by considering the coastline of Norway. If Norway did not have fjords, its coastline would then be rather small (i.e., approximately 1600

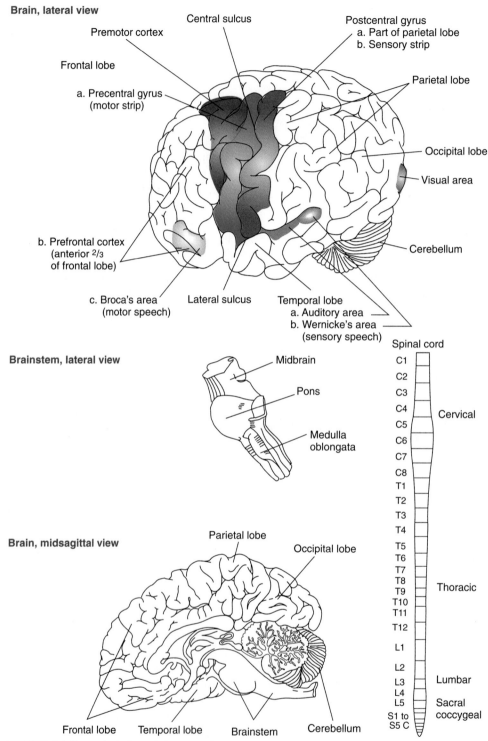

**FIGURE 6-1** Expanded view of the central nervous system. This illustrates the major components (components are not to scale). *(From Sugerman RA, Edmundson MJ, Robinson S: Human anatomy, Edina, MN, 1979, Burgess.)*

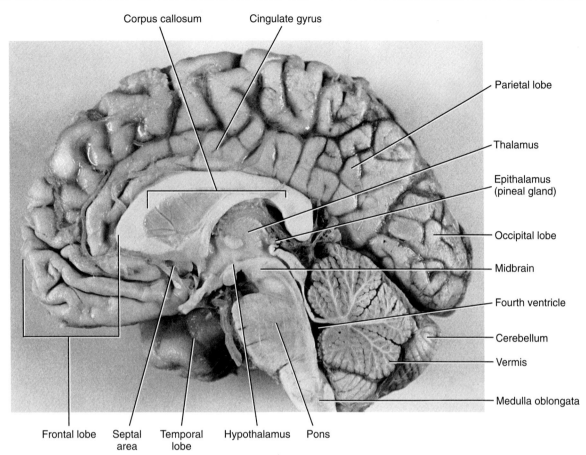

**FIGURE 6-2** Midline view of right hemisphere. Anatomic sites are labeled. *(Photograph by Berto Tarin, Multimedia Department, Western University of Health Sciences, Pomona, CA.)*

miles). However, because of the fjords, the actual coastline of Norway is extraordinarily long for a country of its size (i.e., approximately 12,500 miles). The gyri and sulci of the cerebral cortex can be considered as the *fjords* of the brain. The indentations provide for a much larger coastline of working gray matter than would be the case if the brain's surface were smooth. The four lobes of the cerebral cortex are divided by three sulci.

### Frontal Lobes

The frontal lobes are divided into the *motor* (also called the *motor strip*), *premotor,* and *prefrontal areas.* The motor cortex lies immediately rostral to (in front of) the central sulcus (see Figure 6-1), which separates the frontal and parietal lobes. Because it lies in front of the central sulcus, the motor strip is also called the *precentral gyrus.* The motor cortex controls voluntary motor activity, and the pathway (see Figure 6-4) from this area descends through the corona radiata and the inter-

nal capsule, crosses in the caudal brainstem, and synapses in the spinal cord. Approximately 80% of the corticospinal tract crosses over at the level of the lower brainstem (medulla oblongata), whereas the remaining 20% of the neurons descends down the spinal cord ipsilaterally (same side) before crossing over to the opposite side of the spinal cord. This remaining 20% of the corticospinal tract might be theoretically responsible for some limited motor recovery in patients with hemisected spinal cords; but the incidence of any actual recovery is rare at best. From the spinal cord, spinal nerves branch out into the periphery and connect to muscles. This system of voluntary movement is referred to as the pyramidal system or the *corticospinal tract* (pathway). The term *pyramidal* is used because most neurons in this tract pass through the pyramids of the lower (or caudal) brainstem (medulla oblongata). The extrapyramidal motor system lies outside the pyramids.

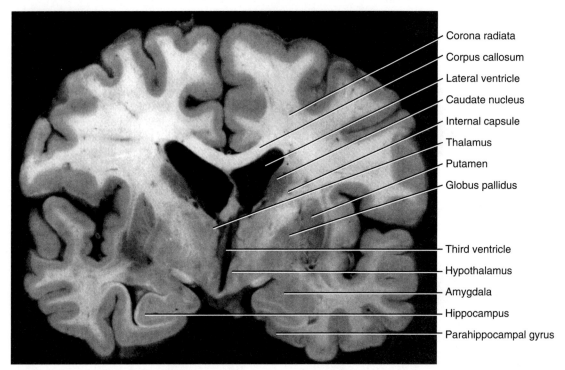

Corona radiata
Corpus callosum
Lateral ventricle
Caudate nucleus
Internal capsule
Thalamus
Putamen
Globus pallidus

Third ventricle
Hypothalamus
Amygdala
Hippocampus
Parahippocampal gyrus

**FIGURE 6-3** Coronal section of the cerebrum. The level of the hypothalamus is shown. *(Courtesy of Richard E. Powers, MD, University of Alabama, Birmingham, AL, Brain Resource Program.)*

## CLINICAL EXAMPLE

Think about wiggling your right big toe and then wiggle it. It is not known how a thought is translated into muscle movement, but what is known is that this voluntary movement is a two-neuron system; that is, neurons from the motor cortex descend as described and synapse with spinal neurons. The spinal neurons project as a spinal nerve from the spinal cord and descend to the toe. The neurons from the motor cortex to the spinal cord are called *upper motor neurons* (see Figure 6-4). The neurons that project from the spinal cord down to the toe are *lower motor neurons*. Whether a disease is an upper motor neuron disease (e.g., stroke) or a lower motor neuron disease (e.g., polio) is clinically significant. An upper motor lesion normally results in a contralateral (body side opposite of the lesion) Babinski's sign. A lower motor neuron lesion normally results in flaccid paralysis.

The premotor area is associated with programmed movement patterns for voluntary motor activity and with inhibiting lower motor neurons from overreacting to stimuli (Kandel et al, 2000). This area is not under conscious control. Many movement disorders, including those associated with psychotropic drug use, arise from the premotor cortex and extrapyramidal system. Both the motor cortex and premotor cortex are organized systematically (Kandel et al, 2000). This arrangement is referred to as *somatotropic organization,* meaning simply that the area of the motor strip that controls a certain part of the body is relatively specific. This biologic reality has been visually depicted as a little person or, more commonly, as a homunculus (Figure 6-5). Perhaps a word picture can best describe this specific pattern of voluntary motor localization. Think of a child hanging on the monkey bars with head down and feet hanging over the bar. Think of the top of the hemisphere as the bar, with the head hanging down laterally and one foot hanging down between the hemispheres. The area of the motor strip where the head is located controls head movements, the area where the foot hangs controls foot movements, and so on.

A health professional can give a physical examination to a person with a neurologic lesion (e.g., stroke, gunshot wound) and, using knowledge of the corticospinal tract and homunculus (see Figures 6-4 and 6-5), can often predict the site of cortical

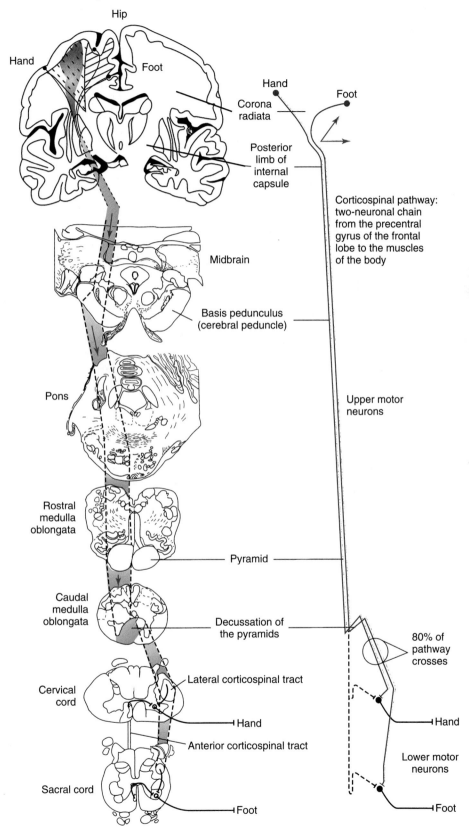

**Cerebral hemispheres: frontal section**

Hip

Hand

Foot

Hand

Foot

Corona radiata

Posterior limb of internal capsule

Corticospinal pathway: two-neuronal chain from the precentral gyrus of the frontal lobe to the muscles of the body

Midbrain

Basis pedunculus (cerebral peduncle)

Pons

Upper motor neurons

Rostral medulla oblongata

Pyramid

Caudal medulla oblongata

Decussation of the pyramids

80% of pathway crosses

Lateral corticospinal tract

Cervical cord

Hand

Hand

Anterior corticospinal tract

Lower motor neurons

Sacral cord

Foot

Foot

**FIGURE 6-4** Distribution of the corticospinal tract. *Left,* Actual representation; *right,* schematic representation.

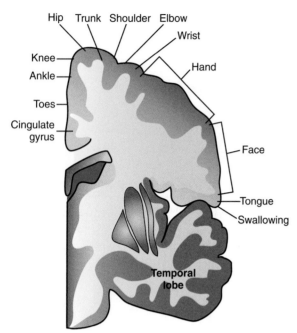

**FIGURE 6-5** Homunculus of the precentral gyrus. This frontal section depicts the relative amount of cortex subserved in controlling the motor functions of various body areas.

lesions in the CNS. Knowing the location of the cranial nuclei allows the examiner to localize brainstem lesions. Two classic vascular lesions (Kiernan, 2005) in the brainstem illustrate how a health care professional can diagnose a lesion site by understanding the location of brainstem structures. A patient who presents with ipsilateral paralysis of at least four of the six extraocular eye muscles and contralateral hemiparesis (weakness of all body muscles on the opposite side) most likely had a vascular accident on one side of the midbrain toward the midline (see Figure 6-4, midbrain, and Figure 6-6B). A lesion affecting half the midbrain can affect the oculomotor nerve (lower motor neuron) and the corticospinal pathway (upper motor neuron), causing the observed signs. In a second example, a patient who presents with contralateral hemiparesis, ipsilateral loss of sensory position and discriminative touch, and ipsilateral paralysis of the tongue most likely had a vascular lesion on one side of the rostral medulla oblongata toward the midline (see Figure 6-4, rostral medulla oblongata). In both cases, the specific cranial nerves that have been damaged indicate the CNS level of these vascular accidents.

The prefrontal area of the cerebral cortex is responsible for thought, goal-oriented behavior, and inhibition. The frontal poles represent the seat of the personality; injuries in this area result in personality changes.

### Temporal Lobes

The temporal lobes lie inferior to the *lateral sulci* (the *lateral fissures of Sylvius*). Each temporal lobe is divided into an olfactory area, a primary auditory receptive area, a secondary auditory association area, and a visual association area (Bear et al, 2001). Aphasias, both visual and auditory, are the result of damage to the temporal lobe. Individuals with visual aphasia cannot recognize words in print that they previously understood; the words are as unrecognizable as printed Russian might be to most people. People with auditory aphasia hear sounds but cannot associate the sounds with meaning.

### Parietal Lobes

The parietal lobes are posterior to the central sulcus. These primarily sensory association areas contain a sensory strip (the postcentral gyrus) that roughly corresponds to the homunculus of the motor strip. The sensory areas interpret sensations. Caudal to this area are the association areas of the parietal lobes.

### Occipital Lobes

The occipital lobes are divided into visual receptive and visual association areas. In contrast to temporal lobe lesions, which can produce various types of visual aphasias, lesions in the occipital lobe's visual association cortex result in loss of vision (blindness) from the contralateral visual field; that is, total damage of the left side of the occipital visual association cortex results in loss of vision from the right visual field. The primary function of the occipital lobes is vision.

## Limbic System

The limbic lobe forms the central core of the limbic system and is composed of the septal area, cingulate gyrus, and parahippocampal gyrus (see Figures 6-2 and 6-3). The limbic lobe is built on the olfactory (smell) system. The *limbic system* is a broad term, referring to the limbic lobe and the structures that function with it: the frontal cortex, hypothalamus, amygdala, hippocampus, numerous tracts, brainstem nuclei, and the autonomic system.

The way in which emotions and motivation are generated in the limbic system remains unclear. No specific anatomic areas exist that can be correlated for emotions such as love, hate, and dislike. Each emotion is likely diffusely linked to different limbic and nonlimbic areas. The limbic system controls the four F's (feeding, fighting, fleeing, and fornicating)—memory, sense of pleasure, emotions, and motivation.

### Limbic Olfactory Function

The first pathway discussed is the olfactory pathway, which is involved with odor detection, feeding, and feeling pleasure. This chapter does not discuss odor detection beyond its relationship to limbic functions. Understanding how significant smell relates to emotion is important. Large department stores have recognized for years that having a perfume display sells more than perfume alone.

Olfactory information is picked up by receptor neurons in the nasal cavity and transmitted to the olfactory bulbs, which are located directly under the surface of the frontal lobes. The olfactory bulbs project axons that synapse in the parahippocampal gyrus and in a subdivision of the amygdala (see Figure 6-3).

### Feeding Functions

The septal area, which connects neuronally with the hypothalamus, is involved in several aspects of feeding (e.g., hypothalamic feeding and satiety centers). Experimentally, researchers can electrically stimulate or destroy these hypothalamic areas and affect whether an animal overeats or stops eating.

### Fight-or-Flight Limbic Function

The fight-or-flight pathway is composed of three major areas: amygdala, hypothalamus, and midbrain. Electric stimulation of these areas elicits either rage behavior or flight. Bilateral destruction of the amygdala and selected areas in the hypothalamus can have a calming effect.

### Memory Limbic Function

The limbic system is crucial to memory. The amygdala and hippocampus, located deep in the temporal lobe, are key structures in the transfer of information from short-term to long-term memory (Bear et al, 2001). The *Papez circuit* consists of brain structures involved in the complex process whereby memories are made and stored. Discussion of the Papez circuit is beyond the scope of this book; however, the reader should recognize that lesions along this circuit cause memory problems. For example, a bilateral lesion of the hippocampus nuclei can be the result of anoxia from near-drowning, and lesions of the mamillary bodies resulting in memory problems can occur in alcoholics because of a thiamine deficiency. These individuals frequently maintain long-term memory, but cannot make new memories.

Amnestic states, amnestic dementias, punch-drunk syndrome, herpes encephalitis, and Alzheimer's disease involve dysfunction of the hippocampi and possibly other limbic structures (Boss and Stowe, 1986).

### Pleasure

Electric stimulation of the reward pathway can cause animals and people to feel pleasure. Rats will press a bar repeatedly to receive electric stimulation to this pathway. The dopaminergic neurons projecting from the ventral tegmental area (VTA) (Figure 6-6) are of particular importance. These brainstem neurons project rostrally to the cortical and limbic areas, particularly the nucleus accumbens. Investigators have hypothesized that cocaine and many other drugs produce their effects by increasing the action of dopamine in the nucleus accumbens (Figure 6-7), which is said to be one of the brain's key pleasure centers. The nucleus accumbens is located in the septal area (see Figure 6-2). Additionally, electric stimulation of the septal area elicits sexual arousal in both animals and people. The nucleus accumbens is probably the nucleus responsible for sexual arousal (Heath, 1972).

### Emotions and Motivation Functions

The emotions and motivation component includes the feelings about people, institutions, and life that affect behavior. For example, feelings help determine whether an act is right or wrong and good or bad, and whether a particular act will be performed. Most authors refer to these feelings as *visceral aspects of behavior.*

## Basal Ganglia

The basal ganglia (see Figure 6-3) are made up of three major nuclei: the caudate nucleus, the putamen, and the globus pallidus. These structures

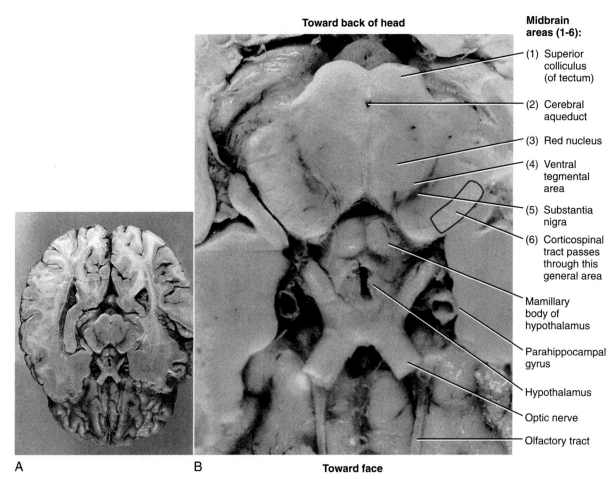

**Toward back of head**

**Midbrain areas (1-6):**

(1) Superior colliculus (of tectum)

(2) Cerebral aqueduct

(3) Red nucleus

(4) Ventral tegmental area

(5) Substantia nigra

(6) Corticospinal tract passes through this general area

Mamillary body of hypothalamus

Parahippocampal gyrus

Hypothalamus

Optic nerve

Olfactory tract

A          B          **Toward face**

**FIGURE 6-6 A,** Brain is sectioned transversely through the midbrain and parahippocampal gyri. **B,** Enlargement of the area through the midbrain is shown. *(Photographs by Berto Tarin, Multimedia Department, Western University of Health Sciences, Pomona, CA.)*

are also involved in motor functions. The putamen and globus pallidus together are referred to as the *lentiform* (lens-shaped) *nucleus*. The basal ganglia, or extrapyramidal system, including the substantia nigra (see Figure 6-6), resides between the midbrain and cerebral cortex and communicates back and forth about ongoing motor activity from the body. The basal ganglia system complements the pyramidal system. The pyramidal (or corticospinal) tract transmits commands for voluntary movement, and the basal ganglia system modulates these movements, maintains appropriate muscle tone, and adjusts posture. For example, when the hand is extended and the fingers are held still, slight oscillations of the fingers occur. The basal ganglia system, which includes some motor pathways, works with the pyramidal system to keep these movements small.

The basal ganglia system balances excitatory and inhibitory neurons that have different neurotransmitters. Acetylcholine is the primary excitatory neurotransmitter. Gamma-aminobutyric acid (GABA) is an important inhibitory neurotransmitter in this system. Dopamine can be either excitatory or inhibitory. It modulates neuronal membranes, and its action depends on the receptors of the neuron it contacts. Any significant decrease or increase in the level of these neurotransmitters can result in basal ganglia (extrapyramidal) motor signs.

The basal ganglia system affects the contralateral side of the body. (A basal ganglia stroke affects the opposite side of the body.) Because this system maintains muscle tone and posture, movements are most noticeable during rest. For instance, Parkinson's disease, an extrapyramidal disorder,

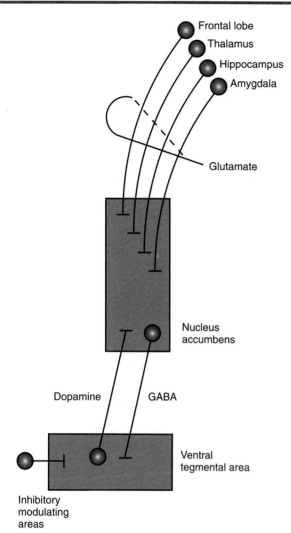

Frontal lobe
Thalamus
Hippocampus
Amygdala

Glutamate

Nucleus accumbens

Dopamine          GABA

Ventral tegmental area

Inhibitory modulating areas

**FIGURE 6-7** Mesolimbic pathway (system). This is identified as the primary pathway involved in substance abuse and in feeling pleasure. The ventral tegmental area (VTA) projects dopamine neurons to the nucleus accumbens. Opioids inhibit the modulating areas that affect the VTA and allow increased amounts of dopamine to be released into the nucleus accumbens, enhancing the reward aspects of the opioids. Glutamate neurons from the prefrontal cortex, thalamus, amygdala, and hippocampus project to the nucleus accumbens and are excitatory. A GABA pathway also exists from the nucleus accumbens to the VTA. The mesolimbic pathway includes many limbic structures. *GABA*, Gamma-aminobutyric acid.

manifests with a resting tremor. These unwanted movements diminish with concentration and intentional movement and are absent during sleep.

In summary, the pyramidal tract or corticospinal tract *controls* precise, voluntary movements; the basal ganglia, in conjunction with the cerebellum, *stabilize* motor movements. Lesions of the basal ganglia result in abnormal motor movements, such

as those present in Parkinson's disease, resulting from decreased dopamine bioavailability from the substantia nigra, and Huntington's disease (chorea), resulting from alterations in the GABA level and in the cholinergic system. All the basal ganglia areas receive, integrate, and transmit motor information.

| CRITICAL THINKING QUESTION | 1 |
|---|---|

1. What disease do you produce when you block the substantia nigra's dopamine from crossing the synapse at the next brain site (basal ganglia)?
2. What might happen to a person with an overproduction of cerebral dopamine?
3. How might a pituitary gland tumor affect a person's hormone production, body development, and behavior?
4. What signs or symptoms are used to differentiate a left- or right-sided cerebral hemisphere stroke?

## Diencephalon

The diencephalon (see Figures 6-2, 6-3, and 6-6) is made up of the thalamus, hypothalamus, epithalamus (including the pineal gland), and subthalamus. Although all the nuclei of the diencephalon are important, only a brief review of the thalamus and the hypothalamus is provided here in this text. The thalamus is the major sensory basal ganglia relay nuclear area to and from the cerebral cortex. All sensory pathways, except the olfactory pathways, synapse in the thalamus (Kiernan, 2005). Sensory fibers ascend to and synapse in the thalamus and are then relayed to the cerebral cortex via the internal capsule and corona radiata (see Figure 6-3). The hypothalamus maintains homeostasis and is the controller of the autonomic nervous system. The hypothalamus (Kiernan, 2005) is a tiny, 4-g structure positioned below the thalamus, which modulates visceral functions such as body temperature regulation, gastrointestinal activity, and cardiovascular functions. The hypothalamus also serves as a chemoreceptor by sampling cerebrospinal fluid and blood. It controls and influences functions such as food and water intake and endocrine secretion. The hypothalamus has two modes for affecting the pituitary gland (the following numbers refer to Figure 6-8). The first mode is through the production of releasing and inhibiting hormones

**Two hypothalamic neurons**

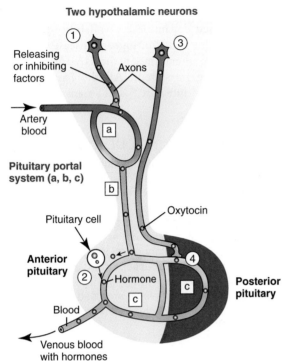

**FIGURE 6-8** Pituitary portal system (PPS). The PPS has a capillary bed *(a)* at the base of the hypothalamus, a capillary bed *(c)* in the pituitary gland, and a portal vein *(b)* in between. Hypothalamic neurons *(1, 3)* make hormones (i.e., neurotransmitters). Neuron *(1)* releases its hormone into capillary bed *(a)*, and the hormone descends through the portal vessel *(b)* into the pituitary gland capillary bed *(c)*. The hormone leaves the capillary bed and causes anterior pituitary gland cells to release specific hormones back into the capillary *(2)* for transport to glands or cells elsewhere in the body. A few hormones from the hypothalamus inhibit the production of pituitary gland cell hormones. Neuron *(3)* directly releases its hormone (e.g., oxytocin) into the posterior pituitary portion of the capillary bed *(c)*. The hormone again leaves in the blood *(4)* and travels to glands or cells elsewhere in the body.

or factors that pass into the pituitary portal system (PPS), such as thyrotropin-releasing hormone or prolactin-releasing factor (PRF) (1). These factors are transmitted to the anterior pituitary (2), where they cause the release or inhibition of anterior pituitary hormones into the blood of the PPS. The second mode is by the direct projection of hypothalamic neurons (3) into the posterior pituitary, where the neurons release their hormones (e.g., oxytocin) directly into the pituitary blood supply (4). Table 6-1 summarizes the hormonal cascade from the hypothalamus and some of the resulting clinical effects. As in the age-old question, "What came first, the chicken or the egg?" an increase or decrease in a specific hormone level during

mental illness fails to explain whether the changes are a cause or a result of the illness. Normally, all hormones are in careful balance.

## BRAINSTEM

The brainstem, cerebellum, and spinal cord are located beneath the cerebrum (see Figure 6-1). The brainstem is a collective term for the midbrain, pons, and medulla oblongata. The cerebellum is an expansive area attached to the posterior surface of the pons and resembles its Latin name, which means "little brain." The most caudal portion of the CNS is the spinal cord (not discussed in this chapter). The reticular formation is an important functional area that spans the brainstem.

### Midbrain

The midbrain (see Figure 6-6), which represents the continuation of the CNS below the cerebrum, is approximately 1.5 cm in length and is relatively narrow. The red nuclei and substantia nigra are large structures in the midbrain that can be easily distinguished on gross examination. The red nuclei in freshly cut brains are large, reddish, round balls; the substantia nigra, as its name implies, is black. This black coloration is the result of melanin pigment found in neurons in the substantia nigra. Most of the brain dopamine is synthesized from these dark cells. In Parkinson's disease, these cells are depigmented, and less dopamine is produced. Dopamine deficiency causes the extrapyramidal motor disorders associated with Parkinson's disease. The VTA, which projects dopaminergic tracts to the limbic and cortical areas, is a midline structure medial and rostral to the red nucleus.

### Pons

The *pons* (literally means bridge) forms a link between the midbrain and the medulla oblongata. The pons is a bulbous area approximately 2.5 cm in length that lies between the midbrain and the medulla oblongata and is anterior to the cerebellum. Some pathway fibers descending from the cerebrum pass through the midbrain and terminate in the pons. The pontine nuclei project motor and posture information to the cerebellum.

**Table 6-1   Hormonal Cascade From the Hypothalamus to Behavioral Effects***

| Hypothalamus-Made Hormones | Pituitary Gland | Target Gland or Hormone | Behavioral Effect |
|---|---|---|---|
| CRH | Stimulates production of two hormones:<br>1. ACTH<br>2. β-Endorphin | Adrenal gland—produces cortisol and cortisol-related hormones<br>ACTH drives cortisol production | 1. Stress causes the release of cortisol<br>2. Depressed children have decreased diurnal cortisol secretory pattern<br>3. Depressed adolescents have increased cortisol around sleep onset<br>4. CRH increases in patient with PTSD<br>5. Patients with PTSD have a blunted ACTH response to CRH<br>6. β-Endorphin is involved in the endorphin pleasure pathway and thus feeling good |
| TRH | Stimulates production of TSH | Thyroid gland produces thyroxine and $T_3$ | 1. Adding $T_3$ to an antidepressant regimen may potentiate medication's response<br>2. In PTSD, $T_3$ level is increased |
| GH-IH (somatostatin) | Inhibits GH | GH stimulates body growth | Depressed children have blunted GH response to some drugs |
| ADH (vasopressin) | Released in pituitary portal system in pituitary | ADH affects renal tubules in kidneys for water retention | 1. Involved in memory acquisition, storage, and retrieval<br>2. May be linked to polydipsic behavior in patients with schizophrenia |
| Oxytocin | Released in pituitary portal system in pituitary | Affects myoepithelial cells in mammary glands for milk release | Involved in memory consolidation and retrieval |
| PRF | Stimulates production of prolactin | Mammary glands—produce milk | No significant effects |
| LH-RH | Stimulates the production of two hormones:<br>1. LH<br>2. FSH | LH:<br>1. Stimulates corpus luteum (female) to produce progesterone<br>2. Stimulates interstitial cells (male) to produce testosterone<br>FSH:<br>1. Stimulates follicle (female) to produce estrogen<br>2. Stimulates seminiferous tubules (male) to facilitate testosterone production | No significant effects |

*This table lists the following: (1) hypothalamic hormones—states whether they are releasing or inhibiting; (2) the specific hormones that they affect in the anterior pituitary gland (Griffin and Ojeda, 2000); (3) the way in which they affect hormone production; (4) the target glands or body cells affected; and (5) the proposed effects of these hormones on behavior (Charney et al, 1999). Antidiuretic hormone and oxytocin are released directly into the blood; thus, they do not affect pituitary gland cells.

*ACTH,* Adrenocorticotropic hormone; *ADH,* antidiuretic hormone; *CRH,* corticotropin-releasing hormone; *FSH,* follicle-stimulating hormone; *GH,* growth hormone; *GH-IH,* growth hormone–inhibiting hormone (somatostatin); *LH,* luteinizing hormone; *LH-RH,* luteinizing hormone–releasing hormone; *PRF,* prolactin-releasing factor; *PTSD,* posttraumatic stress disorder; *TRH,* thyroid-releasing hormone; *TSH,* thyroid-stimulating hormone; $T_3$, triiodothyronine.

### Medulla Oblongata

The medulla oblongata is approximately 3 cm in length and narrows until it becomes continuous with the cervical spinal cord. Many cerebral cortex motor fibers that are in the midbrain and travel through the pons continue their descent on the anterior surface of the medulla oblongata; these fibers collectively form pyramid-shaped bulges known as the *pyramids*. The decussation of the pyramids—that is, the crossing over of the lateral corticospinal motor pathway contralaterally—takes place at the lower end of the medulla oblongata (see Figure 6-4). This crossing over is why a right brain stroke results in left-sided impairment. The medulla oblongata is responsible for many important functions, including respiration, regulation of blood pressure, partial regulation of heart rate, vomiting, and swallowing.

### Reticular Formation

A multineural functional area called the *reticular formation* resides within the brainstem. This area is composed of a series of large nuclei, beginning within the midbrain and extending through the pons and the medulla oblongata. The reticular formation can be thought of as a primitive brain buried deep within the brainstem. Input from most sensory pathways passes into the reticular formation, where it is integrated and then projected to areas such as the thalamus and hypothalamus. The reticular formation affects motor, sensory, and visceral functions.

The reticular activating system (RAS), part of the reticular formation, serves as a screening device that allows individuals to tune out some stimuli and attend to other stimuli. The ability to tune out is fortunate; otherwise, studying or even sleeping in some environments might be impossible. The RAS allows humans to fall asleep. It is activated by sensory stimuli, pain, movement, feedback from the cortex, muscle tone, and sympathomimetic drugs (stimulants). Any of these factors can help a person remain awake. Because of its many synapses, the RAS can be depressed easily. When a disruption occurs in the RAS and a person cannot sleep, psychosis can occur. When the RAS is turned off, however, coma results. Some people have had their RAS deactivated, but how to reactivate it is as yet unknown.

## CEREBELLUM

The cerebellum (see Figures 6-1 and 6-2) consists of two hemispheres separated by a central portion called the *vermis*. The cerebellar hemispheres and most of the vermis simultaneously receive sensory input from muscles and joints and motor signals from the cerebral cortex, indicating how muscles are to be directed. Most of the cerebellum then communicates with the cerebral cortex through the thalamus to coordinate the final motor activity. Writing with a pen, reading a book, shooting a basketball, and climbing a mountain are possible because of a functioning cerebellum. Most of the cerebellum coordinates muscle synergy and activity but does *not* initiate movement. The second function of the cerebellum is maintenance of equilibrium. Differences among movement disorders associated with cerebellar dysfunction and those associated with basal ganglia dysfunction are found in Box 6-1.

---

**Box 6-1    Differences Among Basal Ganglia and Cerebellar Movement Disorders**

**General Difference**
- Cerebellar dysfunction: Awkwardness of intentional movement
- Basal ganglia dysfunction: Meaningless, unintentional movement that occurs unexpectedly

***Cerebellar Disorders***
- Ataxia: Awkwardness of posture and gait; lack of coordination; overshooting the goal when reaching for an object; inability to perform rapid, alternating movements, such as finger tapping; awkward use of speech muscles, resulting in irregularly spaced sounds
- Decreased tendon reflexes on affected side
- Asthenia: Muscles tire easily
- Intention tremor: Noticed when intending to do something, such as reaching for a pencil
- Adiadochokinesia: Inability to perform fine, rapidly repeated coordinated movements

***Basal Ganglia Disorders***
- Parkinsonism: Rigidity, bradykinesia, resting tremor, masklike face, shuffling gait
- Chorea: Sudden, jerky, and purposeless movements (e.g., Huntington's disease, Sydenham's chorea)
- Athetosis: Slow, writhing, snakelike movements, especially of fingers and wrists
- Hemiballismus: A sudden, wild flailing of one arm

Modified from Goldberg S: *Clinical neuroanatomy*, Miami, 2003, MedMaster.

Cerebellar dysfunction can produce intention tremors on the same side of the body as the lesion. Dissimilar to basal ganglia resting tremors, which occur at rest, intention tremors occur when a person is asked to touch something, such as their own nose or a doctor's moving finger. Such individuals have tremors when they attempt to concentrate on moving a limb.

## NEURONS AND NEUROTRANSMITTERS

Neurons are the basic subunit of the nervous system. The brain contains *100 billion* neurons. The neuron is composed of a cell body with a large nucleus. The cell body and dendrites of the neuron make up the gray matter of the cortex and brain nuclei. Neurons transmit information by sending action potentials, or waves of electric depolarization, down their processes to other neurons. Two processes project from the cell body, *dendrites* and *axons*. The dendrites receive impulses from other neurons and transmit these impulses to the cell body. Axons carry impulses away from the cell body to another neuron, muscle, or gland. Each neuron usually projects only one axon. Some axons are up to 3 feet in length but are microscopically thin. Some axons can synapse with thousands of dendrites, and the dendrites of one neuron can receive impulses from the axons of thousands of other neurons (Bear et al, 2001). The brain is extremely complex, and information about this intricate wiring schematic continues to be the subject of research.

Neurons can be divided into three basic types: (1) sensory neurons (or afferent neurons), which send messages to the CNS, (2) motor neurons (or efferent neurons), which send messages from the CNS to the periphery, and (3) association neurons (or interneurons), which lie between sensory and motor neurons. The vast majority of CNS neurons are association neurons. Most impulses (action potentials) travel from one neuron to another by sending a chemical called a *neurotransmitter* across a 20-nm space (the synaptic cleft), which separates these cells, to evoke the next action potential. The junction between two neurons, including two cell membranes and a synaptic cleft, is called a *synapse*. Many drugs have their site of action in the nervous system in or around the synapse.

Neurotransmitters are divided into four major groups or systems—cholinergics, monoamines, neuropeptides, and amino acids. Table 6-2 summarizes these four major groups. Specific examples for each group, where these specific transmitters are concentrated in the brain, and major brain pathways that use these neurotransmitters are indicated in this table. Neurotransmitters are thought to play major roles in some mental disorders (Table 6-3).

## AUTONOMIC NERVOUS SYSTEM

The autonomic nervous system (Figure 6-9) is divided into the parasympathetic (craniosacral) and sympathetic (thoracolumbar) nervous systems. The parasympathetic nervous system, which is a cholinergic system, conserves energy and is divided into cranial and sacral portions. The cranial part has neuronal components in the oculomotor (cranial nerve [CN] III), facial (CN VII), glossopharyngeal (CN IX), and vagus (CN X) nerves; the sacral part is composed of neuronal elements located in the sacral spinal cord areas S2 through S4. Parasympathetic neurons are of particular interest to psychiatric nurses because of the many psychotropic drugs that have anticholinergic properties. Anticholinergic drugs block the function of these nerves; for example, CN III affects pupil and ciliary body constriction, CN VII affects tearing and salivation, CN IX affects salivation, and CN X affects the heart, gastrointestinal tract, and urinary system. Thus, anticholinergic effects on these nerves cause dilated pupils, decreased lacrimation, dry mouth, tachycardia, and slowing of the bowels and bladder.

The sympathetic nervous system expends energy and forms a continuous column that runs from the first thoracic (T1) to the third lumbar (L3) spinal cord areas. Although sympathetic neuron cell bodies are confined within portions of the thoracic and lumbar spinal cord, sympathetic neurons innervate effector organs throughout the body.

Both the sympathetic and the parasympathetic systems contain two neurons between the spinal cord and the effector organs. The first neuronal cell body is in the spinal cord, and its myelinated axon extends from the spinal cord to synapse with a peripheral neuron. The first neuron in the

| Table 6-2 | Classification of Neurotransmitters and Pathways* | | |

| Neurotransmitter | Chemical Transmitter | Location | Major Pathways |
| --- | --- | --- | --- |
| Cholinergics | Acetylcholine | Myoneural junctions, autonomic ganglia, parasympathetic postganglionic neurons | Basal nucleus of Meynert to cerebral cortex, septal area (rostral to hypothalamus) to hippocampus |
| Monoamines | Dopamine | Substantia nigra<br>Ventral tegmental area<br>Hypothalamus | Nigrostriatal tract<br>Mesolimbic tract<br>Mesocortical tract<br>Tuberoinfundibular tract |
| | Norepinephrine | Locus ceruleus | Locus ceruleus (in pons) to thalamus, cerebral cortex, cerebellum, and midbrain to spinal cord; lateral hypothalamus and basal forebrain |
| | Serotonin | Raphe nuclei | Central brainstem nuclei up to cerebral cortex and down to spinal cord |
| Neuropeptides | Enkephalins<br>Endorphins<br>Substance P | Spinal cord, hypothalamus, midbrain<br>Spinal cord, hypothalamus, midbrain<br>Spinal cord, hypothalamus, and many other places | |
| | Somatostatin, VIP, CCK, ACTH, neurotensin, angiotensin II, and others | | |
| Amino acids | GABA | Most common transmitter in brain | |
| | Glycine | Spinal cord, brainstem, and many other CNS areas | |
| | Glutamate | Widely distributed in the CNS | |
| | Aspartate | Hippocampus, dorsal root ganglion | |

*This table presents a simplified summary of many of the better known neurotransmitters and the general location where they are produced and released in the nervous system.
*ACTH*, Adrenocorticotropic hormone; *CCK*, cholecystokinin; *CNS*, central nervous system; *GABA*, gamma-aminobutyric acid; *VIP*, vasoactive intestinal polypeptide.
From Keltner NL, Folks DG: *Psychotropic drugs*, ed 3, St. Louis, 2005, Mosby.

| Table 6-3 | Neurotransmitters and Related Mental Disorders* |

| Neurotransmitter | Mental Disorder |
| --- | --- |
| Increase (↑) in dopamine | Schizophrenia |
| Decrease (↓) in norepinephrine | Depression |
| Decrease (↓) in serotonin | Depression |
| Decrease (↓) in acetylcholine | Alzheimer's disease |
| Decrease (↓) in GABA | Anxiety |

*This is a simplified explanation. A more detailed explanation is offered in appropriate chapters.
*GABA*, Gamma-aminobutyric acid.

system is referred to as the *preganglionic neuron;* the second is the *postganglionic neuron.* Preganglionic neurons secrete acetylcholine as their neurotransmitter (see Figure 6-9). Postganglionic neurons send their unmyelinated axons to their effector organs—smooth muscle, cardiac muscle, or glands. Generally, parasympathetic postganglionic neurons secrete acetylcholine and sympathetic postganglionic neurons secrete norepinephrine as their neurotransmitters.

The hypothalamus has both sympathetic and parasympathetic functions and is considered to be

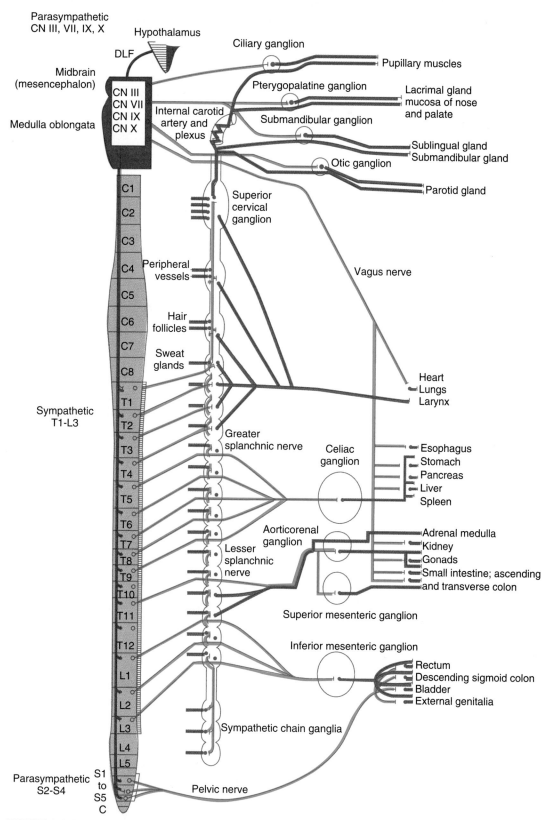

**FIGURE 6-9** Diagram of the entire autonomic nervous system. Preganglionic neurons are represented as green lines; the postganglionic neurons are represented as blue lines. The dorsal longitudinal fasciculus (DLF) (represented as a red line) interconnects the hypothalamus with parasympathetic and sympathetic autonomic neurons down to the sacral spinal cord level.

the highest autonomic center in the CNS. The hypothalamus can drive both systems selectively (see Figure 6-9).

## VENTRICULAR SYSTEM

The brain floats in approximately 140 ml (about the volume of a small cup of coffee) of cerebrospinal fluid (CSF); however, the CNS produces approximately 800 ml of fluid per day. CSF circulates around the brain in the subarachnoid space and inside ventricles in the brain. Three connective tissue layers, known as meninges, cover the brain. The subarachnoid space is a narrow space between the middle meningeal layer (arachnoid) and innermost layer (pia mater), which adheres to the brain. The thick outer layer, the dura mater, attaches to the inner surface of many bones of the skull. The ventricles form four spaces within the brain (see Figure 6-3). One large ventricle resides in each cerebral hemisphere, and small third and fourth ventricles are located, respectively, in the diencephalon and between the pons and the cerebellum. The fourth ventricle communicates with the subarachnoid space. Eventually, the CSF in the subarachnoid space enters the vascular system through arachnoid villi that protrude into the superior sagittal sinus on the superior surface of the brain. If the arachnoid villi are compromised for some reason, such as from a head trauma or meningitis, the CSF then builds up quickly.

Enlargement of the ventricles occurs because of (1) blockage of the CSF outflow within or from the brain, (2) overproduction of CSF, (3) brain atrophy resulting from the death of large numbers of cortical neurons, and (4) neurodevelopmental problems. The first two problems are causes of hydrocephalus, whereas brain atrophy (neurodegeneration) is commonly found in chronic alcoholics and patients with Alzheimer's disease. Neurodevelopmental problems resulting in ventricular variance are thought to be associated with schizophrenia (Charney et al, 1999). In the case of neurodegeneration, creation of new space results in the ventricles enlarging to fill the void.

## CLINICAL APPLICATION

As stressed throughout this text, many mental disorders have biologic bases. A brief overview of these biologic influences is presented here, but the major discussion of these issues is found in the chapter dealing with the respective disorder. This approach is in agreement with our belief that the biologic context of mental disorders is intricately linked to symptoms and behaviors and is part of a holistic approach to understanding psychiatric patients. Placing most of the specific discussion of the psychobiologic parameters of mental disorders in a separate chapter titled "Psychobiology" reinforces the perception that this etiologic view is only one of many from which the student can select. We believe differently. Thus, the student is urged to use this chapter to review brain anatomy and physiology and to apply this information to other chapters.

## SCHIZOPHRENIA

Several psychobiologic influences on schizophrenia have been proposed. First, researchers have noted that an increase in ventricular size is apparent in many people with schizophrenia (Charney et al, 1999). As mentioned, ventricles enlarge for one of four reasons. In schizophrenia, increased ventricle size is most likely related to neurodevelopmental factors; that is, the brain around the ventricles has failed to develop, and the ventricles have enlarged to fill the empty space. This phenomenon is referred to as an increase in *ventricular brain ratios* (VBRs). Furthermore, in many individuals with schizophrenia, a decrease in the gray matter of the cortex and in the major subcortical nuclei is evident.

Other biologic differences found in people with schizophrenia include a decrease in cerebral blood flow, particularly in the prefrontal areas of the cortex. The term used to describe this condition is *hypofrontality* (Charney et al, 1999). Imaging technology that tracks blood flow and glucose metabolism has substantiated this physiologic change. These brain changes result in a decline in frontal cognitive functions, such as organizing, planning, learning, problem solving, and critical thinking.

By far, the most celebrated and widely known biologic theory for schizophrenia is the dopamine hypothesis. According to this theory, schizophrenia is caused by alterations of dopamine levels in the brain. Chapter 28 provides an elaboration of this theory and of the biologically related genetic theory of schizophrenia. Antipsychotics are discussed in Chapter 18.

In some patients with schizophrenia, a decrease in blood flow has been detected in the dorsolateral prefrontal area. Because this site is in the frontal lobe, what type of symptoms might you expect to see in general?

## DEPRESSION

Mood disorders are also thought to have a biologic basis. Decreased amounts of norepinephrine and serotonin, two important brain neurotransmitters, are thought to play a role in depression (see Table 6-3). Apparently, an overall deficiency exists in the concentration of these neurotransmitters, and psychopharmacologic treatment is based on restoring them to optimal levels. More recent findings suggest that other neurotransmitters might also be factors in depression. For example, some researchers have found evidence for the involvement of acetylcholine, dopamine, and GABA.

Chapter 29 presents a discussion of these neurotransmitters, as well as the roles of receptor, thyroid, hypothalamic, and pituitary function in depression.

## ANXIETY DISORDERS

Anxiety disorders appear to have a biologic basis as well. Research has indicated that drugs that activate GABA receptors, causing an inhibitory effect, can calm anxious patients. Other neurotransmitters, such as norepinephrine, dopamine, and serotonin, might also have roles in anxiety. Certainly, stimulation of the sympathetic system, accomplished by epinephrine, norepinephrine, and dopamine (see Table 6-2), causes an anxiety-like reaction. Anxiety disorders are discussed in Chapter 31.

## DEMENTIAS

Dementias are directly related to brain pathology. Alzheimer's disease (AD), the leading cause of dementia in the United States, is caused by brain atrophy, which has been demonstrated microscopically as neurofibrillary tangles and amyloid plaques. Patients with AD tend to have enlarged ventricles, narrowing of the cortical ribbon (gray matter), widening of the sulci, and decreases in the width of the gyri. Furthermore, a loss of cho-

linergic pathways is found in patients with AD, contributing to memory problems. Patients affected with AD forget facts, how to use words, and how to use common objects. AD and other dementias are discussed in Chapter 32.

## DEGENERATIVE DISEASES

Parkinson's disease is an example of a degenerative disease that affects both motor function and emotional stability. In parkinsonism, microscopic examination of the basal ganglia, specifically the caudate nucleus and globus pallidus, reveals degenerative changes. The most significant change, however, is the deterioration of the substantia nigra, the primary site of synthesis of dopamine in the brain. The decreased availability of dopamine in the extrapyramidal system leads to tremor, bradykinesia, and rigidity. Parkinsonism is discussed in Chapters 17 and 32.

## DEMYELINATING DISEASES

Multiple sclerosis is an example of a demyelinating disease. In this disorder, both the myelin and eventually the axons break down (Brodal, 2004). This degeneration of myelin causes various problems, including loss of sensation, muscle weakness, fatigue, double vision, and tingling in the extremities. People with multiple sclerosis also experience psychological symptoms, undoubtedly related to demyelinization that occurs in the brain.

## ANOREXIA NERVOSA

Anorexia nervosa, a disorder characterized by the refusal to eat, appears to be associated with hypothalamic dysfunction. Anorexia nervosa is discussed in Chapter 37.

## TRAUMA

Individuals who have experienced CNS trauma can experience brain insults similar to those found in dementia or parkinsonism. Victims of automobile accidents or gunshot wounds, as well as boxers, can exhibit symptoms based on the nature of the injury. Individuals with an injury to the temporal lobe might experience memory loss or aphasia; those with a prefrontal lobe injury might experience personality changes or psychosis. Dementia pugilistica (punch-drunk syndrome, boxer's disease), a dementia syndrome with the same molecular pathology as that of AD, can result from repeated blows to the head—for example, in the sport of boxing (Kiernan, 2005).

## CHEMICAL DEPENDENCY

The biologic pathways that might be responsible for the control that addictive substances have on people are just beginning to be understood. Research studies have suggested that the nucleus accumbens might be an important part of the addiction puzzle. Charney and associates (1999) have presented a discussion of studies of mechanisms involved in motivation and addiction.

## MITOCHONDRIAL DEOXYRIBONUCLEIC ACID PROBLEMS

Most people are familiar with a large number of genetic diseases that affect the psychological health of individuals, such as Huntington's disease. Many other diseases have been found to have a genetic predisposition similar to that of AD. These problems arise in the deoxyribonucleic acid (DNA) of the chromosomes in each cell of our bodies. In 1988, scientists found that the DNA of mitochondria, the powerhouses of the human body, can mutate and give rise to physical and psychological problems (Wallace, 1997). These mutant mitochondria have been implicated in AD—*m*itochondrial *e*ncephalopathy, *l*actic *a*cidosis, and *s*trokelike episodes (MELAS)—and in diabetes mellitus, among others. Dissimilar to chromosomes, mitochondria are passed to the ovum only by the mother. Various mutant mitochondria can result in a number of diseases. The mechanism involved is that the mutant mitochondria, which fail to produce the energy that cells need to function properly, increase in number over time and damage particular cells and body organs.

---

### CRITICAL THINKING QUESTION    3

From what you have read in this chapter, can you defend Kraepelin's view of schizophrenia as a dementia? Explain.

---

## EARLY LIFE STRESS AND TRAUMA

Another psychobiologic issue worth contemplating is the effects attributed to early life trauma or significant stress that have become increasingly recognized. As noted, the brain continues to develop after birth; hence, the brain becomes larger, more sophisticated, and more efficient. One aspect of that continued development is ongoing myelination. As individuals age, myelin thickens around axons, improving the precision and efficacy of connections among neurons. Myelination continues throughout the teenage years (Herrman, 2005), while at the same time pruning eliminates about 40% of synapses (Miller, 2005a). This suggests that, even at this late age, parents and others should be aware of the possibilities, good and bad, of dynamic brain processes. Some of the very last connections are those that help individuals use good judgment, solve problems, and develop self-regulation (Miller, 2005a). Prolonged stress or significant trauma can compromise these processes.

At an even earlier age, stress and trauma increase cortisol levels. Excessive cortisol levels can cause atrophy of the hippocampus, impairing such hippocampal activities as memory and learning. Animal models consistently demonstrate that maternal deprivation and/or rejection cause profound behavioral changes in the animal's later life. Animals nurtured in good environments have lifelong advantages over deprived animals. Furthermore, early life stressors, if sustained or overwhelming, can lead to an increase in hypothalamic-pituitary-adrenal (HPA) activity. Increased hypothalamic release of corticotropin-releasing factor causes increased release of adrenocorticotropic hormone from the anterior pituitary and results in a subsequent elevation of systemic cortisol. An elevated cortisol level is associated with increased heart rate, muscle tension, anger, anxiety, fear, and depression (Miller, 2005b). When adulthood is reached, this person is left with a hypersensitive HPA system that overreacts to stress and often leads to a life of depression and anxiety. To summarize, stress, maternal behavior, and maltreatment during childhood and adolescence are mental health issues because they have the potential to alter the structure and chemistry of the brain.

## ◾ Study Notes

1. The brain is a complex organ composed of 100 billion neurons, and changes in its anatomy or physiology affect behavior. Holistic nursing

## Highlighting the Evidence

**Are the Brains of Men and Women the Same?**

Men and women possess differences in their brains in terms of the relative size of their anatomic structures, levels of neurotransmitters and hormones, and how various neural structures function. For example, a few structural differences are that men have some larger areas in the parietal lobes, which are involved in spatial perception, whereas women have some larger areas in the frontal lobes and limbic areas, which are concerned with higher cognitive functions. The hippocampus, a structure involved with memory, is larger in women than in men. The neurotransmitter serotonin, a major chemical involved in setting moods, is 52% higher in men than in women. Could this be why women have a higher incidence of depression? The last point is an example of differences in brain function. In a positron emission tomography (PET) study on recall of disturbing films, subjects demonstrated that the right amygdala in men and the left amygdala in women were selectively activated 1 week after testing. These findings indicate that a patient's gender can be a factor in treatment for such problems as addiction, schizophrenia, depression, and posttraumatic stress disorder (Cahill, 2005).

---

care requires an understanding of the impact of brain dysfunction on behavior.

2. Many mental disorders that were formerly thought to have psychological etiologic factors are now known to be influenced by brain dysfunction.

3. The nervous system is divided into the CNS and the PNS.

4. The CNS is divided into the brain and the spinal cord.

5. The nervous pathways in the brain are composed of myelinated axons (white matter) that connect and communicate among brain nuclei (gray matter).

6. The cerebral cortex is the outer layer of gray matter of the brain. The gray matter consists of neuronal cell bodies and is responsible for the work of the brain.

7. The two major neurotransmitters in the extrapyramidal system are dopamine (inhibitory and excitatory) and acetylcholine (excitatory).

8. The pyramidal motor system controls precise movement; the basal ganglia motor system stabilizes motor movement.

9. The RAS involves degrees of consciousness. Sensory stimuli received in this system are forwarded to the thalamus. As stimulation of the RAS increases, the level of alertness increases.

10. Neurons are the basic subunits of the nervous system. The neuron consists of a cell body, *dendrites* that send information to the cell body, and a process called an *axon,* which transmits impulses away from the cell body.

11. Impulses travel from one neuron to another by sending a chemical called a *neurotransmitter* across a microscopic gap, known as a *synaptic cleft.*

12. The dopamine hypothesis postulates that schizophrenia results from increased levels of brain dopamine. Treatment is aimed at reducing those levels through the use of antipsychotic drugs. This broad view of causation is refined in Chapter 28.

13. The neurotransmitter theory of depression states that depression is related to decreased levels of norepinephrine, serotonin, or both. This broad view of causation is refined in Chapter 29.

14. Anxiety disorders might be related to alterations in GABA levels.

15. Dementias, specifically AD, are related to brain atrophy and are characterized by microscopic changes in the cortical neurons, neurofibrillary tangles, and amyloid plaques. A deficiency in the neurotransmitter acetylcholine also occurs.

## ■ References

Bear MF, Connors BW, Paradiso MA: *Neuroscience: exploring the brain,* ed 2, Philadelphia, 2001, Lippincott Williams & Wilkins.

Boss BJ, Stowe AC: Neuroanatomy, *J Neurosci Nurs* 18:214, 1986.

Brodal P: *The central nervous system,* ed 3, New York, 2004, Oxford University Press.

Cahill L: His brain, her brain, *Sci Am* 292:5, 2005.

Charney DS, Nestler EJ, Bunney BS: *Neurobiology of mental illness,* New York, 1999, Oxford University Press.

Griffin JE, Ojeda SR: *Textbook of endocrine physiology,* ed 4, New York, 2000, Oxford University Press.

Heath RG: Pleasure and brain activity in man, *J Nerv Ment Dis* 154:3, 1972.

Hermann JW: The teen brain as a work in progress: implications for pediatric nurses, *Pediatr Nurs* 31:144, 2005.

Kandel ER, Schwartz JH, Jessell TM: *Principles of neural science,* ed 4, New York, 2000, Elsevier.

Keltner NL, Folks DG: *Psychotropic drugs,* ed 4, St. Louis, 2005, Mosby.

Kiernan JA: *Barr's: the human nervous system: an anatomical viewpoint,* ed 8, Philadelphia, 2005, Lippincott.

Miller CM: The adolescent brain: beyond raging hormones, *Harv Ment Health Lett* 22:1, 2005a.

Miller CM: The biology of child maltreatment, *Harv Ment Health Lett* 21:12, 2005b.

Sugerman RA, Edmundson MJ, Robinson S: *Human anatomy,* Edina, MN, 1979, Burgess.

Wallace DC: Mitochondrial DNA in aging and disease, *Sci Am* 277(2):40, 1997.

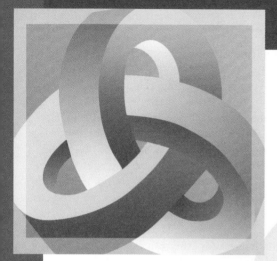

# Chapter 7

# Nurse-Patient Communication

*Lee H. Schwecke*

## Learning Objectives

*After reading this chapter, you should be able to:*
- Understand major influences on communication.
- Distinguish between social and therapeutic communication.
- Identify goals of therapeutic communication.
- Discuss critical therapeutic communication issues.
- Describe various techniques that facilitate patient-centered communication.
- State common causes of interference with therapeutic communication.

**M**ost communication is a two-way process between two or more individuals. In nursing, this process is focused on patients' needs and problems. Professional or therapeutic communication is one of the means whereby the nursing process is implemented to achieve quality patient care. In psychiatric nursing, therapeutic communication is one of the most important tools that nurses can use for building trust, developing therapeutic relationships, providing support and comfort, encouraging growth and change, and implementing patient education.

Nurses rely on verbal, written, telephone, and electronic (computer) communication for sharing information, analyzing data, collaborating with other disciplines, and delivering services. Consequently, nursing requires a solid foundation in effective communication concepts and skills. For nurses who work with psychiatric patients (patients with alterations in thinking, feelings, and behavior), the challenge of communicating is even greater. The goal is not only to understand patients and ensure that they understand the nurse, but also to teach patients more effective communication skills for interaction with those in mainstream society.

## CATEGORIES OF COMMUNICATION

Communication is an interaction between two or more people that involves the exchange of information between a sender and a receiver. The product of communication is the message, which is to be interpreted by the receiver. Words (verbal or written) and behaviors (nonverbal) are the primary channels for communication.

### WRITTEN COMMUNICATION

Because written material is a primary means of acquiring and sharing information, all professions require some form of written reports, instructions, or sharing of findings and ideas. The skill of mastering vocabulary, grammar, and organization of ideas is critical.

**Norm's Notes**

*How important is clear communication? Well, go visit a divorce court or human relations department hearing, or be involved in a malpractice lawsuit ("Hey doc, was that clonidine or Clonopin?"). In many of these cases, poor or lousy communication can be identified. Poor communication is a major enemy of human happiness and well-being. Now, when you add a person with a mental disorder or an emotional problem to the equation of human interaction, even more "stuff" can be misconstrued or damaging. Take a good look. You can't go wrong if you thoroughly understand this material.*

## TELEPHONE COMMUNICATION

Telephones have provided patients access to crisis and suicide services (hot lines) for many years. Community mental health centers also might provide their patients with phone numbers so they can call in between visits to the center or for information or emergencies. Dealing with patients' perceived or real emergencies by telephone often prevents an inpatient admission. A variation of the concept is the use of the telephone for case management for high-risk patients to facilitate discharge planning and increase adherence to follow-up appointments and treatment, thus reducing recidivism (Taylor et al, 2004).

## ELECTRONIC COMMUNICATION

Electronic communication requires special attention. Unfortunately, the ability to send an e-mail quickly can lead to less careful attention to the tone of the message and provides an easy way to avoid sensitive issues that are best handled face to face (Simpson, 1999). In contrast, a study by Leong and associates (2005) found that patient satisfaction with services increased significantly when patients were able to contact their physicians by e-mail. The physicians were not equally satisfied; security and privacy concerns, legal and ethical issues, guidelines and standards, and managing the volume of e-mail were some of the problems identified. Long distance therapy has been implemented for patients who do not live near a therapist's office. Patients visit a satellite clinic and interact with the therapist via computer video contact (Miller, 2005). This does provide an improvement over phone therapy, because nonverbal behaviors can be seen.

Eventually, all patient records will be in electronic form, necessitating care in *not* reducing patient data to "checks in a box" (White, 2005). Check marks do not convey the perceptions, emotional distress, fears, and individual needs of patients. Extra precautions are required to preserve privacy and confidentiality. Internet access to consumer health information presents new challenges for the nurse's role as patient educator. Nurses serve as patient advocates to offer help in accessing and interpreting health information and determining its accuracy (Grace, 2004).

## SPEECH AND BEHAVIOR

In addition to sound, oral communication includes the mannerisms and emotional tone that modify the message. The timbre and tone of the voice have meaning. The rate and emphasis of speech affect the message. Body language can enhance or change the meaning of words. Verbal and nonverbal communication must match. Behaviors can negate a verbal message; for example, a patient is not likely to (nor should) believe a nurse who says "Yes, I will help you" with a frown and an angry tone of voice.

## DYNAMICS OF THERAPEUTIC COMMUNICATION

Therapeutic communication requires attention to multiple, interacting factors. At the core of therapeutic communication are the words and nonverbal behaviors that relate to patients' health needs and are exchanged between patients and the nurse. Figure 7-1 illustrates key variables in communication for the patient and the nurse. Viewing the patient and the nurse as a whole that operates within an environmental context is important. Communication is influenced by the following: (1) an individual's personal experiences, gender, culture, values, and beliefs; (2) the purpose of the interaction; and (3) the physical and emotional context of the interaction. The nurse must communicate on patients' levels (according to their vocabulary, educational backgrounds, and the effects of their illnesses) without using a patron-

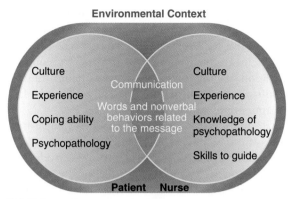

**FIGURE 7-1** Essential and influencing variables of the therapeutic communication environment.

izing, condescending, or stigmatizing manner. Prejudice, stereotyping, and discrimination have no place in quality patient care (White, 2004).

"Elderspeak" is a style of discrimination used with elderly patients based on stereotyping older adults as less competent. It usually involves changes in the rate, tone, and volume of speech and a simpler vocabulary and grammar, which are perceived as demeaning or like baby talk (Talerico, 2005).

## Interpretation of Communication

Interpretation of a message is filtered through an individual's knowledge, experience, and biases. Some aspects of communication are more commonly understood than others. Words are generally understood more precisely than behaviors. Anyone who has studied a foreign language, however, appreciates that nuances are often lost in translation because of the limitations of words. Both the nurse and the patient bring their own experiences to the relationship, which are different lenses through which each views an event. Having a broad knowledge of the effects of cultures is important if the nurse is to interpret accurately and respond appropriately to patient communications. (See Chapter 14 for a discussion of cultural competence in psychiatric nursing.)

## Themes in Patient Communications

Patient communications often convey indirect messages or underlying themes about content, mood, or interaction issues. Themes are reflected in patients' thoughts, which engender feelings and then produce behaviors. *Content themes* go beyond the words that a patient is saying and examine underlying messages about patients' perceptions of themselves and their problems over time. Their messages might relate to beliefs and values, self-concept and self-esteem, a sense of helplessness and hopelessness, suspiciousness, risk for suicide, and disturbances in thinking or processing of information and beliefs. *Mood themes* relate to affect and the feelings conveyed while patients discuss their issues and concerns. Feelings often reflect shame, guilt, anger, sadness, and fear, which might or might not match the content theme. Affect can be flat, blunted, euphoric, labile, or incongruent. Assessing for *interaction themes* involves examining the ways in which patients relate to family, friends, other patients, and staff. A patient might call the crisis center each time her roommate is out of town to complain about nervousness and loneliness. When her roommate returns, the patient is once again comfortable. The interaction theme might be assessed as one of dependency. The patient who plays one staff member against another and seeks attention by complaining about all the other patients might be showing an interaction theme of manipulation.

In another example, a patient might spend 30 minutes describing his divorce of 3 years ago, two other broken relationships since then, having been laid off from his job, having to sell his house, and feeling as though he is a failure. The underlying *content theme* might be interpreted as a series of major losses. As he describes all these losses, he might convey anger, guilt, or both. These *mood themes* would be congruent with the content theme. Feelings do not always match the content theme. If the patient were laughing as he described his losses, then his happiness would be considered as an *incongruent mood theme*. The *interaction theme* might be abandonment or social isolation.

Themes are frequently the source of nursing diagnoses on which care plans are based, such as hopelessness, powerlessness, chronic low self-esteem, risk for suicide, denial, anxiety, fear, interrupted family processes, risk for loneliness, noncompliance, or impaired social interaction.

## Environmental Considerations

The environment can facilitate or impede therapeutic communication. Factors such as noise level, privacy, type of furniture, space, and temperature can affect the quality of communication.

Proxemics refers to the way in which people perceive and use environmental, social, and personal space during interactions. Typically, boundaries of personal space for public and social communication are more distant compared with those for intimate or therapeutic communication. However, illness and emotional factors such as suspiciousness, anxiety, perceptual distortions, aggressiveness, the genders of the two parties, and personal comfort also influence the amount of space needed between the patient and the nurse. Patients are generally more comfortable when the nurse is at their eye level rather than standing over them. Some patients might require sitting at an angle to the nurse or might need a table or empty chair between themselves and the nurse to feel safe enough to talk.

## Physical Considerations

Patients with certain physical problems might experience communication difficulties. Patients with certain sensory limitations, such as hearing loss, might have compromised communication necessitating compensatory measures such as slow, face-to-face speech for lip reading. Developmental disabilities might seriously limit the ability of patients to comprehend and remember. Simple sentences with a single main idea might have to be repeated several times. Speech impediments or other problems might interfere with understanding patients' messages. Asking for repetition, clarification, and validation is important, but this can increase a patient's frustration when the practice becomes excessive. Having patients write their answers is an alternative when they are able to read and write. Physical pain often interferes with patients' abilities to think clearly and concentrate and might affect the sense of priority regarding problems to be addressed. Physical deformities and injuries, particularly facial ones, might inhibit the ability to talk and interfere with the nurse's ability to concentrate on other problems.

## Kinesics Considerations

Kinesics is the study of body movements. Culturally based body language indicates an individual's feelings. Avoiding prolonged eye contact is often used to disengage or ignore communication. Crossing the arms over the chest often occurs when a person feels defensive (however, this also might occur when a person is cold). The nurse must be sensitive to these cues and interpret them in a global context of therapeutic communication. If the message appears inconsistent or confusing, exploring the meaning of body language might then be useful. For example, the nurse might say, "Many times, when people back away from someone, it is because they are afraid. What are you afraid of right now?" Body language might communicate feelings or merely reflect a habit. Behaviors in the nurse that communicate caring, confidence, and calmness should be cultivated.

### CRITICAL THINKING QUESTION    1
Ann Williams has multiple facial injuries, with both eyes patched, is breathing with a ventilator, and has been sedated. In what ways would you modify your techniques to facilitate communication with her?

## THERAPEUTIC COMMUNICATION

## THERAPEUTIC VERSUS SOCIAL COMMUNICATION

The focus of therapeutic communication is on helping patients. Social communication involves equal disclosure of personal information and intimacy, and both parties enjoy equal opportunities for spontaneity, with the expectation of mutual confidentiality. Therapeutic communication focuses on the patient but is planned and directed by the professional. During social exchanges, both participants seek to have personal needs met, whereas the needs of the patient are the focus of therapeutic communication. Therapeutic communication relies on patients' disclosures of personal and occasionally painful feelings with the professional at a calculated emotional distance, near enough to be involved but objective enough to be helpful. In therapeutic communication, although confidentiality must be respected outside the treatment setting, a professional is obligated to share information with the treatment team. The nurse is a patient's advocate, not a patient's friend, so the nurse is not able to keep secrets for the patient (Grace, 2004).

# THERAPEUTIC USE OF SELF

In psychiatric nursing, the nurse, using verbal and nonverbal communication, is the primary therapeutic agent with psychiatric patients (as compared with treatment procedures and physical interventions used by a medical-surgical nurse). The nurse's communication is a major vehicle that helps patients achieve productive thinking, emotional, and behavioral outcomes. Use of self, medications, and the environment are the major components of psychotherapeutic management (see Chapter 2).

Using silence and therapeutic listening are important components of the therapeutic use of self with patients; these are crucial for getting to know patients as individuals, as well as their needs and concerns. Therapeutic listening has been described as being composed of the following attributes (Kemper, 1992):

- Being actively alert
- "Hearing" with all the senses
- Using eye contact
- Exhibiting an attending posture
- Ensuring concentration
- Being patient
- Displaying an openness to receive information
- Offering empathy and support
- Asking questions
- Assimilating verbal and nonverbal information
- Organizing, synthesizing, and interpreting information
- Validating and clarifying information
- Responding verbally and nonverbally to encourage patients to continue
- Summarizing important points
- Giving feedback appropriately

## CRITICAL THINKING QUESTION    2

Select three or four of the previous behaviors and communicate with a friend. What difference do you see in the way in which your friend responds?

Therapeutic use of the self requires the sensitivity to recognize important cues and make decisions about the priority of these cues. Objectivity is the process of remaining open to as many aspects of patients, their problems, and potential solutions as possible. Objectivity requires self-awareness by nurses to decrease their self-consciousness, blaming themselves (Horton-Deutsch and Horton, 2003), and blind spots. Nurses must not allow their own issues and biases to influence their interactions with patients and should avoid being swept away by patients' emotions and perceptions.

Communicating empathy is an essential skill of the nurse. Empathy is the ability to recognize and understand the patient's feelings and point of view objectively. Empathy, expressed verbally and nonverbally, conveys caring, compassion, and concern for patients but never implies that the nurse can fully experience patients' feelings. Empathy helps patients be more accepting of their feelings and express them more readily.

Being therapeutic includes being genuine and sincere, as conveyed by congruent verbal and nonverbal behaviors, authenticity, and honesty (without total self-disclosure by the nurse). Patients must feel respected, valued, and accepted by the nurse, even when all their behaviors are not tolerated. The nurse should not evaluate patients' thoughts, feelings, and behaviors as right or wrong; rather, the nurse helps patients evaluate the effects or consequences of these factors. However, the nurse must also set limits on destructive behaviors to protect the integrity and dignity of patients, as well as the safety and rights of others.

Touching is a complex issue. The meaning of touch varies widely among cultures, individuals, and patients with different diagnoses. Touching a patient's hand or shoulder or giving a light hug can convey caring, empathy, support, and acceptance. On the other hand, touching can be misinterpreted as a violation of personal space or privacy, or as a sexual gesture or aggressive move. Therefore, the use of touch with patients must be approached with caution. Patients' behaviors can provide clues to their ability to tolerate and benefit from touch. For example, a patient who is unable to sit close to the nurse is less likely to want to be touched. A patient who is quite trusting of the nurse is more likely to accept being touched. A patient who is sexually preoccupied might misinterpret any type of touch. With many patients (particularly those who have been sexually or physically abused), asking permission before giving a gentle hug is appropriate: "What do you think about getting a hug from me?"

## TECHNIQUES

Therapeutic techniques are a means of helping patients toward productive goals but are not goals in themselves. The communication techniques presented in Table 7-1 are arranged in a way that facilitates patients' learning, problem solving, and change. Interactions with patients do not involve using all these techniques sequentially. Many nurse-patient interactions do not use a complete nursing process in a single session, but they always involve using therapeutic techniques. Occasionally, interactions have primarily a social or recreational focus rather than being a problem-solving process, but these might still be beneficial to the patient. Every encounter with a patient can be therapeutic with or without full use of the nursing process (see Chapters 8 and 9).

## INTERFERENCE WITH THERAPEUTIC COMMUNICATION

In the same manner that therapeutic communication guides the patient toward goals, certain messages and behaviors interfere with reaching these goals. Some behaviors occur frequently because of nervous mannerisms or result from social expectations in the therapeutic situation. The nurse must recognize and overcome any habitual communication problems that might interfere with effective therapeutic communication.

### NURSE'S FEARS AND FEELINGS

Because therapeutic communication involves the use of self, many personal feelings are naturally evoked and can be disturbing. A nurse might easily develop a feeling of fear when communicating with individuals who are experiencing severe psychic or physical distress. Fear compromises therapeutic communication. The nurse might have concerns such as, "Could this be me someday?" or "My brother does this sometimes; does that mean he's crazy?" or "What if this patient gets angry with me?" Therapeutic communication relies on coming to terms with these types of issues. Individuals become patients because of serious and ongoing difficulties in functioning, not because of an occasional dysfunctional behavior. The nurse should avoid personalizing what patients say and do. Patients who abruptly end a

conversation with a nurse are probably responding to their own thoughts or anxieties rather than to something the nurse said. Nurses can benefit not only from analyzing the technique and content of interactions with patients, but also from analyzing their own feelings and reactions. (See Chapter 11 for further discussion of self-awareness.)

Occasionally, a nurse is afraid of harming patients by saying the wrong thing. Patients do not fall apart or act out because of a nurse's single mistake, particularly when the nurse's overall attitude is positive and helpful; however, patients are sensitive to malicious intent and rejection. A mistake can actually become a therapeutic encounter, because the nurse can represent a role model for the proper way to admit and apologize for an error. Many people, including psychiatric patients, have trouble recognizing and correcting mistakes with those who are significant to them. In many situations, a sincere apology, when warranted, can strengthen the relationship.

Another concern is invasion of privacy. Psychiatric nurses investigate personal areas of patients' lives intensely, such as values, beliefs, feelings, intimate relationships, and sexuality, or legally sensitive areas, such as incest, partner abuse, and drug use. Although patients must address these issues, they are not easy to discuss. The nurse can enhance patients' abilities to be open and honest by explaining the need to know about a sensitive area, by asking questions in a kind and matter-of-fact manner, by conveying empathy, and by reiterating a desire to help.

### NURSE'S LACK OF KNOWLEDGE AND INSECURITY

A lack of knowledge about psychiatric illnesses, defense mechanisms, medication responses, and the dynamics of behaviors and relationships on the nurse's part causes insecurity and diminishes patients' confidence in the nurse. Patients are usually more accepting, however, when the nurse is honest about not knowing an answer and expresses a willingness to find the answer, "I don't know, but I'll find out."

In an attempt to achieve a sense of security, the nurse might assume a parental type of role toward the patient that can be nontherapeutic for the patient. Parental responses also can maintain illness behaviors and are disconfirming, artificially nurturing, critical, or condescending; for example,

## Table 7-1   Therapeutic Techniques in Psychiatric Nursing

### Techniques Fostering Description

*Offering self:* Making self available and showing interest and concern

"I'll sit with you for a while."
"I'll stay with you."

*Active listening:* Paying close attention to verbal and nonverbal communications, patterns of thinking, feelings, and behaviors

Face the patient; maintain eye contact; be open, alert, and patient; respond appropriately.

*Silence:* Planned absence of verbal remarks to allow patients to think and say more

Maintain eye contact; convey interest and concern in facial expressions.

*Empathy:* Recognizing and acknowledging patients' feelings

"I can hear how painful it is for you to talk about this."

*Questioning:* Using open-ended questions to achieve relevance and depth in discussion (not closed/yes-no questions)

"Who?"
"What?"
"Where?"
"What did you say?"
"What happened?"
"Tell me about it."

*General leads:* Using neutral expressions to encourage patients to continue talking

"Go on, I'm listening."
"I hear what you are saying."

*Restating:* Repeating the exact words of patients to remind them of what they said, to let them know that they are heard

"You say you are going home soon."
"Your mother wasn't happy to see you?"

*Verbalizing the implied:* Rephrasing patients' words to highlight an underlying message

*Patient:* "There is nothing to do at home."
*Nurse:* "It sounds as if you might be bored at home."

*Clarification:* Asking patients to restate, elaborate, or give examples of ideas or feelings

"What do you mean by 'feeling sick inside'?"
"Give me an example of feeling 'lost.'"

### Techniques Fostering Analysis and Conclusions

*Making observations:* Commenting on what is seen or heard to encourage discussion

"You seem restless."
"I noticed you had trouble making a decision about . . ."

*Presenting reality:* Offering a view of what is real and what is not without arguing with the patient

"I know the voices are real to you, but I don't hear them."
"I don't see it the same way."

*Encouraging description of perceptions:* Asking for patients' views of their situations

"What do you think is happening to you right now?"
"What do you think is the issue with your wife?"

*Voicing doubt:* Expressing uncertainty about the reality of patients' perceptions and conclusions

"Is that the only way to interpret it?"
"What other conclusion could there be?"

*Placing an event in time or sequence:* Asking for relationships among events

"When did you do this?"
"Then what happened?"
"What led up to . . .?"
"What is the connection between . . .?"

*Encouraging comparisons:* Asking for similarities and differences among feelings, behaviors, and events

"How does this compare with the last time?"
"What is different about your feelings today?"

*Identifying themes:* Asking patients to identify recurrent patterns in thoughts, feelings, and behaviors

"What do you do each time you argue with your wife?"
"What feeling do you get when you see your father?"

*Summarizing:* Reviewing main points and conclusions

"Let's see, so far you have said . . ."

### Techniques Fostering Interpretation of Meaning and Importance

*Focusing:* Pursuing a topic until its meaning or importance is clear

"Explain more about . . ."
"What bothers you about . . .?"
"What happens when you feel this way?"

*Interpreting:* Providing a view of the meaning or importance of something

"It sounds as if this is very important to you."
"You seem to get in trouble when you . . ."

*Encouraging evaluation:* Asking for patients' views of the meaning or importance of something

"So what does all this mean to you?"
"How serious is this for you?"
"How important is it to change this behavior?"

*Continued*

| Table 7-1 | Therapeutic Techniques in Psychiatric Nursing—cont'd |
|---|---|

**Techniques Fostering Problem Solving and Decisions**

| | |
|---|---|
| *Suggesting collaboration:* Offering to help patients solve problems | "I can help you understand this better." "Let's see if we can find an answer." |
| *Encouraging goal setting:* Asking patients to decide on the type of change needed | "What do you think needs to change?" "What do you want to do differently?" |
| *Giving information:* Providing information that will help patients make better choices | "I can tell you about your medicines." "There are self-help groups available." |
| *Encouraging consideration of options:* Asking patients to consider the pros and cons of possible options | "What would be the advantage of trying . . .?" "What might happen if you tried . . .?" |
| *Encouraging decisions:* Asking patients to make a choice among options | "Which is the best alternative for you?" "What would work best?" |
| *Encouraging the formulation of a plan:* Probing for step by step actions that will be needed | "What exactly will it take to carry out your plan?" "What else do you need to do?" |

**Techniques Fostering the Completion of Plans**

| | |
|---|---|
| *Testing out new behaviors and evaluating outcomes:* | |
| *Rehearsing:* Requesting a verbal description of what will be said or done | "Tell me exactly what you will say to your wife on Friday." |
| *Role playing:* Practicing behaviors; the nurse plays a particular role | "I'll play your wife. What do you want to say to me?" |
| *Supportive confrontation:* Acknowledging the difficulty in changing, but pushing for action | "I know this isn't easy to do, but I think you can do it." "It's hard but give it a try." |
| *Limit setting:* Discouraging nonproductive feelings and behaviors, and encouraging productive ones | "You're slipping into your aggressive tone again. Try it again . . ." "That is a negative comment about yourself. Tell me something positive about yourself." |
| *Feedback:* Pointing out specific behaviors and giving impressions of reactions | "I thought you conveyed anger when you said . . ." "When you said . . . I felt . . ." |
| *Encouraging evaluation:* Asking patients to evaluate their actions and the outcomes | "How well did it work when you tried . . .?" "What was your husband's reaction?" |
| *Reinforcement:* Giving feedback on positive behaviors | "This new approach worked for you. Keep it up." |
| *Repeating steps of the nursing process if needed:* Using the steps of the nursing process to get a description of what happened, the degree of success, and ideas for change | "What would help you do even better next time?" "If things didn't go well, what do you want to do differently this time?" |

"Now honey, you know that you shouldn't do that."

## INEFFECTIVE RESPONSES

Learning and consistently using effective communication techniques take practice. This is especially true when trying to decrease the number of yes–no questions (closed questions) asked of patients. Yes-no answers provide little new information and necessitate asking more questions. The nurse's response to messages should be based on assessment and knowledge of the situation, as well as the dynamics of patients' illnesses and problems.

However, beginning nurses might not always interact as effectively as desired. A nurse might become defensive and withdraw from patients who are cursing angrily, rather than discussing the behavior. A patient might pick up on a nurse's anxiety and say, "Are you scared of crazies?" There is a tendency to deny this instead of being more truthful and saying, "I am afraid of saying something that might upset you."

Nurses might get caught up in the unfounded fears and accusations of paranoid patients and inadvertently reinforce the symptoms. Distinguishing between fact and distortion in what patients say is often difficult; thus, the nurse must avoid premature conclusions. For example, staff members did not believe a patient who said he had written the theme song for a popular play. The patient finally brought in his original hand-

## Box 7-1   Ineffective or Inappropriate Responses and Behaviors

Not fully listening, not paying attention
Looking too busy, ignoring the patient
Seeming uncomfortable with silence, fidgeting
Being opinionated, arguing with the patient
Avoiding sensitive topics, changing the topic
Being superficial or using clichés
Having a closed posture, avoiding eye contact with patient
Making false promises or reassurances
Giving advice or talking too much
Laughing or smiling inappropriately
Showing disapproval or being judgmental
Belittling feelings or minimizing problems
Being defensive or avoiding the patient
Making flippant or sarcastic remarks
Lying or being insincere

written sheet music and the list of credits from the play's manuscript for the staff to see. Obtaining information from family members to validate information or waiting until medications help clear delusional thinking is occasionally helpful.

Nurses might be preoccupied with what they want to say next rather than with listening to patients or they might be listening to, but not really hearing or understanding, what the patient is really saying. Nodding one's head as a patient talks might convey, "I hear you" or "I agree with you"—an important difference.

Overuse of one or two therapeutic skills, such as reflecting or restating, can stagnate communications when no movement toward analyzing and problem solving is evident. Giving advice to patients rather than helping them evaluate and choose their own solutions can also impede problem solving. False reassurances, such as, "Everything will be all right" or "Things are bound to get better" are basically promises that the nurse cannot keep. Box 7-1 lists other responses and behaviors that are generally ineffective or inappropriate. Mistakes by the nurse can generally be corrected, explanations given, and damage to the relationship reversed. Patients usually evaluate nurses by their overall attitude of caring and concern rather than by a single inappropriate response.

## Study Notes

1. Therapeutic techniques are skills to help people, but are not goals in themselves.
2. Therapeutic communication occurs with a plan and a purpose, whereas social communication involves equal levels of intimacy, sharing, and the opportunity for spontaneity.
3. Therapeutic communication differs from social communication because the focus is on the patient rather than on a give and take experience.
4. Goals of psychiatric nursing are to understand patients, ensure that patients understand the nurse, and teach more effective communication skills.
5. Listening is a therapeutic communication technique that requires careful concentration to guide the conversation toward a goal.
6. Nurses are responsible for therapeutic communication and must recognize communication interferences that they might be causing.
7. Some common causes of interference with therapeutic communication are fear, lack of knowledge, insecurity, and inappropriate responses.

## References

Grace PJ: Ethical issues: patient safety and the limits of confidentiality, *Am J Nurs* 104:33, 2004.

Horton-Deutsch SL, Horton JM: Mindfulness: overcoming intractable conflict, *Arch Psychiatr Nurs* 17:186, 2003.

Kemper BJ: Therapeutic listening: developing the concept, *J Psychosoc Nurs Ment Health Serv* 30:21, 1992.

Leong SL, Gingrich D, Lewis PR, et al: Enhancing doctor-patient communication using email: a pilot study, *J Am Board Fam Pract* 18:180, 2005.

Miller MC, editor: Long-distance psychotherapy, *Harv Ment Health Lett* 21:7, 2005.

Simpson RL: High touch vs. high tech: rediscover the human element, *Nurs Manag* 30:33, 1999.

Talerico KA: Enhancing communication with older adults: overcoming elderspeak, *J Psychosoc Nurs* 43:12, 2005.

Taylor CE et al: Best practices: Reducing rehospitalization with telephonic targeted care management in a managed health care plan, *Psychiatr Serv*, 2004. Available at http://www.psychservices.psychiatry online.org. Accessed June 29, 2005.

White RF: How stigma interferes with mental healthcare: an expert interview with Patrick W. Corrigan, PsyD, *Medscape Psychiatry Ment Health* 9(2), 2004. Available at http://www.medscape.com/psychiatryhome. Accessed January 27, 2005.

White RF: Patient-centered care and communication: an expert interview with Tom Delbanco, MD, *Medscape Psychiatry Ment Health* 10(1), 2005. Available at http://www.medscape.com/psychiatryhome. Accessed February 28, 2005.

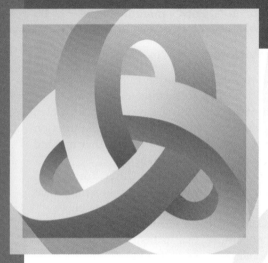

# Chapter 8

# Nurse-Patient Relationship

*Lee H. Schwecke*

## Learning Objectives

*After reading this chapter, you should be able to:*
- Describe the meaning of being therapeutic.
- Describe the stages of a therapeutic nurse-patient relationship.
- Identify the major tasks of each stage of the nurse-patient relationship.
- Recognize verbal strategies in interacting with patients with selected behaviors.

Hildegard Peplau defined nursing as "a significant, therapeutic, interpersonal process. Nursing is an educative instrument, a maturing force, that aims to promote forward movement of personality in the direction of creative, constructive, productive, personal, and community living" (Peplau, 1952). The nurse's relationship with patients consists of a series of goal-directed interactions through which the nurse assesses patients' problems, elicits patient input, selects interventions, and evaluates the effectiveness of care. In psychiatric nursing, the nursing process is grounded in the knowledge of the nature of therapeutic relationships, psychopharmacology, and milieu management, all of which are based on an understanding of concepts and processes of psychopathology. Developing the nurse-patient relationship is the first, and often the most pivotal, step in effective psychotherapeutic management (see Chapter 2). Building this relationship (or therapeutic alliance) is vital, especially in the early phases of treatment (Bender, 2005).

## THERAPEUTIC RELATIONSHIPS

Many factors influence the relationship between the nurse and the patient, and various therapeutic activities can be used within the relationship to facilitate successful patient outcomes. Even patients with the same psychiatric diagnosis will have somewhat different manifestations of symptoms, depending on their history, current life situation, and emerging needs. Each person is a unique, worthwhile, holistic individual who is struggling with internal needs and external realities (Klagsbrun, 2001). The nurse should approach each patient individually by tailoring selected strategies to each patient's problems and needs. Caring is an essential component of nursing that promotes patients' growth (Thomas et al, 2004).

### BRIEF THERAPEUTIC RELATIONSHIPS

Brief therapeutic relationships are not as formalized as therapy but are planned, patient-centered,

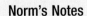

**Norm's Notes**

*This chapter takes the material presented in Chapter 7 and amplifies it within the context of the nurse-patient relationship. Between your instructor and this textbook, you should learn to be therapeutic—not a therapist, mind you, but therapeutic. Learning to be therapeutic is an enormous gift, and you can use it in all types of situations. For example, how do you react to an angry person or someone who is actively hallucinating? How do you react when a friend learns that her husband is leaving her? This chapter provides some time-tested ideas for common situations that you might face as a nurse and as a friend.*

and goal-directed. The nurse purposefully and carefully guides conversations with patients toward the exploration of problems, issues, and needs. The nurse then selects therapeutic strategies to facilitate awareness, decisions, changes, and comfort. Concern, compassion, and interest are demonstrated while the nurse is maintaining an objectivity that patients might lack. The nurse might share some personal data such as age, marital status, or title but should rarely disclose personal problems. Occasionally, a *brief self-disclosure* might help patients clarify specific issues, feel less vulnerable, or feel more normal: "When I feel depressed, it's usually because I'm angry and not talking about it. What kinds of things do you get angry about?" or "Sometimes I'm afraid to tell my wife something because I don't know how she will react. What is hard for you to talk about with your wife?" Therapeutic self-disclosure facilitates comfort, honesty, openness, and risk taking but never burdens patients with the nurse's problems (Haddad, 2001).

## SOCIAL VERSUS THERAPEUTIC RELATIONSHIPS

The nurse-patient relationship is not a social relationship (see Chapter 7). Although the nurse might relate informally with patients, the maintenance of objectivity and goal-directedness is crucial. Patients, particularly those with a history

of unsatisfying relationships, might misinterpret the nurse's interest and concern. Patients often ask (or wish to ask) the nurse to be a friend or to go out on a date. When this occurs, reminding the patient of the nurse's role and taking the opportunity to discuss the need for friendship, love, and support becomes necessary—for example, "I realize you would like to date. As a nurse I can help you find ways to form friendships that can offer you emotional support."

## COLLABORATION

Patients have a right to make decisions about their care. When patients recognize their problems, needs, and desire to change, and when they ask for assistance, the nurse is able to work with them on goals and plans. Collaboration generally produces more effective and enduring change than coercion or simple compliance. Unfortunately, situations arise during which this is not possible, such as when patients have an obvious disturbance in their thought processes (e.g., severe hallucinations or delusions). Patients might be incapable of collaborating with the nurse in their care until these problems subside. Occasionally, the only goal to which a patient will agree is "to get out of the hospital." Even this goal, however, provides an opening for discussion of behavioral changes that are necessary before discharge can occur. Patients with chronic illnesses might be able to agree to only small changes. Unless the nurse is tolerant, flexible, and realistic, the patient might feel overwhelmed.

### CLINICAL EXAMPLE

Jason Schmidy has had four admissions in 3 years, with a diagnosis of paranoid schizophrenia. During each admission, he had achieved new, small goals. Initially, his suspicion was such that he talked only to his sister and refused medications "because they were poison." At the end of his second admission, he talked with staff members and agreed to monthly injections of a long-acting antipsychotic medication. During the third admission, he related that he enjoyed helping a neighbor in his garden. At Mr. Schmidy's last discharge, he expressed interest in attending a self-help group for chronically ill patients.

## BEING THERAPEUTIC VERSUS PROVIDING THERAPY

The nurse's basic education provides the knowledge and skills for being therapeutic in encounters with patients. Psychotherapists and clinical nurse specialists (CNSs) receive specialized training that might be focused on a particular therapeutic model that attempts to explain the causes of mental illness or offers specialized techniques for achieving desired outcomes. CNSs or psychotherapists are also more interested in formalized, ongoing sessions that have a specified time, place, and length. These professionals are selective in their choice of patients and are restrictive in the sense that they have rules for conducting sessions.

In contrast, nurses who engage in therapeutic activities, in an inpatient setting or outpatient program, recognize that each encounter with patients is part of an overall therapeutic picture—a therapeutic milieu. Patients discuss real problems and practical solutions, and practice skills needed in real-life situations to enhance their functioning in the real community. Brief encounters offer an opportunity for patients to process feelings and thoughts as they occur. Validation and feedback from the nurse are available quickly. Many patients cannot tolerate intense, ongoing therapy but can benefit from consistent therapeutic encounters with nurses, even when their hospitalization lasts only a few days or when their attendance at an outpatient program is sporadic.

Informal or recreational encounters with patients (e.g., card games, craft classes, holiday parties) might be spontaneous but must be therapeutic. For example, the nurse might observe inappropriate social behaviors or a lack of social skills. Helping the patient develop appropriate social and verbal skills, test reality, and solicit feedback and support for new behaviors is then appropriate for the nurse. These informal activities also help patients reduce anxiety and body tension, develop a sense of competence, and take risks. Informal encounters are also opportunities for the nurse to demonstrate ways of handling situations: "Well, we didn't win this hand, but I'm enjoying the game anyway." "I've made that mistake before too. I can show you how to correct it." "Everyone has a right to his or her opinion. I'll listen to yours and then you can hear mine."

## STAGES OF DEVELOPMENT OF A THERAPEUTIC RELATIONSHIP

When psychiatric care was provided primarily in long-term hospitals, Peplau believed that the nurse and the patient begin as strangers and move in stages to become collaborators in problem solving. The stages in the nurse-patient relationship have been given various names, but Peplau's concepts remain valid. In the *stage of orientation,* patients recognize needs and seek help. The nurse helps patients understand their problems and accept the help that is available. The nurse works actively to foster trust and to develop the relationship. In the *identification and exploration stage,* or *working stage,* clarification of perceptions and expectations about the relationship takes place. Problems and identification of tentative solutions are further defined. Patients become more motivated to take advantage of available resources to resolve problems. Patients might test the nurse and might fluctuate between dependence and independence. Peplau believed that the *resolution stage,* or *termination stage,* needs close attention to avoid destroying the benefits gained from the relationship. Focus in this stage is on the growth that occurred and on helping the patient develop self-responsibility for setting new goals. The entire relationship is viewed as promoting growth and as a learning experience for the nurse and for patients (Peplau, 1952).

Therapeutic relationships vary in depth, length, and focus. A brief therapeutic encounter might last only a few minutes, focusing on patients' *immediate needs, current feelings,* or *observed behaviors.* In a longer term hospitalization or program, the relationship might last 1 to 3 months with regular meetings that focus on underlying causes of behaviors, developmental issues, or long-term problems. In an acute care setting or outpatient program, patients relate to many nurses and staff members each day. In this situation, progress in the nurse-patient relationship is the responsibility of every nurse with whom the patient has contact. One nurse admits the patient to the unit or program and begins the relationship. Another nurse might discharge the patient and complete termination. Shift reports, team meetings, care plans, and progress notes help each nurse work with the patient toward the same goals.

In this era of brief hospitalization and time-limited outpatient care, the phases of the nurse-patient relationship are not a sequence of processes; rather, they are a matter of different emphases or goals. The nurse concentrates on nursing approaches in a particular phase, depending on the status and needs of individual patients. For example, approaches used in the orientation phase have priority when the patient is highly suspicious because a need exists to develop trust with the patient. For the patient with good insight and motivation, approaches in the working phase are most important because they concentrate on problem solving and change. If the patient is to be admitted for only 3 days, then approaches used in the termination phase are critical because of the need for formalizing plans for follow-up care and referrals to other services along the continuum of care (see Chapter 3).

Moving in and out of the three phases might depend on the patient's ability to cope with various issues (Gauthier, 2000). The patient might be ready to work on divorce issues but might not be able to process incest issues until more trust has been established. Regardless of the phase of the relationship that is most appropriate at any given time, events can alter the patient's situation, necessitating a major change in the nurse-patient relationship. For example, if the patient experiences a crisis event, then the nurse must employ crisis intervention strategies. (See Chapter 10 for information on crisis issues and interventions.)

## STAGE I: ORIENTATION STAGE

The orientation stage involves nurses learning about patients and their initial concerns and needs (Gauthier, 2000). Patients also learn about the roles of the nurse during this first stage. Patients are informed about the general purpose of talking with the nurse. The initial purpose might be stated as broadly as "identifying a problem on which you want to work," "helping you figure out what has been happening to you lately," or "getting to know what has been bothering you." After the problems become more evident, the nurse collaborates with patients to define more specific areas to pursue—for example, learning to be assertive or processing feelings about a divorce. Patients must realize that nurses cannot solve problems or make decisions for their patients. Rather, nurses help patients look at realistic options so that patients can make their own decisions.

In a longer term outpatient relationship between the patient and the nurse, arrangements are made about the time, length, and frequency of meetings. The session might be for 30 to 60 minutes once a week in a clinic or office, or in the patient's home. Even in brief encounters in an outpatient setting or on an inpatient unit, nurses should be aware of the need for privacy and might suggest moving to an uncrowded area to talk. It is helpful for patients to know the length of time the nurse can spend with them (usually 20 minutes or less), and that the relationship will end at the time of discharge or transfer to another level in the continuum of care.

### Building Trust

Regardless of the formality or length of the relationship, each nurse actively encourages patients to feel comfortable in the relationship. An effective connection is based on the patient and the nurse getting to know each other. The nurse conveys concern for and caring about the patient. Trustworthiness is built when the nurse is honest regarding intentions, is consistent, and keeps promises. Mutual respect and trust are crucial goals. Warmth, interest, and concern are conveyed with words and congruent body language. Clear, specific communications decrease confusion and suspiciousness. Confidentiality is explained in terms of patient information being shared *only* with the immediate unit or program staff and not with anyone outside the treatment setting without the patient's consent (Grace, 2004). (See Chapter 5 for legal issues related to confidentiality.)

Many patients are afraid or unable to approach the nurse; thus, reaching out and initiating conversations is important. Quiet, withdrawn patients are often overlooked because they cannot ask for assistance. An offer to listen and help conveys to patients that they are worthwhile individuals who are respected. Initially, the nurse is nonconfrontational by not openly challenging statements that the patient makes. Such a challenge would interfere with trust and with data collection. (Supportive confrontation is discussed later in "Stage II: Working Stage.")

### Beginning Assessment

The initial sessions, including intake interviews, provide an opportunity to begin an assessment of patients' needs, coping strategies, defense mechanisms, and adaptation styles. Patients' recurring thoughts, feelings, and behaviors (*themes*) are clues to problem areas. Assessing the degree of a patient's awareness of problems and the ability and motivation to change is important. Although assessment is ongoing and progresses over time, tentative goals are based on the most immediate needs or problems—for example, suicidal or homicidal thoughts, hallucinations, self-mutilation, or acting out. (For many facilities and programs, the initial care plan must be written within 24 hours of admission.)

Many opportunities are available between interviews (e.g., during activities, meals, free time with other patients, medication times) to observe patients and their behaviors. The family might contribute information as well. Assessment tools might be used, such as a depression scale or personality test.

### Managing Emotions

At the time of admission to a unit or a program, patients typically experience painful thoughts and emotions such as fear, grief, anger, ambivalence, confusion, shame, embarrassment, and guilt. Patients are often afraid of losing control of themselves or of being viewed as weak for expressing their feelings. A way to keep patients' feelings from escalating is to talk about them directly. Because patients are likely to try to conceal or minimize feelings, the nurse must be alert to indirect references, nonverbal cues, and voice tones. The nurse can then identify the feeling and ask for validation: "Your voice is loud. You sound angry. What are you feeling right now?"

To cope effectively with feelings, particularly anger, the nurse should remember that the feeling is created not by the nurse, but by some situation or significant person in the patient's life. A patient might displace anger onto the nurse at first. If questioned about the anger, however, the patient is then more likely to recognize the real source of his or her emotions. Patients must understand that feelings are natural, but that the way they are expressed can cause a problem. Belittling or minimizing a patient's emotions is inappropriate, as is false reassurance—for example, saying that "Everything will be all right." In fact, patients might feel worse for a while as they begin to face their prob-

lems and feelings; thus, such reassurance is dishonest, as well as inappropriate.

Empathy is an objective understanding of the way in which patients see their situation. Conveying empathy is a way of helping patients deal with emotional pain throughout the relationship. Empathy can also convey a hope for improvement: "I hear how painful this is for you and would like to try to help you deal with the situation in a productive way." Sympathy, by contrast, is the nurse having the same feelings as the patient, and objectivity is therefore lost. Sympathy often leads to comforting, reassuring, or pitying patients. The outcome for patients might be a sense of "Poor me; I guess I'll always be this way."

After patients are able to talk directly about emotions, the focus can be on coping more effectively with them. In the orientation stage, resolving the problem that created the feelings is not possible, but temporarily reducing the feelings to a tolerable level by using palliative coping mechanisms is possible (see Chapter 10). Explaining the experiences and feelings to an empathic listener helps but, when ventilation intensifies the feelings, distracting patients from that topic for a while might become necessary.

Adequate rest and nutrition reduce the impact of tension on the body. Physical exercise, meditation, imagery, and relaxation techniques also alleviate some tension that patients might feel (Folsom, 1999). Although in the long run these palliative mechanisms are less desirable than adaptive mechanisms, the goal at this stage is to prevent loss of control or total retreat from emotional pain.

### Providing Support

Support, similar to empathy, begins in the orientation stage and continues throughout the nurse-patient relationship. Support confirms patients' worth and rights as human beings and includes the nurse avoiding value judgments of patients (as bad, stupid, crazy, lazy), even when patients have made poor choices. Support acknowledges that no one is perfect, that making mistakes is human, and that learning from mistakes is beneficial. Support focuses realistically and concretely on patients' abilities and strengths; for example, the nurse would not say, "You're a good person" but rather, "I'm glad you were able to share your feelings in group today." Patients need recognition of their healthy actions and feelings. Patients' dependence is tolerated until they are capable of being more independent, but any independent actions are pointed out. Support includes realistic hope and promises, such as, "I don't have an answer right now, but I will work with you to find one."

## Providing Structure

A major strategy in the orientation stage is to provide structure for patients. When patients lose control of their thoughts, feelings, or behaviors, the nurse has the responsibility for taking temporary control. The action might mean offering a prn medication; directing patients to a quieter, less stimulating place; or staying with patients at a comfortable distance. If these measures are ineffective, seclusion or restraints might then be indicated (see Chapter 11). However, providing structure also includes decreasing the withdrawal and isolation of quiet, nonparticipating patients. Spending time with these patients, even in silence, is important. The nurse can also suggest activities, such as watching television or taking a walk with the patient. A major facet of providing structure is *limit setting*. Decreasing or stopping dysfunctional behaviors is in the best interest of patients. The nurse accepts patients as human beings while discouraging self-defeating behaviors. Patients' rights and self-esteem need protection, but those of others who are around the patients need protection as well (Grace, 2004). Limit setting involves pointing out behaviors and their negative effects and suggesting alternative behaviors. For example, when a patient is self-deprecating, the nurse points out the negative comments and how they affect the patient's self-esteem, and then suggests that the patient identify something positive about himself or herself.

Behaviors that typically require immediate intervention are verbal and physical aggression, self-destructive behaviors, setting fires, noncompliance with rules and medications, alcohol or drug abuse, manipulation of others, inappropriate touching of others, indecent exposure, attempts to leave the hospital without permission, and failure to eat or sleep. Continuous rumination over painful feelings or disturbed thought processes is nonproductive and self-perpetuating. The nurse first listens to the content and the process of negative feelings or thoughts long enough to understand the messages or themes they convey, but then distracts the patient with more productive

suggestions. Limit setting is a kind but firm strategy. "I know you are angry right now, but I'm having trouble understanding the situation because of all the swearing; please stop" or "I realize that these thoughts are really important to you, but there are other areas I need to know about so I can help you."

The transition from the orientation stage to the working stage is not smooth or firmly defined. Patients' anxiety might increase when they are working on issues, and they might return to more superficial matters for a while. Some patients with chronic illnesses or multiple hospitalizations might need more of a focus on orientation stage interventions because of their difficulty in forming relationships.

## STAGE II: WORKING STAGE

When patients are ready, the work toward changing their thoughts, feelings, and behaviors can begin. However, drastic changes might not be the goal for some patients, particularly the chronically ill. Stabilization with medications, reduction of symptoms, and development of supportive relationships are valid goals; thus, the planting of the seeds for change can occur (Miller, 2005). For patients with chronic schizophrenia in particular, the ability to relate to someone is an important goal. Some patients might be hospitalized several times before they can accept the painful fact that they have a chronic illness and need ongoing treatment (McGorry and McConville, 2000). Most patients have sufficient awareness, motivation, and trust in the nurses to begin to explore problems, identify possible solutions, and test new behaviors (Gauthier, 2000).

### Process of Learning

Changing behavior is difficult. Peplau (1963) identified the process of learning as necessary for change. (See Chapter 7 for therapeutic techniques that facilitate learning.) Peplau's process closely parallels the process of change described by Rew (2004) in Chapter 4.

The first step, *observation,* is a prerequisite because, without awareness of a problem, motivation to change cannot exist (*precontemplation*). The nurse learns the extent to which patients understand their problems by asking for in-depth, detailed descriptions of situations, thoughts, feelings, and behaviors. The *analysis* step is then necessary to encourage accuracy in patients' conclusions about their problems (*contemplation*). For a patient to describe the type and sequence of arguments she has had with her husband is one process; to conclude that she is afraid of losing control over her husband is another. Even when patients can identify problems accurately, they might not automatically decide that their behavior is worth changing. The *interpretation* step leads to a decision that change is necessary and appropriate (*contemplation*).

Problem solving is the crux of the *planning* step (*preparation*). Patients are guided in decisions about change, in developing and considering alternative solutions, and in formulating a method for carrying out the plan. The nurse does not give advice but helps patients solve their own problems. The nurse encourages short-term, realistic, and achievable daily goals.

The *testing out* step involves trying the new behavior or solution in a safe environment first (e.g., with the nurse) and then in a real situation (*action*). The nurse asks patients to rehearse the things they will say and do in an upcoming situation: "Tell me what you will say to your daughter tomorrow." Practice allows the patient to obtain feedback and modify the plan. Role playing is another way of practicing behaviors. The nurse plays the roles of those with whom patients are having difficulty and assesses the patients' communication and behavior patterns. This approach helps patients learn to handle situations more effectively.

The objectives of the *evaluation* step are to assess the success of new behaviors or solutions to problems and to determine whether modification or a different approach is needed. The nurse provides feedback in a constructive manner and helps patients learn to ask for and use feedback appropriately. Effective behaviors are more likely to continue when their benefits are discussed and reinforcement is given (*maintenance*). Destructive behaviors are more likely to be identified when patients are taught to evaluate the effects of their actions on themselves and others.

### In-depth Data Collection

Nurses facilitate awareness, analysis, and interpretation through in-depth (but selective) exploration

of issues and by identifying priority issues. Focusing on too many problems at once might overwhelm patients. The nurse directs the data collection and focuses on manageable and changeable issues, thereby helping patients make sense out of their confusion. Spending time and energy exploring an unchangeable problem is frustrating, both to patients and the nurse—for example, rehashing what the patient *could have* done to prevent the divorce rather than focusing on activities he *can do* now to adjust to being single. In-depth data collection increases the nurse's knowledge of patients' strengths, needs, and problems, and of factors that can enhance or interfere with treatment. Assessments include estimating the tasks that can and cannot be accomplished during the expected length of care and identifying the types of referrals likely to be needed at the next level of treatment within the continuum of care.

### Reality Testing and Cognitive Restructuring

*Reality testing* is an important strategy in the analysis, interpretation, and planning steps. Reality testing helps patients see reality more clearly and objectively compared with the past, when distortions or inaccuracies were present. Reality testing is not a matter of arguing with a patient's point of view; rather, it presents a new reality that allows the patient to consider another option. Reality testing is constructive, not destructive, feedback: "I know the voices seem real to you, but I don't hear any" or "You sound as if you think all women are alike; that has not been my experience."

The goal of reality testing is *cognitive restructuring*—helping patients cope with negative thoughts and beliefs and recognizing other viewpoints that will help them come to more realistic conclusions (Wells-Federman et al, 2001). Patients might need to redefine the way in which they interpret a situation, or they might need to change their perception of another person's behavior. Patients might need to give up an irrational belief in favor of a more rational one—for example, changing from "I have to be perfect" to "It's okay to make mistakes; I can learn from them." This approach might also mean giving up an unrealistic goal for a more appropriate one. The redefinition of emotions might involve discovering that sadness is concealing anger.

## Writing and Journaling

Having patients write down their thoughts and feelings each day is often useful. This exercise can be a release for emotions and can facilitate a more objective analysis of issues (Wells-Federman et al, 2001). The nurse asks patients to write a homework assignment between sessions—for example, making a list of their positive qualities and strengths. Patients might also write letters (that are *not* sent) to others with whom they are having problems (Day, 2001). In some instances, a letter might be reworked several times and the message eventually shared with the person to whom the patient is writing.

## Supportive Confrontation

Supportive confrontation is similar to reality testing but has a broader focus. Supportive confrontation is aimed at contradictions, discrepancies, responsibility, accountability, independence, and behavioral change; it combines support with encouragement for constructive, productive action. The support acknowledges fears, pain, ambivalence, and the difficult process of change, whereas the confrontation includes hope and confidence that an action is possible:

- "Giving up alcohol is a scary idea, but in this program, you can get the information and support you need to do it."
- "I hear your reluctance, but taking the risk has much to offer."
- "We all like to be taken care of once in a while, but making our own decisions helps our self-esteem."

Supportive confrontation challenges patients to meet their own needs appropriately and to be accountable for their own decisions, feelings, and behaviors. Confrontation without support is generally perceived as an attack, which is what patients experience at home, school, or work.

## Promoting Change

In addition to problem solving and supportive confrontation, several other important strategies facilitate change as well. One strategy is to change the balance of the *risk-benefit ratio*, because all change has a risk of failure (Rew, 2004). For example, change might mean the loss of a comfortable habit,

the fear of rejection, or worry about the creation of new problems. The potential benefits might be growth, self-satisfaction, improved relationships, and a healthier self-esteem. For everyone, change is more likely to occur when the risks are low and the potential for benefits is high. For example, a patient with alcoholism is at risk for losing his family, yet still values taking care of and staying with his family. The nurse can help decrease risks by discussing ways to overcome them. Short-term and long-term benefits also need to be discussed. Change can be difficult, but several approaches increase the likelihood for success. For example:

1. Carefully considered rational decisions are more likely to result in healthy changes than decisions that are hasty and emotional.
2. Patient-initiated change (with specific plans and actions) tends to be more successful than change that others impose.
3. Practicing or rehearsing changes with the nurse builds confidence for trying new behaviors with others and increases success.
4. Support and acceptance of change by patients' friends and families encourage and help maintain the change.
5. Support groups can reinforce new behaviors.
6. Patients are likely to change when they are ready and motivated.
7. Pushing for change too quickly is frustrating for all concerned.

## Teaching New Skills

The desire to change is insufficient; the patient must know the proper way to change (Klagsbrun, 2001). For example, patients cannot change from being passive to being assertive if they do not understand the meaning or cannot cite examples of assertiveness. Some patients might not have learned skills that a nurse takes for granted. Common skills that patients need to learn are relaxation, stress, conflict, and anger management techniques; assertiveness; problem-solving processes; symptom management; coping skills; stress reduction; and communication, social, and community living skills (Hogarty, 2000). Occasionally, skill training must begin at a basic, concrete level. One patient's first exercise was to approach another patient and read from his 3- × 5-inch card: "Hi, my name is Bill, and I'm from Greenfield. What's your name?" Skills are taught in small steps, with frequent intermittent opportunities for practice and feedback. Again, homework assignments can be used; for example, the nurse might suggest that between sessions the patient practice a particular skill and report the results at the next session.

## STAGE III: TERMINATION STAGE

In acute inpatient settings and short-term outpatient programs, the patient's work and changes are rarely completed. Patients are discharged or transferred to another level of care, and nurses change units or jobs. If all the nurses involved with the patient are not available to discuss termination, then the nurse who is assigned to discharge or transfer the patient can implement the strategies.

### Evaluation and Summary of Progress

The nurse guides discussions to help patients identify *for themselves* the specific changes in thoughts, feelings, and behaviors that have occurred. Even small steps toward long-term goals are discussed. Reinforcing the changes in and strengths of patients is important. Areas or issues that need more work are outlined, cautioning patients to avoid trying to change everything at once. Patients are encouraged to set priorities for these issues and to establish reasonable time frames for action.

### Synthesizing the Outcomes

Synthesizing focuses on the more indirect outcomes of the nurse-patient relationship, such as more open communications or more appropriate expression of feelings. As a result of the relationship, patients often feel more comfortable with initiating interactions, making requests, and expressing opinions, even when these behaviors have not been discussed during the nurse-patient encounters. Increased participation and socialization must be recognized as well. As the nurse points out the benefits from the relationship, patients are encouraged to form other relationships with future nurses, counselors, and new friends.

### Referrals

For problems that need continuing attention after discharge, referrals to appropriate resources are finalized (see Chapter 3). The resources provide support, foster treatment compliance, and promote continued growth. Receiving written discharge instructions, which list medications, dosages, and times, as well as phone numbers, addresses, dates, and times of appointments and self-help meetings, is helpful for patients. Also important is assessing patients' ability to read these instructions; if they cannot, then someone in the patient's support systems who can read the instructions should be found (Atreja et al, 2005). If the patient speaks a language other than English, then the instructions can be translated into the patient's native language.

### Discussion of Termination

Regardless of the length, frequency of contact, or intensity of the nurse-patient relationship, discussing the participants' reactions to the relationship is important. Feelings might be positive, ambivalent, or negative and vary in degree. Superficial relationships are likely to produce mild reactions. However, even in brief relationships, the relationship might mean more to the patient than it does to the nurse; therefore, the loss of contact with the nurse might be significant to the patient. Patients might experience anger or fear related to losing the support and acceptance that the nurse provides. Some patients might avoid any discussion of termination. Nonetheless, the nurse should attempt to make it official by saying "goodbye" and stating his or her feelings about the relationship—for example, "I'm glad I had a chance to work with you."

---

### CRITICAL THINKING QUESTION    1

John Slider is suspicious, is denying his illness, and is hyperactive. What combination of nursing interventions would you use in working with him?

---

## INTERACTIONS WITH SELECTED BEHAVIORS

The purpose of this section is to discuss interventions in regard to specific troublesome behaviors that are appropriate in brief encounters with patients. The behaviors included here are those the nurse might encounter with any patient, regardless of the patient's diagnosis. Certain problem behaviors, such as anger and withdrawal, have already been discussed. Details on the specific behaviors are addressed in more depth elsewhere in the text in the chapters focusing on psychiatric disorders.

## VIOLENT BEHAVIOR

Fear of violent behavior and of being injured is a concern with the few patients who do not respond to staff efforts at verbal diffusion of anger or defensiveness (usually because of internal thought disturbances). The following are a few precautions that can be taken for protection:

- Stay out of striking distance (this also reduces the threat to the patient).
- Avoid touching patients without approval.
- Change the topic temporarily if a patient's behavior is escalating.
- Suggest time out for the patient in a quiet area with fewer stimuli.
- Avoid entering a room alone with a patient who is not in control of his or her behavior.
- Leave temporarily if the patient is agitated and asking to be left alone.
- Call for staff assistance if the patient is losing control.

Chapter 11 focuses on working with patients who are aggressive.

## HALLUCINATIONS

Interventions with a patient with hallucinations generally occur in a sequence with newly admitted patients:

1. The initial approach with patients who appear to be listening to or talking with voices is to comment on their behavior: "You look as if you are listening to something. What do you hear?"
2. If the patient acknowledges hearing something that the nurse cannot hear, the nurse can then say, "I don't hear anything. Tell me what you hear."
3. The next step is assessment of hallucinations based on the content of the messages, which often reveals the dynamics of the patient's illness and typically revolves around *themes* of powerlessness, hatred, guilt, or loneliness.

4. After the content is known, focusing on the hallucinations is unnecessary; doing so might reinforce them: "I know the voices are important to you, but let's talk about your loneliness right now."
5. Eventually, the hallucinations are ignored and the patient is distracted to become engaged in more productive activities or is taught how to distract himself or herself with activities, music, or interactions with others.

The exception is with hallucinations that command patients to harm themselves or others or to do other destructive acts. In such a case, the nurse should contract with patients to avoid acting on the commands they hear and to tell the staff. Another exception is with patients with dementia or severe cognitive impairments. These patients are not likely to be able to process the content or themes of the hallucinations. For them, the strategy of "ignore and distract" is more useful.

## DELUSIONS

The initial approach with respect to delusions is clarification of meanings (Beck and Rector, 1998)—for example, "Who do you think is trying to hurt you?" or "Tell me about this power you think you have." Similar to hallucinations, delusions are not discussed after the meanings are clarified. Arguing with a patient about delusions is ineffective and inappropriate, and might strengthen the patients' belief in them. The underlying *themes* reflected in the delusions are more appropriately addressed in interventions that help the patient, who for example says she is a queen, feel important in realistic ways. Careful monitoring is needed if the delusions might lead patients to harm themselves or others; for example, a patient does not want to eat because he believes all the food is poisoned. Again, with patients with dementia or severe cognitive impairments, ignore and distract might be more effective.

## CONFLICTING VALUES

Occasionally, nurses and patients encounter conflicts with their beliefs or values. Both participants can state their views in a discussion, but arguing is inappropriate. A better approach is to help patients examine the effects or outcomes of their beliefs on their lives, relationships, and happiness.

For example, a patient might believe that she has the right to drink as much and as often as she wants because drinking is legal. Supportive confrontation can help her examine the effects of drinking on her marriage, job, health, and economic status.

Agreeing with every patient's beliefs, values, or behaviors is not necessary for the nurse to be effective. Nurses must be aware of their own stance on issues and understand the patient's point of view *as the patients see them.* Usually, patients need not change a belief or behavior that is not causing problems for them or for others around them. Beliefs and behaviors that have positive effects need reinforcement.

## SEVERE ANXIETY AND INCOHERENT SPEECH PATTERNS

Disturbed thought processes are occasionally evident in speech, especially with patients who are upset, confused, or psychotic. When these processes occur, the typical approach is to clarify the meaning of the communications. However, severely ill and/or anxious patients might be unable to be clearer and repeated questions only increase anxiety. It is more effective to key into their feelings and underlying *themes,* rather than trying to make sense of the content of their speech. Medications often decrease the anxiety and then clear the thought disturbances rather quickly. Until then, the nurse spends frequent, brief time with these patients (without pressuring or frustrating them), offers support, and builds trust.

## MANIPULATION

Common manipulations are a means to gain attention, sympathy, control, and dependence. Manipulation is not often recognized until it has already worked. The nurse might then experience anger or embarrassment. The initial approach is to address what is happening (or has happened):

- "I'm getting the impression that you would like me to tell you what to do. What scares you about this decision?"
- "You are experiencing a lot of emotional pain and would like me to relieve it for you. Let's talk about what *you* can do to relieve it."
- "I see you asking for a lot of attention. What is it that you really want?"

Limit setting is useful with manipulative patients. A power struggle with the patient is useless. Helping patients to express their needs directly to others is more productive.

## CRYING

Unless crying is a manipulative gesture or is prolonged and unproductive, it should be allowed and even encouraged, verbally and nonverbally. By saying, "It's okay to cry" or quietly offering a tissue, the nurse gives patients permission to cry and relieve tension. Privacy should be provided. The nurse should be as quiet and unobtrusive as possible until the crying has ceased. The patient is then offered an opportunity to discuss the circumstance that precipitated the tears.

## SEXUAL INNUENDOS OR INAPPROPRIATE TOUCH

Patients generally stop these behaviors when asked and should be reminded that these actions are inappropriate. The nurse then discusses the underlying need. If the behaviors continue, then setting limits can be stronger: "I want to talk to you but not if you continue to touch me." "If you don't stop, I will have to leave and come back later." The nurse should refrain from touching patients with sexual or boundary issues. The nurse is responsible for maintaining professional boundaries in the relationship, especially when the patient is having difficulty with his or her own boundaries (Gutheil, 2005). Pairing patients who act out sexually and have poor impulse control with staff members of the same gender might also help until these patients are further along in treatment. This strategy, however, might be ineffective with homosexual patients.

## DENIAL AND LACK OF COOPERATION

Many reasons exist that cause patients to be uncooperative with the nurse in working toward treatment goals. A common reason is severe disturbances in thought processes (e.g., hallucinations, delusions, disorientation, and confusion) that interfere with patients' understanding of the nature of the problems and the changes that are needed. With some patients, the disturbances are less evident, but denial of any problems remains and insight into their problems and recognition of the need for treatment is lacking (McGorry and McConville, 2000). In fact, these patients might be angry about being forced into treatment. Reality testing and supportive confrontation with denial focuses on the outcomes of the patient's behavior over time. Occasionally, a patient might admit to the need for help but disagrees with the type of treatment offered. Other patients might be afraid of changing, even though they realize that their behaviors are nonproductive or harmful. Listening, clarifying, and verbalizing thoughts that have been implied are appropriate for identifying the underlying causes of a lack of cooperation. Then, to the greatest extent possible, the causes, fears, and outcomes of patients' behaviors are discussed directly. "What are you afraid will happen if you have to give up alcohol as a way of avoiding your problem?" Trust is often an issue for these patients (Bender, 2005); thus, measures to increase trust and a great deal of patience from the nurse will be needed.

## DEPRESSED AFFECT, APATHY, AND PSYCHOMOTOR RETARDATION

When patients express sadness, helplessness, hopelessness, lack of energy, or a negative attitude about everything, the nurse typically experiences sadness, helplessness, sympathy, or frustration. Patience, frequent contact, and empathy are more effective ways for dealing with these feelings. Even when patients realize the change that must be made, they do not always have the energy to make the adjustment quickly. The nurse acknowledges feelings but discourages rumination: "You are so focused on your sadness that you are stuck. Come take a walk with me for a few minutes." Improvement in personal hygiene, proper nutrition, and a gradual increase in activities are encouraged. Major decisions are postponed until emotions have subsided and thinking is more logical.

## SUSPICIOUSNESS

When patients are suspicious, they might be afraid of everyone, everything, and every interaction around them. The nurse must therefore communicate clearly, simply, and congruently. Misinterpretations by patients are clarified, but arguments over differences in opinion are avoided. Simple rationales or explanations for rules, activities, occurrences, noises, and requests are offered regularly. Patients' participation is encouraged but not forced, thus avoiding an increase in their fears.

## HYPERACTIVITY

Excessive physical and emotional activity of patients is upsetting to the staff, to other patients, and often to the hyperactive patients themselves. Even unintentionally, patients might harm themselves or others (see the previous discussion of violence). These patients should be in a quiet area, with minimal auditory and visual stimulation. Physical activity such as walking or using a stationary bicycle might help drain excess energy. The nurse must remain calm, speak slowly and softly, and respect patients' personal space. Directions are given in a kind, simple, but firm manner. Occasionally, prn medications are required, including one to promote sleep.

## TRANSFERENCE AND COUNTERTRANSFERENCE

*Transference* involves the unconscious emotional reaction that patients have in a current situation that is actually based on previous, even childhood, relationships and experiences (Jones, 2004). For example, a patient perceives the nurse as acting the way that his mother did, regardless of how the nurse is truly acting. Common issues in transference are the wish to be taken care of, have needs met by someone else, and express unresolved emotions. Transference might be severe, in the form of delusions, or they might be subtle, as in stereotyping all males as aggressive and all females as submissive. Transference can be positive if patients view the nurse as helpful and caring. Negative transference is more difficult because of unpleasant emotions that interfere with treatment, such as anger and fear.

Nurses might experience transference reactions with patients, coworkers, and physicians. Guilt or anger about not helping a particular patient or anger toward a demanding physician might be an unconscious transference response. *Countertransference* might occur in response to a patient's transference (Jones, 2004). For example, when a patient criticizes the nurse, the nurse might relive feelings that were experienced when a teacher gave negative feedback to him or her in class. Another nurse might remember a favorite teacher who challenged him or her to improve. These feelings interfere with the nurse's ability to be therapeutic. A reaction might lead to avoidance or rejection of the patient. Another reaction might lead to the nurse becoming sympathetic and unable to confront the patient appropriately. In either case, the nurse's behavior is not therapeutic.

The first intervention is to recognize the transference or countertransference, which is difficult because of the unconscious processes involved. Coworkers are more likely than others to recognize the phenomenon initially and give feedback to the nurse about it. Nurses must examine their strengths, weaknesses, prejudices, and values before they can interact more appropriately with patients. The transference reactions of patients must also be examined, gently but directly. Nurses must be open and clear about their genuine reactions when patients misperceive behavior. Nurses should also state actions that they can and cannot take to meet patients' needs. Limit setting is useful when patients act inappropriately toward the nurse. Redirection of needs to more appropriate people can also be a helpful intervention—for example, "I can't be your girlfriend, but let's talk about making new friends at home."

## Study Notes

1. To be therapeutic, the nurse uses verbal and nonverbal communications to convey a willingness to listen, genuine respect, desire to help, and understanding of the patient as a person with unique problems and needs.

2. The nurse-patient relationship is a series of goal-directed interactions that focus on the patient's thoughts, feelings, behaviors, and potential solutions to problems.

3. The nurse-patient relationship is a tool that the nurse can use to assess each patient's problems, select and carry out specific interventions, and evaluate the effectiveness of care.

4. Each stage of the nurse-patient relationship (orientation, working, termination) involves specific tasks that are used according to the

needs and problems of each patient at a given time.

5. Issues and patient behaviors that interfere with the progress of the nurse-patient relationship must be addressed by the nurse.

## References

Atreja A, Bellam N, Levy SR: Strategies to enhance patient adherence: making it simple, *Medscape Gen Med* 7(1), 2005. Available at http://www.medscape.com/medgenmed. Accessed September 1, 2005.

Beck AT, Rector NA: Cognitive therapy for schizophrenic patients, *Harv Ment Health Lett* 15:4, 1998.

Bender DS: The therapeutic alliance in the treatment of personality disorders, *J Psychiatr Pract* 11:73, 2005.

Day AL: The journal as a guide for the healing journey, *Nurs Clin North Am* 336:131, 2001.

Folsom D: Nursing the patient within, *Am J Nurs* 99:80, 1999.

Gauthier PA: Use of Peplau's interpersonal relations model to counsel people with AIDS, *J Am Psychiatr Nurs Assoc* 6:119, 2000.

Grace PJ: Patient safety and the limits of confidentiality, *Am J Nurs* 104:33, 2004.

Gutheil TG: Boundary issues and personality disorders, *J Psychiatr Pract* 11:88, 2005.

Haddad A: Ethics in action, *RN* 64:25, 2001.

Hogarty GE: Cognitive rehabilitation of schizophrenia, *Harv Ment Health Lett* 17:4, 2000.

Jones AC: Transference and countertransference, *Perspect Psychiatr Care* 40:13, 2004.

Klagsbrun J: Listening and focusing: holistic health care tools for nurses, *Nurs Clin North Am* 36:115, 2001.

McGorry PD, McConville SB: Insight in psychosis, *Harv Ment Health Lett* 17:3, 2000.

Miller MC, editor: Motivational interviewing, *Harv Ment Health Lett* 21:5, 2005.

Peplau HE: *Interpersonal relations in nursing,* New York, 1952, Putnam.

Peplau HE: A working definition of anxiety. In Burd SE, Marshall MA, editors: *Some clinical approaches to psychiatric nursing* (pp. 323-327), Toronto, 1963, Macmillan.

Rew L: Contemplation: A vital step in the process of change, *J Holistic Nurs* 22:3, 2004.

Thomas JD, Finch LP, Schoenhofer SO, et al: The caring relationships created by nurse practitioners and the ones nursed: implications for practice, *Topics Adv Pract Nurs eJournal* 4(14), 2004. Available at http://www.medscape.com. Accessed September 3, 2005.

Walker KM, Alligood MR: Empathy from a nursing perspective: moving beyond borrowed theory, *Arch Psychiatr Nurs* 15:140, 2001.

Wells-Federman CL, Stuart-Shor E, Webster A: Cognitive therapy: applications for health promotion, disease prevention, and disease management, *Nurs Clin North Am* 36:93, 2001.

# Chapter 9

# Nursing Process

*Lee H. Schwecke*

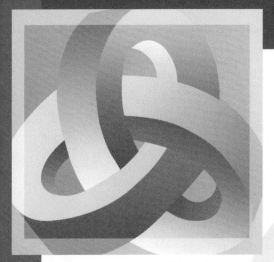

## Learning Objectives

*After reading this chapter, you should be able to:*
- Relate the nursing process to psychiatric nursing practice.
- Identify the components of an initial holistic patient assessment.
- Describe the components of the mental status examination.
- Describe the importance of writing a specific nursing diagnosis and care plan.
- Understand the importance of discharge planning.
- Recognize the value of process recordings for professional growth.

The use of the nursing process (Figure 9-1) has the same goal in psychiatric nursing as it has in other areas of nursing: patient-centered, goal-directed action that facilitates health promotion, primary prevention, treatment, and rehabilitation. Care is adapted to patients' unique needs. Individualized care begins with a detailed assessment.

## ASSESSMENT

### INITIAL PATIENT ASSESSMENT

This phase begins on admission to a unit or program with a nurse. Each psychiatric hospital, unit, clinic, and program has its own version of an intake or nursing assessment form. Box 9-1 provides a sample of the type of information included in the initial assessment.

The multidisciplinary team includes at least the nurse, psychiatrist, psychologist, social worker, pharmacist, and dietitian. A chaplain also might be included on the team to add the component of a spiritual assessment (O'Reilly, 2004). The staff uses all information that the team members collect to confirm the patient assessment while minimizing the need for the patient to repeat information. Because most facilities use intake forms or checklists, the results of the interviews do not have to be written in narrative form. Summarization of the critical content as an admission note included in the progress notes might be expected.

### MENTAL STATUS EXAMINATION

In psychiatric settings, an important component of patient assessment is the mental status examination (MSE), which focuses on the patient's current state in terms of thoughts, feelings, and behaviors. The categories of the MSE help organize a summary of the information gathered during the initial patient assessment. The information related to each of the categories includes the following:

## Norm's Notes

*Well, you might have seen this before, but now the good old nursing process is applied to psychiatric nursing. Can you ever escape it? Of course, it makes perfect sense to use it. You have to go through these steps—and you would want someone to do the same if the patient were you or one of your loved ones. It is a disciplined way of thinking that helps you become competent and helps the patient with minimal omissions in care. Learn it again for the first time (!).*

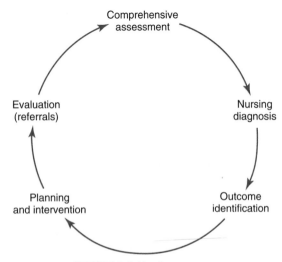

**FIGURE 9-1** Nursing process.

- General appearance: Type, condition, and appropriateness of clothing (for age, season, setting), grooming, cleanliness, physical condition, and posture
- Behaviors during the interview: Degree of cooperation, resistance, or evasiveness
- Social skills: Friendliness, shyness, or withdrawal
- Amount and type of motor activity: Psychomotor agitation or retardation, restlessness, tics, tremors, hypervigilance, or lack of activity
- Speech patterns: Amount, rate, volume, tone pressure, mutism, slurring, or stuttering
- Degree of concentration and attention span
- Orientation: To time, place, person, and level of consciousness
- Memory: Immediate recall, recent, remote, amnesia, and confabulation
- Intellectual functioning: Educational level, use of language and knowledge, abstract versus

### Box 9-1    Initial Patient Assessment

- **Demographic data:** Full name, gender, age, date of birth, address, marital status, and family members', partner's, or significant other's names and ages
- **Admission data:** Date and time of admission and type of admission (voluntary or committed)
- **Reason for admission:** Current problems as perceived by the patient; include stressors, difficulty with coping, developmental issues, "emergency behaviors" (suicidal or homicidal ideas and attempts, aggression, destructive behaviors, risk of escape), and family history
- **Previous psychiatric history:** Dates, inpatient or outpatient, reasons for and types of treatment and their effectiveness, current medications, and compliance
- **Current medical problems and medications:** Allergies, results of laboratory tests, x-rays, examinations
- **Drug and alcohol use or abuse:** Amount, frequency, duration of past and present use of legal and illegal substances, date and time of last use, potential for withdrawal symptoms
- **Disturbances in patterns of daily living:** Sleep, intake, elimination, sexual activity, work, leisure, self-care, and hygiene
- **Culture and spirituality:** Ethnicity, beliefs, practices, and religious preference
- **Support systems:** Amount of contact, nature and quality of relationships, and availability of support

concrete thinking (proverbs), and calculations (serial sevens)
- Affect: Labile, blunted, flat, incongruent, or inappropriate affect
- Mood: Specific moods expressed or observed—euphoria, depression, anxiety, anger, guilt, or fear
- Thought clarity: Coherence, confusion, or vagueness
- Thought content: Helplessness, hopelessness, worthlessness, suicidal thoughts or plans, homicidal thoughts or plans, suspiciousness, phobias, obsessions, compulsions, preoccupations, poverty of content, denial, hallucinations (auditory, visual, olfactory, gustatory, tactile) or delusions (of reference, influence, persecution, grandeur, religious, nihilistic, somatic)
- Thought processes reflected in speech: Ambivalence, circumstantiality, tangentially, thought blocking, loose associations, flight of ideas, perseveration, neologisms, or word salad

- Insight: Degree of awareness of illness, behaviors, problems, and their causes
- Judgment: Soundness of problem solving and decisions
- Motivation: Degree of motivation for treatment

Some patients are too ill to participate in or complete the assessment interview. In these cases, objective data such as patient behaviors and reports by family members are used. In some cases, information from staff in the outpatient setting that the patient attends is available. During the initial assessment, behaviors can be described without knowing or identifying their causes—for example, anxiety level, degree of withdrawal, thought disturbances reflected in speech, voice tone, and general appearance. Causes and dynamics can be elicited later to form a strong basis for a treatment plan.

## CLINICAL EXAMPLE

Anita Jarvis, a 46-year-old patient, is separated from her husband, who asked for a divorce and left her 1 week ago. Her son and daughter brought Anita to the hospital after they visited her and found that she had not been getting out of bed to shower or eat. They reported that their mother stated that she wished she were dead. Anita admits to feeling suicidal but denies having any suicide plans. She has no history of medical or psychiatric illnesses and takes no medications. Anita stated that she stopped seeing her friends 1 month ago and does not want to do anything anymore. She is not close to her parents, who live out of state. She called the school in which she teaches 4 days ago and said she was sick. She admits to staying in bed "all the time" but sleeping only 3 to 4 hours a night. Anita was admitted to the hospital with an initial diagnosis of depression.

Mrs. Jarvis and her situation are used in the chapter examples of a process recording (see Table 9-1), MSE (see Box 9-2), progress note (see Box 9-3), and Care Plan (at the end of the chapter). The process recording is an example of part of an initial assessment with Mrs. Jarvis (see below for an explanation of the purpose of process recordings).

## ONGOING ASSESSMENTS

Even when the initial assessment is complete, each encounter with a patient involves a continuing assessment that might or might not be congruent with the initial assessment. No one acts or feels the same way 24 hours a day, 7 days a week. The ongoing assessment often involves an investigation of patients' statements and actions at the moment: "You have been sitting alone for a while. What have you been thinking about?" or "You mentioned being worried; what about?" When the nurse decides to investigate a patient's specific behavior, exploring the following might be valuable:

- Context or situation that precipitated the behavior
- Patient's thoughts at the time
- Patient's feelings then and now
- Whether the behavior makes sense in that context
- Whether the behavior was adaptive or dysfunctional
- How this episode fits with the total picture of the patient
- Whether a change is needed

A sample MSE with Mrs. Jarvis is given in Box 9-2.

## NURSING DIAGNOSIS

A nursing diagnosis is the identification of patients' problems based on conclusions about the dynamics evident in verbalizations and behaviors. It is directly related to the content, mood, and interaction themes described in Chapter 7. Emergency behaviors (e.g., suicidal or homicidal ideas or attempts, aggression, destructive behaviors, risk of arson or escape) are given priority in establishing nursing diagnoses and in negotiating no-harm contracts with patients. (An in-depth discussion of the risks and benefits of these contracts is found in Reid [2005].) Regardless of the format or style of nursing diagnosis in a particular setting, the diagnosis should be specific and indicate a desired outcome for the patient. In this text, NANDA International diagnoses are used because they are the most widely accepted and commonly used nursing diagnoses. NANDA International diagnoses suggest a statement format that has three components:

1. Potential or actual problems
2. Contributing or causative factor
3. Defining characteristic or behavioral outcome

| Table 9-1 | Sample Process Recording With Mrs. Jarvis |
|---|---|

Nurse introduces himself to Mrs. Jarvis and leads the way to the office, walking slowly but slightly ahead of the patient. The patient follows without looking at the nurse. In the office, the nurse sits in a chair at a desk and opens a folder of papers. The patient sits in a chair at the side of the desk, holding her purse with both hands on her lap.

| NURSE | | PATIENT | | ANALYSIS | |
|---|---|---|---|---|---|
| Verbal | Nonverbal | Verbal | Nonverbal | Themes | Therapeutic Techniques |
| What do you prefer to be called, Mrs. Jarvis or Anita? | Has pen in hand, other hand is flat on desk; is looking at patient. | *(pause)* Anita. | Is looking at floor. | Content—oriented to person. | Questioning, active listening |
| Anita, we will be better able to help you if we know more about you. What has happened in your life recently? | (Same as above.) | *(pause)* I couldn't get out of bed. *(pause)* I was so tired. | Is turning head slightly, still looking at the floor; is not smiling or frowning. | Content—describes fatigue and effects. Mood—sadness. Interaction—opens up with nurse. | Giving information, questioning |
| How long have you been feeling so tired? | Is writing, then looking at patient. | I don't know. *(pause)* A week, I guess. | (Same as above.) | Content—unsure of time frames, marital separation, possible divorce. | Placing event in time or sequence, active listening |
| What happened a week ago? I can see this is difficult for you to talk about. *(pause)* What did he say when he left? | Leans toward patient. Moves tissue box. Looks at patient; both arms are on lap. | *(pause)* My husband *(pause)* left. That he was fed up. *(pause)* That he wanted a divorce. | Tears are in eyes; tries to open purse. Is nodding head; raises eyes slightly; is still not looking at the nurse. Starts to cry; gets tissue. Sobs occasionally. | Mood—sadness, guilt. Interaction—in conflict with husband, is more trusting of nurse. | Focusing Using empathy, and silence, questioning |
| What did you say to him? | Leans slightly toward patient. One arm is on lap, the other is on arm of chair. | I don't know. I don't remember. *(pause)* Maybe I asked him to stay. | Is crying quietly. | Content—difficulty describing situations, short-term memory disturbance. | Focusing, active listening |
| Then what happened? | (Same as above.) | It's all a blur; I think I cried all day. | (Same as above.) | Mood—sadness, guilt. Interactions—abandonment, loneliness. | Focusing |
| Who did you talk to? | (Same as above.) | No one. *(pause)* My kids are married and gone. I just stayed in bed. | Is the same but crying less often. | Content—did not ask for help, avoidance of divorce issue. Mood—sadness. Interaction—perceived lack of support. | Focusing |

| Table 9-1 | Sample Process Recording With Mrs. Jarvis—cont'd |

| NURSE | | PATIENT | | ANALYSIS | |
|---|---|---|---|---|---|
| **Verbal** | **Nonverbal** | **Verbal** | **Nonverbal** | **Themes** | **Therapeutic Techniques** |
| When you were feeling so tired, did you have thoughts of killing yourself? | (Same as above.) | *(pause)* I was so scared of being alone. I thought I'd rather be dead. | Looks at nurse for the first time; both hands are in lap. | Content—aware of fears, suicidal ideation but no plan, difficulty with problem solving. | Questioning |
| How did you think about killing yourself? | (Same as above.) | I couldn't think of anything. I didn't know what to do. | Looks at floor again; fumbles in purse. | Mood—sadness, depression. Interaction— abandonment, lack of support, open with nurse. | Focusing |
| Are you still thinking about suicide? | Hands patient a tissue. | Not really, But *(pause)* I still wish I were dead. I don't know what to do. | Blows nose and then puts hands in lap; looks at nurse. | Content— minimizing suicidal ideation but ambivalent, helplessness. Mood—sadness. | Focusing |
| While you are here, we are going to help you consider some options about what to do so you won't feel so alone and scared. *(pause)* | Leans forward. Looks at patient. Both hands on lap. | (Silence) | Looks at floor; crying has stopped; looks at nurse. | Interaction— asking for help. | Suggesting collaboration, verbalizing the implied, active listening |
| It will help us if I ask you some questions. | Turns back to papers. Is ready to write. | Okay. | Looks at nurse. | | Giving information |

The statement is typically written as follows: (Problem) related to (contributing factor) as evidenced by (behavioral outcome)—for example, "Anxiety, moderate, related to marital problems as evidenced by ineffective problem solving."

Actual or potential problems are identified from the list approved by NANDA International (see the inside back cover). Contributing or causative factors can include stressors, losses, past experiences, developmental issues, environmental circumstances, relationship issues, and self-perceptions. Defining characteristics or behavioral outcomes are the verbal and nonverbal cues that reflect the patient's actual or potential problems. These dysfunctional behaviors or cues are the focus of the nursing interventions, behaviors that it would be helpful to change. Being specific when describing the dysfunctional behaviors or cues is useful in providing direction for selecting desirable or adaptive behaviors identified in the patient's desired outcomes. Nursing diagnoses do not include medical diagnoses in any of the three parts of the diagnostic statement.

## OUTCOME IDENTIFICATION

A goal or outcome specifies an adaptive behavior to replace one that is dysfunctional. Expecting patients to change a negative self-image to a positive self-image during a short inpatient stay or outpatient program is unrealistic. A more realistic behavioral goal would be to ask patients to write a list of their strengths, abilities, and positive qualities. This goal is achievable and measurable.

---

### Box 9-2    Mental Status Examination With Mrs. Jarvis

- **General appearance:** Dressed appropriately for season; clothes are clean but not pressed; hair is unwashed and uncombed; slouched shoulders; pale; blank expression
- **Behaviors during interview:**
  - **Cooperation-resistance-evasiveness:** Slow to respond but cooperative
  - **Social skills:** Withdrawn; no unusual habits; reduced socialization
- **Motor activity:** Slowed; crying at times; no tics or tremors noted
- **Speech patterns:** Amount is reduced with slowed rate and soft tone
- **Concentration-attention span:** Decreased concentration; easily distracted by stimuli; slight shortening of attention span
- **Orientation:** Aware of person, place, and time; responsive
- **Memory:**
  - **Immediate recall:** Remembers nurse's name.
  - **Recent:** Difficulty organizing sequence but mostly complete, except for last week
  - **Remote:** Good detail on birth of children
- **Thought clarity:** Clear, coherent
- **Thought content:** Expressing helplessness, hopelessness, and suicidal thoughts without a plan; fears being alone; no evidence of hallucinations or delusions
- **Thought process:** No disturbances noted
- **Intellectual functioning:** College education evident in vocabulary; calculations and proverbs were not done; abstract thinking evident in discussion of love and fidelity
- **Affect:** Blunted
- **Mood:** Depressed; anxiety level is moderate; guilt and covert anger expressed
- **Insight:** Aware of problems in facing divorce but not yet able to describe factors leading to separation
- **Judgment:** No impairment until last 2 weeks when she became unable to make decisions, take action, or seek support
- **Motivation for treatment:** Wants help with depression, tiredness, and handling divorce; unable to state what type of help she needs

---

Short-term goals or outcomes are those achievable in perhaps 4 to 6 days for hospitalized patients and perhaps somewhat longer for patients in other settings. Long-term goals or outcomes relate to issues that require follow-up counseling after discharge to another type of service within the continuum of care. For example, a female patient's short-term goal might be to identify her fears about relationships with men. The longer term goal is to practice how to respond to potential dating situations; thus, her fears might decrease and enable her to handle these types of situations.

In establishing goals and outcomes *with* a patient (*collaboration*), the nurse must understand the problems that the patient wants to address and the goals that the patient wants to achieve. Patient desires and motivation play a major role in attaining outcomes (Atreja et al, 2005). Patient support systems and resources might also facilitate outcome achievement (Walden-McBride and McBride, 2000). Outcome achievement can also be used to help evaluate the quality and effectiveness of nursing care (Oermann and Huber, 1999).

## PLANNING AND INTERVENTION

### NURSING CARE PLANS

Nursing staff, on units or in programs, often develop standardized care plans with expected outcomes for certain types of patient problems. These care plans might focus on psychiatric diagnoses (e.g., major depression) or more specific problems (e.g., self-mutilation). Standardized care plans can also be called clinical pathways, critical pathways, or multidisciplinary care plans. The initial care plan might be updated at any time but begins with one or two behavior-oriented problems to be addressed immediately (e.g., suicide, aggression, arson, escape, withdrawal or isolation, delusions, hallucinations, impulsive or compulsive acts, suspiciousness, uncooperativeness, or altered thought processes). For example, a patient who has suicidal ideations (problem) would be expected to sign a no-harm contract (outcome) within 24 hours (time constraint) and to verbalize a plan for dealing with suicidal ideation (outcome) by day 3 of admission (time constraint). Related nursing interventions would include (1) a contract with the patient for safety, (2) removal of dangerous objects from the patient and the patient's room, and (3) assessment for suicidal ideation during every shift.

Given the current managed care climate, a goal of standardized care plans is to expedite treatment activities to achieve patient outcomes in a cost-effective manner (i.e., quickly). Nursing interventions focus particularly on "safety, structure, support, and symptom management" (Delaney et al, 2000). However, the nurse must remember that each patient is an individual, even when some of the patient's problems fit into a standardized plan. A patient's unique problems and needs must not be ignored when formulating the plan of care (Benner, 2000).

Psychiatric nursing interventions involve few hands-on activities other than minor treatments, monitoring vital signs, and giving medications. Rather, the focus is on the verbal strategies (discussed in Chapters 7 and 8) that are used to guide patients in solving problems for themselves and in achieving desired outcomes. Psychiatric nurses are primarily facilitators and educators. Solving problems and changing behaviors are never quite as easy as they sound. Patients might need help with developing specific and concrete plans for reaching their goals. For example, a patient might set a goal of finding a new apartment but needs assistance in locating rental options and in evaluating the pros and cons of each apartment option.

## PROGRESS NOTES AND SHIFT REPORTS

The style of charting progress notes (written or electronic) varies in each setting, but the components are basically the same: the patient's statements and the nurse's observations, analyses, and plans. Charting and shift reports are important ways of communicating with team members to ensure continuity of care. These reports are also ways of evaluating the effectiveness of treatment plans and progress toward patient short-term and long-term outcomes (Martin and Street, 2003). Patients must also be kept informed of their progress toward their goals. The nurse must remember that the entire chart is a legal document subject to review by peer review agencies, quality improvement staff, and accreditation bodies (Oermann and Huber, 1999). Box 9-3 details the components of a progress note and provides a sample note for Mrs. Jarvis. Shift reports are a concise, focused, and abbreviated list of the items included in the progress notes.

## EVALUATION

### PATIENT PROGRESS

The more realistic and measurable are the goals, the greater is the likelihood that patients and nurses will have a sense of progress. A major problem arises with evaluating care in psychiatric

---

### Box 9-3    Progress Note Components

- **Subjective content:** The patient's statements about his or her own thoughts, feelings, behaviors, and problems.
- **Objective data:** The nurse's observations or measurements, such as the patient's appearance, nonverbal behaviors, and vital signs.
- **Analysis or conclusions:** The nurse's impressions of what the patient is experiencing or demonstrating in behavioral or descriptive terms (not medical diagnoses); defenses, mood, and issues are identified; depressed mood and paranoid ideas can be discussed, but "depression" and "paranoia" are not listed as illnesses; conclusions about changes (regression or progression) in the patient and medication responses are described.
- **Plans:** Actions that the nurses or other team members can take to intervene with the problems described in the progress note.

**Sample Progress Note for Mrs. Jarvis**
Date and time: 11/10/06, 1600.

**S:** Patient states that she is a little less tired. States she is still unsure of what led to the separation and cannot face living alone. Still has thoughts of suicide but no plan: "I still wish I were dead." A "no-suicide contract" was verbalized by the patient. Verbalizes that she still doesn't know what to do about impending divorce and being alone in the future. Said she called her school to extend her sick leave and called her son and daughter, who now will visit this evening.

**O:** Exhibits blunted, depressed affect, slowed motor activity and speech. Attended one therapeutic group and a craft activity, but only participated briefly. Napped for only 2 hours this shift.

**A:** Patient cannot describe her thoughts and feelings, but guilt, helplessness, and hopelessness are evident. Anger is barely evident at this point. Suicidal but lacks energy to plan. Support is available from her adult children.

**P:** 1. Approach and sit with patient frequently.
2. Encourage verbalization of feelings, especially anger.
3. Monitor energy level and suicidal ideation.
4. Continue medications as ordered.
5. Encourage participation in group meetings and activities.

---

nursing when too much change is expected too soon. When the patient or nurse becomes aware of a lack of progress toward goals, evaluation should lead to reassessment. Using the nursing process leads to a reformulation of the nursing diagnoses and the establishment of more realistic, appropriate outcomes. Even when short-term goals are met, patients have other unsolved problems. If the short-term goals were related to learning better skills (e.g., communication, problem solving, social skills), then patients can continue to progress after discharge.

Evaluating patient progress is important in determining patient referrals to other levels of care and supervision within the continuum of care (see Chapter 3). The issue of prior noncompliance with medications and treatments needs to be addressed early in the admission. This might affect the type of referrals made for outpatient supervision (Atreja et al, 2005). In addition to evaluating the progress of patients, nurses evaluate the quality of their interventions and their professional behaviors.

## DISCHARGE SUMMARIES

Many facilities and programs expect nurses to participate in writing transfer or discharge summaries and discharge instructions that will be given to patients. Summaries usually identify outcomes that the patient has achieved and outcomes that must still be addressed. The following information is usually included in the discharge instructions: medication (including dosages and times), follow-up appointments (with dates and times), and referrals to other services in the continuum of care. As discussed in Chapter 8, assessing the patient's ability to read and understand the discharge instructions is important (Atreja et al, 2005).

## Care Plan

Name: Anita Jarvis                                                                          Admission Date: 11/10/06

DSM-IV-TR Diagnosis: Depressive episode

| | |
|---|---|
| Assessment | **Areas of strength:** Has family who cares; had good work record; has asked for help; is thinking abstractly. |
| | **Problems:** Is unable to get out of bed and care for self; has suicidal thoughts but no plan; exhibits decreased socialization and support; impending divorce. |
| Diagnoses | • Risk for suicide related to impending divorce, as evidenced by a wish to be dead. |
| | • Moderate anxiety related to anger and fear of living alone, as evidenced by expressed helplessness. |
| | • Hopelessness related to lowered self-esteem, as evidenced by not caring for self. |

| Outcomes | *Short-term goals:* | *Date met* |
|---|---|---|
| | • Patient will agree to talk with staff when she thinks about wanting to be dead. | _____ |
| | • Patient will verbally express anger at husband and situation | _____ |
| | • Patient will telephone friend, employer, and children for assistance. | _____ |
| | *Long-term goals:* | |
| | • Patient will state where she will live after discharge. | _____ |
| | • Patient will verbalize confidence in ability to support self. | _____ |
| | • Patient will describe resources available to her, especially if she becomes suicidal again. | _____ |

| | |
|---|---|
| Planning and Interventions | **Nurse-patient relationship:** Initiate suicide precautions as a nursing measure; monitor energy level and suicidal ideas; encourage activities of daily living (ADLs); teach relaxation techniques; offer support as feelings are expressed; reinforce strengths; assist in compiling list of resources. |
| | **Psychopharmacology:** Fluoxetine 20 mg PO every morning. |
| | **Milieu management:** Encourage patient to stay out of room; request patient attendance at grief and loss, self-esteem, assertiveness, problem-solving, and recreational groups. |
| Evaluation | Patient will stay with daughter after discharge; patient called employer and requested extended sick leave. |
| Referral | Patient made appointment for outpatient counseling; patient has information on divorce recovery group and a 24-hour crisis and suicide hotline. |

## PROCESS RECORDINGS

Peplau (1968) used process recordings in her writings to show applications of concepts and examples of interventions. The use of communication skills is emphasized as a means of helping patients learn and solve problems. Process recordings are tools for the nurse, particularly for the student nurse, to learn about working with patients effectively.

This method provides a means of assessing and analyzing communication skills, identifying patient themes, and evaluating the effectiveness of interventions (Festa et al, 2000). Audiotape or videotape recordings are more accurate compared with written reports, but are not always possible to obtain in most settings or with many patients. Written process recordings might begin with notes taken during the interview or might be completely assembled by recall afterward. A process recording is a record of an encounter with a patient that is as verbatim as possible. The recording generally includes the nonverbal behaviors of the nurse and the patient, as well as the verbal interaction.

Analysis of content, mood, and interaction themes (see Chapter 7) might be included next to each written statement or summarized at the end of the process recording. The process recording might be analyzed by the nurse or shared with a colleague who can provide constructive feedback on problem areas and strategies for improvement. Videotaped nurse–patient clinical simulations can also be used (Festa et al, 2000). The recording is a learning tool, not an end in itself, that can be used periodically for professional growth. A sample written process recording with Mrs. Jarvis was presented earlier in the chapter (see Table 9-1).

### CRITICAL THINKING QUESTION    1

For the patient, Mrs. Jarvis, can you identify two additional nursing diagnoses, two short-term goals, two long-term goals, and four nursing interventions?

### ■ Study Notes

1. The nursing process (a systematic approach to treatment) is relevant in psychiatric nursing practice.
2. The nursing process is a tool used by the nurse to assess each patient's problems, select and carry out specific nursing interventions, and evaluate the effectiveness of these interventions on patient outcomes.
3. The initial patient assessment is holistic and includes data from all members of the multidisciplinary team.
4. Written patient assessments, care plans, and progress notes provide an important means of ensuring consistency and continuity of care.
5. Evaluation of patient progress is a foundation for discharge planning and for referrals to other services within the continuum of care.
6. Process recordings are learning tools used to facilitate professional growth.

### ■ References

Atreja A, Bellam N, Levy SR: Strategies to enhance patient adherence: making it simple, Available at http://*Medscape Gen Med*(1), 2005. Available at http://www.medscape.com. Accessed July 15, 2005.

Benner P: The wisdom of our practice, *Am J Nurs* 100:99, 2000.

Delaney KR, Pitula CR, Perraud S: Psychiatric hospitalization and process description: what will nursing add? *J Psychosoc Nurs Ment Health Serv* 38:7, 2000.

Festa LM, Baliko B, Mangiafico T, Jarosinski J: Maximizing learning outcomes by videotaping nursing students' interactions with a standardized patient, *J Psychosoc Nurs Ment Health Serv* 38:37, 2000.

Martin T, Street AF: Exploring evidence of the therapeutic relationship in forensic psychiatric nursing, *J Psychiatr Ment Health Nurs* 10:543, 2003.

Oermann MH, Huber D: Patient outcomes: a measure of nursing's value, *Am J Nurs* 99:40, 1999.

O'Reilly ML: Spirituality and mental health clients, *J Psychosoc Nurs* 42:44, 2004.

Peplau HE: Psychotherapeutic strategies, *Perspect Psychiatr Care* 6:264, 1968.

Reid WH: Contracting for safety redux, *J Psychiatr Pract* 11:54, 2005.

Walden-McBride DL, McBride JL: Listening for the patient's story, *J Psychosoc Nurs Ment Health Serv* 38:26, 2000.

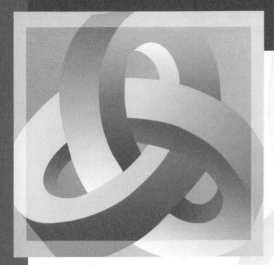

# Chapter 10

# Stress, Anxiety, Coping, and Crisis

*Lee H. Schwecke*

## Learning Objectives

*After reading this chapter, you should be able to:*

- Explain the relationships between anxiety and the neurochemical, emotional, and physiologic responses to anxiety.
- Explain the relationships among stress, anxiety, coping, and crisis.
- Identify common stressors that are likely to cause anxiety.
- Distinguish symptoms reflective of each of the four levels of anxiety.
- Match appropriate nursing interventions to each level of anxiety.

- Describe criteria for evaluating coping mechanisms.
- Identify differences among adaptive, palliative, maladaptive, and dysfunctional coping mechanisms.
- Describe characteristics and effects of crisis situations.
- Outline major crisis intervention goals and strategies.

## STRESS AND ANXIETY

Anxiety in response to stress is inevitable in everyday life. The way in which individuals cope with anxiety and stress is important in understanding the quality with which individuals are functioning in their personal, social, and occupational roles. For nurses in any setting, including nonpsychiatric ones, understanding the nature of anxiety, its causes, the reasons that make it difficult to manage, and the way in which individuals normally cope with it is crucial (Figure 10-1).

## COMMONLY PERCEIVED STRESSORS

The stressor that precipitates anxiety is whatever the individual perceives as a danger, a loss, or a threat to safety and security. The way in which individuals perceive an event depends on their background, needs, desires, self-concept, resources, knowledge, skills, personality traits, and maturity. For example, a skilled athlete might perceive a competitive event as an exciting challenge with a high probability of success. An athlete who is less skilled might perceive the same event as an overwhelming test with a high probability of failure. Each athlete, on the basis of his or her perception of the situation, has different emotional and physical responses (i.e., a different level of anxiety).

Commonalities exist among perceptions of what constitutes a threat, loss, or danger. Individuals typically feel anxious when they perceive a *loss of or threat* to the following:

## Norm's Notes

*I have anxiety and stress, and you have anxiety and stress. Everyone does! The key is to learn how to manage them in your own life and how to help patients both minimize stressors and cope with the stress they have. Anxiety can be miserable and contagious. A good foundation is presented in this chapter for helping you understand these important concepts.*

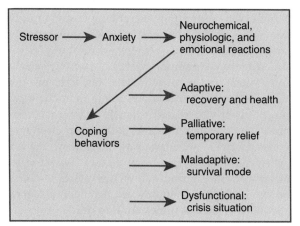

**FIGURE 10-1** Process of anxiety.

1. Health or the ability to perform and function
2. Self-esteem or self-respect
3. Self-control
4. Control or power over one's life
5. Status or prestige
6. Resources (emotional, physical, financial, spiritual, social, cultural)
7. Loved ones
8. Freedom or independence
9. Needs, goals, desires, and expectations

Some threats or losses are external and visible to observers (objective); others are internal and less evident to observers (subjective). The perception of a threat or loss might not seem valid to others; anyone's perceptions can be inaccurate, misinterpreted, exaggerated, or unjustified. For example, a best friend turns down an invitation to dinner, saying that she has to visit her grandmother, who is ill. The best friend has always been honest, but false doubts begin to surface as to whether the friend really cares anymore.

> ### NANDA International Diagnoses Related to Anxiety, Coping, and Crisis*
>
> Adjustment, impaired
> Anxiety
> Breathing pattern, ineffective
> Communication, verbal, impaired
> Conflict, decisional (specify)
> Coping, ineffective
> Fear
> Injury, risk for
> Post-trauma syndrome
> Powerlessness, risk for
> Role performance, ineffective
> Self-esteem, chronic low
> Sensory perception, disturbed
> Sleep patterns, disturbed
> Social interaction, impaired
> Social isolation
> Spiritual distress
> Suicide, risk for
> Thought processes, disturbed
> Violence, other-directed, risk for

*From NANDA International: *NANDA nursing diagnoses: definitions and classifications, 2005-2006,* Philadelphia, 2005, NANDA International.

Stressors might also be classified as maturational or situational. Maturational stressors are experiences that are expected as part of the normal processes of growth and development for most individuals in a particular society (see discussion of Erikson in Chapter 4). For example, in the United States, most individuals start school, leave school, develop relationships, become employed, support families, lose loved ones, and prepare for their own deaths. To varying degrees, these stressors can be anticipated and plans can be made.

Situational stressors are less predictable, and specific actions are taken only when the threat is eminent or after the event has occurred. General precautions might be possible. For example, most individuals recognize that acute illnesses and accidents can happen, so they purchase health, life, and car insurance but they do not know exactly when, where, or how serious the illness or accident will be. Natural disasters and disasters of human origin, such as hurricanes, tornadoes, earthquakes, terrorist attacks, and explosions, fall into this category. Some situational stressors have early warning signs that an individual might ignore until the threat is more eminent or obvious, such as war, divorce, layoff from work, and chronic illness.

## RECURRING THEMES OF ANXIETY

Anxiety as a concept and process has been studied, defined, and described by many respected authors such as Peplau (1952), Sullivan (1953), Lazarus (1966), Levitt (1967), Beck and Clark (1997), and Aguilera (1998). Anxiety has been described as:

- Subjective experience that can be detected only by objective behaviors that result from it
- Emotional pain
- Apprehension, fearfulness, or a sense of powerlessness resulting from a threat that is less visible or definable than is fear that has a visible object or trigger
- Warning sign of a perceived danger or threat
- Emotional response that triggers behaviors (automatic relief behaviors) aimed at eliminating the anxiety
- Alerting an individual to prepare for self-defense
- Occurring in degrees
- Contagious; communicated from one person to another
- Part of a process, not an isolated phenomenon

## GENERAL ETIOLOGY OF ANXIETY

### Psychodynamic Model

Freud viewed the ego as the part of the personality that develops defenses to help individuals to control or cope with anxiety (see Chapter 4). The need to control anxiety stems from conflicts between the id (instincts) and the superego (conscience) (Freud, 1936). Feelings, which are connected with early conflicts, are repressed.

Later in life, as conflicts are once again experienced, the defenses fail, and these feelings emerge, causing anxiety and discomfort. Freud (1936) viewed unrealistic or neurotic anxiety as the fear that instincts will cause the individual to do something that results in punishment.

### Interpersonal Model

Sullivan (1953) examined interpersonal relations and the socialization process, which are important to how individuals feel about themselves (see Chapter 4). Sullivan regarded individuals as striving for security and relief from anxiety to protect their self-systems. In childhood, individuals take on the values of their parents and family to receive approval and to feel good about themselves. Later in life, a threat to the self is based on how individuals perceive the danger or threat and on how they were taught early in life to handle conflict. Issues of dependency, control, and security, and related conflicts, form the basis of handling anxiety.

### Biologic Model

Selye (1956) found that the effects of stress might be observed by the objective measurement of structural and clinical changes in the body. Selye called these changes the *general adaptation syndrome* (see Chapter 4). More recent research on the effects of anxiety and the resulting neurochemical reactions has centered on the hypothalamic-pituitary-adrenal axis, the hypothalamic-pituitary-gonadal axis, and the limbic system reward pathway. The information in this section is meant to convey the significance of the effects of stress on the body. It is complex and detailed, and goes beyond the level of understanding needed by psychiatric nursing students. For those particularly interested in psychobiology, however, the material here can be related to the information in Chapter 6.

Major neurochemical changes identified as affected by stress include the following (Aguilera, 1998; Charney, 2004; Eisner, 2004; Hoffart and Keene, 1998; Taylor et al, 2001):

- Increased regional epinephrine and norepinephrine turnover in the locus ceruleus, limbic regions, and cerebral cortex
- Increased corticotropin-releasing hormone (CRH) and dehydroepiandrosterone (DHEA)
- Increased adrenocorticotropic hormone (ACTH) and corticosterone levels
- Increased dopamine release in the prefrontal cortex and decreased release in the nucleus accumbens
- Increased endogenous opiate release
- Increased glucocorticoid (cortisol) levels
- Increased thyrotropin-releasing hormone (TRH)
- Increased thyroid-stimulating hormone (TSH)
- Increased peripheral sympathetic nervous system activity

- Altered function of the serotonin receptors
- Decreased benzodiazepine receptor binding
- Decreased testosterone levels
- Increased estrogen levels

Anxiety-related responses are critical for surviving and tolerating dangerous situations. Increased noradrenergic and dopaminergic system activity (leading to central nervous system [CNS] hyperarousal and hypervigilance) facilitates rapid behavioral reactions. Tolerating fear and pain associated with serious injuries is enhanced by increased release of endogenous opiates (allowing emotional blunting and physical analgesia). Increased cortisol levels, resulting in metabolic activation, facilitate increased physical activity (Charney, 2004). However, the effectiveness of these responses fades if the individual is continuously exposed to the stressor (Clements and Turpin, 2000). This decrease in effectiveness is related to the alterations in the catecholamine and thyroid systems and the depressed immune system. These effects and a deficiency in serotonin might increase the risk of suicide (Jiwanlal and Weitzel, 2001).

If the threshold set point for anxiety is changed and the allostatic load (a burden with long-term physiologic and psychological effects) occurs, then the individual becomes increasingly sensitive to subsequent stressors, which more easily reactivate the anxiety-related response. The locus ceruleus–norepinephrine system plays a role in chronic anxiety, intrusive memories, and fear (Charney, 2004; Hoffart and Keene, 1998). This tendency is discussed in relation to acute stress disorder (ASD) and posttraumatic stress disorder (PTSD) in Chapter 31. A stress cycle can begin to occur in which physical and psychological symptoms cause additional stress, negative thinking, and fears. These reactions lead to reactivation of the stress response, resulting in increasingly severe or frequent symptoms, or both. Eventually, other symptoms, such as irritability, muscle tension, headaches, back pain, insomnia, gastrointestinal disturbances, hypertension, palpitations, insulin resistance, decreased immune function, increased abdominal fat, and cardiovascular disease, might develop (Charney, 2004; Eisner, 2004; Hoffart and Keene, 1998; Soderstrom et al, 2000). In contrast, if the original stress is resolved, the body can return to normal (a relaxation response) through activation of the parasympathetic nervous system and the decreased activity in the hypothalamus and pituitary. Galanin (a peptide) and neuropeptide Y play a role in decreasing anxiety responses (Charney, 2004; Hoffart and Keene, 1998; Jech, 2001; Taylor et al, 2001).

## LEVELS OF ANXIETY

To assess how patients are responding to the feeling of anxiety generated by a stressor, the nurse should assess patients' perceptions of and reactions to the stressor (subjective). Another way of assessing the severity of responses to a stressor is to observe behaviors (objective). Table 10-1 describes the psychomotor, emotional, and cognitive symptoms of four levels of anxiety, as well as the nursing interventions for each level.

Even a moderate level of anxiety (+2) is uncomfortable and difficult to tolerate. As anxiety increases, a drive to relieve the anxiety as soon as possible develops. Converting anxiety to anger to regain a sense of powerfulness is a common coping method (Rioch, 2003). Selye's stress model, included in Chapter 4, identifies stages of responses that result from the feeling of anxiety. Long-lasting high levels of anxiety (+3 and +4) are physically and emotionally draining to the extent that an individual will do almost anything to escape the pain, such as becoming ill (physically or emotionally) or, in rare instances, even committing suicide. Fortunately, many less debilitating and more productive ways to cope with anxiety are available.

## COPING WITH ANXIETY

Methods of coping with anxiety and the resulting neurochemical, emotional, and physiologic reactions can be divided into four categories, according to the degree of *effectiveness* in decreasing anxiety or eliminating the source of anxiety (Table 10-2).

Although effectiveness is the primary criterion for evaluating a coping method, *outcomes* must also be considered. Sometimes, coping reduces the anxiety and solves the problem but, at the same time, creates other significant problems. Stealing class notes from a friend might result in both an examination score of an A and permanent damage to the friendship. *Duration* and *frequency* of coping methods must be also considered. Prolonged late-night studying might yield an A on a test, but might result in reduced resistance to a virus and

## Table 10-1    Levels of Anxiety

| Levels of Anxiety and Interventions | SYMPTOMS | | |
| --- | --- | --- | --- |
| | **Psychomotor** | **Emotional** | **Cognitive** |
| **Mild: +1**<br>Discuss source of anxiety (steps of learning)<br>Problem solve<br>Accept anxiety as natural; tolerate and benefit from it | Preparation of body for constructive action<br>Slight muscle tension<br>Slight fidgeting<br>Energetic<br>Good eye contact | Occasional slight irritability<br>Feeling challenged<br>Confident<br>(Use of adaptive coping mechanisms) | Alertness<br>Awareness of surroundings<br>Concentration<br>Accurate perceptions<br>Attentiveness<br>Logical reasoning and problem-solving skills |
| **Moderate: +2**<br>Decrease anxiety—ventilation, crying, exercise, relaxation techniques<br>Refocus attention; relate feelings and behaviors to anxiety; then use problem-solving techniques; give oral medication, if needed | Preparation of body for protective action<br>Moderate muscle tension<br>Increased blood pressure, pulse, and respirations<br>Startle reflex<br>Slight perspiration<br>Difficulty sitting still<br>Repeated fidgeting<br>Periodic slow pacing<br>Increased rate of speech<br>Sporadic eye contact | Feeling uncomfortable, on edge, keyed up<br>Motivated to decrease anxiety<br>Increased irritability<br>Decreased confidence<br>(Use of palliative coping mechanisms) | Difficulty in concentrating<br>Easily distracted, can focus with assistance<br>Circumstantiality<br>Tangentiality<br>Loose associations<br>Narrowed perceptions<br>Decreased attention span<br>Misperception of stimuli<br>Problem solving and reasoning skills with effort, or assistance |
| **Severe: +3**<br>Decrease anxiety, stimuli, and pressure<br>Use kind, firm, simple directions<br>Use time out (seclusion)<br>Give intramuscular medications, if needed | Preparation of body for flight or fight<br>Extreme muscle tension<br>Increased perspiration<br>Continuous and rapid pacing<br>Reflex responses<br>Loud or rapid speech, or both<br>Poor eye contact<br>Somatic symptoms<br>Sleep disturbance | Extreme discomfort<br>Feeling of dread<br>Hypersensitivity<br>Defensiveness with threats and demand<br>(Use of maladaptive coping mechanisms) | Distorted perceptions<br>Difficulty focusing, even with assistance<br>Flight of ideas<br>Ineffective reasoning and problem-solving skills<br>Disorientation<br>Delusions and hallucinations, if prolonged<br>Suicidal or homicidal ideations, if prolonged |
| **Panic: +4**<br>Guide firmly, or physically take control<br>Give intramuscular medication<br>Order restraints, if needed | Actual flight, fight, or immobilization<br>Suicide attempts or violence<br>Depletion of body resources<br>Eyes fixed<br>Hysterical or mute<br>Incoherent | Feeling overwhelmed and out of control<br>Rage<br>Desperation<br>Feeling totally drained<br>(Use of dysfunctional coping mechanisms) | Disorganized perceptions<br>Disorganized or irrational reasoning and problem solving<br>Neologisms<br>Clang associations<br>Word salad<br>Out of contact with reality<br>Personality disorganization |

Data from Longo D, Williams R: *Clinical practice in psychosocial nursing: assessment and intervention*, New York, 1986, Appleton-Century-Crofts; Peplau HE: *Interpersonal relations in nursing*, New York, 1952, Putnam; Selye H: *The stress of life*, New York, 1956, McGraw-Hill; Sullivan HS: *The psychiatric interview*, New York, 1954, Norton.

an episode of influenza. Excessive studying might lead to a poorly balanced life of work, love, and play. Thus, a coping method must be examined for its primary effectiveness and for its consequences on the patient's well-being and relationships.

### CRITICAL THINKING QUESTION    1

What symptoms of each level of anxiety have you experienced at different times? Match these with various coping mechanisms you have used to deal with the anxiety levels.

**Table 10-2   Coping With Anxiety**

| Type of Coping | Description | Common Use | Patient Example |
|---|---|---|---|
| Adaptive | Solves the problem that is causing the anxiety, so the anxiety is decreased. The patient is objective, rational, and productive. | Anxiety about an upcoming examination is reduced by studying effectively and passing the examination with a grade of A. | Anxiety about the discharge from the hospital is handled by writing down medications, dates and times of follow-up appointments, and self-help meetings in a calendar. The patient keeps appointments and attends two self-help meetings, takes medications, and returns to work. |
| Palliative | Temporarily decreases the anxiety but does not solve the problem, so the anxiety eventually returns. Temporary relief allows the patient to return to problem solving. | Anxiety about the examination is temporarily reduced by jogging for half an hour. Effective studying is then possible and a grade of A is still achievable. | Anxiety about the discharge is handled by watching television in the evening. In the morning, the patient takes the discharge instructions written by the nurse and puts them in his pocket. He keeps his first follow-up appointment and attends one self-help meeting. He takes his medications and is able to return to work. |
| Maladaptive | Unsuccessful attempts to decrease the anxiety without attempting to solve the problem. The anxiety remains. | Anxiety about the examination is first ignored by going to a movie and then handled by frantically cramming for a few hours. A passing grade of C is obtained. | Anxiety about the discharge is handled by saying that he remembers all the appointments and meetings, and that directions for the medications will be on the bottles. He misses the meetings and his appointment, but makes another appointment when called. He takes his AM and PM medication but forgets the noon dose all week. He goes to work but complains of being anxious all day. |
| Dysfunctional | Is not successful in reducing anxiety or solving the problem. Even minimal functioning becomes difficult, and new problems begin to develop. | Anxiety about the examination is first ignored by going out drinking with friends and then escaped by passing out for the night. A grade of F results and the course has to be repeated. | Anxiety about the discharge is handled by ignoring the nurse and starting an argument with another patient. When asked to take a time out, the patient leaves the hospital without being discharged; his bill is not paid by insurance. He does not get his prescriptions and is brought back to the hospital in 3 weeks. |

A major role of psychiatric nurses is to help patients learn or regain highly effective coping strategies and avoid ineffective or destructive strategies, including most defense mechanisms. To do this, the nurse must identify the strategies that the patient knows and is using, those that the patient knows but is not using, and those that the patient does not know. The nurse often assumes that patients know more about adaptive coping than they really do. The most common *adaptive* coping techniques taught and encouraged include:

- Problem solving
- Assertiveness
- Positive self-talk and self-acceptance
- Stress and anger management
- Learning skills needed for communication and relationships
- Conflict resolution
- Time management
- Community living skills

Strategies are also available for temporarily tolerating and decreasing the effects of anxiety, although these *palliative* techniques do not directly manage the cause of the stress and anxiety (Flannery, 2004; La Torre, 2003; Miller, 2005; O'Haver Day and Horton-Deutsch, 2004; O'Reilly, 2004; Ott, 2004; Washington and Moxley, 2004; Webster et al, 2005); These strategies include:

- Visualization, guided imagery, prayer, and mindfulness-based meditation: creating a safe, relaxing place, using some or all of the five senses, which enhances a sense of security and decreases tension and worry
- Concentrating on breathing and striving for slow, long, deep breathing
- Relaxation training for decreasing tension and increasing muscle relaxation
- Engaging in stretching exercises, such as yoga
- Adopting a healthy lifestyle, such as a balanced diet, quality sleep, and exercise routine
- Avoiding smoking, alcohol, and other substances
- Decreasing unhealthy and self-destructive behaviors or coping, such as avoidance of issues
- Engaging in laughter, hobbies, and noncompetitive activities that are fun
- Spending time with caring, supportive, and optimistic people for social support
- Reducing competing activities and commitments, when possible
- Living within one's means, avoiding debt
- Using cognitive restructuring to decrease a negative view of self, others, problems, and life; replacing these with affirming, positive, and empowering thoughts
- Striving to increase a sense of self-confidence and mastery in solving problems
- Engaging in personal growth activities and increasing self-awareness
- Listening to favorite calming and positive music
- Getting a massage (body, hands, and feet), with or without aromatherapy

Coping strategies take time to learn and use consistently. During a short-term hospitalization or program, the nurse begins the education process, but this should be continued in an after-care program. New skills need ongoing reinforcement until they become habits. (See Chapter 31 for "Key Nursing Intervention to Reduce Anxiety" and "Key Nursing Interventions in Problem-Solving.")

## CLINICAL EXAMPLE

Latasha was admitted to the hospital after a suicide attempt. She said that she was overwhelmed with problems and work, as well as with taking care of her aging parents in her home. "I just couldn't take any more stress. I'm not sleeping or eating right. I never have time for myself. My new boss is a demanding bitch who wants us to do all of her work for her." After affirming that she actually did not want to die, she agreed to make a list of the three most important stressors that she wanted to confront in the next 2 days. For each of these stressors, she identified a realistic goal and initial steps to take toward resolving the problems they cause, along with a reasonable time frame for accomplishing the goal. Latasha then listed three activities that might be put on hold. Latasha began practicing relaxation and visualization techniques to use periodically during the day and at bedtime to decrease body tension and anxiety. She agreed that she needed to resume her exercise routine and eating healthy meals while listening to her favorite music.

## RELATIONSHIP BETWEEN ANXIETY AND ILLNESS

Individuals feel increasing pain and discomfort as anxiety escalates from moderate to severe and then to panic levels. To feel better, these individuals might use behaviors and defense mechanisms to protect themselves. Such behaviors are individualized. For instance, biologic and genetic endowments influence reactions to stress. An individual is born with unique personality traits, predispositions, and physiologic and neurologic systems. If long-term palliative, maladaptive, or dysfunctional coping behaviors are displayed, then an anxiety-related disorder, a physiologic health problem, or even a psychosis might develop. For example, the stress-vulnerability model has been one explanation for the development of schizophrenia: "genetic, physiological, psychological and social predispositions" cause vulnerability under stress, which can lead to the illness (Rathod and Turkington, 2005).

## CRISIS

Any stressful event or hazardous situation has the potential for precipitating a crisis (Lindemann, 1956). Just as with types of stress (see earlier discussion of losses and threats), crises can be maturational or situational, but also might affect a family, a community, or a nation (e.g., as in response to September 11 or Hurricane Katrina). The event or situation that comes at the end of a series of stressors might appear minor, but it can make the situation more than the individual can handle (i.e., the proverbial "straw that breaks the camel's back"). A crisis differs from stress in that a crisis results in a period of severe disorganization resulting from the failure of an individual's usual coping mechanisms, the lack of usual resources, or both. The feeling of being totally out of control, and being unable to function on a daily basis, is extremely frightening and motivates individuals to take measures to escape the situation and pain (Caplan, 1961).

## INDIVIDUAL REACTIONS

Anxiety generally rises to a severe or panic level during a crisis (see Table 10-1). Individuals feel a sense of overwhelming helplessness and hopelessness when nothing appears to be working; they might feel immobilized and either give up or keep trying the same, ineffective coping methods. Individuals in a crisis need and are generally receptive to help. During the period of disorganization, being dependent on others for guidance and assistance is a natural tendency. (Trust is less of an issue at this time.) The right type of help at the right time generally enables individuals to overcome the problem, regain equilibrium, and return to normal. It is common for individuals to learn new coping skills and/or develop new or improved relationships with others, so they might begin functioning better than they did before the crisis occurred. This tendency is why a crisis is said to have growth-promoting potential (Aguilera, 1998).

The disorganization period of a crisis is distressing in that it usually cannot be tolerated emotionally or physically for more than 4 to 6 weeks. If the right type of help is unavailable and the crisis is not successfully resolved during that period, then the individual in crisis might become exhausted and physically ill, adopt dysfunctional coping patterns that manage the intense feelings without solving the problems (i.e., become emotionally ill), become violent, or attempt suicide to escape the pain. Suicide assessment for those in crisis, especially if there is a history of self-harm behaviors, is essential (Cassells et al, 2005). (See Chapter 29 for details on suicide assessment and

intervention.) Dysfunctional patterns of coping tend to persist unless the individual seeks intensive counseling for a prolonged period. Intervening during the crisis to prevent the development of dysfunctional coping patterns, rather than intervening after the crisis has occurred, takes less time and is more effective.

---

**CRITICAL THINKING QUESTION**    **2**

You are seeing a patient in an obstetrician's office. She has been complaining of anxiety and lack of sleep for 2 weeks. What list of questions would you ask to assess her stressors, level of anxiety, and coping mechanisms? List the type of intervention needed.

---

## STRATEGIES OF CRISIS INTERVENTION

Crisis intervention is appropriate whenever a crisis occurs for an individual in any setting. Crisis strategies begin with identifying the point at which the crisis began in response to the stressor or series of stressors, and the resultant way in which the individual's life is being affected. The initial focus is on immediate actions needed to prevent harm to self, harm to others, or further decompensation (survival, safety, and security). In comparison to working with stressed individuals, the nurse using crisis intervention strategies is more active and directive. It might be necessary to make decisions on behalf of the individual and provide concrete instructions on what to do next, whom to call, and where to go. The nurse might call emergency services or family and friends to come to help or to talk individuals through actions step by step until they are able to make decisions or take actions on their own. Box 10-1 presents specific crisis intervention strategies. Also, refer back to Chapters 7 and 8 for specific details and techniques.

Working with an individual in crisis is demanding and intense for a short period, usually a few days to a few weeks. Therefore, the nurse must involve the individual's significant others, who can help over time. With the trend of shorter hospital stays and patients being managed primarily in outpatient treatment settings, patients are admitted to the hospital only when they cannot function (to meet their basic needs for food, clothing, and shelter) or are at risk of harming

## Box 10-1  Crisis Intervention Strategies

1. Focus on survival, safety, and security:
   a. Assess for and prevent suicide, violence, decompensation, and reactivation of serious medical or psychiatric problems.
   b. Arrange for urgent medical care if needed.
   c. Allow for expression of feelings, especially fear and anger, without allowing a loss of control.
   d. Assess for the effects of the crisis on thinking and functioning (e.g., decision making, sleeping, eating).
   e. Validate reactions and feelings as normal—as typical reactions to an atypical situation.
   f. Decrease the sense of loss of control and overwhelming helplessness, hopelessness, and powerlessness by providing specific information about assistance available.
   g. Identify immediately available family and/or friends who can provide support and assistance, especially for food, shelter, and clothing.
   h. If the individual is hospitalized, offer prn medications if appropriate.
2. Reestablish equilibrium and stabilization:
   a. Use quick anxiety reduction strategies.
   b. Offer support, realistic reassurance, information, and education.
   c. Facilitate a sense of control over self and the situation.
   d. Intervene with dysfunctional coping mechanisms.
   e. Counteract irrational thinking and negativity.
3. Focus on strengths and adaptive coping:
   a. Encourage use of adaptive coping and personal, spiritual, family, and community resources.
   b. Involve available support systems as soon as possible and assist them with education and in accessing resources.
   c. Use techniques for reframing, cognitive restructuring, and reality testing.
4. Offer suggestions for concrete, specific problem solving:
   a. Focus on here and now reality, rather than underlying or long-term issues.
   b. Assist in decisions and setting priorities for immediate actions needed.
   c. Encourage activities of daily living, especially food and fluids.
   d. Encourage use of prescribed medications, as directed, if there are medical or psychiatric illnesses.
   e. Arrange for assessment of the need for hospitalization if indicated.
5. Make provisions for follow-up care:
   a. Arrange for monitoring for 2 to 3 months, because the risk for suicide can persist.
   b. Assess for underlying needs and problems requiring short-term counseling and make referrals, as needed.
   c. Teach and encourage use of adaptive coping strategies.
   d. Encourage use of personal and community resources for prevention of future crises.
   e. Make long-term counseling referrals if the crisis is not resolving or for chronic issues or illnesses.
   f. Refer to support or self-help groups, as appropriate.

Data from Bilsker and Forster, 2003; Cassells et al, 2005; Everly, 2004; O'Haver Day and Horton-Deutsch, 2004; O'Reilly, 2004.

themselves or others. Although patients might be in crisis for 4 to 6 weeks, they are not hospitalized for this length of time. Therefore, ideally, the nurse collaborates with and makes referrals to an outpatient treatment facility or to other community resources within the continuum of care.

Crisis intervention can be offered in various ways. Walk-in crisis units, teams in a mental health center, or mobile crisis teams who see individuals in their homes, in community clinics, or in hospital emergency departments are available. Many communities and mental health centers offer 24-hour telephone crisis support (hotlines). Mobile disaster teams are often sent to areas in which tragedies have occurred, such as hurricanes, floods, earthquakes, tornadoes, or the bombing of a building. These disaster teams might use one of several models for assisting individuals and groups of victims to talk about their experiences and deal with acute crisis reactions in an effort to prevent PTSD (Mitchell, 2004; see Chapter 31).

## CLINICAL EXAMPLE

Jalen, 19 years old, was admitted after an episode of acting out that involved breaking light fixtures and furniture in his room. His father called the police when he threatened to get his friend's gun and "kill everyone in sight." His father said Jalen has not been sleeping well, has been staying in his room too long, and has been refusing to eat for the last 3 days, since his best friend was killed in a gang-related drive-by shooting. Jalen signed a no-harm contract. He refused to complete the admission interview but agreed to take an oral antianxiety medication. He went to sleep for 14 hours. After awakening, Jalen was tearful at times, but still extremely angry. Jalen admitted he needed help to deal with the "senseless murder" of his friend. He chose to use a punching bag each time his anger got out of control. Afterward, he was able to talk about his sadness and guilt about not protecting his friend. Within 2 days, Jalen made a list of ways to deal with his anger and grief, including visiting his friend's family (because he had missed the funeral), seeing an outpatient counselor, and attending a meeting of the Survivors of Homicide support group.

## Study Notes

1. A stressor is any event or circumstance that an individual perceives as a threat, loss, or danger.
2. Anxiety has been described in a variety of ways and can generate a variety of responses.
3. Based on Peplau's model, four levels of anxiety have been identified: mild, moderate, severe, and panic.
4. Nursing interventions vary according to the patient's level of anxiety.
5. Evaluating patients' adaptive, palliative, maladaptive, and dysfunctional coping mechanisms is crucial.
6. A crisis results in a period of severe disorganization resulting from the failure of an individual's usual coping mechanisms, the lack of usual resources, or both.
7. Crisis intervention strategies concentrate on the immediate precipitant, as well as on the individual's physical safety and emotional security.

## References

Aguilera DC: Crisis intervention: theory and methodology, ed 8, St. Louis, 1998, Mosby.

Beck AT, Clark DA: An information processing model of anxiety: automatic and strategic processing, Behav Res Ther 35:49, 1997.

Bilsker D, Forster P: Problem-solving interventions for suicidal crises in the psychiatric emergency service, Crisis 24:134, 2003.

Caplan G: An approach to community mental health, New York, 1961, Grune & Stratton.

Cassells C, Paterson B, Dowding D, Morrison D: Long- and short-term risk factors in the prediction of inpatient suicide: a review of the literature, Crisis 26:53, 2005.

Charney DS: Psychobiological mechanisms of resilience and vulnerability: Implications for successful adaptation to extreme stress, Am J Psychiatry 161:195, 2004.

Clements K, Turpin G: Life event exposure, physiological reactivity, and psychological strain, J Behav Med 23:73, 2000.

Eisner R: Stresses stress in his research: a profile of Bruce McEwen, Ph.D., NARSAD Research Newslett 16(3):1, 2004.

Everly GS: Pastoral crisis intervention: a word of caution, Int J Emerg Ment Health 6:211, 2004.

Flannery RB: Managing stress in today's age: a concise guide of emergency services personnel, Int J Emerg Ment Health 6:205, 2004.

Freud S: The problem of anxiety, New York, 1936, Norton.

Hoffart MB, Keene EP: The benefits of visualization, Am J Nurs 98:44, 1998.

Jech AO: (2001, September 30). Calming the cognitively impaired, Nursing Spectrum (Metro edition).

Jiwanlal SS, Weitzel C: The suicide myth, RN 64:33, 2001.

La Torre MA: The use of music and sound to enhance the therapeutic setting, Perspect Psychiatr Care 39:129, 2003.

Lazarus RS: Psychological stress and the coping process, St. Louis, 1966, McGraw-Hill.

Levitt E: The psychology of anxiety, Indianapolis, 1967, Bobbs-Merrill.

Lindemann E: The meaning of crisis in the individual and family, Teachers College Record 57:310, 1956.

Mitchell JT: Characteristics of successful early intervention programs, Int J Emerg Ment Health 6:175, 2004.

Miller CM, editor: Meditation in psychotherapy, Harv Ment Health Lett 21:1, 2005.

O'Haver Day P, Horton-Deutsch S: Using mindfulness-based therapeutic interventions in psychiatric nursing practice—part II: Mindfulness-based approaches for all phases of psychotherapy—clinical case study, Arch Psychiatr Nurs 18:170, 2004.

O'Reilly ML: Spirituality and mental health clients, J Psychosoc Nurs 42:44, 2004.

Ott MJ: Mindfulness meditation: A path of transformation and healing, J Psychosoc Nurs 42:23, 2004.

Peplau HE: Interpersonal relations in nursing, New York, 1952, Putnam.

Rathod S, Turkington D: Cognitive-behavioral therapy for schizophrenia: A review. Available at http://www.medscape.com. Accessed August 12, 2005.

Rioch DM: Reflections on Sullivan and the language of psychiatry, Psychiatry 66:89, 2003.

Selye H: The stress of life, St. Louis, 1956, McGraw-Hill.

Soderstrom M, Dolbier C, Leiferman J, Steinhardt M: The relationship of hardiness, coping strategies, and perceived stress to symptoms of illness, J Behav Med 23:311, 2000.

Sullivan HS: Interpersonal theory of psychiatry, New York, 1953, Norton.

Taylor SE, Klein LC, Lewis BP, et al: Biobehavioral responses to stress in females: tend-and-befriend, not fight-or-flight, Psychol Rev 107:411, 2001.

Washington OGM, Moxley DP: Using scrapbooks and portfolios in group work with women who are chemically dependent, J Psychosoc Nurs 42:42, 2004.

Webster S, Clare A, Collier E: Creative solutions: Innovative use of the arts in mental health settings, J Psychosoc Nurs 43:42, 2005.

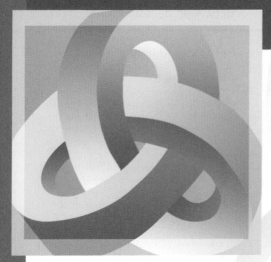

# Chapter 11

# Working With the Aggressive Patient

*Lee H. Schwecke*

## Learning Objectives

*After reading this chapter, you should be able to:*
- Describe the differences among anger, aggression, passive aggression, and assertiveness.
- Recognize the individual, sociocultural, and social-psychological models of aggression.
- Describe the five stages of the assault cycle.
- Recognize the characteristics of intermittent explosive disorder.
- Explain the verbal nursing interventions for anger and nonviolent aggression.
- Recognize the external control interventions appropriate with the escalation and crisis phases of the assault cycle.
- Describe the nursing care of patients in seclusion and restraints.
- Explain the interventions needed to support a staff victim of patient assault.

## ANGER AND RELATED CONCEPTS

### ANGER

Anger is a normal human emotion crucial for individual growth; it is a factor present in all relationships, as is conflict. When handled appropriately and expressed assertively (directly, without violating the rights of the self or others), anger and conflict are positive creative forces that lead to problem solving and productive change (Horton-Deutsch and Horton, 2003). When channeled inappropriately and expressed as verbal aggression (verbal attacks on others) or physical aggression, anger is a destructive and potentially life-threatening force. Anger might be expressed indirectly as passive aggression (e.g., sarcasm, pouting), or it might be passively internalized and lead to unpleasant emotional and physical problems. All of these can lead to difficulties in communication and destructive conflicts with others (Horton-Deutsch and Horton, 2003).

The focus of this chapter is on the individual patient's expressions of anger with the nursing staff and individuals in inpatient or outpatient psychiatric settings. However, it is important for nurses to recognize that anger and aggression occur in any setting, including emergency rooms, medical and surgical units, nursing homes, community health settings, and clinics. Non-psychiatric staff might be less familiar with anticipating, preventing, and managing aggression compared with psychiatric nursing staff members, who are trained in assessing and defusing anger and in safely managing aggressive behaviors.

### AGGRESSION

Everyone experiences feelings of anger, but aggressive displays of anger are considered socially

## Norm's Notes

*If there is one aspect of psychiatric nursing that most students (and many practicing RNs) fear, it is confrontation with an angry, aggressive, and/or violent mentally ill person. I don't blame you for feeling that way—in some ways it is good, because it can motivate you to learn the material in this chapter. Aggressive outbursts, both verbal and physical, do happen, but the good news is that it is not nearly as often as you might have imagined. This chapter provides important concepts on how to prevent (i.e., de-escalate) aggressiveness and how to deal with aggression when it occurs.*

inappropriate and are discouraged in American society. When adults in this culture aggressively express their anger toward someone, the recipient generally responds with fear, frustration, and avoidance of the aggressor, when possible. The recipient of anger might also feel helpless, guilty, defensive, or angry. Occasionally, the recipient might retaliate, seek revenge, or hold a grudge.

Visibly angry behaviors span a continuum from mild irritation and arguing to verbal or physical abuse of the self or others to uncontrolled violence (Table 11-1). Externally expressed anger might lead to assault (any behavior that is physically or verbally aggressive and presents an immediate threat of physical injury to a person or property). Carrying out the threat of injury is defined as battery and includes actions such as hitting, kicking, pulling hair, throwing a chair, biting, and scratching, but does not include verbal abuse.

Nurses have the right and responsibility, both professionally and legally, to use physical restraint to prevent patients from injuring themselves and others. Nursing interventions are based on the principle of the least restrictive alternative, meaning that the nurse will first try to set limits in a humane and least restrictive manner (e.g., talking and oral medications) to ensure the safety and security of patients and others. Physical restraint cannot be used unless eminent danger of physical injury exists (see discussion in Chapter 5).

In psychiatric settings, assault is never tolerated, but normal procedure might allow controlled physical aggression, such as using a punching bag

or foam bats or hitting a bed pillow, but the individual would be stopped from damaging furniture or hitting others. If a patient hits a staff member, the staff member is not allowed to strike back, but the patient might then be restricted with seclusion or restraints. Nurses must be familiar with regulations that govern the use of seclusion and restraints in their state and facility.

## VERBAL AGGRESSION OR ABUSE

Verbally aggressive attacks on others tend to have a repetitive pattern and indicate a major warning sign of assault and battery. Verbal aggression tends to provoke unproductive counterreactions that seldom result in constructive solutions to problems. (Reactions tend to be the same as the recipient's reactions to physical aggression described earlier.)

Social norms influence the degree and amount of verbal aggression that are tolerated. At a sporting event, fans are allowed to scream, swear, and be verbally abusive, especially toward referees and umpires. However, the same behaviors toward an employer are not tolerated. (Note that society does seem to be getting tougher on decreasing physical aggression at sporting events, especially those involving youth sports.) A brother might verbally pick on his sister, but he stops the same behavior of another child toward his sister. In a psychiatric setting, the quiet mumbling or swearing by a patient with schizophrenia or an organic brain syndrome might be ignored. The louder swearing of a patient who is in contact with reality is not tolerated, especially if directed toward a patient who is unable to respond assertively. If two relatively competent patients are arguing, staff members might not intervene, except with brief suggestions, to allow patients to undergo the positive experience of conflict resolution. If one of those patients is less competent, though, staff members might stop the argument as soon as it begins.

## PASSIVE AGGRESSION AND PASSIVITY

Passive-aggressive individuals express their anger indirectly and undermine others in various subtle, evasive ways (see Table 11-1). They tend to deny the anger and its source, even when confronted about their behaviors, because they are afraid of rejection or punishment. A passive-aggressive person has difficulty discussing issues and maintaining a

| Table 11-1 | Possible Sources and Expressions of Anger | | |
|---|---|---|---|
| **TURNED OUTWARD** | | **TURNED INWARD** | |
| **Overt Anger** | **Passive Aggression** | **Subjective Signs** | **Objective Signs** |
| Verbalization of anger | Impatience, intolerance | Feeling upset, tense | Crying |
| Irritation, hostility | Pouting, sulking | Unhappiness | Self-destructive behavior |
| Pacing with agitation | Frustration, annoyance | Feeling hurt | Self-mutilation |
| Swearing, verbal abuse | Tense facial expressions | Disappointment | Substance abuse |
| Contempt | Pessimism | Guilt, inferiority | Suicide |
| Clenched fists | Resentment, jealousy | Low self-esteem | Self-sabotage |
| Insulting remarks | Bitterness, complaining | Sense of failure | Sabotaging offers of |
| Intimidation | Deceptive sweetness | Humiliation | assistance |
| Bragging about violent acts | Resistance, stubbornness | Somatic symptoms | Undermining relationships |
| Sadistic, malicious acts | Cynicism, sarcasm | Sense of harassment | |
| Verbal abuse | Intentional forgetting | Envy | |
| Temper tantrums | Noncompliance | Alienation | |
| Violation of others' rights | Procrastination | Demoralization | |
| Deviance, defiance | Belittling remarks | Depression | |
| Screaming | Faultfinding | Resignation, apathy | |
| Rage, assault | Manipulation | Powerlessness | |
| Argumentativeness | Power struggles | Helplessness | |
| Threats: words or weapons | Unfair teasing | Desperation | |
| Damage to property | Sabotage of others | | |
| Rape, homicide | Domination | | |

quality relationship; they are often inefficient in accomplishing tasks and frustrate those around them.

Passive individuals turn their anger inward (see Table 11-1), might be unaware of their underlying anger, and see themselves as good, kind, congenial, and helpful. They replace their anger with fear and indirectly damage, destroy, or avoid relationships and intimacy. Passive individuals are unable to say "no" and believe that others take advantage of them. Passive individuals waste energy, seldom achieve their goals, and show signs of distress through low self-esteem, depression, substance abuse, physical illnesses, and suicide attempts.

## ASSERTIVENESS

One of the widely accepted methods for replacing aggressive, passive–aggressive, and passive behaviors is healthy assertiveness—the direct expression of feelings and needs in a way that respects the rights of others and the self (Dunbar, 2004). Assertive individuals use their energy constructively to achieve goals and build productive relationships. Assertiveness training is aimed at teaching individuals the behavioral skills needed

to interact successfully with others. Training uses various behavior modification techniques, such as relaxation training, homework assignments, and role playing with feedback.

## ETIOLOGY OF AGGRESSION

## INDIVIDUAL, SOCIAL-PSYCHOLOGICAL, AND SOCIOCULTURAL MODELS

Individual models explain violence using stress models (see Chapter 4) and biologically based explanations of aggression (Miczek et al, 2002). Research continues to focus on areas of the limbic system, the frontal lobe, and the temporal lobe. The neurotransmitters—serotonin, gamma-aminobutyric acid (GABA), and dopamine—influence the expression or suppression of aggressive behaviors (Charney, 2004; Hawkins and Trobst, 2000; Miczek et al, 2002; Teichner and Golden, 2000; see also Chapter 6). Common problems related to aggression include:

- Bifrontal head injuries, damage to the frontal and prefrontal cortex

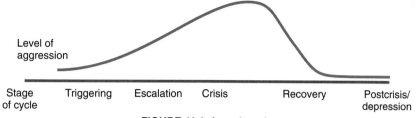

**FIGURE 11-1** Assault cycle.

- Damage to hippocampus, amygdala, and limbic system
- Temporal-parietal lobe dysfunctions
- Early dysfunctions of subcortical areas
- Alzheimer's disease
- Multi-infarct dementia
- Decreased serotonin, GABA, or acetylcholine levels
- Increased dopamine and norepinephrine levels
- Imbalances in hormone levels
- Alcohol and drug use or abuse, especially amphetamines, cocaine, morphine
- Alcohol and drug withdrawal
- Nutritional deficiencies: tryptophan, thiamine, niacin, lecithin
- Medication noncompliance

Social-psychological models focus on the interaction of individuals with their social environment and locate the source of violence in interpersonal requirements and frustrations, such as chaotic families and forms of abuse (Teichner and Golden, 2000). Sociocultural models focus on social structures, norms, values, institutional organizations, and systems' operations to explain individual violence, such as gang activity, poverty, welfare, and availability of drugs and guns (Ollendick, 1996).

## ASSAULT CYCLE

Smith's stress model (1981) includes the assault cycle, with five stages of a predictable pattern or chain of aggressive responses to emotional or physical stress (Figure 11-1). Patients who are repeatedly assaultive exhibit behavior patterns that are ritualistic, stereotypical, and automatic. As the acuity of the aggressive response increases, a comparable decrease occurs in patients' problem-solving abilities, creativity, spontaneity, and behavioral options. Interventions in each stage of the cycle are discussed later in this chapter. The five-phase assault cycle adapted from Smith (1981) includes the following:

1. *Triggering phase.* The stress-producing event occurs, initiating the stress responses.
2. *Escalation phase.* Responses represent escalating behaviors that indicate a movement toward the loss of control.
3. *Crisis phase.* During this period of emotional and physical crisis, loss of control occurs.
4. *Recovery phase.* In this period of cooling down, the person slows down and returns to normal responses.
5. *Postcrisis depression phase.* in this period, the person attempts reconciliation with others.

## INTERMITTENT EXPLOSIVE DISORDER

Intermittent explosive disorder (IED) is included in this chapter because its primary symptom is aggression, but it is one of the impulse control disorders described later in this section. The DSM-IV-TR criteria (APA, 2000) are the following:

1. There are several discrete episodes of failure to resist aggressive impulses, which result in serious assaultive acts or destruction of property.
2. The degree of aggressive episodes expressed during the episodes is grossly out of proportion to any precipitating psychosocial stressors.
3. The aggressive episodes are not better accounted for by another mental disorder (e.g., antisocial personality disorder, borderline personality disorder, psychotic disorder, manic episode, conduct disorder, or attention-deficit/hyperactivity disorder) and are not the result of the direct physiologic effects of a substance (e.g., drug of abuse, medication) or a general medical condition (e.g., head trauma, Alzheimer's disease).

Prior to these aggressive episodes, individuals might experience head pressure, palpitations or chest tightness, tingling or tremors, or sounds, such as an echo. During the episodes, they might experience an "adrenaline rush." IED typically begins in childhood, adolescence, or early adulthood (Olvera, 2002). These episodes are not intentional and are very distressing to the individual. They can lead to interpersonal, social, and occupational difficulties, such as divorce, job loss, car accidents, injuries in fights, financial problems, and arrests, convictions, or other legal outcomes. Impulsiveness, chronic anger, and less destructive aggression might occur in between explosive episodes (APA, 2000). In addition to conditions listed in the criteria above, other factors might cause aggression and impulsivity, such as anxiety, childhood abuse, and eating disorders and cerebral dysfunction, seizures, and migraines. However, these conditions should be diagnosed as such and not confused with IED (APA, 2000).

Research on interventions with IED is focusing on cognitive, behavioral, and psychotherapeutic techniques, social skills training, relaxation techniques, problem solving, and stress management. (See Chapters 4 and 10 for further discussion.) Medications might be of some benefit. Psychopharmacologic research has focused on anticonvulsants, GABA-type mood stabilizers, anxiolytics, atypical antipsychotics, selective serotonin reuptake inhibitors (SSRIs), and beta blockers (carbamazepine [generic], 2004; Miczek et al, 2002; Olvera, 2002).

The other impulse control disorders are not related to anger or vengeance or to another mental disorder, substance abuse, or general medical condition. These disorders can be described as follows (APA, 2000):

*Kleptomania* is characterized by the recurrent failure to resist impulses to steal objects not needed for personal use or monetary value.

*Pyromania* is characterized by a pattern of fire setting for pleasure, gratification, or relief of tension.

*Pathologic gambling* is characterized by recurrent and persistent maladaptive gambling behavior.

*Trichotillomania* is characterized by recurrent pulling out of one's hair for pleasure, gratification, or relief of tension that results in noticeable hair loss.

## ASSESSING KEY VARIABLES OF AGGRESSION

### NURSE (SELF-ASSESSMENT)

Working with psychiatric patients who might act out requires nurses to be aware of their own aggressive impulses, the way in which they deal with their anger, and the methods they use to channel their anger into constructive, productive actions. Knowing how nurses respond to patients who show anger, anxiety, fear, panic, and assaultive behaviors is important (Eckroth-Bucher, 2001). Nurses cannot defuse patients' anger or aggression when they are in a similar state, and their anger might actually intensify patients' emotions; additionally, nurses are ineffective if they withdraw from hostile or demanding patients.

When patients become aggressive, nurses might experience frustration, a feeling of professional inadequacy, or a sense of failure. They might become overly controlling and engage in power struggles with patients. Some nurses believe that their participation in physically controlling acting-out patients damages the chances of developing or continuing a therapeutic relationship; in most cases, however, the opposite is true. If patients' behaviors are viewed as a form of communication, then escalating anger should alert the staff to the fact that patients' inner controls are failing and that assistance is needed to regain impulse control. Nurses have the opportunity to convey to patients that help is available to regain control and deal more constructively with the environmental stresses that caused the initial problems and hospitalization.

## ENVIRONMENT (MILIEU)

Variables in the milieu of a facility might contribute to the development and escalation of aggression and include the following: (1) an environment with excessive stimuli and noise; (2) overcrowding and lack of sufficient space; (3) lack of resources for energy-draining activities, such as exercise equipment and sports areas; (4) patients' perceived lack of control of life and freedom; (5) lack of structured and unstructured diversionary activities, such as movies, games, cards, calming music, crafts, television, and therapeutic and recreational reading materials; and (6) lack of quiet rooms and spaces (Allen, 2000; Bluebird, 2004; Champagne and Stromberg, 2004; Jech, 2001; Johnson, 2004; Lee et al, 2003; McCloskey, 2004).

Staff might need to guide patients in selecting appropriate activities. For example, watching television violence, including sexual aggression, might increase aggressiveness in some patients. Staffing must be sufficient for monitoring patients and supervising activities. Tolerance of a degree of pacing might reduce tension, but an excess of this activity might disturb other patients. Nurses can be instrumental in groups to help patients learn assertiveness, rage prevention, anger management, self-awareness, social skills, cognitive restructuring, and positive coping behaviors (Allen, 2000; Jonikas et al, 2004; Thomas, 2001).

The biases and attitudes of the staff, as well as the philosophies and policies of a facility, affect both the milieu and patients' behaviors. An overly controlled environment, such as excessive or unfair restriction of rights and privileges, might lead to aggression and rebellion. Reasonable yet flexible rules reduce the risk of power and control issues between staff and patients. Policies and rules can contribute positively to the structure, predictability, and consistency of the milieu (Huckshorn, 2004; Johnson, 2004; Jonikas et al, 2004).

## PATIENT

Triggers for aggression are the same threats and losses listed in Chapter 10. At specific times, patients are more likely to become aggressive or assaultive: at change of shifts, at mealtimes, at visiting hours, in elevators, while being escorted to outside areas during invasive procedures, in the evening, and during periods of change (Johnson, 2004; McCloskey, 2004; Secker et al, 2004).

Change is especially unnerving for patients who have dependency needs and/or shaky impulse control. Even positive changes in a patient's status might be experienced as a loss of support, care, and protection—for example, when a patient is transferred to a less restrictive unit or discharged back to the community. All physical moves, status changes, and changes in treatment, such as medications, should be carefully explained in advance. Rapid changes cause the most anxiety, and the nurse must convey support and confidence that the patient has the coping skills to deal with the event. Acting-out behavior is one way patients have of telling the staff that change is highly threatening. Fear of change might be the reason patients do not ask for more freedom, such as going off the unit with visitors. Requests for more freedom might be a way of testing the staff.

Hospitalization itself might escalate patients' anger, anxiety, and symptoms, especially if it is not a voluntary admission. For example, paranoid patients might see the nursing staff as part of a plot to restrict them, whereas compulsive patients might become more stereotyped and rigid when they cannot repeat compulsive behavior as frequently. Many aspects of admission are threatening and can undermine the little amount of impulse control that patients have. The admission process unavoidably involves focusing on emotionally charged issues, explaining rules and policies, personal searches, the removal or restricted use of personal items, physical examinations, and meeting unfamiliar professionals and patients (Joseph-Kinzelman et al, 1994). Nurses must be sensitive to these stresses and integrate patients slowly into the unit. When patients have a history of assault or are currently agitated, delaying all but essential procedures and decreasing the stimuli and stress as much as possible might be important.

Patients might be disruptive to each other, especially those who are hyperactive, intrusive, openly sexual, manipulative, threatening, or exhibiting bizarre behaviors. Staff members are responsible not only for helping these patients control their behaviors, but also for helping the other patients learn assertive responses for handling such situations.

Patients' ages and coexisting medical conditions might provide clues to potential aggression, such as severe pain, confusion, disorientation, malnutrition, infection, physical incapacities, medication toxicity, liver or kidney insufficiency, exhaustion, brain injury, and brain dysfunction. Patients who suffer from dementia or from intellectual or impairments or disorders, which limit their abilities to communicate with or understand others, are at high risk of assault (Johnson, 2004; Mawson, 2005).

Patients with a diagnosis of psychosis, schizophrenia (especially paranoid), schizoaffective disorder, mania, substance abuse disorder, or an organic brain disorder have an increased incidence of aggression after admission. Patients with antisocial, passive-aggressive, and borderline traits might also have aggressive tendencies (Aviram et al, 2004; Krakowski and Czobor, 2004; Kraus and Sheitman, 2004).

Factors in patients' backgrounds that are particularly relevant when assessing for aggressive potential include a history of family (or cultural) violence, abuse, and gross disorganization. Other indicators are histories of truancy, setting fires, promiscuity, impulsivity, thrill-seeking behaviors, drug trafficking, gang membership, easy access to weapons, previous assaults, and destruction of property. A particularly relevant indicator is a specific threat of violence made within approximately 2 weeks before admission (Delaney and Fogg, 2005; Johnson, 2004; Krakowski and Czobor, 2004; Mawson, 2005).

Trauma-informed care requires that staff ask all patients about their history of traumatic events at any point in their lives, and determine how these might affect patients' reactions to staff control, seclusion, and restraints (Champagne and Stromberg, 2004). It is also important to assess patients' perceptions of what triggers their anger and aggression and what helps calm then down (i.e., adaptive and palliative coping strategies, Chapter 10). Documentation in progress notes should include these habitual coping patterns and personal eccentricities. Specific examples of communications that alert staff to potential triggers of aggression include the following: "thinks all female nurses are going to be mean to him, like his mother"; "abuses men as his father abused him"; "gets upset whenever the female physician is here"; "is terrified whenever men are around." Other information includes the times and places when patients appear to be especially vulnerable, such as in large groups, when alone with a staff member of the opposite sex, or when in the bathroom.

It is common practice for facilities to present information in writing to patients and families about the possibility of using seclusion and restraints in the inpatient setting. This information includes rationales for using these procedures as safety precautions with risks and benefits, less restrictive alternatives that will be attempted first, and an explanation that these procedures will be ended as soon as the patient is safe from risk of self-injury or risk of injuring others.

## NURSING INTERVENTIONS FOR ANGER AND NONVIOLENT AGGRESSION

These interventions have the overall goal of preventing violence in psychiatric settings (Huckshorn, 2004). Three factors to consider in intervening with anger and nonviolent (or verbal)

aggression are (1) the *source* and (2) the *target* of the patient's anger, and (3) the *likelihood of* escalation. For example, a patient might be angry about a situation or person outside the psychiatric setting but is directing her anger inward as depression or suicidal ideation. Another patient, angry at a situation or person outside, might show his anger as passive aggression and aim it at no one in particular. A third patient might express anger openly and loudly. In these instances, the anger is likely to be defused by discussing the situation directly each time the anger occurs.

In other situations, the possibility that the patient will lose control of the anger might increase. For example, a patient might be angry at a situation or person in the treatment setting, angry about an outside situation but displacing it onto the staff, or threatening suicide with an available object, or responding to internal stimuli, such as hallucinations, delusions, or physiologic disruptions.

Nursing interventions in both escalating and nonescalating anger begin with an assessment at a safe distance. Chapter 8 describes normal precautions to take with any patient in a potentially unpredictable situation; for example, the nurse stays between the patient and an exit without blocking the exit and uses body language that is the least threatening to the patient. Warmth and empathy are essential, but a need for firm limit setting might also help patients contain their behavior at a safe level (ED Nursing, 2001): "I want to talk, but put the ashtray down first" or "Stay here in your room, I'll be back."

If patients are less verbal, less direct, or overly controlling of their anger, the nurse must take an active, supportive, and directive role. Initially, the nurse might have to point out specific behaviors and ask patients to explain the situation. For example, the nurse might say, "I hear a lot of sarcastic remarks. What happened during your phone call?" or "You look so down right now. What are you thinking about?" Obtaining a complete description of situations, thoughts, and feelings requires thorough questioning and patience. Patients who turn their anger inward should also be asked whether they are thinking about suicide.

The process of asking patients to describe their thoughts, feelings, and situations allows them to ventilate and diffuse some of the emotion. As the anger subsides, problem solving can focus on more effective ways of handling situations and feelings.

Asking patients to assess their own potential for acting on anger can be helpful. For example, the nurse might say, "How likely are you to try to hurt your wife when you are angry?" or "How serious are you about killing yourself?" The nurse might contract with patients to approach the staff and talk about their feelings each time they feel angry. If the anger does not gradually diffuse during the assessment and ventilation processes, or if patients begin to become irrational and out of control, then interventions based on the assault cycle become necessary.

## NURSING INTERVENTIONS BASED ON THE ASSAULT CYCLE

The goal of all interventions based on the assault cycle (Table 11-2) is to strengthen patients' control of feelings and impulses. Nurses should document attempts to use less restrictive measures (talking and oral as-needed [prn] medications, if ordered) before the more restrictive interventions of seclusion and restraints are used, except in rapidly escalating situations. Nurses should strive to achieve a balance between giving the least restrictive care and the restriction of rights to protect the patient and others, while providing quality care (APNA, 2001; Jones et al, 2000; Terpstra et al, 2001). Calm, positive approaches convey to patients that they are expected to cope, and that this attitude supports healthy functioning.

## TRIGGERING PHASE

In the triggering phase, patients' responses are nonviolent and present no danger to others. The behavior reflects patients' usual coping and defense mechanisms. Importantly, the nurse must know how patients perceive the nurse and the environment during the triggering phase and the likelihood that patients will act on these perceptions. If a patient's stressor is another individual in the immediate environment, then the two patients can be separated and nurses can talk with each patient individually to promote safe ventilation of emotions.

To facilitate ventilation of anger, emphasis is on being supportive by using an empathic, nondirective, yet concerned technique. The nurse speaks softly in calm, clear, simple statements, avoiding any challenge to the patient. Aggressive, confron-

tational, or threatening approaches at this time usually result in escalation. Although ventilation is encouraged, patients are reminded to stay in control of themselves and to use relaxation techniques, such as deep breathing. Patients' loss of control is socially embarrassing for them and counterproductive, leaving them with feelings of vulnerability and loss of autonomy. To protect the dignity of patients and the rights and safety of others, patients can be asked to take a time out in their rooms or at least move to a quieter area; other patients might be asked to leave the scene (Kozob and Skidmore, 2001a). When the anger subsides, a problem-solving approach can begin to identify alternative solutions.

If, however, the ventilation has not been successful, patients must be offered alternatives that allow them to express threatening emotions safely, while helping them regain control (ED Nursing, 2001). Common approaches include journal writing, exercising, punching pillows, tearing up telephone books, pounding clay, or walking up and down the hall. Oral antianxiety or antipsychotic medications can also be given, if ordered (Kozob and Skidmore, 2001b).

### CLINICAL EXAMPLE

John Henderson has been a patient on the unit for 3 days. While talking to his wife on the telephone, he becomes upset and raises his voice to her. The nurse calmly suggests that he tell his wife that he will continue their conversation later. He hangs up the telephone and starts pacing in the hallway. The nurse says, "Tell me what you are upset about." For 15 minutes, he describes the telephone conversation in detail, expresses anger toward his wife, and says he is afraid she will divorce him. As he visibly calms down, the nurse asks, "What would be most helpful in handling the situation with your wife?"

## ESCALATION PHASE

When verbalization and tension reduction strategies fail and patients become irrational (e.g., they begin to swear, scream, threaten), the nurse must take control of the situation. For example, at a safe distance, the nurse calls the patient by name and states in a calm, firm manner that the patient's behaviors indicate a loss of control. The nurse does not threaten punishment or engage in power

| Table 11-2 | Interventions Based on the Assault Cycle | |
| --- | --- | --- |
| **Phase** | **Behaviors** | **Nursing Interventions** |
| Triggering phase: +1 to +2 level of anxiety | Muscle tension, changes in voice quality, tapping of fingers, pacing, repeated verbalizations, noncompliance, restlessness, irritability, anxiety, suspiciousness, perspiration, tremors, glaring, changes in breathing | Convey empathic support. Encourage ventilation. Use clear, calm, simple statements. Ask patient to maintain control. Facilitate problem solving by discussing alternative solutions. If needed, ask the patient to go to a quiet area. Offer safe tension reduction measures. If needed, offer oral medications (prn). |
| Escalation phase: +2 to +3 level of anxiety | Pale or flushed face, screaming, anger, swearing, agitation, hypersensitivity, threats, demands, readiness to retaliate, tautness, loss of reasoning ability, provocative behaviors, clenched fists | Take charge with calm, firm directions. Direct patient to a quiet room for "time out." Give oral medications (prn), if ordered. Ask the staff to be on standby at a distance. Prepare for a "show of determination" or "show of force" to take control. |
| Crisis phase: +3 to +4 level of anxiety | Loss of self-control, fighting, hitting, rage, kicking, scratching, throwing things | Use involuntary seclusion, restraints, or IM medications (prn), if ordered. Initiate intensive nursing care. |
| Recovery phase: +3 to +2 level of anxiety | Accusations, recriminations, lowering of voice, decreased body tension, change in conversational content, more normal responses, relaxation | Continue intensive nursing care. Process the incident with the staff and other patients. Assess patient and staff injuries. Evaluate patient's progress toward self-control. |
| Postcrisis depression phase: +2 to +1 level of anxiety | Crying, apologies, reconciliatory interactions, repression of assaultive feelings (which might later appear as hostility, passive aggression) | Process incident with patient. Discuss alternative solutions to the situation and feelings. Progressively reduce the degree of restraint and seclusion. Facilitate reentry to unit. |

*IM,* intramuscular; *prn,* if needed or as needed.
Data from Maier GJ: Managing threatening behavior: the role of talk up and talk down, *J Psychosoc Nurs Ment Health Serv* 34:25, 1996; Smith P: Empirically based models for viewing the dynamics of violence. In Babich K, editor: *Assessing patient violence in the health care setting,* Boulder, CO, 1981, Western Interstate Commission for Higher Education; Stevenson S: Heading off violence with verbal de-escalation, *J Psychosoc Nurs Ment Health Serv* 29:6, 1991.

struggles, but offers help by taking charge on behalf of the patient, who is unable to do so at the time (ED Nursing, 2001; Kozob and Skidmore, 2001a and b). The nurse avoids sudden movements and loud tones so as not to appear to be attacking.

If the patient has orders for prn antianxiety or antipsychotic medications, an oral dose can be offered early in the escalation phase. If the oral dose is refused, or if the escalation is rapid, an intramuscular (IM) medication might be necessary and the nurse might require help from other staff members. Among the oral antianxiety medications, lorazepam (Ativan) and alprazolam (Xanax) are often the drugs of choice because they take effect rapidly and have relatively few side effects.

These medications might occasionally lower a patient's inhibitions and aggravate behaviors. Lorazepam might be given IM. Among the antipsychotic medications, the medications that can be given orally (quetiapine [Seroquel]) or orally or IM (haloperidol [Haldol] and ziprasidone [Geodon]) have lower sedating effects but help decrease agitation.

Given the principle of the least restrictive alternative, a time out in a quiet room is first offered by the nurse in a kind but firm manner. If this measure is ineffective, then more restrictive measures might be instituted when the patient actually begins to lose control. Other staff members might be called to be on standby, but should initially try to remain out of the patient's view. When patients are potentially violent, their physical proximity to others is perceived as being much closer than it actually is, and they might feel threatened.

The nurse who has been talking with the patient decides whether the patient can respond to directions in a reasonable time. If the patient does not respond to directions for self-control or to move to a quiet, safe place, the nurse then asks for staff assistance for a stronger "show of determination" or "show of force" to take control. This action involves having four to six staff members within sight of the patient, but at a greater distance from the patient than the primary nurse; thus, they do not appear ready to attack the patient. Frequently, when the patient becomes aware of the other staff members and is informed that the staff will take control (if the patient does not comply with directions), the patient can gain reasonable composure, cooperate with the nurse's request, take the medications, and go to a quieter room with or without staff escort (Kozob and Skidmore, 2001b) If not, the patient is usually close to entering the crisis phase.

## CLINICAL EXAMPLE

For the second time this shift, John Henderson is talking on the telephone with his wife. He is now shouting, making threats, and demanding that she come to the hospital immediately. The nurse again asks him to end the call and talk about what is happening. As he describes this call, he gets more agitated and yells that he wants to go home immediately. The nurse calmly and firmly says, "I can hear how angry you are. (*Pause.*) You cannot go home now. (*Pause.*) I want you to go to your room and I will bring you an Ativan." Mr. Henderson does not respond immediately, but he stops yelling. The nurse says, "Please go to your room. I will get the Ativan." He goes to his room and slams the door. The nurse alerts other staff members about the plans for Mr. Henderson. The nurse asks them to stay outside of his room until an assessment can be made as to whether a time out is going to be helpful for him, and whether he is willing to take the medication.

## CRISIS PHASE

The crisis phase is reached when the patient is approaching an attack on the environment, self,

other patients, or staff. Verbal limits are ineffective, and external control by the staff is essential. In these emergency or crisis situations, immediate seclusion, restraint, or the administration of stat medications becomes necessary. The patient has the right to refuse medication, but staff might give it in the presence of an *immediate* physical threat to others. These actions should be supported by emergency protocols that have been approved by the physicians and hospital, and any actions taken should be carefully and thoroughly documented in the patient's records.

Psychiatric emergencies must be dealt with in coordinated and organized ways, and the staff must have the opportunity to role-play their approach in advance of a crisis. All staff members should master self-protection techniques against behaviors such as kicking, hitting, and biting. Facilities usually provide aggression management programs for staff members; they are required to update these skills periodically, similarly to other emergency skills, such as cardiopulmonary resuscitation. Staff members who are well trained in preventing and managing aggression are less likely to be victims of patient assaults.

### Seclusion

Seclusion is the process of placing the patient alone in a specially designed, lockable room equipped with a security window or a camera for observation. Nurses usually make the decision to initiate and terminate the seclusion of patients according to established protocols and are almost always involved in the care of patients during seclusion. The principle of seclusion is *containment*: restricting patients so that they do not hurt themselves or others, decreasing stimulation, and increasing intensive nursing care. Agitation and disruptive or inappropriate sexual behaviors are other reasons for seclusion. Seclusion might be viewed as a preventive strategy to *avoid* aggressive assaults, as well as a responsive action. Time out, closer supervision, quiet interactions, and medication are therapeutically effective when used appropriately for brief periods.

The degree of seclusion depends on the patient's current status. The patient who is able to choose time out voluntarily, especially if that patient is already taking prescribed medication, might stay voluntarily in his or her room without a locked door. This degree of seclusion might be relatively brief. The less cooperative patient might be escorted by two staff members, without bodily contact, to a seclusion room that contains only a bed (bolted to the floor) and a mattress, or just a mattress on the floor. This type of room decreases stimuli, protects the patient from injury, prevents destruction of property, and provides for the patient's privacy. The door, lockable from the outside, keeps the patient from leaving the room, if needed. Dangerous articles (e.g., belts, sharp objects such as pens and keys, shoes, and eyeglasses) are taken away from the patient.

## Restraint

The staff must take immediate action when assaults occur. Six to eight staff members (including hospital security officers, if insufficient unit staff members are available) are needed to *safely* control a patient and ensure that no injuries to the staff, patient, or other patients on the unit occur. The number of staff needed should not be underestimated because of the size, age, or gender of the patient. Some agencies include information about patients' previous athletic interests and accomplishments, such as weight lifting and a black belt in karate, on the admission form.

Details of restraint procedures, including therapeutic holds for children, are not described here, but a general outline is presented. To prepare for control of a patient, staff members remove their own glasses, rings, earrings, pens, watches, keys, and anything else that might cause injury to the patient or staff. Furniture and objects that can be used as weapons are removed from the area. One staff member becomes the team leader to organize and direct the planned, coordinated approach, while the original staff member continues talking with the patient. At least one staff member takes the other patients to a safe place and stays with them.

The team approaches the patient calmly, in a show of force or determination, to take control. The patient is told that the team is here to help, will not hurt the patient, and will not allow the patient to hurt anyone. Two team members approach from each side and take control of the patient's arms. Simultaneously, three other staff members quickly take control of the patient's legs and head so that the patient can be carried to the room or held on the floor until a bed is brought to the patient. Physical contact is protective and

defensive, not aggressive. One staff member brings the restraint cuffs, opens doors, and moves obstacles. A nurse prepares the IM medication (or calls to get an order if no routine prn order exists).

Once in the seclusion room, the patient is usually placed on the bed on his or her back. Four or more staff members hold the patient's extremities and head securely, without hyperextending the patient's joints. Wrist and ankle restraints are applied to all four extremities and secured to the frame of the bed. The patient's arms are tied in a position at the side, not above the head. The restraints are tight enough to inhibit slipping out of them but not tight enough to interfere with circulation. The patient should be free of all belongings that might be used to cause harm to self or others. Medications might be administered at this time. A waist restraint, a restraint between the ankles, or a restraint blanket (or any combination of these) is applied *only* if the patient is at risk of injury because of fighting the restraints. Before staff members leave, the patient is checked for injuries and observed for the ability to move safely in the restraints.

Within 1 hour, an order to restrain the patient must be obtained and a physician must perform a face to face evaluation of the patient. Federal, state, and hospital regulations or policies govern the extent to which the patient must be evaluated by the nurse and physician for the need to continue the restraints, by the physician in a face to face examination, and in the progress notes by the nurse and physician (Huckshorn, 2004).

### CRITICAL THINKING QUESTION    1

A visitor to the unit begins to hit a patient. How would you handle this situation?

## Care of Patients in Seclusion or Restraints

When a patient is placed in seclusion or restraints, intensive nursing care is instituted. The patient is continuously observed directly or by video monitor. Other patients are not allowed to be near a restrained patient. The patient's mental status, response to and side effects of medications, hydration, nutrition, elimination, range of motion, vital signs, and hygiene are monitored. Immediate attention to any injuries resulting from the incident or from the restraints is critical and requires documentation. Every 2 hours, with two staff members present, the restraints are removed one at a time, for 10 minutes each, to allow range-of-motion activities. Change of position and skin care are also important. Restricting visitors, telephone calls, and diversional materials, such as radios and magazines, reduces stimuli; however, regular staff contact decreases the patient's sense of isolation and loneliness.

## RECOVERY AND POSTCRISIS DEPRESSION PHASE

In this phase, patients are assured that they are not being punished while in seclusion and that they will be allowed back in the milieu as soon as possible. Patients must be assisted in relaxing, sleeping, and benefiting from these phases of cooling down and reconciliation. The time that patients are in restraints or seclusion should be a supportive, restorative time. Otherwise, patients might remain afraid, frustrated, and angry, possibly leading to future aggression. After patients are calm and in control, they are encouraged to discuss the circumstances during which they lost control, as well as alternatives for handling similar situations in the future (Kozob and Skidmore, 2001a).

Patients are ready to be released from restraints when they show signs of self-control, decreased anxiety and agitation, a stabilized mood, increased attention span, reality orientation, and sound judgment. Patients might be kept in the seclusion room briefly to assess their reaction to release from the restraints. Patients need assistance to reenter the unit with as little fear and embarrassment as possible. The nurse should try to help other patients accept these patients back into the unit.

Immediately after a patient has been secluded and restrained, the staff should meet, ensure that no staff injuries have occurred, evaluate the way in which they handled the situation, and give each other mutual support and feedback. Feelings and attitudes are discussed, along with suggestions for improved use of procedures. These debriefing meetings provide the unit staff with ongoing, in-service opportunities to monitor their reactions, as well as to augment their skills for preventing escalation of anger (Huckshorn, 2004). Careful documentation of patients' behaviors before, during, and after the incident and a rationale for physical control interventions, seclusion, and restraint are essential legal protections for the staff. Documentation might be recorded as incident reports and should be written after everyone concerned has calmed down. Staff perceptions are compared for accuracy. Documentation is descriptive, sequential, organized, and specific about what was seen, heard, and felt; what was said and by whom; who was notified; and what actions were taken and are to be taken. The request for and granting of a physician's order for seclusion and/or restraint are also recorded.

Other patients' reactions to restraint and seclusion situations should be discussed openly and explored in a special meeting with staff. The reasons for and the purpose of seclusion and restraint need to be discussed in a matter of fact and honest manner. Patients must have the opportunity to share their concerns, reactions, and fears of losing control and be reminded to approach staff if they begin feeling upset and angry. Also, patients must be told that staff members are providing control and care (not punishment) until the patient who has lost control regains it.

| CRITICAL THINKING QUESTION | 2 |

Why is it important for other patients to share their opinions and reactions about the seclusion and restraint of another patient?

## STAFF MEMBERS AS VICTIMS OF ASSAULT

Most incidents of patients' outbursts of anger do not result in restraint procedures but, when they occur, the process is always difficult for the staff and patient. The staff and patient are understandably drained, physically and emotionally. The process of debriefing and recovery is complicated when a staff member has been injured.

Being injured by a patient is similar emotionally to being a victim of crime (Chapter 41). This type of occurrence can destroy the staff member's sense of trust in others and sense of control of his or her life, and can result in a loss of self-esteem. The staff member often expresses feelings of guilt and of being vulnerable, irritable, depressed, and anxious; nightmares, grief, symptoms of acute stress disorder (ASD), and fear of the patient who caused the injury may be present. The assault might be minimized and feelings might even be denied if emotional support and debriefing are not provided after the medical examination and treatment have been completed. If the injured staff member is away from work for a while, the rest of the staff might be unaware that their emotions have subsided much more than did those of their injured colleague. To ensure that the staff victim achieves emotional resolution of the incident, some facilities have developed a formalized process of follow-up. A peer support program that understands the dynamics of assault and the common responses of victims is important. Supportive interventions should be available to the person who was injured (Poster, 1996; Whitney et al, 1996). The needs of the victim determine the frequency and number of meetings. A counselor might facilitate meetings between the victim and staff and between the victim and the assaultive patient to facilitate the victim's return to work. Victims are encouraged to share their feelings with family or significant others. The goal of this process is to facilitate emotional resolution, help the person remain productive, and decrease the chance of resignation and development of PTSD (Poster, 1996; Whitney et al, 1996). Whether staff members who are assaulted by patients can or should take legal action against the patient is currently being debated. The hospital might pursue legal action on behalf of the staff.

## Study Notes

1. Anger is a normal human emotion that might be expressed assertively, passively, passive aggressively, and aggressively.
2. Verbal and physical aggression, especially assault and battery, require safe, immediate interventions based on the principle of the least restrictive alternative.
3. The individual, social-psychological, and sociocultural models of aggression offer explanations for the development of aggression.
4. Intermittent explosive disorder is one cause of episodes of aggression.
5. Factors regarding the nurse, the environment, and the patient affect the development and expression of anger.
6. The assault cycle describes the predictable phases of aggression: triggering, escalation, crisis, recovery, and depression.

7. Nursing interventions with anger and nonviolent aggression concentrate on ventilation to defuse the anger and then on problem solving to identify ways of handling the causes of the anger appropriately.
8. Tension reduction, medications, physical control, seclusion, and/or restraints become necessary in the escalation and crisis phases of the assault cycle.
9. Patients in seclusion and restraints require intensive physical and emotional nursing care.
10. Staff members who are injured by a patient might require assistance in recovering.

## References

Allen JJ: Seclusion and restraint of children: a literature review, *J Child Adolesc Psychiatr Nurs* 13:159, 2000.

American Psychiatric Association: *Diagnostic and statistical manual of mental disorders, ed 4, text revision.* Washington, DC, American Psychiatric Association, 2000.

American Psychiatric Nurses Association (APNA): American Psychiatric Nurses Association position statement on the use of seclusion and restraint, *J Am Psychiatr Nurs Assoc* 7:130, 2001.

Aviram RB, Hellerstein DJ, Gerson J, Stanley B: Adapting supportive psychotherapy for individuals with borderline personality disorder who self-injure or attempt suicide, *J Psychiatr Pract* 10:145, 2004.

Bluebird G: Redefining consumer roles: changing culture and practice in mental health care settings, *J Psychosoc Nursing* 42:46, 2004.

Carbamazepine (generic), *Brown Univ Psychopharmacol Update* 15:9, 2004.

Champagne T, Stromberg N: Sensory approaches in inpatient psychiatric settings: innovative alternatives to seclusion and restraint, *J Psychosoc Nurs* 42:35, 2004.

Charney DS: Psychobiological mechanisms of resilience and vulnerability: implications for successful adaptation to extreme stress, *Am J Psychiatry* 162:195, 2004.

Delaney KR, Fogg L: Patient characteristics and setting variables related to use of restraint on four inpatient units for youths, *Psychiatr Serv* 56:186, 2005.

Dunbar B: Anger management: a holistic approach, *Am Psychiatr Nurs Assoc* 10:16 2004.

Eckroth-Bucher M: Philosophical basis and practice of self-awareness in psychiatric nursing, *J Psychosoc Nurs* 39:32, 2001.

ED Nursing: Let agitated patients know they have choices, *RN* 64:24, 2001.

Hawkins KA, Trobst KK: Frontal lobe dysfunction and aggression: conceptual issues and research findings, *Aggression Violent Behav* 5:147, 2000.

Horton-Deutsch SL, Horton JM: Mindfulness: overcoming intractable conflict, *Arch Psychiatr Nurs* 17:186, 2003.

Huckshorn KA: Reducing seclusion and restraint use in mental health settings: core strategies for prevention, *J Psychosoc Nurs* 42:22, 2004.

Jech AO: Calming the cognitively impaired, *Nurs Spectrum* (Metro ed) September:30, 2001.

Johnson ME: Violence on inpatient psychiatric units: state of the science, *Am Psychiatr Nurs Assoc* 10:113, 2004.

Jones J, Ward M, Wellman N et al: Psychiatric inpatients' experience of nursing observation: a United Kingdom perspective, *J Psychosoc Nurs Ment Health Serv* 38:10, 2000.

Jonikas JA, Cook JA, Rosen C, et al: Brief reports: A program to reduce use of physical restraint in psychiatric inpatient facilities, *Psychiatr Serv* 55:818, 2004.

Joseph-Kinzelman A, Taynor J, Rubin WV, et al: Clients' perceptions of involuntary hospitalization, *J Psychosoc Nurs Ment Health Serv* 32:28, 1994.

Kozob ML, Skidmore R: Seclusion and restraint: understanding recent changes, *J Psychosoc Nurs* 39:25, 2001a.

Kozob ML, Skidmore R: Least to most restrictive interventions, *J Psychosoc Nurs* 39:32, 2001b.

Krakowski M, Czobor P: Suicide and violence in patients with major psychiatric disorders, *J Psychiatr Pract* 10:233, 2004.

Kraus JE, Sheitman BB: Characteristics of violent behavior in a large state psychiatric hospital, *Psychiatr Serv* 55:183, 2004.

Lee S, Gray R, Gournay K, et al: Views of nursing staff on the use of physical restraint, *J Psychiatr Ment Health Nurs* 10:425, 2003.

Mawson AR: Intentional injury and the behavioral syndrome, *Aggression Violent Behav* 10:376, 2005.

McCloskey RM: Caring for patients with dementia in the acute care environment, *Geriatr Nurs* 25:139, 2004.

Miczek KA, Fish EW, De Bold JF, De Almeida RM: Social and neural determinants of aggressive behavior: pharmaco-therapeutic targets at serotonin, dopamine and gamma-aminobutyric acid systems, *Psychopharmacology* 163:434, 2002.

Ollendick TH: Violence in youth: where do we go from here? Behavior therapy's approach, *Behav Ther* 27:485, 1996.

Olvera RL: Intermittent explosive disorder: epidemiology, diagnosis and management, *CNS Drugs* 16:517, 2002.

Poster EC: A multinational study of psychiatric nursing staffs' beliefs and concerns about work safety and patient assault, *Arch Psychiatr Nurs* 10:365, 1996.

Secker J, Benson A, Balfe E, et al: Understanding the social context of violent and aggressive incidents on an inpatient unit, *J Psychiatr Ment Health Nurs* 11:172, 2004.

Smith P: Empirically based models for viewing the dynamics of violence. In Babich K, editor: *Assessing patient violence in the health care setting,* Boulder, CO, 1981, Western Interstate Commission for Higher Education.

Teichner G, Golden CJ: The relationship of neuropsychological impairment to conduct disorder in adolescence, *Aggression Violent Behav* 5:509, 2000.

Terpstra TL, Terpstra TL, Pettee EJ, Hunter M: Nursing staffs' attitude toward seclusion and restraint, *J Psychosoc Nurs* 39:20, 2001.

Thomas SP: Teaching healthy anger management, *Perspect Psychiatr Care* 37:41, 2001.

Whitney GA, Jacobson GA, Gawrys MT: The impact of violence in the health care setting upon nursing education, *J Nurs Educ* 35:211, 1996.

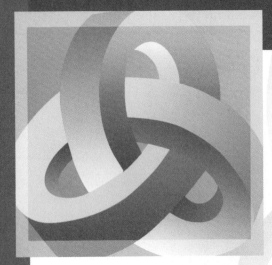

# Chapter 12

# Working With Groups of Patients

*Carol E. Bostrom*

## Learning Objectives

*After reading this chapter, you should be able to:*
- Describe specific therapeutic benefits of groups.
- Identify the major purpose of each type of group.
- Recognize qualities that the nurse leader of groups should have.
- Identify intervention strategies for common management issues in groups.

**W**orking with groups of patients is an integral component of both inpatient and outpatient psychiatric care. Nurses have 24-hour accountability for patient care on the inpatient psychiatric unit and are responsible for leading patient groups. This responsibility dictates economic use of nursing personnel; hence, working with groups of patients addresses staff concerns while providing a proven therapeutic intervention. Similarly, working with groups in the community or outpatient arena has increased because of brief inpatient psychiatric hospitalization and the demand of managed care for the least expensive, most effective care. Therapies that help the patient stabilize quickly and function optimally are currently used (Potter et al, 2004).

Patients with mental illnesses face problems in their daily living similar to those of others but with the complication of symptoms of mental illness. Although mental illness interferes with the way patients can cope with their problems, conflicts, and interpersonal relationships, patients have the capacity to learn techniques to cope with and negotiate life's problems. Groups deal with current here and now issues and stressors whether patients are in or out of the hospital. Patients gain awareness and knowledge about their behaviors and how these behaviors impede communication and coping; they become aware of alternatives that help them make better decisions and choices. On inpatient units and in community settings, nurses lead numerous educational and skill development groups. Nurses also lead groups for patients' families to teach them about mental illness and help them cope with the mentally ill family member. This chapter addresses two questions:

1. Given a patient population that has serious interpersonal and cognitive disturbances, how does group work benefit the individual?
2. What can the nurse realistically expect to accomplish through formal and informal group work with patients?

Because groups typically have short-term, goal-oriented sessions and are composed of acutely ill patients or patients with persistent and severe mental illness, nurses must have relevant information for developing group strategies. Issues

## Norm's Notes

*You will frequently work with groups of patients—it is economical, practical, and has therapeutic advantages. Although a traditional group therapy session is rarely seen these days, psychoeducational and support groups are very common. Beyond such relatively formal atmospheres, you will have many opportunities for informal group activities as patients, clients, or consumers congregate in gathering places. A subtle message given in this chapter is that you are always on duty. Even in a dayroom environment, where patients are mingling casually, your interactions are important and should be therapeutic.*

regarding benefits of groups, types of groups, leadership of groups, and common group management are addressed to provide this information. Because working effectively with groups of patients is inextricably related to milieu management, the nurse is encouraged to read Chapters 23 through 26.

## BENEFITS OF GROUPS

Benefits that patients receive from any group experience include the following:

- Patients gain knowledge about ways to relate to and communicate with others (Yalom, 1995).
- Patients gain acceptance, reassurance, and support from their peers and the group leader.
- Patients gain feelings of hopefulness and a sense of power regarding their ability to help themselves and others in the group.
- Patients are provided the opportunity to *test out* new behaviors with others during their treatment.
- Patients can share their feelings, problems, concerns, and ideas with others in a safe and structured environment.
- Patients' strengths that can enhance self-esteem are affirmed and further developed.
- Patients experience a sense of importance and an increased sense of worth.

### Box 12-1    Yalom's Therapeutic Factors

- **Instillation of hope.** Patients receive hope from observing others who have benefited from the group experience.
- **Universality.** Patients experience relief in knowing that they are not alone and unique, but that others experience similar problems, feelings, and concerns.
- **Imparting of information.** Patients learn or are provided information about areas related to their needs.
- **Altruism.** Patients experience themselves as helpful or useful to others.
- **Corrective recapitulation of primary family group.** Patients review previous dysfunctional family patterns and learn that these patterns can be changed to meet their present needs effectively.
- **Development of socializing techniques.** Patients are taught appropriate social skills.
- **Imitative behavior.** Patients selectively model healthy behaviors of the leader and other group members.
- **Catharsis.** Patients are not only allowed to express feelings, but are also taught ways to express them appropriately.
- **Existential factors.** Patients share feelings about "ultimate concerns" of existence, such as death or isolation, and learn to accept that there is a limit to their control of these issues.
- **Cohesiveness.** Patients experience feelings of being accepted, valued, and part of a group experience.
- **Interpersonal learning.** Patients learn how their behaviors affect others and more appropriate ways of relating in the supportive atmosphere of the group.

From Yalom I: *The theory and practice of group psychotherapy,* ed 4, New York, 1995, Basic Books.

These benefits might occur at different times for individual patients and in different group situations. Each group, depending on its goal or purpose, might focus on one particular outcome. For example, an activity group for art might focus on acceptance; no matter what the patients paint, they will be accepted and praised for their work.

## THERAPEUTIC FACTORS

Yalom has described 11 therapeutic factors that help patients, regardless of the therapeutic group (Box 12-1). Patients experience certain factors or benefits, depending on the type of group in which they participate; the patients as individuals deem these to be beneficial and important to them. Yalom originally related the therapeutic factors to psychotherapy groups but has developed their application to brief, one time–only groups along the continuum of care. The meaning of these therapeutic factors and their significance to patients are important for the nurse to understand. The nurse who understands the ways groups help patients will be more likely to initiate, lead, and participate in formal and informal groups. Nurses do not make therapeutic factors happen, but they facilitate the development and occurrence of these factors for patients.

## TYPES OF GROUPS

Making the inpatient group a positive, beneficial experience for patients is of primary importance. Each session should be treated as a separate entity, with the patient feeling that something positive has been attained during the group session (Yalom, 1995). Patients must believe that they have gained something for themselves during their hospitalization. A positive inpatient group experience favorably predisposes patients to seek treatment on an outpatient basis. After discharge, follow-up care in the community is the setting in which most ongoing treatment occurs.

Numerous types of groups can be offered in both inpatient and outpatient settings: psychoeducational, maintenance, and activity. Self-help or special problem groups and multifamily or couple groups are also available in some treatment settings. Traditional therapy groups, such as insight-oriented groups and psychodrama, are no longer offered today because of brief inpatient stays and reimbursement issues. Frequent patient turnover necessitates focusing on topics that can stand independently and focus on patients' immediate needs (Potter et al, 2004). Psychoeducational groups, activity groups, maintenance groups, and self-help groups are currently offered within the continuum of care.

## PSYCHOEDUCATIONAL GROUPS

Nurses who work in inpatient and outpatient settings lead groups to offer patients and their families a variety of content and skills. Typically,

groups deal with medication, the dynamics and management of illness, problem solving, stress management, anger management, social skills, basic living skills, and relapse prevention (Table 12-1). The reduction in inpatient hospitalization has increased the need for patients to learn skills that help them manage their illnesses and their lives in the community.

Group sessions might vary in length, but typically include 30 to 60 minutes for content presentation and discussion. How long the group meets varies, depending on the patients' level of cognitive and behavioral impairment. One inpatient group might be a 40-minute discussion of medication management, whereas an outpatient group on social skills might be 60 minutes in length. Patients from a variety of health care settings identified having a nurse teach about the illness, medications, treatments, and staying healthy as areas indicative of quality nursing care (Oermann and Templin, 2000). Nurses must collaborate with patients in treatment planning and developing educational programs based on the patients' needs and interests. A study conducted by Payson and associates (1998) found that patients are interested primarily in medication and side effects, obtaining necessary care from the mental health system, and learning ways to solve problems. The nurse's expertise, empathy, and support help patients learn that they themselves can successfully take care of their illnesses and themselves.

Nurses also provide psychoeducational programs for families of mentally ill individuals. Families are interested in the content on illnesses, medication benefits and side effects, communication with the ill family member, ways to manage crisis situations with patients, and ways to negotiate with the mental health system and managed care to have needs met. Families benefit not only from the information they receive in groups, but also from the high level of support that these groups provide. The benefits that families receive from group participation are similar to the patient benefits discussed earlier. Additionally, families experience less anger and have improved relationships with family members as they learn new family communication skills. Families also learn about available sources along the continuum of care and look to the nurse as an advocate and expert to help them arrange for needed services.

| Table 12-1 | **Psychoeducational Groups** |

| Type | Nurse's Purpose or Role | Examples |
|---|---|---|
| Illness | Teach patients and families content related to dynamics of illness, symptoms of illness, signs of relapse, management of illness, and dealing with crises. | Addiction processes, coping with symptoms, management of moods, causes and treatments of illnesses, relapse prevention, community resources |
| Medication | Dispense medications. Assess symptoms and side effects. Explain type and purpose of medication, dosage, therapeutic effects and side effects. Support measures to prevent relapse. | Groups based on category of medications (e.g., antipsychotics versus antidepressants, intramuscular versus oral) |
| Problem solving | Help identify and describe current problems; discuss and develop solutions and their effects; decide on an alternative method and how to try it. Evaluate and choose another method, if necessary. | Milieu issues, conflict resolution, job concerns, relationship issues, discharge planning |
| Stress management | Teach and facilitate adaptive coping behaviors. | Lifestyle balance and management, relaxation training, tension reduction strategies, and anger management |
| Social skills | Teach, develop, and practice skills to enhance interactions with others. Focus on realistic, day-to-day patient needs. | Assertiveness training, handling social interactions (e.g., meeting new people, going on interviews, negotiating the return of a purchase) |

## MAINTENANCE GROUPS

The very nature of nursing implies support. The nurse supports patients in therapeutic interactions. Support means accepting, empathizing, and showing concern while listening and talking with patients. The nurse focuses on responding to patients' needs. The nurse's presence, interest, and encouragement facilitate the expression of patients' feelings and concerns. The nurse is then instrumental in helping patients cope with their feelings and situations. Support is useful in many types of group situations.

The support group is a maintenance group; its purpose is to reinforce or maintain existing strengths and behaviors of patients, rather than to confront or change behaviors or defenses. Patients in a support group can be acutely or chronically ill. Group members might need a great deal of reassurance and emotional support during their hospitalization. These patients also need to reduce their anxiety to mild or moderate levels.

The reality orientation group is an example of a support group frequently found in inpatient settings. Patients who exhibit confusion and short attention spans resulting from some psychopatho-

logic factor can benefit from participation in this type of group. The nurse must provide an atmosphere of safety and security, because these patients might be frightened, unsure, anxious, uncomfortable, and isolated. The reality orientation group can assist patients with decreasing isolation and increasing their self-esteem. Focusing on the here and now provides a framework with structure, social support, and reality testing. The nurse, as leader of this group, facilitates orientation to time, person and place, rules and routines of the unit, and behavioral expectations, including some limit setting. Feeling valued, respected, and important as human beings is a feeling these patients might not have experienced for some time.

## ACTIVITY GROUPS

Activity groups use a variety of techniques to facilitate self-expression, interaction, and acceptance of self and others (McGarry and Prince, 1998). For example, some groups might use art or music to motivate patients to interact and promote socialization. Withdrawn, depressed, and regressed patients benefit from these groups, because these individuals have experienced isolation and lack interpersonal relationships. The general goals of these groups are to help patients increase self-esteem, openness, and the expression of feelings, and decrease isolation. When interpersonal communication increases, focus on the activity per se decreases. The activity is a vehicle or means to facilitate: self-expression of both positive and negative feelings in a creative way, patient interaction, and enjoyment.

Recreation groups provide the opportunity for fun and relieve tension. These groups enable patients to experience a sense of participation, acceptance, and accomplishment. Creative expression groups facilitate expression of feelings, communication with others, and socialization. They allow for creativity, self-expression, and praise for accomplishments.

Exercise or groups that foster physical activity benefit individuals mentally and physically by improving physical health and psychiatric and social disability, resulting in improved quality of life. Individuals with serious mental illness often have sedentary lifestyles and possibly comorbid physical health problems. Some experience weight gain as a side effect of their psychotropic medications. Integration of a structured program, such as a walking group or exercise group, can be helpful. Individuals with serious mental illness value exercise as a component of their treatment (Richardson et al, 2005).

## SELF-HELP AND SPECIAL PROBLEM GROUPS

Many groups focus on helping individuals with special problems—for example, child abuse, anorexia and bulimia, and diabetes. These groups are homogeneous, meaning that all group members share the same problem. Members feel accepted and understood by the group and are therefore more willing to share concerns and ask questions. Information is shared, as well as personal feelings and difficulties. Members assist each other with helpful strategies; they do not feel alone or isolated, but learn that others with the same problem or need are coping effectively. The nurse who leads special problem groups is interested, knowledgeable, and skilled in working with patients with specific problems.

Traditional self-help groups are also homogeneous, but are not professionally organized and led. Self-help groups are organized and led by group members who share a similar problem. Self-help is based on the belief that an individual with a problem can be truly understood and helped only by others who have the same problem. Millions of people participate in hundreds of self-help groups. In some groups, such as Alcoholics Anonymous, individual 24-hour support is available. Members of self-help groups understand each other's lifestyles and needs, help each other solve problems and cope with stress, and confront each other about dysfunctional behaviors.

Professionals might be invited to a self-help group for a specific purpose, such as providing an educational program. Nurses commonly refer individuals to self-help groups and must therefore be knowledgeable about the self-help groups in their area. Interested individuals can call their local mental health organization for information about the availability of groups such as the National Alliance for the Mentally Ill (NAMI), Recovery Incorporated, and Incest Survivors Anonymous.

## GROUP MANAGEMENT ISSUES

### GROUP LEADERSHIP

Group leadership functions range from the formal to the informal. The inpatient psychiatric nurse might engage in spontaneous, informal interactions with a group of patients in a card game or participate formally in a planned, structured group session in a special setting. An informal card game provides the nurse with an opportunity for therapeutic interpersonal interaction, socialization, and role-modeling behavior. Another example might be responding to medication questions that arise in small informal groups; the nurse reinforces compliance with medication and attempts to alleviate anxiety or concerns. These informal, spontaneous interventions with groups of patients occur repeatedly during the course of a day on an inpatient unit.

Brief clinical group encounters are also known as fluid groups. Fluid groups allow the nurse to facilitate interpersonal competencies and learning in informal, 24-hour contacts with patients in the inpatient milieu (Echternacht, 2001).

Although degrees of formality and types of patients vary, the nurse invariably uses group leadership skills to meet patients' needs in the therapeutic milieu. As managers and providers of patient care (24 hours a day), nurses intervene with groups of patients. Consequently, nurses must use effective communication skills to interact with groups of patients (described later in this chapter).

Nurses on inpatient units should be aware of factors that influence the clinical setting. Short-stay inpatient hospitalization affects group work in many ways. For example, short hospitalizations result in a rapid turnover of patients in groups; thus, expecting a high level of trust and cohesion to develop in such a group is unrealistic. Patients might also have various serious illnesses. The nurse must quickly assess the mental status of patients to determine how long it will take before patients can enter groups or whether they can tolerate a group at all. The nurse also assesses the appropriate placement of patients in specific groups based on their level of functioning and the ability to tolerate particular groups. Charting patient progress in the group is an important nursing responsibility for both therapeutic and legal reasons.

Similarly, in outpatient care and in the community, nurses must consider realistic factors that impinge on treatment. Patients might be limited to a specific number of visits because of payment providers, or participation in day treatment or substance-related programs might be limited to a specific number of days during the course of a year.

Confidentiality must be explained to group participants; that is, patients must understand that what is said or takes place in the group setting must remain private. However, statements within group sessions might be shared with staff members or the treatment team because of their responsibility for patient care. Personal information *is* shared in the group, but should not leave the unit or care facility. In reality, group confidentiality can be difficult to ensure because trust and cohesion might not be fully developed. Content, or what is learned in group settings, such as information about medication, can be shared outside of the treatment setting.

## PHYSICAL SETTING

Physical arrangements are important considerations in creating an atmosphere that is conducive to group work. Finding adequate space or a private room is often difficult but is nevertheless important to ensure privacy and a quiet atmosphere. Adequate lighting, comfortable temperature, ample seating, and proper equipment also contribute to successful group functioning. Forming a circle of chairs allows patients to see each other and indicates an expectation that patients will relate to the leader and other group members. Chairs in rows might be appropriate for a didactic group. A blackboard, dry marker board, projector, or video recorder might be necessary. Handouts or printed materials might be useful for patients and families.

Nurse leaders must be active, structured, and empathic. Because of time constraints, leaders cannot afford to be nondirective or to allow the group to be free floating. The nurse must be goal directed and focus on the here and now in each inpatient or outpatient group session. The leader succinctly states the group's purpose at the beginning of the session, and most of the session is spent on the work to be accomplished. Patients generally prefer leaders who provide the group "with an active structure" (Yalom, 1995). The final 5 to 10 minutes is used to summarize and close the session. The summary should have a positive focus and include information that the patients have learned or gained from the group. The leader gives positive feedback to the group regarding progress during the session.

Patients are expected to arrive at the group session on time. Patients remain for the entire group session, if possible. The group leader might permit patients to pace or leave the room and then return when they are able. The inability to sit still for an extended period might be the result of anxiety or medication side effects (usually akathisia). The decision to exclude patients from the group should be made carefully. The nurse might exclude patients who are acutely manic, disoriented, and too psychotic to benefit from group. Patients who are hostile and verbally threatening are also not appropriate candidates for group sessions.

## COMMON MANAGEMENT ISSUES

Basic interventions for groups are based on facilitative communication techniques (see Chapter 7). Nurses use these skills with patients individually and within groups. Nurses who facilitate group interactions on a therapeutic level help enable patients to share thoughts, feelings, and problems. Some basic communication skills useful for nurse leaders are detailed in Table 12-2. These skills are not unique to the group setting, but are skills that nurses use on a daily basis. These general interventions are therapeutic, regardless of the type of group. The use of positive feedback helps patients in their attempt to use new skills. For example, in an attempt to use a particular assertiveness skill, the patient goes off on a tangent. The nurse might say, "You have done well, Sam. When you gave us the example of saying to your boss, 'I need to talk with you about my work schedule,' you used an excellent example of 'I' statements." The nurse chooses to repeat the portion of Sam's statement that is realistic and is a correct example of an "I" statement for emphasis and clarity. As a result, the patient feels a sense of accomplishment and increased self-esteem.

For the group experience to be successful, the nurse leader must recognize and manage process and content areas (Rindner, 2000). The combination of teaching didactic material (psychoeducation) along with managing process issues requires knowledge and skill. The structure of the group session must include a balance between content to be taught and group process for the group experience to be beneficial.

## TYPES OF PATIENTS IN GROUPS

### DOMINANT PATIENT

The dominant patient monopolizes the entire group session to the extent that other patients might believe that they do not have the opportunity to participate. The nurse uses gatekeeping techniques to offer all patients the opportunity to contribute to the group. For example, the nurse can say, "Cathy, you are doing well in contributing to our session today, but I would like to hear what others are thinking about at this time." This intervention can forestall monopolization of the group by a single patient without putting her down, while providing others with the opportunity to express themselves. The other patients in the group might be unable to handle this patient or might be too afraid. If the group leader is afraid

or cannot control the patient, the integrity of the group is compromised.

### UNINVOLVED PATIENT

The uninvolved patient presents another challenge to the nurse leader. The patient might be quiet because of anxiety or fear. Patients with chronic schizophrenia find relating in group sessions to be difficult and threatening. The nurse can say, "It's hard to talk about ourselves in the group, but I know that everyone here has something to share that can help someone else." The nurse recognizes that patients are mistrustful and anxious but can relate the message that each individual is important and capable of helping another.

Some patients who are uninvolved in the group might believe themselves to be at a higher level of functioning than the other members. These patients might believe that they are not as sick as the others, do not belong in the group, and will not benefit from the session. The nurse leader might give attention to these members by giving them a job to perform for the group—for example, arranging chairs for the session. Respect and recognition by the nurse is therapeutic for these patients because they will believe that they can contribute to the group.

| CRITICAL THINKING QUESTION | 1 |
|---|---|

During a group session on medication management, a patient states, "I learn more by listening." How would you involve this patient in the group discussion?

| CRITICAL THINKING QUESTION | 2 |
|---|---|

During group, the nurse observes two patients whispering and snickering to each other. Which communication skills would the nurse use in this situation?

### HOSTILE PATIENT

Hostility might mask a patient's fear, self-anger, or unresolved anger toward others. To help this patient verbalize feelings of anger appropriately, the nurse can say, "Melody, you sound angry today. What happened?" or "Tell us about it." The nurse directly confronts this patient in a supportive manner and attempts to help the patient deal with her feelings. Allowing verbal or

| Table 12-2 | Communication Skills: Eliciting, Qualifying, and Clarifying Communication | |
| --- | --- | --- |
| **Techniques of the Leader(s)** | **Group Member Response** | **Outcome** |
| 1. **Giving information**: "My purpose in offering this group experience is . . ." | Further validates his assumptions: "How is this going to happen?" | Leader(s) and member(s) enter into a dialogue in which member(s) get more information that helps them make decisions and build trust in group experience. |
| 2. **Seeking clarification**: "Did you say you were upset with John because he said that?" | Might try to restate his thoughts or feelings: "Yes, I guess I was upset." | Member becomes aware that he was not clear and learns to identify thoughts and feelings more precisely, at the same time taking responsibility for them. |
| 3. **Encouraging description and exploration** (delving further into communication or experiences): "How did you feel when Joann said that to you?" | Elaborates on his message: "I was angry." | Member deals in great depth with an experience in the group and again takes responsibility for his reactions. (This example also places events in time or in sequence, lending further perspective to group events.) |
| 4. **Presenting reality**: "Would other members think Joann was unstable if they interviewed her for a job? You don't appear shaky to me." | Listens and considers other possibilities. | Member compares perception of self with others' perceptions of him. |
| 5. **Seeking consensual validation** (seeking mutual understanding of what is being communicated): "Did I understand you to say that you feel better now than you did last week?" | Further clarification: "Well, yes, I'm better than last week but not as good as I'd like to be." | Group and leader(s) learn how member views his progress and how they should receive his evaluation of himself. |
| 6. **Focusing** (identifying a single topic to concentrate on): "Could we identify one problem you have and talk more about that?" | Channels thinking: Members might think of the most puzzling problem they have. | Group leader(s) identify specific topics that they can resolve before the meeting ends. They increase their understanding of one problem before jumping to others. |
| 7. **Encouraging comparison** (asking members to compare and contrast their experiences with others in the group): "How did the rest of the group handle this problem?" | Group members share their experiences as they relate to the topic. | Leader(s) and members gain greater insight into their commonalities and differences and learn from one another alternative ways of responding to problems. |
| 8. **Making observations**: "You look more comfortable now, John, than you did at the beginning of the meeting." *or* "The group has been silent for the last 5 minutes." | Group members have something to respond to: "I feel more at ease now." *or* "I think we are quiet because we are bored." | Group members and leader(s) place attention on significant events and can elaborate on their meanings. |
| 9. **Giving recognition or acknowledging**: "John, you are new to the group. Perhaps we can introduce ourselves." | Feels acknowledged and included: "Yes, I'm John, and I came here because . . ." | Members view specific instances as important, and the leader(s) reinforce the behavior or event that they choose to notice—in this case, the desire to come to group. |

*Continued*

| Table 12-2 | **Communication Skills: Eliciting, Qualifying, and Clarifying Communication—cont'd** |
| --- | --- |

| Techniques of the Leader(s) | Group Member Response | Outcome |
| --- | --- | --- |
| 10. **Accepting** (not necessarily agreeing with but receiving communication with openness): "Yes, I hear you say that you don't know if you want to be in the group or not." | Feels heard and understood without fear of attack. | Members learn that even "nonacceptable" attitudes can be talked about, and perhaps any thought is not so horrible that they cannot share it. |
| 11. **Encouraging evaluation** (asking the group as a whole or individual members to judge their experiences): "When Marilyn gives you support, do you feel better?" *or* "How did we do in helping Joann with her problem?" | Member reflects on progress made: "Not exactly, because I don't know if I can trust her to be honest." *or* "It was hard. I'd like to know from her." | The criteria for success become clearer to members, and new directions might be formulated as a result of the discussion. |
| 12. **Summarizing** (encapsulating in a few sentences what has occurred): "The group discussed several issues and problems today. They were . . ." | Members recall significant points events and close off consideration of new or extraneous topics. | Members and leader(s) place in perspective and identify salient points of a group session. Such a summary can lead to a better understanding of group process. |

From Van Servellen G: *Group and family therapy,* St. Louis, 1983, Mosby.

nonverbal hostility to continue jeopardizes the progress of the group session. Unchecked hostility causes discomfort and uneasiness and impairs the ability of other patients to attend to the group's work. Patients might also mistakenly interpret anger as being directed toward them.

## DISTRACTING PATIENT

At times, some patients' behaviors and verbalizations can be very distracting to other members of the group. Others become distracted when inappropriate comments are made and when delusions are voiced or someone hallucinates in group. For the patient who has verbalized a delusion, the nurse could use empathy, focus on the underlying need, present reality, and refocus the group. For example, the patient could state, "Everyone here is against me." The nurse could reply, "It must upset you to feel that way. I don't think that anyone here is against you." The nurse ultimately brings the group members back to the topic being presented and discussed.

For the patient who is hallucinating, the nurse directs the patient to focus on reality and the topic of discussion. A simple statement to the group

such as, "We are talking about side effect management of atypical antipsychotics. Let's review what we've talked about so far." The nurse does not confront the individual in group but meets with the patient after group for one-to-one interaction.

The patient who verbalizes a sexually inappropriate comment can be handled by the nurse using limit setting. For example, the nurse could state, "Jim, that comment is inappropriate. We are discussing symptoms that could indicate relapse."

These group interventions will help the nurse develop as a group leader. Patients quickly recognize the group leader's empathy, understanding, and respect for each patient as caring behaviors. Even though some patients make only minimal progress toward their individual treatment goals, interacting with the nurse who possesses and exhibits these traits can increase the patients' feelings of worth as human beings.

## ■ Study Notes

1. The psychiatric nurse interacts and intervenes with patients and families in informal groups, as well as in formally structured sessions in inpatient and community settings.

2. Patients benefit from group experiences by gaining acceptance, hopefulness, and support from others. Through mutual sharing of feelings and problems, patients learn how their communication methods and behaviors interfere with relationships. Their strengths are reinforced and accumulated.

3. Families of the mentally ill benefit from the information and support they receive in a group.

4. Nurse leaders must be active, empathic, and goal directed and deal with the here and now in each group session.

5. Various types of groups exist in inpatient and outpatient settings that can benefit the acutely and chronically ill. Typical of these are psychoeducational, maintenance, activity, and self-help or special problem groups. Psychoeducational and self-help groups are available for families of mentally ill patients.

6. As group leaders, nurses use facilitative communication techniques and role-modeling behaviors.

7. The nurse leader structures the group session by attending to content and process issues.

8. The nurse leader intervenes therapeutically with dominating, uninvolved, hostile, and distracting patients.

## References

Echternacht M: Fluid group: concept and clinical application in the therapeutic milieu, *J Psychiatr Nurs Assoc* 7:39, 2001.

McGarry T, Prince M: Implementation of groups for creative expression on a psychiatric inpatient unit, *J Psychosoc Nurs* 36:19, 1998.

Oermann M, Templin T: Important attributes of quality health care: consumer perspectives, *J Nurs Scholarship* 332:167, 2000.

Payson A, Wheeler K, Wellington T: Health teaching needs of clients with serious and persistent mental illness: client and provider perspectives, *J Psychosoc Nurs* 36:32, 1998.

Potter M, Williams R, Costanzo R: Using nursing theory and a structured psychoeducational curriculum with inpatient groups, *J Am Psychiatr Nurs Assoc* 10:122, 2004.

Richardson CR, Faulkner G, McDevitt J, et al: Integrating physical activity into mental health services for persons with serious mental illness, *Psychiatr Serv* 56:324, 2005.

Rindner E: Combined group process-psychoeducation model for psychiatric clients and their families, *J Psychosoc Nurs Ment Health Serv* 38:34, 2000.

Van Servellen G: *Group and family therapy,* St. Louis, 1983, Mosby.

Yalom I: *The theory and practice of group psychotherapy,* ed 4, New York, 1995, Basic Books.

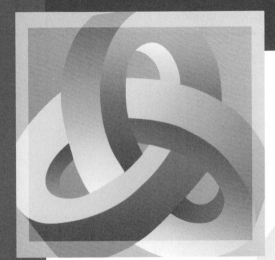

# Chapter 13

# Working With the Family

*Sandra J. Wood*

## Learning Objectives

*After reading this chapter, you should be able to:*
- Define the term *family* and discuss characteristics of contemporary families.
- List the factors to assess when working with families.
- Describe the skills necessary for working therapeutically and collaboratively with families.
- Describe the effects of mental illness on families.
- Discuss the issues associated with caring for psychiatric patients in a family context.

Throughout history, the family unit has functioned to perpetuate society and provide the nurturing, education, values development, and protection needed by children to survive and thrive. Even after reaching adulthood and living independently, most individuals' ties to their family of origin remain intact as they develop their own families or other kinship ties. When individuals become ill or frail in their elder years, families generally supply required care and support to them. Thus, when a family member experiences a mental illness, the family is likely to be the major source of assistance for the mentally ill member. Families are affected by the mental illness of their family member. They have observed the changes in behavior accompanying the illness, have been confused and concerned by their family member's actions, and often have tried desperately to obtain care for their ill family member. Nurses who care for mentally ill individuals need to understand family functioning, work collaboratively with families of patients to promote family adjustment to the illness(es) involved, and improve chances for illness amelioration or effective long-term illness management if the illness is chronic.

This chapter explores characteristics of families, the effects of mental illness on families, and strategies for working therapeutically with families in various settings. Understanding and assessing families as a basis for therapeutic interactions, family conferences, education, support, and referrals rather than family therapy are emphasized.

## DEFINITION OF FAMILY

Over the years, definitions of the word *family* have changed from two or more related people living together who are committed to each other to include unrelated individuals choosing to live together and assume the roles and functions of a family. McGoldrick and Carter (2003, p. 376) have stated that "Families comprise persons who have a shared history and a shared future." This

## Norm's Notes

*Where would you be without your family? I would not want to consider such a life, and you might not either. When a family member develops mental health problems, other family members are affected. Helping families deal with and help a mentally ill family member, and helping them better understand how they have contributed to the problem, if at all, is a fundamental role of nurses and other psychiatric professionals. Remember this, because I think it is humbling: when you have done what you know how to do, the family will almost always still be there dealing with the outcomes, whether good or bad.*

speaks to the permanence of families, regardless of the family form or structure.

## CONTEMPORARY FAMILIES

The extended family of past generations and the nuclear family common during the 1940s and 1950s, although still present, are no longer the predominant family structures in contemporary life. Divorce, remarriage, and the rise of same-sex marriages have led to single-parent families, blended families, and families with two parents of the same gender. Some believe that these changes undermine the integrity of the family, whereas others believe that these new structures demonstrate the flexibility of the family system, allowing the family to remain viable and effective as a vehicle for raising children and maintaining family interpersonal support amid the stresses of modern life (Walsh, 2003a).

Alterations in family structure parallel other societal changes that have affected how families function. Economic pressures have led to major increases in two–wage earner families, necessitating out of home care for children and leaving a gap in the supervision of older children and adolescents after school. Additionally, in families in which there is divorce and/or remarriage, the presence of parents, stepparents, grandparents, and stepgrandparents, not to mention half-siblings and stepsiblings, makes family interaction more complex and difficult than in the past.

For economic reasons, young adults might continue living in their parents' home after completing school and beginning work or return home after having lived on their own because of divorce, job loss, or financial hardship. Relationships between parents and adult children living in the same household can become strained and, even if cordial, require significant effort to remain harmonious and stable over time as roles and functions shift from what they had been while the children were growing up. Young adults who choose to live independently of their parents often live with a roommate or partner for economic as well as personal reasons (Walsh, 2003a).

In today's complex society, parents might be unable to raise their children as a result of their illness, substance abuse, financial strain, or death. Grandparents are increasingly stepping in to assume childrearing responsibilities for their grandchildren in such situations. This role alteration and economic burden profoundly alter family dynamics. Although children benefit greatly from being parented by a family member when their parents cannot assume this role, the practice often robs grandparents of their retirement and forces them to expend energy and money that might be in short supply. The fact that grandparents assume such roles at significant cost to themselves is a testament to the flexibility and strength of family ties (Leder et al, 2003).

Longer life expectancy means that many adults are caring for their aging parent(s) in their homes or monitoring their care in a facility. The economic burden of such care can be overwhelming, especially if the elderly person(s) reside in a facility. Furthermore, the role reversal caused by the physical and mental decline of an aged parent or parents, although necessary, is difficult for all involved and can put a strain on family relationships (Walsh, 2003a).

Society has become more culturally diverse as a result of immigration, intermarriage, and cross-cultural adoption. Issues of assimilation, integration, and maintaining one's cultural identity all affect the structure and function of families. In regard to immigration, cross-cultural marriage, and adoption, the involved parties must balance allegiance to their cultural heritage against the values, norms, and behavior of the new culture in which they find themselves. Parents who adopt a child of another race or culture are faced with decisions regarding how much to focus on their own culture and how to give their adopted child some ties to his or her culture of origin. Over time, the children of immigrants adopt the customs of the culture in which they are living, often causing distress and feelings of loss in their immigrant parents. Assimilation of the younger generation into the new society is necessary for them to fit into the new culture and feel successful, but might come at a price in terms of their cultural identity (Walsh, 2003a). Discrimination and racism are faced by many immigrants, especially if their cultural norms and appearance are very different from the dominant culture in their new country. Lack of familiarity with the culture, possible inability to speak the language, and lack of job skills in a highly technical society can cause a ripple effect of low wages and economic hardship that can weaken the family structure.

Alterations in family structure and function, along with societal changes, can create stress in the family. In today's world, communications technology makes everyone constantly aware of world events, which can fuel fear about the future and one's own personal safety, and make it more difficult for families to feel secure. The subway and bus bombings in London on July 7, 2005 left people in large cities all over the world who use public transportation wary about the safety of using mass transit, possibly resulting in individuals and their families restricting their daily activities. Such restriction makes it more difficult for families to function optimally, although most have shown great resiliency in dealing with such threats (Walsh, 2003a).

Nurses working with families must recognize that the families they encounter are less likely to fit the traditional model of the past and more likely to be negatively affected by external stresses in their work and family life. In addition, they are more likely to be culturally diverse, requiring the nurse to find out about the values, beliefs, and customs of families from another culture. Information in this chapter and in Chapter 14 should provide assistance to nurses in understanding and responding to culturally diverse families.

## FAMILY CHARACTERISTICS

The varied definitions and forms of family structure might prompt the questions, "What is a normal family? What does a normal family look like and how do they act?" Walsh (2003a) has addressed the issue of family normalcy:

> Societies worldwide are experiencing rapid transformation and uncertainties about the future. Amid the turmoil couples and families have been forging new and varied arrangements as they strive to build caring and committed relationships. These efforts are made more difficult by questions about their normalcy (p. 4).

Thus, when conceptualizing beliefs about normal family processes, professionals must consider the rapid pace of change in the world and the need for families to adapt to such changes. If Walsh's advice is followed, new family types can be perceived as adaptive rather than dysfunctional. Perhaps the term *normal,* with its limits on form and function and on what is most common rather than what is most helpful, is not best for characterizing families. The terms *healthy* or *functional* seem more in tune with the type of family functioning we wish to describe (Walsh, 2003a).

To define a healthy or functional family, it is necessary to consider what is done by successful families of all types. Healthy, well-functioning families nurture and support their members and provide stability and cohesion in a rapidly changing world. It is often said in families that "Home is the place you can go and be accepted when the rest of the world rejects you." In today's fast-paced, high-stress society, such nurturing is invaluable. Everyone needs someone to care and help them when facing challenges. Knowing that the family will remain together and provide predictability in an unpredictable world can buffer the stresses that individuals face every day.

Successful families also protect their members from dangers by caring for vulnerable members whose age or condition renders them unable to care for themselves independently; for example, infants and children require many years of parental care and supervision. Family members who experience acute injury or illness or chronic conditions benefit from family care and support. Elderly individuals experiencing physical and mental decline also receive care that is generally provided by family members.

The family provides the first education for children. It is where family members initially learn what is needed to function in the world, from communication and socialization to values and roles required within the family and in the outside world. Children learn language, communication skills, and religious and secular beliefs, as well as how to be a child, sibling, student, and parent from interactions within the family. In healthy, functional families, communication is open, lines of authority are clear, socialization is encouraged, and respect for self and others is taught, as well as how to relate to each other and those outside the family. When external assistance is needed, it is sought and accepted rather than denying that problems exist. In such an environment, whether a nuclear family, an extended family, or a single-parent household, members are cared for, valued, and prepared to cope with the society in which they live. The nurturing of individuals as they grow and develop leads to the achievement of autonomy as a well-functioning, healthy adult.

These characteristics provide the basis for the family to cope effectively with internal pressures, such as the illness of a member, or external pressures, such as the loss of a job by a parent. During times of stress, a family might experience disruption in one or more of these desirable characteristics; however, the retention of others and the support of caregivers and the extended family can help the family weather the disruption and remain resilient. Job loss by the father causes an initial economic and personal crisis. However, if his wife can move to full-time employment and the family can problem solve the crisis together, the father can return to school to retrain for a better position to improve the family's long-term stability.

## STAGES OF FAMILY DEVELOPMENT

Duvall and Miller (1985) defined stages of family development based on the people and events involved in a family at different periods of life. Initially, the single individual marries and becomes part of a "beginning family" (a couple). If a child enters the family, the stage changes to the "early childbearing family" when the oldest child is a toddler or preschooler and the family concentrates on incorporating the child into the family, introducing him or her to the outside world but controlling contact with others. As the oldest child enters elementary school—"families with school-children"—parents must accept increased contact

of their children with the outside world and focus on education, socialization, and monitoring contact with the outside world. "Families with teenagers" have their oldest child encountering increasing independence and planning for the future as the child negotiates high school and work or college. After the oldest child reaches the end of the teenage years, plans are made for the child to begin a life on his or her own— "launching center families." This is followed by "families in midlife," in which the couple readjusts to life without children (the empty nest). In the final stage, "families in retirement," the couple deals with issues of adjusting to retirement, becoming grandparents, and facing the eventual death of spouse and friends (McGoldrick and Carter, 2003).

Knowing the stage of family development with which a family is dealing can give the nurse an idea of potential issues and problems that the family might be facing. If a family has children of widely varying ages, the family might be dealing with developmental tasks at several levels at the same time. For example, in a blended family, one or both spouses might have adolescents and schoolage children from a previous marriage while also dealing with a newborn from their current union. Nurturing an infant and simultaneously guiding an adolescent to self-sufficiency requires different parenting techniques and might create stress in the family. Knowledge of appropriate child behavior at each developmental stage of childhood is also an important part of successful parenting that can contribute to the strength of family ties.

### CRITICAL THINKING QUESTION    1
Can healthy families have mentally ill members?

## EFFECTS OF MENTAL ILLNESS ON THE FAMILY AND INDIVIDUAL

Mental illness is a particularly stressful event in a family's life. The diagnosis of a mental illness in a family member can elicit feelings of guilt over possible genetic transmission of the disease to the ill family member by parents, concern over the prognosis and course of the disease, worry among other family members that they might become mentally ill, and shame or embarrassment in the family about how people outside the family will view the family and the ill member. Also, the ill family member might experience feelings of sadness, anger, or resentment about being ill or about the intervention of other family members, guilt about the difficulties caused to the family by his or her mental illness, or resignation and hopelessness about the prognosis of the illness (Oyebode, 2003). In addition to the feelings engendered by the diagnosis, the ill member might display unusual or dangerous behavior, such as making suicidal or homicidal threats or actions. The family must deal with the ill member's behavior as well as with agencies and institutions available to assist the ill family member. Law enforcement agencies, courts, social service agencies, schools, hospitals, clinics, and churches are among the many agencies having differing rules and procedures with which the mentally ill person and family must negotiate. These agencies might be consulted in the process of obtaining needed care, or contacts might be made as a result of dangerous behavior related to the family member's mental illness. For example, the mentally ill family member who is paranoid might believe that the neighbor is planning to harm him or her and, as a result, might make a threat against the neighbor. This action will bring the family into contact with the local law enforcement agency and the courts. If the ill family member is committed for treatment, mental health agencies and hospitals might become involved in the person's care. Issues that might surface as a result of a family member's mental illness include the following:

- Medication compliance, presence and treatment of side effects of medication
- Lack of energy to complete activities of daily living (ADLs)
- Social isolation, avoidance of contact with others
- Acting-out behaviors, particularly threatening or paranoid behavior
- Mood swings
- Denial of illness, lack of appropriate reasoning or judgment
- Inappropriate or incomprehensible communication
- Persistence of dangerous behavior (e.g., drug or alcohol abuse)
- Manipulation of others to achieve desired goals

When a family member is diagnosed as mentally ill, the ill person and family must deal with grief issues, which include the loss of individual and family functioning because of the illness of the mentally ill member. Income might be lost if the family member has been a wage earner. Stress on the ill member and others in the family can increase and affect everyone's school or work performance. Stigma from inside or outside the family related to being mentally ill can affect the ill individual and other family members. The future of both the individual and family might also be jeopardized (Conn and Marsh, 1999). The diagnosis of a mental illness can break apart a family—for example, when a spouse can no longer live with and subject children to an alcoholic or abusive partner—or it can bring family members together. Kay Redfield Jamison, a professor of psychiatry who also has manic-depressive illness, spoke of her mother in her autobiography (1995) in the following terms:

> She could not have known how difficult it would be to deal with madness: had no preparation for what to do with madness—none of us did—but, consistent with her ability to love and her native will, she handled it with empathy and intelligence (p. 9).

## CRITICAL THINKING QUESTION    2

If the family of a mentally ill child is told that the child's mental illness has a biologic-genetic component, what effect will that statement likely have on the thoughts and feelings of the parents and siblings of the child?

## FAMILY REACTIONS TO PSYCHIATRIC TREATMENT AND HOSPITALIZATION

When a family member is diagnosed with a mental illness and possibly hospitalized in a psychiatric facility, patients and families react in various ways. Relief might be felt among family members and, at times, by the patient. The patient might not want others to know about the illness, fearing a negative reaction from family and friends. The family might be exhausted because of difficulty in coping with the patient's bizarre behavior or be concerned about the safety of the patient or others related to suicidal or homicidal threats or actions.

When the ill individual must be involuntarily committed to a facility, conflicting emotions can arise on the part of the family. The family might want the person admitted, but not agree with any coercion used to force the patient into admission. The patient might desire help and agree to be admitted, or the patient might want help, but refuse to be admitted to an inpatient facility.

Frequent admissions might cause the family to experience burnout. When stress in the family is high, the family might wish the mentally ill family member to be hospitalized to provide relief for the family system. Admission might be helpful to the entire family if the treatment provided meets the current safety and security needs of the patient and family. However, if a family hospitalizes a patient for his or her problems when only the family unit is experiencing difficulties, the patient is made to feel responsible for the mental health of the entire family and is burdened beyond the stress of his or her illness. Family therapy might be indicated for all or some members of the family when conflict between the patient and family cannot be mediated by the nurse or other health care staff (Merrell, 2001). Family therapy should be carried out by a professional who has been prepared at the master's or doctoral level because of the complexity of the issues and the skills needed to carry out the treatment. Professionals who are qualified for family therapy are social workers, marriage and family therapists, psychologists, and advanced practice psychiatric nurses. Family therapy is beyond the scope of practice of the baccalaureate-prepared nurse.

Psychiatric admissions in which abuse or assault is discovered in the family are problematic for caregivers, patients, and others in the family, as well as the nurse. Abused members might experience relief that the *secret* has finally been revealed but might also experience anger, rejection, or humiliation from exposure of abuse. Fear about the future, fear of retribution, or fear of legal consequences of the abuse might be of concern to family members who have been victimized by another family member. Ensuring the safety of abused family members is necessary for them to confront the pain and suffering caused by the abuse. See Chapter 41 for further information.

## NURSE RESPONSE TO PATIENTS AND FAMILIES SEEKING TREATMENT

When a family seeks treatment for any of the problems listed in Box 13-1 or for other problems, the nurse must listen to all parties involved and withhold judgment until all points of view have been examined. The nurse should refrain from perceiving one family member or an entire family as problematic. The nurse and other caregivers must refrain from giving the impression that the family caused the problems of an individual member, or that the ill individual is responsible for the problems that the family is experiencing. Family members who become emotionally ill might not be the sickest members of the family. Scapegoating the ill family member as the cause of all family problems might be tempting, but is inaccurate. Often, the ill family member is the one who is most sensitive to the disruptions in family life and most desirous of obtaining help to overcome the problem (Walsh, 2003b). The nurse can ameliorate some of the scapegoating that might be occurring in a family by consulting directly with the patient and other family members during assessment and treatment. The nurse can offer positive reinforcement about the patient's willingness to engage in the treatment process. Even if the patient is only minimally cooperative with treatment, positive reinforcement can serve to improve the patient's cooperation and boost his or her self-esteem.

---

**Box 13-1    Reasons for a Family to Seek Treatment for Mental Health Issues**

- Situational crises, such as loss of job, divorce
- Developmental crises, such as a child leaving home for the first time
- Relationship problems and conflicts, such as abuse of one or more family members
- Conflicts between families of origin and current family (family of marriage)
- Addition of family members through remarriage, adoption, and foster care
- Family conflicts over treatment when a family member has another type of illness
- Custody conflicts and issues
- Family exploitation of an ill family member
- Family confrontation or conflict with caregivers
- Acute or chronic mental illness of a family member

## ABILITIES NEEDED WHEN WORKING WITH FAMILIES

To work constructively with patients and their families, the nurse must possess important characteristics: self-knowledge, spirituality, and the ability to assess, communicate therapeutically, collaborate with patients, families, and other caregivers, and provide appropriate referrals to patients and families.

## SELF-KNOWLEDGE

The nurse must recognize and accept his or her own values, beliefs, and biases related to the importance of families and their involvement in the care of their mentally ill member. The nurse must also avoid allowing personal concerns to become involved with the problems of patients and families. To do this, the nurse must be aware of and acknowledge his or her own family history and appreciate that all families have strengths and needs (Walsh, 2003b). The nurse must model adaptive self-care and stress management techniques, such as regular exercise, healthy eating, and strong support and nurturance from friends and family. Such self-care activities prepare the nurse to assist patients and families in learning better coping skills to manage their problems.

## ASSESSMENT

Interactions among all family members are the raw material for problem solving by the family and nurse. The nurse must become the family's partner in assessment and decision making so that the family can own and be invested in problem solving (Johnson et al, 2002). A family assessment guide (Box 13-2) can help the nurse obtain information about family strengths and the problem(s) for which they seek assistance, so that the nurse can base problem solving on these and available resources while addressing family needs. Individual and family strengths are used to overcome deficits, helping the family see themselves as capable of change rather than feeling at the mercy of their circumstances and problems. Additionally, by participating in assessment of their problems, the family learns valuable skills for managing future problems that they might encounter.

Assessments include the following:

---

### Box 13-2   Family Assessment Guidelines: Possible Questions to Ask

**Family membership and development**

- "Tell me about the members of your immediate (nuclear) family, including ages and gender (male or female)."
- "What other relatives do you have? How are they involved with your immediate family?"

**Family strengths and needs**

- "What do you think is a strength of your family?"
- "What is something you would like to change about your family?"

**Family coping**

- "Describe a problem that your family has dealt with successfully."
- "What helped you to deal with this problem successfully?"

**Family problem identification**

- "What is your perception of the current family problem?"
- "How do you think the current problem should be resolved?"

**Family use of resources**

- "What resources or agencies have you used in the past in dealing with this type of problem?"
- "What does your family do to stay healthy? What does your family do to treat or control mental, emotional, and physical illness?"
- "What type of help would you like from me (the nurse) in resolving the current problem?"

---

- Family characteristics in both the family of origin and the present family
- Developmental stage of the family at the present time
- Family's accomplishment of developmental and daily tasks
- Patient's and family's reasons for seeking treatment and reactions to care
- Effects of mental illness on family members and on the family as a whole
- Family strengths
- Family's understanding of the illness and current coping skills for managing the illness and its attendant behaviors
- Other health problems of the patient, family members, or significant others that might affect care

The nurse's observational skills are important when interacting with members of the family. The nurse should observe the behavior and words of all family members and consider how members relate to each other and to the nurse, rather than focusing on the actions of one individual (the patient) alone. The nurse must consider all available information, its relevance, and impact before arriving at conclusions about a family. If conclusions are drawn too quickly and with too little information, the solution is not likely to be effective; this might discourage the family from seeking help with family problems in the future.

## THERAPEUTIC COMMUNICATION

Therapeutic interactions should be based on the nurse's understanding of the following: families are generally functioning as well as possible, in view of their available resources and abilities; families are capable of solving their problems with the guidance and support of caregivers; all families have strengths that can be applied to solving their problems; placing blame does nothing to solve the family's problems and serves only to diminish the self-esteem of family members and the family as a whole; and family members act out frustration or pain when they are unable to face their problems directly (Conn and Marsh, 1999). Nurses should also remember that every interaction with a patient and family represents an opportunity to be therapeutic. Therapeutic interviewing skills include the ability to display respect for all family members and an ability to be nonjudgmental about the family, its members, and the problems they face.

Specific therapeutic communication techniques used with families by the nurse vary depending on the stage of the relationship with the family, but are likely to include active listening, eye contact, expressions of empathy and support, sensitivity to verbal and nonverbal cues, validating and clarifying information, summarizing, and reinforcing the family's efforts. Chapter 7 presents more information concerning therapeutic communication.

## FAMILY EDUCATION

Nurses, who have always educated patients and families, can serve as a support to families in both treating and preventing mental health problems. For at-risk families, preventive education can enhance functioning and prevent the occurrence of mental health problems. Nardi (1999) demonstrated that a parenting education program such as *S*ystematic *T*raining for *E*ffective *P*arenting (STEP) can diminish the use of harsh discipline, promote parent-child attachment, and encourage parents in a low-income, high-violence geographic area to play with their children. Nurses can promote a therapeutic partnership by acting as a family educator about topics of interest and need for specific families. Wilson and Hobbs (1999) have described this type of nursing role with newly diagnosed psychotic patients and their families. The nurse explains the disorder and symptoms that might be frightening to patients and their families, which eases the shock and distress that occurs when patients begin to act and talk in strange ways. This role involves partnership and advocacy of the family with the treatment team and community, reinforcement of family strengths, and facilitation of transition to postdischarge rehabilitation. Programs of family education, such as those presented by Wilson and Hobbs (1999), are similar to the rehabilitation programs that patients and family members go through in medical settings after a family member experiences a stroke or heart attack. Such programs not only speed recovery from acute episodes of the illness but also enable the patient and family to manage the ill member's chronic illness better, with fewer relapses.

Effective education of patients and families requires knowledge of learning styles and the ability to present information in a variety of ways, such as through oral and written communication, pictures, and stories. The most successful educators adapt information to the patient's and family's preferred method of learning. For example, if the nurse must educate a family whose members have a low level of formal schooling, pamphlets written at an elementary school reading level with pictures to illustrate important information can be helpful. Interpreters or pamphlets written in Spanish are helpful for a family who has just arrived from Mexico. The proliferation of information on the Internet provides rich educational resources for the nurse and family, although the nurse must evaluate the quality and accuracy of Internet information and determine whether it comes from reliable sources before offering it to the patient and family.

The National Alliance for the Mentally Ill (NAMI) and other groups such as the National

Mental Health Association advocate effectively for the rights of patients and their families. These groups also provide information about the availability of new treatments, effectiveness of certain treatments, risks and benefits of specific treatments, cost-benefit ratio of specific services, availability of services such as mutual support groups, and assistance in negotiating insurance, mental health systems, and other bureaucracies. The NAMI Family to Family program is a good example of an effective educational and support program for families of mentally ill individuals (Dixon et al, 2001).

## SPIRITUALITY

By demonstrating caring, empathy, support, patience, and hope, the nurse facilitates care and provides a spiritual dimension to treatment, enriching interventions that have been implemented (Sperry, 2000). Because of their close and frequent contact with patients and families, nurses are adept at providing spiritual care by partnering with the patient and family, sharing their pain and joy, and respecting the values and beliefs of the patient and family. The nurse should also consider making a referral for a spiritual guide, such as a minister, priest, or rabbi, when needed or desired by the patient or family. If a family's spiritual beliefs conflict with the prescribed treatment, the nurse should accommodate the beliefs whenever possible, unless doing so would hinder the patient's care. For example, some patients and families are wary of using medication to alter mental function and prefer to rely on prayer as a treatment. However, when a patient is experiencing psychosis, a reduction in symptoms is not likely to occur without the aid of antipsychotic medication. The nurse, other caregivers, and patient and family must then collaborate on the cost-benefit ratio of accommodating the family's spiritual beliefs versus the needed medical treatment and decide on the best action in view of the conflict of values and beliefs. In this example, a compromise incorporating both prayer and medication might resolve the conflict in a manner that acknowledges the value of prayer while also using the physical benefits of medication (Sperry, 2000).

## COLLABORATION

The nurse must work with patients, families, and colleagues in providing care for families and helping families reach their goals. This requires that nurses collaborate with multidisciplinary teams and agencies to advocate for patients and achieve positive family outcomes.

Competencies of mental health care workers have been identified by members of the Adult Panel of the Managed Care Initiative coordinated by the Center for Mental Health Policy and Service Research at the University of Pennsylvania (Coursey et al, 2000). Three of the 12 competencies developed by the panel relate to collaboration. The first competency mentions engaging seriously mentally ill adults as full collaborators in planning, delivering, and evaluating their care. The second indicates that family members and others who care about the seriously mentally ill adult should be involved in all aspects of care. The ninth directs caregivers to work collaboratively with all sectors of the service delivery system. The focus on collaboration in this article demonstrates that interdisciplinary collaboration is essential for the delivery of quality mental health care.

To collaborate successfully with all stakeholders in providing comprehensive mental health care, nurses need to recognize their skills; acknowledge the contributions of other team members; involve the patient, family, and other health care workers in problem identification and problem solving; be knowledgeable about resources; and work cooperatively with all involved to attain quality mental health care for the patient and family.

## REFERRALS AND FAMILY SUPPORT

Referrals are helpful when working with families who have unmet needs. The nurse must have the knowledge and skills to support families as they enter the health care system to ensure that they can receive the assistance they require for their specific problems. The nurse must be knowledgeable about the resources to which he or she refers families. The referral is most effective when the patient and family know where to go, whom to meet, the reason for the referral, and what to expect when they get there. If the nurse merely gives the patient and family the name and address of a facility or support person, the probability that the patient and family will follow up is low. The family might not know how to get to the location, might be afraid that the treatment will be harmful or costly, or might fear that the ill family member will be taken away from them and hospitalized against their wishes. The extra effort made by the nurse to personalize and individualize a referral will pay dividends in better continuity of care and better mental health for the entire family.

## APPLICATION OF THE NURSING PROCESS TO THE FAMILY

### ASSESSMENT

The assessment process begins within the context of the nurse-patient-family relationship. Assessment provides the nurse, patient, and family an opportunity to discuss how problems are viewed. Questions might be asked when the patient and the family are together, when only some family members are present without the patient, or when only the patient is available. Obtaining the viewpoint of as many family members as possible greatly enhances treatment.

Patients who seek treatment might live with their intact family of origin, a parent who has remarried, adoptive parents, foster parents, other relatives, a spouse or significant other, by themselves, or in a residential facility. The nurse must consider living arrangements and the person(s) supporting the patient who are involved in his or her treatment. Current problems might be an extension of problems that began with the original family or might represent new issues not related to the family of origin.

An assessment should also consider other physical and mental health problems within the family that might be a result of dealing with the mentally ill member or those that might impinge on care given to this individual. Families dealing with a seriously mentally ill member can lose sleep, fail to eat healthy meals, and be susceptible to stress related to dealing with the behavior of the ill family member. All these can lead to headaches, indigestion, ulcers, hypertension, and other stress-related physical problems. Puchelak (2003) has indicated that, among parents of mentally ill adults in the Family Association in Poland, the most distressing and burdensome feelings include feeling helpless and fearful, losing dreams for the future of their mentally ill child, and the necessity of changing plans they had made prior to the illness. Another source of stress for elderly parents and siblings is the care of their mentally ill child or

sibling after they die (Lively et al, 2004; Smith et al, 2000).

A family assessment guideline can help the nurse think of the family as a system when conducting a family assessment. Examples of questions that the nurse might wish to ask are listed in Box 13-2. These questions are designed as triggers to help the family tell their story, rather than respond to standardized questions that might not reflect the family's problems and concerns. Through nurse-guided discussions, families can be actively engaged in decision making regarding health priorities.

### NURSING DIAGNOSIS

Based on the family assessment, the nurse develops priority nursing diagnoses from those approved by the NANDA International classification system. Examples of some typical diagnoses are ineffective family therapeutic regimen maintenance, impaired parenting, interrupted family processes, and risk for caregiver role strain. These nursing diagnoses help define the problems that the family is facing, thus providing a foundation for outcome identification. Although nursing diagnoses are generally stated in terms of deficits, the nurse needs to remember that the assessment should include a determination of patient and family strengths that can be used to help overcome deficits and/or prevent risks for deficits from becoming actual patient problems (NANDA International, 2005).

### OUTCOME IDENTIFICATION

The nurse works with patients and their families to establish goals to be accomplished during treatment based on the family assessment. These goals might be individual goals for a specific family member, goals for the family as a whole, or both. The outcomes or goals identified must be specific, measurable, and achievable within a time frame appropriate to the period of contact of the nurse, patient, and family. When establishing goals with very troubled families, the nurse must consider how other agencies will be involved in the treatment process. Agency contact might focus on economic issues, protection for one or more family members, reporting of abuse to a state agency, contacts with police, or actions of a court order.

---

## Key Nursing Interventions *for Working With Families*

- Provide respect, empathy, support, and acceptance to patients and families.
- Advocate for patients and families in their interactions with other providers, institutions, and organizations.
- Help families build patients' self-esteem, yet be realistic in their expectations of the patient, themselves, and others.
- Facilitate resolution of normal developmental problems of individuals and families.
- Help the family use more adaptive coping skills, thereby facilitating future problem solving.
- Provide referrals to support groups and resources for families who are experiencing normal developmental issues of family life, as well as families dealing with more serious crises.
- Empower the family by teaching problem solving, limit setting, and conflict resolution skills.
- Help families validate, clarify, negotiate, and communicate feelings appropriately.
- Assist families in recognizing and coping with abuse issues to maintain safety of all family members.
- Offer feedback to patients and families concerning their progress in dealing with their problems.
- Negotiate role flexibility between patients and their families in response to family needs.
- Provide support for families through referral to brief, problem-focused, and psycho-educational groups.
- Be honest with patients and families if abuse must be reported.
- Teach communication and parenting skills.
- Teach families about the causes, manifestations, and treatment of psychiatric illnesses.
- Teach about the desired effects and side effects of medications and symptoms to report to professionals to prevent or minimize relapse.
- Teach and model the management of difficult behaviors of patients.
- Include the patient and family in goal setting and treatment planning.
- Teach and encourage family members to practice self-care as well as care for the patient.

---

## PLANNING AND IMPLEMENTATION

The skills needed for therapeutic interactions have already been specified earlier in this chapter. Other interventions that the nurse might use when working with patients and their families individually and in groups are listed in the Key Nursing Interventions for Working With Families box. Through the process of understanding the patient's and family's perspective concerning the stresses of living with a mental illness, the nurse can help develop interventions helpful for all parties involved. Parents in the Mental Health Family Association in Poland determined that relief of caregiver burden involved providing information to help them understand the mentally ill family member, hope that the ill family member's life could improve, and supportive family, friends, and professionals to talk to about their concerns (Puchelak, 2003).

## EVALUATION

Outcomes of working with patients and their families can be measured by determining whether treatment goals have been met and whether patients and families have developed solutions for current problems. Periodically, throughout treatment, the nurse and family must evaluate progress toward the resolution of problems defined by the nurse, patient, and family. When appropriate, the nurse can assist patients and families in reformulating goals and creating post-treatment goals toward which the family can work after the patient's discharge from an inpatient unit or outpatient program. Ongoing nursing evaluation of patient progress and outcome achievement is essential for successful treatment and represents one of the most important phases of the nursing process.

## RESOURCES AVAILABLE TO FAMILIES

The nurse can assist families in finding helpful resources and arranging for services. These services might include medical services, social welfare agencies, churches, emergency food services, voluntary agencies, support groups, community health services, and psychiatric home-care services. Some resources for families include the following:

- Al-Anon/Al-A-Teen: Available @ http://www.al-anon.org

- Alcoholics Anonymous: Available @ http://www.alcoholics-anonymous.org
- Families Anonymous: Available @ http://www.familiesanonymous.org
- Narcotics Anonymous: Available @ http://www.na.org
- NAMI and NAMI-CAN (Child/Adolescent Network): Available @ http://www.nami.org
- Parents Anonymous: Available @ http://www.parentsanonymous.org
- Alzheimer's Association: Available @ http://www.alz.org
- National Mental Health Association: Available @ http://www.nmha.org

## CRITICAL THINKING QUESTION    3

What family-oriented approaches would you use with a family having difficulty adjusting to the increasing dependence of an older adult member with physical and psychological impairments who is becoming less able to function independently but resents being dependent on other family members? What referrals might you make as part of treatment?

## Study Notes

1. The nurse who works with families will see many types of contemporary families and should respect their diversity and resilience.
2. Difficulties in accomplishing family tasks and developmental stages reflect the complexities and issues of modern life in a family.
3. The family of origin influences the communication skills, self-esteem, and coping skills that a person brings to the current family. However, healthy problem-solving and interaction skills can be developed, with the assistance of health care professionals and community resources, when an individual's skills are lacking.
4. Having a family member who is mentally ill inalterably changes the dynamics and communication within a family.
5. The nursing process with families requires that the nurse possess self-knowledge, assessment, therapeutic communication, spiritual, and collaboration skills, and skills regarding referrals and family support to help families deal with their mentally ill member.

6. The nurse must collaborate with the family to assess the function of the identified patient and family and refer the family to the most appropriate resource for assistance.

## References

Conn VS, Marsh DT: Working with families. In Shea CA, Pelletier LR, Poster EC, et al, editors: *Advanced practice nursing in psychiatric and mental health care* (pp. 371-385), St. Louis, Mosby, 1999.

Coursey RD, Curtis L, Marsh DT, et al: Competencies for direct service staff members who work with adults with severe mental illness: specific knowledge, attitudes, skills, and bibliography, *Psychiatr Rehabil J* 23:370, 2000.

Dixon L, McFarlane WR, Lefley H, et al: Evidence-based practices for services to families of people with psychiatric disabilities, *Psychiatr Serv* 52:903, 2001.

Duvall E, Miller B: *Marriage and family development,* ed 6, New York, 1985, Harper & Row.

Jamison KR: *An unquiet mind,* New York, 1995, Vintage.

Jensen LE: Mental health care experiences: listening to families, *J Am Psychiatr Nurs Assoc* 10:33, 2004.

Johnson LN, Wright DW, Ketring SA: The therapeutic alliance in home-based family therapy, *J Marital Fam Ther* 28:93, 2002.

Leder S, Grinstead LN, Jensen S, Bond L: Psychotherapeutic treatment outcomes in grandparent-raised children, *J Child Adolesc Psychiatr Nurs* 16:5, 2003.

Lively S, Friedrich RM, Rubenstein L: The effect of disturbing illness behaviors on siblings of persons with schizophrenia, *J Am Psychiatr Nurs Assoc* 10:222, 2004.

McGoldrick M, Carter B: The family life cycle. In Walsh F, editor: *Normal family processes,* ed 3 (pp. 375-398), New York, 2003, Guilford.

Merrell J: Social support for victims of domestic violence, *J Psychosoc Nurs* 39:30, 2001.

Nardi DA: Parenting education as family support for low-income families of young children, *J Psychosoc Nurs* 37:7, 1999.

NANDA International: *NANDA nursing diagnoses: definitions and classifications, 2005,* Philadelphia, 2005, NANDA International.

Oyebode J: Assessment of carer's psychological needs, *Adv Psychiatric Treat* 9:45, 2003.

Puchelak R: The face of family burden, *Newsletter of the World Fellowship for Schizophrenia and Allied Disorders,* First Quarter, 10, 2003.

Smith GC, Hatfield AB, Miller DC: Planning by older mothers for the future care of offspring with serious mental illness, *Psychiatr Serv* 51:1162, 2000.

Sperry L: Spirituality and psychiatry: incorporating the spiritual dimension into clinical practice, *Psychiatr Ann* 3:518, 2000.

Walsh F: Changing families in a changing world: reconstructing family normality. In Walsh F, editor: *Normal family processes,* ed 3 (pp. 3-26), New York, 2003a, Guilford.

Walsh F: Clinical views of family normality, health, and dysfunction: From deficit to strengths perspective, In Walsh F, editor: *Normal family processes,* ed 3, New York, 2003b, Guilford.

Wilson JH, Hobbs H: The family educator: a professional resource for families, *J Psychosoc Nurs Mental Health Serv* 37:22, 1999.

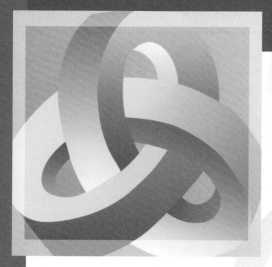

# Chapter 14

# Cultural Competence in Psychiatric Nursing

*Barbara Jones Warren*

## Learning Objectives

*After reading this chapter, you should be able to:*
- Understand the importance of the effect of cultural variables on health and health care.
- Describe the components of cultural competence.
- Describe the factors involved in patients' and nurses' cultural perspectives.
- Articulate the differences in and the importance of worldview.
- Explain how incorporation of cultural competence can enhance psychiatric nursing clinical excellence.
- Analyze the symptomatology suggestive of culture-bound syndromes.
- Apply understanding of ethnopharmacology as it might relate to a specific drug and a specific ethnic group.

Culture is a critical component of patients' lives that affects their health care attitudes and actions as well as their ability to understand and use the interventions that psychiatric nurses develop (Campinha-Bacote, 2003, 2005; Warren, 1999, 2000). *Culture* is the internal and external manifestation of a person's, group's, or community's learned and shared values, beliefs, and norms used to help individuals function in life and understand and interpret life occurrences (Leininger, 2002). The cultural perspectives and patterns of both the nurse and patient influence the nurse-patient interaction. These perspectives and patterns also affect a patient's level of mental health. For example, a patient's behaviors might be labeled as *pathologic* if a nurse misinterprets the patient's normal or culturally relevant beliefs and health care actions (Warren, 2000, 2003). Furthermore, a patient labeled as *noncompliant* might not be receiving culturally competent care (Purnell and Paulanka, 2003). The purpose of this chapter is to explain the role of the nurse and the connection between culture and cultural competence as they relate to psychiatric nursing.

## BASIC CONCEPTS

### IMPORTANCE OF CULTURAL COMPETENCE

*Cultural competence* is the process whereby the nurse shows proficiency in developing cultural awareness, knowledge, and skills to promote effective health care. A culturally competent psychiatric nurse not only possesses knowledge about the process of cultural competence, but also incorporates the process into interactions with peers, students, patients, families, and communities. The

## Norm's Notes

*Nurses must be culturally relevant. In many parts of the United States, nurses might work with five or more distinct cultural groups on an ongoing basis. How can you do this and provide the type of nursing care that takes into account the various cultural backgrounds? Dr. Warren has spent many years helping nurses learn this. This chapter outlines some basic nursing behaviors to help you help all patients.*

use of cultural competence, in conjunction with the psychotherapeutic management model, can enhance clinical excellence and promote recovery of psychiatric patients. Research on the use of culturally competent mental health strategies has indicated that cultural competence is key to patients' recovery process (Anthony, 1993; Warren, 2000, 2002; Warren and Lutz, 2000).

## CULTURE AND PSYCHIATRIC NURSING

The U.S. Surgeon General's report on mental health has emphasized the need for culturally competent mental health care (U.S. Surgeon General, 2001). Nurses provide services to a multitude of patients from diverse cultures. The term *cultural diversity* might encompass areas such as age, gender, socioeconomic status, religion, race, ethnicity, mental illness, and physically challenging conditions (Andrews and Boyle, 2002; Campinha-Bacote, 2003; Comas-Diaz and Green, 1994; Giger and Davidhizar, 2003; Institute of Medicine [IOM], 2003; Leininger, 2002; Spector, 2004). The *Diagnostic and Statistical Manual of Mental Disorders-IV-Text Revision (DSM-IV-TR)* has incorporated additional information regarding specific cultural features for each diagnostic category and includes an appendix, Outline for Cultural Formulation and Glossary of Culture-Bound Syndromes (American Psychiatric Association [APA], 2000).

## BARRIERS TO CULTURALLY COMPETENT CARE

A growing knowledge and research base has indicated that patients' adherence to treatment increases when cultural needs are incorporated into health care planning (APA, 2000; U.S. Surgeon General,

2001; Warren, 2001). Because nurses are often the gatekeepers for health care systems, knowledge of cultural factors related to psychiatric care is important.

The most common barrier to the delivery of culturally competent nursing care involves miscommunication between nurses and patients. A nurse might lack knowledge and sensitivity regarding a patient's cultural beliefs and practices; hence, the nurse might not recognize the importance and value of these beliefs to the patient as they relate to health care practices. Similarly, patients might be unaware of the nurse's cultural perspectives and misinterpret health care recommendations from the nurse (Diala et al, 2001). Consequently, to facilitate successful relationships with their patients, the nurse must understand his or her own cultural beliefs and values and how these beliefs and values influence patient care. This cultural awareness facilitates the psychotherapeutic relationship and the nursing process (Quander, 2001).

### CRITICAL THINKING QUESTION    1

Mr. James, a 40-year-old African-American man, comes into the medical clinic for his 6-month checkup. The nurse who assesses him notices that there is no information in his chart regarding cultural issues. How would she gather this information?

Another barrier to culturally competent care results from failure to assess the patient's cultural perspective. A variety of clinical cultural assessment tools and models are available for assessing cultural perspective. Some of these tools can be found in Tables 14-1 through 14-4 (Berlin and Fowkes, 1982; Chong, 2002; Hicks et al, 2004; Warren et al, 1994).

Finally, barriers to culturally competent nursing care are primarily grounded in differences between nurses and patients' cultural worldviews. These differences can increase miscommunication and thus affect the nurse-patient relationship and interaction negatively.

## CULTURAL ETIOLOGY OF ILLNESS AND DISEASE

Nurses' and patients' health care actions and beliefs are generally formulated by three factors:

(1) their definition of health; (2) their perception of the way in which illness occurs; and (3) their cultural worldview (Carter, 1995; Chong, 2002; Diala et al, 2001; Herrera et al, 1999). Nurses and patients might define *health* quite differently.

Closely connected to a nurse or patient's definition of health is his or her belief of how illness and disease occur. The nurse or patient might believe that illness and disease are created by natural, unnatural, or scientific causes. For example, a person who believes in the concept of natural cause of illness or disease believes that everyone and everything in the world is interrelated and that a disruption of this connectedness (e.g., a tornado) causes an illness or disease (Giger and Davidhizar, 2003; Spector, 2004). Conversely, nurses or patients might believe that *unnatural* or outside forces create illness and disease. An individual might believe that another person enlists the services of a magician, witch, ghost, or supernatural being to cast a spell or hex on him or her. Finally, nurses or patients might believe in the scientific cause of illness—specific, concrete explanations exist for every illness and disease (i.e., the entrance of pathogens such as viruses, bacteria, and germs into the body) (Campinha-Bacote, 2003; Warren, 1999). The scientific model is the typical model taught in most Western culture schools of nursing. However, many non-Western cultures acknowledge and teach health care providers the importance of the natural and unnatural causes of illness.

Patients' health care beliefs and actions are related not only to the way in which health, illness, and the cause of illness are defined but also to individual worldviews. There are four primary worldviews: (1) analytic, (2) relational, (3) community, and (4) ecologic. This primary worldview is often the one that individuals express or are comfortable with when they are with family or significant others, or during stressful times. Many individuals use a mixture of the four worldviews or adopt another worldview when they are in another environment, such as a work or business setting. The nurse's failure to understand the patient's primary worldview might negatively affect the nurse-patient relationship and impede successful interventions and mental health outcomes. Overarching worldviews that can be associated with ethnic populations are presented in Tables 14-1 through 14-4.

## CRITICAL THINKING QUESTION    2

Mrs. Gomez comes to a community health clinic with complaints of headache, nausea, and vomiting. She is accompanied by her daughter, Leticia, who is a nursing student at the local college, who says, "I have been worried about her and wanted her to come in for treatment." Mrs. Gomez states that she has had her symptoms for 2 days and believes that she was hexed by someone at work who was very angry with her. The nurse practitioner conducts a complete assessment of the patient, finds no other symptoms, and makes the initial diagnosis of a viral infection that is currently affecting many people in the community. The nurse practitioner prescribes medication and advises that Mrs. Gomez needs to rest at home until she feels better. The nurse also requests that Mrs. Gomez return to the clinic for a follow-up appointment in 1 week. Mrs. Gomez says that is not needed, because she has a *curandera* and will see her after leaving the hospital. How should the nurse handle informing Mrs. Gomez about her symptoms and supporting the prescribed treatment protocol?

## FOUR WORLDVIEWS

A person who expresses the analytic worldview values detail to time, individuality, and possessions. A person with this view also prefers to learn through written, hands-on, and visual resources. The relational worldview is grounded in a belief in spirituality and the significance of relationships and interactions between and among individuals. The preferred learning style is through verbal communication. An individual who expresses the community worldview believes that community needs and concerns are more important than individual ones. Quiet, respectful communication, as well as meditation and reading, are valued as a learning style. The ecologic worldview is based on a belief that a form of interconnectedness exists between human beings and the earth, and that individuals have a responsibility to take care of the earth. Learning is accomplished through quiet observation and contemplation, and verbal communication is minimized.

Worldviews form the basis for the expression of culturally bound mental health and wellness issues. For example, a patient or nurse using an analytic worldview perspective might espouse specific detail to time, calculations, individuality, and

## Table 14-1   European-American Worldview

| Component | Perspective |
| --- | --- |
| Cultural value | Value is placed on the member or object or on the attainment of the object. |
| Knowledge | Knowledge is acquired according to proof of the existence of anything—that is, the ability of an individual to see, hear, touch, taste, or smell it. |
| Logic | Dichotomous mode of reasoning is used. |
| Relationship | Relationships are developed, based on the perceived need for them. |

## Table 14-2   African, African-American, Hispanic, and Arabic Worldview

| Component | Perspective |
| --- | --- |
| Cultural value | Value is placed on the development and maintenance of interpersonal relationships. |
| Knowledge | Knowledge bases are developed through the use of the affective or feeling senses. |
| Logic | Reasoning ability is based on the union of opposites. |
| Relationship | Development of interpersonal relationships is based on the fact that all relationships are interrelated across all continua. |

## Table 14-3   Asian, Asian-American, and Polynesian Worldview

| Component | Perspective |
| --- | --- |
| Cultural value | Value is placed on the balance between member and group interactions. |
| Knowledge | Knowledge bases are developed in striving for transcendence of the mind and body. |
| Logic | Reasoning ability is based on the belief that the mind and body can exist independently of the physical world. |
| Relationship | Development of relationships is grounded in the belief that everyone and everything in the physical and spiritual worlds are related. |

## Table 14-4   Native-American Worldview

| Component | Perspective |
| --- | --- |
| Cultural value | Value is placed in the context of a person's relationship to a Greater or Supreme Being. |
| Knowledge | Knowledge bases are developed on the basis of a person's understanding of an individual's relationship with the Greater or Supreme Being. |
| Logic | Reasoning ability is grounded in the belief that every person is innately good and has no evil within. |
| Relationship | Development of relationships with another person, group, or community is grounded in the idea that the Greater or Supreme Being is in every person; hence, all persons should be valued. |

the importance of acquiring material objects. Being on time for appointments, immediately getting to the purpose of a health visit, and using printed pamphlets and books for health education are valued. Nurses and other health care professionals must be extremely accurate and precise when providing care for these patients. The example of individuality and valuing material goods is often embodied in traditional American society's values, beliefs, and actions.

The individual with a relational worldview values the development of interactions and relationships, usually prefers learning through verbal communication, and views spirituality as an important context for living life. These individuals might want to chat for a moment before getting to the heart of the health visit. They might desire the involvement of relatives, friends, or spiritual and religious advisors during the health visit or during the nurse's development of the nursing process. The relational worldview might be noted in certain individuals from African-American, Latino (Latina), or Hispanic cultures (Plummer, 1996; Warren, 1999).

Individuals with a community worldview value the importance and needs of the community over the individual. People with this perspective often use meditation and contemplation techniques. A patient with this view is respectful and polite regarding health care advice and might not want to question a nurse or physician. This reticence might occur even if the patient does not understand the nurse's recommendation. People from some Asian cultural groups often embody these philosophies (Warren, 1999).

Finally, a patient or nurse with an ecologic worldview values an interconnectedness with other people and the universe, takes responsibility for others and the world, and feels a need to maintain peace and tranquility. These individuals prefer a quiet, restful approach in interactions with others. Conversation is respectful, concise, and often kept to a minimum. Individuals from some of the indigenous or Native-American cultures might embrace this worldview.

### CRITICAL THINKING QUESTION    3

Why is it important for nurses to understand worldview perspectives for themselves and their patients? What are some questions that a psychiatric nurse might ask to find out about a patient's world perspective?

## CULTURE-BOUND MENTAL HEALTH ISSUES

Culture-bound syndromes are recurring patterns of behavior that create disturbing experiences for individuals (APA, 2000). These behaviors might or might not be congruent with symptomatology presented in the *DSM-IV-TR* for various diagnostic categories. However, because these behaviors can be culture-based, nurses must be aware of the symptoms to assess patients who are from racially and ethnically diverse cultures accurately.

People from racially and ethnically diverse cultures often use culturally specific language to describe mental distress that they experience (Ross, 2001; Taylor, 2003). One example involves the description of depressive symptoms and the actual symptomatology (Baker, 2001; Delahanty et al, 2001; Pouissaint and Alexander, 2000). Native Americans might state that they are "having heart pain" or are "heartbroken" when they experience depressive symptomatology (Warren, 1999). A person of Hispanic descent might say that his or her "soul was lost" *(susto)* because of another person's ability to cause a frightening experience or to place an "evil eye" *(mal ojo)* on them (APA, 2000; Campinha-Bacote, 2003). Someone who is experiencing a lost soul might be lethargic, have appetite and sleep changes, and have multiple physical complaints. Because good health is contingent on the restoration of a person's equilibrium, an ill person might initially consult a healer or root doctor to help break the spell of the evil eye and return the lost soul (Giger and Davidhizar, 2003). Traditional Western health care might be the last resource that the person contacts. Nurses must be knowledgeable about and sensitive to these beliefs.

People from diverse cultural groups often describe psychotic symptomatology differently. Individuals from Malaya and Laos use the term *running amok.* People from certain Native-American nations might use the term *ghost sickness.* African- and Appalachian-American individuals might say a *spell* has been cast on them. A more inclusive description of culture-bound syndromes can be found in Appendix I of the *DSM-IV-TR* (APA, 2000).

### CLINICAL EXAMPLE

Mr. Kilm is a 33-year-old Caucasian man with a history of paranoid delusions and congruent auditory hallucinations. He is estranged from his mother and father, who raised him in a very religious culture that interpreted his psychotic symptoms as "possession of the devil." Both his parents and his pastor believe that Mr. Kilm's sinfulness and failure to attend church on a regular basis are the causes of his behavior. With a certain level of insight, Mr. Kilm states, "I don't blame them no more. They don't know no better. They're just ignorant people."

The assessment of possible culture-bound syndromes and the cultural expression of psychiatric symptomatology must be part of the psychotherapeutic and nursing processes. This additional assessment can provide important information that the nurse must have to provide culturally competent services for patients.

## ALTERNATIVE THERAPIES

People from racially and ethnically diverse groups often use alternative therapies. These treatments might include the use of acupuncture, acupressure, nutritional therapies, skin scraping, moxibustion, and cupping. Acupressure and acupuncture use linear and circular lines throughout the body, known as meridians, which are stimulated to restore balance through the use of needles *(acupuncture)* or pressure *(acupressure)* (Giger and Davidhizar, 2003). *Nutritional therapies* might include the use of certain foods or herbs. *Skin scraping* or *coining, moxibustion,* and *cupping* are used to restore balance by bringing heat to the skin surface, which allows the release of the toxin or evil spirit from the affected body area (Giger and Davidhizar, 2003). In the case of skin scraping or coining, a person, generally a healer in the community, uses a coin and briskly rubs or scrapes the skin surface. In moxibustion, a cotton ball containing a substance known as *moxa* is ignited with a match in a small glass or cup, which is then placed on the skin above a meridian. The belief is that the illness or evil is released from a person's body when heat is generated within the meridians. However, skin abrasions and contusions, often occurring on the skin as a result of skin scraping or coining, moxibustion, or cupping, might provide a climate for infection.

Certain cultural groups (e.g., Hispanic, South American) believe that certain liquids, foods, or medicines must be taken in balance to restore health (Fontaine, 2000; Spence and Jacobs, 1999). A medicine might be labeled as being *hot* and might need to be taken in conjunction with a *cold* liquid or food to be effective. The terms *hot* and *cold* have nothing to do with temperature but are indicative of how the substance reacts within the body to restore equilibrium.

## ETHNOPHARMACOLOGY

Ethnopharmacology is the study of pharmacogenetic, pharmacodynamic, and pharmacokinetic influences based on different ethnic, racial, and cultural groups (Herrera et al, 1999; Warren, 1999). Culturally competent care is enhanced when this type of cultural knowledge is incorporated into patient care.

Individuals react to pharmacologic interventions based on their normal biologic makeup, environmental influences, and cultural influences (Herrera et al, 1999; Keltner and Folks, 2005). Specific ethnic, racial, and cultural differences affect a patient's medication options and dose requirements.

Variation in metabolism is most often cited as the cause of cross-ethnic differences in response to medications. Herrera and associates (1999) have indicated that individuals from certain racial and ethnic groups have a genetically based pharmacokinetic variation, which causes them to be fast or slow metabolizers. Drugs might accumulate in a patient's body when medications are metabolized too slowly. For example, people of Asian (about 50%) and Native-American descent are more sensitive to the effects of alcohol than people from other ethnic and racial backgrounds. This sensitivity is based on their relative deficiency of aldehyde dehydrogenase, resulting in slowed metabolism of the highly toxic intermediate product, acetylaldehyde (Herrera et al, 1999). Symptoms include a reddened flush to the neck and face, tachycardia, and a burning sensation in the stomach.

Most psychotropic drugs are metabolized by the cytochrome P-450 system (Ruiz, 2000). Basically, only two cytochrome P-450 enzymes (see Chapter 16 for this discussion), 2D6 and 2C19, appear to have extensive cross-ethnic variability. Substrates of these enzymes (again, see Chapter 16) are metabolized more slowly (poor metabolizers) in a certain percentage of each of these cultural groups (Keltner and Folks, 2005), as shown in Table 14-5.

Other enzymes also vary substantially across ethnic groups. For example, alcohol dehydrogenase, aldehyde dehydrogenase, butylcholinesterase, catechol O-methyltransferase, dopamine β-hydroxylase, and monoamine oxidase all have

| Table 14-5 | Metabolism by 2D6 and 2C19 Enzymes: Cross-Ethnic Variability | |
|---|---|---|
| Ethnic Group | 2D6-Poor Metabolizers (%) | 2C19-Poor Metabolizers (%) |
| African Americans | ~2 | ~19 |
| Caucasians | 3–9 | 2.5–6.7 |
| Hispanics | | |
| Native Americans | 1–4.5 | ~5 |
| | 0 | ~21 |
| East Asians | 0–2.5 | 17–22 |

Modified from Keltner NL, Folks DG: *Psychotropic Drugs*, ed 4, St. Louis, 2005, Mosby.

interethnic and intraethnic variabilities of expression.

## NURSE'S ROLE IN CULTURAL ASSESSMENT

Nurses should not only use the process of cultural competence in their practice settings, but also help others understand the need for culturally competent health care. One skill every nurse must develop is the ability to integrate cultural factors into the health assessment (Munoz and Luckmann, 2005; Warren, 2005).

### CULTURAL ASSESSMENT ISSUES

Nurses must include some basic elements within their cultural assessments of patients. These elements include communication, orientation, nutrition, family relationships, health beliefs, education, spiritual or religious views, and biologic or physiologic elements. Table 14-6 provides a handy assessment sheet to consider when evaluating culturally relevant information.

Questions and observations relative to cultural issues must be smoothly and sensitively incorporated into the nursing assessment process to ensure that the nurse does not appear rude or intrusive. Including someone from the patient's community or from the same cultural background during the assessment interview might also be appropriate. Cultural preservation, cultural negotiation, and cultural repatterning are other culturally competent techniques that nurses might use during assessment and in care planning.

*Cultural preservation* is the nurse's ability to acknowledge, value, and accept a patient's cultural beliefs. *Cultural negotiation* is the nurse's ability to work within a patient's cultural belief system to develop culturally appropriate interventions. *Cultural repatterning* is the nurse's ability to incorporate cultural preservation and negotiation to identify patient needs, develop expected outcomes, and evaluate outcome plans (Leininger, 2002). The critical thinking questions and clinical example in this chapter provide examples of how these three techniques might be incorporated into the care of a patient.

## SUMMARY

Cultural competence is an important part of effective psychiatric nursing. Important components for the development of culturally competent nursing care include the nurse's understanding of the concepts of a worldview, culture-bound syndromes, ethnopharmacology, and the nurse's role in assessing patients for cultural variables that might affect patient care.

### Study Notes

1. Culture is the manifestation of an individual's, group's, or community's beliefs, values, and norms used for daily life functioning.
2. Cultural competence is the process whereby the nurse develops cultural awareness, knowledge, and skills to promote effective health care for patients.
3. Cultural diversity refers to unique differences in areas such as age, gender, socioeconomic status, religion, race, and ethnicity.
4. A person's worldview is a perspective of what people value in how they function and interact with others on a daily basis.
5. Barriers to culturally competent care include miscommunication, failure to assess for a cultural perspective, and differences in worldview.
6. Illness can be viewed as resulting from natural, unnatural, or scientific (i.e., explainable) causes.
7. Four worldviews are the analytic, relational, community, and ecologic worldviews.
8. Culture-bound syndromes are recurring patterns of behavior that create disturbing experiences for people.

| Table 14-6 | Cultural Assessment Worksheet |
| --- | --- |

| Assessment Area | Questions or Areas of Inquiry |
| --- | --- |
| Communication | 1. Do you speak any foreign languages?<br>2. Is English your first language?<br>3. Does the patient speak English fluently?<br>4. Does the patient prefer an interpreter?<br>5. Does the patient believe that appropriate touching is acceptable?<br>6. Are there ethnic behaviors that the patient uses? |
| Orientation | 1. How long have you lived where you now live?<br>2. Where were you born?<br>3. With which ethnic, racial, or cultural group do you identify yourself?<br>4. How closely do you follow the traditional values, beliefs, and practices of your self-identified group?<br>5. What are the patient's thoughts on the following: human nature, development of knowledge, work ethic, relationship with nature? |
| Nutrition | 1. Do you have certain foods you prefer?<br>2. What kind of foods do you eat when you are ill?<br>3. Do you avoid certain foods because of your beliefs? |
| Significant others and family | 1. Who do you consider as important to you?<br>2. Is there anyone that you would like me to contact or not contact while you are here for treatment?<br>3. How are decisions made in your home environment?<br>4. In your home, what are the roles for children, women, and men?<br>5. What are some of the social customs or practices that you do at home?<br>6. Share with me three of your most important values. |
| Health | 1. What brought you here for treatment today?<br>2. What do you think will help you feel better or get well?<br>3. Have you used treatments in the past that were helpful for you?<br>4. What type of treatments don't you like or feel uncomfortable receiving?<br>5. Is there something you think I can assist you with to help you improve?<br>6. Who do you usually go to for help or treatment when you are ill?<br>7. What do you think causes physical and mental problems? |
| Education | 1. How do you prefer to learn new things and tasks (e.g., reading, watching television or videos, talking with someone)?<br>2. How have you received your education (e.g., in school, by self-instruction)?<br>3. How would you prefer to pay for your treatment? |
| Spirituality and religion | 1. Do you consider yourself spiritual or religious? If so, what does that mean to you?<br>2. Do you have a religious preference?<br>3. Are there certain individuals you like to talk with regarding your spiritual views, religious beliefs, or health care? Are there certain practices in which you like to participate? |
| Biology and physiology | 1. Do you have any specific health problems or disease conditions in your family of origin?<br>2. Are there certain medications, herbs, or therapies that you avoid because they make you ill?<br>3. Are there specific skin, hair, grooming, or health care needs that you prefer?<br>4. Are you taking any medications now? (Include an examination of vitamin, nutritional, and herbal approaches.)<br>5. How many cigarettes do you smoke every day?<br>6. How many glasses of wine do you drink per week?<br>7. How many cans or bottles of Coke, root beer, or beer do you drink per week?<br>8. How many cups of tea or coffee, or both, do you drink every day?<br>9. Are there any other beverages that you drink every day?<br>10. How many bars or pieces of chocolate do you eat every day? |

From Warren BJ, Campinha-Bacote J, Munoz C: *Cultural assessment worksheet,* Columbus, OH, 1994, Authors.

9. Patients from non–Western cultures might use acupuncture, acupressure, nutritional therapies (e.g., herbal remedies), skin scraping, moxibustion, and cupping to treat illness.

10. Ethnopharmacology involves the study of genetic and culture-related factors that can affect metabolism of medications.

11. An important nursing role is the incorporation of cultural knowledge into addressing health and health care.

## References

American Psychiatric Association (APA): *Diagnostic and statistical manual of mental disorders-IV—text revision [DSM-IV-TR],* ed 4, Washington, DC, 2000, APA.

Andrews MM, Boyle JS: *Transcultural concepts in nursing care,* ed 4, Philadelphia, 2002, Lippincott.

Anthony WA: Recovery from mental illness: the guiding vision of the mental health services in the 1990's, *Psychiatr Rehabil J* 2:17, 1993.

Baker FM: Diagnosing depression in African Americans, *Community Ment Health J* 37:31, 2001.

Berlin J, Fowkes W: A teaching framework for cross-cultural health, *West J Med* 139:934, 1982.

Bloch B: Bloch's assessment guide for ethnic/cultural variations. In Orque M, Monry L, editors: *A multicultural approach,* St. Louis, 1983, Mosby, pp. 49-75.

Campinha-Bacote J: *The process of cultural competence in the delivery of healthcare services: a culturally competent model of care,* ed 4, Cincinnati, 2003, Transcultural C.A.R.E. Associates.

Campinha-Bacote J: *A biblically based model of cultural competence in the delivery of healthcare services,* Cincinnati, 2005, Transcultural C.A.R.E. Associates.

Carter RT: *The influence of race and racial identity in psychotherapy: toward a racially inclusive model,* New York, 1995, Wiley & Sons.

Chong N: *The Latino patient: A cultural guide for health care providers,* Boston, 2002, Intercultural Press.

Comas-Diaz L, Green B: *Women of color: integrating ethnic and gender identities in psychotherapy,* New York, 1994, Guilford.

Delahanty J, Ram R, Postrado L, et al: Differences in rates of depression in schizophrenia by race, *Schizophr Bull* 27:29, 2001.

Diala CC, Muntaner C, Walrath C, et al: Racial/ethnic differences in attitudes toward professional mental health care and the use of services, *Am J Public Health* 91:805, 2001.

Fontaine KL: *Healing practices: alternative therapies for nursing,* Upper Saddle River, NJ, 2000, Prentice-Hall.

Giger JN, Davidhizar RE: *Transcultural nursing: assessment and intervention,* ed 4, St. Louis, 2003, Mosby.

Herrera JM, Lawson WB, Sramek JJ: *Cross cultural psychiatry,* New York, 1999, Wiley & Sons.

Hicks PL, et al: *Creating a culturally competent mental health system: consolidated culturalogical assessment tools.* Columbus, OH, 2004, Ohio Department of Mental Health.

Institute of Medicine (IOM): *Unequal treatment: confronting racial and ethnic disparities in healthcare,* Washington, DC, 2003, National Academy Press.

Keltner NL, Folks DG: *Psychotropic drugs,* ed 3, St. Louis, 2005, Mosby.

Leininger M: *Transcultural nursing: concepts, theories and practices,* New York, 2002, McGraw-Hill.

Munoz C, Luckmann J: *Transcultural communication in nursing,* New York, 2005, Thomson Delmar.

Plummer P: Developing culturally responsive psychosocial rehabilitative programs for African Americans, *Psychiatr Rehabil J* 19:38, 1996.

Pouissaint AF, Alexander A: *Lay my burden down: unraveling suicide and the mental health crisis among African Americans,* Boston, 2000, Beacon Press.

Purnell LD, Paulanka BJ: The Purnell model for cultural competence. In Purnell, LD, Paulanka P, editors: *Transcultural health care: a culturally competent approach,* Philadelphia, 2003, FA Davis, pp. 8-39.

Quander L: Let's talk: answers to your questions about cultural competency, *HIV Impact* 7, Winter, 2001.

Ross H: Office of Minority Health publishes final standards for cultural and linguistic competence, *Closing the Gap* February/March:1, 2001. Accessed January 20, 2006. Available at http://www.omhrc.gov/assets/pdf/checked/Final%20 Standards%20for%20Cultural%20and%20Linguistic%20 Competence.pdf

Ruiz P: *Ethnicity and psychopharmacology,* Washington, DC, 2000, American Psychiatric Press.

Spector R: *Cultural diversity in health and illness,* ed 6, Upper Saddle River, NJ, 2004, Prentice-Hall Health.

Spence JW, Jacobs JJ: *Complementary/alternative medicine: an evidence-based approach,* St. Louis, 1999, Mosby.

Taylor JS: The story catches you and you fall down: tragedy, ethnography, and "cultural competence," *Med Anthropol Q* 17:159, 2003.

U.S. Surgeon General: *Mental health: culture, race, and ethnicity, a supplement to mental health: a report of the Surgeon General,* Washington, DC, 2001, U.S. Department of Health and Human Services. Accessed January 20, 2006. Available from http://www.surgeongeneral.gov/library/mentalhealth/cre/

Warren BJ: The cultural expression of dying, *Case Manager* 16:44, 2005.

Warren BJ: Cultural and ethnic considerations. In Antai-Otong D, editor: *Psychiatric nursing: biological and behavioral concepts,* New York, 2003, Delmar.

Warren BJ: Interlocking paradigm of cultural competence: a model for psychiatric mental health nursing practice, *J Am Psychiatr Nurs Assoc* 8:209, 2002.

Warren BJ: The rainbow approach for culturally competent care of people of African-American heritage, *Case Manager* September/October:2:52-55, 2001.

Warren BJ: Point of view: a best practice process for psychiatric mental health nursing, *J Am Psychiatr Nurs Assoc* 6:135, 2000.

Warren BJ: Cultural competence in psychiatric nursing: an interlocking paradigm approach. In Keltner NL, Schwecke LH, Bostrom CE, editors: *Psychiatric nursing,* ed 3, St. Louis, 1999, Mosby, pp. 199-218.

Warren BJ, Campinha-Bacote J, Munoz C: *Cultural assessment worksheet,* Columbus, OH, 1994, Authors.

Warren BJ, Lutz W: A consumer-oriented practice model for psychiatric mental health nursing, *Arch Psychiatr Nurs* 14:117, 2000.

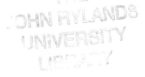

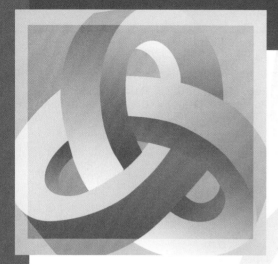

# Chapter 15

# Spirituality

*Gordon I.G. Pugh*

## Learning Objectives

*After reading this chapter, you should be able to:*

- Describe two general uses of the term *spirituality*.
- Identify the four largest religious groups in the United States.
- Explain three helpful theoretical constructs regarding spirituality.
- Discuss and evaluate benefits and concerns of including spiritual care in patients' treatment.
- Be familiar with the *Diagnostic and Statistical Manual of Mental Disorders,* 4th edition, Text Revision (DSM-IV-TR) (APA, 2000) and the NANDA International (NANDA International, 2005) diagnoses of spiritual care issues.

- Know two pieces of practical advice from psychiatric patients themselves regarding communication about spiritual concerns.
- Practice spiritually sensitive things to say to bereaved individuals (and know what things to avoid saying).
- Identify how the nurse can intervene, including using the HOPE Questions.
- Convey two stories about the way in which spirituality can be understood (Native American and pediatric)
- Know how and when to make a referral to a spiritual care professional.

One criticism of some psychological theories (Jung, 1984) is that they are psychology without the psyche, and this suits people who think they have no spiritual needs or aspirations. But here both doctor and patient deceive themselves. . . . In a word, they do not give enough meaning to life, and it is only meaning that liberates (p. 198).

NANDA International (NANDA International, 2005) and the American Psychological Association's *DSM-IV-TR* (APA, 2000) have categories for spiritual concerns. Cultural diversity is another reason to be aware of patients' spiritual concerns or spirituality. When people hear the term *spirituality,* they frequently assume the meaning of the term based on their own experience. In North America, the most common understandings of spirituality are tied to people's experiences of religion. These experiences with particular religions can be positive or negative or both. People hold to their opinions about spirituality quite tenaciously. In 2001, most religious adherents in the United States (about 78%) identified with a monotheistic religion (Adherents.com, 2002). Hence, the language used in this chapter will be familiar to most nurses and their patients. It should be noted

| Table 15-1 | Top Ten U.S. Religious Affiliations—2001* | | | |
|---|---|---|---|---|
| Religion | 1990 Estimated Adult Population | 2001 Estimated Adult Population | Percentage of U.S. Population (2000) | Percentage of Change (1990-2000) |
| Christianity | 151,225,000 | 159,030,000 | 76.5% | +5% |
| Nonreligious; secular | 13,116,000 | 27,539,000 | 13.2% | +110% |
| Judaism | 3,137,000 | 2,831,000 | 1.3% | −10% |
| Islam | 527,000 | 1,104,000 | 0.5% | +109% |
| Buddhism | 401,000 | 1,082,000 | 0.5% | +170% |
| Agnostic | 1,186,000 | 991,000 | 0.5% | −16% |
| Atheist | — | 902,000 | 0.4% | — |
| Hinduism | 227,000 | 766,000 | 0.4% | +237% |
| Unitarian Universalist | 502,000 | 629,000 | 0.3% | +25% |
| Wiccan/Pagan/Druid | | 307,000 | 0.1% | — |

*Unlike some countries, the United States does not include a question about religion in its census and has not for over 50 years. Religious adherents statistics in the United States are obtained from surveys and organizational reporting. From http://www.adherents.com/rel_USA.html. Accessed June 26, 2005.

### Norm's Notes

*Spiritual care—what is it? We all have a spirit and we can feel it. Spiritual care attempts to go beyond the facts of psychiatry and brain biology and deal with that intangible part of our being that we call a spirit, but it can get tricky. You cannot impose your spiritual worldview on a patient, but how can you talk about spiritual issues without bringing your own values to the discussion? This chapter attempts to show how these competing forces can be dealt with—without reducing spiritual care to a meaningless behavior.*

People born between 1945 and 1980 (baby boomers and Generation Xers) have likely heard someone say that he or she is "spiritual but not religious." Alcoholics Anonymous, for example, talks of a spiritual awakening, but maintains that it is not a religious organization. In their National Study for Religion and Youth, Smith and Denton (2005) found that most modern American teenagers they interviewed, however, "had never heard this phrase before, and the vast majority, even if they had heard this phrase, said that they had no clue what it meant." Their research indicates that most teens in the United States are "rather positive about and conventional in living out religion" (Smith and Denton, 2005).

that approximately 13% of Americans identify themselves as nonreligious or secular (Table 15-1). Thus, the second largest religious group in the United States is those who self-report having no religious affiliation.

In the past, the term *spirituality* was understood by most Americans to be roughly equivalent to overt religious expression, such as attendance at worship services and prayer. Today, however, the term is understood more broadly than it was in the past. Even among people who identify themselves as belonging to a particular religion (or subgroup within a religion), diverse (and divergent) expressions of spirituality exist. The term has taken on a variety of meanings, particularly in light of postmodern culture.

## TOWARD A DEFINITION OF SPIRITUALITY

### PSYCHIATRY BASED ON GREEK *PSYCHE* (THE SOUL)

The word *psychiatry* comes from two Greek words, *psyche* (soul) and *iatreia* (healing)—thus, healing of the soul. *Psyche* has a variety of meanings: the breath of life, the seat of feelings and emotions, and the part of humans that transcends the earthly. Spirituality means the things beyond mere biologic existence. Spiritual concerns are considered when advanced directives and quality of life issues are considered.

## COMMON UNDERSTANDINGS OF SPIRITUALITY

The variety of ways in which the word *spirit* is used underscores an important problem in understanding what is meant by spirituality. This ambiguity has existed for a long time and continues today. Not surprisingly, when people talk of spirituality, definitions are personalized, nebulous, and subjective.

Most people will agree, however, that spirit means something not material, which gives life, depth, and meaning to existence (Jung, 1980). Common understandings of spirituality have to do with making sense of life; with hopes, plans, and fears; with things that people value; with the way in which individuals relate to others; and with issues of meaning and belonging. The word *spirituality* is generally used in two ways. The first sees the human spirit as inextricably connected to a transcendent source, or higher power, and is often expressed within the individual's religious community. The second seeks to distinguish itself from a religious perspective by emphasizing aspects of the human spirit and its relationship to other human spirits.

### Spirituality in Relation to a Transcendent Spirit (Theistic View)

The first view is exemplified in the creation story of the world's three largest monotheistic religions (Christianity, Islam, and Judaism). In short, God constructed the world, including human beings. God molded dirt to form a human body and breathed life into a human being; thus, it became a living soul. The first understanding, therefore, is that human lives are inspired (literally, breathed into) by a Supreme Being. This view is often marked by a sense of gratitude for basic existence. Although this view is theistic—that is, it includes a concept of God—it is not necessarily an exclusively religious view.

### Spirituality in Relation to Human Spirit (Humanistic View)

Jung (1980) also considered the second general understanding of the word *spirituality*, describing spirituality as "the sum total of intellectual and cultural possessions...." This understanding includes the way in which people attempt to bring meaning in their lives in secular ways, apart from a religious community or from traditional understandings of God. The emphasis is on the human spirit. These two understandings (theistic and humanistic) are not necessarily mutually exclusive; however, the latter understanding deemphasizes (and sometimes completely rejects) the theistic approach. This understanding emphasizes not a transcendent source but self-transcendence in particular.

## CLINICAL UNDERSTANDING

Xavier (1987), a clinical psychiatrist, made a similar distinction between spirituality and religion and offered a useful vocabulary from his psychiatric experience between "healthy spirituality" and "sick religiosity." People who generalize institutional religion (e.g., church, synagogue, mosque) as only negative have often had some painful, dehumanizing experience at the hands of those who practice sick religiosity. William James (1958) stated that this sick religiosity comes from a lack of balance. Xavier (1987) said that sick religiosity is also marked by a "lack of openness to other possibilities, a sense of exclusiveness and absolutism." Xavier recognized, however, that many religious expressions are healthy. This reminder is especially important to his fellow psychiatrists, who appear to see a greater amount of psychopathology characterized by manifestations of sick religiosity than would presumably be found in the general population.

## OTHER MEANINGFUL THEORETICAL CONSTRUCTS FOR THE PSYCHIATRIC NURSE

Having explored a basic definition of spirituality as that part of humans that is not merely physical, and learning the two general views (a theistic approach and a humanistic approach), some meaningful theoretical constructs are called for. I have found the following theoretical constructs, or models, to be especially helpful in understanding how spiritual concerns are demonstrated.

### Construct 1: Making Meaning Through Freedom to Choose

The first model is derived from a notable psychiatrist's reflection on his own experience of intense suffering. Viktor Frankl, a psychiatrist, was a prisoner in the Nazi concentration camps of Dachau and Auschwitz during World War II. His understanding of meaning in the face of brutality is based on the philosophy of existentialism (Frankl, 1967). Frankl recognized that, although individuals cannot always choose the circumstances within which they find themselves, people always have a choice, at least in the attitudes they have toward their experiences. This view was forged in the midst of the helplessness he witnessed at the death camps. Prisoners who had no desire to live first gave up hope, then life. Prisoners who did not exchange their cigarettes for food, for example, "were those who had lost the will to live and wanted to 'enjoy' their last days" (Frankl, 1984). Many of the prisoners who found a reason to live, however, maintained hope and were able to survive.

Frankl's primary emphasis was on finding meaning in a person's life, beginning with the question of who the person is. Frankl believed that an individual cannot search for his or her identity directly. To do so would be a futile effort. Humans find meaning when they commit themselves to something beyond themselves, to a cause greater than themselves. A person must still decide what sort of something outside the individual is worth living for. Obviously, a risk of choosing badly, of making a commitment to an unworthy cause, is present. However, without this risk, no freedom would exist. In contemplating the meaning of existence and trying to live out this meaning, Frankl said that a connection is established between the way in which a person constructs meaning and the person's mental health. In other words, people who have something to live for outside of themselves experience better mental health.

## Construct 2: Higher Power, Higher Purpose, Higher Principles

The second helpful model comes from the clinical reflections of another psychiatrist, N.S. Xavier (1987), who made the distinction between healthy spirituality and sick religiosity. Xavier liked the distinction that Alcoholics Anonymous (AA) makes between religion and spirituality. AA asserts belief in "a power greater than ourselves" that can restore the alcoholic to sanity. AA calls this power "God as we understood God" or a "Higher Power." Xavier spent his childhood in the state of Kerala in southern India, where Hinduism, Christianity, and Islam, as well as other religions, have

peacefully coexisted for centuries. His discussion of the psychopathology of sick religiosity from a cross-cultural perspective is especially insightful. He noted three essential by-products of mature, healthy spirituality: *courage, love,* and *wisdom.*

Xavier (personal communication, March 1, 1994) has seized on AA's wording of Higher Power and expanded that understanding, saying that spiritual maturity is marked, quite simply, by three higher elements: higher power, higher purpose, and higher principles.

### Higher Power

Spiritually mature people know healthy ego boundaries; they display a humility that comes from an inner strength in being comfortable with who they are. Thus, spiritually mature people see themselves as part of something bigger than they are, before which or to whom they are responsible.

### Higher Purpose

Spiritually mature people understand that life has meaning and that their individual lives have a purpose in the grand scheme of the universe; thus, they can experience deep satisfaction in living out their responsibilities *vis-à-vis* their higher power.

### Higher Principles

Understanding that a higher power exists, a source of life to which or to whom they give gratitude, and understanding that each individual's life has meaning within the context of responsibility to a higher power, spiritually mature people seek to live their lives by ethical standards that incorporate these values and ideals. Xavier (1987) found this view mentally healthy.

## Construct 3: Acknowledging a Presence That Orders the World

The third helpful model involves a simplified form of Loder's (1989) research into the relationship between theology and psychiatric theory. James E. Loder was a professor at Princeton Theological Seminary who specialized in interdisciplinary studies combining theology and science, especially the human sciences and psychology. Loder postulated that early developmental experiences set the stage for later spiritual dynamics within the individual. In the biblical languages, the words for "face" also mean "presence." At the age of 3 months, infants begin to recognize faces. The most important face, at least insofar as the development of trust is considered, is the primary caregiver, typically the mother. The primal response to this presence is a smile. At this point in the infant's development, a concept of time has yet to develop. By the age of 9 months, the child will understand that times occur when the mother is not present and will experience anxiety at her absence, because the mother meets the child's basic needs. For the 3- to 6-month-old child (who has not yet developed a sense of time or absence), these basic needs are met by one whose presence is always assumed, who loves unconditionally (or at least appears to), and who orders the child's whole world. The child experiences no shame when gazing at this face.

Loder (1989) has described the way in which the child's burgeoning capacity to trust is strengthened by the presence (face) of this nurturing person. The infant's experiences are thus a model for the adult's search for spiritual fulfillment. "I suggest that what is established in the original face-to-face interaction is the child's sense of personhood and a universal prototype of the Divine Presence" (Loder, 1989). Loder also contended that the spiritual search that many people later experience is connected with the desire to experience in a new way the nature of being "given a place in the cosmos, confirmed as a self, and addressed by the presence of a loving other." Loder's model can be useful in helping deal with the spiritual issues of abandonment and shame.

Frankl's search for meaning in the midst of suffering, Xavier's distinction between sick religiosity and healthy spirituality, as well as Loder's notion that nurturance in infancy provides a prototype for later seeking and recognizing connection with a presence that orders one's world, have all been examined. These three perspectives are meant to provide the nurse with ways of looking at patients as spiritual beings and helping to see their spiritual struggles and concerns from more than one perspective.

## PATIENT SPIRITUALITY AND THE PSYCHIATRIC NURSE

### EVIDENCE SUPPORTING THE IMPORTANCE OF SPIRITUAL CARE

Aside from the implicit importance of that which gives meaning and principles to guide human lives, other reasons exist as to the importance of addressing issues of spirituality within the health care setting. Nursing, medical, and accrediting groups have recognized this importance. For example, the NANDA International nursing diagnoses (NANDA International, 2005) include "Spiritual distress," "Spiritual distress, risk for" and "Spiritual well-being, readiness for enhanced." The *DSM-IV-TR* (APA, 2000) has a diagnostic category dedicated to a "Religious or Spiritual Problem" (see *DSM-IV-TR* and NANDA International box). Furthermore, the Canadian Council on Health Services Accreditation has noted that, "When developing the service plan, the team considers the client's physical, mental, spiritual, and emotional needs. The team respects the clients' cultural and religious beliefs and enables them to carry out their usual cultural or religious practices as appropriate" (VandeCreek and Burton, 2001). The Joint Commission on the Accreditation of Healthcare Organizations (JCAHO, 1998) has maintained that patients have a basic right to care that respects their cultural, psychosocial, and spiritual values. Worth noting is that for both of these accreditation groups, the spiritual aspect is viewed as unique and separate from the cultural, mental, emotional, psychosocial, and religious aspects.

The nurse must remember that, although many people identify themselves as part of a religious tradition, "evidence suggests that . . . the percentage of people with a deep, transforming, lived-out [religious] faith is far smaller than the overall percentage of religious belief would seem to indicate" (Gallup Organization, 2001). Barrett and associates (2001) found a similar phenomenon by noting the number of unaffiliated Christians as 15.8%. Hence, having a broader view of patients' spirituality than reported by their religious affiliation alone can be especially helpful and can serve the patient well (Box 15-1).

## CLINICAL ATTENTION TO SPIRITUAL CONCERNS

Despite the declared validity of spirituality, spiritual concerns are rarely the focus of clinical attention. Given the importance of patients' spirituality, and its declared recognition by health care professionals from a clinical perspective, one might think that spirituality is often a focus of clinical attention, but this notion does not appear to be the case. One study found that 60% of adolescent psychiatric inpatients

### DSM-IV-TR and NANDA International: Religious or Spiritual Problem

This category can be used when the focus of clinical attention is a religious or spiritual problem. Examples include distressing experiences that involve loss or questioning of faith, problems associated with conversion to a new faith, or questioning of spiritual values that might not necessarily be related to an organized church or religious institution.*

**SPIRITUAL DISTRESS (DISTRESS OF THE HUMAN SPIRIT)**

*Definition*
Disruption in the life principle that pervades a person's entire being and that integrates and transcends one's biologic and psychosocial nature.

*Defining Characteristics*
Expresses concern with the meaning of life or death and belief systems; anger toward God; questions meaning of suffering; verbalizes inner conflict about beliefs; verbalizes concern about relationship with deity; questions meaning of own existence; unable to participate in usual religious practices; seeks spiritual assistance; questions moral and ethical implications of therapeutic regimen; gallows humor; displacement of anger toward religious representatives; description of nightmares and sleep disturbances; alteration in behavior and mood evidenced by anger, crying, withdrawal, preoccupation, anxiety, hostility, apathy, and so forth.

*Related Factors*
Separation from religious and cultural ties; challenges belief and value system (e.g., resulting from moral and ethical implications of therapy, intense suffering).

**POTENTIAL FOR ENHANCED SPIRITUAL WELL-BEING†**

*Definition*
Spiritual well-being—process of an individual's developing and unfolding of mystery through harmonious interconnectedness that springs from inner strengths.

*Defining Characteristics*
*Inner strengths:* A sense of awareness, self-consciousness, sacred source, unifying force, inner core, and transcendence
*Unfolding mystery:* One's experience about life's purpose and meaning, mystery, uncertainty, and struggles
*Harmonious interconnectedness:* Relatedness, connectedness, harmony with self, others, higher power or God, and the environment

*American Psychological Association (APA): *Diagnostic and statistical manual of mental disorders-IV—text revision [DSM-IV-TR]*, ed 4, Washington, DC, 2000, APA.
†NANDA International: *Nursing diagnoses: definitions and classifications 2005-2006*, Philadelphia, 2005, NANDA International.

reported that they had never been asked about their religious or spiritual beliefs by any mental health professional (other than the chaplain) (Grossoehme, 2001). Grossoehme made the following observation concerning the disparity between the professed importance of spiritual care and the actual treatment that psychiatric patients generally receive:

> A study of the relationship between psychiatrists' religious beliefs and their practice documented that the majority of them believe spirituality to be an area with which psychiatrists may appropriately be concerned. However, over half of the psychiatrists in that study inquired about their patients' religious beliefs "occasionally" or even less frequently; those that did assess this area generally did not have any interventions based upon their findings (p. 139).

Community clergy are frequently not prepared to address the spiritual needs of psychiatric patients.

Möller (1999) reported on an adult group of psychiatric inpatients from widely diverse religious backgrounds, discovering that only 12.3% of participants reported receiving any spiritual care during an inpatient psychiatric hospitalization. Patients' heartbreaking stories centered around fumbling attempts of community clergy, which were often offensive and proved to do more harm than good. Only 12.5% of these patients (1.5% of the total group) reported a positive experience with community clergy. Despite the paucity of spiritual care that these patients were offered, Möller noted that 40% of people with mental illness call on their religious leaders. Participants describe significant resistance on the part of the hospital staff when they have tried to talk about spiritual concerns. The staff labeled these desires as religious delusions. Some facilities have even removed bibles from the patients' rooms after these conversations.

## Box 15-1 Ojibway Indian Smudging in an Intensive Care Unit

Mike McLemore, an elder of the Native American Ojibway Nation, has given the reminder that many Native Americans count themselves as adherents of Christianity, yet they continue to practice what he calls "the traditional ways." He relates the story of being called on to perform a **smudging** in an intensive care unit. With his smudge pot and eagle feather, he entered the unit, as requested by the patient. The nurses, seeing the smoke, were understandably concerned; their lack of knowledge about the patient's spiritual practices might have proved to be a problem. They might have made lots of assumptions based on the fact that the patient listed her religious affiliation as Catholic. The nurses were, however, open to helping address the patient's spiritual needs. When the elder explained the spiritual significance of the healing ritual and told the nurses of its importance to the patient (and assured them that there was no open flame!), the nurses allowed him to provide the cultural and spiritual practice that the patient had requested.

From McLemore M: Personal communication, July 14, 2001.

One community minister reported praying with a Muslim family member and further reported being surprised when the family member was offended. "But I've been praying in the name of Jesus all of my life!" the minister said. Stories abound of well-meaning clergy who tell psychotic patients to resist the devil, that people who commit suicide automatically go to hell, or that their illness has come about because of a lack of piety or faith. It is no wonder, then, that people want to make a distinction between sick religiosity and healthy spirituality, and that mental health professionals are hesitant to call on clergy.

Given staff concerns about psychiatric patients' religious delusions, and given patient reports that they desire competent spiritual care (in addition to the fact that JCAHO considers spiritual care as a fundamental patient right), having a clinically trained professional chaplain be an integral component of the health care team makes sense (Box 15-2). Psychiatric health care settings do a terrible disservice to patients when they leave "untrained and insensitive clergy to provide pastoral care" (Post and Whitehouse, 1999).

## EVIDENCE OF CLINICAL BENEFITS OF HEALTHY SPIRITUALITY

Wallace and Forman (1998) studied the relationship between religion and health among adolescents. Although most research of adolescents' religious practices has described their religion as a social control against deviant behavior, these researchers examined the secondary benefits of religious practice as a primary factor that effects tendencies to engage in dangerous (or at-risk) behaviors. The study noted that strongly religious high school seniors tend to begin sexual activity later and have fewer sexual partners, are less likely to be involved in drug use, and are less given to interpersonal violence compared with less religious students. The preventive health issues related to these avoidance behaviors are obvious. These religiously oriented adolescents benefit not only from the deterrent aspects of negative lifestyle choices, but also are more apt as a group to engage in behaviors that promote health, such as eating more healthily, exercising more regularly, and getting adequate sleep, the study says.

Harris and associates (1999) recounted that cardiac patients who were prayed for experienced "a measurable improvement in the medical outcomes." The authors also cited a 6-month trial of "distant healing" in which patients with acquired immunodeficiency syndrome (AIDS) who were prayed for experienced "statistically significant benefits." Ellison and Levin (1998) maintained that

> Contrary to the assertions of critics, who base their claims primarily on anecdotal accounts of religion's pathological effects, systematic reviews of the research literature over the years have consistently reported that aspects of religious involvement are associated with desirable mental health outcomes (p. 702).

These associations might exist because of lifestyle practices of highly religious people as a group or possibly because the practice of a person's spirituality through religious practices "may lead to the experience or expression of certain emotions that, through psychoneuroimmunologic or neuroendocrine pathways, could affect physiological parameters" (Ellison and Levin, 1998). The authors also noted that these practices "may lead to positive emotions such as forgiveness, contentment, and love, as well as to negative emotions such as guilt and fear" and cautioned that "overinterpretation [of the data] must be discouraged to eliminate unrealistic assumptions" about the connections between spirituality and health.

Additionally, it is clear that some beliefs, those that Xavier (1987) identified with sick religiosity,

---

### Box 15-2 Making a Referral to a Professional Chaplain

1. **Definition of a professional chaplain:** Over 10,000 professional chaplains serve in North America, from Catholic, Jewish, Muslim, Protestant, and other traditions. When religious beliefs and practices are tightly interwoven with cultural contexts, professional chaplains constitute a powerful reminder of the healing, sustaining, guiding, and reconciling power of religious faith.

   *What is required of a professional chaplain?* Graduate theologic education; endorsement by a faith group; 1 year of postgraduate clinical pastoral training; demonstrated clinical competency; annual continuing education; adherence to a code of ethics for health care chaplains; and professional growth in competencies demonstrated in peer review.

   *What do professional chaplains do?* They serve as a member of the interdisciplinary health care team; reach across faith group boundaries; do not proselytize; seek to protect patients in their institutions from being confronted by other, unwelcome, forms of spiritual intrusion; participate in interdisciplinary education regarding the interface of religion and spirituality with medical care; point to human value aspects of institutional policies and behaviors; interpret and analyze multifaith and multicultural traditions as they influence clinical services; offer patients, family members, and staff an emotionally and spiritually safe professional from whom they can seek counsel or guidance; and establish and maintain important relationships with community clergy.

2. **When to consult a professional chaplain:** When patients, family members, or staff need time-tested spiritual resources that help them focus on transcendent meaning, purpose, and value; when a religious or spiritual leader is needed to fill the special requirements involved in intense medical environments when local religious leaders cannot (e.g., when patient confidentiality is considered, especially with minors, substance abusers, and psychiatric patients); when one of these people needs someone who can take the time to listen; when people ask spiritually relevant questions; when a patient's religious or cultural requirements appear to be in conflict with institutional policy; when someone is being proselytized by an unwelcome intrusion; when the institution fails to consider the human value aspects of care; when a new diagnosis is made; when a more in-depth spiritual assessment or intervention is needed; when an ethical consultation is needed; and when a crisis, death, or impending death occurs.

3. **How to consult a professional chaplain:** Depending on the structure of the hospital, contacting a chaplain, if one is available in the institution, can be performed in a variety of ways. One way is to ask the nursing supervisor or hospital telephone operator. Asking to meet a chaplain can be helpful if the patient has not already met him or her. The nurse generally spends more time with a given patient than anyone else in a health care setting. The nurse's being attuned to spiritual needs and communicating these to the spiritual care provider of the patient's choice (within the policies and procedures of the institution) is vitally important to the spiritual care of patients.

   If the chaplain is a part of the health care team, the nurse might sometimes make a referral without asking the patient. An important point to remember, however, is that patients have a right to decline pastoral services. It is best not to say to the patient a statement such as, "You don't want me to call the chaplain, do you?" A better way to approach the patient is to say, "Have you met our Chaplain, Terry Smith? I have found her to be really helpful with people who are asking these kinds of questions [or who are going through these kinds of difficult times]. May I call her for you?"

Modified from VandeCreek L, Burton L, editors: *Professional chaplaincy: its role and importance in healthcare.* Available at http://www.healthcarechaplaincy.org/publications/publications/white_paper_05.22.01/index.html. Accessed January 18, 2006.

---

are correlated with increased risk for mortality. A study reported at the Annual Meeting of the American Psychological Association identified three beliefs that increase the risk of death by 19% to 28% (Anonymous, 2001): (1) feeling separated from God, (2) feeling unloved by God, or (3) attributing illness to the devil. This view illustrates the importance of health care professionals being attentive to patients' spiritual concerns.

Although evidence of the clinical benefits of addressing spirituality is growing, some research-

ers have raised the concern that improved medical outcomes do not mean that prescribing spiritual practices will bring about a specific healing function in a given patient. Sloan and colleagues (1999) feared that some patients might feel that "illness is the result of insufficient faith." This view might reflect the very overinterpretation against which Ellison and Levin (1998) cautioned.

Chamberlain and Hall (2000) have given a similar caveat. Their comprehensive research documented over 300 published scientific studies

---

Box 15-3    **Who to Call?**

Physicians are not trained to engage in in-depth conversations with their patients about their spiritual concerns. Such discussions are not the sole domain of any one profession, but many health care facilities have chaplains or other community clergy who have received systematic postseminary training and clinical supervision in such areas as pastoral psychology, ethics, and multicultural pastoral care and who are endorsed by their denominations. Thus, patients who seek spiritual support can be appropriately referred to these professionals.

From Sloan RP, Bagiella E, VandeCreek L, et al: Sounding board: should physicians prescribe religious activities? *N Engl J Med* 342:1913, 2000. Copyright © 2000, Massachusetts Medical Society. All rights reserved.

---

that examined Christianity, Judaism, Islam, and Hinduism. Most studies showed that beliefs and practices of these religions appear to have a positive influence on depression, anxiety, suicide rates, and promotion of a healthy lifestyle. Other researchers have found a weak connection or none at all, explaining that prescribing religious activities to achieve health benefits assumes too strong of a cause-and-effect relationship and might therefore be ineffective in these cases.

I recommend that patients with these types of concerns should be referred to a clinically trained spiritual care professional, and that this person should be part of an interdisciplinary health care team (see Box 15-2).

## HEALTH CARE APPLICATIONS

### IS SPIRITUALITY A VALID OR REALISTIC NURSING CONCERN?

VandeCreek (2001) reported that, although many health care professionals want to engage in spiritual care and assessment, most are simply too overwhelmed to do so (Box 15-3). VandeCreek (2001) cited a 1998 survey completed by readers of the *American Journal of Nursing*, and contended that the survey demonstrates that nurses have little time or energy to conduct meaningful spiritual assessments or to provide spiritual care. The reasons cited include more patients, more cross-training responsibilities, higher patient acuity, more work-related injuries, unexpected readmission of patients, workplace violence, family complaints, and medi-

cation errors. These nurses reported decreased continuity of care, time to comfort and talk to patients, time to provide basic nursing care, and time to teach patients and their families. Of the nurses surveyed, 57% answered "No" when asked if the quality of health care they provide meets their professional standards. These are serious considerations to ponder.

### SUFFERING AND ILLNESS ELICIT CRISES

In the wake of people's worry and confusion following the terrorist attacks of September 11, 2001, many Americans began realizing how short, precious, and unpredictable life can be. The number of new wills and life insurance policies has reportedly surged as a result. A major life crisis such as facing an individual's own mortality is among the most difficult points in a person's life. Suffering, distress, illness, and death can induce an existential urgency that causes people to consider their own mortality. However, although this type of crisis might be common, it almost always comes unexpectedly. At these critical life junctures, people have the opportunity to become more acutely aware of and interested in issues of meaning and their place in the world (Box 15-4).

### SUFFERING PHYSICAL DISTRESS AND DEATH

Physical suffering, such as that which often accompanies terminal or chronic illness, can lead to a realization of life's brevity. People with severe back pain, who have had multiple surgeries with little pain relief, sometimes report being ready to die. Patients who battle terminal illness frequently take great spiritual comfort in the words of St. Paul, "I have fought the good fight," of the Koheleth in Ecclesiastes, "For everything there is a season and a time for every purpose under heaven" including "a time to die," or in the hymn "Amazing Grace." This hymn, written in 1779, remains so popular that journalist Bill Moyers has made a television documentary about it and its powerful words: "Through many dangers, toils and snares I have already come; 'Tis grace has brought me safe thus far and grace will lead me home."

People who have not experienced a physical disability are sometimes referred to as "the

## Box 15-4    A Story of Spirituality in a Pediatric Setting

Reverend Doreen M. Duley is Director of Pastoral Care at Children's Hospital in Birmingham, Alabama. A board-certified chaplain and pediatric chaplain, she related the following story:

"Tracy" was a 7-year-old boy with leukemia who was completing a 3-year cycle of treatment and was now in remission. He was going to another state, north of the hospital, for a bone marrow transplant. The health care staff worked with Tracy's mother to help make arrangements and to prepare for being away from home for 3 months. Tracy was an active part of his faith community, and had a keen sense of spirituality. He loved the Power Rangers; they were his favorite toys.

The day before Tracy was supposed to leave the state to go up north for the bone marrow transplant, his hospital room was a flurry of activity. Lots of last minute preparations for air travel and treatment were being finalized with the physicians, nurses, social workers, and others on the team. Chaplain Duley took Tracy out of the room so as not to disrupt the preparations but also to assess his own understanding of the treatment that Tracy was about to undertake.

Tracy and the chaplain went to play and talk next to a large picture window overlooking the city below. Tracy had his Power Ranger toys with him. "Tomorrow is a big day for you," the chaplain said. "What's going to happen?" Tracy responded: "I'm going to fly up *really high,* higher even than this," he explained, looking out the window at the ground below. "Higher than I've ever been before." This was the way he interpreted what he had heard about his first ride in an airplane.

"And then what?" the chaplain asked.

"Then I fall into a deep, deep pit, lower than the ground—real far down," Tracy answered. This is the way he understood what he had heard about his counts going so low and the way he would be "down" emotionally and physically. Tracy would be sicker than he had ever been before, close to death because of the virtual erasure of his immune system.

"What will happen then?"

"I don't know."

"How will you get out?"

"A Power Ranger will get me. It will be a Power Ranger, dressed in white, but not *this* one (as he showed her his white Power Ranger). It will be a different one. It will come and get me, bring me back to my mom, and I'm going to be OK."

"Do you know the Power Ranger's name?"

"Maybe Jesus? I think it is. It's Jesus."

When Tracy and the chaplain returned, Tracy's mother was frightened. She had pulled away from her faith of origin and was afraid that she had not taught him enough of her religious tradition. She was concerned that Tracy did not understand the journey he was about to undertake. "I think he does understand," the chaplain said and explained what Tracy had told her.

From Duley DM: Personal communication, 2001.

temporarily abled" (Little, personal communication, October 15, 2001), clearly suggesting that most people will eventually face their own mortality in some way. Those with chronic illness are sometimes forced to confront the fragility of life before others of their own age. Many patients who grow up with cystic fibrosis form close friendships with one another during their long and frequent hospitalizations. For these individuals, seeing their friends die as they grow into adolescence and young adulthood becomes common. By the age of 15 years, some of these patients have had to make life and death decisions for themselves, such as whether to consent to lung transplantation. For many people, these experiences of death, and decisions about their own health care, raise spiritual questions that they have been considering for as long as they can remember.

Dying patients report that they find value in praying and coming to peace with God. In fact, "coming to peace with God and pain control were nearly identical in importance for [dying] patients and bereaved family members" (Steinhauser et al, 2000).

Death and other tragedies, and their accompanying grief, can arouse symptoms of depression and other profound spiritual crises in patients, family members, and health care professionals. The nurse's first experience with the death of a patient can be sad, disturbing, sacred, and beautiful at the same time. Most people, however, do not have much experience with the dying; their first encounter can be frightening. The experience with death can leave them feeling inadequate, even speechless. In our own efforts at finding meaning in someone else's tragedy, we might say things that are inappropriate. The nurse's efforts at making sense of a tragedy can be vastly different from those of others touched by this type of calamity. Most people genuinely want to be helpful, but in the chaos of their emotions and in coming face to face with the realization that they, too, will die one day, they might say things that are amazingly insensitive. Even nurses, known for their deep commitment to care for the sick and injured, can be at a loss and make inappropriate statements. Because the fear of death raises deeply spiritual issues, not only for the dying and their loved ones who might seek psychiatric assistance but also for health care professionals, a reminder of what not to say and some guidelines about what can be truly helpful are provided in Box 15-5. Although a grieving person might find meaning in a loved one's injury, illness, or death with a statement such as those found in Box 15-5, any conclusion must belong to the one experiencing the grief and not to the one attempting to provide comfort. Of special note is the use of religious language in many of these efforts at creating meaning from the death experience.

---

**Box 15-5 Dos and Don'ts in a Death Situation**

**What Not to Say**
Grieving family members have offered this partial list of wrong and right things to say. As inappropriate as these might look in print, a great many people who want to offer comfort (including health care professionals who should know better) frequently make discounting or patronizing statements such as these:
"I know how you feel."
"It is time to get on with your life."
"God needed her (more than you did) [or God needed another angel in heaven, or another flower in his garden]."
"It must have been his time."
"God won't put on you any more than you can bear."
"It was God's will."
"You can (or still do) have other children [in event of miscarriage, stillbirth, loss of child]."
"It was for the best."
"Good will come out of this."
Any statement that begins with "At least . . ."

**What to Say or Do (especially for the health care professional)**
A heartfelt "I'm so sorry."
"They did everything they could to save him."
"It's harder than most people think."
"I'm here for you" [and then *be available*].
"What questions do you have?" [Or, in some cultures, it is better to ask, "What concerns can I answer for you?"]
Be sure to answer all questions honestly.
Listen carefully. Ask questions. Check out all your assumptions.

Modified from Reverend James Woodson (speech), April 25, 2001, Thanatology Workshop, University of Alabama, and my interview with Melissa Wallace of Mercy Medical Hospice Grief Group, Mobile, Alabama, September 7, 2001 (personal communication).

---

Serious illness can also present loved ones with equally difficult dilemmas that evoke questions of meaning. Religious activities are important coping mechanisms for African-American caregivers of older adult patients. Post and Whitehouse (1999) have indicated that religious practice has a bearing on reducing rates of depression, noting that depression is especially marked among caregivers of patients with Alzheimer's disease (AD). Individuals who suffer from AD or traumatic brain injury often find comfort in the religious rituals they recall from their youth, such as hearing or reciting prayers or songs from their own religious tradition.

---

**CRITICAL THINKING QUESTION** 1

Psychiatric patients describe concrete thinking during a psychotic episode. How can these patients be open to spiritual care when spiritual language is by nature symbolic?

---

## INTERSECTION OF SPIRITUALITY AND MENTAL OR EMOTIONAL DISTRESS

Mental illness is a distressing factor that can give rise to important spiritual questions. Jung (1984) asserted that "A neurosis must be understood, ultimately, as the suffering of a soul which has not discovered its meaning." Oates (1978) has recounted that some influential religious figures in the history of the Christian tradition experienced symptoms of clinical depression, including St. Augustine, Martin Luther, John Bunyan, Jonathan Edwards, and Henry Emerson Fosdick. Oates (1978) asserted that suicide is a spiritual question, because the question is not ultimately whether to believe in the existence of God but whether to accept our own humanity.

Oates (1978) identified how aspects of schizophrenia affect the patient's spiritual care. The incapacity to symbolize—that is, the patient's concrete thinking—can cause special problems, because "religious language is symbolic by nature." Oates related the story of a schizophrenic patient who decompensated while at a Pentecostal religious gathering: "She was terrified at the thought of Jesus 'entering her heart.' To her this was a literal invasion of her body."

Möller's (1999) participants reported being especially frustrated by their concrete thinking and with the clergy's lack of understanding of this phenomenon. To a psychotic patient, a prayer such as "Hold Susan close" might be less than therapeutic.

Oates (1978) discussed the incapacity to accept human limitations of the body, noting that the patient's history often includes "dreadfully distorted" religious teaching and a "wretched exploitation of the body." Oates further discussed blunted affect, the incapacity for commitment, and ascetic tendencies—that is, the way people separate themselves from the world. Some people separate themselves for religious reasons, as in the case of certain hermits, but this phenomenon can also exist among the mentally ill. Oates (1978) said that, although religion can be a common theme in hallucinations and delusions and that these vary among cultures, the diminished capacity for trust tends to be consistent cross-culturally. This trust is built on consistently demonstrated, genuinely compassionate behavior on the part of the caregiver. The most practical advice is from patients themselves, who reported that they want most of all for their spiritual care provider to (1) be authentic, caring, and respectful and (2) speak slowly and in concrete terms.

A study by Fitchett and associates (2004) confirmed the association between religious struggle and emotional distress in three groups of medical patients: (1) diabetics, (2) congestive heart failure patients, and (3) oncology patients. Patients who experience religious struggle might experience transformation or distress and despair. Their study suggested that as many as 15% of these patients could have significant levels of spiritual distress, putting them at risk for "poor physical or mental health outcomes." The interdisciplinary group of authors suggested that clinicians ought to look for signs of what they call "religious struggle" in their patients, and consider referring such patients to a professional chaplain.

## HOW CAN THE NURSE ASSESS AND INTERVENE IN A REALISTIC WAY?

The issue of trust is at the core of providing quality spiritual care. Möller (1999) stated that her group of psychiatric inpatients cited a primary need for their spiritual advisor, imam, pastor, or rabbi not to abandon them. Patients with no formal religious affiliation strongly wanted at least to be asked whether they had a religious preference and wanted the nurse to contact a member from the group they identified. Möller found four essential spiritual themes that arose—namely, the patients' desire for:

1. Comfort
2. Companionship
3. Conversation
4. Consolation

Many spiritual assessment tools of different lengths and complexity are available from a variety of disciplines. Among the simplest and easiest to use is the HOPE questions. Two physicians at Brown University School of Medicine have developed a tool that can provide the health care professional with four concepts to discuss with patients, given the easy to remember mnemonic HOPE (Anandarajah and Hight, 2001). The answers can be an opportunity for further exploration of the spiritual issues involved.

**H:** Sources of *h*ope, strength, comfort, meaning, peace, love, and connection
**O:** The role of *o*rganized religion for the patient
**P:** *P*ersonal spirituality and *p*ractices
**E:** *E*ffects on medical care and *e*nd-of-life issues

The reference for this source at the end of this chapter (see reference list) provides the Internet address for this brief article. A link to a patient information handout is also available there. The reader is encouraged to consult the article before using the HOPE questions.

### CRITICAL THINKING QUESTION    2

How do you think the HOPE questions can provide an opportunity for further exploration of spiritual issues for a patient who is not involved with organized religion?

### FINAL THOUGHT

It has been said that the professional's best friend is a Rolodex—that is, knowing one's strengths and limitations, as well as the proper time to refer to someone else, and knowing to whom to refer that person, is an important mark of personal and professional maturity. I hope that patients' spiritual concerns will continue to receive attention and that health care professionals will make their patients' spiritual considerations an important adjunct to conventional therapies.

CRITICAL THINKING QUESTION   3

Why do you think so many people want to draw a distinction between religion and spirituality?

## Study Notes

1. It is generally understood that spirituality is a major component of mental health and psychiatric care.
2. Spirituality is more broadly defined today in the postmodern culture than it was in the past.
3. At its most basic, spirituality has to do with making sense of life, with hopes, plans, and fears; with things that people value; with the way in which individuals relate to others; and with issues of meaning and belonging.
4. There are two basic views of spirituality: (1) transcendent view, in which life is ordered and given meaning by a source greater than humankind; and (2) humanistic view, in which life is ordered and given meaning by humankind.
5. The chapter discusses three different models for clinical application: (1) making meaning through freedom to choose; (2) higher power, higher purpose, higher principles; and (3) acknowledging a presence that orders the world.
6. NANDA International *DSM-IV-TR*, JCAHO, and the Canadian Council on Health Services Accreditation all recognize the importance of and encourage a spiritual component to nursing care.
7. Some nurses and other professionals believe that nurses are not prepared to provide in-depth spiritual care.
8. Although often discussed by clinicians, spiritual care remains a neglected component of psychiatric care. Nurses should not be afraid of patients' desires to discuss these issues.
9. There is evidence of the clinical benefits of a healthy spirituality.
10. There is evidence of the harmful consequences of sick religiosity.
11. A clinically trained spiritual care professional should be part of the health care team.
12. Patients suffering physical distress and facing death often find comfort in the transcendent view of spirituality, although these issues can arouse a sense of discomfort for health care providers.
13. Patients suffering from psychiatric disorders frequently present conditions with spiritual themes.
14. Nurses can provide comfort, companionship, conversation, and consolation.
15. Nurses can use a spiritual assessment tool to help patients explore spiritual issues. A brief tool is included in the text, and many facilities have their own approach to spiritual assessment.

## References

Adherents.com, 2002. Available at http://www.adherents.com/rel_usa.html. Accessed June 26, 2005.

American Psychological Association (APA): *Diagnostic and statistical manual of mental disorders-IV—text revision* [DSM-IV-TR], ed 4, Washington, DC, 2000, APA.

Anonymous: Beliefs that make you sick, *Spirituality and Health* 3(4):16, 2001.

Anandarajah G, Hight E: Spirituality and medical practice: using the HOPE questions as a practical tool for spiritual assessment, *Am Fam Physician* 63:81, 2001.

Barrett DB, Kurian GT, Johnson TM: The world by countries: religionists, churches, ministries. In Barrett DB, Kurian GT, Johnson TM, editors: *World Christian encyclopedia: a comparative survey of churches and religions in the modern world*, Oxford, England, 2001, Oxford University Press.

Chamberlain TJ, Hall CA: *Realized religion: research on the relationship between religion and health*, Radnor, PA, 2000, Templeton Foundation Press.

Ellison CG, Levin JS: The religion-health connection: evidence, theory, and future directions, *Health Educ Behav* 25:700, 1998.

Fitchett G, Murphy P, Kim J, et al: Religious struggle: prevalence, correlates and mental health risks in diabetic, congestive heart failure and oncology patients, *Int J Psychiatry Med* 34:179, 2004.

Frankl VE: *Man's search for meaning*, New York, 1984, Touchstone.

Frankl VE: *Psychotherapy and existentialism*, New York, 1967, Washington Square Press.

Gallup Organization: *Easter season finds a religious nation*, April 13, 2001. Available at http://www.gallup.com/poll/releases/pr010413.asp. Accessed September 1, 2001.

Grossoehme DH: Self-reported value of spiritual issues among adolescent psychiatric inpatients, *J Pastoral Care* 55:139, 2001.

Harris WS, Gowda M, Kalb JW, et al: A randomized, controlled trial of the effects of remote, intercessory prayer on outcomes in patients admitted to the coronary care unit, *Arch Intern Med* 159:2273, 1999.

James W: *The varieties of religious experience*, New York, 1958, New American Library.

Joint Commission on the Accreditation of Healthcare Organizations (JCAHO): *CAMH refreshed core*, Oakbrook Terrace, IL, January, RI1, 1998, Author.

Jung CG: *Psychology and Western religion* (trans. Hull RFC), New York, 1984, Princeton University Press.

Jung CG: *The archetypes and the collective unconscious* (trans. Hull RFC), New York, 1980, Princeton University Press and Bollingen Foundation.

Loder JE: *The transforming moment,* Colorado Springs, CO, 1989, Helmers & Howard.

Möller MD: Meeting spiritual needs on an inpatient unit, *J Psychosoc Nurs* 37:5, 1999.

NANDA International: *Nursing diagnoses: definitions and classifications 2005-2006,* Philadelphia, 2005, NANDA International.

Oates WE: *The religious care of the psychiatric patient,* Philadelphia, 1978, Westminster Press.

Post SG, Whitehouse PJ: Spirituality, religion and Alzheimer's disease, *J Health Care Chaplain* 8:45, 1999.

Sloan RP, Bagiella E, Powell T: Religion, spirituality, and medicine, *Lancet* 353:664, 1999.

Smith C, Denton ML: *Soul searching: the religious and spiritual lives of American teenagers,* New York, 2005, Oxford University Press.

Steinhauser KE, Christakis NA, Clipp EC, et al: Factors considered important at the end of life by patients, family, physicians, and other care providers, *JAMA* 284:2476, 2000.

VandeCreek L: Spiritual assessment and care by nurses? *APC News* 4:18, 2001.

VandeCreek L, Burton L, editors: *Professional chaplaincy: its role and importance in healthcare.* Available at http://www.healthcarechaplaincy.org/publications/publications/white_paper_05.22.01/index.html. Accessed January 18, 2006.

Wallace JM, Forman TA: Religion's role in promoting health and reducing risk among American youth, *Health Educ Behav* 25:721, 1998.

Xavier NS: *The two faces of religion: a psychiatrist's view,* Tuscaloosa, AL, 1987, Portals Press.

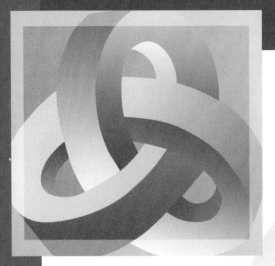

# Chapter 16

# Introduction to Psychotropic Drugs

*Norman L. Keltner*

## Learning Objectives

*After reading this chapter, you should be able to:*

- Define the role of psychopharmacology in psychotherapeutic management.
- Identify the nurse's responsibilities in administering psychotropic drugs.
- Describe pharmacokinetic and pharmacodynamic processes as they relate to clinical practice.
- Describe the function and inactivation of neurotransmitters.
- Discuss the function of the blood-brain barrier and the significance of lipid solubility.
- State the benefits of teaching patients about psychotropic drugs.
- Describe common reasons why psychiatric patients might not comply with prescribed drug regimens.

*Telling me that I have a brain disease and that I should take medications does not solve my problems.*
                                                   *Dr. N.W. Riffer (1997)*

T he United States is a drug-taking society. People take all types of drugs: drugs to sleep, drugs to wake up, drugs to fight infections, drugs to lower blood pressure, drugs to lower cholesterol, drugs to lose weight. People take drugs for all types of reasons. People take prescription drugs, over-the-counter drugs, legal drugs, and illegal drugs. Drugs, drugs, drugs! Drugs are taken to fix things, including mental and emotional problems.

Among these drugs are those that treat delusions and hallucinations (antipsychotics), slow down runaway thinking (mood stabilizers, or antimanic agents), improve mood (antidepressants), calm nerves (antianxiety drugs), improve thinking (drugs for Alzheimer's disease), and even drugs to correct problems caused by some of the drugs just listed (e.g., antiparkinsonian drugs).

The introductory quote from Dr. Riffer, when coupled with the pejorative tone of the opening paragraph, would suggest a negative view of psychotropic drugs by the authors of this text. Nothing could be further from the truth. However, the following points must be made:

1. Psychotropic drugs are not always effective.
2. Not every patient needs psychotropic drugs.
3. Even when psychotropic drugs are effective, best outcomes typically occur when other interventions (e.g., counseling, therapy) are co-administered.
4. Psychotropic agents can be used (by both patients and clinicians) to avoid the hard work of getting better.

### Norm's Notes

Take a good look at this chapter. If you read it thoroughly, it will help you really understand psychotropic drugs. If you don't understand such basics as pharmacokinetics and pharmacodynamics, though, you will have to memorize each drug. You shouldn't have to do that! You have often heard that nurses need to know the reason for some treatment, side effect, or adverse response. The basics found in this chapter form the foundation for understanding a drug's actions. So, take your time—Norm's key to learning important information is repetition, repetition, repetition.

| Table 16-1 | Success of Treatment for Selected Mental Disorders |
|---|---|

| Disorder | Patients Demonstrating Some Improvement (%) |
|---|---|
| Panic disorder | 80 |
| Bipolar disorder | 80 |
| Major depression | 65 |
| Schizophrenia | 60 |
| Obsessive-compulsive disorder | 60 |

Data from National Mental Health Advisory Council: 1993 Health Care Reform in Americans With Severe Mental Illness, *Am J Psychiatry* 150(10):1447-1465. The Winds of Change: *Treatment Works!: Mental Disorder Treatment Success Rates.* Available at: http://www.thewindsofchange.org/old/rates.html. Accessed February 1, 2006. *Journal of Psychiatric Nursing* summarization of National Institutes of Health data; and Portrait of schizophrenia, *J Psychosoc Nurs Ment Health Serv* 35:5, 1997. Treatment can include all treatment modalities.

5. Many psychotropic drugs have significant or even life-threatening side effects, drug interactions, or both.
6. Unfortunately, finding the right drug regimen is often a trial-and-error exercise.

Ideally, psychotropic drugs should be prescribed based on an accurate diagnosis and then taken until an acceptable mental or emotional state can be maintained (Table 16-1). At this point, the patient can hopefully be withdrawn from the medication and proceed with his or her life. Unfortunately, this scenario does not always occur.

Some individuals recover and never need medications again, others become dependent on psychotropic agents to function, thus finding it difficult to quit, and still others might need the chemistry-correcting properties of these drugs for the remainder of their lives. Tragically, some individuals, especially those referred to as the severely mentally ill, might improve enough to warrant drug continuation but never improve enough to be functionally independent.

In Chapter 1, a brief historical review of the development of psychotropic drugs was presented. Box 16-1 summarizes significant points during the evolution of psychopharmacology. A careful reading of this information reveals that antipsychotics, antidepressants, and antimanic agents were all discovered, serendipitously, before 1960. Although many related drugs were eventually synthesized from the prototypes of each class, the clones were remarkably similar to the original. However, since the 1990s, several substantially different types of drugs have emerged. Clozapine (Clozaril) and other atypical antipsychotic medications are different from the traditional antipsychotics (see Chapter 18), and selective serotonin reuptake inhibitors (SSRIs, [e.g., Prozac]) and other new antidepressants (e.g., Effexor) are quite different from the earlier antidepressants (see Chapter 19). Finally, newer drugs in the treatment of Alzheimer's disease (e.g., Aricept, Exelon, Namenda) are providing hope and encouragement to many patients and families plagued by this illness. These examples point to the continuing effort by clinicians and researchers to address the mental, emotional, and addictive disorders afflicting approximately 25% of Americans effectively. These exciting developments in psychopharmacology should challenge every nurse to understand psychopharmacologic concepts and apply them to practice.

## NURSING RESPONSIBILITIES

Psychopharmacology is the second component of the psychotherapeutic management model (see Chapter 2 to review this model, if needed). The effectiveness of treatment with antipsychotic, antidepressant, antimanic, and antianxiety drugs has been well established. These drugs have enabled millions of individuals to live increasingly satisfying and productive lives. The least restrictive

---

### Box 16-1  Significant Points in the Evolution of Psychotropic Drugs

| | | | |
|---|---|---|---|
| 1930s | Sternbach first synthesizes benzodiazepines. | 1958 | Kuhn publishes the first article on tricyclic antidepressants in the *American Journal of Psychiatry.* |
| 1948 | Rapport, Green, and Page isolate "serotonin" from beef serum. | | |
| 1949 | John Cade, an Australian psychiatrist, reports on the efficacy of lithium in mania. | 1960 | Harris presents the first paper on the effectiveness of benzodiazepines in the *Journal of the American Medical Association.* |
| 1949 | The U.S. Food and Drug Administration bans lithium because of deaths of patients with cardiac disease. | 1970 | The ban on lithium is lifted in the United States. |
| 1951 | Chlorpromazine is developed as a nonsedating antihistamine. Laborit and others report diminished surgical anxiety in conscious patients. | 1980s | A new class of antidepressants, selective serotonin reuptake inhibitors (SSRIs), is developed. The first SSRI marketed is Prozac. |
| 1952 | Iproniazid, a derivative of the antituberculosis agent isoniazid, is identified as a monoamine oxidase inhibitor (MAOI). | 1980s | The antiepileptic drugs carbamazepine and valproate are reported to have mood-stabilizing properties. |
| 1953 | Bein isolates reserpine from rauwolfia. Reserpine, effective in treating psychosis, causes severe depression related to depletion of norepinephrine. | 1990s | Clozapine (Clozaril), the first truly new antipsychotic agent in 40 years, is released in the United States. Risperdal, Zyprexa, Seroquel, Geodon, and Abilify follow over the next 10 years or so. |
| 1954 | Lehman publishes the first article in the United States on chlorpromazine in the *Archives of Neurology and Psychiatry.* | 1990s | Other SSRIs are developed—Zoloft, Paxil, Celexa, Lexapro. A report linking Prozac to suicidal behavior is published in 1990. |
| 1955 | Researchers alter the molecular structure of chlorpromazine and begin developing new antipsychotic agents. | 1990s | Drugs used to treat patients with Alzheimer's disease are made available. |
| 1957 | The first papers appear on MAOIs as antidepressants. | 2004 | Concerns arise about the linkage of SSRIs to violent and suicidal behavior. |
| 1957 | Haldol is developed. | | |

From Ayd FJ: The early history of modern psychopharmacology, *Neuropsychopharmacology* 5:71, 1991; Kuhn R: The treatment of depressive states with G 22355 (imipramine hydrochloride), *Am J Psychiatry* 115:459, 1958; Gunnell D, Saperia J, Ashby D: Selective serotonin reuptake inhibitors (SSRIs) and suicide in adults: meta-analysis of drug company data from placebo-controlled, randomised controlled trials submitted to the MHRA's safety review, *BMJ* 330(7488):385, 2005; and Rifkin A: Extrapyramidal side effects: a historical perspective, *J Clin Psychiatry* 48:3, 1987.

---

alternative or environment, a concept that reflects the community mental health effort to allow individuals to live their lives in an unrestrictive atmosphere, has largely evolved as a result of the impact of these drugs.

Because nursing provides 24-hour care, the nurse is responsible for assessing drug side effects, evaluating desired effects, and applying preventive care to reduce potential problems. Additionally, the nurse usually makes decisions concerning as-needed (prn) medications. The nurse must therefore understand key dimensions of psychotropic drug use. Box 16-2 outlines nursing responsibilities for psychotropic drug administration based on the American Nurses Association's (ANA) guidelines on psychopharmacology (Laraia et al, 1994).

Each chapter in Unit III: Psychopharmacology provides a discussion of pharmacologic effects (desired effects), pharmacokinetics (i.e., absorption, distribution, metabolism, excretion), admin-istration, side effects (undesired effects), and drug interactions. Equally important, a discussion of nursing implications emphasizes nursing interventions related to therapeutic versus toxic drug levels, use during pregnancy, use for older adults, side effects, interactions, and teaching patients.

Understanding psychopharmacology involves more than memorizing facts. It should be noted that *memorization* is not a dirty word. Some basics of pharmacology must be memorized, but the nurse who tries to get by on memorization alone is a medication error waiting to happen. Because of our strong belief in the importance of nurses' (and nursing students') understanding of the basics of psychopharmacology, several important concepts will be reviewed. These concepts are:

• Pharmacokinetics
• Pharmacodynamics
• Blood-brain barrier

## Box 16-2    Nursing Responsibilities for Psychotropic Drug Administration*

The psychiatric mental health nurse can do the following:

1. Describe psychopharmacologic agents based on similarities and differences.
2. Discuss actions of psychopharmacologic agents from global responses to cellular responses.
3. Differentiate psychiatric symptoms from medication side effects.
4. Apply basic principles of pharmacokinetics and pharmacodynamics.
5. Identify appropriate use of psychopharmacologic agents in special populations.
6. Involve clients and their families.
7. Identify factors that might prevent the active involvement of clients in their care.
8. Describe appropriate nonpsychopharmacologic interventions.
9. Discuss the use of standardized rating scales.
10. Demonstrate the knowledge necessary to develop psychopharmacologic education and treatment plans.

*Objectives based on the American Nurses Association Guidelines on Psychopharmacology.
Modified from Laraia MT, Beeber LS, Callwood GB, et al: *Psychiatric mental health nursing psychopharmacology project,* Washington, DC, 1994, American Nurses Association.

- Neurons and neurotransmitters
- Receptors

This chapter concludes with a few general strategies for helping patients and families understand important considerations in regard to psychotropic drug use. Drug-specific patient teaching content is presented in each chapter.

### CRITICAL THINKING QUESTION    1

Some nurses might have little knowledge about some drugs they administer. Do you consider this unethical, unprofessional, unsafe, or simply a reality of the nursing profession? Because no one can know every drug, what basic information should a nurse know before giving medication?

## PHARMACOKINETICS

Pharmacokinetics is defined as the effects that the body has on a drug. The four aspects of pharmacokinetics are the following:

- *Absorption,* or getting the drug into the bloodstream
- *Distribution,* or getting the drug from the bloodstream to the tissues and organs
- *Metabolism,* or breaking the drug down into an inactive and typically water-soluble form
- *Excretion,* or getting the drug out of the body

## ABSORPTION

Drugs taken orally must get out of the gastrointestinal (GI) tract and into the bloodstream to have an effect. For a drug to get out of the GI tract, the drug molecule must pass through the stomach or small intestinal wall into blood vessels. Molecules pass through cell membranes (composed of a phospholipid bilayer) in three ways:

1. Small molecules can fit through pores or channels in the membrane.
2. Some drug molecules have special transport systems to ferry them across the membrane.
3. Lipid-soluble drugs (and most drugs are lipophilic) can pass through phospholipid membranes.

Only a certain percentage of an oral drug reaches the systemic circulation, whereas approximately 100% of a drug given intravenously reaches the systemic circulation. The percentage that reaches the systemic circulation is said to be a drug's bioavailability. Bioavailability is only a fraction of the dose for many drugs given orally because of incomplete absorption and first-pass metabolism. First-pass metabolism is the enzymatic breakdown of drugs before they reach systemic circulation. This occurs during passage through the gut wall and in a presystemic hepatic exposure. The latter occurs because the capillaries in the GI tract do not behave as do most capillaries (i.e., dumping into venules) but, instead, connect with hepatic portal veins, shunting drugs through the *liver* before reaching the general system. Some drugs are substantially metabolized in this manner. For example, buspirone (BuSpar), an antianxiety drug, has a bioavailability of 1% to 4%, which means that most of this drug is metabolized before it gets into general circulation. If, by some mechanism, the first pass through the liver could be eliminated for buspirone, its dose would have to be dramatically reduced.

*Clinical relevance:* Only absorbed drugs can have an effect. Drugs with a high first-pass metabolism and low bioavailability after oral ingestion must be significantly reduced in dose level if given intramuscularly or intravenously.

## DISTRIBUTION

Distribution is the process of the body getting the drug out of the bloodstream and to tissues and organs. If a psychotropic drug cannot leave the bloodstream, it cannot have a therapeutic effect. Lipid-soluble molecules can penetrate capillary membranes as easily as they can penetrate other cell membranes. However, water-soluble (or polar) molecules also leave circulation because of significant gaps between the cells of the capillary wall. Essentially, because molecules are innately active, water-soluble molecules bounce around inside the capillary until they hit a gap and move into extracellular fluid. Another distribution issue involves protein binding. Most drugs bind to plasma proteins (mostly albumin) to some degree or another.

For example:

| Familiar Psychotropic Drug | Protein Binding (%) |
| --- | --- |
| Zoloft | 99 |
| Valium | 98 |
| Prozac | 95 |
| Ativan | 92 |
| Lexapro | 55 |
| Effexor | 23 |

Protein binding is important because molecules that are bound to proteins cannot leave circulation—that is, the protein is simply too large to pass through the gaps. Hence, protein-bound drugs do not have a pharmacologic effect, cannot be metabolized, and cannot be excreted. Specifically, Valium, which has a calming (or anxiolytic) effect, produces its results because of the 2% or so of active drug. Other drugs that can reduce Valium's protein binding to 96% would literally double its effect.

*Clinical relevance:* Effects, both desired and undesired, of highly protein-bound drugs result from the activity of the few free drug molecules in circulation. Drug combinations that compete for binding sites have the potential of causing significant increases in levels of the free or active drug.

## METABOLISM

Metabolism is the process whereby the body breaks down a drug molecule. Most drugs are metabolized to inactive and water-soluble states in preparation for excretion from the body in the urine. An important point to note is that not all drugs are broken down into inactive forms, nor are all drugs converted into water-soluble particles, nor are all drugs eliminated via the renal system. More detailed descriptions of metabolism can be found in a general pharmacology text.

Most metabolism occurs in the liver, but it is not the only site; some metabolic activity occurs in the kidneys, lungs, GI tract, and plasma. Enzymes facilitate the metabolic processes and are said to be catalysts because they provoke yet are unaffected by the biochemical reaction. An enzyme is much larger (perhaps one hundred times larger) compared with the drug molecule and is configured in such a way that only those molecules matching that specific configuration (i. e., the enzyme's substrates) can be metabolized (Keltner et al, 2001c). A single enzyme performs its metabolic task over and over and, in the case of cholinesterase, metabolizes 5000 molecules of acetylcholine per cholinesterase molecule per second (Purves et al, 1997).

Two enzyme systems of particular importance to nurses who administer psychotropic drugs must be mentioned here: (1) the monoamine oxidase (MAO) system and (2) the cytochrome P-450 system. The MAO system metabolizes monoamines, which include dopamine, norepinephrine, and serotonin. The other system, cytochrome P-450, breaks down most psychotropic drugs.

### Monoamine Oxidase System

MAO is the enzyme that rapidly inactivates monoamines (e.g., serotonin, dopamine, norepinephrine) and slowly metabolizes noncatecholamines (e.g., ephedrine, phenylephrine). MAO is located in the liver, intestinal wall, and central nervous system (CNS) in the terminals of neurons containing serotonin, norepinephrine, or dopamine. In the liver, MAO inactivates tyramine, which is found in many foods, and the biogenic amines found in some drugs. When liver MAO is prevented from metabolizing these amines, serious sympathetic effects can develop. MAO is present in two forms: (1) MAO-A, which inactivates norepinephrine and serotonin, and (2) MAO-B, which inactivates dopamine. Some psychotropic drugs inhibit both MAO-A and MAO-B and are correctly described as *nonselective* MAO inhibitors (these are the agents warned about on many over-the-counter drug containers). A few drugs are highly selective and inhibit either MAO-A or MAO-B. These agents are described as *selective* MAO inhibitors. MAO inhibitors are discussed in Chapter 19.

---

**Dopamine**

**Activation**
Positive symptoms of schizophrenia
Psychoses
Dyskinesias
Hallucinations
Delusions
Nausea
Vomiting
Addictive behaviors
Sexual function enhancement

**Antagonism**
Antipsychotic effect for positive symptoms of
    schizophrenia
Negative symptoms of schizophrenia
Temperature dysregulation
Antiemetic effect
Parkinson's and related disorders
Dystonias
Akathisias
Cognitive problems
Sexual dysfunction
Neuroendocrine dysregulation
Depression, anhedonia
Lack of energy, motivation

---

### Cytochrome P-450 Enzyme System

Beyond being involved in the metabolism of psychotropic drugs, the cytochrome P-450 system is said to be the point at which most drug interactions occur (Cozza et al, 2003). Box 16-3 presents a list of psychotropic drugs that are substrates for these enzymes and a broad list of inhibitors.

The cytochrome P-450 enzyme (P-450 enzyme) system has been traditionally referred to as the hepatic microsomal enzyme system (Lehne, 2004). This complex name can be broken down as follows: *cyto* stands for microsomal vesicles, *P* stands for pigmentation (because the enzymes contain red-pigmented heme), and *450* refers to the wavelength

(in nanometers) at which light absorption occurs (Cozza et al, 2003). Although this much information is probably more than you want to know, it is included here for two reasons: (1) this is the same system that older texts refer to as the hepatic microsomal system, and (2) it outlines the reasoning behind an otherwise intimidating name.

P-450 enzymes contain 12 families, with over 40 individual enzymes found in humans (Lehne, 2004). Six enzymes account for approximately 90% of P-450 enzymes in humans: 1A2, 3A4, 2C9, 2C19, 2D6, and 2E1 (Cozza et al, 2003). These enzymes are sometimes referred to as *isoenzymes* or *isozymes*. This text will use only the more generic but equally accurate term, *enzymes*.

*Clinical relevance:* Most drugs must be metabolized to an inactive and water-soluble form to be excreted from the system. Certain conditions (e.g., liver disease, kidney disease) or drug combinations that inhibit metabolism can lead to significant, and even deadly, results.

---

**CRITICAL THINKING QUESTION**    2

As stated, most psychotropic drug interactions occur as a result of the effects on the P-450 system. If an inhibitor of the P-450 3A4 enzyme is to be given (e.g., grapefruit juice), which psychotropic drugs will be affected? What is the effect? (Refer to Box 16-3 to answer this question.)

---

### Half-Life of Drugs

The half-life of a drug is the amount of time required for 50% of the drug to disappear from the body. If drug X has a half-life of 4 hours, then 50% of the drug will be out of the system in 4 hours. In another 4 hours, only 25% of the original dose will remain. In most cases, it will not matter whether the patient took 100 mg or 300 mg; the amount of drug in the body will decrease by 50% every 4 hours. This action is referred to as *linear kinetics,* and most drugs follow this pattern. This rule has exceptions, most notably alcohol, in which only a set amount of the drug is metabolized in a given period, regardless of the amount ingested (i.e., nonlinear kinetics). If the nurse gives the same drug dose (e.g., 100 mg) at the same time (e.g., three times a day), a steady state is achieved in four to five half-lives. When discontinuing a drug, four to five half-lives are

**Box 16-3   Psychotropic Substrates and General Inhibitors of Selected Cytochrome P-450 Enzymes**

**2D6 Substrates**

*Antidepressants*
Some tricyclic antidepressants (e.g., desipramine, nortriptyline)
Venlafaxine
Fluoxetine
Paroxetine
Trazodone
Mirtazapine

*Antipsychotics*
Thioridazine
Risperidone
Haloperidol
Clozapine

**2D6 Inhibitors**
Paroxetine
Fluoxetine
Fluphenazine
Sertraline (>100 mg)
Quinidine
Haloperidol
Cimetidine
Thioridazine
Amitriptyline
Oral contraceptives
Clomipramine
Desipramine

**1A2 Substrates**

*Antidepressants*
Amitriptyline
Imipramine
Fluvoxamine
Mirtazapine
Clomipramine

*Antipsychotics*
Clozapine
Haloperidol
Olanzapine
Phenothiazines

*Other Drugs*
Caffeine
Tacrine

**1A2 Inhibitors**
Fluvoxamine
Fluoroquinolones
Beta-estradiol
Ciprofloxacin
Erythromycin
Grapefruit juice

**3A4 Substrates**

*Antidepressants*
Amitriptyline
Imipramine
Clomipramine
Sertraline
Mirtazapine
Nefazodone
Bupropion

*Antipsychotics*
Clozapine
Haloperidol
Quetiapine

*Benzodiazepines*
Alprazolam
Diazepam

**3A4 Inhibitors**
Nefazodone
Fluvoxamine
Sertraline (>100 mg)
Cimetidine
Diltiazem
Verapamil
Ketoconazole
Erythromycin
Fluoxetine
Progestagens
Grapefruit juice
Paroxetine

**Psychotropic Drug Inhibitors of 2C9**
Fluoxetine
Fluvoxamine
Paroxetine
Sertraline

**2C19 Substrates**

*Antidepressants*
Amitriptyline
Citalopram
Clomipramine
Imipramine
Moclobemide

**2C19 Inhibitors**
Fluvoxamine
Fluoxetine
Paroxetine

From Keltner NL, Folks DG: *Psychotropic drugs,* ed 4, St. Louis, 2005, Mosby.

required to eliminate 96% of the drug. This period is referred to as the *washout period.*

## EXCRETION

The kidney excretes most drugs, but other routes of excretion exist, such as breast milk, bile, feces, saliva, sweat, and the lungs. Factors that can affect excretion include kidney disease, age, and drug competition for active tubular transport.

*Clinical relevance:* Drugs that are not adequately excreted (e.g., because of kidney disease), particularly drugs excreted unchanged (i.e., drugs that are not metabolized, such as lithium and amphetamines), have a more pronounced effect compared with drugs that are excreted.

## PHARMACODYNAMICS

Pharmacodynamics is the effect that a drug has on the body. The two global responses to drugs are the desired effects and side effects. Drugs that activate receptors are termed *agonists,* and drugs that block receptors are named *antagonists.* Some psychotropic drugs are agonists, whereas many others are antagonists. Pharmacodynamic effects of particular interest to this discussion are down-regulation of receptors and pharmacodynamic tolerance.

## DOWN-REGULATION

Down-regulation of receptors is an important concept, primarily because chronic exposure to certain psychotropic drugs causes receptors to change. For example, consistent use of antidepressants causes postsynaptic receptors to decrease in number. Because this down-regulation occurs at about the same time that the antidepressant effect develops (approximately 2 to 4 weeks), it is thought that reduction in postsynaptic receptors might provide a better explanation for mood elevation than increases in neurotransmitters.

## PHARMACODYNAMIC TOLERANCE

Pharmacodynamic tolerance is a term used to describe a reduction in receptor sensitivity. A good example is the chronic drinker of alcohol. When the newspaper reports a person driving a car with a blood alcohol level (BAL) of 0.35, the story is likely about a case of pharmacodynamic tolerance. This person's receptors are no longer responding to the ethanol in the way a normal person's receptors would respond. Although at first glance this idea might appear appealing, it really is not. Tolerance to a BAL that could cause deadly respiratory depression does not occur. Hence, a person who is functioning at an elevated BAL can drink only a little more alcohol and die.

*Clinical relevance:* Knowledge of down-regulatory functions helps the nurse explain the lag time between initiating drug therapy and clinical improvement. Knowledge of pharmacodynamic tolerance aids in teaching patients and families about drug tolerance to some drug effects but little, if any, tolerance to some lethal effects (e.g., respiratory depression) at just slightly higher doses.

## BLOOD-BRAIN BARRIER

The blood-brain barrier is also an important concept for understanding psychotropic drug activity. The brain, more than other organs of the body, requires a constant internal milieu. Whereas other parts of the body experience fluctuations in body chemistry, even small changes in the brain produce serious problems. The brain is protected from fluctuations by the blood-brain barrier. This barrier regulates the amount and speed of substances in the blood entering the brain. Water, carbon dioxide, and oxygen readily cross the barrier; other substances are excluded from the brain.

The blood-brain barrier has three dimensions: (1) an anatomic dimension, (2) a physiologic dimension, and (3) a metabolic dimension. The anatomic dimension is the structure of the capillaries that supply blood to the brain and prevent many molecules from slipping through. There are no gaps.

The physiologic dimension is a chemical and transport system that recognizes and then allows certain molecules into the brain. Lipid solubility is the most important of the chemical properties that determine whether a molecule can pass through the blood-brain barrier. Highly lipid-soluble substances pass the blood-brain barrier with relative ease. Highly water-soluble substances penetrate this barrier slowly and in insignificant amounts. Nicotine, ethanol, heroin, caffeine, and diazepam (Valium) are examples of highly lipid-soluble substances. This characteristic is clinically important, because only drugs that can pass through this barrier in significant amounts are effective in treating a psychiatric or medical disorder of the brain. Certain nonlipid-soluble substances such as glucose, which is the brain's primary energy source, and essential amino acids, which are needed for the synthesis of neurotransmitters, are required for normal brain function. Special transport systems carry these essential substances across the blood-brain barrier.

The metabolic barrier prevents molecules from entering the brain by enzymatic action within the endothelial lining of the brain capillaries. For example, levodopa can pass the blood-brain barrier, but much of it is changed to dopamine before it can pass completely through the capillary wall into the brain. The metabolic product, dopamine, does not readily pass this barrier, thus illustrating the third way that the brain protect humans from substances in peripheral circulation.

Understanding the blood-brain barrier helps the nurse conceptualize, administer, and monitor drug therapy accurately, as well as understand addiction to highly lipid-soluble substances such as alcohol and heroin. A comparison of systemic penicillin and dopamine serves as an example for understanding this important principle. For example, if penicillin were the only antibiotic available (which was true at one time), large doses would then be needed to treat a CNS infection, because this water-soluble drug does not pass through the blood-brain barrier easily. When a large dose of penicillin is given, only a fraction of that dose enters the brain. Most of the penicillin stays in the peripheral system, which does not cause alarm because penicillin has relatively few adverse effects. On the other hand, dopamine (and many other drugs) has many adverse effects on the body. The dose needed to penetrate the blood-brain barrier and thus affect the brain adequately (a central effect) is so large that it would have serious adverse effects on the rest of the body (e.g., cardiac stimulation, a peripheral effect).

## NEURONS AND NEUROTRANSMITTERS

Nerve cells, or neurons, comprise the basic unit of the nervous system. Nerve cells are designed to receive and give information. Dendrites are the projections from the neuron that receive information and transmit it to the cell body. Axons send information from the nerve cell to the dendrites, axons, or cell bodies of other neurons. Axons of one cell are separated from the dendrites, axons, or cell body of another by a microscopic space known as a synapse (Figure 16-1). Figure 16-2

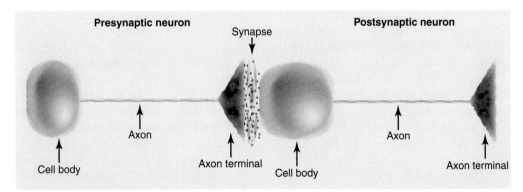

**FIGURE 16-1** Two-neuron chain shows the presynaptic and postsynaptic neurons interconnected by a synapse. The synapse is composed of a synaptic bouton (*triangle*) or presynaptic terminal, the synaptic cleft, and the postsynaptic membrane, which, in this example, is the dendrite or cell body (*circle*) of the postsynaptic neuron. (From Keltner N, Folks D: *Psychotropic drugs*, St. Louis, 1997, Mosby.)

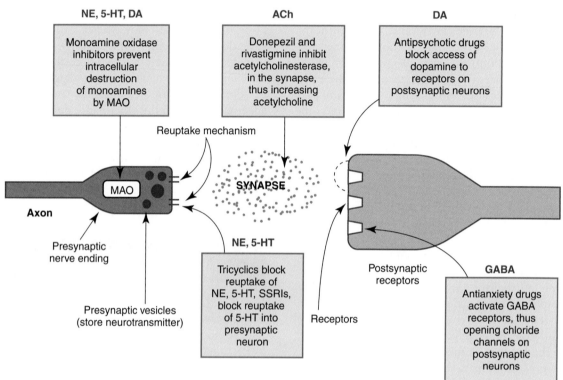

**FIGURE 16-2** Explanation of the way psychotropic drugs affect five major neurotransmitters. (Modified from Stuart G, Sundeen S: *Principles and practice of psychiatric nursing,* ed 5, St. Louis, 1995, Mosby.)

depicts the relationships among neurotransmitters, neurons, and psychotropic drugs.

Information, in the form of an electrochemical excitation, is communicated between cells in a specific manner. An electrochemical impulse runs from the cell body through the axon to the synaptic terminal. Neurotransmitters are stimulated and released from the synaptic terminal into the synaptic cleft and combine with receptors on the postsynaptic neuron, evoking a neuronal response. Remember, though, that neurons are not strung throughout the brain end on end. The neuronal system is highly complex, with most neurons receiving input from thousands of other neurons. Furthermore, the arborization, or branching, of dendrites continues into late adolescence and early adulthood. It is when most of these connec-

tions are finally complete that who we are truly emerges.

Neurotransmitters are synthesized from natural precursors (e.g., amino acids) in the body (Box 16-4). These precursors are extracted from the bloodstream and synthesized in the cell into neurotransmitters. Neurotransmitters are stored in storage vesicles in the presynaptic terminals of the cell. Neurotransmitters come in many forms, and they combine with specific receptors. For example, the neurotransmitter norepinephrine combines with a norepinephrine receptor. After norepinephrine electrochemically stimulates the norepinephrine receptor, information is transmitted to the cell body, which, in turn, communicates to the next neuron, and so on. After it is in the synaptic cleft, the neurotransmitter can, until it is inacti-

## Box 16-4   Four Categories of Neurotransmitters

**Monoamines**
Dopamine (a catecholamine)
Norepinephrine (a catecholamine)
Serotonin (an indolamine)
**Cholinergic**
Acetylcholine
**Amino Acids**
Gamma-aminobutyric acid (GABA)
Glutamate
**Peptide**
Enkephalins

## Box 16-5   Most Important Neurotransmitters That Psychiatric Nursing Students Should Know

Psychotropic drugs work by affecting neurotransmitter systems. We believe that the foundation for understanding psychotropic drugs rests on knowledge of only six neurotransmitters. Although a great deal is to be learned, we are satisfied that understanding the way psychotropic drugs affect acetylcholine, dopamine, gamma-aminobutyric acid (GABA), glutamate, norepinephrine, and serotonin is the starting point. As the following chapters will discuss:

- Acetylcholine is important in conceptualizing the pathology and treatment of Alzheimer's disease and parkinsonism.
- Dopamine is important in conceptualizing the pathology and treatment of schizophrenia and parkinsonism.
- GABA is important in conceptualizing the pathology and treatment of anxiety.
- Glutamate is an excitatory neurotransmitter and might be important in conceptualizing the pathology and treatment of Alzheimer's disease.
- Norepinephrine is important in conceptualizing the pathology and treatment of mania and depression.
- Serotonin is important in conceptualizing the pathology and treatment of mania and depression.

## Table 16-2   Neurotransmitters and Related Mental Disorders*

| Neurotransmitter-Related State | Mental Disorder |
| --- | --- |
| Increase in dopamine level | Schizophrenia |
| Decrease in norepinephrine level | Depression |
| Decrease in serotonin level | Depression |
| Decrease in acetylcholine level | Alzheimer's disease |
| Decrease in GABA level | Anxiety |
| Increase in glutamate level | Excitotoxicity leading to neuronal death |
| Decrease in glutamate level | Can lead to psychotic thinking |

*GABA,* Gamma-aminobutyric acid.
*I realize that this explanation is overly simplistic, but the information given here nevertheless serves to convey the basic neurotransmitter theories for the related mental disorder.

## RECEPTORS

Receptors are proteins on cell surfaces that respond to endogenous ligands or to drug molecules. A ligand is a transmitter substance or molecule that fits and evokes a response from a receptor. Examples of ligands include drugs, neurotransmitters, hormones, prostaglandins, and leukotrienes. Receptors are configured so that only precisely shaped molecules can fit and subsequently cause or prevent a response. For example, the neurotransmitter serotonin fits serotonin receptors, but acetylcholine molecules do not fit serotonin receptors.

Four primary receptor processes exist (Lehne, 2004). The two most commonly addressed processes in psychopharmacology literature are the ligand-gated ion channel (or first-messenger) process and the G-protein–coupled (or second-messenger) process. When the ligand-gated receptor is activated, an ion channel such as a sodium, calcium, or chloride channel opens, and the respective ion flows through into the cell. Depending on the ion, this action causes cell depolarization (the cell fires) or hyperpolarization (cell firing slows down, or the cell does not fire). The process is extremely rapid, usually occurring within milliseconds. Acetylcholine (at nicotinic receptors only), gamma-aminobutyric acid (GABA), glycine, and glutamate use the first-messenger system. The G-protein–coupled receptor is a more complex

vated, continue to stimulate the postsynaptic receptor. Neurotransmitters are inactivated by enzymes in the synaptic cleft or by enzymes in the presynaptic terminal, and/or are taken up into surrounding glial cells. Knowledge of this inactivation process has facilitated the evolution of psychopharmacology. The most important neurotransmitters for psychiatric nursing students to understand, and related mental disorders, are presented in Box 16-5 and Table 16-2.

### Box 16-6   Results of Activation or Antagonism of Selected Receptors

**Serotonin Activation**
Antidepressant effect
Anxiety
Migraine headaches
Nausea
Vomiting
Other GI disturbances
Sexual dysfunction
Decrease in penile erection capability
Reduced appetite and weight loss
Insomnia
Movement disorders
Temperature dysregulation
Psychotic thinking (e.g., hallucinations)

**Serotonin Antagonism**
Depression
Dysthymia
Suicidality
Aggressiveness
Obsessive thinking
Sleep-wake cycle disruption
Pain
Compulsive behavior
Anxiety
Migraine headaches
Panic

**Acetylcholine Activation**
Pupil contraction
Decreased heart rate
Constriction of bronchi

Increased respiratory secretions
Increased voiding
Salivation
Increased gastric secretions
Increased defecation
Sweating
Enhancement of cognitive processes

**Acetylcholine Antagonism**
Dilated pupils
Increased heart rate
Dilation of bronchi
Decreased respiratory secretions
Decreased voiding
Dry mouth
Decreased gastric secretions
Constipation
Decreased sweating
Cognitive slowing

**Norepinephrine Activation**
Antidepressant effect
Vasoconstriction (alpha-1)
Increased heart rate (beta-1)
Bronchial dilation
Other physical effects

**Norepinephrine Antagonism**
Depressive effect
Vasodilation (alpha-1 antagonism)
Decreased heart rate (beta blocker)
Sexual dysfunction
Other physical effects

Modified from Keltner NL, Zielinski AL, Hardin MS: Drugs used for cognitive symptoms of Alzheimer's disease, *Perspect Psychiatr Care* 37:31, 2001; Keltner NL, Hogan B, Guy DM: Dopaminergic and serotonergic receptor function in the CNS, *Perspect Psychiatr Care* 37:65, 2001; and Keltner NL, Hogan B, Knight T, Royals LA: Adrenergic, cholinergic, GABAergic, and glutaminergic receptor function in the CNS, *Perspect Psychiatr Care* 37:140, 2001.

process—a biologic cascade of intracellular reactions develops—and is slower compared with the first-messenger system (Piercey, 1998). Norepinephrine, serotonin, dopamine, acetylcholine (at muscarinic receptors only), and peptides couple with G-protein or second-messenger receptors. Consequences of selected receptor activation or antagonism are listed in Box 16-6.

Psychotropic drugs can affect neurotransmitters in several ways:

1. Prevent metabolism (e.g., some antidepressants and drugs for Alzheimer's disease)
2. Prevent reuptake (e.g., SSRIs and other antidepressants)
3. Block postsynaptic receptors (antagonists) (e.g., antipsychotic drugs)
4. Activate or block autoreceptors (see discussion on autoreceptors later in this chapter)

5. Block calcium channels (calcium channel blockers are occasionally used in psychiatry)

The following terms relating to receptors are defined to facilitate understanding of information presented in the drug chapters (Keltner, 2000; Keltner et al, 2001a).

*Receptor antagonism.* Receptor antagonism is the process in which receptor function is compromised related to blocking of that receptor by a psychotropic drug. Antagonists prevent the endogenous ligand from activating the receptor.
*Receptor agonist.* A receptor agonist is a drug that fits and activates the receptor in the same manner as the naturally occurring ligand.
*Autoreceptor.* An autoreceptor is the feedback mechanism that neurons use to increase or decrease the release of a neurotransmitter; they are typically, but not always, found on the pre-

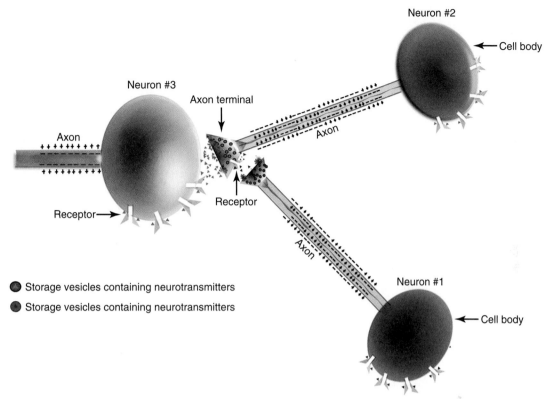

**FIGURE 16-3** Neuronal modulation. (Courtesy of Vicki Johnson, Assistant Professor, University of Alabama School of Nursing.)

synaptic neuron. Autoreceptor agonists tell the neuron that enough of the neurotransmitter is present; hence, a decrease in the release of the neurotransmitter occurs. Autoreceptor antagonists tell the receptor to release more of the neurotransmitter.

*Receptor affinity.* Receptor affinity is the attraction or strength of attraction between neurotransmitters and receptors.

*Receptor life cycle.* Receptors are continually being formed and continually breaking down. The life cycle of the average receptor is short (Lehne, 2004).

*Receptor modulation.* Some neurotransmitters do not have a direct effect but modify (or modulate) the effect of another neurotransmitter. The following scenario might help in the understanding of receptor modulation. Picture, if possible, one neuron (#1) synapsing with the synaptic terminal of a presynaptic neuron (#2), which is synapsing in the traditional way with a third neuron (#3). Neuron #1 influences the release of neurotransmitter from #2, which then will affect the amount of neurotransmitter released

into the synapse between #2 and #3. Neuron #1 is modulating neuron #2 (Figure 16-3).

## PATIENT EDUCATION

The importance of patient and family education cannot be overemphasized. Historically, many psychiatric patients and their families demonstrated little understanding of their medications. Although the emphasis on education has partially remedied this problem, teaching about these potent drugs will always be a nursing priority. Furthermore, many rehospitalizations are related to patients' nonadherence to medication schedules. As knowledge deficits are removed, better compliance can be anticipated.

Despite a certain risk associated with discussing medications and side effects with patients, nurses have a professional duty to do so with knowledge and sensitivity—that is, with balance. The nurse might frighten patients with too much or inappropriate information. Good professional judgment is important, including teaching patients about what effects are visible, what can be felt, and what the possibilities are of becoming drug-dependent. The nurse should also emphasize regular checkups and tests. Specific areas of education include the following (Malone et al, 2004):

1. Discussion of side effects:
   - Side effects can directly affect the patient's willingness to adhere to the drug regimen; for example, the SSRIs, such as Zoloft, are known to reduce libido and sexual functioning. Thus, these drugs indirectly affect spouses as well.
   - Side effects can cause medical problems, or even cause death.
   - Some drugs cause patients to experience emotional flattening, thus dulling responses to the environment, counseling, and family.
   - Some drugs cause cognitive slowing.
   - The nurse should always inquire about the patient's response to a drug, both therapeutic responses and adverse responses.
2. Discussion of safety issues:
   - Does the patient take the drug as prescribed?
   - Do the patient and family know which effects should be reported to the nurse or physician?
   - Because some drugs, such as tricyclic antidepressants, have a narrow therapeutic index, thoughts of self-harm must be discussed.
   - Does the drug have potential for abuse or dependence?
   - Can the drug be discontinued abruptly without effect? Patients should know that many drugs must be tapered gradually.
   - Because many psychotropic drugs cause sedation or drowsiness, discussions concerning use of hazardous machinery, driving, and so forth must be reviewed.
3. Attitudes of patient and nurse about medications:
   - Because many patients and families believe that the use of medications is a sign of weakness or lack of faith in God, the nurse must discuss these issues.
   - Some nurses do not really believe in psychotropic medications either. These nurses must examine their own views and perhaps work in areas of nursing that do not involve psychotropic drugs.
   - For patients and families who are resistant to the use of psychotropic agents, the nurse must discuss the potential ramifications of noncompliance.

- Issues of dependence and long-term medication use must be discussed.
- Because many patients and families do not want to become addicted, the nurse must point out the specific addiction potential of any specific drug. Most psychotropic drugs are not addicting.

4. Drug interactions:
   - Patients and families must be taught to discuss the effects of the addition of over-the-counter drugs, alcohol, and illegal drugs to currently prescribed drugs.
   - Patients who meet with more than one clinician must make potential prescribing professionals aware of all drugs that are currently being taken.
5. Instructions for older adult patients or children of older adult patients:
   - Because older individuals have a different pharmacokinetic profile than younger adults, special instructions concerning side effects and drug-drug interactions should be tailored for this population.
6. Instructions for pregnant or breast-feeding patients:
   - Because pregnant or breast-feeding patients have special risks associated with psychotropic drug therapy, special instructions should be tailored for these individuals.

Teaching patients about their medications enables them to be mature participants in their own care and decreases undesirable side effects. Furthermore, effective teaching can reduce noncompliance, or the failure to take medications as prescribed. Box 16-7 lists common

---

**Box 16-7    Common Reasons for Patients Not Taking Medication as Prescribed**

Sexual dysfunction
Specific side effects—dry mouth, insomnia, sleepiness
Other side effects
Emotional dulling
Cognitive slowing
Denial of need
Fear of becoming addicted
Religious reasons
Interference with work
Inability to use alcohol or other recreational drugs
Pregnancy
Illness (suspiciousness, delusions of conspiracy)

reasons that patients give for not taking their medication as prescribed. Each chapter in this unit outlines patient education issues specific to each class of drugs discussed.

## CRITICAL THINKING QUESTION    4

In this chapter, I state that the nurse should use balance when giving information to a patient about a drug. What is the balance between arousing unneeded apprehension in a patient who is vulnerable to suggestion (i.e., giving complete information) and treating that adult patient as a child (i.e., withholding information to protect the patient)? Obviously, in your role as student and later as nurse, you would not want to do either.

## Study Notes

1. Psychopharmacology is the second component of psychotherapeutic management. Psychotropic drugs have enabled millions of people to live more productive lives in the least restrictive environment.
2. Nurses assess for drug side effects, evaluate desired effects, and make decisions about prn medications. Thus, nurses must understand general principles of psychopharmacology and have specific knowledge concerning frequently used psychotropic drugs.
3. Pharmacokinetic processes include the absorption, distribution, metabolism, and excretion of drugs.
4. Absorption is the process whereby drugs leave the GI tract and get into the bloodstream.
5. Bioavailability is the percentage of a drug that reaches the systemic circulation.
6. Distribution refers to the process of drug molecules leaving the bloodstream to reach tissues and organs. Drugs that do not leave the bloodstream cannot have a psychiatric effect.
7. Lipid solubility is a property that affects both absorption and distribution. Highly lipid-soluble drugs easily penetrate the blood-brain barrier.
8. Protein binding—that is, the propensity of a drug to bind to serum proteins—also affects drug distribution. Drugs bound to serum proteins cannot leave the bloodstream.
9. Metabolism is the process whereby the body breaks down a drug so as to remove the drug from the body.
10. The liver is the site of most drug metabolism.
11. The two major enzyme systems associated with psychotropic drugs include the MAO system and the cytochrome P-450 system.
12. An individual enzyme breaks down thousands of drug molecules per second.
13. The P-450 system is mentioned often in current psychotropic drug literature. Older texts referred to the P-450 system as the hepatic microsomal enzyme system.
14. Most drug-drug interactions are related to interference with the P-450 system.
15. The half-life of a drug is the length of time required for the body to remove 50% of the original dose. If a single dose of a drug is given and the drug has a half-life of 4 hours, 50% of the drug will remain in the body after 4 hours, 25% of the drug will remain after 8 hours, and 12.5% of the drug will remain after 12 hours.
16. Excretion is the removal of drug from the body through the kidneys via the urine.
17. Pharmacodynamics involves the effects of the drug on the body.
18. Drug effects are typically categorized as desired effects or side effects.
19. Down-regulation of a receptor refers to a decrease in receptor numbers.
20. Pharmacodynamic tolerance is a state in which receptors become less sensitive to agonists.
21. Highly lipid-soluble drugs, such as ethanol, heroin, and diazepam (Valium), pass the blood-brain barrier with ease. This characteristic partially accounts for the widespread abuse of these drugs.
22. Only drugs that pass the blood-brain barrier can affect the CNS.
23. Neurotransmitters, which are neurochemical substances in the brain, evoke a neuronal response, are synthesized by cytoplasmic enzymes, and are usually stored in storage vesicles in the presynaptic terminals of the neuron.
24. Because both neurotransmitter deficiency and excess are related to mental disorders, psychotropic drugs are effective because they cause an increase or decrease in the brain's ability to use a specific neurotransmitter.
25. Receptors are proteins on the cell surface that respond to specific ligands.

26. The two receptor processes most important for psychiatric nurses to understand are the first-messenger system and the second-messenger system.

27. The first-messenger system causes a cellular response when a ligand couples with the receptor, which, in turn, immediately opens an ion channel.

28. The second-messenger system is more complex compared with the first-messenger system. The initial ligand-receptor coupling initiates a series of events that culminate in a neuronal response.

29. The blood-brain barrier protects the brain from the physiologic fluctuations that the body experiences and regulates the amount of substances entering the brain and the speed with which they enter.

30. Teaching patients can decrease the incidence of side effects while increasing compliance with the drug regimen. The nurse should use good clinical judgment when deciding what to share with patients and their families.

## References

Cozza KL, Armstrong SC, Oesterheld JR: *Drug interaction principles for medical practice,* Washington, DC, 2003, American Psychiatric Publishing.

Keltner NL: Neuroreceptor function and psychopharmacologic response, *Issues Ment Health Nurs* 21:31, 2000.

Keltner NL, Hogan B, Guy DM: Dopaminergic and serotonergic receptor function in the CNS, *Perspect Psychiatr Care* 37:6568, 2001a.

Keltner NL, Hogan B, Knight T, Royals LA: Adrenergic, cholinergic, GABAergic, and glutaminergic receptor function in the CNS, *Perspect Psychiatr Care* 37:140, 2001b.

Keltner NL, Zielinski AL, Hardin MS: Drugs used for cognitive symptoms of Alzheimer's disease, *Perspect Psychiatr Care* 37:31, 2001c.

Lehne RA: *Pharmacology for nursing care,* Philadelphia, 2004, WB Saunders.

Malone K, Papagni K, Ramini S, Keltner NL: Antidepressants, antipsychotics, benzodiazepines, and the breastfeeding dyad. *Perspect Psychiatr Care* 40:133, 2004.

Piercey MF: Pharmacology of pramipexole, a dopamine $D_3$-preferring agonist useful in treating Parkinson's disease, *Clin Neuropharmacol* 21:141, 1998.

Purves D, Augustine GJ, Fitzpatrick D: *Neuroscience,* Sunderland, MA, 1997, Sinauer Associates.

Riffer NW: It's a brain disease, *Psychiatr Serv* 48:773, 1997.

## Bibliography

Cozza KL, Armstrong SC: *The cytochrome P450 system,* Washington, DC, 2001, American Psychiatric Publishing.

Cozza KL, Armstrong SC, Oesterheld JR: *Drug interaction principles for medical practice,* Washington, DC, 2003, American Psychiatric Publishing.

Keltner NL, Folks DG: *Psychotropic drugs,* ed 3, St. Louis, 2005, Mosby.

Lehne RA: *Pharmacology for nursing care,* Philadelphia, 2004, WB Saunders.

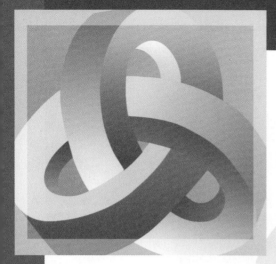

# Chapter 17

# Antiparkinsonian Drugs

*Norman L. Keltner*

## Learning Objectives

*After reading this chapter, you should be able to:*
- Differentiate between Parkinson's disease and parkinsonism.
- Discuss the causes and symptoms of parkinsonism.
- Identify the two neurotransmitters primarily associated with Parkinson's disease.
- Describe the biochemical relationship between Parkinson's disease and extrapyramidal side effects (EPSEs).
- Discuss side effects of antiparkinsonian drugs.

## PARKINSON'S DISEASE AND EXTRAPYRAMIDAL SIDE EFFECTS

Extrapyramidal side effects (EPSEs) are serious and sometimes dangerous complications of treating people with psychotropic drugs. Antipsychotic agents typically cause these adverse responses (see Chapter 18), but other drugs can also produce EPSEs. EPSEs are the result of the biochemical alterations related to those found in Parkinson's disease (PD) (Keltner and Folks, 2005).

PD is a progressive, chronic, degenerative disease of unknown cause that involves the area of the brain called the extrapyramidal system. A well-regulated extrapyramidal system is needed for normal coordination of involuntary movement, which, in turn, supports voluntary movement. For example, when a person walks down the street, a host of involuntary movements facilitate the voluntary movements associated with walking. PD is characterized by four cardinal symptoms: (1) tremors, (2) bradykinesia, (3) rigid-

ity, and (4) postural instability (Pennachio, 2000). A balance of two neurotransmitters, acetylcholine (ACh) and dopamine, is required for normal functioning of the extrapyramidal system. The four primary symptoms and other associated symptoms (e.g., difficulty in swallowing, drooling, weight loss, choking, impaired breathing, urinary retention, constipation) occur when these two neurotransmitters are out of balance.

### CRITICAL THINKING QUESTION 1

How are the associated or secondary symptoms linked to the primary symptoms?

Dopamine is synthesized in the midbrain by pigmented cells in an area called the substantia nigra (black substance). Cell bodies are located in the substantia nigra, and their axons project to the basal ganglia (a major component of the extrapyramidal system), where they release dopamine, which, in turn, activates dopamine receptors. This

**Norm's Notes**

As you might have guessed, I love understanding how drugs work and how a certain category of drug helps treat a specific mental disorder. I always start teaching my students about psychotropic drugs by discussing the antiparkinsonian drugs. Studying these drugs, and Parkinson's disease itself, provides a perfect vehicle for explaining neurotransmitter imbalance (and balance) and neuronal tract degeneration. In some ways, Parkinson's disease could be considered the opposite of schizophrenia, and overtreating schizophrenia can cause Parkinson's disease–type side effects. This is a great place to start.

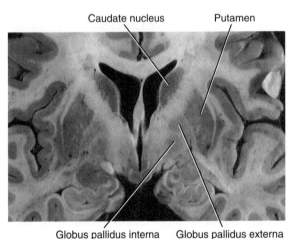

FIGURE 17-1 Basal ganglia. The basal ganglia are composed of several subcortical (below the surface of the outer brain gray matter [or cortex]) nuclei, including the caudate nucleus, the putamen, and the globus pallidus. The globus pallidus can be further divided into the globus pallidus externa and the globus pallidus interna. (Courtesy of Richard E. Powers, Director, Brain Resource Program, University of Alabama at Birmingham.)

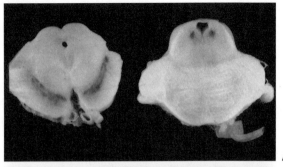

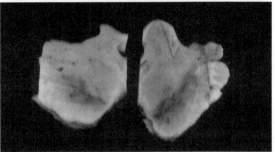

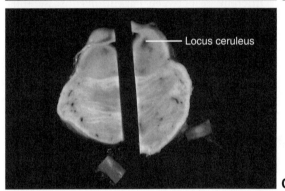

FIGURE 17-2 The effects of aging and disease on catecholamine centers in the brainstem. **A,** Normal pigment in the substantia nigra (*left*) and locus ceruleus (*right*) of a young man. **B,** Mild age-related loss of pigment in the brainstem of a normal individual (*right*) and loss of pigmented neurons in the brainstem of an individual with Parkinson's disease (*left*). **C,** Mild depigmentation of the locus ceruleus (site of norepinephrine synthesis) in an aged individual (*right*) and severe depigmentation in Parkinson's disease (*left*). (Courtesy of Richard E. Powers, Director, Brain Resource Program, University of Alabama at Birmingham.)

pathway, from the midbrain to the basal ganglia, is known as the nigrostriatal tract. In PD, the pigmented neurons of the substantia nigra lose their pigmentation, indicating a decline in dopamine production. A deficiency in dopamine and a subsequent decrease in dopamine transmission to the basal ganglia result in an imbalance with ACh in the basal ganglia. The basal ganglia are shown in Figure 17-1 in what is referred to as a coronal cut of the brain (a cut that runs from side to side).

Figure 17-2 illustrates the depigmentation occurring in PD by comparing the substantia nigra and locus ceruleus (where norepinephrine is synthesized) of a young man (Figure 17-2, *A*) with those of an older man without PD (on the right) and an older man with PD (on the left). This figure clearly shows normal aging, which results in a loss of pigmented neurons, and demonstrates that PD dramatically accelerates the process (Keltner et al, 1998).

EPSEs are also caused by an imbalance between ACh and dopamine (Figure 17-3), but with one important difference. Whereas PD is related to neurodegeneration of the substantia nigra at the beginning of the dopamine tracts, EPSEs are caused by the blockade of dopamine receptors in the basal ganglia at the end of the dopamine tracts.

PD is treated with antiparkinsonian agents that increase dopamine (or dopaminergic) levels, such as Sinemet and levodopa, with anticholinergic agents (e.g., benztropine [Cogentin]), or with both. EPSEs are treated only with anticholinergics because psychosis is thought to be related to an increase in dopamine levels. To give a dopamine-enhancing drug to a patient suffering from schizophrenia might cause psychotic symptoms to increase. A careful review of Table 17-1 will facilitate your understanding of the central point of this chapter.

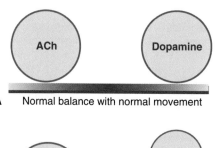

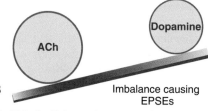

**FIGURE 17-3 A,** Balance between ACh and dopamine, resulting in normal movement. **B,** Imbalance (too little dopamine) results in extrapyramidal side effects (EPSEs).

> **CRITICAL THINKING QUESTION**   2
>
> What is the connection between PD and schizophrenia from a neurotransmitter perspective? (*Hint:* You might need to look at the next chapter.)

## SPECIFIC EXTRAPYRAMIDAL SIDE EFFECTS

Although EPSEs are biochemically related to PD, they are not the same as PD. EPSEs are divided into at least seven distinct types. Table 17-2 provides further information on these disorders.

- *Akathisia.* Akathisia is a subjective feeling of restlessness that elicits restless legs, jittery feelings, and nervous energy. Akathisia is the most common EPSE and responds poorly to treatment.
- *Akinesia.* Akinesia refers to an absence of movement, but a slowed movement (i.e., bradykinesia) is more likely. Symptoms include weakness, fatigue, painful muscles, and anergia. Akinesia responds to anticholinergics.
- *Dystonia.* Dystonias are abnormal postures (i.e., muscle freezing) caused by involuntary muscle spasms. Symptoms manifest as sustained, twisted, and contracted positioning of the limbs, trunk, neck, or mouth. Dystonias tend to appear early in treatment (within about 3 days) and respond to anticholinergic drugs. These agents must occasionally be given parenterally because of the gravity of the situation. Types of dystonias include:
  - Torticollis—contracted positioning of the neck
  - Oculogyric crisis—contracted positioning of the eyes upward

| Table 17-1 | **Model for Drug-Induced Parkinsonism** | | |  |
|---|---|---|---|---|

| Clinical Manifestation | Theoretical Understanding | Intervention | Possible Effect of Intervention |
|---|---|---|---|
| Positive symptoms of schizophrenia | Increased levels of dopamine given | Antipsychotic drug(s) given (dopamine antagonists) | Improvement of psychotic symptoms and possible development of EPSEs |
| EPSEs (e.g., parkinsonism, akathisia) | Drug-induced imbalance between ACh and dopamine has occurred | Anticholinergic drug added to treatment regimen | Continued improvement in psychotic symptoms and amelioration of EPSEs (restored balance between dopamine and ACh) |

*ACh,* Acetylcholine; *EPSEs,* extrapyramidal side effects.
From Keltner NL, Folks DG, Palmer CA, et al: *Psychobiological foundations of psychiatric care,* St. Louis, 1998, Mosby.

| Table 17-2 | Extrapyramidal Side Effects (EPSEs) Caused by Antipsychotic Drugs and Their Nursing Interventions |  |
|---|---|---|

| EPSE | Nursing Interventions |
|---|---|
| Akathisia | Be patient and reassure patient who is "jittery" that you understand the need to move and that appropriate drug interventions can help differentiate akathisia and agitation. Because akathisia is the chief cause of noncompliance with antipsychotic regimens, switching to a different class of antipsychotic drug might be necessary to achieve compliance. |
| Dystonias | If a severe reaction (e.g., oculogyric crisis, torticollis) occurs, give antiparkinsonian drug (e.g., benztropine [Cogentin]) or antihistamine (e.g., diphenhydramine [Benadryl]) immediately, as needed; offer reassurance. If an order for intramuscular administration has not been written, call the physician at once to obtain the order. When an order for an antiparkinsonian drug is warranted for less severe dystonias, notify the physician. |
| Drug-induced parkinsonism | Assess for the major parkinsonism symptoms: tremors, rigidity, and bradykinesia; report to physician. Antiparkinsonian drugs will probably be indicated. |
| Tardive dyskinesia | Assess for signs by using the abnormal inventory movement scale. Drug holidays might help prevent tardive dyskinesia. Anticholinergic agents will worsen tardive dyskinesia; therefore, question their indiscriminate prophylactic use. |
| Neuroleptic malignant syndrome | Be alert for this potentially fatal side effect. Routinely take temperatures, and encourage adequate water intake for all patients on a regimen of antipsychotic drugs; routinely assess for rigidity, tremor, and similar symptoms. |
| Pisa syndrome | Treat with higher doses of antiparkinsonian drugs. |
| Akinesia | May respond to anticholinergics. May want to reduce dose or change antipsychotics. |

- Writer's cramp—fatigue spasms affecting a hand
- Laryngeal-pharyngeal constriction (potentially life-threatening)
- *Drug-induced parkinsonism.* The cardinal symptoms of PD are experienced.
- *Tardive dyskinesia (TD).* Tardive means "late appearing." This EPSE tends to develop late, after about 6 months of antipsychotic therapy. It is not the dopamine-ACh imbalance per se that causes tardive dyskinesia; as a result, anticholinergics are not administered for treatment. In fact, anticholinergics generally worsen TD. Chronic use of antipsychotics is thought to cause dopamine receptors in the basal ganglia to become hypersensitive. Symptoms are bothersome and can be embarrassing. Typical symptoms include tongue writhing, tongue protrusion, teeth grinding, and lip smacking. TD stops with sleep. Although TD movements can be suppressed willfully for a short time, they soon reappear. TD is often irreversible. No satisfactory pharmacologic treatment has yet

been developed; however, the atypical antipsychotic clozapine has been used with some success (Bassitt and Louza Neto, 1998; Casey, 1998).
- *Neuroleptic malignant syndrome (NMS).* NMS is a potentially lethal side effect of antipsychotic agents. Fewer than 1% of patients taking antipsychotics will develop this problem, but 5% to 20% of those untreated will die (Pelonero et al, 1998). The incidence was much higher in the past, but careful scrutiny of patients by nurses and physicians has reduced both incidence and mortality. Cardinal symptoms include hyperthermia, rigidity, and autonomic dysfunction. NMS can be treated with muscle relaxants (e.g., dantrolene [Dantrium]) and with centrally acting dopaminergics (e.g., bromocriptine [Parlodel]).
- *Pisa syndrome.* Pisa syndrome is a condition marked by the patient leaning to one side. It can be acute or tardive, with elderly patients more vulnerable.

Some people are simply more vulnerable to developing EPSEs than others. Box 17-1 lists those at a higher risk for developing EPSEs from antipsychotics (Avron et al, 1994; Sweet and Pollock, 1998).

## ANTICHOLINERGICS TO TREAT EXTRAPYRAMIDAL SIDE EFFECTS

Anticholinergic drugs are used to treat EPSEs and work by restoring the imbalance caused by antipsychotic drugs. As noted in this chapter and in Chapter 18, antipsychotic agents block (or antagonize) dopamine receptors. This dopamine-receptor antagonism causes an artificial or iatrogenic parkinsonian-like syndrome, the aforementioned EPSEs. However, restoring the balance with a dopaminergic is inappropriate because, as the chapter on schizophrenia emphasizes (Chapter 28), the most compelling hypothesis for schizophrenia is the presence of excessive amounts of dopamine. Hence, anticholinergics (drugs that block cholinergic receptors) are used to restore the balance.

Box 17-1   **Populations at Higher Risk for EPSEs**

1. Women
2. First episode of schizophrenia
3. Older people
4. Patients with affective symptoms

From Avorn J, Monane M, Everitt DE, et al: Clinical assessment of extrapyramidal signs in nursing home patients given antipsychotic medication. *Arch Intern Med* 154:1113, 1994; Sweet R, Pollock B: New atypical antipsychotics. Experience and utility in the elderly, *Drugs Aging* 12:115, 1998.

The following outline is repetitive but might be helpful:

1. Individuals with schizophrenia have excessive amounts of dopamine.
2. Antipsychotic agents (particularly those referred to as high-potency antipsychotics) block dopamine receptors.
3. When dopamine receptors are blocked in the basal ganglia, a drug-induced parkinsonism can develop.
4. An antiparkinsonian drug is needed to fix the problem that antipsychotics create.
5. However, if dopaminergic antiparkinsonian drugs are given, schizophrenia might worsen.
6. Therefore, anticholinergic drugs are given to restore ACh-dopamine balance.

Several anticholinergic drugs are available to treat EPSEs. These drugs' site of action for relieving EPSEs is the central nervous system (CNS). They also have pronounced peripheral effects. The prototype drug for this class of drugs is atropine, but it is not used to treat EPSEs. Atropine is most commonly used to reduce aspiration during surgery. Benztropine (Cogentin) is the most commonly prescribed anticholinergic for EPSEs. The relative anticholinergic potency of selected psychotropic drugs is found in Table 17-3. (Table 17-4 lists the adult dosages of anticholinergics.)

## PHARMACOLOGIC EFFECTS

Primarily, anticholinergic drugs inhibit ACh, thus preventing its stimulation of the cholinergic

| Table 17-3 | **Anticholinergic Effect of Frequently Prescribed Psychotropic Drugs Compared With Benztropine (Cogentin)** |  |
|---|---|---|

| **Drug** | **Equivalent (in mg)** | **Typical Use** |
|---|---|---|
| Atropine | 0 | Given before surgery |
| Benztropine (Cogentin) | 1 | Antiparkinson |
| Trihexyphenidyl (Artane) | 2 | Antiparkinson |
| Biperiden (Akineton) | 1 | Antiparkinson |
| Amitriptyline (Elavil) | 10 | Antidepressant |
| Nortriptyline (Pamelor) | 60 | Antidepressant |
| Imipramine (Tofranil) | 75 | Antidepressant |
| Desipramine (Norpramin) | 150 | Antidepressant |
| Clozapine (Clozaril) | 15 | Antipsychotic |
| Chlorpromazine (Thorazine) | 370 | Antipsychotic |
| Diphenhydramine (Benadryl) | 50 | Antihistamine |

Note: According to this table, 50 mg of Benadryl has the same anticholinergic effect as 1 mg of benztropine.
Modified from de Leon J, Canuso C, White AO, Simpson GM: A pilot effort to determine benztropine equivalents of anticholinergic medications, *Hosp Community Psychiatry* 45:606, 1994.

excitatory pathways. Anticholinergics are used alone in the treatment of EPSEs.

Antipsychotic drugs block dopamine receptors, frequently causing EPSEs. Many of the symptoms associated with naturally occurring PD—tremors, rigidity, and bradykinesia—are present in drug-induced parkinsonism, along with related symptoms such as akathisia, dystonia, and dyskinesia. Blockade of dopamine receptors in the basal ganglia (i.e., nigrostriatal tract) produces EPSEs. High-potency antipsychotic agents such as haloperidol cause EPSEs more often than low-potency or atypical agents. Additionally, several nonneuroleptic drugs cause EPSEs. These symptoms contribute to the discomfort, anxiety, and frustration of this already troubled population and are major contributors to noncompliance. Patients taking antipsychotic drugs can experience a gradual or sudden onset of EPSEs.

| Table 17-4 | Anticholinergic Adult Drug Dosages for EPSEs |  |
|---|---|---|

| Anticholinergic | Dosage |
|---|---|
| Benztropine (Cogentin) | 1-4 mg, qd or bid; PO, IM, or IV *For acute dystonic reactions:* 1-2 mg IM, then 1-2 mg PO bid |
| Biperiden (Akineton) | 2 mg qd or tid |
| Trihexyphenidyl (Artane) | Start with 1 mg daily, then increase Usual dosage range: 5-15 mg/day |

**CRITICAL THINKING QUESTION**　**3**

Although you have not read the chapter on antidepressants yet (Chapter 19), it is known that selective serotonin reuptake inhibitors (SSRIs, [e.g., Prozac, Paxil]) can cause EPSEs. Can you figure out why that is so? This question will be repeated in that chapter.

## SIDE EFFECTS

Anticholinergic drugs produce both CNS and peripheral nervous system (PNS) side effects, listed in Table 17-5. CNS effects include confusion, cognitive impoverishment, agitation, dizziness, drowsiness, and disturbances in behavior. Because the cholinergic system contributes to memory and learning, anticholinergic drugs affect these cognitive functions as well (Keltner et al, 2001). Ingesting drugs with anticholinergic properties can often explain recent changes in cognition in older adults.

PNS anticholinergic effects such as dry mouth, blurred vision, nausea, and nervousness occur in 30% to 50% of these patients. Basically, peripheral anticholinergic side effects result from blocking the parasympathetic system (a cholinergic [ACh] system) (Table 17-6). For example, blurred vision results from pupils that dilate because of the blocking of ACh receptors of the third cranial nerve (oculomotor nerve). The third cranial nerve constricts the pupil; when it is blocked, the pupil dilates. Dry mouth results when cranial nerves VII and IX (facial and glossopharyngeal nerves) are

| Table 17-5 | Side Effects and Nursing Interventions for Anticholinergics |  |
|---|---|---|

| Side Effects | Nursing Interventions |
|---|---|
| Dry mouth | Offer sugarless hard candy and chewing gum; encourage frequent rinses; take medication before meals. |
| Nasal congestion | Recommend over-the-counter nasal decongestant, if approved by physician. |
| Urinary hesitation | Introduce running water, privacy, warm water over perineum. |
| Urinary retention | Catheterize for residual fluids; encourage frequent voiding. |
| Blurred vision, photophobia | Provide reassurance (normal vision typically returns in a few weeks); encourage sunglasses; advise caution when driving (tolerance develops). |
| Constipation | Give laxatives, as ordered; encourage diet with roughage; recommend 2500 to 3000 mL of water daily. |
| Mydriasis | If eye pain develops, undiagnosed narrow-angle glaucoma might be the cause; immediate attention is warranted. |
| Decreased sweating | Decreased sweating can lead to fever; take temperature; if fever occurs, reduce body temperature (e.g., sponge baths). |
| Fever | Advise limited strenuous activity; encourage patient to wear appropriate clothing. |

| Table 17-6 | Anticholinergic Effects on Cranial Nerves With Parasympathetic Functions | |  |
|---|---|---|---|

| Cranial Nerve | Parasympathetic Function | Anticholinergic Effect |
|---|---|---|
| III | Constricts pupils | Mydriasis (dilates pupils), blurred vision |
| | Alters shape of lens | Impairs accommodation |
| VII | Salivation | Dry mouth |
| | Lacrimation | Decreased tearing |
| | Nasal mucous secretion | Dry nasal passage |
| IX | Salivation | Dry mouth |
| | Nasal mucous secretion | Dry nasal passage |
| X | Slows heart rate | Tachycardia |
| | Promotes peristalsis | Slows peristalsis; constipation |
| | Constricts bronchi | Dilates bronchi |

### Norm's Notes

*The sinoatrial (SA) node has a rhythm of 100 to 120 impulses per minute. Hearts do not beat this fast, because the parasympathetic system provides a braking action. When anticholinergic drugs are given, part of the brake is removed, which can result in major problems, particularly for older individuals.*

| Box 17-2 | Risks Associated With Anticholinergic Use |  |
|---|---|---|

1. Might be lethal in overdose
2. Might induce dependence
3. Might exacerbate tardive dyskinesia
4. Might induce psychosis

From Houltram B, Scalan M: Extrapyramidal side effects, *Nurs Standard* 18:39, 2004.

blocked from causing salivation. Decreased tearing is related to blockage of cranial nerve VII. Although these problems are annoying, they are not usually major health hazards. On the other hand, when cranial nerve X (vagus nerve) is blocked, tachycardia can occur and cause serious problems. Why?

Constipation, a problem with parkinsonism patients because of rigidity, can be worsened by anticholinergics as well. Urinary hesitance and retention and decreased sweating are other PNS effects. Interestingly, patients who drool or perspire excessively might welcome dry mouth and decreased sweating.

Box 17-2 lists the more serious risks associated with anticholinergic use.

## NURSING IMPLICATIONS FOR ANTICHOLINERGIC DRUGS

### Therapeutic Versus Toxic Dose Levels

Therapeutic dose ranges are found in Table 17-4. Doses above this range can cause toxic effects.

Overdose might result in CNS hyperstimulation (confusion, excitement, hyperpyrexia, agitation, disorientation, delirium, or hallucinations) or CNS depression (drowsiness, sedation, or coma). The cardiovascular, urinary, and gastrointestinal systems are particularly involved. The eyes are also affected. High fevers are the result of the CNS effects of anticholinergics and their ability to decrease sweating.

### Use During Pregnancy

Anticholinergics should be used cautiously during pregnancy. Theoretically, these drugs will decrease milk flow during lactation.

### Use in Older Adults

As this chapter and other chapters in this text have emphasized, older individuals are particularly sensitive to anticholinergic agents. Cognitive, cardiovascular, and gastrointestinal side effects are more pronounced in this age group compared with the younger population. Older men with prostatic enlargement can have these difficulties exacerbated with the use of these agents.

### Side Effect Interventions

Numerous annoying side effects are associated with anticholinergic drugs (see Table 17-5). Several nondrug alternatives to help the patient are listed in this table.

### Interactions With Anticholinergic Drugs

The nurse should alert the patient to the dangers of over-the-counter drugs and other prescription drugs that intensify the atropine-like effects of centrally acting anticholinergics. Other interactions include an intensification of sedative effects when combined with CNS depressants and a decrease in absorption when combined with antacids and antidiarrheal drugs.

### Teaching Patients

In addition to teaching appropriate information about side effects, the nurse should also emphasize certain points. The patient and family should be advised of the following:

- Avoid discontinuing these drugs abruptly. Tapering off over a 1-week period is advised.
- Avoid driving or other hazardous activities until tolerance develops and drowsiness and blurred vision diminish.
- Avoid over-the-counter medications (e.g., cough and cold preparations) that have anticholinergic or antihistamine properties; alcohol, which will exacerbate CNS depression; and antacids, which will interfere with the absorption of anticholinergics.

## SELECTED ANTICHOLINERGIC DRUGS

### Benztropine (Cogentin)

Benztropine is used to treat all parkinsonian-like disorders, including drug-induced EPSEs. Benztropine, which is the most frequently prescribed anticholinergic antiparkinsonian drug, is usually given orally but can be given intramuscularly for noncompliant psychotic patients and intramuscularly or intravenously for acute dystonic reactions.

### Biperiden (Akineton)

Biperiden is used adjunctively in all parkinsonian-like disorders, including drug-induced EPSEs.

### Diphenhydramine (Benadryl)

Diphenhydramine, the prototype antihistamine, is effective for most parkinsonian-like disorders. Diphenhydramine can cause considerable sedation in some individuals and little in others; it is considerably less potent than benztropine (see Table 17-3).

### Trihexyphenidyl (Artane)

Trihexyphenidyl was the first anticholinergic used extensively for EPSEs. Trihexyphenidyl is not available in a parenteral form; thus, its use for acute dystonias is limited.

## OTHER TREATMENT OPTIONS FOR EXTRAPYRAMIDAL SIDE EFFECTS

### DRUGS

Although anticholinergic agents are the mainstay of treatment and prophylaxis of EPSEs, several other agents are available as well. Included among those drugs are the following:

- Dopamine agonist: Amantadine (Symmetrel)
- Antihistamine: Diphenhydramine (Benadryl)
- Beta blocker: Propranolol (Inderal)
- Benzodiazepine: Diazepam (Valium), lorazepam (Ativan), clonazepam (Klonopin)

### VITAMINS

Both vitamins E and $B_6$ have some empirical support for their abilities to diminish symptoms associated with TD (Barak et al, 1998). Anecdotal evidence also suggests that a substantial minority of patients benefit from vitamin E. Whether this vitamin actually reduces TD symptoms or prevents further deterioration has been debated (Houltram and Scalan, 2004).

## PREVENTION

The best approach to treating EPSEs is prevention. By following a few simple guidelines, both the prescriber and nurse can reduce EPSE incidence (Houltram and Scalan, 2004). Enhanced patient care requires the following (in about this order):

1. Establish whether patient is from a high-risk group (review Box 17-1).
2. Obtain baseline information about EPSEs using a validated tool.
3. Choose an antipsychotic with a lower probability of causing EPSEs:
   a. High-risk agents: Haldol, Prolixin, other traditional antipsychotics
   b. Lower-risk agents: Zyprexa, Risperdal (at lower doses), Seroquel, and other atypical antipsychotics.
4. Monitor the patient on a regular basis.
5. If EPSEs develop, consider switching to an atypical drug or, if on an atypical drug, lower the dose or change to another atypical with a better side effect profile. Add an antiparkinsonian agent.

## CASE STUDY

A 25-year-old woman who is taking an antipsychotic drug (haloperidol) starts to experience psychomotor slowing as she walks down the hallway of the hospital. Before she reaches the end of the hall, she requires assistance. Within 2 minutes of sitting down, her neck becomes rigidly hyperextended, and her eyes roll upward in a fixed stare. Her breathing becomes labored because of the position of her neck, and she is frightened. Because she is also delusional, what this frightening side effect of her medication represents to her is difficult to imagine. Benztropine (Cogentin), 2 mg, is given intramuscularly and then repeated in 15 minutes, because she did not respond as quickly as was hoped. Within another 5 minutes, she was back to her "normal" self.

## Study Notes

1. PD is related to degeneration of the substantia nigra, the dopamine-generating portion of the brain; however, the cause is unknown.
2. EPSEs, a type of parkinsonism (cause known), develop when dopamine receptors in the basal ganglia are blocked by antipsychotic or other drugs.
3. Normal muscle activity requires a balance between dopamine and ACh; consequently, a dopamine deficiency is responsible for symptoms of PD.
4. The four primary symptoms associated with PD include tremors, bradykinesia, rigidity, and postural instability.

5. Drug treatment of PD is based on reestablishing a balance between dopamine and ACh.
6. Drug treatment for EPSEs is based on blocking ACh receptors. Administering a dopaminergic drug could exacerbate psychotic symptoms.
7. The two major anticholinergic antiparkinsonian drugs are benztropine (Cogentin) and trihexyphenidyl (Artane).
8. Anticholinergic drugs have many side effects. Older individuals are particularly sensitive to these side effects.

## References

Avorn J, Monane M, Everitt DE, et al: Clinical assessment of extrapyramidal signs in nursing home patients given antipsychotic medication, *Arch Intern Med* 154:1113, 1994.

Barak Y, Swartz M, Shamir E, et al: Vitamin E (alpha-tocopherol) in the treatment of tardive dyskinesia: a statistical meta analysis, *Ann Clin Psychiatry* 10:101, 1998.

Bassitt DP, Louza Neto MR: Clozapine efficacy in tardive dyskinesia in schizophrenic patients, *Eur Arch Psychiatry Clin Neurosci* 248:209, 1998.

Casey DE: Effects of clozapine therapy in schizophrenic individuals at risk for tardive dyskinesia, *J Clin Psychiatry* 59(Suppl 3):31, 1998.

de Leon J, Canuso C, White AO, Simpson GM: A pilot effort to determine benztropine equivalents of anticholinergic medications, *Hosp Community Psychiatry* 45:606, 1994.

Houltram B, Scalan M: Extrapyramidal side effects, *Nurs Standard* 18:39, 2004.

Keltner NL, Folks DG, Palmer CA, et al: *Psychobiological foundations of psychiatric care*, St. Louis, 1998, Mosby.

Keltner NL, Folks DG: *Psychotropic drugs*, ed 3, Philadelphia, 2005, Mosby.

Keltner NL, Zielinski AL, Hardin MS: Drugs used for cognitive symptoms of Alzheimer's disease, *Perspect Psychiatr Care* 37:31, 2001.

Pelonero AL, Levenson JL, Pandurangi AK: Neuroleptic malignant syndrome: a review, *Psychiatr Serv* 49:1163, 1998.

Pennachio DL: Parkinson's disease: progress along the continuum of care, *Patient Care Nurs Pract* 3:26, 2000.

Sweet R, Pollock B: New atypical antipsychotics. Experience and utility in the elderly, *Drugs Aging* 12:115, 1998.

## Bibliography

Agid Y: Parkinson's disease: pathophysiology, *Lancet* 337:1321, 1991.

Bezchlibnyk KZ, Jeffries JJ: *Clinical handbook of psychotropic drugs*, ed 14, Seattle, 2004, Hogrefe & Huber.

Keltner NL: Neuroreceptor function and psychopharmacological response, *Issues Ment Health Nurs* 21:31, 2000.

Keltner NL, Folks DG: *Psychotropic drugs*, ed 3, Philadelphia, 2005, Mosby.

Lehne RA: *Pharmacology for nursing care*, ed 4, Philadelphia, 2004, WB Saunders.

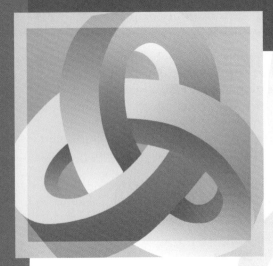

# Chapter 18

# Antipsychotic Drugs

*Norman L. Keltner*

## Learning Objectives

*After reading this chapter, you should be able to:*
- Explain the concept of neurotransmitters, specifically dopamine, in relation to psychosis.
- Identify the clinical uses of first-, second-, and third-generation antipsychotic drugs.
- Recognize differences between high-potency and low-potency traditional antipsychotic drugs.
- Identify a representative high-potency, low-potency, and atypical antipsychotic drug, including the specific side effects and interactions of each drug.
- Describe signs and symptoms associated with extrapyramidal side effects.
- Describe potential interactions of antipsychotic drugs.
- Discuss implications for teaching patients about antipsychotic drugs.

Antipsychotic drugs are used to treat schizophrenia, bipolar disorder, and other psychoses. Additionally, various other manifestations of mental illness are amenable to treatment with these agents.

Antipsychotics were discovered accidentally around 1950. A French scientist was hoping to develop a new antihistamine and, in the process, formulated chlorpromazine, which was initially used to calm presurgery jitters but was soon found to possess antipsychotic properties. Chlorpromazine is considered the first antipsychotic drug.

Before the introduction and acceptance of chlorpromazine and of many related drugs, hundreds of thousands of patients with severe psychiatric disturbances were hospitalized, many never to be released. These patients were isolated, physically restrained, and occasionally subjected to psychosurgery (lobotomy). These treatments rarely restored patients to a state that enabled them to function productively or to interact in a reasonably normal way with others.

Although all the hopes for antipsychotic drugs have not been realized, these drugs have had a dramatic impact on psychiatric care. The use of antipsychotic drugs resulted in the abandonment of most of the ineffective treatments while dramatically reducing long-term hospitalizations.

The drugs discussed in this chapter are generally called antipsychotic agents, but historically they have also been referred to as major tranquilizers, ataractics (drugs that produce calmness or serenity), and neuroleptics (because they can produce neurologic symptoms).

### Norm's Notes

*There are two categories of drugs that dominate psychiatric care, antipsychotics and antidepressants. I think that the antipsychotics are the more important. Many years ago, when I worked in a large state hospital, the antipsychotics had only recently been discovered. Some of the staff had worked there since the 1930s, and I was fascinated with their stories of the pre-Thorazine days, when the hospital could only be described as a madhouse—so much pain, so much agony. Although not without some problems, what a difference antipsychotics have made in some people's lives.*

## CLASSIFICATION SYSTEMS

Antipsychotic drugs are generally conceptualized in three ways: (1) traditional antipsychotics, or first-generation drugs, (2) atypical antipsychotics, or second-generation drugs, and (3) novel antipsychotics, or third-generation drugs. Antipsychotic drugs are listed under these headings in Table 18-1. Antipsychotics have diverse chemical properties but all effectively reduce various psychiatric symptoms. The type, intensity, and frequency of side effects vary among these drugs because of intrinsic differences.

Traditional antipsychotic drugs, developed from 1950 to 1990, are further divided based on potency (Box 18-1). Subclassification based on potency has

**Table 18-1    Major Traditional and Atypical Antipsychotic Drugs**

| Drug | Usual Adult Maintenance Range (mg/day) | Rate of EPSEs | Rate of Anticholinergic Effects | Rate of Orthostasis | Rate of Sedation | Rate of Weight Gain |
|---|---|---|---|---|---|---|
| **Traditional (First Generation)** | | | | | | |
| ***High-Potency Drug*** | | | | | | |
| Fluphenazine (Prolixin) | 0.5-40 | High | Low | Low | Low | Low |
| Haloperidol (Haldol) | 1-15 | High | Low | Low | Low | Low |
| ***Moderate-Potency Drug*** | | | | | | |
| Pherphenazine (Trilafon) | 12-64 | High | Low | Low | Moderate | Low |
| ***Low-Potency Drug*** | | | | | | |
| Chlorpromazine (Thorazine) | 200-1000 | Moderate | Moderate | High | Moderate | High |
| Thioridazine (Mellaril) | 200-800 | Low | High | High | High | High |
| **Atypical (Second Generation)** | | | | | | |
| Clozapine (Clozaril) | 75-900 | Low | High | High | High | High |
| Risperidone (Risperdal) | 0.5-6 | Low* | Low | Moderate | Moderate | Moderate |
| Olanzapine (Zyprexa) | 5-20 | Low | Moderate | Low | High | High |
| Quetiapine (Seroquel) | 200-800 | Low | Low | Moderate | Moderate | Moderate |
| Ziprasidone (Geodon) | 40-160 | Low | Low | Low | Low | Low |
| **Novel (Third Generation)** | | | | | | |
| Aripiprazole (Abilify) | 10-30 | Low | Low | Low | Low | Low |

*However, EPSEs develop at high doses.
*EPSEs,* Extrapyramidal side effects.

support because of its clinical utility. Essentially, the effects of traditional antipsychotics are related to the blockade of a specific type of dopamine receptor ($D_2$) (Box 18-2). Clinical effectiveness occurs when 60% to 70% of these receptors are blocked in a certain area of the brain (to be discussed later). For example, approximately 100 mg of chlorpromazine (a low-potency drug) is required to achieve the same clinical effect as 2 mg of haloperidol (a high-potency drug). This classification system is not perfect. A few traditional drugs do not fall comfortably into either high- or low-potency groups (i.e., moderate potency). Nonetheless, this dichotomy is clinically significant because low-potency drugs tend to cause more intense anticholinergic effects (e.g., dry mouth, blurred vision) and antiadrenergic effects (e.g., orthostatic hypotension), whereas high-potency drugs cause more extrapyramidal side effects (EPSEs). Knowing this difference prepares the nurse for the most likely set of side effects. For example, as a general rule, drugs with increased anticholinergic effects produce fewer EPSEs (see Table 18-1). Table 18-2 outlines the theoretical effects of specific receptor blockade (Jibson and Tandon, 1998).

A second category is based on typicality. That is, drugs developed between 1950 and 1990 are considered as traditional or typical antipsychotics. The newer agents (from 1990 on) are referred to as atypical because of the following characteristics:

1. Reduced or no risk for EPSEs
2. Increased effectiveness in treating negative (Box 18-3) and cognitive symptoms
3. Minimal risk of tardive dyskinesia (TD)
4. Absence of prolactin level elevation and associated side effects

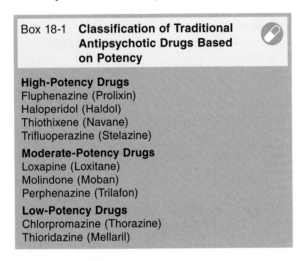

**Box 18-1  Classification of Traditional Antipsychotic Drugs Based on Potency**

**High-Potency Drugs**
Fluphenazine (Prolixin)
Haloperidol (Haldol)
Thiothixene (Navane)
Trifluoperazine (Stelazine)

**Moderate-Potency Drugs**
Loxapine (Loxitane)
Molindone (Moban)
Perphenazine (Trilafon)

**Low-Potency Drugs**
Chlorpromazine (Thorazine)
Thioridazine (Mellaril)

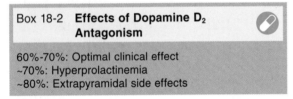

**Box 18-2  Effects of Dopamine $D_2$ Antagonism**

60%-70%: Optimal clinical effect
~70%: Hyperprolactinemia
~80%: Extrapyramidal side effects

| Table 18-2 | Theoretical Effects of Receptor Blockade |
| --- | --- |

| Receptor | Effects |
| --- | --- |
| $D_2$ | Mesolimbic tract: antipsychotic effect (all antipsychotic drugs antagonize $D_2$)<br>Nigrostriatal tract: EPSEs<br>Tuberoinfundibular tract: Prolactin level elevation<br>Mesocortical tract: Might cause secondary negative symptoms (symptoms caused by antipsychotic drugs themselves) |
| $5\text{-HT}_{2a}$* | Antipsychotic effect on negative and cognitive symptoms; decreased EPSEs |
| $5\text{-HT}_3$ | Nausea |
| $M_1$ | Can restore acetylcholine (Ach)-dopamine balance for EPSEs (i.e., anticholinergics)<br>Anticholinergic side effects |
| $H_1$ | Sedation, orthostasis, weight gain |
| Alpha-1 | Orthostasis, dizziness, sedation |
| Alpha-2 | Sexual dysfunction |
| GABA | Lowers seizure threshold; produces anxiety |

*$5\text{-HT}_2$ receptors are subdivided (e.g., $5\text{-HT}_{2A}$, $5\text{HT}_{2c}$). Here, $5\text{-HT}_{2a}$ would be most specific.
*EPSEs,* Extrapyramidal side effects; $M_1$, cholinergic muscarinic receptors.
From Bezchlibnyk-Butler KZ, Jeffries JJ: *Clinical handbook of psychotropic drugs,* ed 14, Seattle, 2004, Hogrefe & Huber; Jibson MD, Tandon R: New atypical antipsychotic medications, *J Psychiatr Res* 32:215, 1998; and Keltner NL: Neuroreceptor function and psychopharmacologic response, *Issues Ment Health Nurs* 21:31, 2000.

The third category is currently composed of just one drug, aripiprazole, which has a novel pharmacologic approach.

## NEUROCHEMICAL THEORY OF SCHIZOPHRENIA

The neurochemical theory affords the best explanation for the effectiveness of antipsychotic agents. This theory states that increased levels of dopamine in the limbic area of the brain cause schizophrenia and its psychotic symptoms (e.g., hallucinations, delusions). Because antipsychotic drugs are dopamine blockers, it follows that their effectiveness can be attributed to this dopamine-blocking activity. Furthermore, this theory of schizophrenia is supported by clinical observations and clinical research, both of which demonstrate that high doses of the dopaminergic drugs levodopa and amphetamine can produce schizophrenic symptoms.

This explanation, however, does not answer all the questions surrounding the issue, most specifically those regarding negative symptoms. Figure 18-1 provides additional useful information. As shown in this figure, the brain has four major dopaminergic tracts. Dopamine is synthesized primarily in the substantia nigra and ventral tegmental area and is delivered to distant sites via dopaminergic tracts. To appreciate the complexity of psychopharmacologic treatment of schizophrenia fully, the student must recognize the existence of dopamine-dependent areas of the brain that communicate with dopamine-synthesizing areas (substantia nigra and ventral tegmental areas in the midbrain) via different neuronal tracts.

Tract 1: The nigrostriatal tract is involved in movement. Traditional antipsychotic blockade can cause EPSEs.

Tract 2: The tuberoinfundibular tract modulates pituitary function. Traditional antipsychotic blockade can lead to elevation in prolactin levels.

Tract 3: The mesolimbic tract is involved in emotional and sensory processes. Traditional antipsychotic blockade normalizes these processes in individuals with schizophrenia, relieving or eliminating hallucinations and delusions.

Tract 4: The mesocortical tract is involved in cognitive processes. Traditional antipsychotic blockade can intensify negative and cognitive problems.

Traditional antipsychotics can do all of the above, but this is a high price to pay to be free of hallucinations and delusions.

The ultimate antipsychotic agent might be one that blocks dopamine receptors in the mesolimbic area (decreasing hallucinations and delusions) and liberates dopamine in the mesocortical area (treating negative and cognitive symptoms), while not obstructing the function of the nigrostriatal tract (hence, not causing EPSEs) nor blocking receptors in the tuberoinfundibular tract (i.e., not elevating prolactin levels). Atypical antipsychotics *can* do this.

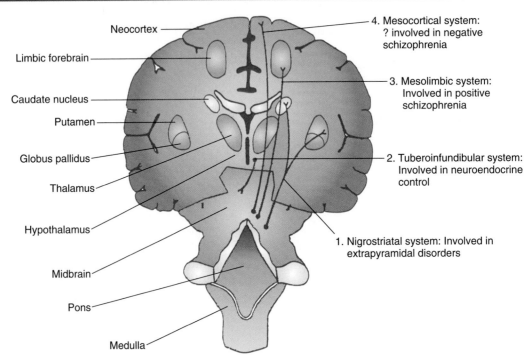

Neocortex

Limbic forebrain

Caudate nucleus

Putamen

Globus pallidus

Thalamus

Hypothalamus

Midbrain

Pons

Medulla

4. Mesocortical system:
? involved in negative
schizophrenia

3. Mesolimbic system:
Involved in positive
schizophrenia

2. Tuberoinfundibular system:
Involved in neuroendocrine
control

1. Nigrostriatal system: Involved in
extrapyramidal disorders

**FIGURE 18-1** Four dopaminergic tracts are important for understanding the actions of antipsychotic drugs. *1,* Nigrostriatal system. When antipsychotic drugs antagonize this system, a pseudoparkinsonism or extrapyramidal effect occurs. *2,* Tuberoinfundibular system. When antipsychotic drugs antagonize this system, the dopamine inhibition of the pituitary hormone prolactin is lifted and can lead to gynecomastia and galactorrhea. *3,* Mesolimbic system. When antipsychotic drugs antagonize this system, a decrease in the symptoms of schizophrenia occurs (primarily positive symptoms). This particular effect makes these drugs antipsychotic. *4,* Mesocortical system. When antipsychotic drugs antagonize this system, the disorder can worsen in some patients. Atypical antipsychotics are thought to antagonize serotonin receptors in the cortex that, in turn, liberate dopamine there; that is, theories suggest that a mesocortical hypodopaminergic state might contribute to negative symptoms. Much remains to be understood about the role, if any, of the mesocortical dopaminergic tract in schizophrenia. (From Roberts GW, Leigh PN, Weinberger DR: *Neuropsychiatric disorders,* London, 1993, Wolfe.)

## OVERVIEW

### PHARMACOLOGIC EFFECTS

Antipsychotic drugs are used primarily to treat psychotic disorders—specifically, schizophrenia, bipolar disorder, and other chronic mental illness. Tolerance to their antipsychotic effect is uncommon.

Central nervous system (CNS) effects include emotional quieting and sedation, which explains why these drugs were once generally referred to as *major tranquilizers.* Emotional quieting enables the patient to take advantage of other forms of therapeutic intervention—for example, the therapeutic nurse-patient relationship and the well-managed milieu.

Sedation decreases insomnia, a frequent complaint of psychotic patients. Whether this is a result of the sedating effect itself or of being freed from disturbing thoughts (or a combination of the two) is not fully understood. Not all antipsychotic drugs are significantly sedating but are still therapeutic. The conclusion that the effectiveness of antipsychotic agents results from more than their tranquilizing qualities alone is reasonable.

### PSYCHIATRIC SYMPTOMS MODIFIED BY ANTIPSYCHOTIC DRUGS

A tranquilizing effect occurs within an hour or so after ingestion. Antipsychotic effects are often observed within a few weeks, with improvement continuing for up to 6 to 8 weeks or longer. Antipsychotic drugs are most effective in treating what have been called the positive symptoms of schizophrenia (see Box 18-3). Positive symptoms include hallucinations and delusions. Negative symptoms are less responsive to antipsychotic drugs and include those developed over an extended period, such as a flattened affect, verbal paucity, and a lack of drive or goal-directed activity. Referring once again to Figure 18-1, the student can infer that positive symptoms arise from too much dopamine in the limbic area (hyperactive mesolimbic tract), and that negative symptoms arise from too little dopamine in the cortex (hypoactive mesocortical tract). It stands to reason, then, that antipsychotic drugs that are strictly dopamine antagonists are better at decreasing the effect of dopamine in the limbic area than they are at increasing the effect of dopamine in the cerebral cortex. As discussed later, atypical agents can increase the dopamine level in one area of the brain while decreasing it in another.

Ultimately, improvement in objective and subjective or positive and negative symptoms is the measurement of progress. Psychotic symptoms associated with other mental disorders, such as bipolar disorder and cognitive disorders, also improve with these drugs.

## Alterations of Perception

As a rule, the more bizarre the behavior of a person experiencing psychotic symptoms (the more positive symptoms), the more likely that an antipsychotic drug will be beneficial. Hallucinations and illusions are reduced with these drugs. Even when the symptoms are not fully eradicated, antipsychotic drugs might enable the person to understand that hallucinations and illusions are not real, which is an improvement.

## Alterations of Thought

Antipsychotic drugs improve reasoning, decrease ambivalence, and decrease delusions. Because clouded reasoning, ambivalence, and delusional thoughts are frustrating and, at times, frightening, antipsychotic agents can free the patient to think more clearly and communicate better with others.

## Alterations of Activity

Individuals with schizophrenia are often hyperactive because of their internal turmoil and, perhaps, their neurochemical state. Antipsychotic drugs slow psychomotor activity.

## Alterations in Consciousness

Mental clouding and confusion are anxiety-producing symptoms associated with **psychosis.** Some mental health professionals believe that these disorders are the most disabling. Antipsychotic drugs are effective in decreasing confusion and clouding.

## Alterations in Personal Relationships

Patients with schizophrenia often have histories of social withdrawal and might have few, if any, close personal relationships. If relationships with family members exist, they are often strained. Individuals with schizophrenia might invest little effort in their appearance and might not be particularly careful about their behaviors. The combination of introspection, rumination, and self-focused speech produces ineffective communication patterns that reinforce isolation and alienation. In the give-and-take atmosphere of society, individuals with schizophrenia often have little to give and, as a result, are basically socially unattractive to most people. Antipsychotic drugs potentially can enable patients to become less focused on themselves and more focused on others. The socially damaging, self-absorptive thinking experienced by patients with schizophrenia might be a result of the considerable energy they must expend to maintain some degree of equilibrium in the face of psychological turmoil. This is similar to the way many people give less attention to their appearance or behavior during an acute illness. Antipsychotic drugs reduce the inner turmoil, freeing psychic energy for normal interpersonal relationships and for the therapeutic nurse-patient relationship.

---

### CRITICAL THINKING QUESTION    1

If the following are true:

1. Excessive bioavailability of dopamine causes the positive symptoms of schizophrenia.
2. Antipsychotic drugs are effective because they block dopamine receptors.
3. Decreased dopamine levels contribute to EPSEs.

then why is it that not all patients who receive antipsychotic drugs develop EPSEs? (Hint: review the four major dopaminergic tracts in the brain.)

## Alterations of Affect

Affective flattening, blunting, inappropriateness, and lability are affective symptoms sometimes associated with schizophrenia and often respond to antipsychotic drugs. However, a flat affect is a cardinal symptom of negative schizophrenia and might respond only to an atypical antipsychotic drug.

## PHARMACOKINETICS

A detailed pharmacokinetic discussion of each antipsychotic agent is beyond the scope of this text. Rather, an overview of significant pharmacokinetic mechanisms is presented.

Absorption for these drugs is variable. Oral drugs are absorbed in 1 to 6 hours, whereas the newer disintegrating tablets are absorbed within 2 minutes. These highly lipid-soluble drugs accumulate in fatty tissue and are released slowly, which might explain why patients who abruptly stop taking their medications continue to experience an antipsychotic effect for some time. This slow release from fatty stores might also account for nonadherence, because the patient who stops taking this medication does not experience an immediate return of symptoms. The following clinical example probably represents this phenomenon.

### CLINICAL EXAMPLE

Bob, a 58-year-old military veteran with a long history of mental illness, has been taking chlorpromazine for 30 years. Over that time, the nursing staff at the Veterans' Administration hospital has gotten to know Bob well because he periodically requires hospital-based intervention. One day, Bob calls the nursing office on the psychiatric floor and tells the nurse that he believes that he can conquer his problems by using "mind over matter." He is going to stop all psychotropic medications. Bob appears to do quite well for a couple of weeks, causing some of the nursing staff to wonder about the new approach. At the end of 3 weeks, Bob is brought to the hospital in a highly disturbed psychotic state. His medication is reinstituted, and Bob's delusional thoughts subside.

Antipsychotics are highly bound (most between 90% and 99%) to plasma proteins. Physiologic changes that even slightly disrupt this level of protein-binding action might increase the percentage of free drug and potentially have a greater effect. As with most highly protein-bound drugs, a greater effect might occur in older adults (who more often experience a decline in serum protein levels).

Antipsychotics are metabolized in the liver by the cytochrome P-450 system. Their average half-life ranges from 10 to 30 hours. Impaired hepatic function extends the half-life and effect of these drugs.

Many antipsychotic drugs are available in both oral and parenteral forms. Oral administration is the preferred route for a variety of reasons, including the fact that patients generally prefer this route. Tablets, however, have consistently created a problem because they are so easy to "cheek." Cheeking occurs when patients place the tablet to one side of the mouth and pretend to swallow it. Nonadherence is thought to be the single most important cause of symptom exacerbation and rehospitalization. Psychiatric patients might not want to take their medication for several reasons, including the admission of illness that taking oral medication might imply, paranoid fears of poisoning, or unpleasant reactions or side effects. A few oral versions of these agents dissolve instantly when placed in the mouth.

Parenteral drugs are usually used to treat acutely disturbed individuals or patients who represent significant compliance risks. Long-acting injectable forms are also available and require injection only once every 2 to 4 weeks or less frequently. These long-acting injections prove beneficial for outpatients or for patients who are nonadherent. Some long-acting agents are:

1. Fluphenazine decanoate (Prolixin Decanoate)
2. Haloperidol decanoate (Haldol Decanoate)
3. Risperidone (Risperdal Consta)

When a patient does not respond to antipsychotic drug therapy, the nurse's assessment of the patient might be quite helpful to the prescriber. Two considerations should be kept in mind when assessing a patient's response:

1. Is the patient actually taking the drug?
2. Has the drug been given a fair trial (usually 3 to 6 weeks)?

## SIDE EFFECTS

Antipsychotic drugs produce numerous side effects because of peripheral nervous system (PNS) and CNS actions (Box 18-4; also see Table 18-1).

---

| Box 18-4 | Major Adverse Responses to Antipsychotic Drugs in Summary |

**Neuroleptic Malignant Syndrome (NMS)**
Cause: Blockade of $D_2$ receptors
Offending agents: Typically, high-potency antipsychotics

*Signs and symptoms*
Altered levels of consciousness
Autonomic hyperactivity
Elevated enzyme levels (CPK)
Hyperreflexia
Hyperthermia
Intense sweating
Rigidity
Rhabdomyolysis, leading to acute myoglobinuric renal failure

**Anticholinergic Side Effects**
Cause: Blockade of cholinergic receptors (muscarinic receptors)
Offending agents: Anticholinergic drugs such as the low-potency antipsychotics and anticholinergic-antiparkinson drugs

*Signs and symptoms*
Blurred vision
Constipation
Decreased sweating
Diminished lacrimation
Dry mouth
Mydriasis
Tachycardia
Urinary hesitancy

**Extrapyramidal Side Effects (EPSEs)**
Cause: Blockade of $D_2$ receptors
Offending agents: Typically, high-potency antipsychotics

*Signs and symptoms*
Akathisia
Akinesia
Dystonia
Drug-induced parkinsonism
Pisa syndrome
Tardive dyskinesia*

*Tardive dyskinesia is thought to be caused by dopamine hypersensitivity rather than by a hypodopaminergic state.

## Anticholinergic Effects

PNS anticholinergic effects are a result of the blocking of cranial nerves (CNs) with parasympathetic components. For example:

- CN III: Oculomotor nerve blockade results in mydriasis and impaired accommodation. Blurred vision might result.
- CN VII: Facial nerve blockade results in dry mouth, decreased tearing, and dry nasal passage.

- CN IX: Glossopharyngeal nerve blockade results in dry mouth and dry nasal passage.
- CN X: Vagus nerve blockade results in tachycardia, constipation, and urinary hesitation.

*Nursing Alert: Anticholinergic Effects*
1. Can increase intraocular pressure, aggravating narrow-angle glaucoma
2. Can intensify prostatic hypertrophy, making urination more difficult
3. Can trigger arrhythmias and cause death

## Antiadrenergic Effects

Hypotension is the major antiadrenergic effect of antipsychotic drugs. The blocking of alpha-1 receptors is the primary cause of hypotension. Blocking these sympathetic receptors on peripheral blood vessels prevents these vessels from responding (constricting) automatically to changes in position. Hypotension occurs most often in older adults. Hypotension often occurs when the individual stands or changes positions suddenly (orthostatic hypotension); thus, precautions against falls must be instituted. In a healthy, younger person, accommodation usually occurs within a few weeks; however, many patients cannot tolerate orthostatic hypotension for that long. Hypotension also causes a reflex tachycardia that can, in turn, cause general cardiovascular inefficiency. A reflex tachycardia is, by definition, tachycardia that automatically occurs as an adaptive function to compensate for lower extremity vasodilation. Antipsychotic drugs are prescribed cautiously for individuals with severe hypotension, heart failure, or a history of arrhythmias.

## Cardiac Effects

A growing concern among clinicians prescribing antipsychotics is that these drugs have a potential for lengthening the QTc interval. Lengthening the QTc interval can be associated with a fatal arrhythmia known as torsades de pointes (Welch and Chue, 2000). Because of this concern, electrocardiographic monitoring is becoming increasingly important.

## Extrapyramidal Side Effects

The following formula traces the most familiar path leading to rehospitalization:

EPSEs → nonadherence → relapse →
rehospitalization

Hence, preventing or minimizing EPSEs whenever possible is important. It has been estimated that most patients receiving antipsychotic medications have EPSEs and, in turn, EPSEs account for many readmissions. High-potency traditional antipsychotics are most likely and atypical antipsychotics are least likely to cause EPSEs. Abnormal involuntary movement disorders develop because of drug-induced imbalances between dopamine and acetylcholine (ACh) in a specific part of the brain. EPSEs can be grouped as follows: akathisia, akinesia, dystonia, TD, drug-induced parkinsonism, Pisa syndrome, and neuroleptic malignant syndrome. TD, a late-appearing dyskinesia, can be irreversible. Guidelines for minimizing EPSEs are found in Box 18-5.

### Akathisia

**Akathisia** is a subjective feeling of restlessness demonstrated by restless legs, jittery feelings, and nervous energy. Akathisia is the most common EPSE and responds poorly to treatment. It is a major reason why patients stop taking medications.

### Akinesia and Bradykinesia

Akinesia refers to an absence of movement; however, slowed movement, or bradykinesia, is more likely. Symptoms include weakness, fatigue, painful muscles, and anergia. Akinesia responds to anticholinergics.

### Dystonia

Dystonias are abnormal postures caused by involuntary muscle spasms. They elicit a sustained, twisted, and contracted positioning of the limbs, trunk, neck, or mouth. Dystonias tend to appear early in treatment. Types of dystonias include:

- Torticollis—contracted positioning of the neck
- Oculogyric crisis—contracted positioning of the eyes upward
- Writer's cramp—fatigue spasms affecting a hand
- Laryngeal-pharyngeal constriction (potentially life-threatening)

Dystonias respond to anticholinergic drugs, which must occasionally be given parenterally because of the gravity of the situation.

### Drug-induced Parkinsonism

The cardinal symptoms of Parkinson's disease (PD), which include tremors, bradykinesia, and rigidity, are present.

### Tardive Dyskinesia

Tardive means *late appearing*. Tardive dyskinesia (TD) is an EPSE that tends to develop after approximately 6 months or more of antipsychotic therapy and is not caused by the dopamine-ACh imbalance per se; consequently, anticholinergics are ineffective. In fact, anticholinergics typically worsen the symptoms of TD. Chronic use of antipsychotics is thought to cause dopamine receptors in the basal ganglia to become hypersensitive to dopamine. Symptoms are bothersome and can be embarrassing. Typical symptoms include tongue writhing, tongue protrusion, teeth grinding, and lip smacking. The symptoms stop with sleep. Although TD movements can be suppressed willfully for a short time, they eventually reappear. Up to 35% of individuals on chronic traditional antipsychotic therapy develop TD. Often, TD is irreversible. No satisfactory pharmacologic response has yet been developed, but anecdotal reports suggest that a substantial minority of patients improve with vitamin E. However, there have been reports of spontaneous remission in up to 25% of patients after 5 years of symptoms (Bezchlibnyk-Butler and Jefferies, 2004).

### Pisa Syndrome

Older individuals are particularly susceptible to this effect of leaning to one side. Higher doses of antiparkinsonian drugs may be helpful.

---

**Box 18-5    Guidelines for Minimizing Extrapyramidal Side Effects (EPSEs)**

1. Antipsychotic drugs should not be used for nonapproved indications; for example, they should not be used to treat simple anxiety.
2. The dose for certain groups should be limited. Older adults, for instance, are especially susceptible to hypotension and tardive dyskinesia (TD).
3. As is the case with all drugs, but especially because of the apparent dose-EPSE relationship, the lowest effective dose of an antipsychotic drug should be given.

### Neuroleptic Malignant Syndrome

NMS is a potentially lethal side effect of antipsychotic agents. Fewer than 1% of patients taking antipsychotics develop this problem, but up to 5% to 20% of those will die without treatment (Pelonero et al, 1998). The incidence was formerly much higher, but careful scrutiny of patients by nurses and physicians has reduced both its incidence and mortality. NMS occurs most often when high-potency antipsychotic drugs are prescribed (e.g., haloperidol). NMS is not related to toxic drug levels and might occur after only a few doses. Typically, onset is within a week or so after initiation of an antipsychotic. NMS symptoms include muscular rigidity, tremors, impaired ventilations, muteness, altered consciousness, and autonomic hyperactivity. Perhaps the cardinal symptom is high body temperature. Temperatures as high as 108°F (42.2°C) have been reported, although temperatures are more likely to be 101° to 103°F. Because an increased temperature is the chief sign of NMS, nurses should monitor temperatures closely.

Dantrolene (Dantrium), a skeletal muscle relaxant, and bromocriptine (Parlodel), a dopamine agonist, are drugs of choice for treating NMS. Antipsychotics should not be reinstituted for at least 2 weeks after complete resolution of NMS symptoms.

### Endocrine Side Effects

Traditional antipsychotics elevate prolactin levels by blocking $D_2$ receptors (at about 70% occupancy). Dopamine inhibits prolactin and, when dopamine receptors are blocked, prolactin levels rise. A number of bothersome side effects occur because of chronic prolactin level elevation (Table 18-3). Traditional agents are much more likely to cause hyperprolactinemia.

| Table 18-3 | Consequences of Chronic Prolactin Elevation  |
| --- | --- |

| Women | Men |
| --- | --- |
| Amenorrhea | Impotence |
| Loss of libido | Loss of libido |
| Galactorrhea | Gynecomastia |
| Long-term risk for osteoporosis | Lowered sperm count |
| Changes in menstrual cycle | Feminization |

Metabolic syndrome, or insulin resistance syndrome, presents as a reduced metabolism of glucose and resistance to insulin by insulin receptors on cells. This can result in type 2 diabetes with the associated problems of hyperglycemia, obesity, elevated lipid levels, coagulation abnormalities, and hypertension. Atypical antipsychotics are more likely to cause metabolic syndrome. Accordingly, the U.S. Food and Drug Administration (FDA) requires drug manufacturers to include a warning about this problem.

### Sexual Side Effects

Decreased libido, impotency, and impaired ejaculation occur with significant regularity. $D_2$, 5-$HT_2$, and alpha-2 blockade, as well as the aforementioned elevated prolactin levels, are thought to be responsible for this syndrome (Bezchlibnyk-Butler and Jeffries, 2004).

### Gastrointestinal Effects

Weight gain can be significant, particularly for patients taking the newer agents. This phenomenon is probably related to blockade of $H_1$, 5-$HT_{2c}$, and other receptors. Insulin resistance is an outcome and a cause of excessive weight gain. Carbohydrate craving is a common feature (Bezchlibnyk-Butler and Jeffries, 2004).

> #### CLINICAL EXAMPLE
> Bud, a 23-year-old with a diagnosis of schizophrenia, gained 105 pounds in less than 1 year on a particular atypical drug. He was finally switched to another agent and, when I last saw him, eventually lost about 75 pounds of the extra weight.

### Other Side Effects

Other side effects that might occur in patients taking antipsychotic drugs include jaundice, rare but serious blood dyscrasias, susceptibility to hyperthermia, sun-sensitive skin, nasal congestion, wheezing, and memory loss. Because the cholinergic system is implicated in memory and learning, low-potency antipsychotic drugs might play a role in the cognitive symptoms. Clozapine (Clozaril) causes agranulocytosis in 1% of patients and is potentially fatal. Agranulocytosis will be discussed later in this chapter.

## NURSING IMPLICATIONS

### Therapeutic Versus Toxic Levels

Overdoses of antipsychotic drugs are seldom fatal. An overdose can cause severe CNS depression, hypotension, and EPSEs. Restlessness or agitation, convulsions, hyperthermia, increased anticholinergic symptoms, and arrhythmias are other indicators of an overdose.

### Use During Pregnancy

Antipsychotics pose few risks during pregnancy; nonetheless, they should be avoided during the first trimester (Richards et al, 1999). These drugs readily pass the placental barrier, reach significant levels in the fetus, and have been documented to cause EPSEs in some newborns (Arana and Hyman, 1991).

### Use in Older Adults

Because older individuals have decreased hepatic metabolism capability, reducing the dose in this age group is prudent. Furthermore, age-related nigrostriatal and cholinergic degeneration cause pharmacodynamic responses that are more intense than those experienced by younger individuals. Hence, both extrapyramidal and anticholinergic effects can be heightened. Older adults are also at higher risk for TD (Jeste et al, 1999). Furthermore, a black box warning for the atypical agents was issued in 2005, indicating that elderly patients with dementia-related psychosis were at increased risk of dying from sudden death or pneumonia when treated with these drugs (Janssen Pharmaceutica, 2005).

### Side Effects

PNS anticholinergic and antiadrenergic effects of antipsychotic drugs are troublesome but not always as serious or as disturbing to the patient as are CNS EPSEs. The nurse can provide several specific interventions to ameliorate side effects or to prevent serious consequences (PNS and Nursing Interventions table; EPSEs and Nursing Intervention table).

### Interactions

Antipsychotic drugs interact with many other drugs. Because these interactions can be serious, the nurse must review offending agents and then advise the family and patient accordingly. CNS depressants such as alcohol, antihistamines, antianxiety drugs, antidepressants, barbiturates, meperidine, and morphine have additive effects that can cause profound CNS depression. A few of the most common adverse interactions are found in Table 18-4.

Peripheral Nervous System (PNS) Effects and Nursing Interventions

| PNS Side Effects | Nursing Interventions |
| --- | --- |
| Constipation | Encourage high dietary fiber and increased water intake; give laxatives as ordered. |
| Decreased sweating | Avoid exposure to extreme heat, if possible. |
| Dry mouth | Advise patient to take sips of water frequently; provide sugarless hard candies, sugarless gum, and mouth rinses. |
| Blurred vision | Advise patient to avoid potentially dangerous tasks. Reassure patient that normal vision typically returns in a few weeks, when tolerance to this side effect develops. Pilocarpine eyedrops can be used on a short-term basis. |
| Mydriasis | Advise patient to report eye pain immediately. |
| Photophobia | Advise patient to wear sunglasses outdoors. |
| Orthostatic hypotension | Ask patient to get out of bed or chair slowly. If hypotension is a problem, measure blood pressure before each dose is given. |
| Tachycardia | Tachycardia is usually a reflex response to hypotension. When intervention for hypotension is effective, reflex tachycardia usually decreases. |
| Urinary retention | Encourage frequent voiding and voiding whenever the urge is present. Older men with benign prostatic hypertrophy are particularly susceptible to urinary retention. |
| Urinary hesitation | Provide privacy, run water in the sink, or run warm water over the perineum. |
| Sedation | Help patient get up early and get the day started. |
| Weight gain | Help patient order an appropriate diet; diet pills should not be taken. |

## Extrapyramidal Side Effects (EPSEs) and Nursing Interventions

| EPSE | Nursing Interventions |
|---|---|
| Akathisia | Be patient and reassure the patient who is jittery that you understand the need to move. Because akathisia is the chief cause of nonadherence with antipsychotic regimens, a drug change is often necessary |
| Dystonias | If a severe reaction such as oculogyric crisis or torticollis occurs, give benztropine [Cogentin]) or diphenhydramine (Benadryl) immediately, as needed, and offer reassurance. For some situations, IM administration of benztropine is required because of the seriousness of the dystonic reaction. |
| Drug-induced parkinsonism | Antiparkinsonian drugs are probably indicated. |
| TD | Assess for signs and symptoms by using the AIMS. Anticholinergic agents worsen TD. |
| NMS | Be alert for this potentially fatal side effect. Routinely take temperatures and encourage adequate water intake for all patients on a regimen of antipsychotic drugs; routinely assess for rigidity, tremor, and similar symptoms. |

*AIMS,* Abnormal involuntary movement scale; *NMS,* neuroleptic malignant syndrome; *TD,* tardive dyskinesia.

| Table 18-4 | **Adverse Interactions of Antipsychotics With Some Other Drugs** |  |
|---|---|---|

| Drug | Effect of Interaction |
|---|---|
| Amphetamines | Decreased antipsychotic effect |
| Barbiturates | All cause respiratory depression and increase sedation; all decrease antipsychotic serum levels; hypotension |
| Benzodiazepines | Increased sedation; respiratory depression with lorazepam and loxapine |
| Cigarette smoking | Decreased serum levels of some antipsychotic drugs |
| Insulin, oral hypoglycemics | Control of diabetes is weakened |
| L-Dopa | Decreased antiparkinsonian effect of L-dopa; might exacerbate psychosis |
| Lithium | Decreased antipsychotic effect; lithium toxicity might be masked by antiemetic effect of antipsychotic drugs; increased EPSEs |
| Narcotics | Increased sedation; respiratory depression augmented |
| Tricyclics | Possible increased blood serum levels of both; hypotension; sedation; anticholinergic effect; increased risk of seizures |

*EPSEs,* Extrapyramidal side effects.
From Keltner NL, Folks DG: *Psychotropic drugs,* ed 3, St. Louis, 2005, Mosby.

### Prescription Drugs

The nurse should review prescriptions to serve as a safety net for the prescriber who might make an inadvertent error. This safety measure is also important because nurses often act as case managers or advocates for patients who are seeing many caregivers and receiving prescriptions from multiple providers.

### Nonprescription Drugs

Many nonprescription drugs have potentially harmful interactive effects with antipsychotic drugs. CNS depressants such as alcohol, cold and influenza agents, and sleep aids can have additive effects. Other drugs decrease the effect of antipsychotics. For instance, antacids decrease absorption of antipsychotic drugs.

### Teaching Patients

Teaching patients is an important dimension of nursing care for patients who are taking antipsychotic drugs. The nurse should use discretion in selecting the content of educational sessions, because some patients have a tendency to become anxious and paranoid about potential side effects. The nurse should focus on symptoms that can be seen or felt. The patient should be given a simply written description of drug benefits and side effects, with instructions on how to cope with the side effects. Having this information in a written format helps the patient and family be more in control and able to act as collaborators in treatment.

In addition to the education issues already mentioned, the patient and family should be taught the following:

- Avoid immersion in hot water because hypotension might occur, causing falls.
- Avoid abrupt withdrawal of medication, because EPSEs can occur.
- Use a sunscreen to prevent sunburn and use a maximum-strength variety when sunbathing.
- Take the drug as prescribed. Nonadherence is the leading cause of the return of symptoms and a leading cause of readmission.
- Immediately report signs of a sore throat, malaise, fever, or bleeding. These signs might indicate a blood dyscrasia.
- Dress appropriately in hot weather and drink plenty of water to avoid heatstroke.

---

### CRITICAL THINKING QUESTION    2

The chapter states that low-potency antipsychotic drugs have fewer EPSEs than do high-potency drugs. Why might this be true? (Hint: the answer is related to the type of effects that are more prominent with low-potency drugs and the kind of drugs that are used to treat EPSEs.)

---

### CRITICAL THINKING QUESTION    3

Clozapine remains an expensive drug and can cause fatal agranulocytosis. It is easy to say that everyone who needs clozapine should have it. Focus on the population who is most resistant to traditional drugs, as well as on the compliance problems among this population. Consider a delivery system for getting this drug to the people who need it. How can this goal be accomplished? What role can nursing play in the solution to this problem?

---

## TRADITIONAL (FIRST-GENERATION) DRUGS: INTRODUCED IN 1950

This section provides additional details about the traditional antipsychotics. Traditional antipsychotics account for only 3% of market sales but about 20% of prescriptions (IMS Health, 2002). These drugs are effective but have a higher risk for adverse effects. It should be noted that some patients do very well on these drugs. They remain viable options because they are effective

and incredibly cheaper for patients and payors. Because schizophrenia can be viewed as a lifetime illness, the difference in cost over many years dictates that traditional drugs be at least considered. For example, a month's supply of haloperidol costs less than $20, whereas a month's supply of olanzapine (Zyprexa) costs several hundred dollars.

## LOW-POTENCY TRADITIONAL ANTIPSYCHOTICS

Only the most prescribed traditional antipsychotics will be discussed here; Box 18-1 provides a broader list of these agents.

### Chlorpromazine (Thorazine)

Chlorpromazine was the first antipsychotic developed. When it became available to state hospitals in the United States, workers viewed it as a godsend. Some patients dramatically improved. Chlorpromazine is a low-potency agent and thus results in anticholinergic and antiadrenergic effects. It is also sedating and causes significant weight gain. EPSEs are moderately produced.

### Thioridazine (Mellaril)

Thioridazine is almost as old as is chlorpromazine and was the best-selling antipsychotic in the United States at one time (Wysowski and Baum, 1989). A few patients tend to respond to thioridazine better than to any other drugs. Unfortunately, in the past few years, cases of sudden death have been linked to thioridazine (Hennessy et al, 2004).

Thioridazine has been therapeutic in children with severe behavioral problems marked by combativeness. This drug has a maximum upper limit of 800 mg/day because of the possibility of pigmentary retinopathy, which decreases visual acuity, impairs night vision, and is characterized by pigment deposits on the fundus.

## MODERATE-POTENCY TRADITIONAL ANTIPSYCHOTICS

Some drugs do not fit into the high- versus low-potency conceptual framework. Loxapine (Loxitane) and molindone (Moban) are two of these drugs but perhaps the most important moderate-potency drug is perphenazine (Trilafon). Recent evidence (Lieberman et al, 2005) suggests that perphenazine, when compared with the second-generation antipsychotics, was as effective as all of them except olanzapine. (It should be noted that clozapine was not included in this trial.) Because perphenazine is so much less expensive, this research could have significant impact on prescribing patterns in the future.

## HIGH-POTENCY TRADITIONAL ANTIPSYCHOTICS

### Fluphenazine (Prolixin)

Fluphenazine, a high-potency antipsychotic, is commonly prescribed and considered to be an effective medication. Fluphenazine decanoate (Prolixin Decanoate), the long-acting form, is beneficial for patients who do not comply with a daily oral medication regimen. This injection can be given every 2 to 3 weeks.

### Haloperidol (Haldol)

Haloperidol is a high-potency drug that tends to cause more EPSEs and fewer anticholinergic side effects than low-potency drugs. Haloperidol accounts for about 7% of all antipsychotic drugs prescribed and is by far the most frequently prescribed traditional drug (IMS Health, 2002). It is used extensively in older adults (because of fewer anticholinergic effects) and in pediatric psychiatry (see Chapters 42 and 43).

A problem of ongoing concern to psychiatric nurses is the threat of aggressive behavior of psychiatric patients. Chemical restraint, an unfortunate choice of words for describing psychopharmacologic intervention of this type, is a means of relieving a patient of distressing symptoms that lead to aggressive behavior. Parenteral haloperidol alone or in combination with the benzodiazepine lorazepam (Ativan) is an excellent approach for helping patients stay in control. These two agents can be drawn up in the same syringe and administered as a single injection.

Haloperidol decanoate, which is a long-acting form and can be given at 2- to 4-week intervals (or longer), is particularly beneficial for individuals who struggle with compliance.

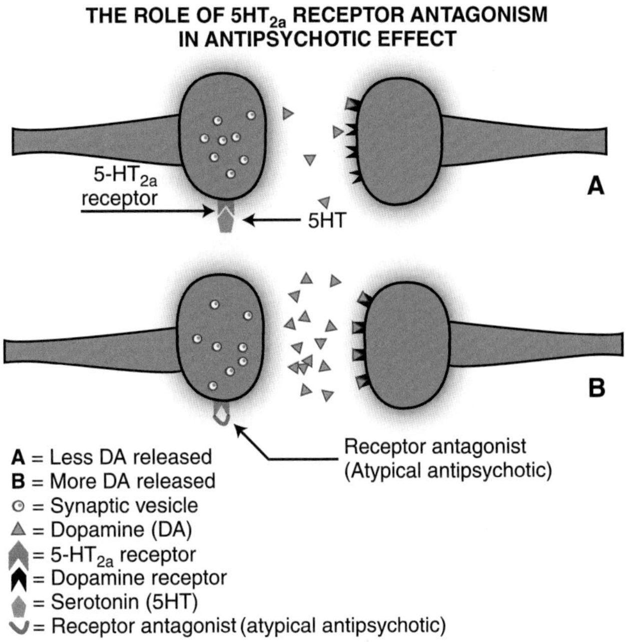

## THE ROLE OF 5HT$_{2a}$ RECEPTOR ANTAGONISM IN ANTIPSYCHOTIC EFFECT

A = Less DA released
B = More DA released
⊙ = Synaptic vesicle
△ = Dopamine (DA)
⬆ = 5-HT$_{2a}$ receptor
⋀ = Dopamine receptor
⬥ = Serotonin (5HT)
⌄ = Receptor antagonist (atypical antipsychotic)

**FIGURE 18-2** The role of 5-HT$_{2a}$ modulation of dopaminergic neurons and the role of atypical antipsychotics. **A,** The 5-HT$_{2a}$ receptor inhibits the presynaptic dopamine neuron. When serotonin fits this receptor, it down-regulates dopamine release and thus can contribute to extrapyramidal side effects (EPSEs) (nigrostriatal tract), hyperprolactinemia (tuberoinfundibular tract), and negative and cognitive symptoms (mesocortical tract). **B,** An atypical antipsychotic has blocked the 5-HT$_{2a}$ receptor. This antagonism increases release of dopamine into the synapse, thus decreasing EPSEs, stabilizing prolactin, and improving negative/cognitive symptoms. (From Keltner NL, Folks DG: *Psychotropic drugs,* ed 4, St. Louis, Mosby, 2005.)

## ATYPICAL ANTIPSYCHOTIC (SECOND-GENERATION) DRUGS: INTRODUCED IN 1990

Chlorpromazine, the first antipsychotic, was developed around 1950. Atypical agents were not marketed until 1990. During this 40-year period, hundreds of antipsychotic formulations were developed, although the drugs were not terribly different; they were all traditional or typical. Atypical antipsychotics are atypical because they work differently (have a different mechanism of action) than the traditional drugs and have a greater effect on negative symptoms. They block 5-HT$_2$ receptors (Figure 18-2). Because this receptor is thought to inhibit dopamine, by blocking it, dopamine is liberated. As previously noted and repeated here, these drugs have the following features that make them atypical:

1. Reduced or no risk for EPSEs: $5\text{-}HT_2$ blockade prevents $D_2$ blockade.
2. Increased effectiveness in treating negative and cognitive symptoms: Dopamine is increased.
3. Minimal risk of TD: Without dopamine blockade in the nigrostriatal tract, dopamine receptors do not become hypersensitive.
4. Absence of prolactin level elevation and the associated side effects: Prolactin-inhibiting factor (i.e., dopamine) is still available.

Each of the four differences is produced by the blockade of serotonin $5\text{-}HT_2$ receptors, which putatively liberates dopamine. The reasoning is as follows (a rationale for the claims of atypicals is underlined for each):

*If* EPSEs are caused by dopamine $D_2$ blockade, *atypicals* keep dopamine available and highly competitive for those receptors.

*If* negative and cognitive symptoms are caused (at least partially) by decreased dopamine in the cortex, *atypicals* increase dopamine in the cortex.

*If* prolactin level elevation is caused by a deficiency in dopamine, *atypicals* increase dopamine in this tract.

*If* TD is caused by irritation of $D_2$ receptors being continually "grasped" by $D_2$ antagonists, *atypicals* prevent this from occurring.

In the years since their introduction, atypical drugs have totally dominated the market. Atypical antipsychotic drugs account for 97% of market sales (in dollars) and over 80% of prescriptions written (IMS Health, 2002) (Figure 18-3).

In general, these agents have a broad affinity for several neurotransmitter systems thought to be implicated in schizophrenia (Tollefson, 1997). Addi-

tionally, they appear to demonstrate regionally specific activity in the brain. For example, they can modulate mesolimbic function without a significant effect on the nigrostriatal tract. Because of the complexity of these pharmacologic effects, a more refined receptor affinity profile could be developed for each of these drugs. However, I believe that it is beyond the scope of an introductory undergraduate text to do so. The atypical antipsychotics are treated as $D_2$–$5\text{-}HT_2$ antagonists, except in the case of several drugs; doing so in such cases would cloud their distinctiveness. A companion textbook, *Psychotropic Drugs* (Keltner and Folks, 2005), provides more detail for those students seeking an in-depth study.

The first atypical agent to be marketed was clozapine.

### Clozapine (Clozaril)

Clozapine, released to the retail market in 1990, was the first truly new antipsychotic agent to be introduced into the United States in 40 years. Clozapine has been referred to as the gold standard in the management of refractory schizophrenia (Oyemumi, 1999). Although clozapine had been used in Europe and China for some time, it was not approved in the United States because of the seriousness of a major side effect, agranulocytosis. Because of this, clozapine is indicated only after severely mentally ill patients with schizophrenia have failed to respond to other antipsychotic drugs. The following summary underscores the severity of this adverse effect.

In Finland, during June and July 1975, 9 out of 18 patients who developed clozapine-induced agranulocytosis died (Idanpaan-Heikkila et al, 1975). This alarming event sent shudders through the psychiatric community; thus, clozapine was not approved in the United States for another 15 years. By the mid-1980s, studies revealed a more optimistic picture of this drug and its effects. However, this was still tempered by an excessively high morbidity rate of 1% to 2% for agranulocytosis and a mortality rate of approximately 33% for those developing this blood dyscrasia (Keltner, 1997). Current investigations have indicated a slightly lower morbidity rate of less than 1%, and the mortality rate has also declined significantly. If deaths related to agranulocytosis do occur, they tend to occur early in treatment (Micromedex, 2002).

Clozapine's side effects result from its antagonism of cholinergic, alpha-1, alpha-2, and histamine $H_1$

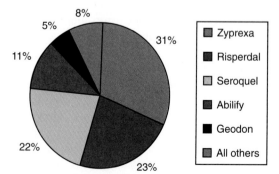

**FIGURE 18-3** Sales for antipsychotics in 2004. (From *Clin Psychiatry News* 33:1, 2005.

receptors. As demonstrated from comparing clozapine's receptor-antagonism profile with those shown in Table 18-2, clozapine causes significant anticholinergic effects, orthostasis, sexual dysfunction, sedation, and weight gain. Sexual dysfunction and weight gain are particularly troublesome and have social implications.

Clozapine is primarily metabolized by P-450 1A2. This is important, because most patients with schizophrenia smoke, and cigarette smoking induces 1A2, causing a decreased level of clozapine (Keltner et al, 2000b).

---

**CLINICAL EXAMPLE**

During a group therapy session in a state public hospital, Bill continually stands up and cannot sit down for long. The moment the group leader instructs Bill to sit down, he does so but immediately stands up again. The group leader misinterprets Bill's behavior as defiance. This misinterpretation escalates into a confrontation that culminates when Bill is forcibly restrained and given a prn injection of an antipsychotic agent.

Had the group leader been more aware of EPSEs, he would have suspected akathisia and would have further recognized that an antipsychotic would only make the patient worse.

---

**CLINICAL EXAMPLE**

Fred White is a 45-year-old man who has struggled with schizophrenia since late adolescence. Because his illness was not manageable at times, he experienced several short hospitalizations. He was eventually placed involuntarily in the state hospital and was living there in 1990 when clozapine became available. After 4 months of taking clozapine, Fred was discharged from the state hospital. After 3 years, Fred's WBC count began to drop, and he was withdrawn from clozapine and placed on large doses of haloperidol. He was hospitalized "locally" on several occasions, and then, as a "last-ditch effort," the psychiatrist rechallenged Fred with clozapine after gaining approval from the manufacturer. Fred improved but was hospitalized several months later for a decreased WBC count. Fred's presenting symptoms were sore throat (to the extent that he gave up eating and had trouble speaking), malaise, and a high temperature (103°F). He was withdrawn from clozapine again, never to be rechallenged, and remains in the state hospital.

Agranulocytosis is clinically defined as an absolute neutrophil count (ANC) below 500/mm$^3$ (Novartis, 2000) and might be caused by bone marrow suppression. Because of its life-threatening potential, the manufacturer of Clozaril requires that its representative closely monitor patients. Box 18-6 outlines the protocols for clozapine therapy.

Clozapine is associated with several other important side effects, including dose-related seizures (5% at higher doses) and excessive salivation (about 30%). Some patients carry paper cups to hold excessive saliva. Myocarditis is another significant side effect. Patients should be instructed to report dyspnea, fever, chest pain, palpitation, tachycardia, and other symptoms of heart failure immediately. Fatal overdoses (e.g., more than 2500 mg) have been associated with clozapine (Keck and McElroy, 2002).

### Risperidone (Risperdal)

Risperidone, approved in 1994, is the most frequently prescribed antipsychotic (IMS Health, 2002) and is atypical but different from clozapine. Risperidone has a greater affinity for dopamine D$_2$

---

**Box 18-6   Protocols for Clozapine Therapy**

1. The normal white blood cell (WBC) count is above 3500/mm$^3$ and the absolute neutrophil count (ANC) is 2000/mm$^3$ or higher.
2. If the baseline WBC and ANC counts are lower than 3500/mm$^3$ and 2000/mm$^3$, respectively, do not start clozapine.
3. Once started, monitor the WBC count weekly.
4. If WBC and ANC levels are normal for 6 months (i.e., WBC of 3500/mm$^3$ or higher and ANC of 2000/mm$^3$), monitor level every 2 weeks.
5. If WBC and ANC levels are normal for 1 year, monitor monthly.
6. If WBC levels drop below 3000/mm$^3$, or the ANC is below 1500/mm$^3$, clozapine should be discontinued. Monitoring the WBC count and ANC should be performed daily.
7. If no sign of infection is present, clozapine therapy can be resumed once the WBC count is higher than 3000/mm$^3$ and the ANC is higher than 1500/mm$^3$.
8. If the WBC count drops below 2000/mm$^3$ and the ANC is below 1000/mm$^3$, clozapine should be permanently discontinued.

Modified from Mechcatie E: FDA approves two monitoring changes for clozapine patients. *Clin Psychiatry News* 33:8, 2005.

receptors and a similar antagonism of serotonin 5-HT$_2$ receptors compared with clozapine; thus, risperidone theoretically has a favorable receptor profile for both positive and negative schizophrenia (Keltner, 1995). Risperidone's lack of serious side effects make it a well-tolerated drug as well. Risperidone has little affinity for muscarinic (i.e., cholinergic) receptors, so anticholinergic side effects are minimized (see Table 18-1). In addition, risperidone does not appear to cause agranulocytosis, TD, or NMS. Moreover, risperidone appears to be a safe drug, with patients surviving amounts many times higher than therapeutic doses (Brown et al, 1993). Nonetheless, risperidone significantly blocks alpha-1 and H$_1$ receptors, resulting in orthostatic hypotension, sedation, and appetite stimulation, respectively. At higher doses, patients taking risperidone have experienced EPSEs and hyperprolactinemia. Other side effects include insomnia (in some patients), agitation, headache, anxiety, and rhinitis.

A long-acting, intramuscular version (Risperdal Consta) is available.

### Olanzapine (Zyprexa)

Olanzapine (Zyprexa), which was released to the market in 1996, is comparable to risperidone in efficacy and side effect profile, and does not cause agranulocytosis. Olanzapine is the highest selling antipsychotic, accounting for 46% of market sales (IMS Health, 2002). Olanzapine blocks 5-HT$_2$ and D$_2$ receptors significantly (Keltner et al, 2000a). It also has high affinity for cholinergic, H$_1$, and alpha-1 receptors, resulting in anticholinergic effects, sedation, weight gain, and orthostasis (Ganguli, 1999; Sussman and Ginsberg, 1999; Wirshing et al, 1999). Olanzapine normalizes N-methyl-D-aspartate (NMDA) receptor function in the glutaminergic system, thus blocking some signs and symptoms associated with schizophrenia. It has a favorable side effect profile, with few incidents of EPSEs. Olanzapine causes considerable weight gain in some patients (National Alliance for the Mentally Ill, 2001). In a recent study, 30% of patients who had been prescribed olanzapine gained at least 7% of their body weight during the trial (Lieberman et al, 2005).

Olanzapine has proven effective in treating acute mania (Keck and McElroy, 2002; Tohen et al, 1999) and is an FDA-approved drug for monotherapy for bipolar disorder. An intramuscular formulation is available.

The following clinical example illustrates how olanzapine made a significant difference in one man's life.

### CLINICAL EXAMPLE

Bill, a man in his early 30s, was first diagnosed with schizophrenia when he was 19 years of age. He experienced a sudden onset and was hospitalized locally five times in 6 months. In the early 1990s, he was admitted to the state hospital; clozapine was prescribed within a few weeks, and he responded favorably. Bill was discharged from the hospital after 5 months to a day-treatment program and did well in that program while on a regimen of clozapine. As protocols required, he was monitored for blood work on a weekly basis and after several years experienced a drop in his WBC count. Clozapine therapy was discontinued, and olanzapine therapy was started. Bill is doing well with olanzapine. His parents have described him as being as well or better than he was before he became ill. After years in the day-treatment program and only a few months on olanzapine therapy, he was discharged and now lives on his own.

### Quetiapine (Seroquel)

Quetiapine (Seroquel) was made available in 1997. Quetiapine, similar to clozapine, has a lower affinity for dopamine D$_2$ receptors than for serotonin 5-HT$_2$ receptors (McManus et al, 1999). Quetiapine has little affinity for muscarinic cholinergic receptors; therefore, few anticholinergic side effects are expected. However, quetiapine antagonizes alpha-1 receptors, which leads to orthostatic hypotension, and antagonizes H$_1$ receptors, which leads to sedation and appetite stimulation. Clinically, quetiapine is effective for both positive and negative symptoms, provokes few EPSEs, does not significantly increase serum prolactin levels, and appears to improve elements of cognitive function. Current formulations must be titrated slowly over a 4- to 5-day period. Anecdotal reports suggest that the effective dose range is higher than manufacturer's recommendations.

### Ziprasidone (Geodon)

Ziprasidone is effective for both positive and negative schizophrenia (Blin, 1999). Ziprasidone acts on several neurotransmitter systems (Tandon, 1997), has a high affinity for 5-HT$_2$ receptors and for dopamine D$_2$ receptors, moderately blocks the reuptake of serotonin and norepinephrine, and is an agonist for the serotonin 5-HT$_{1a}$ receptor. These pharmacologic properties suggest a drug that has the potential to ameliorate depression and anxiety, which are commonly associated with schizophrenia (Keck et al, 2000). Ziprasidone causes few EPSEs, few anticholinergic side effects, and mild antihistaminic effects. Common side effects include nausea, dyspepsia, abdominal pain, constipation, somnolence, insomnia, and coryzal symptoms. Ziprasidone appears to cause less weight gain than some other atypical agents. Ziprasidone has been linked to potential cardiac problems related to lengthening of the QTc interval. Studies have indicated a low potential for drug-drug interactions. An intramuscular form is available. Absorption is increased when ziprasidone is given with food.

### Effects of 5-HT$_{1a}$ Agonism by Ziprasidone

- Decreased anxiety
- Decreased depressive symptoms
- Improvement in negative symptoms

## NOVEL ANTIPSYCHOTIC (THIRD-GENERATION) DRUG: INTRODUCED IN 2002

A relatively new drug, aripiprazole (Abilify), is referred to as a dopamine system stabilizer (DSS) and represents what has been called the third generation of antipsychotics. DSSs are thought to balance the dopamine systems by increasing dopamine in brain areas in which dopamine is deficient and decreasing dopamine in brain areas in which dopamine is overactive. Figure 18-4 contrasts the blockade of dopamine D$_2$ receptors by traditional drugs (Figure 18-4, *A*) with the partial agonism of those same receptors by a drug such as

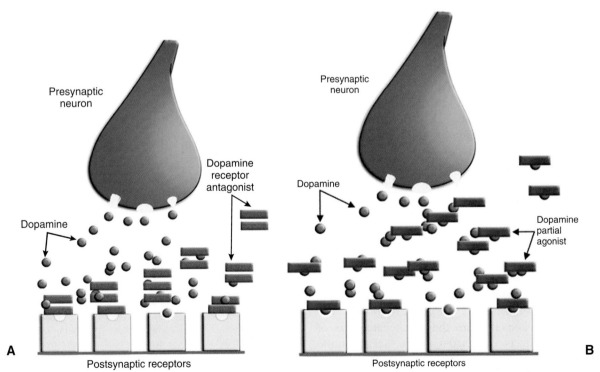

**FIGURE 18-4 A,** Dopamine receptor antagonism. **B,** Dopamine system stabilization. (From Keltner NL, Johnson VY, Aripiprazole: A third generation of antipsychotics begins?, *Perspec Psychiatr Care* 38(4):157-159, 2002.)

aripiprazole (Figure 18-4, *B*). Aripiprazole accomplishes this because it is a partial dopamine agonist, producing activation where lower dopamine tone exists and inhibition at brain sites with high dopaminergic tone (Stahl, 2001). Areas with too much dopamine begin to stabilize because the aripiprazole molecule is less potent than the dopamine molecule; this effect reduces positive symptoms. Mesocortical areas also begin to stabilize from the opposite direction. Patients begin to feel better, with more energy as negative symptoms subside. Aripiprazole also antagonizes 5-HT$_2$ receptors, as do other atypical drugs (Keltner and Johnson, 2002), and is a partial agonist at the 5-HT$_{1a}$ receptor. Clinical studies have suggested a very good side effect profile.

## CRITICAL THINKING QUESTION   5

Some clinicians believe that, unless a patient has some level of EPSEs, the patient is not receiving enough medication. What might the rationale be for this view?

## Study Notes

1. The dopamine hypothesis of schizophrenia states that an excessive level of dopamine in the brain causes schizophrenia.
2. Antipsychotic drugs block dopamine receptors, reducing the effect of excessive availability of dopamine in the brain, specifically in the mesolimbic tract.
3. Antipsychotic drugs are classified in three ways: traditional, atypical, and novel.
4. The traditional agents are further divided into high- and low-potency drugs.
5. Desired effects of antipsychotic drugs include sedation, emotional quieting, psychomotor slowing, and alleviation of major symptoms of schizophrenia (e.g., alterations in perceptions, thoughts, consciousness, interpersonal relationships, affect).
6. Anticholinergic side effects (e.g., dry mouth, blurred vision, constipation) and EPSEs, including akathisia, akinesia, dystonic reactions, drug-induced parkinsonism, Pisa syndrome, and TD, are the major categories of side effects associated with antipsychotic drugs.
7. High-potency antipsychotic drugs, such as haloperidol and fluphenazine, tend to cause more EPSEs. Low-potency antipsychotic drugs, such as chlorpromazine and thioridazine, tend to cause more anticholinergic and antiadrenergic side effects.
8. NMS is a serious adverse effect of antipsychotic drugs (primarily high-potency drugs).
9. Overdoses of antipsychotic drugs are seldom fatal.
10. Antipsychotic drugs interact with other CNS depressants such as alcohol, meperidine, and morphine, thereby increasing CNS depression.
11. Patient teaching should focus on recognizing side effects and on avoiding CNS depressants.
12. The nurse should routinely assess for NMS by taking the patient's temperature and evaluating for rigidity and tremors.
13. Clozapine (Clozaril), introduced into the United States in 1990, was the first truly new antipsychotic drug in 40 years.
14. Other atypical antipsychotics have a great affinity for dopamine D$_2$ and serotonin 5-HT$_2$ receptors, produce few EPSEs, and have had remarkable success in treatment-resistant patients.
15. Clozapine causes agranulocytosis, a potentially fatal illness.
16. The other atypical antipsychotics do not cause the life-threatening agranulocytosis.
17. Weight gain can be a particularly troublesome side effect of atypical agents.
18. Aripiprazole is called a novel or third-generation antipsychotic. Its mechanism of action is unique—partial agonism of dopamine D$_2$ and 5-HT$_2$ receptors.

## References

Arana GW, Hyman SE: *Handbook of psychiatric drug therapy*, ed 2, Boston, 1991, Little Brown.

Bezchlibnyk-Butler KZ, Jeffries JJ: *Clinical handbook of psychotropic drugs*, ed 14, Seattle, 2004, Hogrefe & Huber.

Blin O: A comparative review of new antipsychotics, *Can J Psychiatry* 44:235, 1999.

Brown K, Levy H, Brenner C, et al: Overdose of risperidone, *Ann Emerg Med* 22:1908, 1993.

Ganguli R: Newer antipsychotics versus older neuroleptics. Is weight gain still a problem? *Ther Adv Psychoses* 6:8, 1999.

Hennessy S, Bilker WB, Knauss JS, et al: Comparative cardiac safety of low-dose thioridazine and low-dose haloperidol, *Br J Clin Pharmacol* 58(1):81-87, 2004.

Idanpaan-Heikkila J, Alhava E, Olkinuora M, Palva I: Clozapine and agranulocytosis (letter), *Lancet* 2:611, 1975.

IMS Health: *Antipsychotic market sales,* 2002, IMS Health.

Jannsen Pharmaceutica: *Important drug warning,* Titusville, NJ, May 2005, Janssen Pharmaceutica.

Jeste DV, Rockwell E, Harris MJ, et al: Conventional vs. newer antipsychotics in elderly patients, *Am J Geriatr Psychiatry* 7:70, 1999.

Jibson MD, Tandon R: New atypical antipsychotic medications, *J Psychiatr Res* 32:215, 1998.

Keck PE, McElroy SL: Clinical pharmacodynamics and pharmacokinetics of antimanic and mood-stabilizing medications, *J Clin Psychiatry* 63(Suppl 4):3, 2002.

Keck P, Strakowski S, McElroy S: The efficacy of atypical antipsychotics in the treatment of depressive symptoms, hostility, and suicidality in patients with schizophrenia, *J Clin Psychiatry* 61(Suppl 3):4, 2000.

Keltner NL: Catastrophic consequences secondary to psychotropic drugs. Part II, *J Psychosoc Nurs Ment Health Serv* 35:48, 1997.

Keltner NL: Risperidone: the search for a better antipsychotic, *Perspect Psychiatr Care* 31:30, 1995.

Keltner NL, Folks DG: *Psychotropic drugs,* ed 3, St. Louis, 2005, Mosby.

Keltner NL, Johnson V: Aripiprazole: A third generation of antipsychotics. *Perspect Psychiatr Care* 38:157, 2002.

Keltner NL, Coffeen H, Johnson JE: Atypical antipsychotics: part I, *Perspect Psychiatr Care* 36:139, 2000a.

Keltner NL, Coffeen H, Johnson JE: Atypical antipsychotics: part II, *Perspect Psychiatr Care* 36:101, 2000b.

Lieberman JA, Stroup S, McEvoy JP, et al: Effectiveness of antipsychotic drugs in patients with chronic schizophrenia. *N Engl J Med* 353:1209, 2005.

McManus DQ, Arvanitis LA, Kowalcyk BB: Quetiapine, a novel antipsychotic: experience in elderly patients with psychotic disorders, *J Clin Psychiatry* 60:292, 1999.

Micromedex: *Drug information for the health care professional,* Englewood, CO, 2002, Micromedex:.

National Alliance for the Mentally Ill: Things to watch, *Advocate* winter/spring:18, 2001.

Novartis: *Clozaril,* East Hanover, NJ, 2002, Novartis.

Oyemumi LK: Does lithium have a role in the prevention and management of clozapine-induced granulocytopenia? *Psychiatr Ann* 29:597, 1999.

Pelonero AL, Levenson JL, Pandurangi AK: Neuroleptic malignant syndrome: a review, *Psychiatr Serv* 49:1163, 1998.

Richards SS, Musser WS, Gershon S: *Maintenance pharmacotherapies for neuropsychiatric disorders,* Philadelphia, 1999, Brunner/Mazel.

Stahl SM: Dopamine system stabilizers, aripiprazole, and the next generation of antipsychotics: part I, "Goldilocks" actions at dopamine receptors, *J Clin Psychiatry* 62:841, 2001.

Sussman N, Ginsberg D: Effects of psychotropic drugs on weight gain, *Psychiatr Ann* 29:580, 1999.

Tandon R: Ziprasidone (Zeldox), *The decade of the brain* 8:13, 1997.

Tohen M, Sanger TM, McElroy SL, et al: Olanzapine versus placebo in the treatment of acute mania. Olanzapine HGEH Study Group, *Am J Psychiatry* 156:702, 1999.

Tollefson GD: Olanzapine (Zyprexa), *The decade of the brain* 8:7, 1997.

Welch R, Chue P: Antipsychotic agents and QT change, *J Psychiatry Neurosci* 25:154, 2000.

Wirshing DA, Wirshing WC, Kysar L, et al: Novel antipsychotics: comparison of weight gain liabilities, *J Clin Psychiatry* 60:358, 1999.

Wysowski DK, Baum C: Antipsychotic drug use in the United States, 1976-1985, *Arch Gen Psychiatry* 46:929, 1989.

## Bibliography

Ayd FJ: The early history of modern psychopharmacology, *Neuropsychopharmacology* 5:71, 1991.

Bezchlibnyk-Butler KZ, Jeffries JJ: *Clinical handbook of psychotropic drugs,* ed 14, Seattle, 2004, Hogrefe & Huber.

Fuller MA, Sajatovic M: *Psychotropic drug information handbook,* ed 3, Cleveland, 2002, American Pharmaceutical Association.

Keltner NL, Folks DG: *Psychotropic drugs,* St. Louis, 2005, Mosby.

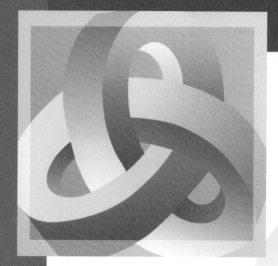

# Chapter 19

# Antidepressant Drugs

*Norman L. Keltner*

## Learning Objectives

*After reading this chapter, you should be able to:*

- Understand neurobiologic concepts of depression.
- Describe the differences among the three major classes of antidepressant drugs: (1) tricyclic antidepressants, (2) selective serotonin reuptake inhibitors, and (3) monoamine oxidase inhibitors.
- Explain the mechanism of action of antidepressant drugs, including the novel antidepressants.

- Discuss side effects of antidepressant drugs.
- Identify symptoms of toxicity for tricyclic antidepressants and monoamine oxidase inhibitors.
- Describe potential interactions of antidepressant drugs.
- Discuss the implications of teaching patients about antidepressant drugs.

Antidepressants are used in the treatment of depressive and other disorders. This chapter will focus on the psychopharmacologic classes of drugs used to treat depression (Box 19-1). A complete discussion of depressive disorders is found in Chapter 29. Goals of antidepressant medications are to:

Alleviate depressive symptoms
Restore normal mood
Prevent recurrence of depression
Prevent a swing into mania for bipolar patients

## BIOCHEMICAL THEORY OF DEPRESSION

A number of theories exist concerning the cause of depression, but the efficacy of antidepressants is best understood from a neurochemical perspective that had its genesis 50 years ago. In the early 1950s, Bein isolated reserpine from rauwolfia serpentina, a naturally occurring medicinal agent that had been used to treat hypertension (Ayd, 1991). Reserpine was found to have additional value in the treatment of psychosis, but some patients developed profound depression and became suicidal. The researchers related this action of reserpine to norepinephrine depletion. From this early linking of neurotransmitter depletion to depression, scientists began conceptualizing pharmacologic interventions. The crucial step in the development of antidepressant drugs was the synthesizing of agents that would increase the intrasynaptic availability of certain neurotransmitters, such as norepinephrine, serotonin, and dopamine (Anand and Charney, 2000; Hirshfeld, 2000).

Complementary views suggest that changes in receptors and genes might be an important aspect

## Norm's Notes

*These drugs are everywhere and probably overprescribed. I'd be very surprised if you didn't know someone on one of the SSRIs (e.g., Prozac, Paxil, Zoloft). These are great drugs when really needed, but just numbing oneself to avoid some pain is not always best. So, even though I think highly of these drugs, I also think that they are overused, when working through a problem might have been the better option. Read this chapter carefully. I guarantee you will need to know this information—it could help someone you know.*

### Box 19-1    Antidepressant Drugs Based on Traditional Classifications

**Selective Serotonin Reuptake Inhibitors**
Citalopram (Celexa)
Escitalopram (Lexapro)
Fluoxetine (Prozac)
Fluvoxamine (Luvox)
Paroxetine (Paxil)
Sertraline (Zoloft)

**Novel Antidepressants**
Bupropion (Wellbutrin)
Duloxetine (Cymbalta)
Mirtazapine (Remeron)
Venlafaxine (Effexor)

**Tricyclic and Related Nonselective Cyclic Antidepressant Drugs**
Amitriptyline (Elavil)
Amoxapine (Asendin)
Desipramine (Norpramin)
Doxepin (Sinequan)
Imipramine (Tofranil)
Maprotiline (Ludiomil)
Nortriptyline (Aventyl, Pamelor)
Protriptyline (Vivactil)
Trimipramine (Surmontil)

**Monoamine Oxidase Inhibitors**

***Reversible Inhibitor of MAO-A (RIMA)***
Moclobemide (Manerex)

***Irreversible Nonselective Inhibitors of MAO***
Phenelzine (Nardil)
Tranylcypromine (Parnate)

of antidepressant activity. This is bolstered by the observation that antidepressants usually require 2 to 4 weeks for a clinical response. Elevations in these neurotransmitter levels occur within hours

of treatment initiation, whereas receptor changes take approximately 2 to 4 weeks and genetic changes even longer.

Antidepressant-mediated genetic modification might be the most important current hypothesis describing antidepressant action. This view states that reregulation of the complex workings of the second messenger system is the key to antidepressant effectiveness (Stahl, 2000a). Figure 19-1 illustrates an important schematic of the second messenger system. In depression, key genetic products are undersynthesized, and thus depression occurs. Of particular interest is a potential deficiency of brain-derived neurotropic factor (BDNF) that would, at normal levels, oppose cellular apoptotic forces (genetically programmed cell death). Left unopposed, apoptosis is accelerated. Depression might well be caused by actual neuronal death, which, in turn, is caused by dysregulated monoaminergic systems. Antidepressants' efficacy is probably related to regulation of the second messenger system (Stahl, 2000a).

Psychopharmacologic treatment is based on the restoration of normal levels of these neurotransmitters and the consequent neuronal changes (Figure 19-2). Available antidepressants achieve this goal in several distinct ways (Bezchlibnyk-Butler and Jeffries, 2004; Keltner, 2000; Stahl, 2000b). Although the following list might appear complex, understanding these mechanisms will provide a firm understanding of how antidepressants work (also see Box 19-1).

1. *Selective serotonin reuptake inhibitors (SSRIs).* SSRIs selectively block the uptake of serotonin. These drugs are first-line agents for treatment of depression. SSRIs are effective and have a good side effect profile. Unfortunately, SSRIs cause significant sexual dysfunction and gastrointestinal (GI) symptoms.

2. *Norepinephrine and dopamine reuptake inhibitors (NDRIs).* Bupropion (Wellbutrin, Zyban) is the only drug in this category and is unique in two ways: it is the only antidepressant that primarily inhibits dopamine uptake and the only one that does not affect serotonin systems. Bupropion also inhibits norepinephrine uptake and is considered a novel antidepressant.

3. *Selective serotonin-norepinephrine reuptake inhibitors (SNRIs).* Venlafaxine (Effexor) and duloxetine (Cymbalta) are in this category, and inhibition activity is dose dependent. At lower doses, they

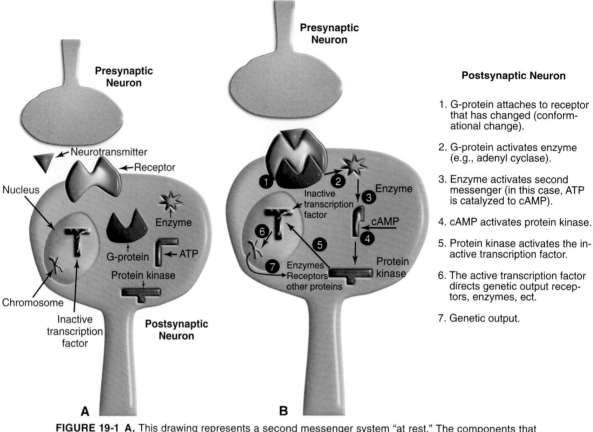

**FIGURE 19-1 A,** This drawing represents a second messenger system "at rest." The components that will be affected by neurotransmitter activation of the second messenger system are labeled. **B,** This drawing represents the sequence of events that transpires with second messenger activation. Steps 1-7 indicate the sequence, with step 7 providing the genetic output: enzymes, receptors, and other proteins. It is thought that in depression, key genetic products are undersynthesized. Antidepressants "reregulate" the second messenger system.

**Postsynaptic Neuron**

1. G-protein attaches to receptor that has changed (conformational change).

2. G-protein activates enzyme (e.g., adenyl cyclase).

3. Enzyme activates second messenger (in this case, ATP is catalyzed to cAMP).

4. cAMP activates protein kinase.

5. Protein kinase activates the inactive transcription factor.

6. The active transcription factor directs genetic output receptors, enzymes, ect.

7. Genetic output.

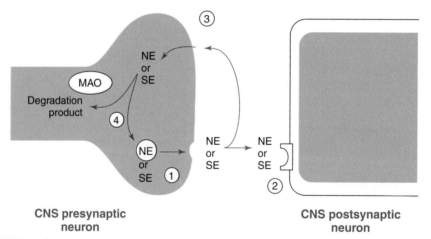

**FIGURE 19-2** Depression results from an amine (e.g., norepinephrine, serotonin) concentration that is too low to activate sufficient receptors; mania results from overabundance of amines acting at receptors. The biogenic amine theory of depression is applied to actions of antidepressant drugs, tricyclic antidepressants (TCAs), selective serotonin reuptake inhibitors (SSRIs), and monoamine oxidase inhibitors (MAOIs), and to the action of lithium, which is used to treat mania. *1,* Lithium inhibits release of norepinephrine and serotonin; *2,* TCAs and MAOIs increase receptor sensitivity to norepinephrine and serotonin; *3,* TCAs block reuptake of norepinephrine and serotonin; SSRIs block reuptake of serotonin; lithium enhances reuptake of norepinephrine and serotonin; *4,* MAOIs prevent degradation of norepinephrine and serotonin. NE, Norepinephrine; SE, serotonin. (From Clark J, Queener S, Karb V: *Pharmacologic basis of nursing practice,* ed 4, St. Louis, 1993, Mosby.)

inhibit serotonin uptake; at moderate to high doses, norepinephrine reuptake is inhibited; at higher doses, dopamine uptake is added. They are considered novel antidepressants.

4. *Alpha-2 antagonism with 5-HT₂ and 5-HT₃ antagonism.* Mirtazapine (Remeron), also referred to as a noradrenergic-specific serotonergic agent (NaSSA), increases the availability of both serotonin and norepinephrine by its antagonism of alpha-2 autoreceptors. This antagonism triggers the feedback system to increase norepinephrine and serotonin activity. By blocking 5-T₂ receptors, mirtazapine does not have the side effects associated with this receptor (i.e., sexual dysfunction) and, by blocking 5-HT₃, it produces no GI symptoms, as do the SSRIs. Mirtazapine is considered a novel antidepressant.

5. *Nonselective inhibition of norepinephrine and serotonin.* The tricyclic antidepressants (TCAs) block the reuptake of both norepinephrine and serotonin. Some TCAs are more potent norepinephrine uptake inhibitors and some are more potent serotonin uptake inhibitors. Because of their nonselectivity, TCAs cause many side effects. Until the development of SSRIs, TCAs were the gold standard for treatment of depression.

6. *Inhibition of enzymes.* The monoamine oxidase inhibitors (MAOIs) are the only antidepressants that inhibit neurotransmitter breakdown as their primary mechanism of action.

It should be noted that all but the last mechanism work by blocking the reuptake of neurotransmitters (see Figure 19-1).

Antidepressants are not always indicated when individuals report being depressed (e.g., grief); however, when antidepressants are indicated, approximately 90% of patients respond to treatment if the clinician is persistent (Stahl, 2000b). Technically, treatment response means that the patient has experienced a 50% reduction in depression severity as measured by a standardized depression scale (Gumnick and Nemeroff, 2000). These drugs do not cure depression, but long-term use has been successful in reducing symptoms. Most relapses are associated with patient–initiated tapering off or discontinuance. However, up to 20% of patients who are compliant with these medications experience antidepressant "poop out." Whether this is related to a tolerance developing or worsening of the depression is not known.

Box 19-2   **Antidepressant Treatment Strategies**

**First-line agents:** SSRIs, novel antidepressants
**Second-line agents:** TCAs
**Third-line agents:** MAOIs, ECT

*ECT,* Electroconvulsive therapy; *MAOIs,* monoamine oxidase inhibitors; *SSRIs,* selective serotonin reuptake inhibitors; *TCAs,* tricyclic antidepressants.

TCAs have been around for some time and are still the first choice of some clinicians. However, SSRIs and the novel antidepressants (Box 19-2) are the first-line agents selected by most prescribers for several reasons (discussed later in this chapter). MAOIs are usually the last choice because of their serious side effects. Another effective treatment approach, electroconvulsive therapy (ECT), is discussed in Chapter 39. Obviously, consideration of various forms of psychotherapy and other psychotherapeutic interventions is always indicated.

## SELECTIVE SEROTONIN REUPTAKE INHIBITORS

SSRIs are effective antidepressants that have fewer side effects than TCAs and are far less dangerous than MAOIs. Accordingly, they are first-line drugs for treatment of depression (Table 19-1). SSRIs have fewer anticholinergic, cardiovascular, and sedating side effects. Fluoxetine (Prozac) was the first SSRI marketed in the United States. Stories of near-miraculous recoveries were followed by reports of major problems associated with this drug. Early anecdotal information, coupled with some research findings, associated fluoxetine with suicidal and homicidal behaviors. Interestingly, antidepressants now carry a black box warning cautioning clinicians about the risk of suicidal thinking and behavior when these drugs are prescribed to children and adolescents. Whether this increase in suicidal ideation is a product of the energizing effects of these drugs (e.g., fluoxetine is an *activating* drug) or is related to more basic mental processes has been debated by clinicians.

Another recognized phenomenon related to SSRIs is a high level of apathy that is apparently induced by these drugs. The antidepressant apathy syndrome (AAS) presents as lack of motivation, indifference, disinhibition, and poor attention. Lee and Keltner (2005) wondered whether some suicides and homicides that have occurred might

| Table 19-1 | Comprehensive Table of Antidepressants |
| --- | --- |

| | DOSAGES AND PHARMACOKINETICS | | | SPECIFICITY FOR NT REUPTAKE | | |
| --- | --- | --- | --- | --- | --- | --- |
| | Daily Dosage Range (mg) | Half-Life* (hr) | Protein Binding (%) | NE | 5-HT | DA |
| **Tricyclic Antidepressants (TCAs)** | | | | | | |
| Amitriptyline (Elavil) | 75-300 | 31-46 | 97 | 1 | 3 | 1 |
| Clomipramine (Anafranil) | 75-300 | 19-37 | 97 | 1 | 4 | 1 |
| Desipramine (Norpramin) | 75-300 | 12-24 | 90-95 | 5 | 1 | 1 |
| Imipramine (Tofranil) | 75-300 | 11-25 | 89-95 | 2 | 3 | 1 |
| Nortriptyline (Pamelor, Aventyl) | 50-150 | 18-44 | 92 | 4 | 2 | 1 |
| **Selective Serotonin Reuptake Inhibitors (SSRIs)** | | | | | | |
| Citalopram (Celexa) | 10-60 | 23-45 | 80 | 1 | 4 | 1 |
| Escitalopram (Lexapro) | 10-20 | 27-32 | 55 | 1 | 4 | 1 |
| Fluoxetine (Prozac) | 10-80 | 48-216 | 95 | 1 | 3 | 1 |
| Fluvoxamine (Luvox) | 50-300 | 15-19 | 80 | 1 | 4 | 1 |
| Paroxetine (Paxil) | 10-60 | 3-21 | 95 | 1 | 5 | 1 |
| Sertraline (Zoloft) | 25-200 | 26-98 | 98 | 1 | 4 | 2 |
| **Novel Antidepressants** | | | | | | |
| Bupropion (Wellbutrin) | 150-450 | 8-15 | 80 | 1 | 0/1 | 2 |
| Duloxetine (Cymbalta) | 20-60 | 8-17 | 90 | 3 | 2 | 1 |
| Mirtazapine (Remeron) | 7.5-45 | 20-40 | 85 | 1 | 1 | 0 |
| Trazodone (Desyrel) | 150-600 | 4-9 | 89-95 | 0 | 2 | 1 |
| Venlafaxine (Effexor) | 75-225 | 5-11 | 25 | 2 | 4 | 1 |
| **Monoamine Oxidase Inhibitors (MAOIs)** | | | | | | |
| ***Irreversible MAOIs*** | | | | | | |
| Phenelzine (Nardil) | 30-90 | 2-3 | ? | — | — | — |
| Tranylcypromine (Parnate) | 20-60 | 2-3 | ? | — | — | — |
| ***Reversible Inhibitor of MAO-A (RIMA)*** | | | | — | — | — |
| Moclobemide (Manerex) | 300-600 | 1-3 | 50 | — | — | — |

*With active metabolite.
Scale for receptor antagonism specificity: 1, low; 5, high.
Severity of side effects: 0, none; X, low; XX, moderate; XXX, high; XXXX, very high.
*5-HT,* serotonin; *ACh,* acetylcholine; *DA,* dopamine; *NE,* norepinephrine; *NT,* Neurotransmitter.
Modified from Bezchlibnyk-Butler KZ, Jeffries JJ: *Clinical handbook of psychotropic drugs,* ed 16, Seattle, 2006, Hogrefe & Huber; and Crutchfield DB: Review of psychotropic drugs, *CNS News Special Edition* 6:51, 2004.

be related to antidepressant-induced indifference and disinhibition. They discussed the following media-followed events in their article:

- July 2003: Jake Steinberg, a college student with the habit of biting his nails, was prescribed paroxetine (Paxil) to curb this anxious habit. A little over a month later, he jumped 24 floors to his death. His mother states that the drug killed her son.
- February 2004: Kara Jayne-Anne Otter, 12, taking Paxil for depression, killed herself.

Her mother, Shannon Baker, blamed the SSRI.

- February 2005: A 15-year-old boy in Charleston, SC, killed his grandparents. He claimed that the antidepressant Zoloft drove him to it.
- March 2005: Jeff Weise, 16 years old, opened fire on faculty and students at Red Lake High School in Minnesota, killing nine. His family has wondered aloud if his medication (Prozac) might have contributed to his loss of control.

| Orthostatic Hypotension | Anticholinergic Effects | Insomnia | Sedation | Sexual Dysfunction | GI Effects |
|---|---|---|---|---|---|
| XXXX | XXXX | X | XXXX | XX | X |
| XX | XXX | XX | XXX | XXX | XX |
| X | X | X | X | XX | X |
| XX | XX | X | XXX | XXX | XX |
| X | XX | X | XX | X | X |
| | | | | | |
| X | X | X | XX | XXXX | XXX |
| X | X | X | X | X | XXX |
| XX | X | XXXX | XX | XXXX | XXX |
| X | X | XX | XX | XXXX | XXXX |
| X | X | XX | XX | XXXX | XXX |
| XX | XX | XX | XX | XXXX | XXX |
| | | | | | |
| X | X | XXXX | X | 0 | X |
| X | X | XX | X | XX | XXX |
| XX | XX | 0 | XXXX | X | X |
| XX | XX | X | XXXX | X | XX |
| X | X | X | XX | XXX | XXX |
| | | | | | |
| XX | XX | X | XX | XXX | XX |
| XX | XX | XXXX | X | XX | X |
| | | | | | |
| XX | XX | XX | XX | XXX | XX |

## PHARMACOLOGIC EFFECT

The antidepressant effect of SSRIs is thought to be linked to their inhibition of serotonin reuptake into neurons. These drugs do not bind significantly to histaminic, cholinergic, dopaminergic, or adrenergic receptors, thus reducing many of the side effects that plague people who are taking TCAs.

## PHARMACOKINETICS

SSRIs are absorbed in the GI tract. Peak plasma levels are achieved for most of these drugs between 4 and 6 hours. SSRIs are metabolized in the liver and have relatively long serum half-lives. The long half-lives allow once-daily dosing schedules. Both fluoxetine and sertraline have active metabolites that significantly extend their half-lives. Abrupt cessation is associated with the development of specific signs and symptoms (Box 19-3).

## SIDE EFFECTS

As previously noted, SSRIs have relatively few anticholinergic, antihistaminic, or antiadrenergic effects; thus, they do not cause the same intensity of side effects associated with TCAs. Dry mouth, blurred vision, sedation, and cardiovascular symptoms are not as common with these agents as with TCAs; however, these side effects do occur and can be very bothersome for some patients. However, GI symptoms such as nausea, diarrhea, loose stools, and weight loss or gain are relatively common. It is believed that activation of $5\text{-}HT_3$ receptors by the elevated levels of serotonin causes these GI symptoms. Furthermore, hyponatremia has occurred with these drugs, mostly in older patients.

### Box 19-3    Is There an SSRI Withdrawal Syndrome?

A question many people have about SSRIs is whether a withdrawal syndrome develops on abrupt cessation of these drugs. The answer to this question is yes. Abrupt discontinuation of SSRIs might cause the following symptoms.

*Somatic Symptoms:* Dizziness, lethargy, nausea, vomiting, diarrhea, flulike symptoms (e.g., headache, fever, sweating, chills, malaise), insomnia, vivid dreams

*Psychological Symptoms:* Anxiety, agitation, irritability, confusion, slowed thinking

Fluoxetine, because of its long half-life, is less likely to cause a withdrawal syndrome.

Modified from Bezchlibnyk-Butler KZ, Jeffries JJ: *Clinical handbook of psychotropic drugs,* Seattle, 2004, Hogrefe and Huber.

### Box 19-4    Sexual Dysfunctions Associated With SSRIs

| Sexual Sequence | SSRIs Can Cause Any or All of the Following |
|---|---|
| Desire | Decreased libido |
| Arousal | Erectile dysfunction or lack of vaginal lubrication |
| Orgasm | Inability to achieve orgasm |

*SSRIs,* Selective serotonin renptake inhibitors.

Central nervous system (CNS) effects include headache, dizziness, tremors, anxiety, insomnia, decreased libido, impotence, ejaculatory delay, and decreased orgasm. Up to one third or more of patients prescribed SSRIs experience sexual dysfunction (Boxes 19-4, 19-5, and 19-6). Anxiety, insomnia, and sexual dysfunction are thought to be related to serotonin 5-HT$_2$ receptor activation. Anecdotal reports from some practitioners suggest that as many as 70% of these patients suffer some form of sexual dysfunction. Obviously, for many individuals, sexual dysfunction is a major factor in decisions about compliance. Nonetheless, because of this overall side effect profile, SSRIs are frequently prescribed. Conversely, the incidence of premature ejaculation seems to be increasing, and some SSRIs are used to delay orgasm in these men.

## INTERACTIONS

SSRIs interact with several drugs (Table 19-2), and some of these interactions are related to SSRI inhibition of the cytochrome P-450 enzyme system. Combining SSRIs and MAOIs has proven

### Box 19-5    Treatment Strategies for SSRI Sexual Dysfunction

1. Wait and see if improvement in patient occurs naturally.
2. Decrease dosage of SSRI.
3. Time SSRI dose to maximize probability of sexual satisfaction.
4. Change antidepressants.
5. Augment with other drugs:
   Amantadine: Dopaminergic that inhibits prolactin
   Amphetamines: Increase dopamine
   Bupropion: Increases dopamine
   Buspirone: Binds to histamine, serotonin and dopamine receptors
   Methylphenidate: Stimulant
   Sildenafil (Viagra): Enhances erections

Modified from Keltner NL, McAffee K, Taylor C: Mechanisms and treatments for SSRI-induced sexual dysfunction, *Perspect Psychiatr Care* 38:111-116, 2002.

### Box 19-6    SSRIs Most Likely to Cause Sexual Dysfunction*

Paroxetine
Fluoxetine
Citalopram
Sertraline
Escitalopram

*In descending order.

### Table 19-2    Some Significant Drug Interactions With SSRIs

| Drug | Effect of Interaction |
|---|---|
| Irreversible MAOIs | *Avoid;* this combination can be fatal (i.e., serotonin syndrome) |
| Lithium | Increased lithium levels, increased serotonergic effect |
| Antipsychotics | Increased EPSEs |
| Benzodiazepines | Increased benzodiazepine half-life |
| TCAs | Increased TCA serum levels → toxicity |
| | Displacement of TCAs from serum proteins → toxicity |
| Carbamazepine, phenytoin | Increased anticonvulsant serum levels |

*EPSEs,* Extrapyramidal side effects; *MAOIs,* monoamine oxidase inhibitors; *SSRIs,* selective serotonin reuptake inhibitors; *TCAs,* tricyclic antidepressants.

## Box 19-7   Serotonin Syndrome

Serotonin syndrome can occur if an SSRI is combined with the following:

- MAOIs: Phenelzine, tranylcypromine
- MAOIs (selective): Selegiline, moclobemide
- Tryptophan: Serotonin precursor
- St. John's wort

Signs and symptoms of serotonin syndrome (most to least frequent):

- Mental status changes, including confusion or hypomania
- Restlessness or agitation
- Myoclonus
- Hyperreflexia
- Diaphoresis
- Shivering (or shaking chills)
- Tremor
- Diarrhea, abdominal cramps, nausea
- Ataxia or incoordination
- Headaches

From Keltner NL, Folks DG: *Psychotropic drugs*, Philadelphia, 2005, Elsevier.

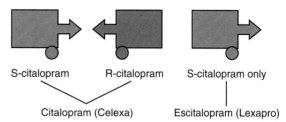

FIGURE 19-3 Model demonstrating the mirror image S and R isomers of citalopram and the S-only isomer of escitalopram.

to be fatal, a phenomenon is called the *serotonin syndrome* (Box 19-7).

## NURSING IMPLICATIONS

### Therapeutic Versus Toxic Drug Levels

SSRIs have a low potential for overdose. Even high doses have not resulted in fatalities. Toxic symptoms include nausea, vomiting, tremor, myoclonus, and irritability. Treatment is symptomatic and supportive.

### Use During Pregnancy

SSRIs are pregnancy category B drugs (meaning that risks to the fetus have not been established). However, these drugs should be avoided during the first trimester as a prudent precaution. The long half-lives of fluoxetine and sertraline might also be significant factors in treating the pregnant patient. Malone and associates (2004), in a thorough review of the literature, found that SSRIs were not associated with teratogenicity. Hence, these antidepressants are frequently continued during pregnancy. Keltner and Hall (2005), however, have reported on the recently recognized neonatal serotonin syndrome (NSS). Neonates who have been exposed to SSRIs in utero, and who are not breast-fed, suffer a withdrawal

syndrome. This syndrome includes respiratory depression, hypoglycemia, tremor, and lower birth weight. These symptoms seem to have a short half-life and all affected are typically symptom-free within 2 weeks. Nonetheless, pregnant women prescribed SSRIs should be well informed about this possibility.

### Use in Older Adults

SSRIs are safe for use in older adults because of the good side effect profile of these drugs. As with most medications, SSRI dosage levels should be reduced in older adults. However, older adults' potential for weight loss must be monitored. The half-life of paroxetine (Paxil) increases two or three times in older adults, so extra precautions are warranted.

## INDIVIDUAL SELECTIVE SEROTONIN REUPTAKE INHIBITORS

### Citalopram (Celexa)

Citalopram, because of its pharmacologic profile (i.e., its weaker inhibition of P-450 enzymes compared with other SSRIs), has fewer serious drug-drug interactions. Citalopram is composed of stereoisomers that are mirror images of each other. For example, your right hand and left hand are exactly alike but backward—that is, your left hand cannot fit into a right-handed glove. The two reverse image isomers in citalopram are called S and R. It is believed that most side effects are caused by the R isomer and most therapeutic benefits are derived from the S isomer. Figure 19-3 illustrates this concept.

### Escitalopram (Lexapro)

Escitalopram is related to citalopram: the "*es*" stands for the S isomer. Theoretically, escitalopram should provide most of the therapeutic benefits of citalopram without all of its side effects. In fact, escitalopram does have a better side effect profile. It has also been approved for treatment of generalized anxiety disorder.

### Fluoxetine (Prozac, Sarafem)

Fluoxetine was the first SSRI developed and is frequently prescribed. Beyond the more typical uses of fluoxetine, it is approved for the treatment of bulimia and premenstrual dysphoric disorder (under the trade name Sarafem). Other uses include pain management and promoting smoking cessation (Bezchlibnyk-Butler and Jeffries, 2004). Fluoxetine has a long half-life, up to 9 days or longer (including its active metabolite). Drugs that have a high probability for serious interactions (e.g., MAOIs) will need to be withheld for up to 5 weeks as fluoxetine is washing out of the system. Prozac is available in a once-weekly formulation for long-term treatment of depression; it is made with a special delayed-release coating.

A unique combination of fluoxetine and olanzapine (Symbyax) is available for individuals suffering from bipolar depression.

### Fluvoxamine (Luvox)

Fluvoxamine is specifically approved for the treatment of obsessive-compulsive disorder (OCD). Fluvoxamine does not have an active metabolite and has a side effect profile similar to that of other SSRIs.

### Paroxetine (Paxil)

Paroxetine is a potent serotonin reuptake blocker and is approved for the treatment of panic attacks. Because its metabolites are not active, paroxetine has a shorter half-life and poses fewer problems than other SSRIs if it needs to be discontinued. A common side effect is nausea, but this effect rarely leads to dose reduction or drug discontinuation. Paroxetine has also been shown to be effective for the prevention of depressive relapse (Nemeroff, 1993). Similar to the other SSRIs, paroxetine can be given on a once-daily basis and causes sexual side effects. It is approved for treatment of premenstrual dysphoric disorder.

All is not good news about paroxetine, however. A December 2005 FDA warning to physicians indicates that Paxil may be teratogenic. Apparently the risk of birth defects doubles for women taking this drug. The manufacturer has been asked to upgrade the pregnancy warning category from C to D (Peck, 2005).

### Sertraline (Zoloft)

Sertraline is a widely marketed SSRI and was the second drug of this class to be used in the United States. Sertraline can also be given once daily, morning or evening, with or without food. Sertraline causes sexual dysfunction in men and women. Sexual function typically returns to normal 2 to 3 days after drug cessation.

## NOVEL ANTIDEPRESSANTS

### Bupropion (Wellbutrin)

Bupropion, an NDRI, is unique in two ways: (1) it is the only antidepressant with dopamine uptake inhibition as a major mechanism of action; and (2) it does not affect serotonin systems. Bupropion has a good side effect profile, as shown in Box 19-8.

Bupropion should not be given in combination with drugs that increase the dopamine level. Bupropion has proven to be an effective replacement for, or as an addition to, SSRIs when these drugs cause sexual dysfunction. In a general sense, it can be said that dopamine enhances sexuality and serotonin inhibits sexual functioning. Because bupropion increases intrasynaptic dopamine, it offsets SSRI-mediated sexual inhibition and is prescribed in low doses along with SSRIs for this reason (Keltner, 2000). Bupropion has a narrow

| Box 19-8  **Bupropion Side Effect Profile** | |
|---|---|
| *Good News About Bupropion* | *Bad News About Bupropion* |
| *Causes minimal:* | *But can cause:* |
| Orthostatic hypotension | Agitation |
| Cardiovascular conduction problems | Seizures (contraindicated in epilepsy patients) |
| Anticholinergic effects | Weight loss (complicating anorexia) |
| Daytime sedation | |
| Sexual dysfunction | |

therapeutic index but is far less lethal than TCAs or MAOIs. Under the trade name Zyban, bupropion is marketed as a smoking cessation agent. It is believed that dopamine counters the craving associated with nicotine withdrawal for smokers who have or who want to quit smoking. Bupropion is contraindicated for individuals with seizure disorders.

## Venlafaxine (Effexor) and Duloxetine (Cymbalta)

Venlafaxine and duloxetine are structurally unrelated to other currently marketed antidepressants. These drugs are classified as SNRIs. At lower doses, venlafaxine causes serotonin to be enhanced, at medium to high doses norepinephrine reuptake is inhibited, and at the highest doses dopamine intrasynaptic levels are increased. These drugs appear to combine the best qualities of TCAs and SSRIs in that they inhibit the reuptake of both norepinephrine and serotonin, as do TCAs and, like SSRIs, do not bind significantly to muscarinic, histaminergic, or adrenergic receptors. Theoretically, few anticholinergic, antihistaminic, or antiadrenergic side effects should occur. Venlafaxine has a lower potential for drug interaction than other antidepressants and does not exaggerate the effects of alcohol. Venlafaxine is effective in treating generalized anxiety disorder, social phobias, SSRI-induced sexual dysfunction, OCD, and panic disorders. Duloxetine is approved for the treatment of diabetic neuropathy pain.

## Nefazodone and Trazodone (Desyrel)

Nefazodone (Serzone) and trazodone (Desyrel) are classified as serotonin reuptake inhibitors–receptor 5-HT$_2$ blockers. However, Serzone was taken off the market in 2004 because of a high incidence of hepatic failure. Although generic nefazodone remains available, this text will not describe the mechanism of action of this drug.

Trazodone is now seldom prescribed as an antidepressant but is frequently prescribed for sleep in nondepressed individuals. It is now the second most commonly prescribed drug for insomnia (Mendleson, 2005). One unusual adverse reaction to this drug is *priapism* (i.e., prolonged penile erection). Surgical intervention has been required in some affected men. If priapism occurs, the nurse should stop the medication and notify the prescriber.

## Mirtazapine (Remeron)

Mirtazapine is an alpha-2 antagonist with 5-HT$_2$ and 5-HT$_3$ antagonism that has been approved for major depression. It is also used to reduce SSRI-induced sexual dysfunction. Mirtazapine's pharmacologic effect is different from that of other antidepressants: it selectively blocks alpha-2 autoreceptors, which increases norepinephrine and serotonin levels by using the presynaptic feedback system; that is, blockade of alpha-2 autoreceptors signals the need for more of these neurotransmitters. Related to its antihistaminic effects, sedation is reported in over 30% of patients taking mirtazapine, and weight gain occurs in approximately 15% of patients (Bezchlibnyk-Butler and Jeffries, 2004). Paradoxically, sedation decreases at higher dosage levels. An increase in the serum cholesterol level occurs in some patients. Mirtazapine's uniqueness is attributable to its antagonism of both 5-HT$_2$ (i.e., reducing sexual dysfunction, anxiety, and insomnia) and 5-HT$_3$ (i.e., reducing GI distress). Remeron is available in an orally dissolvable form under the trade name Remeron SolTabs. It dissolves on the tongue in approximately 30 seconds.

## TRICYCLIC ANTIDEPRESSANTS

## PHARMACOLOGIC EFFECTS

Theoretically, the serum level of **monoamines** (i.e., norepinephrine, serotonin) in the depressed person is so low that achieving a normal mood is impossible. TCAs block the reuptake of these released neurotransmitters, thereby increasing the intrasynaptic levels and alleviating the symptoms of depression.

Because reuptake terminates normal neurotransmitter activity, this blocking causes greater neurotransmitter availability and thus prolongs the stimulating action. As noted, clinical studies have shown that this specific effect occurs quickly, yet there is a lag period of 2 to 4 weeks before an antidepressant effect is experienced.

TCAs can be categorized further as secondary amines or tertiary amines. Drugs that tend to increase the availability of norepinephrine more than serotonin are termed *secondary amines,* and drugs that tend to increase serotonin availability more than norepinephrine are called *tertiary amines.*

| Secondary Amines (Enhance Norepinephrine More) | Tertiary Amines (Enhance Serotonin More) |
|---|---|
| Amoxapine | Amitriptyline |
| Desipramine | Clomipramine |
| Nortriptyline | Doxepin |
| Protriptyline | Imipramine |

Clomipramine (Anafranil), although a strong potentiator of serotonin, is not typically prescribed for depression but is a drug of choice for OCD.

## OTHER THERAPEUTIC EFFECTS OF TRICYCLIC ANTIDEPRESSANTS

*Sedation* is a therapeutic effect of these drugs, because depressed patients commonly experience insomnia and agitation. Tolerance to sedation usually develops.

*Lethargy* is a common symptom of depression. Some TCAs, described as *activating antidepressants,* might alleviate lethargy.

*Improved appetite* is another effect of TCAs. Loss of appetite and a consequent loss of weight are symptoms of depression. This effect is probably related to the TCAs' antihistaminic effect but might be related to improved mood. Unfortunately, weight gain can be significant and might contribute to a new set of problems.

*Anxiety reduction* is another positive effect of TCAs.

*Urinary hesitancy,* although definitely problematic for many patients, can be used therapeutically for childhood enuresis.

## PHARMACOKINETICS AND DOSING

TCAs are absorbed well from the GI tract and are usually given orally (PO). TCAs are metabolized in the liver, and some metabolites have antidepressant effects (e.g., desipramine is a metabolite of imipramine; nortriptyline is a metabolite of amitriptyline).

Peak plasma concentrations are reached in 2 to 4 hours, on average; however, because of a significant first pass through the liver, only about 30% to 70% of an oral dose reaches the bloodstream. TCAs are highly bound to plasma proteins, so their effects are produced by only a small fraction of free drug; even a small increase in free drug is potentially serious. Individuals with diminished liver function (e.g., older adults, children, alcoholics, individuals with a history of hepatitis) or those with decreased plasma protein levels (e.g., older adults) might be at special risk of elevated serum levels. People older than 55 years of age are often started at half the regular adult dose.

The relatively long half-lives of these drugs usually allow once-daily dosing schedules. A steady state is typically reached in approximately 5 days. These drugs are initiated at low doses and increased every 3 to 5 days until the patient becomes intolerant of side effects.

All TCAs appear to be equally effective. Table 19-1 lists several important treatment parameters of antidepressants.

## SIDE EFFECTS

Patients taking TCAs experience undesirable side effects of both the peripheral nervous system (PNS) and the CNS. Tertiary amines (more serotonin enhancing) have more frequent and more severe side effects than secondary amines (more norepinephrine enhancing).

### Peripheral Nervous System Effects

#### Anticholinergic Effects

Anticholinergic effects on the peripheral autonomic nervous system range from annoying to dangerous and include the following:

Dry mouth and anhidrosis (decreased sweating, which impairs cooling)
Visual disturbances (e.g., mydriasis, blurred vision, might precipitate acute attack of glaucoma)
Constipation
Bladder dysfunction (e.g., urinary retention, urinary hesitancy)

Older adults are most susceptible to these side effects, and older men with benign prostatic hypertrophy are at a special risk for bladder problems.

#### Cardiac Effects

Anticholinergic effects on the cardiovascular system are common enough to warrant serious consideration. Essentially, the parasympathetic system serves as a brake for the heart and, when this system is blocked by anticholinergics, the brake is released and the heart speeds up. Tachycardias and arrhythmias can lead to myocardial infarction. TCAs can also have a quinidine-like effect that delays conduction. In susceptible patients, this effect can lead to heart block. Patients with a history of heart problems must be carefully evaluated. Amitriptyline is considered the most cardiotoxic antidepressant and, with its high levels of sedation, anticholinergic activity, and orthostatic hypotension, is a less desirable drug for older adults (Gomez and Gomez, 1992).

Children have shown troublesome cardiovascular responses to TCAs (notably desipramine) that warrant serious consideration. Since these concerns were first noted, several deaths have occurred in children taking these drugs. In each case, sudden death, usually associated with physical activity, was the cause. The serum level might be almost 50% higher in children than in adults at the same dose (Bezchlibnyk-Butler and Jeffries, 2004).

### Antiadrenergic Effects

These drugs also block alpha-1 adrenergic receptors on peripheral blood vessels and inhibit the body's natural vasoconstricting reaction when a person stands. Blood pooling occurs in the lower extremities, leading to inadequate cerebral perfusion. The heart responds with a reflex tachycardia to help the body adapt. Dimming of vision, dizziness, and fainting cause a sense of loss of control and can lead to falls and serious injury. Box 19-9 provides a reference for orthostatic hypotension, a significant and disabling side effect of both antidepressant and antipsychotic drugs. Healthy

individuals frequently make cardiovascular accommodations and this side effect diminishes within a few weeks. Patients with a history of heart problems, however, must be carefully evaluated and closely monitored.

### Central Nervous System Effects

#### Sedation

Sedation is a common side effect and can be helpful, because insomnia is a frequent symptom of depression. Sedation occurs because of histamine $H_1$ antagonism.

#### Cognitive or Psychiatric Effects

CNS effects include confusion, disorientation, delusions, agitation, anxiety, ataxia, insomnia, and nightmares. Blockade of cholinergic receptors accounts for some of these symptoms. These side effects might be found in a significant number of patients treated with TCAs. The effects usually occur when serum TCA levels are elevated and most often affect older adult patients. TCAs might aggravate an existing dementia or mimic dementia.

### Suicide

A clear association exists between suicide and depression. In fact, most individuals who commit suicide are found to have demonstrated characteristics of depression. Consequently, considerable evidence exists to support treating depressed individuals who are suicidal with antidepressants. Paradoxically, however, antidepressants can *energize* patients who have been too depressed to act on their suicidal thoughts. Therefore, depressed individuals who are suicidal warrant special nursing consideration after antidepressant therapy has been initiated. Activating antidepressants such as desipramine and fluoxetine might increase the likelihood of energizing a patient in this manner. Furthermore, as discussed later, TCAs are generally highly toxic, which means that the actual drug that a patient is taking to treat depression could be used to overdose and die. TCAs account for a little less than 10% of all deaths from intentional drug overdose (Zimmermann, 1997). Interestingly, only 21% of all suicide completers testing positive for antidepressants had taken TCAs, whereas 44% tested positive for novel antidepressants and 35% for SSRIs (Jancin, 2005). Although it might seem as if TCAs are more effective at reducing suicide, one must remember that many more individuals

| Box 19-9 | Orthostatic Hypotension (OH) Caused by Antidepressant Drugs |
|---|---|
| Definition | On standing, the patient experiences significant drop in blood pressure |
| Risk factors | Age 65 years or older<br>Dehydration<br>Fluid loss<br>Cardiac medications |
| Interventions | Regularly monitor OH vital signs<br>Caffeine<br>Sodium chloride tablets<br>Support stockings<br>Teach patient the following: to rise slowly, dangle feet before standing; that OH is worse in the morning; the importance of adequate fluids; to avoid hot showers and baths; that symptoms decrease with time |

take novel antidepressants and SSRIs than take TCAs. Nonetheless, the statistics are interesting and worthy of discussion. Figure 19-4 provides a graphic example of the percentages of suicide victims who were taking antidepressants.

Novel antidepressants have a lower potential for lethal overdose than TCAs and might be better suited for actively suicidal patients.

## INTERACTIONS

TCAs are metabolized primarily by P-450 enzymes 2D6, 1A2, and 3A4. Several serious drug interactions occur with TCAs when drugs affecting these

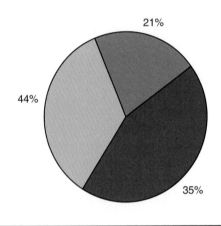

FIGURE 19-4 Suicide completers testing positive for antidepressants: individual agents, in descending order. (Modified from Jancin B: Toxicology shows antidepressants present in 21% of suicide completers, *Clin Psychiatr News* 33:6, 2005.)

same enzymes are used. Other problematic interactions might also occur (Table 19-3).

### Central Nervous System Depression

Increased CNS depression might occur when TCAs are taken with CNS depressants (e.g., alcohol, benzodiazepines).

### Cardiovascular and Hypertensive Effects

Cardiovascular arrhythmias or hypertension can occur when sympathomimetic drugs are given with TCAs. Because TCAs block the reuptake of norepinephrine, sympathomimetic agents cause an increase in norepinephrine in the synaptic cleft. Interactants to avoid include norepinephrine, dopamine, ephedrine, and phenylpropanolamine (found in many over-the-counter stimulants). MAOIs are almost always avoided. Severe reactions, including high fever, seizures, and a fatal hypertensive crisis, can occur. MAOIs are not usually prescribed unless TCAs have failed. When changing to MAOIs, the patient *must discontinue TCAs for 14 days* before the new drug is given.

TCAs block alpha-adrenergic receptors, thus compromising the effectiveness of many antihypertensives to control hypertension.

### Additive Anticholinergic Effects

Additive anticholinergic effects can occur when TCAs are given with other anticholinergic drugs, including antipsychotics, antiparkinsonian drugs, and antihistamines. Older adult patients are especially susceptible. All the PNS and CNS anticholinergic effects mentioned earlier in this chapter can be aggravated.

| Table 19-3 | Some Significant Interactions With TCAs |  |
| --- | --- | --- |

| Drug | Effect of Interaction |
| --- | --- |
| MAOIs | Hyperpyrexia, excitability, muscular rigidity, convulsions, fatal hypertensive crisis, mania |
| Sympathomimetics | Cardiac arrhythmias, hypertension |
| Warfarin | Increased bleeding |
| Barbiturates, carbamazepine, phenytoin | Decreased TCA effect |
| Antipsychotics | Increased extrapyramidal side effects |
| Procainamide, guanidine | Prolongation of cardiac conduction |
| Anticholinergics | Increased anticholinergic effect |
| L-Dopa | Increased agitation, tremor, and rigidity |
| Alcohol, anticonvulsants, benzodiazepines | Increased sedation |

*MAOIs,* Monoamine oxidase inhibitors; *TCAs,* tricyclic antidepressants.

# NURSING IMPLICATIONS

## Therapeutic Versus Toxic Blood Levels

TCAs do not produce euphoria and are not addicting; therefore, the potential for abuse is not great. Overdose, however, is a real issue and accounts for fewer than 10% of intentional suicides (Zimmermann, 1997). The difference between a therapeutic dose and a lethal dose is small. Therefore, outpatients who are at risk for suicide are frequently restricted to a 7-day supply.

Toxic blood levels can result in sedation, ataxia, agitation, stupor, coma, respiratory depression, and convulsions. Exaggeration of side effects previously mentioned can also occur. Cardiovascular reactions can occur suddenly and cause acute heart failure, even several days after the overdose. Furthermore, cardiovascular reactions can be delayed; that is, they can occur after recovery from overdose. Thus, all antidepressant overdoses should be considered serious, and the patient should be admitted to a hospital for monitoring.

The nurse should be aware of several assessment and intervention strategies when a toxic level of TCAs is suspected (see the Key Nursing Interventions for TCA Overdose box).

## Use During Pregnancy

These drugs have not been definitively found to cause teratogenic effects but should be avoided in the first trimester. Because depressive symptoms, such as loss of appetite, can interfere with fetal development by preventing adequate fetal weight gain, antidepressants should be prescribed cautiously to pregnant women. Antidepressants are typically placed in FDA pregnancy categories B or C. During pregnancy, TCAs with low anticholinergic effects (e.g., nortriptyline, desipramine) are preferred to those with high anticholinergic effects. TCAs must be tapered off before delivery to avoid transient perinatal toxicity (Cohen, 1989).

| Depressive Symptoms Associated With Serotonin Deficiencies | Depressive Symptoms Associated With Norepinephrine Deficiencies |
|---|---|
| Anxiety | Fatigue |
| Panic | Apathy |
| Phobias | Cognitive disturbances |
| Posttraumatic stress disorder | Impaired concentration |
| Obsessions | Focusing attention |
| Compulsions | Slowed information processing |
| Eating disorders | Deficiencies in working memory |

Although serotonin and norepinephrine deficiencies are both considered causative for depression, Stahl (2000b) has noted that low levels of these two monoamines produce distinct depressive syndromes.

## Use in Older Adults

TCAs should be given in reduced doses to older adult patients. The maxim "start low and go slow" is particularly true for this population. The secondary amines (e.g., desipramine, nortriptyline, protriptyline) are preferred. Side effects previously mentioned, such as cardiovascular effects, orthostatic hypotension, cognitive impairment, and all peripheral anticholinergic effects, are more pronounced in this age group.

## Side Effects

Selected side effects and appropriate nursing interventions are listed in the Side Effects and Nursing Interventions for Antidepressants box.

---

## Key Nursing Interventions   *for TCA Overdose*

- Monitor blood pressure, heart rate and rhythm, and respirations.
- Maintain patent airway.
- ECG (electrocardiography) is recommended.
- Use cathartics or gastric lavage with activated charcoal to *prevent further drug absorption* (for up to 24 hours).
- The antidote for severe TCA poisoning (anticholinergic toxicity) is physostigmine (Antilirium), an acetylcholinesterase inhibitor *(inhibits the breakdown of acetylcholine)*. It should be given only to patients with life-threatening symptoms (e.g., coma, convulsions) because of risk associated with physostigmine use.

## Side Effects and Nursing Interventions for Antidepressants

| Side Effects | Interventions |
| --- | --- |
| **Peripheral Nervous System** | |
| Dry mouth | Advise frequent sips of water, hard candies, sugarless gum. |
| Mydriasis | Advise wearing of sunglasses outdoors. |
| Diminished lacrimation | Suggest artificial tears. |
| Blurred vision | Caution about driving and potential for falls (usually subsides in 1 to 2 weeks). The patient should remove objects in the house that might be tripped over (e.g., throw rugs, small tables). |
| Eye pain | Advise patient to report eye pain immediately, because it might indicate an acute glaucoma attack. All older adult patients should be screened for glaucoma before treatment with TCAs is initiated. |
| Urinary hesitancy and retention | Monitor fluid intake. Patients should be told to avoid putting off urinating. Catheterization might be needed. |
| Constipation | Monitor fluid and food intake. Urge patients to heed the urge to defecate. A high-fiber diet and large amounts of water (2500 to 3000 mL/day) are helpful. |
| Anhidrosis | Decreased sweating can lead to an increase in body temperature. Adequate fluids, appropriate clothing, and sensible exercise should be stressed. |
| Cardiovascular effects | TCAs are contraindicated during the recovery phase of myocardial infarction. |
| Orthostatic hypotension | See Box 19-9. |
| **Central Nervous System** | |
| Sedation | Caution patient about driving. |
| Delirium or mania | Discontinue the drug and call the physician. |
| Suicidal patients | Observe patients closely, because antidepressants might increase motivation for suicide. |

*TCAs,* Tricyclic antidepressants.

## Interactions

The nurse should be aware of the interactants mentioned in Table 19-3. As a general rule, individuals who are taking TCAs should avoid certain types of drugs, both prescribed and over-the-counter, including the following:

- Drugs that depress the CNS
- Drugs that have anticholinergic properties
- Drugs that stimulate the CNS
- MAOIs (deaths have occurred)

## Teaching Patients

The nurse should discuss side effects and several important principles with patients and their families:

- A lag period of 2 to 4 weeks occurs before full therapeutic effects are experienced.
- Certain drugs must be avoided, including over-the-counter preparations.
- Abrupt discontinuation can cause nausea, headache, and malaise.
- Eye pain must be reported immediately, particularly in older adults, in which undiagnosed narrow-angle glaucoma can lead to an emergency situation.
- Some side effects lessen after patients adjust to the medication.

## INDIVIDUAL TRICYCLIC ANTIDEPRESSANTS

The following are brief descriptive statements about TCAs, but include only unique features of usage and side effects. Uses and side effects common to all the drugs are not discussed nor is information that is given in the tables in this chapter.

### Amitriptyline (Elavil)

Amitriptyline is highly anticholinergic and one of the most sedating and cardiotoxic antidepressants.

### Amoxapine (Asendin)

Amoxapine is a metabolite of the antipsychotic drug loxapine and blocks dopamine receptors. As might be deduced, amoxapine can cause side effects typically associated with neuroleptics (e.g., extrapyramidal side effects [EPSEs], tardive dyskinesia). Amoxapine might be beneficial for patients who are both psychotic and depressed.

### Desipramine (Norpramin)

Desipramine is a secondary amine and a metabolite of imipramine. Desipramine is an *activating antidepressant* and thus might be advantageous for apathetic, lethargic, and hypersomnic patients. Because of its aforementioned effects on children's cardiovascular systems, desipramine should be used with care in this age group.

### Imipramine (Tofranil)

Imipramine is the oldest TCA. None of the newer antidepressants has proven to be more effective. Imipramine, because of its anticholinergic properties, has proven effective in the treatment of childhood enuresis. Imipramine should be used with care in children because of its cardiovascular effects.

### Nortriptyline (Aventyl, Pamelor)

Because nortriptyline, a secondary amine TCA, is somewhat sedating and has a good side effect profile, it is often prescribed for older adult patients who are depressed, agitated, and suffering from insomnia. Nortriptyline is a metabolite of the tertiary amine, amitriptyline.

## MONOAMINE OXIDASE INHIBITORS

MAOIs, the third major class of antidepressants, are usually administered to hospitalized patients or to individuals who can be closely supervised. In brief, these drugs are currently not used much but deserve mention because they have potentially fatal interactions and can help the student conceptualize significant pharmacokinetic processes.

Two MAOIs, phenelzine (Nardil) and tranylcypromine (Parnate), are occasionally used; they are referred to as *irreversible nonselective inhibitors* because they inhibit both variants of monoamine oxidase, MAO-A and MAO-B. Moclobemide (Manerex) is a *reversible selective inhibitor of MAO-A only* (RIMA).

The older irreversible MAOIs are almost always prescribed after other antidepressants have failed because of the serious adverse reactions to these drugs, especially life-threatening hypertension. Although some clinicians believe that MAOIs are particularly effective in treating atypical depression (e.g., hypersomnia, somatic anxiety, excessive eating), they are still seldom prescribed.

Moclobemide does not seem to interact with tyramine-containing foods; thus, it lacks the serious side effects of the older MAOIs.

## PHARMACOLOGIC EFFECTS

MAOIs block monoamine oxidase, a major enzyme involved in the metabolic decomposition and inactivation of norepinephrine, serotonin, and dopamine. This enzyme inhibition lasts for 10 days in the irreversible MAOIs and 24 hours in moclobemide. The enzyme inhibition increases the levels of these neurotransmitters in the PNS and the CNS. According to the neurochemical theory of depression, depressed individuals have lower than normal levels of these neurotransmitters available. MAOIs help in attaining normal levels by slowing the deactivation of these amines. This action is in contrast to that of TCAs, which help attain normal levels by preventing the reuptake of amines by the neurons. Approximately 2 to 4 weeks is required for the antidepressant effect of MAOIs to occur; however, as is the case with TCAs, the inhibition of monoamine oxidase occurs immediately. This suggests that factors other than low levels of specific neurotransmitters are involved in depression.

## ABSORPTION, DISTRIBUTION, AND ADMINISTRATION

MAOIs are well absorbed from the GI tract and are given PO. They are metabolized in the liver. Because monoamine oxidase does not decline with age, MAOIs do not present the same age-related risks associated with other drugs.

Moclobemide has a high first-pass metabolism. Age does not affect moclobemide's pharmacokinetic activities; it has modest protein binding (50%) and a half-life of 1 to 3 hours, and is metabolized by cytochrome P-450 enzymes (Cozza and Armstrong, 2001).

## SIDE EFFECTS

MAOIs cause CNS, cardiovascular, and anticholinergic side effects. Serious life-threatening reactions can occur when irreversible MAOIs interact with certain drugs or foods (see the following discussion on interactions).

Because MAOIs increase the availability of biogenic amines in the brain, CNS hyperstimulation might occur, causing agitation, acute anxiety attacks, restlessness, insomnia, and euphoria. In individuals thought to have quiescent schizophrenia (an unrecognized, latent form), full schizophrenic episodes have erupted. Hypomania (which is less severe compared with full mania) is a more common effect.

Hypotension is a common cardiovascular effect, resulting from the slowdown in the release of norepinephrine. Unlike the effect of TCAs, a reflex tachycardia does not occur, because other adrenergic nerves also experience the slowed release of norepinephrine and the heart does not speed up reflexively. Hypotension, combined with the absence of a compensatory increased heart rate, can lead to heart failure.

MAOIs can cause anticholinergic effects such as dry mouth, blurred vision, urinary hesitancy, and constipation. Hepatic and hematologic dysfunctions can occur and, although rare, are potentially serious. Blood counts and liver function test results should be obtained before therapy begins.

## INTERACTIONS

MAOIs have a number of serious interactions. Potentially lethal interactants include both drugs and foods.

## Drug-Drug Interactions

The nurse should be aware of several types of drug interactions (Table 19-4):

- Those that cause hypertension
- Those that cause severe anticholinergic responses
- Those that can cause profound CNS depression

Sympathomimetic drugs are classified as direct-acting, indirect-acting, and mixed-acting (having both direct and indirect properties) drugs. Indirect-acting and mixed-acting sympathomimetics cause serious and sometimes fatal hypertension. Direct-acting sympathomimetics add new norepinephrine to the body, whereas indirect-acting sympathomimetics release existing norepinephrine from the neurons. Because MAOIs increase the amount of stored norepinephrine in the PNS, a potential exists for indirect-acting and mixed-acting sympathomimetics to induce the release of large amounts of norepinephrine. Therefore, avoiding these interacting drugs is crucial. Even small amounts can trigger a hypertensive crisis. Typical indirect-acting and mixed-acting sympathomimetics include amphetamines, cocaine, methylphenidate (Ritalin), dopamine, mephentermine, and ephedrine. Over-the-counter weight loss and stimulant products contain phenylephrine, phenylpropanolamine, and pseudoephedrine, which are mixed- or indirect-acting sympathomimetics. Theoretically, direct-acting sympathomimetics

| Table 19-4 | Some Significant Drug Interactions With Irreversible Nonselective MAOIs* |  |

| Drugs | Effect of Interaction |
| --- | --- |
| Anticholinergic drugs | Increase anticholinergic response |
| Anesthetics (general) | Deepen CNS depression |
| Antihypertensives (diuretics, beta blockers, hydralazine) | Cause hypotension |
| CNS depressants | Intensify CNS depression |
| Sympathomimetics (*mixed- and indirect-acting*): amphetamines, methylphenidate, dopamine, phenylpropanolamine (in many over-the-counter hay fever, cold, and diet medications) | Precipitate hypertensive crisis, cardiac stimulation, arrhythmias, cerebrovascular hemorrhage |
| Sympathomimetics (*direct-acting*): epinephrine, norepinephrine, isoproterenol; less likely to cause problems | Theoretically should not produce a reaction, but caution is recommended |
| Serotonergic drugs (e.g., SSRIs) | *Avoid.* This combination can be fatal. |

*Less severe interactions with these drugs also occur with the RIMA (reversible selective inhibitor of MAO-A), moclobemide.
*MAOIs,* monoamine oxidase inhibitors; *SSRIs,* selective serotonin reuptake inhibitors; *TCAs,* tricyclic antidepressants.

such as norepinephrine, epinephrine, and isoproterenol should not trigger the release of existing norepinephrine. Moclobemide should not be combined with the irreversible MAOIs or with narcotics. Finally, MAOIs should not be given in combination with TCAs, except in unusually refractory cases, and never in combination with SSRIs.

The initial symptoms of hypertensive crisis are palpitation, tightness in the chest, stiff neck, and a throbbing, radiating headache. Extremely high blood pressure with elevation of the heart rate is common. Cardiovascular consequences have included myocardial infarction, cerebral hemorrhage, myocardial ischemia, and arrhythmias. Diaphoresis and pupillary dilation are also prominent signs.

Anticholinergic effects can be severe if other anticholinergic drugs are given with MAOIs. Typical anticholinergic side effects can be reviewed in the discussion of TCA side effects.

Finally, because MAOIs inhibit monoamine oxidase in the liver, some drugs, particularly CNS depressants, are not rapidly metabolized in the liver and result in serum levels high enough to depress the CNS seriously.

Meperidine (Demerol) is specifically contraindicated. A marked potentiation of this drug can occur, and deaths have been documented. Hypotensive drugs are also enhanced by MAOIs. The nurse should be aware that MAOI inhibition continues for up to 10 days after tranylcypromine and phenelzine are discontinued. In other words, the potential for serious interactions continues for some time after MAOIs are discontinued.

## Food-Drug Interactions

Food-drug interactions center on the amine tyramine, a decarboxylation product of tyrosine, the precursor to dopamine, norepinephrine, and epinephrine. Tyramine is found in many foods commonly consumed in the North American diet (Box 19-10). Aged cheese, bananas, salami, and coffee are a few foods containing tyramine that must be avoided by the patient. In fact, all high-protein foods that have undergone protein breakdown by aging, fermentation, pickling, or smoking should be avoided. Hypertension and hypertensive crisis can develop from this food-drug combination.

---

**Box 19-10    Tyramine-Rich Foods to Avoid With MAOIs**

**Alcoholic Beverages**
Beer and ale
Chianti and sherry wine
Alcohol-free beer

**Dairy Products**
All mature cheese: Cheddar, blue, Brie, mozzarella
Sour cream
Yogurt

**Fruits and Vegetables**
Avocados
Bananas
Fava beans
Canned figs

**Meats**
Bologna
Chicken liver
Fish, dried
Liver
Meat tenderizer
Pickled herring
Salami
Sausage

**Other Foods**
Caffeinated coffee, colas, tea (large amounts)
Chocolate
Licorice
Sauerkraut
Soy sauce
Yeast

---

## NURSING IMPLICATIONS

### Therapeutic Versus Toxic Drug Levels

An intensification of the effects already discussed occurs with overdose. A lethal dose of MAOIs is only 6 to 10 times the daily dose (see Table 19-1 for dosages). Careful monitoring when these medications are given is important. "Cheeking" and hoarding of these drugs can be disastrous. If MAOI overdose is indicated, the nurse should know the following:

- Emesis and gastric lavage might be helpful if performed early.
- Monitoring of vital signs is important.
- External cooling is warranted if high fever occurs.
- Hypotension should be treated in the standard manner.

## Use During Pregnancy

MAOIs should be avoided during the first trimester of pregnancy. Later use is justified only when the anticipated benefit outweighs the potential risk to the fetus.

## Use in Older Adults

MAOIs might be effective in older patients because monoamine oxidase activity increases with age (Bezchlibnyk-Butler and Jeffries, 2004). Precautions for orthostatic hypotension should, however, be observed in this age group.

## Side Effects

The nurse should be familiar with the common side effects of MAOIs and the appropriate nursing interventions (see the Side Effects and Nursing Interventions for MAOIs box).

---

### Side Effects and Nursing Interventions for MAOIs

| Side Effects | Interventions |
| --- | --- |
| CNS hyperstimulation | Reassure the patient. Assess for developing psychosis, hypomania, or seizures. If symptoms warrant, withhold the drug and notify the physician. |
| Hypotension | Monitor blood pressure frequently and intervene to prevent falls and injuries; having patient lie down might help return blood pressure to normal. |
| Anticholinergic effects | See antidepressant side effects for appropriate nursing interventions. |
| Hepatic and hematologic dysfunction | Blood counts and liver function test results should be performed. If dysfunction is apparent, MAOI should be discontinued. |

---

## Interactions and Contraindications

As noted, the nurse must understand that drug-drug and food-drug interactions are serious and potentially fatal. MAOIs should not be given in combination with:

- Other MAOIs
- TCAs or SSRIs
- Meperidine (Demerol)

Hypertensive crisis is a major concern. If it occurs, then the nurse should:

- Discontinue MAOIs and contact the physician.
- Know that therapy to reduce the blood pressure is warranted (e.g., an alpha-1 blocker).
- Monitor vital signs.
- Have the patient walk (which lowers blood pressure slightly).
- Manage fever by external cooling.
- Institute supportive nursing care, as indicated.

## Teaching Patients

The nurse must be persistent in teaching patients and their families about MAOIs and their side effects. Although most of these drugs are administered in a closely supervised setting, the nurse is nonetheless responsible for educating patients. Because patients taking MAOIs can experience serious reactions to some other drugs and foods, the nurse must clearly convey this information.

## APPLICATION OF ESTABLISHED DRUGS TO TREAT DEPRESSION

Mifepristone (Mifeprex), also known as RU-486, an early abortion drug, appears to be beneficial in the treatment of psychotic depression (i.e., delusional depression).

Testosterone might also have a role in treating depression. The idea to use testosterone came from the observation that many depressed men had low levels of testosterone, whereas many body builders who used testosterone to enhance muscle structure developed mania. Furthermore, these body builders became depressed when testosterone was no longer used. Male hormones might thus have limited benefits for some men suffering from depression (Miller, 2003).

## ▌Study Notes

1. According to the neurochemical theory, depression is the result of a decreased availability of the neurotransmitters norepinephrine, serotonin, and possibly dopamine in the brain.

2. The three major classes of antidepressants are SSRIs, TCAs, and MAOIs. An additional major group of agents that cannot be easily categorized are known as novel antidepressants.

3. SSRIs and TCAs block the reuptake of neurotransmitters back into nerve endings, thereby increasing their availability.

4. MAOIs slow the breakdown of these neurotransmitters by inhibiting the enzyme monoamine oxidase, thereby increasing the availability of these neurotransmitters.

5. SSRIs have fewer anticholinergic, antihistaminic, antidopaminergic, and antiadrenergic side effects than TCAs.

6. SSRIs are first-choice drugs for the treatment of depression.

7. SSRIs are highly bound to serum proteins and can displace other protein-bound drugs.

8. All SSRIs affect cytochrome P-450 metabolizing enzymes and the metabolism of other drugs metabolized by this system.

9. Newer novel antidepressants include bupropion, venlafaxine, and mirtazapine. These agents are first-line agents in the treatment of depression.

10. Common side effects of TCAs (e.g., dry mouth, blurred vision, constipation, tachycardia) are associated with their anticholinergic properties.

11. Because TCAs have a narrow therapeutic index, amounts even slightly higher than therapeutic doses can be fatal. TCAs account for approximately 7% of all deaths from intentional overdose.

12. Patients should be taught about the lag time of 2 to 4 weeks that is required for a full therapeutic effect to be experienced with TCAs.

13. MAOIs can cause central (stimulation), cardiovascular (hypotension), and anticholinergic system side effects.

14. Traditional irreversible nonselective MAOIs interact with certain foods that contain tyramine (e.g., aged cheese, bananas, salami) and with indirect- and mixed-acting sympathomimetic drugs (e.g., amphetamines, methylphenidate [Ritalin]) to cause hypertensive crisis. Reversible inhibitors of MAO-A (RIMAs) appear to have minimal interactions with foods containing tyramine.

15. MAOIs have a lag time of approximately 2 to 4 weeks.

16. Mifepristone and testosterone might have unique roles in the treatment of depression.

## References

Anand A, Charney NS: Norepinephrine dysfunction in depression, *J Clin Psychiatry* 61(Suppl 10):16, 2000.

Ayd FJ: The early history of modern psychopharmacology, *Neuropsychopharmacology* 5:71, 1991.

Bezchlibnyk-Butler KZ, Jeffries JJ: *Clinical handbook of psychotropic drugs,* Seattle, 2004, Hogrefe & Huber.

Cohen LS: Psychotropic drug use in pregnancy, *Hosp Community Psychiatry* 40:566, 1989.

Cozza KL, Armstrong SC: *The cytochrome P450 system,* Washington, DC, 2001, American Psychiatric Publishing.

Crutchfield DB: Review of psychotropic drugs, *CNS News Special Edition* 6:51, 2004.

Gomez GE, Gomez EA: The use of antidepressants with elderly patients, *J Psychosoc Nurs Ment Health Serv* 30:21, 1992.

Gumnick JF, Nemeroff CB: Problems with currently available antidepressants, *J Clin Psychiatry* 61(Suppl 6):5, 2000.

Hirshfeld RMA: History and evolution of the monoamine hypothesis of depression, *J Clin Psychiatry* 61(Suppl 1):4, 2000.

Jancin B: Toxicology shows antidepressants present in 21% of suicide completers, *Clin Psychiatr News* 33:6, 2005.

Keltner NL: Mechanisms of antidepressant action: in brief, *Perspect Psychiatr Care* 36:69, 2000.

Keltner NL, Hall S: Neonatal serotonin syndrome, *Perspect Psychiatr Care* 41:88, 2005.

Keltner NL, Folks DG: *Psychotropic drugs,* Philadelphia, 2005, Harcourt.

Keltner NL, McAffee K, Taylor C: Mechanisms and treatments for SSRI-induced sexual dysfunction, *Perspect Psychiatr Care* 38:111, 2002.

Lee SI, Keltner NL: Antidepressant apathy syndrome, *Perspect Psychiatr Care* 41:188, 2005.

Malone KJ, Papagni K, Ramini S, Keltner NL: Antidepressants, antipsychotics, benzodiazepines, and the breastfeeding dyad, *Perspect Psychiatr Care* 40:73, 2004.

Mendleson W: A review of the evidence for the efficacy and safety of trazodone in insomnia, *J Clin Psychiatry* 66:469, 2005.

Miller CM: New treatments for depression with psychosis, *Harv Ment Health Lett* 20:4, 2003.

Nemeroff CB: Paroxetine: an overview of the efficacy and safety of a new selective serotonin reuptake inhibitor in the treatment of depression, *J Clin Psychopharmacol* 13(Suppl 2):10, 1993.

Peck P: *FDA: Paxil linked to birth defects.* Available at: www.medpagetoday.com/ProductAlert/Prescriptions/tb/2293. Accessed February 24, 2006.

Stahl SM: Blue genes and the mechanism of action of antidepressants, *J Clin Psychiatry* 61:164, 2000a.

Stahl SM: *Essential psychopharmacology,* Cambridge, MA, 2000b, Cambridge Press.

Zimmermann PG: Tricyclic antidepressant overdose, *Am J Nurs* 97:39, 1997.

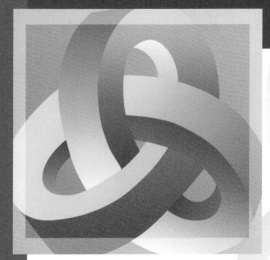

# Chapter 20

# Antimanic Drugs

*Norman L. Keltner*

## Learning Objectives

*After reading this chapter, you should be able to:*

- Explain the mechanism of action of antimanic drugs.
- Discuss the side effects of antimanic drugs.
- Identify therapeutic versus toxic serum levels of lithium.
- Describe potential interactions of antimanic drugs.
- Discuss the implications of teaching patients about antimanic drugs.

*Lithium has a unique and pivotal position in psychopharmacology. It preceded the introduction of chlorpromazine into psychiatry and in fact fired the first barrage that initiated the modern era of psychopharmacology.*

Soares and Gershon (2000, p 16)

**A**ntimanic drugs (or mood stabilizers) include lithium, anticonvulsants, and antipsychotics. No single drug or combination of drugs is always effective, however. The two poles suggested in the term bipolar are dysphoria (or depression) and euphoria (or mania). Although these extremes in emotions are seemingly opposite, they are related. This chapter will primarily focus on the psychopharmacologic classes of drugs used to treat the euphoric end of the bipolar spectrum, the antimanic drugs (Table 20-1). These drug classes include lithium, anticonvulsants, and antipsychotic agents.

There are three overarching treatment issues in treating bipolar disorder:

1. Getting acute mania under control
2. Preventing relapse once remission occurs
3. Returning to the prior level of functioning (i.e., social, occupational, interpersonal)

**Treatment Goals for Bipolar Disorder**
1. Remission
2. Prevention
3. Return to premorbid function

Treating acute symptoms is focused on helping the patient regain control. Box 20-1 lists the typical signs and symptoms associated with acute bipolar disorder (see Chapter 30 for full discussion of bipolar disorders). Maintenance therapy attempts to provide relapse prevention, reduce suicide risks, improve functioning, and reduce what are called *subthreshold symptoms* (symptoms not quite reaching a level of clinical diagnostic significance).

## LITHIUM

Lithium is considered the gold standard by many clinicians for the treatment of bipolar disorder. Lithium, a naturally occurring element, is not much different from sodium. The differences, however, are significant enough to make lithium useful in treating bipolar disorder. Lithium was

| Table 20-1 | Lithium and Anticonvulsants Used for Treatment of Bipolar Disorder |
|---|---|

| Antimanic Drug | Usual Adult Daily Dosage | Half-Life (hr) | Therapeutic Serum Level | Excretion | Common Side Effects | Warnings |
|---|---|---|---|---|---|---|
| Lithium | Acute: 600-1800 mg Maintenance: 900-1200 mg | ~24 | 0.6-1.2 mEq/L | 95% unchanged | N/V, diarrhea, polyuria, polydipsia, weight gain, tremor, fatigue | Lithium toxicity; teratogenicity |
| Carbamazepine | 800-1000 mg and titrated upward until side effects or serum level reached | 12-17; induces own metabolism | 4-12 mcg/mL | P-450 enzymes | N/V, dizziness, sedation, rash, HA | Blood dyscrasias; teratogenicity |
| Divalproex | 1000-1500 mg | 6-16 | 50-115 mcg/mL | P-450 enzymes | N/V, sedation, weight gain, hair loss | Hepatoxicity, teratogenicity, pancreatitis |
| Lamotrigine | Begin at 25-50 mg and increase by 12.5-25 mg a week, up to 250 mg bid | ~24 with chronic use | N/A | Attaches to glucuronic acid by conjugation | HA, sedation, cognitive dulling, insomnia, ataxia, N/V, dizziness, diplopia | Serious rash, e.g., Stevens-Johnson; breast-feeding? |
| Oxcarbazepine | 600-2400 mg in two or three divided doses | 7-20 with active metabolites | 15-35 mcg/mL | Metabolized to an active metabolite | Fatigue, N/V, dizziness, sedation, diplopia, hyponatremia | Teratogenicity; breastfeeding? |
| Gabapentin | 900-4000 mg in three divided doses | 5-7 | N/A | Not metabolized | Sedation, fatigue, tremors, nausea, dry mouth, dizziness, diplopia, hyperthermia | Teratogenicity; breast-feeding? |
| Topiramate | Acute: 200-600 mg Maintenance: 50-400 mg | 19-23 | N/A | 70% unchanged | Sedation, cognitive blunting, anxiety, tremors, weight loss, dizziness | Breast-feeding; cognitive dulling |

*HA,* headache; *N/V,* nausea and vomiting.
Modified from Bezchlibnyk-Butler KZ, Jeffries JJ: *Clinical handbook of psychotropic drugs,* Seattle, 2004, Hogrefe & Huber; and Keltner NL, Folks DG: *Psychotropic drugs,* St. Louis, 2005, Mosby.

discovered in 1817 and named after the Greek word for stone. It came to be touted as a cure for epilepsy, gout, and other problems. In 1949, an Australian, John Cade, reported his research in the *Medical Journal of Australia,* showing lithium to be effective in the treatment of manic depression. Of the manic patients he treated, all demonstrated considerable improvement (Soares and Gershon, 2000). Lithium's effect was so pronounced that Cade (1949) called the illness a "lithium deficiency disease" (McIntyre et al, 2001). In that same year, the March 12th issue of the *Journal of the American Medical Association* reported two accounts of fatal lithium poisoning in cardiac patients who were given lithium chloride as a salt substitute. These deaths led to a 20-year hibernation for lithium in this country (Ayd, 1991). Fears of lithium were compounded by a lack of interest on the part of

### Norm's Notes

*These drugs are a little more challenging. We have the gold standard, lithium, but the antiepileptic drugs are rapidly becoming first-choice agents, particularly divalproex. The trick for knowing the reason for antimanic treatment is to find the similarities in action of both the antiepileptics and lithium. How are these drugs slowing down manic thinking? If you can nail that down, then you are really beginning to learn about psychotropic drugs.*

---

Box 20-1    **Signs and Symptoms of Bipolar Disorder—Mania**

Elevated mood
Increase in activities
Flight of ideas
Racing thoughts
Inflated self-esteem
Decreased need for sleep
Agitation
More talkative than is usual
Pacing, hand wringing
Extreme restlessness
Loses temper often
Significant irresponsible behavior
Increased goal-directed activities (e.g., sexual, social)
Impaired excessive involvement in pleasurable activities, with high potential for painful consequences
Delusions
Hallucinations

---

drug companies. As a natural element, lithium is not patentable and, consequently, a drug company might invest research funds, only to have another pharmaceutical company legally use the findings (Ayd, 1991). Lithium was not made available in the United States until 1970.

Lithium is now used for the treatment and prophylaxis of the manic phase of manic-depressive illness. At one time, 80% to 90% of patients responded to lithium, but today only approximately 50% seem to respond (U.S. Surgeon General, 1999). It is not clear why fewer patients with bipolar disorders are responding to this drug today. Additionally, a growing body of clinical research supports its use as an antidepressant, for augmentation of other antidepressants in refractory depression, and for other disorders. Finally,

for reasons not yet understood, lithium seems to have a greater antisuicide effect than the other antimanic drugs (Dunner, 2004).

## PHARMACOLOGIC EFFECTS

Although exactly how lithium achieves its normalizing effect on mania is unknown (Phiel and Klein, 2001), theories have suggested that the lithium ion substitutes for the sodium ion in neurons. It has been said that the body cannot distinguish lithium from sodium. This exchange compromises the ability of neurons to release, inactivate, and respond to neurotransmitters; facilitates the reuptake of norepinephrine and serotonin into presynaptic terminals; and inhibits their release from these same neurons. Lithium also normalizes a dysfunctional second-messenger system (Manji and Lenox, 2000). This multistep system eventuates in activation of transcription factors that literally instruct genes on what proteins to synthesize (e.g., enzymes, receptors, neurotropic factors). In bipolar disorder, the second-messenger system is too active and lithium (and other antimanic agents) are thought to reset this system. Figure 20-1 (Clark et al, 1993) illustrates some basic mechanisms of action for lithium, although this explanation simplifies what is thought to occur. Lenox and Hahn (2000), after an in-depth review of lithium's mechanism of action, reduced its effect to ". . . the ability of the monovalent cation to uniquely alter signaling in critical regions of the brain."

Using El-Mallakh's (1996) model as an explanatory guide, the information just given can be expanded. Lithium can substitute for sodium, thus normalizing Na,K-ATPase pump activity, and it increases the number of sodium pumps. The net effect is a decrease in the intracellular sodium level, which creates a higher threshold for cell depolarization. Apparently, lithium also accelerates calcium removal from the neuronal terminal, thus normalizing calcium-dependent neurotransmitter release and synthesis, cytoskeletal remodeling, and neuronal excitability (Manji and Lenox, 2000). The overall effect is a reduction in neurotransmitter release. Gamma-aminobutyric acid (GABA) function, an inhibitory neurotransmitter system, is also enhanced (Bezchlibnyk-Butler and Jeffries, 2004).

In summary, it is not clear exactly how lithium is effective. However, at least four hypotheses have been advanced:

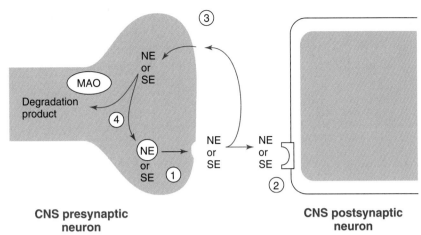

**CNS presynaptic neuron**

**CNS postsynaptic neuron**

**FIGURE 20-1** Depression results from an amine (e.g., norepinephrine [NE], serotonin [SE]) concentration that is too low to activate sufficient receptors; mania results from overabundance of amines acting at receptors. The biogenic amine theory of depression is applied to actions of antidepressant drugs, tricyclic antidepressants (TCAs), selective serotonin reuptake inhibitors (SSRIs), and monoamine oxidase inhibitors (MAOIs), and to the action of lithium, which is used to treat mania. *1,* Lithium inhibits release of norepinephrine and serotonin; *2,* TCAs and MAOIs increase receptor sensitivity to norepinephrine and serotonin; *3,* TCAs block reuptake of norepinephrine and serotonin, SSRIs block reuptake of serotonin, lithium enhances reuptake of norepinephrine and serotonin; *4,* MAOIs prevent degradation of norepinephrine and serotonin. (From Clark J, Queener S, Karb V: *Pharmacologic basis of nursing practice,* ed 4, St. Louis, 1993, Mosby.)

1. Lithium substitutes for sodium.
2. Lithium inhibits the release of and facilitates the reuptake of norepinephrine and serotonin.
3. Lithium regulates the Na,K-ATPase pump.
4. Lithium stabilizes the second-messenger system, thus regulating intracellular signaling.

---

### What Goes Wrong in Bipolar Disorder

What is known about bipolar disorder is that individuals have specific signs and symptoms (e.g., elevated mood, grandiosity, irritability, insomnia, anorexia). What is not known is exactly what causes this disorder to happen. Thus, the question remains: "What goes wrong in bipolar disorder?" El-Mallakh (1996) has proposed a convincing model for the pathology of bipolar disorder, suggesting that a disruption in ion regulation is the cause. Ion regulation is important for normal mood. A key part of ion regulation is the sodium (Na) and potassium (K)–activated adenosine triphosphatase (ATPase) pump. As this chapter explores, bipolar depression and mania are related, and this model proposes a biochemical explanation.

According to this model, both bipolar depression and mania result from a decrease in Na,K-ATPase activity. As activity declines, neuronal membranes become irritable, requiring fewer stimuli to provoke cell firing. Furthermore, as Na accumulates intracellularly because of this faulty pumping action, hyperpolarizing functions of inhibitory neurotransmitters (e.g., GABA) are diminished. Additionally, because neurotransmitter release is calcium dependent, the presynaptic terminals might release more neurotransmitter because of a related deficiency in Na-dependent calcium efflux. All these factors contribute to increased neurotransmitter release and firing—or mania.

However, the very term *bipolar* means two poles—the pole of mania and the pole of depression. These two poles are related. As the Na,K-ATPase pump continues to decrease in activity, neuronal irritability reaches a point whereby less stimulation triggers depolarization. The neuron fires more easily, but the action potential loses amplitude. Hence, this loss of amplitude causes calcium channels to decrease their activity and results in a subsequent reduction in neurotransmitter release. To summarize, mania is the first disorder to occur when ion dysregulation occurs, but as the Na,K-ATPase pump becomes more dysfunctional, the depressive side of bipolar disorder develops. Catatonia might be the ultimate expression of ionic dysregulation (El-Mallakh, 1996).

| Table 20-2 | **Pharmacokinetics of Antimanic Agents** | | | | |
|---|---|---|---|---|---|

| Drug | Absorption | Protein Binding | Active Metabolites | Half-Life |
|---|---|---|---|---|
| Lithium | 100% | 0% | None | 24 hours |
| Depakote | 100% | Up to 95% | Many | 6-16 hours |
| Olanzapine | >99% | 93% | None | 30 hours |

Modified from Keck PE: Pharmacokinetics and pharmacodynamics of antimanic and mood-stabilizing agents, *J Clin Psychiatry Visuals* 4:1, 2002.

## PHARMACOKINETICS

Lithium is well absorbed from the gastrointestinal (GI) tract and is therefore given orally (PO) in tablets, capsules, or concentrate. Peak blood levels are reached in 1 to 3 hours. The kidneys excrete more than 95% of the amount ingested unchanged. Lithium is not metabolized. Hence, renal disease lengthens the half-life, necessitating a reduction in dose. Lithium's typical plasma half-life is approximately 24 hours. The absorption and excretion of lithium and sodium are closely linked. Lithium is reabsorbed with sodium in the proximal tubule. Diuretics, particularly those affecting the loop of Henle and the distal tubule, lead to increased retention of lithium (Horne et al, 1991; Trimble, 1996). If dietary sodium intake increases, plasma lithium levels will likely drop, because lithium is excreted more rapidly. Conversely, if sodium in the diet decreases, or if sodium is lost in ways other than through the kidneys (e.g., sweating, diarrhea), lithium levels increase. These considerations are important; therapeutic serum levels need to be stable, because therapeutic levels of lithium are not much lower than toxic levels. Diet and activity levels should not change abruptly (Keck, 2002) (Table 20-2).

Lithium is effective in about 50% of cases; however, 7 to 10 days is required to achieve a clinical response. Lithium dosage is based on both clinical response and serum lithium levels. The typical dosage for acute mania is 600 mg three times per day, which usually produces a serum level of 1 to 1.5 mEq/L. Desirable maintenance blood levels are 0.6 to 1.2 mEq/L, which can be maintained on a dosage of 900 to 1200 mg/day. Blood levels higher than 1.5 mEq/L can be toxic, but moderate to severe toxicity typically develops only after blood levels exceed 2 mEq/L.

## SIDE EFFECTS

Lithium's side effects are linked to serum blood levels. Blood levels higher than 1.5 mEq/L can be considered toxic. Common side effects are nausea, dry mouth, diarrhea, and thirst. Drowsiness, mild hand tremor, polyuria, weight gain, a bloated feeling, sleeplessness, and lightheadedness are other relatively common side effects. Polyuria and polydipsia occur in up to about 70% of patients taking lithium (Maxmen et al, 2002). Side effects occur at therapeutic levels but usually decrease or cease after 3 to 6 weeks. However, these same side effects increase in severity at toxic serum levels.

Side effects unrelated to serum levels include weight gain, a metallic taste, headache, edema of the hands and ankles, and pruritus. Even at therapeutic levels, lithium can affect thyroid gland function. Approximately 30% of patients develop clinical hypothyroidism, with some needing levothyroxine (e.g., Synthroid) (Bezchlibnyk-Butler and Jeffries, 2004). Lithium can also impair the mental or physical abilities required for driving.

Lithium is generally contraindicated in people with cardiovascular disease. Lithium might also harm the fetus and is a U.S. Food and Drug Administration (FDA) category D drug (evidence of fetal risk has been established). Adverse reactions to toxic blood levels are discussed later. Lithium therapy is contraindicated for individuals with renal disease; if lithium is necessary, close supervision of these patients is recommended. Lithium-induced renal insufficiency (creatinine level consistently over 2 mg/100 mL) is apparently uncommon. However, nephrogenic diabetes insipidus develops in a significant number of patients taking lithium. Nephrogenic diabetes insipidus is caused by inhibition of the action of antidiuretic hormone (ADH) on the kidneys (specifically, the distal tubule and collecting duct cells). When ADH is blocked, the patient experiences polyuria (defined as urinating in excess of 3 L/day). The following clinical example highlights nephrogenic diabetes insipidus and the attempts to treat it.

## CRITICAL THINKING QUESTION    1

If a person taking lithium suffers from serious diarrhea, what will happen to the person's serum level?

## CLINICAL EXAMPLE

Mr. Jones, a 67-year-old man on the geropsychiatric unit, drinks approximately 4 L/day of water. He urinates more than 3 L/day. His creatinine level is 2 mg/dL. Mr. Jones is diagnosed with nephrogenic diabetes insipidus related to long-term lithium treatment. His potassium level is 3 mEq/L. He complains of shakiness, tremors, weakness, and general malaise. He is on daily fluid balance profiles. Treatment follows a stepwise approach:

1. Lithium is discontinued.
2. Potassium supplement is started.
3. Amiloride (Midamor) is begun to enhance ADH activity.

## INTERACTIONS

Familiarity with the drugs that can elevate lithium serum levels is essential. Diuretics (except acetazolamide [Diamox]) decrease lithium excretion and thereby elevate serum lithium levels. Indomethacin and other nonsteroidal antiinflammatory drugs (NSAIDs) reduce renal elimination of lithium, thereby increasing serum lithium levels. Switching to a low-salt diet after treatment commences also elevates serum lithium levels.

Some drugs and other agents decrease serum lithium levels and pose the problem of inadequate treatment and symptom exacerbation. Those that increase lithium excretion decrease lithium levels. Acetazolamide (Diamox), caffeine, and alcohol are included in this group.

Combining lithium with antipsychotic drugs or benzodiazepines is not uncommon. These drugs are ordered with lithium because of lithium's clinical response lag time of 1 to 2 weeks. Antipsychotic agents are prescribed to produce a tran-

quilizing effect until the lithium produces a clinical response.

In summary, diuretics and NSAIDs increase lithium serum levels and toxicity can result. A few other drugs and agents decrease lithium levels, and symptom breakthrough can occur.

## NURSING IMPLICATIONS

### Therapeutic Versus Toxic Drug Levels

Therapeutic serum lithium levels are 0.6 to 1.2 mEq/L. The optimal maintenance level is approximately 0.8 mEq/L (McIntyre et al, 2001). Serum levels higher than 1.5 mEq/L can cause adverse reactions. Typically, the higher serum levels correspond directly to the severity of the reaction. Mild to moderate toxic reactions occur at levels from 1.5 to 2 mEq/L, and moderate to severe reactions occur at 2 to 3 mEq/L. At serum levels higher than 3 mEq/L, multiple organs and organ systems might be involved, leading to coma and death (Sugarman, 1984). Serum levels should be monitored and not be allowed to exceed 2 mEq/L.

No antidote is available for lithium poisoning. Discontinuing the drug might be enough when supportive nursing care is available. Gastric lavage has been used successfully. Parenteral normal saline might provide enough volume and sodium to prevent major problems for serum levels lower than 2.5 mEq/L. For more severe lithium poisoning, forced diuresis or hemodialysis might be needed.

### Use During Pregnancy

Treating bipolar disorder during pregnancy is difficult. Cessation of lithium during pregnancy is suggested because of fetal cardiovascular malformation when lithium is taken in the first trimester and because of neonatal toxicity if taken thereafter. The occurrence of major congenital abnormalities for lithium-taking mothers is 4% to 12% and for pregnant women taking the anticonvulsant alternatives it is 2% to 4% (Bezchlibnyk-Butler and Jeffries, 2004). The risk of congenital abnormalities in the general population is 2% to 4% (Fact Sheet, 1998). Lithium is present in breast milk at 30% to 100% of the mother's serum level; therefore, postnatal treatment also poses problems.

| Therapeutic Serum Levels (0.6-1.2 mEq/L) | Mild to Moderate Toxicity (1.5-2 mEq/L) | Moderate to Severe Toxicity (2-3 mEq/L) | Severe Toxicity (>3 mEq/L) |
|---|---|---|---|
| Hand tremor (fine) | Diarrhea | Previous symptoms and: | Previous symptoms and: |
| Memory problems | Vomiting | Ataxia | Seizures |
| Goiter | Drowsiness | Giddiness | Organ failure |
| Hypothyroidism | Dizziness | Tinnitus | Renal failure |
| Mild diarrhea | Hand tremor (coarse) | Blurred vision | Coma |
| Anorexia | Muscular weakness | Large output of dilute urine | Death |
| Nausea | Lack of coordination | Delirium | |
| Edema | Dry mouth | Nystagmus | |
| Weight gain | | | |
| Polydipsia, polyuria | | | |

## Key Nursing Interventions   *for Patients Taking Lithium*

- Prepare the patient for expected side effects without instilling anxiety.
- Discuss the side effects that should subside (e.g., nausea, dry mouth, diarrhea, thirst, mild hand tremor, weight gain, bloatedness, insomnia, lightheadedness).
- Identify the side effects that require immediate notification of the physician (e.g., vomiting, severe tremor, sedation, muscle weakness, vertigo).
- Suggest taking lithium with meals to reduce nausea.
- Suggest drinking 10 to 12 glasses of water per day to reduce thirst and maintain normal fluid balance.
- Advise the patient to elevate the feet to relieve ankle edema.
- Advise the patient to maintain a consistent dietary sodium intake, but to increase sodium if a major increase in perspiration occurs.

### Use in Older Adults

Older adult patients can benefit from lithium but, because of the severity of side effects and adverse reactions, these patients must be assessed for renal function and dietary history. Most of the lithium-induced reactions are more likely in this age group. Serum levels of 0.4 to 0.8 mEq/L are appropriate for older patients.

### Side Effects

Because lithium has a narrow therapeutic index, serum lithium levels should be determined frequently. After the patient is stabilized, monthly or even less frequent serum level determinations are usually adequate. Blood levels are usually drawn before the first dose in the morning. However, the nurse should not rely on laboratory tests alone and should continue clinical evaluation of the patient. (See the Key Nursing Interventions for Patients Taking Lithium box.)

### Interactions

The nurse should help patients understand the basic mechanisms affecting serum lithium levels. Drug interactions that increase or decrease serum levels should be reviewed. The nurse must impress on patients the necessity for alerting all other health care providers to the lithium treatment, even though some patients might be reluctant to do so.

### Teaching Patients

The nurse should teach patients and their families the following (Box 20-2 provides a complete list of patient guidelines for taking lithium):

- Symptoms of minor toxicity, which include vomiting, diarrhea, drowsiness, muscular weakness, and lack of coordination
- Symptoms of major toxicity, which include giddiness, tinnitus, blurred vision, and dilute urine

- Side effects associated with lithium and the proper time to notify the physician
Avoidance of conception, because lithium might harm the fetus
- Avoidance of driving until stabilized on the lithium

---

## CRITICAL THINKING QUESTION    2

Johnny is a good basketball player. He is 23 years old and is taking lithium. Because Johnny perspires a great deal on the days he plays (approximately four times per week), his nurse is concerned about his serum levels being consistent. What is this nurse considering?

---

| Box 20-2 | Patient Guidelines for Taking Lithium |  |

To achieve a therapeutic effect and prevent lithium toxicity, patients taking lithium should be advised of the following:

1. Lithium must be taken on a regular basis, preferably at the same time daily. For example, a patient taking lithium on a three times daily schedule, and who forgets a dose, should wait until the next scheduled time to take the lithium, but should not take twice the amount at that time, because lithium toxicity could occur.
2. When lithium treatment is initiated, mild side effects such as a fine hand tremor, increased thirst and urination, nausea, anorexia, and diarrhea or constipation might develop. Most of the mild side effects are transient and do not indicate lithium toxicity. Additionally, in some patients taking lithium, some foods such as celery and butter fat have an unappealing taste.
3. Serious side effects of lithium that necessitate its discontinuance include vomiting, extreme hand tremor, sedation, muscle weakness, and vertigo. The prescribing physician should be notified immediately if any of these side effects occur.
4. Lithium and sodium are eliminated from the body through the kidneys. An increase in salt intake increases lithium elimination, and a decrease in salt intake decreases lithium elimination. Thus, the patient must maintain a balanced diet and salt intake. The patient should consult with the prescribing physician before making any dietary alterations.
5. Various situations can require an adjustment in the amount of lithium administered to a patient— for example, the addition of a new medication to the patient's drug regimen, a new diet, or an illness with fever or excessive sweating.
6. For determination of lithium levels, blood should be drawn in the morning approximately 8 to 12 hours after the last dose was taken.

---

## ANTICONVULSANTS

Although lithium is often the first drug prescribed for bipolar disorder, only about 50% of patients respond to it (U.S. Surgeon General, 1999). Approximately 80% of all individuals diagnosed with bipolar disorder also have one or more subsequent bouts with the disorder (Sanger et al, 2001). Because of the seriousness of bipolar disorder, researchers have diligently sought alternatives for patients who do not respond to lithium (Table 20-3). Anticonvulsant alternatives include valproates, carbamazepine, gabapentin, lamotrigine, oxcarbazepine, and topiramate.

### Valproates

Valproic acid (Depakene) and divalproex sodium (Depakote) have been used since the 1960s as antiepileptic agents. In 1995, these drugs were approved for the treatment of mania and are considered first-line agents. Valproates appear to be particularly effective for patients with a rapid cycling variant of bipolar disorder and for those with mania secondary to a general medical condition (Lennkh and Simhandl, 2000).

Advantages of the valproates are that they have a rapid onset, can be used initially without attempting lithium, and are well tolerated, with little effect on cognition. Disadvantages include

---

| Table 20-3 | Agents Used to Treat Bipolar Disorder |  |
|---|---|---|

| | |
|---|---|
| Lithium | *Tablets:* Lithotabs |
| | *Capsules:* Eskalith, Lithane, Lithonate, Carbolith |
| | *Long-acting forms:* Lithobid, Eskalith CR |
| Anticonvulsants | Carbamazepine (Tegretol) |
| | Divalproex sodium (Depakote) |
| | Gabapentin (Neurontin) |
| | Lamotrigine (Lamictal) |
| | Oxcarbazepine (Trileptal) |
| | Topiramate (Topamax) |
| | Valproic acid (Depakene) |
| Antipsychotics | Aripiprazole (Abilify) |
| | Clozapine (Clozaril) |
| | Olanzapine (Zyprexa) |
| | Quetiapine (Seroquel) |
| | Risperidone (Risperdal) |
| | Ziprasidone (Geodon) |

### How Valproates Work

Although the precise nature of the valproates' action is not known, three or four mechanisms might be responsible for their antimanic effect:

1. Increase in GABA either by decreasing GABA metabolism or reducing its uptake
2. Increased postsynaptic response to GABA
3. Increase in the resting membrane potential (the membrane is less irritable)
4. Suppression of calcium influx through specific calcium channels

Modified from Keltner NL, Folks DG: *Psychotropic drugs,* St. Louis, 2005, Mosby.

transient hair loss, weight gain, tremors, GI upset, and dose-related thrombocytopenia.

Bioavailability is approximately 100%, with up to 95% protein binding. The drug can be replaced at binding sites by other drugs such as carbamazepine or warfarin, causing toxic effects. Valproates have a half-life of 6 to 16 hours and reach a steady state in 2 to 5 days. Therapeutic serum levels are from 50 to 115 mcg/mL or levels consistent with their antiepileptic effects.

### Carbamazepine (Tegretol)

Carbamazepine is effective for most patients who do not respond to lithium or to the valproates; it also has a faster onset of action compared with lithium. Patients who are more likely to be unresponsive to lithium and who, in turn, do respond to carbamazepine, are patients with a rapidly cycling bipolar episode. Carbamazepine might, at times, be given in combination with lithium. The concept of kindling can be used to explain seizure activity in the brain, as follows. The effectiveness of carbamazepine might be related to its inhibition of kindling activity in the brain. In other words, just as kindling in the fireplace is the first step in building a fire, some abnormal brain activities might begin as kindling and then spread. Some water can dowse the fire when it first starts but is ineffective in the control of a raging fire. Carbamazepine's probable mechanism of action is related to normalizing sodium channel activity (and sodium influx), thus increasing the threshold of stimulation needed for cell firing. Carbamazepine's therapeutic antimanic serum levels are 8 to 12 mcg/mL.

Although generally well tolerated, side effects include nausea, anorexia, and occasional vomiting. Sedation and drowsiness are other relatively common side effects. The most serious potential side effect of carbamazepine is agranulocytosis. Complete blood counts should be determined weekly when this drug treatment is initiated.

Significant drug interactions with carbamazepine include antibiotics, other anticonvulsants, lithium, calcium channel blockers, and angiotensin-converting enzyme (ACE) inhibitors. Drugs that inhibit the cytochrome P-450 3A4 enzyme, such as the selective serotonin reuptake inhibitors (SSRIs), can cause toxic effects (Cozza et al, 2003).

### Lamotrigine (Lamictal)

Lamotrigine is approved for the prophylaxis of bipolar disorder. Its effectiveness in treating acute mania has not been substantiated by research at this time. Lamotrigine is also effective for the treatment of bipolar depression.

This drug works by manipulating the GABA system, thus inhibiting neuronal firing. Other mechanisms of action include blocking of voltage-gated sodium and calcium channels, further inhibiting neuronal conduction. Finally, lamotrigine is believed to inhibit the excitatory neurotransmitter glutamate.

Similar to the effects of most drugs, lamotrigine causes a number of side effects; however, one particular adverse reaction is especially noteworthy—lamotrigine-induced rash. Lamotrigine can cause somewhat moderate skin rashes (about 10% of patients) and the potentially fatal Stevens-Johnson syndrome (1% to 2% of children and 0.1% of adults). (One infectious disease physician has compared the Stevens-Johnson rash to patients who have been in a severe fire.) Patients should be encouraged to report rashes and nurses must assess for change in skin condition. Ongoing assessment is important, because it is difficult to differentiate between moderate and more serious rashes at onset.

### Oxcarbazepine (Trileptal)

Oxcarbazepine is structurally related to carbamazepine and has similar pharmacologic activity. However, this drug does not cause some of the more serious adverse reactions associated with carbamazepine. Oxcarbazepine is becoming a somewhat commonly prescribed agent for bipolar disorder. Therapeutic serum levels have been determined to be in the range of 15 to 35 mcg/mL.

### Gabapentin (Neurontin)

Gabapentin tends to be used in an adjunctive role and not as monotherapy. As an adjunctive agent, it is believed to be particularly effective if the patient also experiences anxiety. Similar to lamotrigine, gabapentin up-regulates the GABA system, blocks sodium and calcium voltage-gated channels, and inhibits glutamate (glutamate increases cell firing).

### Topiramate (Topamax)

Topiramate has a mechanism of action similar to gabapentin. It increases GABA activity, blocks voltage-gated sodium and calcium channels, and inhibits the excitatory neurotransmitter glutamate.

Interestingly, many patients report weight loss with this drug, the only anticonvulsant known to have this effect. However, whatever positive response this effect has among clinicians and patients is tempered by a cognitive dulling that some patients have reported (Antai-Otong, 2005; Aschenbrenner, 2004).

## ANTIPSYCHOTICS

Antipsychotics are discussed at length in Chapter 18. All atypical antipsychotics except clozapine (although it is effective) have been approved for the treatment of mania. These agents have proven effective for the treatment of bipolar disorder, both as monotherapy and as an adjunct to mood stabilizers. They are particularly beneficial for control of acute mania. A brief description of these drugs is given here.

### Olanzapine (Zyprexa)

Olanzapine is approved as monotherapy for acute and maintenance treatment of bipolar disorder. Studies have shown that olanzapine controls mania and acts as a mood stabilizer (Price, 2000; Sanger et al, 2001). This particular pharmacologic profile might reduce the risk of precipitating a depression after treatment for acute mania. Olanzapine is associated with significant weight gain in some patients.

### Risperidone (Risperdal)

Risperidone has been established as an effective agent for acute bipolar disorder. It does not cause as much weight gain as other mood stabilizers.

### Quetiapine (Seroquel)

Quetiapine has recently received recognition for treatment of bipolar disorders. It can control acute mania and rapidly cycling mania, and is used prophylactically.

### Ziprasidone (Geodon)

Ziprasidone has also recently received approval to be used for treatment of acute bipolar disorder. It causes little or no weight gain and is reported to be well tolerated (Keck et al, 2003).

### Clozapine (Clozaril)

Clozapine is very effective for the treatment and prophylaxis of acute mania; however, the same concern associated with its more conventional antipsychotic use remains problematic—that is, agranulocytosis. Hematologic monitoring is required.

### Aripiprazole (Abilify)

Aripiprazole, the newest antipsychotic, sometimes referred to as a third-generation agent, has also been shown to be effective in the treatment of bipolar disorder (Keck et al, 2003).

## OTHER TREATMENTS FOR BIPOLAR DISORDER

Several benzodiazepines (e.g., clonazepam [Klonopin], lorazepam [Ativan]), and calcium channel blockers (e.g., nimodipine, verapamil) have been used with some success in treating bipolar disorder (Keck and McElroy, 2002). Agitation, insomnia, and anxiety are probably treatable by the benzodiazepines. Finally, electroconvulsive therapy (ECT) has proven useful for bipolar disorder and was used effectively before the discovery of lithium and these other drugs (Geoghegan and Stevenson, 1949). ECT is particularly valuable for pregnant patients, who should avoid medication that is teratogenic (American Psychiatric Association, 2002).

## Study Notes

1. Antimanic or mood stabilizers are used to treat bipolar disorder (i.e., manic depression).
2. There are two overarching treatment concerns: (1) controlling the symptoms of acute mania and (2) maintenance treatment.
3. Goals of maintenance treatment are:
   a. Prevention of relapse
   b. Reduction of suicides
   c. Improvement of functioning
   d. Reduction of subthreshold symptoms
4. Lithium is a naturally occurring element that has been a mainstay of bipolar disorder treatment for over 50 years.
5. Other first-line agents used to treat bipolar disorder are anticonvulsants and antipsychotics.
6. Lithium alters intracellular conductance; the anticonvulsants act on the GABA system and sodium and calcium voltage-gated channels.
7. Clinically therapeutic serum levels of lithium are 0.6 to 1.2 mEq/L; at higher serum levels, serious or even fatal reactions can occur.
8. Common side effects of lithium include nausea, dry mouth, diarrhea, thirst, and mild hand tremor.
9. Lithium has a narrow therapeutic index and a lag time of 7 to 10 days.
10. Valproates are effective, have rapid onset of action, and are relatively well tolerated.
11. Carbamazepine has a more rapid onset compared with lithium and is generally well tolerated.
12. Other anticonvulsants, such as lamotrigine, oxcarbazepine, gabapentin, and topiramate, have proven effective in treating bipolar disorder.
13. Lamotrigine use must be accompanied by close assessment for skin rashes. Some of these rashes, such as the Stevens-Johnson syndrome, have proven fatal.
14. Topiramate causes weight loss and is also associated with cognitive dulling.

15. The antipsychotic drugs control the symptoms of acute mania and act as mood stabilizers (Tables 20-4, 20-5, and 20-6).

| Table 20-4 | Strategy for Treating Mania |  |
| --- | --- | --- |
| First-line treatments | Lithium + atypical antipsychotic Valproates + atypical antipsychotic Carbamazepine ECT | |
| *If inadequate response:* | Optimize the dosage of drugs being used. *Then, if needed:* Add or change mood stabilizer. *or* Add or change atypical antipsychotic. *or* Add lamotrigine. | |

*ECT,* Electroconvulsive therapy.
Modified from American Psychiatric Association: Practice guidelines for the treatment of patients with bipolar disorder, *Am J Psychiatry* 159(Suppl 4):16, 2002.

| Table 20-5 | Treatment Strategies for Bipolar Depression |  |
| --- | --- | --- |
| First-line treatments | Lithium or lamotrigine ECT | |
| *If inadequate response:* | Optimize the dosage of drugs being used. *Then, if needed:* Add another mood-stabilizer. *or* Add atypical antipsychotic. *or* Add antidepressant. | |

*ECT,* Electroconvulsive therapy.
Modified from American Psychiatric Association: Practice guidelines for the treatment of patients with bipolar disorder, *Am J Psychiatry* 159(Suppl 4):16, 2002.

| Table 20-6 | Basic Regimens for Treating Severe Versus Less Severe Bipolar Disorder |  |
| --- | --- | --- |
| Severe acute mania | Lithium or valproate + atypical antipsychotic | |
| Less severe acute mania | Lithium or valproate or atypical antipsychotic | |
| Maintenance Severely ill Less ill | Combination Monotherapy | |

## References

Antai-Otong D: Mitigating cognitive side effects associated with topiramate, *Perspect Psychiatr Care* 41:92, 2005.

American Psychiatric Association: Practice guidelines for the treatment of patients with bipolar disorder, *Am J Psychiatry* 159(Suppl 4):16, 2002.

Aschenbrenner DS: DRUG watch, *Am J Nurs* 104:29, 2004.

Ayd FJ: The early history of modern psychopharmacology, *Neuropsychopharmacology* 5:71, 1991.

Bezchlibnyk-Butler KZ, Jeffries JJ: *Clinical handbook of psychotropic drugs,* Seattle, 2004, Hogrefe & Huber.

Cade JF: Lithium salts in the treatment of psychotic excitement, *Med J Aust* 36:349, 1949.

Clark J, Queener S, Karb V: *Pharmacologic basis of nursing practice,* ed 4, St. Louis, 1993, Mosby.

Cozza KL, Armstrong SC, Oesterheld JR: *Drug interaction principles for medical practice,* Washington, DC, 2003, American Psychiatric Publishing.

Dunner DL: Correlates of suicidal behavior and lithium treatment in bipolar disorder, *J Clin Psychiatry* 65(Suppl):5, 2004.

El-Mallakh RS: *Lithium: actions and mechanisms,* Washington, DC, 1996, American Psychiatric Press.

Fact Sheet: Taking mood stabilizers during childbearing years, *NAMI Advocate* 19:16, 1998.

Geoghegan JJ, Stevenson GH: Prophylactic electroshock, *Am J Psychiatry* 105:494, 1949.

Horne MM, Heitz UE, Swearingen PL: *Fluid and electrolyte balance,* St. Louis, 1991, Mosby.

Keck PE Jr: Pharmacokinetics and pharmacodynamics of antimanic and mood-stabilizing agents, *J Clin Psychiatry Visuals* 4:1, 2002.

Keck PE Jr, McElroy SL: Clinical pharmacodynamics and pharmacokinetics of antimanic and mood-stabilizing medications, *J Clin Psychiatry* 63(Suppl 4):3, 2002.

Keck PE Jr, Versiani M, Potkin S, et al: Ziprasidone in Mania Study Group: Ziprasidone in the treatment of acute bipolar mania: a three-week, placebo-controlled, double-bind, randomized trial, *J Clin Psychiatry* 160:741, 2003.

Keltner NL, Folks DG: *Psychotropic drugs,* St. Louis, 2005, Mosby.

Lennkh C, Simhandl C: Current aspects of valproate in bipolar disorder, *Int Clin Psychopharmacol* 15:1, 2000.

Lenox RH, Hahn C-G: Overview of the mechanism of action of lithium in the brain: fifty-year update, *J Clin Psychiatry* 61(Suppl 6):5, 2000.

Manji HK, Lenox RH: The nature of bipolar disorder, *J Clin Psychiatry* 61(Suppl 13):42, 2000.

Maxmen JS, Ward NG: *Psychotropic drugs: fast facts,* ed 3, New York, 2002, WW Norton.

McIntyre RS, Mancini DA, Parikh S, Kennedy SH: Lithium revisited, *Can J Psychiatry* 46:322, 2001.

Phiel CJ, Klein PS: Molecular targets of lithium action, *Ann Rev Pharmacol Toxicol* 41:789, 2001.

Price PL: Olanzapine to treat the acute mania of bipolar disorder, *S D J Med* 53:523, 2000.

Sanger TM, Grundy SL, Gibson PJ, et al: Long-term olanzapine therapy in the treatment of bipolar I disorder: an open label continuation phase study, *J Clin Psychiatry* 62:273, 2001.

Soares JC, Gershon S: The psychopharmacologic specificity of the lithium ion: origins and trajectory, *J Clin Psychiatry* 61(Suppl 9):16, 2000.

Sugarman JR: Management of lithium intoxication, *Fam Pract* 18:237, 1984.

Trimble MR: *Biological psychiatry,* New York, 1996, John Wiley.

U.S. Surgeon General: *Mental health: a report from the Surgeon General,* Washington, DC, 1999, Department of Health and Human Services.

## Bibliography

Bezchlibnyk-Butler KZ, Jeffries JJ: *Clinical handbook of psychotropic drugs,* Seattle, 2004, Hogrefe & Huber.

El-Mallakh RS: *Lithium: actions and mechanisms,* Washington, DC, 1996, American Psychiatric Press.

Keltner NL, Folks DG: *Psychotropic drugs,* St. Louis, 2005, Mosby.

Maxmen JS, Ward NG: *Psychotropic drugs: fast facts,* ed 3, New York, 2002, WW Norton.

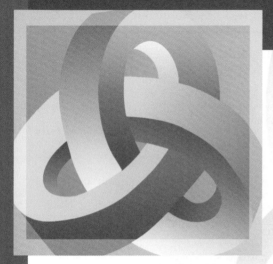

# Chapter 21

# Antianxiety Drugs

*Norman L. Keltner*

## Learning Objectives

*After reading this chapter, you should be able to:*

- Describe the differences between benzodiazepines and buspirone.
- Identify when benzodiazepines are indicated.
- Discuss the side effects of benzodiazepines.
- Identify benzodiazepines appropriate for older adults.
- Identify the specific antidote for benzodiazepine overdose.
- Describe potential drug interactions with benzodiazepines.
- Discuss the implications for teaching patients about antianxiety drugs.

*Case Example* (Keltner et al, 2003)*: Annie dreaded what would happen next—she had been down this road many times before. There she was, minding her own business, just wanting to watch a movie, like any normal person, when she noticed her breathing was off. Immediately she began to monitor her breathing and soon it seemed as if she just could not get enough air. She remembered a recent visit to the ER when the nurse patiently showed her that her oxygen saturation levels were good. She remembered, but it didn't help. It wasn't that she believed that this time was different, that this time she was going to suffocate. No, that might be a textbook explanation, but it wasn't her explanation. She just couldn't breathe, and knowing that "it was all in her head" just didn't seem to help. Soon she would be spiraling into symptoms that, like an Old Testament prophet, would beget more apprehension, which would beget more symptoms—palpitations, dizziness, a fear of fainting, trembling, feeling that things around her were unreal, fear of going crazy—which would beget more dread. Worst of all, she feared looking foolish. What if she lost control and started gulping big chunks of air down? What if she . . . ? What would they think of her?*

People have been seeking relief from anxiety since the beginning of recorded history. Alcohol is the oldest drug used to reduce anxiety, and has been used by countless millions to self-medicate fears, phobias, and nerves. In more recent times, other drugs have been developed to alleviate anxiety. In the early 1900s, bromo seltzers were advertised as having anxiolytic properties but had to be withdrawn from the market because of their addictive qualities (Harvey, 1985). In the 1930s and 1940s, barbiturates were heralded as having potential to treat anxiety, but they too were found to have many adverse effects, including seizures, dependence, addiction, and withdrawal.

The first drug specific for treating anxiety was meprobamate (Miltown, Equanil), developed in 1955 (Ayd, 1991). This drug, with its ability to calm nerves, to blur the reality of stressors and, in

## Norm's Notes

*Can you spell addiction? These are great drugs ("benzos") for a short while, but they can certainly be overprescribed and overused. They are very useful when you are really anxious, but almost anyone can get hooked on these drugs in a short time—and long-term use generally does not lead to anything good. Watch out for your patients, your friends, your family, and yourself. It could happen to your mom or dad. And, it can be hell to come off benzodiazepines.*

general, to make people feel better, was a national sensation. How it was received probably says far more about the American psyche than about the efficacy of meprobamate. Obviously, the United States was ready for a drug to buffer the stressors of a busy society. For several years, meprobamate was a widely prescribed medication but, similar to alcohol, bromo seltzer, and barbiturates, problems surfaced. Individuals using meprobamate were subject to abusing it, developed tolerance, and experienced lethal overdose. Its appeal as an antianxiety agent began to diminish. Fortunately, new agents to calm the trembling hands of a nation besieged with anxiety were waiting in the wings.

Before the end of the 1950s, another class of antianxiety drugs was developed—the benzodiazepines. These drugs had advantages over barbiturates in that they were less likely to be abused and were safer when overdoses occurred. Although first synthesized in the 1930s, benzodiazepines were not discovered to have a psychiatric effect until the late 1950s. Eventually, several thousand benzodiazepine derivatives would be synthesized, including familiar drugs such as diazepam (Valium), lorazepam (Ativan), alprazolam (Xanax), oxazepam (Serax), and clonazepam (Klonopin). However, these drugs were also linked to significant problems. Benzodiazepines were abused, induced tolerance, and implicated in lethal overdoses (although always when combined with other drugs). Over 10% of American adults have admitted using benzodiazepines (Ashton, 2000).

Clinical researchers and drug manufacturers continue to search for the perfect antianxiety drug, the drug that will ameliorate anxiety without significant adverse effects. A nonbenzodiazepine antianxiety agent that has been widely marketed is buspirone (BuSpar). Buspirone does not have the potential for abuse, dependency, and withdrawal associated with the benzodiazepines. The selective serotonin reuptake inhibitors (SSRIs) were developed in the late 1980s. These agents have emerged as a first-line treatment choice for anxiety. Because they are discussed in detail in Chapter 19, this chapter only presents a brief review.

A large group of unrelated drugs appear to have antianxiety properties, or at least have been found useful in the treatment of specific anxiety-like syndromes. Examples of drugs with antianxiety properties include some beta blockers (e.g., propranolol), antihistamines, monoamine oxidase inhibitors (MAOIs), tricyclic antidepressants (TCAs), clonidine (Catapres), phenothiazines, hydroxyzine (Vistaril), and opioids. A brief discussion of some of these is presented at the end of the chapter.

## MODELS OF ANXIETY

Anxiety and its causes are discussed in Chapter 31. Basically, three areas involving causative factors exist:

1. Autonomic system dysregulation
   a. Dysregulation of beta-adrenergic receptors
   b. Inhibition of gamma-aminobutyric acid (GABA) system
2. Neuroendocrine overactivity
3. Faulty thinking

The autonomic system overperforms when the person is anxious (Box 21-1, Figure 21-1). Studies have found that beta agonists, such as isoproterenol, cause anxiety (Keltner et al, 2003). The adrenergic autoreceptors, the alpha-2 receptors, also produce anxiety when blocked by drugs. On the other hand, alpha-2 agonists such as the antihypertensive clonidine have antianxiety properties. The extension of this thinking suggests that individuals with anxiety are believed to suffer

---

**Box 21-1   Autonomic (Noradrenergic System) Symptoms of Anxiety**

Tachycardia
Dilated pupils
Tremor
Sweating

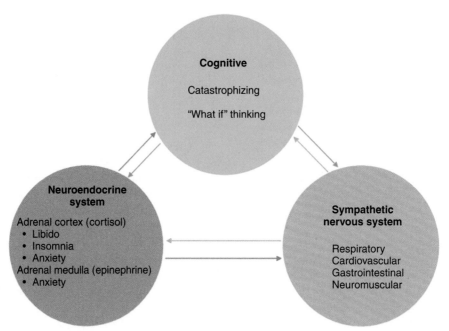

**FIGURE 21-1** Interacting systems of panic attacks. (From Keltner NL, Perrry BA, Williams AR: Panic disorder: a tightening vortex of misery, *Perspect Psychiatr Care* 39:38, 2003.)

from an alpha-2 autoreceptor underfunctioning, which causes the locus ceruleus, the site of norepinephrine synthesis in the brain, to overproduce norepinephrine. As will be seen later in this discussion, serotonin-enhancing agents play a major role in the treatment of anxiety, which is probably related to the putative modulation of adrenergic neurons by serotonin (Stahl, 2000).

GABA inhibition might play a role in anxiety because these neurons synapse with adrenergic neurons in the brain. As GABA inhibition is lifted, there is greater inhibition of the adrenergic system. This view is supported by the fact that GABAergic drugs such as the benzodiazepines decrease anxiety, whereas GABA receptor blockers such as flumazenil cause anxiety.

Increased levels of the hormone cortisol, which is secreted by the adrenal cortex in response to increased hypothalamic release of corticotropin-releasing hormone or increased anterior pituitary release of adrenocorticotropic hormone, are related to increased anxiety and insomnia.

People who suffer with anxiety, particularly those who suffer panic attacks, tend to engage in negative thinking. These negative thoughts (also known as *what if* or *catastrophic* thinking) can trigger anxiety. See Box 21-2 for the symptoms of panic attack.

---

**Box 21-2    Symptoms Associated With Panic Attacks**

Palpitations
Sweating
Trembling or shaking
Shortness of breath
Feeling of choking
Chest pain
Nausea and abdominal distress
Feeling dizzy, unsteady, lightheaded, faint
Derealization
Fear of losing control or going crazy
Fear of dying
Tingling sensations
Chills or hot flashes

Modified from American Psychiatric Association: *Diagnostic and statistical manual of mental diseases,* text revision, ed 4, Washington, DC, 2000, American Psychiatric Association.

---

## BENZODIAZEPINES

Although benzodiazepines are not considered first-line agents by psychiatric professionals, these drugs are still frequently prescribed by clinicians and are extensively discussed in this chapter. Many benzodiazepines are on the market. Table 21-1 presents information on benzodiazepines, includ-

| Table 21-1 | Benzodiazepines | | | | |  |

| Anxiety Drug | Usual Daily Dosage (mg/day) | Equivalent Dose (mg) | Half-Life (hr) | Anxiolytic Effect | Sedative Effect |
|---|---|---|---|---|---|
| **Benzodiazepine** | | | | | |
| Short-acting | Triazolam (Halcion), 01.25-0.5 | 0.25 | 2-5 | X | XXX |
| Intermediate-acting | Alprazolam (Xanax), 0.75-4* | 0.50 | 12-15 | XX | X |
| Intermediate-acting | Halazepam (Paxipam), 60-160* | 40 | 14-100† | XX | — |
| Intermediate-acting | Lorazepam (Ativan), 2-6* (P) | 1 | 10-20 | XXX | XX |
| Intermediate-acting | Oxazepam (Serax), 30-60 | 15 | 5-20 | XX | X |
| Intermediate-acting | Temazepam (Restoril), 10-60 | 10 | 10-15 | X | XXX |
| Long-acting | Chlordiazepoxide (Librium), 15-100* (P) | 25 | 5-30† | XX | — |
| Long-acting | Clonazepam (Klonopin), 0.5-10* | 0.25 | 18-60† | XX | X |
| Long-acting | Clorazepate (Tranxene), 7.5-60* | 10 | 30-100† | XX | — |
| Long-acting | Diazepam (Valium), 4-40* (P) | 5 | 20-80† | XXX | XX |
| Long-acting | Flurazepam (Dalmane), 15-30 | 15 | 3-150† | X | XXX |
| Long-acting | Prazepam (Centrax), 20-40* | 10 | 30-100† | XX | — |
| Long-acting | Quazepam (Doral), 7.5-30* | 7.5 | 30-150† | X | XX |
| **Nonbenzodiazepine** | Buspirone (BuSpar), 15-40* | N/A | 2-11† | XX | — |

*Given in divided doses.
†With active metabolites.
*X,* Mild effect; *XX,* moderate effect; *XXX,* strong effect; *N/A, not applicable; P,* parenteral form available.
Modified from Bezchlibnyk-Butler KZ, Jeffries JJ: *Clinical handbook of psychotropic drugs,* ed 16, Seattle, 2006, Hogrefe & Huber; Lieberman JA, Tasman A: *Psychiatric drugs,* St. Louis, 2000, WB Saunders; Keltner NL, Folks DG, *Psychotropic drugs,* ed 3, St. Louis, 2005, Mosby.

ing duration of effect, the usual adult daily dose, equivalent dose, elimination half-life, anxiolytic effect, and sedative effect. Historically, antianxiety agents have been referred to as anxiolytics or minor tranquilizers. Benzodiazepines are widely used by both psychiatric and general medicine patients (and might be prescribed more often by non–psychiatric clinicians). Major indications for benzodiazepines include chronic anxiety, time-limited treatment for crisis, presurgery jitters, and panic disorder.

Anxiety is a subjective experience, but can be observed by others (Box 21-3). The anxious person feels excessively alert, is easily startled, is restless, might talk too much, visually scans the environment, has tremors, and might have dilated pupils. Although many people use these drugs, as needed, benzodiazepines generally should not be taken for the stresses of everyday life. Benzodiazepines have no therapeutic value in the treatment of psychosis.

## HOW BENZODIAZEPINES WORK

Benzodiazepines enhance the effects of the inhibitory neurotransmitter GABA. GABA attaches to GABA receptors, which trigger the opening of chloride channels. Chloride has a hyperpolarizing effect on the neuron, which makes the neuron less

## Box 21-3 Subjective Symptoms of Anxiety Observable by Others

Patient might be:

- Anxious
- Apprehensive
- Compulsive
- Fearful
- Experiencing feelings of dread
- Irritable
- Intolerant
- Nervous
- Overconcerned
- Panicky
- Phobic
- Preoccupied
- Experiencing repetition in motor activities
- Feeling threatened
- Wound up
- Sensitive to shame
- Worried

responsive to excitatory neurons. The overall effect is one of slowing down or halting neuronal firing (Ashton, 2000). Neuronal inhibition is important, as important to brain function as the brake is to the operation of a car. Driving a car without brakes risks being involved in an accident. A brain without the inhibition of GABA can produce thought acceleration, autonomic dysfunction, excessive anxiety, panic, or even seizure activity or, to stretch the analogy, a runaway brain (Keltner et al, 2001; Sterling, 2001). Benzodiazepines help GABA tone down or inhibit the anxiety response to stressors.

GABA is a product of the Krebs cycle. It is synthesized by the decarboxylation of glutamate (i.e., the acid group of the amino acid glutamate is taken off), an amino acid produced from the Krebs cycle.

GABA receptors are located on approximately 40% of all neurons (Sugerman, 2005). GABA receptors are composed of five subunits and, on a particular receptor complex, these subunits can be arranged in any number of configurations (Seighart, 1995). The composition of these subunits determines the functional characteristics of the receptor (Löw et al, 2001). Because of these unique configurations, some GABA receptors are selective for specific ligands (molecules that bind to and evoke a response from the receptor). Spe-

cific subunit configurations exist for benzodiazepines—a benzodiazepine receptor site. When attaching to these receptor types, benzodiazepines enhance the effects of GABA. Benzodiazepine effects are dependent on endogenous GABA, and these drugs are inactive in the absence of GABA. In other words, the level of endogenous GABA limits the effect of benzodiazepine. Barbiturates, on the other hand, both enhance GABA and mimic GABA. Hence, barbiturates can cause profound central nervous system (CNS) depression and even death from overdose (Lehne, 2004; Williams and Akabas, 2000).

## PHARMACOLOGIC EFFECTS

Benzodiazepines have a generally depressing effect on the CNS, including the limbic system, the thalamus, the hypothalamus, and the reticular activating system (through which incoming sensory information is funneled). Benzodiazepines have five major effects (Ashton, 2000) that are used therapeutically to:

1. Reduce anxiety
2. Promote sleep
3. Relax muscles
4. Prevent seizures
5. Produce amnesia

Because benzodiazepines depress the reticular activating system, incoming stimuli are muted and evoke less reaction. To illustrate the concept of *muting,* two symptoms will be highlighted: hyperalertness and environmental scanning. The anxious person uses these defensive reactions to guard against an environment perceived to be threatening. The stressed out person might overreact to being startled because the body's system is on alert. As the antianxiety agent decreases environmental input, a general relaxing of the anxious posture takes place. The body's reactor is toned down and the environmental stressors are tuned out.

These drugs can cause several levels of CNS depression, from sedation to anesthesia. Benzodiazepines accomplish this by sedating the patient and depressing the inhibitory neurons that affect arousal. The latter effect causes a state of disinhibition, or loosening, of inner impediments to conduct. Disinhibition results in feelings of euphoria and excitement that, in turn, can lead to poor judgment. The natural restraint that minimizes social blunders is depressed.

To visualize the potential allure of benzodiazepines, one might imagine a tension continuum, with anxiety at one end and a carefree sense of being at the other. Benzodiazepines have the potential to move the anxious person from the agony of the anxiety end to the relaxed feeling of the carefree end. In therapeutic doses, this degree of shift from anxiety to disinhibition is not gained or sought but, because of the possibility of reaching a carefree zone, benzodiazepines have become drugs of abuse. Furthermore, many polysubstance abusers also use benzodiazepines because of their ability to increase the high of other drugs.

The inhibiting effect of benzodiazepines also accounts for their anticonvulsive activity. Intravenous diazepam (Valium) and lorazepam (Ativan) are first-line agents for status epilepticus, and clonazepam (Klonopin) is regularly prescribed orally as an anticonvulsant.

### Paradoxical Reactions to Benzodiazepines

A significant number of individuals (about 30% in some studies) have a paradoxical reaction to benzodiazepines (Gutierrez et al, 2001). These symptoms include agitation, emotional lability, and occasionally rage. Children, older adults, patients with poor impulse control, and individuals with organic brain syndrome are most at risk.

## PHARMACOKINETICS

Benzodiazepines are readily absorbed after oral ingestion; however, intramuscular administration produces slow and inconsistent absorption for most of these drugs (lorazepam [Ativan] is an exception). The benzodiazepines are highly lipid-soluble and therefore readily cross the blood-brain barrier. The benzodiazepines are metabolized by the liver but do not significantly induce their own hepatic metabolism (compared with barbiturates), and they are excreted in the urine. The active metabolites can exert an effect for up to 10 days. In fact, a convenient way of categorizing benzodiazepines is to divide them into those with short half-lives (20 hours or less) and those with long half-lives (longer than 20 hours). Of the selected benzodiazepines with short half-lives listed in Table 21-1, lorazepam (Ativan), oxazepam (Serax), and temazepam (Restoril) are preferable for use in older adults. Clorazepate (Tranxene), chlordiazepoxide (Librium), and diazepam (Valium) have long half-lives and therefore have an extended duration of action. Accordingly, these drugs are not suited for use in older patients.

However, considering only the half-life is misleading. An important factor in half-life determination over time is the metabolic process that each benzodiazepine undergoes. Most benzodiazepines are oxidized in the liver to active metabolites but, because hepatic function and hepatic volume change with age, the liver becomes less efficient at metabolizing these drugs over a lifetime. For instance, the half-life of diazepam is approximately 20 hours in a young man but stretches to 80 hours in a man 80 years of age. On the other hand, a few benzodiazepines (e.g., lorazepam, oxazepam, and temazepam) rely on conjugation with glucuronic acid to form inactive metabolites (Keltner and Folks, 2005). This process is not significantly affected by the aging process. Because the half-lives of these drugs remain fairly stable throughout life, and because these drugs have no active metabolites, they are better suited for use in older adults.

Hepatic metabolism is the primary mechanism for drug disposition. Thus, drugs that interfere with liver metabolism (e.g., alcohol) dangerously compound the effect of benzodiazepines.

## SIDE EFFECTS

Commonly, CNS side effects such as drowsiness, fatigue, and decreased coordination are exhibited. A certain mental impairment and slowing of reflexes also occurs. Less frequently, confusion, depression, and headache might be present. Peripheral nervous system (PNS) effects include occasional constipation, double vision, hypotension, incontinence, and urinary retention. Benzodiazepines can exacerbate narrow-angle glaucoma. Older adults with impaired liver or renal function and individuals who are debilitated experience increased side effects and, consequently, should receive a decreased amount of these drugs (see Side Effects and Nursing Interventions for Benzodiazepines box and discussion of pharmacokinetics).

## Side Effects and Nursing Interventions for Benzodiazepines

| Side Effects | Interventions |
|---|---|
| Dry mouth | Advise rinsing mouth with water often, eating sugarless hard candies, and chewing sugarless gum. |
| Ataxia | Provide assistance with ambulation. |
| Dizziness, drowsiness | Assist with ambulation and with getting in and out of bed. Caution about driving. |
| Nausea | Take with food. |
| Withdrawal symptoms (increased anxiety, influenza-like symptoms, tremors) | Contact prescriber. |

## DEPENDENCE, WITHDRAWAL, AND TOLERANCE

In addition to the undesired effects listed above are the triple problems of dependence, withdrawal, and tolerance.

### Dependence

Dependence can be defined as a state in which the body functions normally when the drug is present. The body, in turn, functions abnormally when the drug is absent. Dependence can develop within a few weeks or months of regular use. When benzodiazepine is withdrawn from the dependent person, symptoms such as agitation, tremor, irritability, insomnia, vomiting, sweating, and even convulsions might be experienced. Ashton (2000) has described three types of benzodiazepine dependence:

1. *Therapeutic dose dependence.* These individuals take the drug as prescribed but develop a need for the drug; they have outgrown the original reason for their taking the drug but now need it to get through the day.
2. *Prescribed high-dose dependent.* These individuals are still taking prescribed benzodiazepines but have talked their doctor into escalating the dose. Sometimes, these individuals are receiving prescriptions from more than one clinician.
3. *Recreational benzodiazepine abuse.* These individuals use benzodiazepines outside the traditional medical system. Benzodiazepines are often used

to enhance the effects of other abused substances. Typically, the amount of drug used is significantly greater than the amount prescribed for medicinal purposes. For example, a high-end dose of diazepam is 40 mg/day, but recreational abusers often ingest 100 mg daily. Some abusers take benzodiazepines intravenously.

### Withdrawal

Abrupt withdrawal from benzodiazepines can cause troublesome to serious effects. For example, agitation, tremor, irritability, insomnia, vomiting, sweating, convulsions, and even psychotic episodes have occurred. Thus, gradual tapering of the dose is imperative. Because GABA is an inhibitory neurotransmitter, releasing the inhibition results in the *taking off the brake* phenomenon. Because long-term use of benzodiazepines reduces the number of GABA receptors, an abrupt discontinuation of these drugs leaves the brain unable to fulfill inhibitory functions (Ashton, 2000). Hence, the adverse effects previously mentioned occur. The tapering or withdrawal process is highly individual and can take up to 1 year or longer in some heavily dependent individuals. Table 21-2 provides a more complete list of withdrawal symptoms.

### Tolerance

Tolerance to the effects of benzodiazepines occurs, so individuals need an increasing amount of the drug to achieve the same effect. Tolerance to sedation develops fairly quickly (within weeks), whereas tolerance to antianxiety effects occurs somewhat slowly (over a few months). Anticonvulsive tolerance also develops slowly, so the use of benzodiazepines for epilepsy is probably ill advised for most patients. Cognitive and memory effects appear to continue as long as these agents are used (Ashton, 2000). In review, tolerance develops to some of the desired effects of benzodiazepines (i.e., hypnotic, anxiolytic, anticonvulsive effects), although tolerance does not appear to develop to the unwanted effects of cognitive and memory deficits.

## INTERACTIONS

Benzodiazepines are CNS depressants and interact *additively* with other CNS depressants. Alcohol, TCAs, opioids, antipsychotics, and antihistamines increase the sedative effects of benzodiazepines.

| Table 21-2 | Symptoms Emerging After Withdrawal From Benzodiazepines |
|---|---|

| Neurologic | Gastrointestinal | Psychiatric | Other |
|---|---|---|---|
| Convulsions | Nausea | Anxiety | Tachycardia |
| Insomnia | Vomiting | Irritability | Sweating |
| Lightheadedness | Diarrhea | Cognitive | |
| Involuntary movements | Weight loss | Memory impairment | |
| Headache | Decreased appetite | Depression | |
| Weakness | | Confusion | |

| Table 21-3 | Major Interactions With Benzodiazepines |
|---|---|

| Interactant | Interaction |
|---|---|
| Alcohol and other CNS depressants | Increased sedation, CNS depression |
| Antacids | Impaired absorption rate of benzodiazepine |
| Disulfiram (Antabuse) and cimetidine (Tagamet) | Increased plasma level of benzodiazepines that are oxidized |
| Phenytoin | Increased anticonvulsant serum level |
| TCAs | Increased sedation, confusion, impaired motor function |
| MAOIs | CNS depression |
| Succinylcholine | Decreased neuromuscular blockage |

*CNS*, Central nervous system; *TCAs*, tricyclic antidepressants; *MAOIs*, monoamine oxidase inhibitors.

Furthermore, the common drink, grapefruit juice, can also cause problems, because it inhibits the cytochrome P-450 3A4 enzyme, thus extending the life of several benzodiazepines (Keltner and Opara, 2002). Table 21-3 lists major interactants for the benzodiazepines.

## NURSING IMPLICATIONS

### Therapeutic Versus Toxic Drug Levels

Benzodiazepines taken alone are relatively safe drugs. Overdoses hundreds of times higher than a therapeutic dose have been reported without resulting in death. However, if benzodiazepines are combined with other drugs, such as alcohol, the effect can be fatal. Signs and symptoms of overdose include somnolence, confusion, coma, diminished reflexes, and hypotension. Effective treatment begins with emptying the stomach by induced vomiting and gastric lavage, followed by activated charcoal. The nurse should monitor blood pressure, pulse, and respirations and provide supportive care as indicated.

### Benzodiazepine Receptor Antagonist

Flumazenil (Romazicon) blocks the benzodiazepine-binding site on the GABA receptor. It selec-

tively blocks benzodiazepine receptors but does not block adrenergic or cholinergic receptors. Thus, because flumazenil does not stimulate the CNS and does not block other receptors, it can usually be given when benzodiazepine overdose is suspected without fear of unexpected interactions. A response to flumazenil typically occurs within 30 to 60 seconds. Two important considerations when giving flumazenil are that (1) it does not speed up the metabolism or excretion of benzodiazepines and (2) it has a short duration of action. These considerations present a clinical management problem. If the patient responds to flumazenil, then benzodiazepines are present, but because flumazenil does not speed up metabolism and has a short duration of action, the patient might recover only to return to a preflumazenil state. This problem requires constant vigilance by the nurse and repeated doses of flumazenil as the body eliminates the benzodiazepine from the system. Furthermore, flumazenil might not reverse benzodiazepine-induced respiratory depression and can precipitate seizures (Lehne, 2004).

### Use During Pregnancy

The association of benzodiazepine use and fetal abnormalities has not been not supported (Maxmen and Ward, 2002). Some concern exists that benzodiazepines might be associated with cleft lip and cleft palate in the first trimester, but the evidence has been inconclusive. Even these findings, however, might warrant discontinuance during pregnancy. Furthermore, floppy infant syndrome has been associated with benzodiazepine use during labor (Malone et al, 2004). Benzodiazepines are also known to be found in breast milk, so nursing mothers must be cautious about their usage (Hale, 2002). However, if the drug cannot be discontinued without exacerbation of symptoms, then tapering to the lowest possible dose is desirable, as is the use of shorter acting agents such as alprazolam or lorazepam (Malone et al, 2004).

### Use in Older Adults

As mentioned in the pharmacokinetic discussion, specific benzodiazepines are acceptable for use in older adults, but most are not recommended. This dichotomy is based on metabolic processes. Lorazepam (Ativan) and oxazepam (Serax) are considered to be the best benzodiazepines for older individuals. Temazepam (Restoril), and occasionally alprazolam (Xanax), are also used in this age group. The other benzodiazepines, including diazepam (Valium) and chlordiazepoxide (Librium), have extended half-lives and active metabolites and should not be routinely prescribed for older patients.

### Side Effects

The most common side effects are related to sedation and mental alertness. The patient should be cautioned about driving or operating hazardous machinery. Tolerance to sedation quickly develops. Blood pressure should be monitored routinely, and a 20–mm Hg drop of the systolic level while the patient is standing warrants withholding the drug and notifying the physician.

### Interactions

Benzodiazepines interact with a number of CNS depressants. The nurse should explain this carefully to patients who are taking benzodiazepines. A high percentage of psychiatric patients abuse drugs, so a real potential exists for deadly combinations to be taken. It is also likely that these patients will develop a cross-tolerance to hepatic-metabolized drugs. For example, individuals who develop a

tolerance to alcohol have an increased tolerance to diazepam but not when alcohol and diazepam are taken together. Hearing a patient who is experienced in taking diazepam speak with disdain about typical doses is not uncommon—for example, "Ten mg of Valium doesn't even touch me!" Although diazepam alone might not touch these patients, diazepam combined with alcohol *will*. The nurse should remind these patients that if they mix diazepam with alcohol, they might die.

### Teaching Patients

Patient education is important because benzodiazepines have tremendous potential for abuse or misuse. Consequently, teaching patients and their families about these drugs is important. The nurse should teach the following:

- Benzodiazepines are not intended for the minor stresses of everyday life.
- Over-the-counter drugs might enhance the actions of benzodiazepines.
- Certain herbal preparations such as kava and valerian cause an additive effect.
- Driving should be avoided until tolerance develops.
- The prescribed dose should not be exceeded.
- Alcohol and other CNS depressants exacerbate the effects of benzodiazepines.
- Hypersensitivity to one benzodiazepine might mean hypersensitivity to another.
- These drugs should not be stopped abruptly.

## SELECTED BENZODIAZEPINES

### Alprazolam

Alprazolam (Xanax) is particularly useful for generalized anxiety, adjustment disorders, panic disorder, and anxiety associated with depression. It is also prescribed as an antitremor agent. Alprazolam has been criticized for its potential to cause addiction and dependence and there have been reports of alprazolam-induced violent or aggressive behavior (Glod, 1992; Shelton, 1993). Little risk exists of accumulation of alprazolam during repeated dosing.

### Chlordiazepoxide

Chlordiazepoxide (Librium) is prescribed for anxiety disorders, the relief of the symptoms of anxiety, and acute alcohol withdrawal. Chlordiazepoxide is absorbed well orally. Additionally, chlordiazepoxide can be used as an antitremor agent. Parenteral chlordiazepoxide is used as an antipanic agent. Accumulation occurs with this drug.

## Clonazepam

Clonazepam (Klonopin) is used most often as an anticonvulsant but also has clinical use in the treatment of panic disorder. Clonazepam alone or as an adjunct is useful in the treatment of Lennox-Gastaut syndrome (a petit mal variant) and akinetic, absence, and myoclonic seizures. Patients taking clonazepam over the long term should be slowly tapered off this drug, because evidence suggests that abrupt withdrawal can precipitate status epilepticus. Clonazepam is also used for benzodiazepine withdrawal (Keltner and Folks, 2005).

## Diazepam

Diazepam (Valium) is an often prescribed antianxiety agent that has multiple uses related to its CNS-depressing effect. In addition to treating anxiety disorders and providing short-term relief from symptoms of anxiety, diazepam is used preoperatively to relieve presurgery jitters, for skeletal muscle spasms (e.g., lower back pain), as a drug of choice (IV) for status epilepticus, and as an adjunct for endoscopic procedures. Additionally, diazepam might be useful for symptomatic relief of alcohol withdrawal.

## Lorazepam

Lorazepam (Ativan) is used to treat anxiety disorders and also can be used as an antitremor agent, antipanic agent, anticonvulsant (parenteral only), and antiemetic for cancer patients undergoing chemotherapy. The metabolites of lorazepam are inactive, so the effects of this drug do not persist. Patients with impaired liver function can handle this drug better than most other benzodiazepines, because lorazepam is metabolized to inactive metabolites. Lorazepam is recommended for use in older patients when a benzodiazepine is indicated.

## Oxazepam

Oxazepam (Serax) is similar to lorazepam in that its metabolite is inactive and it is metabolized by

a conjugative reaction. Thus, the drug is effective for a relatively short time (24 hours) and is suitable for patients with liver disorders and for older adults. Oxazepam is used for anxiety associated with depression and relief from acute alcohol withdrawal.

## NONBENZODIAZEPINE: BUSPIRONE

Buspirone (BuSpar) is a first-line agent for anxiety. It is not a benzodiazepine and does not bind to benzodiazepine recognition sites but probably acts as an agonist at the presynaptic serotonin 1A receptor. Considerable interest exists in buspirone because it differs from benzodiazepines in several important ways. Advantages of buspirone are that it:

- Is not sedating
- Does not cause a high, so has almost no abuse potential
- Has no cross-tolerance with sedatives or alcohol
- Does not produce dependence, withdrawal, or tolerance

The disadvantage of buspirone is that it:

- Has a delayed onset of antianxiety effect compared with benzodiazepines (1 to 6 weeks)

Buspirone's effects help distinguish anxiety control from the sedative and euphoric actions of older benzodiazepines. Buspirone is particularly effective in reducing symptoms of worry, apprehension, difficulties with concentration and cognition, and irritability. These subjective symptoms are probably more serotonin-based than the more physical symptoms of anxiety (Stahl, 2000). Buspirone does not depress the CNS, and its lack of a sedative effect makes buspirone less attractive for abuse. Because it has no abuse potential, buspirone is not a controlled substance.

Buspirone provides relief from anxiety within 7 to 10 days, but *maximal* therapeutic gain is not achieved until 3 to 6 weeks after treatment is initiated. Buspirone has a relatively short half-life, so it is usually given in divided doses. Buspirone is extensively metabolized after the first pass; as little as 1% to 4% becomes bioavailable. Foods increase its bioavailability by decreasing first-pass metabolism. Side effects include dizziness, nausea,

| Table 21-4 | Antidepressants Indicated for Anxiety | | |
|---|---|---|---|

| Agent | Class | Dosage Range (mg/day) | Comment (FDA Approval) |
|---|---|---|---|
| Clomipramine (Anafranil) | SRI | 100-250 | Approved for OCD; 250 mg is the maximum dose because of increased risk of seizures |
| Escitalopram (Lexapro) | SSRI | 10-20 | Approved for GAD |
| Fluvoxamine (Luvox) | SSRI | 100-300 | Approved for OCD |
| Paroxetine (Paxil) | SSRI | 40-60 | Approved for panic, OCD, social anxiety, GAD (maximum 50 mg/day), PTSD (maximum 50 mg/day) |
| Sertraline (Zoloft) | SSRI | 50-200 | Approved for panic, OCD, PTSD |
| Venlafaxine (Effexor XR) | SNRI | 75-225 | Approved for generalized anxiety; 150- and 225-mg doses are superior (possibly because of more potent norepinephrine reuptake blockade) |
| Fluoxetine (Prozac) | SSRI | 20-80 | Approved for OCD, panic disorder (maximum 60 mg/day) |

*FDA,* U.S. Food and Drug Administration; *OCD,* obsessive-compulsive disorder; *PTSD,* posttraumatic stress disorder; *SNRI,* selective serotonin-norepinephrine reuptake inhibitor; *SRI,* serotonin reuptake inhibitor; *SSRI,* selective serotonin reuptake inhibitor.
From Keltner NL, Folks DG: *Psychotropic drugs,* ed 3, St. Louis, 2005, Mosby.

headache, nervousness, light-headedness, and excitement. Buspirone is a remarkably safe drug and has few drug interactions.

The nursing student should note that, when switching from a benzodiazepine to buspirone, the benzodiazepine should not be stopped immediately. Because of dissimilarities in their pharmacologic properties, benzodiazepines must be tapered (to prevent withdrawal effects) while buspirone is initiated.

## SELECTIVE SEROTONIN REUPTAKE INHIBITORS

SSRIs are first-line agents for anxiety spectrum disorders, are discussed in detail in Chapter 19, and will only be briefly mentioned here. The fact that these drugs work so well in treating anxiety underscores the overlapping nature of depression and anxiety. SSRIs are prescribed for generalized anxiety disorder (GAD), obsessive-compulsive disorder (OCD), panic attacks, posttraumatic stress disorder (PTSD), and social phobias. OCD is perhaps the most difficult mental disorder to treat satisfactorily. Several SSRIs are considered first-line approaches to the treatment of OCD (Table 21-4). Specifically, fluoxetine (Prozac), fluvoxamine (Luvox), paroxetine (Paxil), and sertraline (Zoloft) are approved for treatment of this disor-

der. SSRIs are probably the most effective, as well as the safest, agents for the prophylaxis and long-term treatment of panic attacks (Black et al, 1993). GABA receptors are thought to be involved in the pathophysiology of panic disorders. It has been theorized that the overwhelming anxiety associated with panic might stem from abnormal serotonin transmission (Sterling, 2001). Saito (2001) has noted that SSRI effectiveness in panic and other anxiety disorders can be partially explained by serotonin's role in up-regulating GABA transmission in the prefrontal cortex. By up-regulating inhibitory neurons, a more inhibitory effect can be expected. This hypothesis agrees with what we know about symptoms of anxiety.

### Venlafaxine

Venlafaxine (Effexor, Effexor XR), a selective serotonin-norepinephrine reuptake inhibitor (SNRI), is approved for GAD and was the first drug approved for both GAD and major depression. This agent offers a dual approach to treatment because it blocks the reuptake of both serotonin (at lower doses) and norepinephrine (at medium to higher doses). Doses at the higher range are believed to be more effective, possibly because of the increased norepinephrine reuptake inhibition at that range.

Table 21-5 outlines pharmacologic interventions for specific anxiety disorders.

## Table 21-5  Pharmacologic Interventions for Specific Anxiety Disorders

| Disorder | Pharmacologic Treatment |
| --- | --- |
| **Panic Disorder** | |
| Exhibited as discrete and intense period of anxiety, apprehension, and distress | SSRIs are perhaps the safest for long-term and prophylactic doses; gradual titration to sertraline 50 mg qd or paroxetine 40 mg qd have proven to be minimum effective dosages. |
| Associated symptoms include palpitations, sweating, trembling, and dyspnea | Benzodiazepines: Clonazepam (average dosage 1.5 mg/day) and alprazolam (average dosage 3 mg/day) can provide more immediate relief. |
| | TCAs: Same dosage as that used in treating depressive syndromes, but dose level should be carefully titrated because of risk of a paradoxical effect. |
| **Phobic Disorder** | |
| *Agoraphobia* | |
| Fear of being away from home or in situations in which escape is inhibited | Alprazolam at the relatively high dosage of 3 to 6 mg/day has proven effective. |
| | TCAs: Dosage typically between 150 and 200 mg/day. |
| | SSRIs and highly serotonergic TCAs (e.g., clomipramine, amitriptyline, trazodone) are effective for agoraphobia. |
| *Social Phobia* | |
| Persistent fears of situations in which the person is exposed to the scrutiny of others (e.g., stage fright) | Beta blockers are often taken in combination with antidepressants or benzodiazepine; propranolol 10 to 20 mg tid or qid. |
| | Benzodiazepines alone or in combination with antidepressants. Clonazepam: 0.5 mg bid. |
| | SSRIs: Low doses initially. |
| **Obsessive-Compulsive Disorder** | |
| Obsessions, compulsions, or both | Clomipramine: 100 to 200 mg/day. |
| | Fluvoxamine: 200 to 300 mg/day. |
| | Other SSRIs or gabapentin (Neurontin) titrated to 1800 to 2400 mg/day. |

*bid,* Twice a day; *qd,* every day; *qid,* four times a day; *SSRIs,* selective serotonin reuptake inhibitors; *TCAs,* tricyclic antidepressants; *tid,* three times a day.

## OTHER DRUGS WITH ANTIANXIETY PROPERTIES

### Clomipramine and Other Tricyclic Antidepressants

Clomipramine (Anafranil) is one of two drugs (the other is the SSRI, fluvoxamine [Luvox]) considered most effective for OCD. Clomipramine is a serotonin reuptake inhibitor (SRI), although it is not as potent as the more traditional SSRIs. The major central side effects of clomipramine include headache, reduced libido, nervousness, myoclonus, and increased appetite. Peripheral effects include dry mouth, constipation, ejaculation failure (42%), erectile dysfunction (20%), and weight gain (Keltner

and Folks, 2005). Imipramine (Tofranil) and desipramine (Norpramin) have proven to be effective for panic-anxiety attacks. Trazodone (Desyrel) has a highly sedative quality and is often prescribed for individuals who are experiencing anxiety, particularly older adults, to facilitate sleep.

### Clonidine

Clonidine (Catapres) is an alpha-2 agonist. Because agonistic stimulation of autoreceptors such as alpha-2 cause a decrease in neurotransmitter production, it follows that this drug typically indicated for hypertension could have antianxiety effects, and it does.

## Gabapentin

Gabapentin (Neurontin) is a commonly used anticonvulsant with antianxiety properties. It has been found effective in the treatment of social phobia and moderately effective in the treatment of OCD, and has been used to augment the antidepressant treatment of PTSD.

## Pregabalin

Pregabalin (Lyrica) is a new agent that is currently under development for the treatment of anxiety spectrum disorders, as well as neuropathic pain and seizures. It is related to gabapentin in that it inhibits neuronal excitability. In a trial comparing pregabalin with lorazepam, pregabalin was better tolerated and demonstrated comparable antianxiety efficacy (Feltner et al, 2003).

## Propranolol

Propranolol (Inderal) is a beta blocker that effectively interrupts the physiologic responses of anxiety related to social phobia. As noted above, autonomic dysregulation is a factor in anxiety. It makes sense, then, that a drug that blocks these receptors could be effective. Propranolol is less effective than the benzodiazepines but is relatively safe and has little abuse potential. Most side effects are transient and mild. However, bradycardia, lightheadedness, and heart block have been reported.

## ▌ Study Notes

1. Antianxiety agents are commonly prescribed psychotropic drugs.
2. SSRIs are first line agents used to treat anxiety. They are discussed in detail in Chapter 19.
3. The nonbenzodiazepine buspirone is also a first-line agent that is relatively safe and interacts with few other drugs.
4. Benzodiazepines are also commonly used.
5. Diazepam (Valium) is the prototype benzodiazepine; however, other benzodiazepines, particularly alprazolam (Xanax) and lorazepam (Ativan), are used extensively.
6. Benzodiazepines have four basic clinical uses: (1) for chronic anxiety, (2) for time-limited periods in people going through crises, (3) for presurgery nervousness, and (4) for the treatment of panic disorder.
7. The ability to mute incoming stimuli gives benzodiazepines a great potential for abuse.
8. Benzodiazepines can cause a physical dependence and produce a withdrawal syndrome. Discontinuance should be tapered gradually.
9. Side effects of the benzodiazepines include drowsiness, fatigue, ataxia, and other peripheral and central effects; however, tolerance to side effects occurs.
10. Benzodiazepines are relatively safe drugs when taken alone but can be deadly if mixed with other CNS depressants (e.g., alcohol).
11. Benzodiazepines that ultimately rely on conjugation with glucuronic acid to inactive metabolites are more appropriate for older adults (e.g., lorazepam [Ativan] and oxazepam [Serax]).
12. Buspirone is a nonbenzodiazepine and has gained extensive use for the treatment of anxiety. Buspirone differs from the benzodiazepines in the following ways:
    • It is not sedating.
    • It is not a drug that causes a high, so it has almost no abuse potential.
    • It has no cross-tolerance with sedatives or alcohol.
    • It takes 1 to 6 weeks to be effective.
    • It does not produce dependence, withdrawal, or tolerance.
    • It does not cause muscle relaxation.
13. Venlafaxine, which has a dual action, was the first drug approved for treatment of both anxiety and depression.

## ▌ References

Ashton CH: *Benzodiazepines: how they work and how to withdraw,* Newcastle, England, 2000, University of Newcastle.

Ayd FJ: The early history of modern psychopharmacology, *Neuropsychopharmacology* 5:71, 1991.

Bezchlibnyk-Butler KZ, Jeffries JJ: *Clinical handbook of psychotropic drugs,* ed 7, Seattle, 2004, Hogrefe & Huber.

Black DW, Wesner R, Bowers W, Gabel J: A comparison of fluvoxamine, cognitive therapy, and placebo in the treatment of panic disorder, *Arch Gen Psychiatry* 50:44, 1993.

Ciraulo DA, Shader RI, Greenblatt DJ, et al: *Drug interactions in psychiatry,* Baltimore, 1989, Williams & Wilkins.

Feltner DE, Crockatt JG, Dubovsky SJ, et al: A randomized, placebo-controlled, multicenter study of pregabalin in patients with generalized anxiety disorder, *J Clin Psychiatry* 23:240, 2003.

Glod CA: Xanax: pros and cons, *J Psychosoc Nurs Ment Health Serv* 30:36, 1992.

Gutierrez MA, Roper JM, Hahn P: Paradoxical reactions to benzodiazepines, *Am J Nurs* 101:34, 2001.

Hale TW: *Medications and mothers' milk,* ed 10, Amarillo, TX, 2002, Pharmasoft.

Harvey SC: Hypnotics and sedatives. In Gilman AG, Goodman LS, Rall TW, editors: *The pharmacological basis of therapeutics,* ed 7, New York, 1985, Macmillan.

Hollister LE: New psychotherapeutic drugs, *J Clin Psychopharmacol* 14:50, 1994.

Keltner NL, Folks DG: *Psychotropic drugs,* ed 3, St. Louis, 2005, Mosby.

Keltner NL, Opara I: Psychotropic drug interactions with grapefruit juice, *Perspect Psychiatr Care* 38:31, 2002.

Keltner NL, Hogan B, Knight T, Royals LA: Adrenergic, cholinergic, GABAergic, and glutaminergic receptor function in the CNS, *Perspect Psychiatr Care* 37:140, 2001.

Keltner NL, Perry BA, Williams AR: Panic disorder: a tightening vortex of misery, *Perspect Psychiatr Care* 39:38, 2003.

Lehne RA: *Pharmacology for nursing care,* Philadelphia, 2004, WB Saunders.

Lieberman JA, Tasman A: *Psychiatric drugs,* St. Louis, 2000, WB Saunders.

Löw K, Crestani F, Keist R, et al: Molecular and neuronal substrate for the selective attenuation of anxiety. Available at http://usm.maine.edu/psy/broida/366/anxietyattenuation.html. Accessed February 8, 2001.

Malone K, Papagni K, Ramini S, Keltner NL: Antidepressants, antipsychotics, benzodiazepines, and the breastfeeding dyad, *Perspect Psychiatr Care* 40:73, 2004.

Maxman JS, Ward NG: *Psychotropic drugs: fast facts,* New York, 2002, Norton.

Saito T: GABA circuitry and the implications for psychiatric and neurologic disorders, XXIInd Congress of the Collegium Internationale Neuro-Psychopharmacologicum, 2001. Available at http://www.medscape.com/viewarticle/420861. Accessed February 8, 2001.

Seighart W: Structure and pharmacology of gamma-aminobutyric acid-A receptor subtypes, *Pharmacol Rev* 47:181, 1995.

Shelton RC: Pharmacotherapy of panic disorder, *Hosp Community Psychiatry* 44:725, 1993.

Stahl SM: *Essential psychopharmacology,* ed 2, New York, 2000, Cambridge University Press

Sterling L: Pharmacologic review of SSRIs in panic disorder, *Clin Rev Suppl* 2001. Available at http://www.medscape.com/CPG/ClinReviews/1999/TherSpot/c03ts.02.ster/c03ts.02.ster-01.html. Accessed February 8, 2001.

Sugerman RA: Functional neuroanatomy. In Keltner NL, Folks DG, editors: *Psychotropic drugs,* ed 4 (pp. 12-38), St. Louis, 2005, Mosby.

United States Pharmacopeia: *Drug information for the health care professional,* Englewood, CO, 2001, Micromedex.

Williams DB, Akabas MH: Benzodiazepines induce a conformational change in the region of gamma-aminobutyric acid type A receptor alpha (1) subunit M3 membrane-spanning segment, *Mol Pharmacol* 58:1129, 2000.

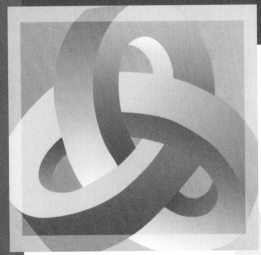

# Chapter 22

# Antidementia Drugs

*Norman L. Keltner*

## Learning Objective

*After reading this chapter, you should be able to:*
- Identify the drugs used in the treatment of Alzheimer's disease and other dementias.

Drugs used for Alzheimer's disease (AD) can be roughly categorized as those used for treatment and those used for prevention. Neither treatment nor preventive drugs provide the definitive approach that patients and families seek. Nevertheless, the available agents provide some relief and might indeed help prevent AD. In addition to the drugs used to treat or prevent, there are a few experimental agents that show promise. Certainly, although significant limitations exist, current approaches target specific physiologic mechanisms; this hardly resembles the serendipitous approach that dominated drug discovery during the early years of psychopharmacology.

## DRUGS USED TO TREAT DEMENTIAS

AD is a degenerative disease that is progressive and brutal. Sufferers lose memory-making ability, experience memory loss, cannot find the right words to express themselves, and have generalized cognitive impairment. The neurobiologic reasons for this are neuronal death and neurotransmitter deficiency. At this point, the most common approach to treatment attempts to restore neurotransmitter loss. The less common drug approach attempts to and might halt neuronal dying. Chapter 32 provides greater detail but, simply, neuronal loss occurs in many places in the brain; however the hippocampus, where memories are made, is never spared. Neurotransmitter restoration focuses on one primary neurotransmitter, acetylcholine (ACh), but other systems are degenerating as well—namely, the dopamine system and the norepinephrine system.

## AGENTS THAT RESTORE ACETYLCHOLINE

### BACKGROUND

To understand the agents used to restore acetylcholine losses completely, it is important to review related concepts. A discussion of cholinergic pathways, enzymes, enzyme inhibition, types of ACh receptors, and types of cholinesterases facilitates understanding how these drugs work.

## Cholinergic Pathways

Cholinergic pathways, although just one of several neurotransmitter systems affected, are selectively destroyed in AD (Keltner et al, 2001a). Most cholinergic fibers (about 90%) arise from one area, the nucleus basalis of Meynert (NBM). As might be suspected, the hippocampus is particularly rich in cholinergic receptors, and loss of ACh in this area causes the aforementioned memory-making loss. The amygdala, the locus of human emotion, is in front of the hippocampus and plays a role in memorization selection (Miller, 2005). Stated another way, many of our memories are linked to emotional events, so we often remember embarrassing or frightening moments. The amygdala apparently drives this type of memory-making selection. Unfortunately, the amygdala is heavily dependent

### Norm's Notes

*There is not a whole lot that our society can do for the patient with Alzheimer's disease today, but it is an area of well-funded research, with some promising answers on the horizon. This chapter takes a slightly different approach than the previous drug chapters. Receptors and enzymes are reviewed, because understanding their actions is critical to knowing the "why." If you study this chapter thoroughly, you will have very useful information for patients' families and maybe even for people you know.*

on ACh for this function and suffers significantly as ACh pathways decline.

## Enzymes

Enzymes are large molecules that are produced according to specific genetic coding. Enzymes provide the catalytic force that drives production of energy and the material required for the building blocks of life itself (Keltner, 2001b).

Enzyme configuration is such that certain molecules, including neurotransmitters and drugs, fit onto the enzyme and then undergo metabolic change. The enzyme is a catalyst of the metabolic change but not a participant. It is not changed itself, but repeats its catalytic activity many times. In the case of cholinesterase (ChE), a single molecule can metabolize 5000 molecules of ACh every second (Purves et al, 1997) (Figure 22-1).

ChE breaks down ACh into inactive metabolites, choline and acetate. Once fragmented, these inactive remnants of ACh can no longer activate cholinergic receptors. Because a loss of ACh is the primary neurotransmitter loss in AD, attempting to prevent the metabolism of ACh has proven to be the most effective means for restoring this neurotransmitter.

## Enzyme Inhibition

The approach to ACh inhibition centers around blocking the enzyme ChE. This is accomplished by introducing molecules into the system that preferentially attach to ChE. When this is accomplished, ACh cannot be metabolized, thus

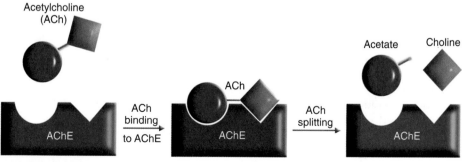

**FIGURE 22-1** Shown are an acetylcholine (ACh) molecule and an acetylcholinesterase (AChE) molecule (*left panel*). AChE binds the ACh molecule (*center panel*) and the products of AChE's metabolic activity, acetate and choline, are illustrated (*right panel*). (Courtesy of Vicki Johnson. Modified from Lehne RA: *Pharmacology for nursing care,* St. Louis, 2003, WB Saunders.)

Box 22-1    **Cholinesterases**

| Site(s) of Action of AChE | Site(s) of Action of BChE |
|---|---|
| Primary site: brain | Primary sites in the periphery |
| | Plasma |
| | Skeletal muscles |
| | Placenta |
| | Liver |
| Other sites | Other site: brain |
| Skeletal muscles | |
| Red blood cells | |
| Lymphocytes | |
| Platelets | |

*AChE,* acetylcholinesterase; *BChE,* butyrylcholinesterase. Modified from Stahl SM: *Essential psychopharmacology,* Cambridge, UK, 2000, Cambridge University Press.

increasing the availability of this neurotransmitter to postsynaptic cholinergic receptors.

### Types of ACh Receptors

Two types of ACh receptors have been identified in humans: nicotinic receptors and muscarinic receptors. The nicotinic receptor is best understood as two subtypes: (1) those on the cell bodies of the postganglionic neurons in the autonomic nervous system, and (2) those on skeletal muscles. Muscarinic receptors are divided into five subtypes; however, for the purpose of this discussion, they will be grouped simply as muscarinic receptors, which are of interest in AD. Although nicotinic receptors are found in the brain, they play a less significant role in treatment.

### Types of Cholinesterase

Just as there are two types of monoamine oxidase enzymes, so there are two types of ChE. Acetylcholinesterase (AChE) is more common in the brain. The other ChE, butyrylcholinesterase (BChE), is more common in the periphery (Stahl, 2000) (Box 22-1). Because a central nervous system effect is required to treat AD, drugs that inhibit both ChEs have greater potential for causing unnecessary and often adverse effects. For example, inhibiting BChE produces nausea and vomiting, diarrhea, facial flushing, sweating, rhinitis, bradycardia, and leg cramps. The ideal drug might selectively inhibit AChE while not inhibiting BChE (Roger et al, 1998).

## CHOLINESTERASE INHIBITORS

There are four drugs, known as cholinesterase inhibitors, that target ACh deficiency. By attaching to and thus blocking ChE, these four drugs substantially increase the amount of intrasynaptic ACh available to cholinergic receptors.

### Tacrine (Cognex)

Tacrine was the first cholinesterase inhibitor available for use. It was marketed as an antidementia drug in 1993 but was actually synthesized much earlier. In fact, in 1945, tacrine plus morphine was heralded as an effective pain management combination for cancer patients (Terpstra and Terpstra, 1998).

Tacrine has an interesting history related to what some have described as sloppy research, but that issue will not be discussed here. It is important to note that, although tacrine does inhibit ChE, its use is also linked to serious hepatic effects and thus it is seldom prescribed (Keltner, 1994).

### Donepezil (Aricept)

Donepezil was approved in 1996 and is a reversible inhibitor of ChE (Nordberg and Svensson, 1998). Whereas tacrine inhibits both AChE and BChE, donepezil is much more selective for AChE (1200 to 1 times more selective), so theoretically its use should cause fewer peripheral side effects (Geldmacher, 1997). Other advantages over tacrine include absence of hepatoxicity, once-daily dosing related to a longer half-life, and 100% bioavailability whether taken with or without food. Some peripheral effects have been reported, including gastrointestinal (GI) problems and bradycardia, suggesting that selectivity for brain AChE is not complete (Keltner and Folks, 2005) (Figure 22-2).

### Rivastigmine (Exelon)

Rivastigmine was approved for treatment of AD in 2000. It also inhibits ChE but does so in a slightly different way than the previously described ChE inhibitors. Whereas tacrine and donepezil are reversible inhibitors of ChE, rivastigmine is said to be irreversible. Stated another way, tacrine and donepezil slip off and on ChE continuously, whereas rivastigmine remains attached and forms a covalent bond with the enzyme. Rivastigmine

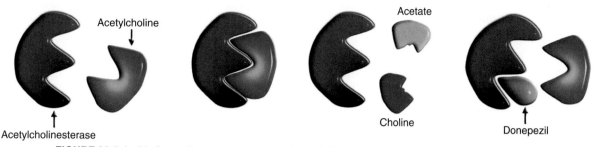

**FIGURE 22-2** In this figure, the same process as shown in Figure 22-1 is illustrated. However, the AChE is inhibited from its metabolic activity by the AChE inhibitor donepezil (*last panel*). Accordingly, ACh survives and builds up in the synapse. (Courtesy of Vicki Johnson. Modified from Lehne RA: *Pharmacology for nursing care,* St. Louis, 2003, WB Saunders.)

remains effective until the life cycle of the enzyme is complete. Rivastigmine has a relatively short plasma half-life (about 2 hours) but has an inhibition half-life of 10 hours. Essentially while attached irreversibly to ChE, rivastigmine is not factored into the plasma level (Keltner and Folks, 2005).

Rivastigmine is not metabolized by the cytochrome P-450 enzymes, so it does not interact with drugs metabolized by this system. In regard to this aspect of drug administration, rivastigmine has an advantage over tacrine and donepezil. Rivastigmine prefers AChE over BChE but produces peripheral side effects (Alagiakrishnan et al, 2000).

### Galantamine (Razadyne)

Galantamine is the last ChE inhibitor to be discussed. It also demonstrates preference for AChE over BChE but presents with typically cholinergic side effects, such as GI symptoms. An added feature with galantamine is its ability to modulate the relatively few nicotinic receptors in the brain. Nicotine receptors are thought to play a role in memory and learning, although their exact mechanism has not been fully elucidated (Tariot et al, 2004).

Furthermore, there is some evidence that galantamine might also provide neuroprotection by upregulating neurotrophic factors such as bcl-2 via nicotinic receptors (Geerts, 2005). Such findings, if replicable, might give galantamine an advantage over other drugs in this class.

Galantamine is readily absorbed; it has a bioavailability of about 85% and a half-life of about 6 hours. It has a relatively high volume of distribution and insignificant protein binding. It is metabolized by the cytochrome P-450 system, so it can interact with drugs catalyzed by this enzyme system (Farlow, 2003).

### Summary of Cholinesterase Inhibitors

Elevating ACh levels does not slow the disease process of AD or the other irreversible dementias. If one of these drugs is discontinued, the patient's cognitive abilities are what they would have been had the drug never been administered. These drugs, all approved for mild to moderate AD, help the patient preserve cognitive performance longer than if he or she had not taken the medication. Eventually, the underlying neurodegeneration becomes so profound that these efforts to bolster ACh no longer mask the devastation of the brain. Obviously, if the observation that galantamine increases neuroprotective factors is correct, it would be the exception related to this non–Ach-boosting mechanism.

## AGENTS THAT RETARD NEURODEGENERATION

AD progressively marches through the brain, leaving dead neurons in its path. Although the analogy of a destroyer marching through does not exactly reflect what occurs, it does come close.

Neurons probably die in several ways. One of these is what has been identified as neuronal excitotoxicity. Excitotoxicity, or very rapid firing of the neuron, is caused by aberrant (i.e., sustained) depolarization of the glutamate–N-methyl-D-aspartate receptor (NDMA) complex. Glutamate is an excitatory neurotransmitter and NDMA is a glutamate receptor. Whenever this coupling causes too many neuronal firings, the neuron can die.

| Table 22-1 | **Antidementia Drugs** | | | | |  |

| Drug | Typical Daily Dosage | Half-Life (hr) | Protein Binding (%) | Cytochrome P-450 Enzymes | Mechanism of Action |
|---|---|---|---|---|---|
| Donepezil (Aricept) | 5-10 mg at bedtime | ~70 | ~95 | 2D6, 3A4 | Cholinesterase inhibitor |
| Rivastigmine (Exelon) | 6-12 mg in two divided doses | ~2 | ~40 | Not metabolized | Cholinesterase inhibitor |
| Galantamine (Razadyne) | 8-16 mg twice a day | ~6 | Insignificant | 2D6 | Cholinesterase inhibitor |
| Tacrine (Cognex) | 40-160 mg in four divided | ~3 | ~55 | 1A2, 2D6 | Cholinesterase inhibitor |
| Memantine (Namenda) | 20 mg in two divided doses | ~60-80 | ~45 | Not extensively metabolized | NMDA antagonist |

*NMDA, N*-methyl-D-aspartate.

One approach to preventing excitotoxicity is to give a drug that blocks NDMA receptors.

### Memantine (Namenda)

Memantine is an NDMA antagonist. By blocking the NDMA receptor, memantine prevents glutamate from overstimulating it. This blockade results in a reduction in depolarizations. Although the manufacturer of Namenda clearly states on the package insert that it does not claim that the drug slows neuronal degeneration, the implication is that it could (Keltner and Williams, 2004).

NDMA receptor antagonists are familiar to nurses in the emergency department because of the use of the drug PCP (phencyclidine). PCP is an NDMA antagonist. Users of the drug exhibit behaviors similar to those of paranoid schizophrenia. They are often violent and then, just as quickly, become nonviolent. The conundrum for the clinician is this: too much NDMA stimulation (i.e., excitotoxicity) can cause neuronal death, whereas too little (i.e., NDMA antagonism) can lead to psychotic behavior. Memantine is formulated so that NDMA stimulation will not occur, yet neither will severe behavioral effects develop. This is a fine line, but it allows the student to appreciate the risks and benefits involved in treating this devastating illness. (Admittedly, PCP-mediated psychotic behavior is probably linked to PCP's dopamine-enhancing effects as well.)

Memantine also has an interesting pharmacokinetic profile. It has a long half-life (60 to 80 hours) but is not metabolized to a great degree (Forest Laboratories, 2003). Most memantine is excreted unchanged. The latter property (i.e., not being metabolized) accounts for few drug interactions with memantine.

Memantine is often co-prescribed with donepezil. Studies have suggested that memantine is effective either in this combination or as monotherapy (Reisberg et al, 2003; Tariot et al, 2004).

In summary, memantine has few side effects of significance, few if any drug interactions and, unlike the ChE inhibitors, is approved by the U.S. Food and Drug Administration (FDA) for moderate to severe AD.

## DRUGS TO PREVENT ALZHEIMER'S DISEASE

Drugs used to treat AD are useful and widely prescribed, but do not stop the destructive onslaught of the disorder. That being the case, it is even more important to find means of preventing AD, if that is possible. Although no one knows with certainty whether the following drugs do, in fact, prevent or forestall AD, evidence has suggested that they might. Because these drugs are relatively benign as far as severe consequences, they might be worth promoting in the hope that they might be preventive.

### NONSTEROIDAL ANTI-INFLAMMATORY DRUGS

Cyclooxygenase (COX) is an enzyme that synthesizes prostaglandins which, in turn, protect the stomach, promote platelet aggregation, and increase renal blood flow, but also cause inflammation, pain, and fever. The positive effects mentioned are attributed to the enzymatic action of COX-1 inhibitors, whereas the negative effects are attributed to the enzymatic action of COX-2 inhibitors. COX-2 inhibitors then have the potential to decrease inflammation and fever. Some researchers believe that one of the ways in which neurons die is related to a low-burner inflammatory process. Other studies have suggested a significant decline in the incidence of AD if these nonsteroidal anti-inflammatory drugs (NSAIDs) are used on a regular basis.

In 2004 and 2005, several COX-2 inhibitors (e.g., Celebrex, Vioxx) were taken off the market because of increased risk of cerebrovascular accidents and heart attacks. Older individuals and their prescribers need to weigh the potential risks versus the benefits of using NSAIDs on a regular basis.

## STATINS

In the last 20 years or so, the use of statin drugs to reduce elevated cholesterol levels has skyrocketed. Some clinicians believe that there is a relationship between high cholesterol levels and AD. If their theory is correct, statins, with their cholesterol-lowering potential, might provide dual benefits. One study has suggested that statins might reduce the risk of AD by about 70% (Wolozin et al, 2000).

## ESTROGEN

Some researchers believe that the decrease in the estrogen level after menopause increases the risk of women developing AD. Studies have suggested that women taking estrogen lower their risk of developing AD; however, other studies have not been able to confirm this effect. Although estrogen might play a role in forestalling AD and has other benefits (e.g., improved bone density), it has been associated with increased risk of heart attacks and other cardiovascular complications.

## B VITAMINS

An elevated serum level of homocysteine, an amino acid, is thought to be associated with AD (Selley, 2004). Furthermore, the higher the blood level of homocysteine, the greater the association. Because deficiency of three B vitamins ($B_6$, $B_{12}$, and folic acid) is linked to an elevated homocysteine level, some clinicians have attempted to prevent AD by prescribing these vitamins. At this time, however, there is no conclusive evidence that taking these B vitamins slows or prevents AD.

## Study Notes

1. Drugs used to treat dementias can be categorized as (1) drugs for treatment of dementia and (2) drugs for prevention of dementia.
2. The causes of AD can be broadly grouped as (1) neuronal death and (2) neurotransmitter deficiency.
3. The most common drug interventions restore deficient neurotransmitters.
4. The primary neurotransmitter deficiency is acetylcholine (ACh).
5. Agents that restore ACh levels do so by blocking the enzyme that metabolizes ACh.
6. Cholinesterases (ChE) breakdown ACh. There are two types: (1) acetylcholinesterase (AChE) and (2) butyrylcholinesterase (BChE).
7. Antidementia drugs attach to ChEs and prevent them from bonding to and then metabolizing ACh.
8. Four drugs are available that are identified as ChE (or AChE or BChE) inhibitors: tacrine, donepezil, rivastigmine, and galantamine.
9. One drug, memantine, has a different mechanism of action. Memantine is an NMDA receptor inhibitor.
10. Theoretically, memantine could prevent neuronal death.
11. Other drugs are used to prevent dementias.
12. NSAIDs, statins, estrogen, and B vitamins might prevent or forestall the development of dementia. Much research remains to be carried out before such claims can be broadly accepted, however.

## References

Alagiakrishnan K, Wong W, Blanchette PL: Use of donepezil in elderly patients with Alzheimer's disease—a Hawaii-based study, *Hawaii Med J* 59:57, 2000.

Farlow MR: Clinical pharmacokinetics of galantamine, *Clin Pharmacokinet* 42:1383, 2003.

Forest Laboratories: *Namenda package insert,* St. Louis, MO, 2003, Forest Pharmaceuticals.

Geerts H: Indicators of neuroprotection with galantamine, *Brain Res Bull* 64:519, 2005.

Geldmacher DS: Donepezil (Aricept) therapy for Alzheimer's disease, *Compr Ther* 23:492, 1997.

Keltner NL: Tacrine: a pharmacological approach to Alzheimer's disease, *J Psychosoc Nurs Ment Health Serv* 323:37, 1994.

Keltner NL, Folks DG: *Psychotropic drugs,* ed 3, St. Louis, 2005, Mosby.

Keltner NL, Hogan B, Knight T, Royals LA: Adrenergic, cholinergic, GABAergic, and glutaminergic receptor function in the CNS, *Perspect Psychiatr Care* 37:140, 2001a.

Keltner NL, Zielinski AL, Hardin MS: Drugs used for cognitive symptoms in Alzheimer's disease, *Perspect Psychiatr Care* 37:31, 2001b.

Keltner NL, Williams B: Memantine: a new approach to Alzheimer's disease, *Perspect Psychiatr Care* 40:123, 2004.

Miller MC: What is the amygdala and what are its functions? *Harvard Ment Health Lett* 21:8, 2005.

Nordberg A, Svensson A: Cholinesterase inhibitors in the treatment of Alzheimer's disease, *Drug Safety* 19:465, 1998.

Purves D, Augustine GJ, Fitzpatrick D, et al: *Neuroscience,* Sunderland, MA, 1997, Sinauer Associates.

Reisberg B, Doody R, Stöffler A, et al, for the Memantine Study Group: Memantine in moderate-to-severe Alzheimer's disease, *N Engl J Med* 348:1333, 2003.

Rogers SL, Doody RS, Mohs RC, Friedhoff LT: Donepezil improves cognitition and global function in Alzheimer's disease, *Arch Int Med* 158:1021-1031, 1998.

Selley ML: Increased homocysteine and decreased adenosine formation in Alzheimer's disease. *Neurol Res* 26:554, 2004.

Stahl SM: *Essential psychopharmacology,* Cambridge, UK, 2000, Cambridge University Press.

Tariot PN, Farlow MR, Grossberg GT, et al: Memantine treatment in patients with moderate to severe Alzheimer disease already receiving donepezil, *JAMA* 291:317, 2004.

Terpstra T, Terpstra T: Treating Alzheimer's disease with cholinergic drugs, part I, *Nurse Pract* 23:90, 1998.

Wolozin B, Kellman W, Ruosseau P, et al: Decreased prevalence of Alzheimer disease associated with 3-hydroxy-3-methyglutaryl coenzyme A reductase inhibitors [see comment], *Arch Neurol* 57:1439, 2000.

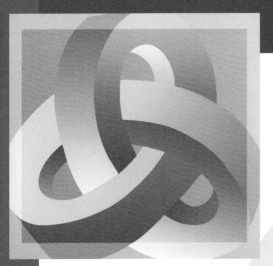

# Chapter 23

# Introduction to Milieu Management

*Beverly K. Hogan and Mona M. Shattell*

## Learning Objectives

*After reading this chapter, you should be able to:*
- Define the terms *therapeutic milieu, therapeutic environment,* and *therapeutic community.*
- Describe the goal of managing the therapeutic environment in the care of psychiatric patients.
- Identify the elements of the therapeutic environment.
- Discuss several ways in which nurses can influence the therapeutic environment.

***Note to Students:*** *Political, social, economic, and other forces have resulted in a health care system that changes quickly. These forces dictate the setting in which care takes place. For example, managed care insurance plans favor the use of less expensive forms of treatment than that of the inpatient unit. Although hospitals used to employ most psychiatric nurses, a great number of psychiatric nurses currently practice in community settings. As the struggle to define a system of mental health care continues, treatment settings continue to emerge and vary; however, treatment principles remain the same when the nurse is guided by the professional definition of nursing—that is, attention to the range of human experiences and responses to health and illness within the physical and social environments (American Nurses Association, 2005). The treatment environment is affected by many variables but it is the nurse's involvement in creating a therapeutic environment that ultimately determines the overall atmosphere of the treatment setting. This role is true in any specialty area, but it is the focus of psychiatric nursing and therefore the purpose for including these chapters. Even if the inpatient environment ceased to be therapeutic, it would be a neglectful omission to exclude the importance of the treatment environment in a psychiatric nursing textbook.*

The purpose of a therapeutic environment is to help patients recover from psychiatric and mental health problems; at the very least, the environment should function to protect the patient from destructive influences and, ideally, it should also maximize opportunities for patients to learn something about themselves and their problems in everyday living. The terms *therapeutic environment* and *therapeutic milieu* are sometimes used interchangeably to describe the atmosphere of a psychiatric unit. Strictly speaking, therapeutic milieu refers to a formalized treatment modality called milieu therapy. Milieu therapy, as it was originally described, has faded in importance as the era of psychobiology has come to dominate psychiatric treatment philosophies and inpatient units have become centers of acute crisis intervention (Norton, 2004; Satcher, 2005). We prefer therapeutic environment, because this term acknowledges that the site of treatment is supposed

**Norm's Notes**

*This gets right back to the beginning of the book and psychotherapeutic management. You cannot work with people without being affected by the environment. When you really understand this, it will change a lot of things about your understanding of nursing and perhaps even your personal life. Here's the question: how can you shape an environment to make it more therapeutic?*

to be therapeutic regardless of the specific treatment modality adopted. Therapeutic environment also avoids conveying the idea that milieu therapy is still practiced as intended. In our opinion, all treatment environments affect patient care; the environment can be therapeutic or nontherapeutic. This is also true in nonpsychiatric patient care environments (e.g., medical surgical, intensive care, postpartum units), even when the environment is not given the primacy given in a psychiatric setting. To say that milieu therapy is not being used might mean that the unit does not formally adopt the principles of milieu therapy, as described in the next section, or that a significant responsibility of psychiatric nursing is being neglected (i.e., managing the environment, one of the three tools of the psychotherapeutic management model described in Chapter 2).

In the sections that follow, a history of the concept of milieu therapy is presented, followed by a discussion of the components essential for creating a therapeutic environment.

## HISTORICAL OVERVIEW

Concepts related to milieu management were originally applied only to inpatient settings. The discussion in this section will therefore focus on *milieu therapy* as it applies to hospital inpatient settings. It is assumed that similar principles could be applied in most treatment settings.

For many years, custodial care was the norm in inpatient settings. Custodial care referred to a *mind-set* in which patient care focused exclusively on the patient's activities of daily living, such as hygiene, nutrition, elimination, and safety needs. Custodial care was a paternalistic system in which

the staff knew best what the patient needed. Few attempts were made to allow the patient to participate in his or her own treatment, and beyond basic needs; there were no efforts to provide structured treatment activities. After World War II, some professionals began to be concerned that an opportunity to enhance treatment was being missed by not taking advantage of potentially therapeutic time. Stanton and Schwartz (1954) noted the discrepancy between "what could be and what was" in the hospital. They believed that a better result from hospitalization might be realized if *all* dimensions of care were focused on their potential for therapeutic benefit.

The most notable figure of this time was Maxwell Jones. In 1953, Jones wrote his landmark book, *The Therapeutic Community,* in which he described the benefits of an environment that was therapeutic in and of itself. Jones (1953) proposed patient involvement in decision making through daily group meetings, termed *therapeutic community meetings.* In these daily meetings, patients participated in planning ward activities. Patient self-responsibility was an important concept in the therapeutic community, whereby patients were expected to take an active role in their treatment. Increasingly, the importance of the patients' contribution to their own treatment replaced the paternalistic system of the treatment team knows best.

For a period of time, milieu therapy and therapeutic community were common names for psychiatric treatment settings. Rarely are these used today and, when they are, the terms hardly reflect the originally conceived idea of comprehensive use of the environment as a tool to facilitate the recovery of patients experiencing psychiatric and mental health problems. Today's inpatient psychiatric units are short-term intensive settings to contain and resolve crises (Satcher, 2005). Even if the type of active patient participation described by Jones in 1953 were still being used today, most patients now admitted to acute inpatient psychiatric units are experiencing a severity of psychiatric illness that often precludes their participation in even basic self-care. It is difficult to apply milieu therapy principles in an inpatient hospital environment in which the primary directive is rapid stabilization of symptoms and return of the patient to a less expensive community-based treatment program. Nonetheless, it is still expected that the inpatient environment should at least offer safety and an opportunity to improve enough to return to community care.

*Note to Students:* *The terms* treatment environment *and* therapeutic environment *are used for the remainder of this chapter. Even if a treatment program is not using milieu therapy, a treatment environment is still supposed to be therapeutic.*

## JOINT COMMISSION ON THE ACCREDIATION OF HEALTHCARE ORGANIZATIONS: ENVIRONMENT OF CARE ISSUES

Environment of care standards require that facilities be designed and constructed to ensure a safe, accessible environment. The Joint Commission on the Accreditation of Healthcare Organizations (JCAHO) requires that institutions routinely evaluate the environment for its ongoing effectiveness for providing care. Additionally, the facility must establish a social environment supporting its basic philosophy. Box 23-1 lists the JCAHO environment of care standards for inpatient psychiatric units. The goal of management of the environment is "to provide a safe, functional, supportive, and effective environment for patients, staff members, and other individuals in the hospital" (JCAHO, 2001). Detailed standards for managing the environment of care are outlined in JCAHO's *Comprehensive Accreditation Manual for Hospitals* (JCAHO, 2001). These standards apply to outpatient clinics and counseling centers as well as to inpatient environments.

### CLINICAL EXAMPLE

A day treatment program for patients with chronic mental illness is housed in a large rustic building in a rural county in a southeastern state in the United States. Within easy walking distance of the day treatment program are two group homes. Many of the residents from the group home are also patients at the day treatment center. The therapeutic environment for the day treatment program includes a range of structured treatment activities, such as educational classes, group and individual therapy, and basic living skills such as making a budget, riding the bus, reading food labels for nutrition, planning meals, and washing clothes. For those patients living in the group home, many of

---

**Box 23-1    JCAHO Environment of Care Standards**

Environmental safety is attained through:

- Ongoing assessment and maintenance of all equipment
- Hazard surveillance
- Reporting and investigation of safety issues
- Monitoring of safety management techniques and procedures
- Orientation programs that address safety issues

A health care facility ensures the security of all people through:

- Mechanisms for addressing security issues
- Provision of appropriate identification for all staff, patients, and visitors
- Security orientation programs
- Mechanisms for handling emergencies
- Mechanisms for interacting with the media

The social environment must provide:

- Space for storage of grooming and hygiene articles
- Closet and drawer space for personal property
- Clothing that is suitable for clinical conditions

The physical setting must provide:

- Adequate privacy to ensure respect for patients
- Door locks consistent with program goals
- Availability of telephones that allow for private conversations
- Sleeping rooms with doors for privacy unless clinically contraindicated
- Furnishings suitable to the population served
- Access to the outdoors unless contraindicated for therapeutic reasons

From Joint Commission on the Accreditation of Healthcare Organizations (JCAHO): *Comprehensive accreditation manual for hospitals,* Chicago, 2001, JCAHO, p EC-1.

---

these activities are enhanced and reinforced by trained staff members who structure the days and evenings at the group home. Both of these treatment settings manage the environment to make it therapeutic for patients.

## NURSING AND THE THERAPEUTIC ENVIRONMENT

Florence Nightingale recognized the importance of the environment on the patient's recovery. Nurses have traditionally been responsible for activities that involve management of the environment. Weekend and late evening or night care

---

**Highlighting the Evidence: Current Research**

**What's Therapeutic About the Therapeutic Milieu?**

Thomas and associates (2002) wanted to know how patients experienced the inpatient acute care psychiatric environment. In their study, eight inpatients, ranging in age from 23 to 58, on the acute psychiatric unit of a metropolitan general hospital participated in interviews about their experience of the environment.

The essential purpose of the hospital was to provide a refuge from self-destructiveness. Prominent aspects of patients' experience within the place of refuge fit into three interrelated themes: (1) like me/not like me, (2) possibilities/no possibilities, and (3) connection/disconnection.

**Refuge from Self-Destructiveness**

In contrast to the chaotic outside world, the hospital was portrayed as a safe house, neutral territory, and a cooling-down place. Hospitalization provided a calming respite from the daily struggle against self-destructive impulses.

*Like Me/Not Like Me*

In the psychiatric unit, identity was affirmed amid kindred souls. There was solidarity among the patients, often referred to as bonding, that most did not experience in the outside world—that is, when not in the hospital.

*Possibilities/No Possibilities*

Hospitalization opened possibilities for the future. Participants described feeling more levelheaded, straightened out, and back in balance again. Despite goals and determination to follow up with aftercare plans, patients feared being released from the safe hospital environment.

*Connection/Disconnection*

The connection/disconnection theme refers to patients' experiences within the milieu of connecting—or failing to connect—with other people. Socialization with other patients was valued by patients. Interactions with professional staff tended to be superficial.

Universally, patients perceived peer-administered therapy as the most beneficial aspect of their hospitalization. They expressed longing for a deeper connection with staff and more insight-oriented therapies.

Although their needs for safety, structure, and medications were met, patients did not gain greater understanding of their dysfunctional patterns of behavior. Renewed emphasis must be placed on the nurse-patient relationship, the therapeutic alliance, and the therapeutic environment.

From Thomas SP, Shattell M, Martin T: What's therapeutic about the therapeutic milieu? *Arch Psychiatr Nurs* 16:99, 2002.

---

have traditionally been the sole responsibility of nursing. Other disciplines have more recently been challenged about the usefulness of their therapies if they can be suspended on the weekend (Norton, 2004). Patients are admitted to inpatient units because they require 24-hour nursing care; if the patient needs additional therapies, most regulatory agencies stipulate that if payment for such therapies is sought, it is not acceptable to waste treatment time over the weekend by suspending therapies or delegating them to nurses.

Patients can benefit from a therapeutic environment because it provides opportunities to try out new behaviors and solve problems in real situations with others. Current research has shown that a therapeutic environment also benefits nurses, because positive nurse-patient relationships contribute to professional satisfaction and the knowledge that she or he has made a difference (Thomas et al, 2005). Nurses draw on their therapeutic relationship with patients to create corrective learning experiences in the treatment environment. Interactions in the treatment environment are opportunities to help patients learn and adapt to their problems in living. Distortions, conflicts, and inappropriate behavior are dealt with in the here and now of each interaction and related back to the patient's treatment plan.

The nurse must work actively to make the environment therapeutic. It is sometimes surprising to novice psychiatric nurses and students that they leave their shift on an inpatient psychiatric unit feeling tired, even though they might not have had a physically demanding day. Those who see psychiatric nursing as not doing much, or as just sitting around talking, would likely also experience this as surprising. What student would deny that mental work, such as writing a paper or pondering creative interventions to patient care problems, requires energy? Mental work is a large part of the work required of psychiatric nurses and is a very active, carefully coordinated and thought-out process. Thoughtful reflection about interactions is also a conscious and deliberate action of the psychiatric nurse done to help make the nurse-patient relationship as therapeutic as possible. Paying attention to one's personal values, reactions, and preconceptions is only one aspect of keeping the environment therapeutic; a number of other elements are also important in the construction of a therapeutic environment. Because nursing has a central role in managing this environment (especially in inpatient settings), it is important to identify these elements to begin to comprehend the types of competencies required of the psychiatric nurse.

A few examples of ineffective nursing care should suffice to exemplify an ineffective environment. A clear signal that the environment is *not* therapeutic can be observed when nurses rarely leave the nursing station, except in the event of a crisis or medically prescribed treatment. The treatment environment cannot be favorably affected from a desk, with a pill, or by spending an inordinate amount of time in staff meetings and administrative care duties. Altering the environment, by definition, requires that the nurse take an active role in the environment. Excessive television watching by patients (Hillbrand et al, 1998), in lieu of structured therapeutic activities or interactions, also suggests an ineffectively managed environment. Thomas and associates (2002) found that, although the inpatient acute care environment of psychiatric units provided a basic structure, it lacked *meaningful* therapeutic activities. Patients expressed a desire for examining their perceptions of the inpatient psychiatric environment, more interaction, and deeper connections with the nurses. Patients reported that their greatest therapeutic benefit was from connections established with other patients (Thomas et al, 2002). Boredom and lack of meaningful activities were found to be common complaints of patients on inpatient psychiatric units (Binnema, 2004).

## ELEMENTS OF THE TREATMENT ENVIRONMENT

For the treatment environment to managed be effectively, we consider several interrelated elements essential. These elements, which provide the foundation necessary for the nurse to manage the environment effectively, include:

- Safety
- Structure
- Norms
- Limit setting
- Balance

## SAFETY

Safety is primary to all other aspects of the environment. Safety includes both physical and psychological protection. Physical protection refers to safety from physical harm through the management of risks in the environment, such as the prevention of physical aggression and the requirement of staff supervision for patients when using potentially unsafe grooming items (e.g., sharps, glass items, and plastic bags). Psychological safety involves the nurses' active intervention to prohibit verbal abuse, ridicule, or harassment of patients. To this end, it might be necessary to restrict visitors known to disparage patients. Intrusive behaviors such as getting in other people's private space or bullying others about personal characteristics need to be dealt with by staff to protect patients from this destructive behavior in the treatment environment. Safety cannot be fully accomplished unless the nurses are regularly out among the patients in the environment.

Psychiatric patients are a vulnerable population because of the ease with which their illness can be blamed for any allegations they might make; thus, it is essential to be attentive to complaints of abuse made by patients. The paranoid, delusional, or personality-disordered patient might distort events as abuse, but all allegations require the attention of the treatment team. Incident reports, follow-up by management, and notification of patient representatives or advocates might be necessary when allegations of abuse are made. Complaints against staff members are especially difficult for staff committed to the care of their patients, but it is important to be attentive to patterns suggestive of patients being exploited by staff and to take action when suspicious or confirmed patterns are discovered. Patients need to know that the staff will not harm them nor will they permit anyone else to do so. Posting patient rights, including telephone numbers to access assistance for violations of these rights, creates feelings of safety by empowering patients in an environment that can leave them feeling unsafe and vulnerable.

Nurses should create and adhere closely to the nursing policies and procedures developed for control of aggression. This usually involves intervening before the aggressive event occurs by such actions as sending a patient to their room, talking one to one with a patient, assisting with problem solving in conflicts between patients, administering prn medications and, as a last resort, the use of seclusion or restraints to control behavior (see Chapter 11 for more information on seclusion and restraints).

Intervening before situations escalate requires that the nurse be aware of the unit environment at all times, either by direct observation or through the reports of psychiatric technicians and aides, during those times when the nurse needs to be outside of the treatment environment. The relationship between the nurse and psychiatric technicians or other unlicensed assistive personnel needs to be an active, team-oriented approach for mutual understanding of goals for the patient. Most psychiatric units require the documentation of safety observations (often termed *rounds*) on patients, at a frequency ranging from hourly checks to constant observation (often termed *one-on-one observation*). Done with the safety of both staff and patients in mind, the routine and prescribed safety observations on a psychiatric unit are essential for maintaining safety of the environment. Safety is important and has a high priority because admission to an inpatient unit is often precipitated by concerns for the safety of the patient or of others who might be harmed by the patient. Safety issues alone can be enough to keep a nurse on a psychiatric unit active and engaged in the environment.

## CLINICAL EXAMPLE

In response to hearing voices, a patient named Tim hits one of the staff nurses. Tim agrees to walk to the seclusion room. At that time, he is given an intramuscular dose of an ordered medication to help control his agitation. Tim is told that the medication is to help him relax and that he will be kept in seclusion until he indicates, and staff members agree, that he can control his behavior. A staff member is either assigned to stay with Tim to reaffirm that he is not being punished or reassures him of frequent observation and attention to the patients' safety, comfort, and physical care needs. The intended message to Tim and other patients on the unit is that the staff is concerned that patients on the unit remain safe.

## CLINICAL EXAMPLE

John is angry with another patient and is threatening him with bodily harm. The nurse intervenes by firmly directing John to go to his room. The nurse stays with John and encourages him to talk about what he is feeling rather than to act on his feelings.

## STRUCTURE

Structure refers to the physical environment, rules, and daily schedules of treatment activities. Structure is an essential component of psychiatric treatment because, without it, there is no justification for the patient being in a treatment environment, particularly if custodial care is outmoded (see Chapter 2). Nurses lead activities such as patient education and social skills training groups. Teaching about medications, side effects, and aftercare support for both patients and families is an important function of the psychiatric nurse in minimizing patient noncompliance.

Opportunities for recreation also help provide structure to the treatment environment. In some cases, exercise therapists or recreation therapists fulfill this function; however, nurses often must complement these activities when other team members are not present.

The physical design of the unit is also an aspect of structure. Once the physical layout of a unit is in place, it is difficult to change in response to varying needs; thus, it is important that preplanning design plans for a psychiatric unit include input from an experienced psychiatric nurse.

Adequate space, areas for socializing and receiving visitors, telephones, and areas for privacy are all required elements of a therapeutic environment and communicate something about the values of the treatment environment. Such factors as furnishings and the color of the walls all reveal facility philosophy to the patients, families, and staff. The physical structure can constrain or enhance nursing care of patients. Much can be surmised about a unit by how it is physically arranged— units without places to sit and talk privately say a lot about how the unit will be run (Cleary and Edwards, 1999). Inaccessible nursing stations with locked doors also send messages to patients. On the other hand, a unit with an attractive décor, access to amenities as needed, and accessible staff can communicate a very different message. Patients need a central location to interact with each other; often, this is the dayroom, a designated smoking or a fresh air room. Research has shown that patients believe that they are truly able to connect with others and work on problems in their inner sanctuary during these informal gatherings (Thomas et al, 2002). Thomas and colleagues (2002) found that even nonsmokers would go into smoking rooms to partake of the gathering because of its perceived therapeutic benefit.

Some elements of structure on a psychiatric unit overlap with the concept of safety. When seclusion rooms are necessary, their design, location, and furnishings must maintain the safety and dignity of patients who might require their use, as well as that of other patients who observe their use and presence. In other words, it is important that the room be seen as a treatment intervention when someone is unresponsive to other nursing interventions and environmental modifications, and not as a place of punishment.

## NORMS

Norms are specific expectations of behavior that permeate the treatment environment; they are intended to promote safety and trust in the environment through the sanctioning of socially acceptable behaviors and consistency about what to expect. For example, a norm of nonviolence provides physical and emotional security in the environment.

Other norms focus on the level of personal control. For example, patients might be required to take a bath; however, the time at which they take their bath might be negotiable. The same is true for other aspects of treatment. Particularly for the involuntary patient, it is important to offer a sense of control whenever possible; this helps preserve the patient's dignity and can avert power struggles with patients whose tolerance for being made to do things is tenuous. Norms attempt to create an environment that is more predictable and applicable to all who share the environment. Norms are well described by what a patient has said about the unit rules and activities, "You might not like some of the thing you have to do and you might not agree with the rules, but you can kinda see how it's best in the long run cause you have so many different people and problems to deal with; I guess it keeps it smooth."

## LIMIT SETTING

Limit setting is an important element of the treatment environment and is related to norms. Limits should be set on acting-out behavior such as self-destructive acts, physical aggressiveness, and sexual behavior. It is also sometimes necessary to set limits on behaviors such as excessive requests, attempts to overly personalize the therapeutic relationship, and refusal to participate in treatment activities. Closely related to limit setting are rules. Limit setting reinforces the norm of making rules and expectations clear and also encourages the milieu therapy concept of *responsibility for self.* It is important that patients be advised of rules on admission or when they are capable of comprehending and attending to advice about unit rules. Written copies of unit rules should be provided to each patient and posted on the unit or in the patient's room. No one likes to be called out on rules unknown to them. The purpose of limit setting is not for the nurse to have the upper hand, but to assist patients with behaviors that get in the way of their recovery (see clinical example below). Often, behaviors such as making excessive phone calls or making frequent visits to the nursing station are defense mechanisms related to anxiety. If the patient can be assisted to deal with underlying anxieties in a more appropriate way, limit setting has served a good purpose. Obviously, some limits are related to the limitations of nursing staff in accommodating certain requests. Limits are part of daily living, and both patients and nurses sometimes need to be reminded about being realistic in their expectations.

### CLINICAL EXAMPLE

Mary, who is attending a partial hospital day program, is very anxious and approaches the nurses' station every 10 minutes, asking to talk with a staff member. Staff members are concerned that they might be encouraging Mary to be too dependent by talking with her each time she approaches. The staff jointly decides to set limits on Mary by telling her that a staff member will meet with her once every 4 hours for a 15-minute period. This approach encourages the patient to limit her demands on others and also to meet some of her own needs between the times she meets with a staff member.

CRITICAL THINKING QUESTION    1

In what ways are the concepts of *norms* and *limit setting* similar? How are they different?

## BALANCE

Balance, perhaps more than any other element of managing the therapeutic environment, represents the value of developing expertise in nursing. Balance involves the process of gradually allowing independent behaviors in a dependent situation. It might be necessary to make specific judgments about a patient's readiness to assume certain responsibilities for his or her own care versus providing assistance when the patient might not be able to act on his or her own behalf. Making this decision requires the nurse to weigh the multiple and competing needs of the patient involved, as well as those of other patients on the unit. Inconsistency in following rules is a major source of problematic interaction on psychiatric units. Bending rules for a patient is something that can really only be done, without creating havoc, by an experienced psychiatric nurse who is well informed about how to balance a number of variables when making exceptions to rules at an appropriate time. Consistency in responding to patients' behaviors and requests is essential if treatment goals are to be met.

The nurse also has to balance the patients' personal rights with those of the other patients. For example, patients have a right to religious expression, but the other patients have a right not to have religious views forced on them or disrupt the treatment environment. Thus, each patient has certain individual rights; however, these rights might be mitigated by the rights of *all* patients to be protected from the symptoms and behaviors exhibited by other patients. The skillful use of balance comes with an understanding of ethical concerns, legal issues, and psychopathology, and represents a progression from novice to expert psychiatric nurse.

CRITICAL THINKING QUESTION    2

In this chapter, *balance* is defined as "... the process of gradually allowing independent behavior in a dependent situation." What is meant by a *dependent situation?*

## THE NURSE AS MANAGER OF THE TREATMENT ENVIRONMENT

Environmental modification is an important intervention of the psychiatric nurse (Baker, 2000; Cleary and Edwards, 1999) and entails using the elements of safety, structure, norms, limit setting, and balance to facilitate meeting patients' treatment goals. Through environmental modification, the nurse can develop a therapeutic environment for the patient. Physical arrangements, safety issues, and other features can create an atmosphere in which patients can learn new behaviors or become aware of their personal strengths. Responsiveness to the needs of patients necessitates that nursing staff continually review environmental norms, rules, and regulations as an important aspect of managing and modifying the environment. Flexibility in maintaining a therapeutic environment is accomplished by this ongoing evaluation of effectiveness. The care plan illustrates how environmental modification is used as a tool for meeting the patients' treatment goals. One of the most challenging and rewarding aspects of psychiatric nursing is the ability to affect the experience of patients in the hospital in a positive, therapeutic, and creative way. Nurses have published both research and anecdotal details of their successes in implementing an improved therapeutic environment in psychiatric care settings (Baker, 2000; Baker et al, 2002; Smith et al, 1996). The psychiatric nurse can often offer insight and assistance to nurse colleagues on other nursing units when environmental management issues or specific behavioral interventions are needed.

CRITICAL THINKING QUESTION    3

A 16-year-old boy with a diagnosis of bipolar disorder has been admitted to the adolescent unit of a psychiatric hospital because of recent fighting at school and threatening his parents at home. How might the use of a therapeutic environment assist this patient in changing his behaviors?

In a review of the changes of the treatment environments of inpatient settings, Norton (2004) summarized significant alterations of the acute psychiatric inpatient unit:

# Care Plan

Name: ZZ                                                              Admission Date: 6-03-05

*DSM-IV-TR* Diagnosis: Major depressive disorder with dependent and narcissistic features

| | |
|---|---|
| Assessment | **Areas of strength:** Asks for help, willing to learn and apply relaxation techniques, work history in health care. |

**Problems:** Patient has been unable to manage her increasing anxiety without calling family six to eight times per day and has called her physician three times per week for the last 2 weeks.

Diagnosis — Anxiety related to ineffective coping skills:
1. Patient states she is "very upset" by "little" things.
2. Patient's affect very unsettled and anxious.
3. Patient makes frequent complaints (up to 10 times per 8-hour shift) of being very hot or cold, wanting more medication, being annoyed by other patients, etc.
4. Patient expresses need for Xanax 1 to 2 hours after AM dose.
5. Patient expresses fearfulness about her anxiety becoming out of control.
6. When out of bed, patient walks the floor of the unit constantly and becomes irritable with other patients.

Outcomes

*Short-term goals:*                                                                   *Date met*

1. Patient will identify feelings of anxiety and explore thoughts/ events preceding anxious feelings.                                    _____
2. Patient will report a decrease in anxiety level on a scale of 1 to 10.                                                              _____
3. Patient will reduce complaints to the nurses to three times per shift.                                                              _____
4. Patient will practice relaxation techniques twice daily and as needed.                                                             _____
5. Patient will manage anxiety without additional doses of medication.                                                               _____
6. Patient will engage in planned exercise and recreational activities as an outlet for increased activity associated with anxiety.       _____

*Long-term goals*

1. Patient will report confidence in ability to manage anxiety without as needed doses of medication.                               _____
2. Patient will participate in follow-up psychotherapy.                              _____

Planning/ Interventions

**Nurse-patient relationship:** Assist patient to identify and explore feelings of anxiety, including the events or thoughts contributing to the development of increased feelings of anxiety; have patient use a written journal to record anxiety levels on an hourly basis using a scale of 1 to 10, with 10 representing the greatest anxiety felt.

**Psychopharmacology:** Paxil 30 mg PO every morning; meet with patient three times per shift to discuss anxiety levels and problems experienced on the unit. Discuss the role of medications and self-care activities in learning to manage anxiety effectively.

**Milieu management:** Assist patient in problem solving to remedy any complaints verbalized. Support the patient's efforts to decrease anxiety level by managing disruptive patients on the unit. Provide a quiet space for patient to work on relaxation techniques and monitor progress in using the techniques and their effectiveness. Involve patient in recreational and exercise activities.

In the 21st century, the environment of the acute inpatient psychiatric ward is significantly different from that of the 1960s and 1970s, to which most of the therapeutic milieu literature refers. The number of wards, hence beds, is much fewer. The patients' average length of stay is greatly reduced. The proportion of psychotic and detained patients is higher, as is the level of risk of violence. All these factors pose a great challenge to staff who are expected, and who themselves expect, to create a therapeutic as well as a safe ward environment for those in their charge. The wide and constantly changing needs and demands of such a rapidly turning over, non-compliant patient group can easily frustrate the efforts of even the most dedicated and professional of multidisciplinary teams (p 280).

The present-day environment of psychiatric units brings to the forefront the need to address variables affecting the therapeutic environment (Chapter 24).

---

### CRITICAL THINKING QUESTION    4

Review Box 1-1: On Being Sane in Insane Places. What were the things that were wrong on the inpatient unit? How should this be corrected to facilitate a therapeutic environment?

---

### ■ Study Notes

1. Environmental modification is the purposeful use of all interpersonal and environmental forces to enhance the mental health of psychiatric patients through the development of a therapeutic environment.

2. Because nurses use environmental modification as a tool for assisting patients, nurses have a significant part of the responsibility for shaping the therapeutic environment.

3. The JCAHO has very clear standards regarding the effects of the environment of care on inpatient psychiatric settings. Safety and a functional environment conducive to patient care are major priorities of the environment of care.

4. Historically, nurses provided only custodial care but, after World War II, Maxwell Jones (1953) and others conceptualized an environment in which all aspects of the psychiatric patient's day would be used to promote mental health. This was termed *milieu therapy*.

5. The therapeutic environment in inpatient settings has diminished as biologically based treat-ments have gained prominence and community care has become the preferred setting for treatment. In inpatient settings, safety is a priority goal.

6. Principles of milieu therapy can also be applied to community settings.

7. All treatment environments can be therapeutic or nontherapeutic.

8. Psychiatric nurses manage the treatment environment by modification of five elements: (1) safety, (2) structure, (3) norms, (4) limit setting, and (5) balance.

9. Creating and managing a therapeutic environment require the psychiatric nurse to be active.

### ■ References

American Nurses Association: *Definition of nursing.* Available at http://www.nursingworld.org/about/faq.htm#def. Accessed May 24, 2005.

Baker JA: Developing psychosocial care for acute psychiatric wards, *J Psychiatr Ment Health Nurs* 7:95, 2000.

Baker JA, O'Higgins H, Parkinson J, Tracey N: The construction and implementation of a psychosocial interventions care pathway within a low secure environment: a pilot study, *J Psychiatr Ment Health Nurs* 9:737, 2002.

Binnema D: Interrelations of psychiatric patient experiences of boredom and mental health, *Issues Ment Health Nurs* 25:833, 2004.

Cleary M, Edwards C: Something always comes up: nurse-patient interaction in an acute psychiatric setting, *J Psychiatr Ment Health Nurs* 6:469, 1999.

Hillbrand M, Waite BM, Young JL: Restricting TV access by forensic patients, *Psychiatr Serv* 49:107, 1998.

Joint Commission on the Accreditation of Healthcare Organizations (JCAHO): *Comprehensive accreditation manual for hospitals,* Chicago, 2001, JCAHO.

Jones M: *The therapeutic community,* New York, 1953, Basic Books.

Norton K: Re-thinking acute psychiatric inpatient care, *Int J Social Psychiatry* 50:274, 2004.

Rosenhan DL: On being sane in insane places, *Science* 179:250, 1973.

Satcher D: *Inpatient hospitalization and community alternatives for crisis care: a report of the Surgeon General.* Available at http://www.surgeongeneral.gov/library/mentalhealth/chapter4/sec5.html#inpatient Accessed May 27, 2005.

Smith J, Gross C, Roberts J: The evolution of a therapeutic environment for patients with long-term illness as measured by the Ward Atmosphere Scale, *J Psychiatr Ment Health Nurs* 5:349, 1996.

Stanton A, Schwartz M: *The mental hospital,* New York, 1954, Basic Books.

Thomas S, Martin T, Shattell M: *Longing to make a difference: nurses' experience of the acute psychiatric inpatient environment.* Presented at the 19th Annual Convention of the Southern Nursing Research Society, Atlanta, February 23, 2005.

Thomas S, Shattel, M, Martin T: What's therapeutic about the therapeutic milieu? *Arch Psychiatr Nurs* 16:99, 2002.

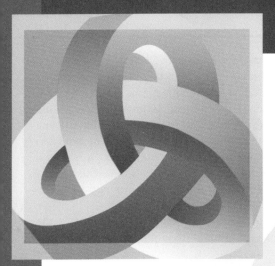

# Chapter 24

# Variables Affecting the Therapeutic Environment

*Beverly K. Hogan and Mona M. Shattell*

## Learning Objectives

*After reading this chapter, you should be able to:*
- Identify variables affecting the creation and maintenance of a therapeutic environment.
- Talk about how staff relationships affect the treatment environment.

- Explain the importance of nursing management to the treatment environment.
- Discuss the impact that nurses have on the therapeutic environment.

In Chapter 23, management of the treatment environment was presented as a process whereby the nurse modifies elements of the treatment environment: safety, structure, norms, limit setting, and balance. Each of these essential components of a therapeutic environment is used by the nurse in making decisions about how to modify various aspects of the environment to meet the treatment needs of patients. Many variables enhance or detract from this process; in this chapter, the focus is on some of the more significant of these variables.

## STAFF RELATIONSHIPS

One of the most important aspects of the treatment environment is the relationships among and between staff members and patients. The nurse-patient relationship is discussed in Chapter 8. This section will mainly focus on staff-staff relations. As is the case with all relationships, the potential for conflict, strained relationships, and dissatisfaction exists. Unresolved conflict and disgruntled

attitudes can permeate the atmosphere of a treatment environment and interfere with the development of a therapeutic environment. Most people can identify with a particular feeling they get when walking into a social, business, or health care setting. The feeling might be one of tension, creating the desire to get away as soon as possible, or it might be a good atmosphere, generating a positive feeling about being there. The latter is sought in creating a therapeutic environment. If one were to examine factors in the environment that make it positive, such features such as how well people get along, whether people smile, and welcoming comments and gestures would likely be present (see the Highlighting the Evidence: Current Research box).

On the other hand, chronic conflict among staff members creates more of the "can't wait to get away from here" feeling. Treatment staff does not have to be drawn to socialize with each other; however, it is a work responsibility in psychiatry to manage one's relations with other treatment team members. This is done not just because it makes for a more harmonious work environment, but because it is critical to making the treatment environment therapeutic as opposed to merely a location for receiving treatment. Nurses are usually aware of the importance of establishing good relationships with colleagues to facilitate a therapeutic

environment for patients (Cleary and Edwards, 1999); however conflictual relations might be promoted by a rigid organizational hierarchy that overrides collaboration and communication among staff (Simms, 1999). Staff members unable to cope with conflict are less effective in their interactions with patients. In such environments, a parental style of communication is prevalent (Cleary and Edwards, 1999), which serves to disempower those lower in the hierarchy.

A potential source of conflict among staff is the model of care adopted by a given treatment facility. The psychiatrist, as head of the treatment team, sets the tone for treatment based on his or her own theoretical perspective about patient care. Some psychiatrists have a purely medical focus and minimize the value of psychosocially oriented interventions. Because nurses are educated to provide holistic care, conflict can erupt in a setting that marginalizes psychosocial intervention. Nurses trapped in a model of care divergent from their

### Norm's Notes

*Each unit or situation has variables affecting the environment. This chapter brings it up a notch by pointing out that staff relationships, management philosophy, and your own work satisfaction can contribute to or detract from the therapeutic effectiveness of the work environment. Some of you, during the course of your career, might have to move to another job because the constraints placed on you by management hinder you from developing an effective environment.*

### Highlighting the Evidence: Current Research

#### "It's the People That Make the Environment Good or Bad:" The Patient's Experience of the Acute Care Hospital Environment

A review of contemporary nursing research reveals a tendency to focus on certain aspects of the hospital environment, such as noise, light, and music. Although studies such as these shed light on discrete aspects of the hospital environment, this body of literature contributes little to understanding the entirety of that world as experienced by the patient. The purpose of our study (Shattell et al, 2005) was to describe the patient's experience of the acute care (medical-surgical) hospital environment. Nondirective, in-depth interviews were conducted, transcribed verbatim, and analyzed for themes. Against the backdrop of "I lived and that's all that matters," there were three predominant themes in patients' experience of the acute care environment: disconnection/connection, fear/less fear, and confinement/freedom.

Patients want interpersonal connections with nurses who are friendly, check in frequently, and are responsive. Some patients seek to be good patients and to make friends with the nurses, which is consistent with findings from a study of

how hospitalized patients solicit nursing care (Shattell et al, 2005). Interpersonal connections to others help decrease patients' fears and feelings of confinement in the acute care hospital environment. As one participant said, "The relationship makes the environment better."

In essence, the global quality of care outcome from the patient's perspective was survival of the hospitalization. Perceived quality of care was determined by the friendliness, attentiveness, and responsiveness of the nurses. Technical skill or competence was rarely mentioned.

In the medical-surgical hospital environment, human-to-human contact increased feelings of security and power in an environment that was described as sterile, disorienting, and untrustworthy. In an environment that produces feelings of fear and confinement, patients focus on their *relationships with nurses*—the people on whom they depend to mediate this stressful environment. In summary, these findings suggest that a focus on therapeutic environments needs to be primarily focused on interpersonal care, not on the physical environment, such as the color of the walls or the architectural design.

From Shattell M, Hogan B, and Thomas S: "It's the people that make the environment good or bad": the patient's experience of the acute care hospital environment, *AACN Clin Issues: Adv Prac Acute Crit Care*, 16:159, 2005.

belief system experience conflict in their provision of care to patients. For instance, milieu therapy might conflict greatly with a purely medical model of care. In a pure medical model, the use of medications and other biologically based interventions is seen as the solution, with psychosocial care being given little importance. Chronic dissonance about the care being provided is one factor leading to burnout and low morale of the nursing staff (Schreiber and Lutzen, 2000).

## NURSING'S INFLUENCE

Nursing's contribution to the treatment environment was addressed in Chapter 24, so it should suffice to reiterate the importance of the nurse in creating a therapeutic environment briefly. The article excerpt, On Being Sane in Insane Places (see Box 1-1), noted that nurses spend little time interacting with patients. More recent studies have documented that less than 50% of the nurses' time is spent in direct patient contact, with the percentage of time devoted to potentially therapeutic interaction being slightly less than 7% (Whittington and McLaughlin, 2000). Other studies have found that patients spend most of their time alone and, although they understand the nurse's time constraints, patients regret the lack of time available to spend with them (Cleary and Edwards, 1999; Shattell, 2002; Thomas et al, 2002, 2005). Patients might interpret this lack of attention as a dismissal or minimization of their symptoms and problems. Cleary (1999) found that patient dissatisfaction with nursing care was related to the quality and time that nurses spent with them. Patients especially valued those nurses who dealt with problem patients, an important function of the nurse in creating safety, as noted in the previous chapter. If nurses were simply available, if they greeted the patients by name and made time to spend with them, patients viewed nurses as valuable (Cleary and Edwards, 1999). Three recent studies of the inpatient acute care psychiatric environment found that both nurses and patients focus more on the interpersonal environment (Shattell, 2002; Thomas et al, 2002, 2005) than on the physical layout of the units. This is consistent with our study on the experience of patients in the medical-surgical environment as well (Shattell et al, 2005). Nursing is such a significant influence on the patient's treatment environment that this documented tendency toward minimal interaction with patients requires attention. Burnout and secondary traumatization represent our theory about the notable distancing from patients occurring on today's inpatient psychiatric units.

### CRITICAL THINKING QUESTION    1

A job title, such as physician extender, even if it is not one's preferred title, appears to be benign. What are the implications for one's professional self-concept and identity?

## BURNOUT AND SECONDARY TRAUMATIZATION

Burnout can be defined as "a state of physical, emotional, and mental exhaustion caused by long-term involvement in emotionally demanding situations" (Pines and Aronson, 1988). Collins and Long (2003) added that burnout is a process "that includes a gradual exposure to job strain, erosion of idealism and a void in achievement." Burnout diminishes the nurse's ability to be effective on a psychiatric unit. Maslach (2001) found that persons use avoidance and distancing themselves as a self-protective reaction to burnout. Younger and less experienced mental health care providers tend to be at greater risk for burnout (Ackerley et al, 1988). Burned-out staff members score high on scales measuring feelings of being emotionally burdened, and they tend to overinterpret patient care failures as their own fault (Schreiber and Lutzen, 2000; Thomas et al, 2005). This tendency leads to a spiraling process of decreased effectiveness in nurse-patient interactions at all levels. Some manifestations of burnout on a psychiatric unit are low morale, passivity, avoidance, disinterest, chronic complaining, and negative, hostile reactions to others (Schreiber and Lutzen, 2000). A more recent study suggested that strong moral sensitivity among nurses accompanied by low organizational support places nurses at risk for health problems (Lutzen et al, 2003).

### CRITICAL THINKING QUESTION    2

How would you use the principles learned in this chapter or course to deal with a co-worker who constantly complains and gossips about other co-workers?

## CRITICAL THINKING QUESTION    3

What might you do, other than transfer or resign, if you found yourself in a work environment in which management was unsupportive of nursing staff?

Working on a psychiatric unit involves emotional labor and can involve high stress, which contributes to burnout. The concept of emotional labor has appeared in the literature since the early 1980s and refers to the emotional effort involved in having to suppress one's usual human reactions to others in the name of social acceptability—that is, professionalism (Mann and Cowburn, 2005). Evers and colleagues (2001) found that staff reporting high levels of emotional exhaustion tended to have cold, insensitive treatment attitudes. Later studies showed a relationship between burnout and being a victim of physical aggression (Evers et al, 2002; Farrell and Cubit, 2005). Dealing with aggressive behavior is stressful to begin with and is certainly made worsen by the burden of burnout. It could be surmised that this results from reduced awareness and responsiveness to personal risk.

## CRITICAL THINKING QUESTION    4

How would you ensure good nurse-patient interaction within a unit?

Many factors operate to add to stress on a psychiatric unit. Apart from the stress of patients' behaviors, nurses are often also conflicted about their reactions to such behaviors, having been socialized in nursing to be nonjudgmental and tolerant (Dinwiddie and Briska, 2004). Additionally, nurses expect themselves to be able to come up with creative solutions to patients' behaviors and problems. Regulatory and accreditation agencies also place nurses under stress to avoid the use of restraints and seclusion to comply with behavioral guidelines; however, restraints and seclusion are sometimes required to control aggression that is unresponsive to less restrictive alternatives. This can result in the nurse feeling like a failure (Cleary, 2003) and also create conflict for the nurse who is, on the one hand, prided for encouraging autonomy and respect for the individual, yet obliged to intervene with force when other measures are ineffective (Johnson, 1998).

Coping with burnout and the continuous exposure to traumatic events inevitably evokes some type of coping response from nurses. Humor is one method used in stressful occupations to help relieve the anxiety, fear, or horror experienced by coping with stressful work. Sayre (2001) studied the use of humor by mental health professionals in psychiatry, categorized humor into types ranging from whimsical to sarcastic or hostile, and examined its influence on patient care. Although whimsical humor (defined as playful, poking of fun) was generally accepted as a way of coping with stress, humor that leans toward the sarcastic (defined as intentional hurt with mocking ridicule) and hostile end of the scale tended to erode professional competence and morale, ultimately affecting patient care. When interactions between staff and patients were perceived as more stressful, staff tended to engage in more of the sarcastic variety of humor. Under the veil of sarcasm, feelings of anger and a discounting of or vengeance for the target of sarcastic humor were evident. The use of sarcastic humor, in particular, creates a type of nontherapeutic distancing, thereby interfering with successful development of a therapeutic relationship with patients. This type of humor is so commonplace in the media that recognizing its antitherapeutic effects might be difficult. Although nurses in Sayre's study (2001) used sarcastic humor about patients quite often, they rarely ridiculed the misfortune of patients directly. Although sarcasm and burnout are understandable responses to underlying distress in nurses' work environments, it is neither acceptable nor effective interpersonal behavior in a health care environment.

For the last several decades, increased attention has been given to the effects of trauma on individuals. The professional literature related to working with trauma began to reveal the phenomenon of vicarious traumatization, also called secondary traumatization, *helper stress,* or *compassion fatigue* (Thomas and Wilson, 2004). Vicarious traumatization "refers to the cumulative effect . . . of working with survivors of traumatic life events. Anyone who engages empathetically with victims or survivors is vulnerable" (Pearlman and Saakvitne, 1995). Secondary traumatization is associated with burnout among nurses (Johnson, 1992); however, some scholars see burnout and secondary trauma as separate entities with different causes, courses, and solutions. It is important to note that exposure to traumatic events does not always result in secondary traumatization (King et al, 1998). The reasons for its occurrence in some nurses but not in others have been related to the presence of certain protective factors, such as "feelings of control, commitment, and change as challenge" (Collins and Long, 2003).

The daily stress of dealing with patients with behavioral problems can be taxing for the nursing staff. This is particularly true when working in a unit that primarily serves patients from the public psychiatric sector. Patients in a public psychiatric hospital are among the sickest, with seemingly limitless needs, poor insight, frequent readmissions, few placement alternatives, and sometimes violent behavior. Stressors such as these take their toll on the nurse. Norton (2004) stated the following about today's inpatient units: "The wide and constantly changing needs and demands of such a rapidly turning over, noncompliant patient group can easily frustrate the efforts of even the most dedicated and professional of multidisciplinary teams."

Often, students in psychiatric nursing express dismay at the minimal amount of interaction observed between nurses and patients. Although not applicable to all cases, we believe that many of the nurses observed sitting in nursing stations rather than being active in the treatment environment are there as a result of secondary traumatization. The term *burnout* is reserved for those who started out on fire, as opposed to those who never even flickered. Many of the nurses who retreat to the nursing station entered their jobs with much enthusiasm and energy; however, the continuous giving of oneself emotionally, without having supports in place, is a recipe for depletion of one's emotional reserves. In the following sections, management's responsibility in supporting staff and creating opportunities to respond to these problems is addressed. Box 24-1 lists some resources for dealing with burnout.

## MANAGEMENT PRACTICES AND ORGANIZATIONAL STRUCTURE

Aside from dealing with conflicting staff relationships, excessive bureaucracy is seen by nurses as a major impediment to their effectiveness (Boey, 1999). Staff requires administrative and management support to deliver the care required on a psychiatric unit (Smith, 1998). As representatives

---

### Box 24-1  Resources for Burnout

It is important that nurses seek out assistance for preventing and recovering from burnout. Examples of potential professional resources are individuals with experience in burnout and professional nursing issues, such as Dr. Marion Conti-O'Hare, author of *The Nurse as Wounded Healer: From Trauma to Transcendence*\* and the American Nurses Association (http://www.nursingworld.org). Involvement in one's professional association can be a great resource for new as well as experienced nurses.

\*2002, Jones and Bartlett.

---

of the model of care of an agency, management influences the practice of nursing. Stated another way, nursing practice can only be as effective as management allows. It is difficult to imagine that nursing management would engage in practices that restrict the practice of good nursing care, but it does occur. Several studies have documented the influence of management on nursing morale and implementation of care (Boey, 1999; Brekke et al, 1997; Graham, 2001; Lutzen, 1998; Schreiber and Lutzen, 2000; Smith, 1998). Nurses cannot practice their profession unless management establishes structures that support and reinforce good patient care.

Institutional restraints and bureaucracy also affect the caring ethic of nurses. In nonsupportive, oppressive atmospheres, nurses might face sanctions for doing the right thing. These sanctions come from peers, or worse, from management. In a study of the moral survival strategies practiced by nurses in environments constrained by excessive bureaucracy, Lutzen (1998) found management practices to be a significant influence on how nurses cope in such environments. Nurses become demoralized when they do not have appropriate support to practice nursing. This type of oppression is harmful not only to the patient, but also to the nurse (Schreiber and Lutzen, 2000).

Ongoing research on how nurses negotiate dealing with such ethical dilemmas raises questions about the responsibility of organizations to nurses in resolving this source of stress. Those who experience a lack of control over their work situation, along with simultaneous high work demands, have been found to have an elevated risk of cardiovascular disease (Lutzen et al, 2003). In an increasingly litigious environment, management would be well served to be aware of the implications of not addressing these hazards; however, protection of health care workers has traditionally awaited the manifestation of risk (Love, 2003). Farrell and Cubit (2005) found that even when workplace safety is addressed by management, organizational costs and emotional effects on staff are rarely addressed.

Cleary (2003) studied psychiatric nurses in their work environment and found that many of the nurses also experienced distress as a result of the time intended for interacting with patients being diverted into other less meaningful tasks. In this study, such devaluing of one's professional responsibilities to patients contributed to being unfulfilled in one's work. Nurses generally know what they need to do but do not always have organizational backing and support. Organizational structures that are rigid and characterized by a high need for efficiency interfere with nursing care. Lack of positive reinforcement and being held accountable for impossible to meet care objectives, with dwindling resources and rigidly burdensome rules that delay patient care, erode the morale and professional competence of nurses (Sayre, 2001). In studies examining strategies for reducing burnout and dissatisfaction in nurses, most researchers concluded that effective management actions can alleviate many of the problems. When organizational support is provided to nurses, psychosocial care interventions can receive their deserved priority in psychiatric settings (Baker et al, 2002).

## CLINICAL SUPERVISION

Clinical supervision is an important aspect of the therapeutic environment. The purpose of clinical supervision is to provide a place for nurses caring for patients to examine attitudes, reactions, and conflicts with patients on the unit and to find new ways of approaching patient problems. This goal requires a commitment by the nurse to a process of self-awareness, openness, and receptiveness to feedback. Providing a structured time for this important process ensures that it will occur. An improvement in staff cohesiveness, morale, and creativity as a result of regular clinical supervision being provided for nursing staff has been demonstrated (Berg and Hallberg, 1999). Activities such as clinical supervision also help nurses develop

sensitivity to the patient. The importance of understanding the patient's distress and providing supportive interpersonal communication has remained unchallenged, even in an era of biologic psychiatry (Reynolds and Scott, 1999).

In the past, clinical nurse specialists (CNSs) fulfilled this role of clinical supervision for staff nurses on psychiatric units. Unfortunately, the role of the CNS has, in many institutions, been changed from directly working with nurses to being a direct agent of psychiatrists. In some agencies, the title of the has been changed to that of *physician extender,* potentially reducing an important source of support for nurses.

Increasingly, studies have emphasized the impact of experiencing trauma secondary to being surrounded by traumatic experiences of others (Ackerley et al, 1988; Cleary, 2003, 2004; Collins and Long, 2003; Johnson, 1992; King et al, 1998; Lutzen et al, 2003; Maslach, 2001; Pearlman and Saakvitne, 1995). Begat (2005) discussed several studies that clearly document the value of CNS-led supervision for reducing stress in nursing staff and improving the ability to provide empathic, compassionate care. Because the consistent experiencing of the trauma of others (i.e., patients) directly affects one's work with patients, it would appear to be a responsibility of the institution to ensure that this type of professional supervision of one's practice is provided.

Today's health care environment, particularly in psychiatry, requires active attention to the effects of a stressful environment on one's own health. When nurses are stressed and kept in crisis mode, it is impossible to provide appropriate and effective psychosocial care. Nurses need clinical supervision to support the work they do with patients, and they also must have very good self-care practices and support in place. In psychiatry, it is particularly important that nursing staff engage in clinical supervision, because it allows others from the same environment to serve as a mirror for staff to see such areas as overidentifying with patients, overreacting to some event, and appearing excessively tired. In psychiatry, it is still important to retain clinical assessment and technical skills, but the primary tool available to psychiatric nurses and their patients is themselves. It is incredibly arrogant to believe that one could work with so much intense human suffering without having checks and balances built in to keep clear on reaction to these various issues. Similarly, it is terribly wrong for management to neglect this needed support for staff.

## AGGRESSION AND VIOLENCE

Probably the greatest concern that students have about psychiatric nursing involves the potential for violence. Safety is an essential component of the therapeutic environment, particularly to the extent that nursing staff is competent in managing potential aggression (and is adequately staffed), aggression on a psychiatric unit is managed by prevention and early intervention (see Chapter 11 for detailed discussion of the aggressive patient). This prevention–early intervention approach to potential aggression is required to maintain the feeling of safety for everyone within the unit (Johnson, 2004). Research has shown that nurses trained in physical and verbal intervention techniques for dealing with aggression have greater confidence and less stress (Evers et al, 2001).

From the patient's perspective, being forced into treatment activities reduces trust in staff, and therefore interferes with the nurse's ability to develop a therapeutic relationship. Often, struggle over rules is the precipitating factor leading to a patient being restrained. Rules on a psychiatric unit are intended for safety, not for a control battle. The way in which nurses enforce rules and norms in a treatment environment affects the nurse-patient relationship and the therapeutic environment. Excessive focus on rules and efficiency might be seen as necessary and desirable to some staff, but is harmful to patients. Abrupt dismissal of the patient's perspective occurs when rules and regulations have a stronger focus than individualized patient care and creativity among the nursing staff. Patients refer to staff members who are more concerned with rules, efficiency, and order as *institutionalized,* a term originally coined by professionals to describe patients with the same characteristics (Wirt, 1999).

### CRITICAL THINKING QUESTION    5

What are the advantages of openness and feedback on a psychiatric unit? Can you think of any drawbacks? Are the nurses "open" on the unit where you do clinical rotations?

### CLINICAL EXAMPLE

The unit routine dictates that patients take a bath in the morning and take medications at 8 AM. A patient recently admitted involuntarily angrily refuses both. The nurse talks with the patient and offers a choice about when to take a bath. The nurse also learns that the patient usually takes medications later in the morning. The nurse negotiates with the treatment team and pharmacy department to change the times of the patient's scheduled medication.

Aside from episodes of restraint or seclusion occurring as a result of conflict related to rules, sometimes patients have episodes of violence that occur without warning or cannot be de-escalated. In such instances, restraints are sometimes the only mechanism available for controlling a patient's behavior. There has been a widespread effort, initiated by regulatory agencies and consumer advocacy groups, to eliminate the use of restraints and seclusion because of the risks involved for patients. When a patient is restrained or secluded, staff must remain within an arm's length of the patient to ensure safety. Restraints and seclusion place a patient in a vulnerable position. The continued presence of the staff averts any danger to the restrained or secluded patient. It is important for patients on the unit to know that the safety of all patients is the primary concern, not punishment or mere control of a patient's behavior. Although restraints and seclusion are sometimes necessary, they still remain a method of last resort.

Expert psychiatric nurses are skilled at managing potentially aggressive patients. Carlsson and colleagues (2004) found that the nurse's presence and ability to be with the patient as a unique person in a unique situation was considered essential by nurses for dealing with potentially violent patients. Johnson and Hauser (2001) found that expert nurses used their skills to find a way to connect with the patient and interpret patient behavior within the context and knowledge of a patient's pathology. Understanding the patient's experience is considered a crucial factor in establishing a less aggressive milieu.

Patients are comforted by the staff's competence in managing stressful situations. An acute psychiatric unit is generally perceived by patients as a very stressful place. In an article examining how patients dealt with fear on an inpatient psychiatric unit, one patient was quoted as follows (Quirk et al, 2004):

> There were ... lots of angry young men (on the ward). The nurses spent their time shut in the office and the door to the ward was locked most of the time. There was much overt racism among the staff. Later I found out that one of the nurses had been badly assaulted by one of the patients, and so the staff were very scared. I was scared; the nurses were scared—it could hardly be a therapeutic environment (p. 2573).

Participants in this study were very clear about using active strategies to manage their perceived risks. Tactics such as avoidance, forming alliances with staff, making their own risk assessments about other patients, seeking places on the unit that felt safer than others, and against-medical-advice discharges were used by patients to manage their fear of the inpatient environment (Quirk et al, 2004).

Although there is no guarantee against the occurrence of violence toward nursing staff, one variable affecting the risk of aggression is staff attitude. A study of attitudinal variables and risk of being targeted for patient aggression found that a higher risk exists for staff with more authoritarian attitudes, an external locus of control (looking outside themselves for blame rather than looking within [i.e., self-reflection]), and a high degree of anxiety (Ray and Subich, 1998). Although it is mandatory for staff to complete annual training about management of violent behavior, Farrell and Cubit (2005) compared the content of 28 aggression management programs for staff in psychiatric treatment settings and found that most of these programs failed to address the emotional impact of violence on the staff. Witnessing violence or being a victim of violence is known to have a tremendously negative effect on staff morale, burnout, absenteeism, and similar issues (Farrell and Cubit, 2005). Springboards for worsening one's own stress derive from the observation that staff in psychiatry are known to be overly dismissive of patients' behaviors, including violence. Even when it is not clear whether the violence was prompted by the patient's illness, staff remain reluctant and conflicted about prosecuting patients for violence, although this might be the appropriate action when it is obvious that the patient could have controlled the behavior (Dinwiddie and Briska, 2004). Some preliminary evidence has

suggested that efforts to decrease seclusion and restraint might be accompanied by an increased risk of harm to psychiatric patients and staff (Khadivi et al, 2004).

The necessity of staff-patient interaction cannot be overemphasized. Although violence cannot always be predicted, it is important to be able to intervene when clear warning signs are evident. Nurses cannot know what is occurring on the unit if they spend most of their time in the nurses' station. Additionally, patients and novice staff or students are likely to feel less fearful when interacting with patients if they see staff and clinical instructors doing so.

## INPATIENT SUICIDAL BEHAVIOR

One of the most frequently reported distressing events on a psychiatric unit is dealing with suicidal behavior. In fact, among a group of forensic psychiatric nurses, dealing with suicidal patients ranked higher than dealing with aggressive behavior (Coffey, 1999). Close observation, also called one-to-one or constant observation, is a common strategy used in psychiatric units for suicidal patients. Fletcher (1999) examined ways in which nurses and patients perceived actions of staff while doing constant observation on a suicidal patient. Staff and patients had divergent perceptions, such as staff thinking that sitting outside the room was therapeutic for the patient, whereas the patient was more likely to perceive it as controlling behavior. Allowing for silence was perceived as therapeutic by staff but as hostile by patients. Patients were more likely to feel cared for when they were informed of the purpose of actions. Initiating a no-suicide contract with patients is also a way for patients to feel in control (Fletcher, 1999), and it is perhaps for this reason that this practice continues, even though most studies have found the no-suicide contract to be ineffective. Clinical supervision, as discussed earlier in this chapter, is a resource for nurses in psychiatry when dealing with stressful patient situations, such as suicidal behavior. (See Box 24-2 for tips from the Joint Commission on Accreditation of Healthcare Organizations [JCAHO] on preventing inpatient suicides.)

The inpatient acute care environment is designed with safety in mind. For example, patient rooms are furnished with materials that could not

## Box 24-2   JCAHO Tips for Preventing Inpatient Suicides

Environmental factors that mitigate inpatient suicides include the following:

- Breakaway bars, rods, showerheads, safety rails, low flush toilets, weight-tested for safety
- Adequate visualization of high-risk areas
- Monitoring use of equipment
- Complete assessment of risk at admission and thereafter
- Standardized assessments, with test possessing known psychometric properties
- Orientation, training, competency review, credentialing, and staffing levels
- Continuity of care on transfer
- Appropriate unit assignment
- Checking for contraband on admission
- Observation at frequency prescribed by risk
- Engagement of family, friends in process
- Identification of high-risk populations
- Prescribed checklists used for observations
- Use of standard vocabulary for communicating
- Consideration of staff assignment, including consideration of circadian rhythms, workloads, and time pressures
- Same personnel providing care should perform reviews and make quality improvement on errors
- Provisions for shift change
- Using medications to treat conditions that contribute to risk
- Safety contract

From Joint Commission on Accreditation of Healthcare Organizations: *Comprehensive accreditation manual for hospitals,* Chicago, 2001, JCAHO.

be used by suicidal patients to harm themselves. Beds, desks, and clothes armoires are often bolted to the floors and/or walls; windows are made with reinforced Plexiglas that cannot be opened or broken; bathrooms are designed with plastic vanity mirrors and breakaway shower curtain rods; and trash cans are lined with paper bags instead of plastic bags. Careful thought is placed on the environment to decrease the possibility of patient suicidal or violent behavior.

## MANAGED CARE

In the past, longer inpatient stays were common, but today's inpatient psychiatric units have high turnover and acuity rates. Patients are often quite ill when admitted to an inpatient psychiatric unit as a result of insurance and managed care restrictions on admissions. Additionally, many psychiatric patients have comorbid medical conditions that further increase problems on the unit, leaving less time for psychosocial intervention. Substance abuse is a common problem among patients admitted to acute psychiatric units. This type of patient acuity, rapid patient turnover, and crisis mode of care make the task of developing and maintaining a therapeutic environment difficult. The cost-efficient managed care approach forces inpatient units into a rapid return of the patient to the community for less expensive treatment options (Satcher, 2001). Lacking time to plan care, nurses find themselves responding only to emerging crises and patients quickly learn that getting the nurses' attention requires a crisis. The combined effect of a lack of improvement in the patient's functioning at discharge, an overreliance on medications, and inadequate time to assess and diagnose patients adequately causes serious disturbances to the purported goal of developing a therapeutic relationship (Grinfeld, 2000).

Cleary's studies (2003, 2004) of psychiatric nurses' work environment in inpatient units have highlighted their frustrations as they attempt to deliver care according to traditional models of psychiatric nursing practice to a widely varied population with multiple competing needs. Although the nurses derived a certain pride from being the backbone of the unit, there remained awareness that the work was much more complex, requiring a faster response (Cleary, 2004). Nurses in the study talked about their perception that nurses need to assert their right to practice their nursing work (presumably having time with patients), albeit in a situation that is increasingly crisis–oriented.

## CONSUMERS AND ADVOCATES ON THE PSYCHIATRIC UNIT

In response to a system that has failed in meeting the needs of the chronically mentally ill and has a history of patients' rights violations, the consumer movement has emerged as a highly active and present voice for recovery from mental illness (Center for Mental Health Services, 1999). Consumers serve on boards of mental health care facilities and are often invited, if not mandated, to be a part of the review process for an agency receiving state funds.

Dialogue among patients (consumers) has provided important feedback to professionals about the experiences and needs of individuals with a mental illness. Patients report that they do not like being labeled; they conceptualize themselves as a person with a mental illness rather than as a mentally ill patient (Center for Mental Health Services, 1999). Increasingly, consumers are establishing a presence within treatment programs for the purpose of increasing staff sensitivity to the patient's perspective. In the *Surgeon General's Report,* better outcomes for patients have been noted with consumers involved in psychosocial rehabilitation programs (Satcher, 2001). Consumers bring a recovery perspective that offers hope and support for integration into the community. For example, consumer-run psychosocial rehabilitation drop-in centers might have staff available for crisis intervention, but the focus is on consumers helping each other reach mutual goals of recovery (Brekke et al, 1997).

Many patients discharged to community care require a tremendous amount of connection to services and support in the community. To assess discharge needs accurately requires time to develop a thorough understanding of the patients' difficulties in adjusting to their psychiatric problems while living in the community.

## EFFECTIVE FUNCTIONING IN THE ACUTE PSYCHIATRIC SETTING

At the close of this chapter, discussing solutions is in order. Norton (2004) has indicated that one way to reduce frustrations is for inpatient units to define how the different parts fit together into a functioning whole. This also applies to other aspects of psychiatric care. Clearly articulating the real purpose of the unit, as opposed to holding to standards of care that cannot be met in this new era of psychiatric care, allows all parties to be more realistic about the intent of the inpatient unit or other treatment setting (Norton, 2004):

> To function effectively, the acute psychiatric ward requires: (1) its therapeutic objectives, and how they are to be achieved, to be clearly articulated and communicated, including to patients; (2) the differing needs of subgroups of patients to be identified and targeted in relation to the therapeutic functions required at that time; (3) inpatient staff to be supported by managers to have time for

supervision and support in respect of team function, not just individual performance; (4) the lead clinician and management to agree [about] the limits of the inpatient ward's role in the overall local mental health service (p. 282).

| CRITICAL THINKING QUESTION | 6 |

How do you think the treatment environment affects the physical and emotional recovery of patients in nonpsychiatric treatment settings?

*Note to Students: A number of variables affecting the therapeutic environment of a psychiatric unit have been presented in this chapter. Although the interpersonal environment might not be the primary focus on other nursing units, these same variables affect these environments as well; it is therefore imperative that students take note of these factors, because this information will certainly enhance your value to the patients you care for in any setting.*

## Study Notes

1. Teamwork in psychiatry is essential in maintaining a therapeutic environment. Staff members must be able to work together and resolve any conflicts that arise. Failure to do so adversely affects the treatment environment.

2. The theoretical model of care adopted by a health care facility affects the type of nursing care provided.

3. Staff burnout negatively affects patient care and the therapeutic environment.

4. Vicarious or secondary traumatization, compassion fatigue, and other similar terms describe the possible negative effects for staff when dealing with the daily traumas in particular patient care areas.

5. Management plays an extremely important role in the type of care nurses are empowered to deliver.

6. The consumer movement has influenced treatment settings by providing feedback to staff about the patients' perspective of the treatment environment.

7. Managed care has led to sicker patients, with a more rapid turnover in patient admissions and discharges, which creates stress for the staff and patients.

8. The use of clinical supervision for nursing staff can be a tool to facilitate improved staff cohe-

sion, morale, and the ability to maintain therapeutic relationships with patients.

## References

Ackerley G, Burnell J, Holder D, Kurdek L: Burnout among licensed psychologists. *Prof Psychol: Res Pract* 19:624, 1988.

Baker JA, O'Higgins H, Parkinson J, Tracey N: The construction and implementation of a psychosocial interventions care pathway within a low secure environment: a pilot study, *J Psychiatr Ment Health Nurs* 9:737, 2002.

Baker JA: Developing psychosocial care for acute psychiatric wards, *J Psychiatr Ment Health Nurs* 7:95, 2000.

Begat I, Ellefsen B, Severinsson E: Nurses' satisfaction with their work environment and the outcomes of clinical nursing supervision on nurses' experiences of well-being—a Norwegian study, *J Nurs Manag* 13:221, 2005.

Berg A, Hallberg IR: Effects of systematic clinical supervision on psychiatric nurses' sense of coherence, creativity, work-related strain, job satisfaction and view of the effects of clinical supervision: a pre-post test design, *J Psychosoc Ment Health Serv* 6:371, 1999.

Boey KW: Distressed and stress resistant nurses, *Issues Ment Health Nurs* 20:33, 1999.

Brekke J, Long J, Nesbitt N and Sobel E: The impact of service characteristics on functional outcomes from community support programs for persons with schizophrenia, *J Consult Clin Psychol* 65:464-475, 1997.

Carlsson G, Dahlberg K, Lutzen K, Nystrom M: Violent encounters in psychiatric care: a phenomenological study of embodied caring knowledge, *Issues Ment Health Nurs* 25:191, 2004.

Center for Mental Health Services, Substance Abuse and Mental Health Services Administration, U.S. Department of Health and Human Services: Consumers and psychiatric-mental health nurses in dialogue July 26-27, 1999, Willard Inter-Continental Hotel, Washington, DC. Available at http://www.mentalhealth.samhsa.gov/publications/allpubs/OEL00-0006/default.asp. Accessed October 13, 2005.

Cleary M: The realities of mental health nursing in acute inpatient environments, *Int J Ment Health Nurs* 13:53, 2004.

Cleary M: The challenges of mental health care reform for contemporary mental health nursing practice: Relationships, power and control, *Int J Ment Health Nurs* 12:139, 2003.

Cleary M, Edwards C: Something always comes up: nurse-patient interaction in an acute psychiatric setting, *J Psychiatr Ment Health Nurs* 6:469, 1999.

Cleary M, Edwards C, Meehan T: Factors influencing nurse-patient interaction in the acute psychiatric setting: an exploratory investigation, *Aust N Z J Ment Health Nurs* 8:109, 1999.

Coffey M: Stress and burnout in forensic community psychiatric nursing: an investigation of its causes and effects, *J Psychiatr Ment Health Nurs* 6:433, 1999.

Collins S, Long A: Working with the psychological effects of trauma: consequences for mental health-care workers—a literature review, *J Psychiatr Ment Health Nurs* 10:417, 2003.

Dinwiddie SH, Briska W: Prosecution of violent psychiatric inpatients: theoretical and practical issues, *Int J Law Psychiatry* 27:17, 2004.

Evers W, Tomic W, Brouwers A: Aggressive behaviour and burnout among staff of homes for the elderly, *Int J Ment Health Nurs* 11:2, 2002.

Evers W, Tomic W, Brouwers A: Effects of aggressive behavior and perceived self-efficacy on burnout among staff of homes for the elderly, *Issues Ment Health Nurs* 22:439, 2001.

Farrell G, Cubit K: Nurses under threat: a comparison of content of 28 aggression management programs, *Int J Ment Health Nurs* 14:44, 2005.

Fletcher R: The process of constant observation: perspectives of staff and suicidal patients, *J Psychiatr Ment Health Nurs* 6:9, 1999.

Graham IW: Seeking a clarification of meaning: a phenomenological interpretation of the craft of mental health nursing, *J Psychiatr Nurs Ment Health Serv* 8:335, 2001.

Grinfeld MJ: Managed care for public mental health yields mixed results, *Psychiatr Times* 17:32, 2000.

Johnson C: Coping with compassion fatigue, *Nursing* 22:116, 1992.

Johnson M: Violence on inpatient psychiatric units: state of the science, *J Am Psychiatr Nurs Assoc* 10:133, 2004.

Johnson ME: Being restrained: a study of power and powerlessness, *Issues Ment Health Nurs* 19:191, 1998.

Johnson ME, Hauser PM: The practices of expert psychiatric nurses: accompanying the patient to a calmer interpersonal space, *Issues Ment Health Nurs* 22:651, 2001.

Joint Commission on Accreditation of Healthcare Organizations: *Comprehensive accreditation manual for hospitals,* Chicago, 2001, JCAHO.

Khadivi AN, Patel RC, Atkinson AR, Levine JM: Association between seclusion and restraint and patient-related violence, *Psychiatr Serv* 55:1311, 2004.

King L, King D, Fairbank H, Adams G: Resilience-recovery factors in post-traumatic stress disorder among female and male veterans: hardiness, post war social support and additional stressful life events, *J Personality Social Psychol* 74:420, 1998.

Love C, Morrison E, American Academy of Nursing Expert Panel on Violence: Policy recommendations on workplace violence, *Issues Ment Health Nurs* 24:599, 2003.

Lutzen K: Subtle coercion in psychiatric practice, *J Psychiatr Ment Health Nurs* 5:101, 1998.

Lutzen K, Cronqvist A, Magnusson A, Andersson L: Moral stress: synthesis of a concept, *Nurs Ethics* 10:312, 2003.

Mann S, Cowburn J: Emotional labour and stress within mental health nursing, *J Psychiatr Ment Health Nurs* 12:154, 2005.

Maslach C: *The truth about burnout,* San Francisco, 2001, Jossey Bass.

Norton K: Re-thinking acute psychiatric inpatient care, *Int J Soc Psychiatry* 50:274, 2004.

Pearlman L, Saakvitne K: *Trauma and the therapist: countertransference and vicarious traumatization in psychotherapy with incest survivors,* New York, 1995, WW Norton.

Pines A, Aronson E: *Career burnout: causes and cures,* New York, 1988, Free Press.

Quirk A, Lelliott P, Seale O: Service users' strategies for managing risk in the volatile environment of an acute psychiatric ward, *Soc Sci Med* 59:2573, 2004.

Ray CL, Subich LM: Staff assaults and injuries in a psychiatric hospital as a function of three attitudinal variables, *Issues Ment Health Nurs* 19:277, 1998.

Reynolds WJ, Scott B: Empathy: a crucial component of the helping relationship, *J Psychiatr Ment Health Nurs* 6:363, 1999.

Satcher D: Mental health: a report of the Surgeon General, 2001. Available at http://www.surgeongeneral.gov/library/mentalhealth/home.html. Accessed May 27, 2005.

Sayre J: The use of aberrant medical humor by psychiatric nursing staff, *Issues Ment Health Nurs* 22:669, 2001.

Schreiber R, Lutzen K: Revisiting nursing in a nontherapeutic environment, *Issues Ment Health Nurs* 21:257, 2000.

Shattell M: "Nurse bait:" strategies hospitalized patients use to entice nurses within the context of the nurse-patient relationship, *Issues Ment Health Nurs* 26:205, 2005.

Shattell M: Eventually it'll be over: the dialectic between confinement and freedom in the world of the hospitalized patient. In Thomas S, Pollio H, editors: *Listening to the patient: existential phenomenology for nursing* (pp. 214-236), New York, 2002, Springer.

Shattell M, Hogan B, Thomas S: It's the people that make the environment good or bad: the patient's experience of the acute care hospital environment, *J Am Assoc Crit-Care Nurses: Adv Pract Acute Critical Care* 16(2):159-169, 2005.

Simms C: Don't become a causality in the war of words, *Nursing* 29:48, 1999.

Smith R: Rehab rounds: implementing psychosocial rehabilitation with long-term patients in a public psychiatric hospital, *Psychiatr Serv* 49:593, 1998.

Thomas RB, Wilson JP: Issues and controversies in the understanding and diagnosis of compassion fatigue, vicarious traumatization, and secondary traumatic stress disorder, *Int J Emerg Ment Health* 6:81,2004.

Thomas S, Martin T, Shattell M: Longing to make a difference: nurses' experience of the acute psychiatric inpatient environment. Presented at the 19th Annual Convention of the Southern Nursing Research Society, Atlanta, February 3, 2005.

Thomas S, Shattell M, Martin T: What's therapeutic about the therapeutic milieu? *Arch Psychiatr Nurs* 16:99, 2002.

Whittington D, McLaughlin C: Finding time for patients: an exploration of nurses' time allocation in an acute psychiatric setting, *J Psychiatr Ment Health Nurs* 7:259, 2000.

Wirt GL: Causes of institutionalism: patient and staff perspectives, *Issues Ment Health Nurs* 20:259, 1999.

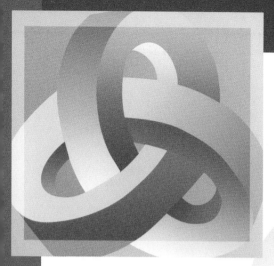

# Chapter 25

# Therapeutic Environment in Various Treatment Settings

*Beverly K. Hogan and Mona M. Shattell*

## Learning Objectives

*After reading this chapter, you should be able to:*

- Describe the treatment environment of inpatient psychiatric settings, including:
  - Open or less acute adult units
  - Adolescent psychiatric units
  - Medical-psychiatric units
  - Acute or intensive care psychiatric units (locked units)
  - Substance abuse units
- Dual-diagnosis units
- Geropsychiatric units
- State psychiatric hospitals
- State forensic psychiatric hospitals
- Describe the treatment environment of community psychiatric settings, including:
  - Outpatient mental health clinics
  - Day treatment facilities
  - Residential care facilities

In the preceding two chapters, discussion focused on the characteristics and variables of a therapeutic environment. The purpose was to define the structure of the treatment environment and factors that enhance or detract from its goals. In this chapter, emphasis is placed on settings of the therapeutic environment and some typical treatment activities.

discipline contributes to the patient's recovery in a way that complements or reinforces treatment efforts of other professionals.

## CRITICAL THINKING QUESTION    1

What is it about a treatment setting that defines its degree of restrictiveness?

## INPATIENT SETTINGS

### TREATMENT ACTIVITIES

Before discussing the various inpatient treatment settings, it is helpful to have a general idea of the types of therapeutic activities offered in a psychiatric setting. Box 25-1 lists a typical inpatient schedule, which includes treatment activities offered by each of the following disciplines. Each

### Occupational Therapy

Occupational therapists (OTs) typically have a baccalaureate degree, although many employed in psychiatry have earned master's degrees. OTs are concerned with functional capabilities of patients as they affect their capacity to work and perform tasks of daily living. OTs assist patients in mastering skills needed for self-care, work, and play. Activities of everyday living are used by the OT

| Box 25-1   Sample Treatment Schedule | | |
|---|---|---|
| Time | Monday Through Friday | Saturday and Sunday |
| 7:00-8:00 AM | Breakfast | Breakfast |
| 8:00-8:45 AM | Therapeutic community | Therapeutic community |
| 9:00-9:45 AM | Patient education | Patient education |
| 10:00-11:00 AM | Meet with treatment team | Physician rounds |
| 11:00-12:00 AM | Occupational therapy | Free time |
| 12:00-1:00 PM | Lunch | Lunch |
| 1:00-2:00 PM | Group therapy | Visiting hours |
| 2:30-3:30 PM | Exercise therapy | Exercise therapy |
| 4:00-5:00 PM | Free time | Spirituality group |
| 5:00-6:00 PM | Dinner | Dinner |
| 6:00-8:00 PM | Visiting hours | Visiting hours |
| 8:30-9:00 PM | Relaxation group | Free time |

### Norm's Notes

*I have mentioned the importance of the environment but, as I noted in Chapter 2, one size does not fit all. How can you apply these concepts to different types of settings? Does it even matter? Both answers are "yes." You can't get away from your environment and neither can the people under your care. This chapter gives some ideas about how the concept of environmental manipulation can foster a therapeutic atmosphere in many diverse settings. And, as you might guess, what might be therapeutic in one setting might not be therapeutic in another.*

| Box 25-2   Psychoeducational Topics |
|---|
| • Medication self-management |
| • Symptom self-management |
| • Recreation for leisure |
| • Grooming and self-care |
| • Money management |
| • Finding employment |
| • Food preparation |
| • Personal effectiveness |

to help people with mental disabilities achieve maximal functioning and independence at home, in the workplace, or both (Box 25-2). Ignorant observers might minimize the therapeutic value of occupational therapy by making references to arts and crafts classes, but these classes are carefully selected based on the OT's functional assessments of patients' deficits and strengths. For example, certain arts and crafts might be selected for their value in improving the patient's attention span and concentration. (See Box 25-3 for a sample of a treatment plan.) Specific therapy approaches selected by OTs and patients are done based on joint decisions in treatment team meetings.

### Recreational Therapy

The use of leisure time is an important intervention for psychiatric patients. Recreational thera-

pists (RTs) assist patients in finding leisure interests that help them learn to balance work and play. Many RTs complete a bachelor's or master's degree program in therapeutic recreation; however, wide variability exists in the level of training of RTs employed at various facilities. RTs are skilled at assessing patients' leisure needs and formulating individualized plans of care that involve recreational therapy. Learning to make time for pleasure and fun can be therapeutic for those dealing with the stress of a mental illness. A skilled RT can make specific assessments and recommendations for a particular patient's needs.

### Exercise Therapy

The benefits of exercise in modulating mood and well-being have been well documented; as patients become withdrawn, their motivation to exercise decreases. Exercise groups counter this tendency somewhat and also provide the added psychological benefit of doing something good for oneself. Exercise therapy is especially important on a psychiatric unit, because it helps channel the negative energy of anxiety or agitation into more appropri-

---

**Box 25-3   Sample Interdisciplinary Treatment Plan**

*Patient Strengths*                                                    *Limitations*

_____          _____
_____          _____
_____          _____

**Support System:**
   Name: _____ Phone number _____

_____

**Advanced Directive for Psychiatric Care: Yes _____ No _____**
**DSM-IV-TR Diagnoses:**
   Axis I   _____
   Axis II  _____
   Axis III _____
   Axis IV  _____
   Axis V   _____

**Discharge Plan:**

_____
_____

Signatures: _____ _____ _____ _____
            _____ _____ _____ _____

_____

| Problem | Goal or Measurable Outcome | Intervention | Evaluation | Signature |
|---------|---------------------------|--------------|------------|-----------|
| Imbalance between work and leisure activity | | | | S Jay, RT |
| Impaired ability to concentrate | Read for 30 minutes and complete assigned tasks. | Engage in activities and tasks for progressively increasing periods of time. | | B Kay, RN |
| Physical inactivity | Attend exercise therapy daily. | Instruct regarding benefits of exercise. | | R Tau, ET |
| Spiritual distress | Attend spirituality group twice weekly. | Explore beliefs and relationship to distress. | | H Yew, MDiv |

---

ate outlets. The level of training or education varies greatly in treatment settings. Ideally, exercise therapists have an educational background incorporating the principles of exercise physiology and its therapeutic application to clinical settings. Exercise therapists often lead group exercise activities and develop individualized plans of care on treatment plans (see Box 25-3). As research on the benefits of particular activities continues to be done, exercise therapists can contribute by ensuring that exercise activities are tailored to patients' needs. For instance, exercise such as strength training is beneficial for patients who are feeling powerless, and aerobic activity is beneficial to patients with depression and certain anxiety disorders On the other hand, some anxiety disorders, such as panic disorders, might be precipitated by strenuous activities, so individualized strategies must be developed.

## PATIENT EDUCATION

Educating patients regarding symptom recognition and management is essential if the patient is to maintain stability outside the treatment environment. Sometimes, the term *psychoeducational group* is used to refer to how patients are educated about psychiatric illness management. Psychoeducational efforts are based on empirical evidence, which has shown that understanding mental illness helps patients and their families cope more positively with the illness. Numerous studies have demonstrated the value of psychoeducation groups in improving quality of life, preventing relapse, and altering negative family reactions (Dixon et al, 2000; Herz, 2000; Motlova, 2000; Pekkala and Merinder, 2000; Schimmel-Spreeuw et al, 2000). Studies generally have shown a high degree of patient satisfaction with such programs (Dowrick et al, 2000). Psychoeducation content rated most helpful by patients is information about diagnosis and medications (Ascher-Svanum et al, 2001). In a study based in Germany (Riedel-Heller et al, 2005), researchers investigated what the lay public believed to be helpful for the treatment of mental disorders. In the case of psychoses, almost all respondents recommended turning to a psychiatrist as the first choice. With regard to depressive symptoms, a psychotherapist or confidant was suggested as the first choice, rated above seeing a psychiatrist. Respondents were more apt to choose psychotherapy, followed by medication as the first line of treatment for either disorder. Natural remedies were also likely to be considered as first-choice options (Riedel-Heller et al, 2005). These studies suggest that mental health professionals need to recognize that noncompliance is more likely a reflection of popular public opinion than a result of a knowledge deficit.

Researchers have found psychoeducation to be very effective for improving treatment adherence rates (Colom et al, 2004; Keller, 2004; Sajatovic, 2004). Clinicians who took time and energy to implement these types of programs transformed their treatment environments from custodial to rehabilitative (Smith, 1998). Because families often assume much of the care burden for chronically mentally ill patients, their inclusion in psychoeducational groups is essential. Box 25-4

lists some topics appropriate for psychoeducational groups. Theoretically, any member of the treatment team could offer psychoeducational groups and, in many cases, the psychiatric nurse uses this format for patient and family teaching, particularly in preparation for discharge.

## GROUP THERAPY

Group therapy might be conducted by advanced practice psychiatric nurses, psychologists, psychiatric residents, licensed professional counselors, or licensed psychiatric social workers. Although the length of time spent by psychiatrists on medication management and coordination of other identified medical problems usually prohibits their leading group therapy sessions, psychiatrists could conduct these groups. University-based teaching hospitals and facilities focusing more on psychotherapies, as opposed to biologically based therapies, are more likely to have group therapies run by psychiatrists. Group therapy is a type of therapeutic environment of its own because it uses many of the principles important to a therapeutic environment: openness, giving and receiving feedback, respect for the patient, privacy, acceptance, independence, and individual responsibility.

In general, the purpose of group therapy is to facilitate awareness and insight about behavior and to develop plans for change or coping. Group therapy can be particularly effective when members are in the group over a long enough period of time, thus allowing some of the unique curative factors of group work to develop. Using a group format to deliver patient education differs from group therapy in that the focus is more on a specific topic and less on the interaction among group members.

## SPIRITUALITY GROUPS

Although spirituality groups are not consistently offered in psychiatric treatment settings, it is likely that the Joint Commission on Accreditation of Healthcare Organizations (JCAHO) will soon specifically mandate formal attention to the spiritual needs of patients. The JCAHO already has standards requiring the assessment and interdisciplinary planning for the spiritual concerns and needs of patients. A chaplain or other mental health treatment team professional conducts these groups; the focus of these groups is usually on

---

**Box 25-4    Examples of Topics for Psychoeducational Groups**

- Recognizing signs of relapse
- Using public transportation
- Talking with your therapist, case worker, psychiatrist
- Coping with stress
- Managing your medications
- Coping with symptoms
- Knowing when to call your physician
- Getting along with family members
- Returning to work
- Anger management
- Interpersonal skills
- Concepts of addiction
- Issues of self-esteem

topics such as forgiveness, grieving, and finding meaning in life. Patients vary in their response to these groups, but the potential for enhancing treatment is available to patients choosing to participate.

The topic of religion and spirituality is often a difficult one on psychiatric units, particularly if there are patients having delusions pertaining to religion. Patients have a right to practice their religion and perhaps attend services, unless there is some particular reason to deny this right. Such decisions obviously have to be very carefully considered within the context of individual rights. When patients cannot leave the unit voluntarily, they do have a right to be visited by their own house of worship members or leaders, or by the hospital chaplain. Unless this is carefully considered, there is great potential for treatment team members to impose their own values on patients when making these decisions.

## THERAPEUTIC GROUPS RELATED TO LIVING SKILLS

Some mental illnesses, such as schizophrenia and Alzheimer's disease, result in an impairment that works against developing meaningful relationships; other mental illnesses have social withdrawal as a characteristic symptom. Social skills groups help psychiatric patients learn, practice, and develop skills for dealing with people in social situations. Skills training might focus on appropriate dress, grooming, or table manners. More advanced efforts address appropriate social and interpersonal verbal skills—for example, meeting new people, initiating conversations, and interviewing for a job.

The opportunity to try out new skills and make mistakes in a safe environment is crucial to learning. Feedback helps patients assess their progress in improving or acquiring social skills.

## THERAPEUTIC COMMUNITY MEETINGS

The therapeutic community meeting consists of all patients, staff, and students in the treatment setting. The community meeting is a regular meeting that all staff and patients attend for the purpose of welcoming new patients, reviewing unit rules, and making general announcements about the day's activities. The community meeting also serves as a forum for patients to initiate discussions of community or individual concerns and to receive feedback from staff and other patients.

A community constitution is a formal, written document that provides the basis for the therapeutic community. It includes definitions, objectives, meetings, responsibilities of patients who are elected as officers, officer approval or removal procedures, and community responses to infractions. A written community constitution is not used in all therapeutic environments, but it is especially appropriate in settings with longer lengths of stay.

Community meetings can also be used to plan activities, such as program picnics or social gatherings. The community meeting provides a forum for exploring the problems of community living. Conflicts between patients or between patients and staff are frequent concerns. Common patient-patient conflicts involve the control of the television, generational issues (e.g., the radio is played too loudly, type of music is not preferred), and personal hygiene (e.g., someone is not bathing regularly).

Patient-staff conflicts are more delicate matters but, in an effective community meeting, they can be handled skillfully. Common conflicts between patients and staff include issues related to how staff

---

### Highlighting the Evidence: Therapeutic Community

Therapeutic community (TC) has been previously shown to be especially effective in substance abuse settings; however, the particular characteristics of individuals who do well with this approach have not been identified. The TC model is distinguished from other types of substance abuse treatment in that it addresses the "whole person" approach and the fact that all interactions are considered for their potentially therapeutic value. This approach was examined with a group of patients, many of whom had criminal behaviors. The results of this study revealed that women tended to have higher scores, suggesting their amenability to the therapeutic community approach.

From Chan KS, Wenzel S, Orlando M, et al: How important are client characteristics to understanding treatment process in the therapeutic community? *Am J Drug Alcohol Abuse* 30:871, 2004.

members act or fail to act with patients. Community meetings are not forums for discussing individual treatment needs and issues of patients; rather, they serve to address daily aspects of being in the treatment environment. (See Chapter 23 for further discussion of the milieu concept of balance.) The skilled group leader will direct patients to discuss personal issues with an appropriate staffperson following the community meeting.

Some acute care inpatient units, residential care programs, and forensic facilities include a level or step system as part of the therapeutic community. This type of system works well on substance abuse units and child-adolescent units, but can potentially be applied in any setting. A step system is a process whereby inpatients gain privileges and responsibilities based on their progress. Through various efforts, individual patients can earn privileges and responsibilities throughout hospitalization. A step system serves as motivation and might be discussed in community meetings. It is important to ensure that patient rights are not withheld as part of the level system of privileges.

## TREATMENT TEAM MEETINGS

Most inpatient settings have a forum for discussing patient treatment issues. One such forum is the treatment team meeting. Psychiatrists, psychologists, psychiatric social workers, pharmacists, occupational therapists, recreational therapists, and psychiatric nurses all provide input about treatment issues. The treatment team meeting is an excellent opportunity to promote collegial relationships with other mental health professionals. In the treatment team meeting, nurses provide patient assessment data and observations about the treatment environment. Most students are positively influenced by this experience and can see the benefit when the team approach is used.

## DIFFERENCES IN INPATIENT UNITS

### OPEN OR LESS ACUTE ADULT PSYCHIATRIC UNITS

An open adult psychiatric unit is the least restrictive of all inpatient psychiatric units; it is the treatment setting of choice for patients with less severe symptoms and some degree of self-control over symptoms. Patients appropriate for an open unit include those with the full range of psychiatric disorders; however, patients on open units are generally able to participate in therapeutic activities and are not actively suicidal (i.e., do not have a definite plan of action for suicide). Most units have admission criteria detailing appropriate patients for the specific treatment environment. Physicians and nurses sometimes disagree about the physician's decision to admit a patient who does not meet the designated criteria. These conflicts are sometimes worked out through discussion and negotiation between the nurse and physician, but might require intervention by administration or management. Although patients on open units might be able to control their symptoms within the safety of the inpatient environment, they are not well; rather, they have active psychiatric symptoms that interfere with their daily functioning outside the hospital.

Activities on the open psychiatric unit tend to focus on developing insight into problems surrounding admission and on problem-solving strategies to avoid re-admission. Less severe symptoms enable the use of more verbal or talk therapies. Generally, patients on open units are more amenable to and cooperative with therapeutic activities. Often, open units serve as a step down, less restrictive treatment setting for patients who will soon be discharged.

### CLINICAL EXAMPLE

Mary is a 37-year-old Caucasian woman who has had severe panic attacks and depression off and on since her early 20s. Mary takes Klonopin 0.5 mg twice daily and Paxil 40 mg four times daily for the panic disorder and depression. A recent series of stressors involving her work and marriage precipitated this admission. Mary is married to a man with an alcohol problem and a pattern of irresponsibility related to family finances. Mary works two jobs to make ends meet; one boss is very demanding, frequently giving her last-minute projects at the end of the day with a deadline the following morning. Recently, Mary has started having panic attacks as she is driving to work. Yesterday, she experienced an especially severe panic attack and pulled over on the side of the road and started crying. After seeing her psychiatrist, she was admitted for medication management and inpatient therapy. In OT, Mary practices relaxation and cognitive behavioral exercises to help her deal with the panic attacks in various situations, such as driving. The RT works with Mary on finding time for activities she once enjoyed, such as camping and reading novels. During group therapy sessions, Mary works on her problem of taking care of others while neglecting her own needs. The nurse works with Mary to reinforce all these therapeutic activities and also identifies problem areas to explore with the patient in their one-to-one therapeutic interactions.

## CRITICAL THINKING QUESTION    2

Physicians and nurses traditionally get along very well in psychiatry. Why might this be true?

## CRITICAL THINKING QUESTION    3

What are the major contributing factors to the trend for hospitalized psychiatric patients to be more medically ill now than they were in the past?

## INTENSIVE OR ACUTE CARE PSYCHIATRIC UNITS (LOCKED UNITS)

The goal of acute care psychiatric units is to provide rapid amelioration of symptoms (U.S. Surgeon General, 2000). Patients on acute locked psychiatric units usually meet criteria for an involuntary admission, even if they are admitted voluntarily. Severity of patients' illnesses tends to be quite high, with the need for close supervision and intervention by nursing staff. The number and restrictiveness of rules is greater on locked units, because of the general safety of all patients and staff. For example, staff might not think a particular patient can be trusted to use a razor, so the safety of the entire unit overrides the individual patient's need to act independently. Many patients, especially on an involuntary unit, look forward to their smoke breaks. As hospitals have increasingly become smoke-free, including psychiatric units, it has become necessary to address nicotine withdrawal, especially for heavy smokers. Because many patients with psychiatric problems are heavy smokers, even adding a patch or using nicotine gum does not fully address withdrawal symptoms, especially agitation and irritability, which can have negative consequences on an involuntary unit (van Weeghel et al, 2005).

How does the patient view the intensive or acute care psychiatric unit? How does staff view this same environment? Research has shown that patients and staff view the same acute care environment quite differently (Miller and Lee, 1980; Moos, 1974; Rossberg and Friis, 2004; Skodol et al, 1980). Staff view treatment environments in a more positive light than patients. For example, staff gave a higher rating on variables such as staff involvement, support, autonomy, practical orientation, personal problem orientation, and programs (Rossberg and Friis, 2004). Basically, psychiatric nursing staff believe that acute care psychiatric environments are more therapeutic than do patients on those units. So, the important question was: "What is important to patients in these environments?" Their answer was this: "A therapeutic relationship is most important to patients in acute care psychiatric settings" (Jackson and Stevenson, 2000; Johansson and Eklund, 2004).

### CLINICAL EXAMPLE

John is a 23-year-old Caucasian man who barricaded himself in his family's home and called the FBI to report that his parents were aliens infiltrating the city government. Although John had not been overtly violent, he had a rifle in his possession and reportedly aimed it at his father. The county sheriff brought John to the emergency room for a psychiatric evaluation. John agreed to be admitted to the psychiatric unit, where he would be "safe" from the alien invasion. John's parents were contacted and agreed to file a petition for involuntary evaluation and treatment in case John should decide to leave against medical advice. John's delusions and agitation about an involuntary admission prohibit his participation in group therapy at this time, so the therapist works with John one to one for brief periods and consults with the treatment team regarding his readiness to participate in group therapy with other patients. John also attends psychoeducational groups to learn about the signs and symptoms of mental illness. One-to-one interactions with John's nurse focus on dealing with other patients on the unit and ways to deal with the resultant anxiety. The nurse also reinforces teaching about mental illness and medication management. John refuses to participate in other therapeutic activities at this time. As John's illness is better controlled and he begins to develop insight, John will work with the OT to determine activities that will help him with his trouble concentrating.

## CHILD-ADOLESCENT INPATIENT UNITS

It has often been said that children are not little adults. The child-adolescent unit must meet specific age-appropriate criteria in terms of the physical environment and the treatment activities offered. See Chapter 42 for further discussion of the child-adolescent population.

Although it is widely accepted that the milieu of child-adolescent psychiatric units is important, little research to date has been conducted into the nature, construction, maintenance, and function of the milieu, especially with regard to how units affect treatment outcomes (Geanellos, 2000).

A number of traditional views about adolescent psychiatric nursing are now being reconsidered. For example, in the past, separating parents from their child during a psychiatric admission was considered essential; this action often communicated that the parent was part of the problem. This approach has shifted in an entirely different direction—it is now realized that parents are essential to the treatment process for the child or adolescent patient.

Another shift concerns the frequently used time-out intervention (Delaney, 1999). The original intent of time-out was to remove the patient from potential reinforcers for inappropriate behavior. Because it is an effective and easily learned intervention, staff tends to rely on time-out as an intervention for any behavioral problem that occurs. For example, if patients break a unit rule, they might be sent to their room for time-out. In contrast, patients who are receiving a lot of attention from peers for their rebellious remarks might also be sent to their room for time-out. The former applies negative sanctions to inappropriate behavior (punishment), whereas the latter is a direct effort to remove the source of reward for inappropriate behavior (operant shaping). The purpose of a time-out must be clear and appropriate; otherwise, it could become another form of punishment. There is a clear need for more active and innovative strategies for dealing with complex problems presented by child-adolescent psychiatric patients. For example, cognitive-behavioral approaches for dealing with aggressive behavior through skills training groups and reinforcement of appropriate behavior have been effective in reducing aggressive behavior in adolescents (Snyder et al, 1999).

When time-out and cognitive-behavioral strategies fail, a more restrictive intervention might be warranted. The use of seclusion might be used when time-out is unsuccessful in protecting patients and staff from aggressive behavior in children and adolescents. Seclusion is much more restrictive than time-out, because it places the child or adolescent in a room where the door is locked. The purpose of seclusion is to protect patients from harming themselves or others. Gullick and colleagues (2005) studied the factors associated with seclusion use in children and adolescents in an eight-bed inpatient child and adolescent psychiatric unit in Australia. Not surprisingly, these researchers found that patients with greater psychopathology and family problems had a higher incidence of seclusion.

A very traditional treatment strategy incorporated into child-adolescent treatment is the level or step system, whereby patients gain privileges based on behavior. Whether this is a viable approach in today's shorter stay environment has been challenged by recent evidence (Mohr and Pumariega, 2004).

Another important aspect of the interpersonal environment on child-adolescent units is the interactions among patients. Peers can unduly influence each other, especially in the case of adolescent patients who are seeking to establish their own identities. Patients can learn self-defeating behavior patterns from each other. Hence, part of the nurse's role in developing a therapeutic environment in a child-adolescent unit is the monitoring of peer relationships and intervening as conditions warrant.

Consistency of staff is important in any psychiatric setting and is especially important on child-adolescent units. Adolescents and children who have grown up entirely in foster care or residential care settings might have difficulty establishing relationships and might have developed a number of defenses counterproductive to forming relationships. Nurses can intervene by being consistent and trustworthy. Nurses who have not successfully mastered the developmental tasks of childhood and adolescence themselves will have great difficulty working on child-adolescent psychiatric units. See Chapter 42 for more information on child and adolescent issues.

### CLINICAL EXAMPLE

Kisha is an 8-year-old African-American girl who has been getting into trouble at school for fighting. She has also been running away from home and setting fires at neighbors' houses. Kisha talks with the nurse about difficulties with peers at school and says that she feels sad all the time. Kisha participates in group therapy by discussing her behavior with her peers and getting feedback about the way she interacts with others. She also attends OT to complete projects that focus on resisting impulsivity. During community meetings, treatment team members and peers point out to Kisha how she has improved since being in the hospital and participating in the unit treatment activities.

## MEDICAL-PSYCHIATRIC UNITS

In recent years, there has been a rekindled interest in the interrelationship between mind and body. It has become increasingly clear that chronic psychiatric patients have a number of unmet medical needs (Koran et al, 2002). An increasing body of research has indicated greater risk for certain chronic physical conditions among patients with psychiatric disorders as compared with patients in the general population (O'Day et al, 2005). Additionally, there has been increasing attention in the media and professional literature to particular risks associated with certain psychotropic drugs. At least 50% of patients admitted to hospitals have comorbid medical and psychiatric problems (Kathol, 1998; O'Day et al, 2005).

Psychiatric comorbidity increases the length of stay for the hospitalized medically ill psychiatric patient (Wancata et al, 2001). Similarly, the medical patient with a psychiatric condition poses a challenge to the traditional medical unit and can be disruptive to the unit routine. A medical unit lacks necessary physical and safety features important for patients with psychiatric problems. Also, psychiatric patients with medical problems might not receive adequate attention to their comorbid medical condition if staff members do not actively maintain their medical nursing skills (Inventor et al, 2005). Medical equipment on a traditional psychiatric unit can also pose a challenge in terms of availability and safety. Although most of these comorbid cases require only a straightforward consideration of factors in care planning, at least 10% of patients require simultaneous specialty care for both conditions. Particularly of concern are the studies that have indicated the failure of psychiatric staff to recognize and fully address medical problems (Koran, 2004; O'Day, 2005; Zun, 2005). It is a challenge to maintain competency in general nursing skills when psycho-

social interventions are the primary interventions used on psychiatric units. Fear of losing one's technical nursing skills has led many nurses interested in psychiatric nursing to pursue other practice areas. As increasing numbers of psychiatric patients are admitted to psychiatric units with medical problems, it becomes likely that a full complement of interpersonal and technical skills will be required.

This high percentage of chronically mentally ill patients with coexisting medical problems and the high prevalence of medical disorders among chronically mentally ill patients have led to the creation of specialized units that can address both problems simultaneously. These units, sometimes called *integrated medicine* psychiatric units, can yield significant savings for the hospital and improve outcomes for patients with psychiatric-medical comorbidity. Understandably, the focus of therapeutic activities will depend on the nature of the medical infirmity. Some geriatric psychiatric units have been reclassified as medical-psychiatric units because of the very large number of medical problems in this population (Inventor, 2005).

Some facilities have tried and abandoned these units because of cost considerations; however, there is a clear need for these facilities, and it is expected these units will continue to be tried and then successfully implemented through the creative planning of administrators. Psychiatric liaison services often refer to themselves as practicing psychological medicine, because they make treatment recommendations on the psychological aspects of care for patients on medical units (Lloyd and Mayou, 2003).

### CLINICAL EXAMPLE

Marvin is a 47-year-old African-American man with a history of bipolar affective disorder, diabetes, and congestive heart failure. He was brought to the emergency room with a blood sugar level of 700 mg/dL, severe dehydration, and cardiac arrhythmia. Marvin stopped taking his medications recently because he believed he was able to handle his problems on his own. He has been walking the streets and preaching to people in fast food restaurants. Last night, the McDonald's store manager found Marvin babbling and acting "drunk." The manager called the police, who then escorted Marvin to the local emergency room. Typically, Marvin's diabetes is difficult to control. After Marvin was rehydrated and his blood sugar level restabilized, Marvin was admitted to the integrated medical-psychiatric unit for close observation of his medical status and simultaneous participation in treatment activities for his mental illness. Marvin attends a psychoeducational group with several other patients who also have problems with medication compliance and exacerbation of serious medical problems. Once Marvin is stabilized medically, he will participate in other treatment activities.

## SUBSTANCE ABUSE UNITS

Although substance abuse treatment requires a specialized, controlled environment for optimal recovery, it is still fairly common for patients with substance abuse problems to undergo initial evaluation and detoxification in open or locked psychiatric units. Therapeutic activities on substance abuse units include rigorous patient education, sensitization groups, and confrontational feedback sessions. Traditionally, substance abuse treatment approaches tend to be more confrontational because of the severity of denial. See Chapter 35 for further discussion of the patient with substance-related problems.

### CLINICAL EXAMPLE

Sara is a 42-year old Caucasian woman who has been drinking alcohol excessively and taking Xanax for the past 3 years. Sara's withdrawal symptoms were managed on the open psychiatric unit, after which Sara was transferred to the substance abuse unit. On the substance abuse unit, Sara attends educational sessions about addiction, alcoholism, and dealing with unhealthy relationships. Sara also attends group therapy, in which she talks about a number of underlying unaddressed feelings of grief about her mother's death. As Sara progresses through treatment, she will participate in a number of therapy groups aimed at helping her avoid relapse after discharge.

## DUAL-DIAGNOSIS UNITS

More than 50% of patients in mental health treatment settings have a coexisting substance-related disorder. Similarly, more than 50% of patients in substance abuse treatment settings have a coexisting psychiatric disorder (Minkoff, 2001). Some hospitals and free-standing psychiatric facil-

ities (not attached to a general hospital) find a dual-diagnosis unit better able to meet the unique needs of this population (Donat and Haverkamp, 2004; Timko and Moos, 1998). Treatment approaches on dual-diagnosis units balance confrontational and supportive approaches. (See Chapter 36 for a discussion of treatment issues of the patient with a dual diagnosis.) Although some agencies have not separated this population, there are some indications that this population has needs that are unique and require a different approach, and that a failure to address this problem of dual diagnosis has deleterious consequences for the treatment outcomes of patients (Donat and Haverkamp, 2004).

### CLINICAL EXAMPLE

Several months after discharge from the substance abuse unit, Sara was diagnosed with panic disorder. Sara relapsed from her commitment to drug and alcohol abstinence and became very depressed. She was admitted to the dual-diagnosis unit for simultaneous management of both disorders. Sara will participate in therapeutic activities with other patients who are dually diagnosed.

## GEROPSYCHIATRIC UNITS

Population demographics reflect an increasingly aging population, and patients on geropsychiatric units have complex medical, psychological, and social needs (Inventor, 2005). A number of differences in the treatment environment are dictated by these complex needs. In particular, the physical structure of geropsychiatric units must be designed with special consideration for safety issues and cognitive limitations. For example, physical space must be less cluttered to address safety, and should be free of unnecessary noise to counter the vulnerability of older patients to sensory overstimulation. A smaller unit with fewer patients has been shown to improve interaction not only among patients, but also between patients and staff (Day et al, 2000; Teresi et al, 2000). Smith and associates (2005) surveyed 31 geropsychiatric units across the United States in search of best nursing care practices and challenges. They found that 22% of respondents who answered the question, "What three things are needed to take your unit and its services to the next level of excellence in care?" made reference to a larger unit with more private rooms.

Older patients, especially those with dementia, might have difficulty navigating the hospital environment without environmental cues. Environmental cues include large orientation boards on which the date, time, and location of daily events are posted; clearly marked names or graphic images (e.g., bathroom, bedrooms with patients' names on the doors); and color-coding of different locations. Just as children are not little adults, geriatric patients are not just chronologically older adults. Older patients are likely to have comorbid medical conditions that could affect mobility, balance, and vision. Increased lighting is needed to counter diminished vision of the older adult. Confusion and disorientation can be exacerbated or helped by environmental interventions.

Falls are of great concern on the geropsychiatric unit, and many of the medications prescribed in this setting might increase the risk of falls.

A patient with dementia needs a different environment than the older patient who is cognitively intact. For example, bathing is considered one of the most stressful events associated with dementia. Design accommodations should include features that maximize the patient's autonomy and independence. Bathrooms should be large enough to accommodate the need for others to assist the patient.

The importance of the environment for the geropsychiatric patient is evident by the increasing numbers of studies on facility design and planning. These studies have shown an association between the environmental design of the unit and patients' level of improvement in regard to variables such as self-care, agitation, and mood. Group therapy, for those able to participate, might involve issues such as grief and loss. For less cognitively functional patients, group therapy might involve orientation, memory enhancement, and reminiscence activities in a more structured format. See Chapters 32 and 43 for discussion of the unique care needs of the geriatric patient.

## CLINICAL EXAMPLE

Ms. Castanada is an 82-year-old Hispanic woman who was admitted to the geriatric unit for increasing confusion and wandering behavior at home. Ms. Castanada is diagnosed with Alzheimer's disease and is started on Aricept. The OT works with Ms. Castanada to help her complete her bathing and dressing with minimal assistance. The nurse works closely with Ms. Castanada and her family members to identify triggers to agitation and strategies for dealing with these episodes. The nurse noticed that Ms. Castanada does very well at dinnertime if her favorite song from her teenage years is played.

## STATE HOSPITALS

### State Psychiatric Hospital Units

The primary difference in the treatment environment between a state hospital setting and other facilities is based on the length of stay, greater degree of restrictiveness, and the need to prepare patients for community placement.

## CLINICAL EXAMPLE

Marvin, who was previously an inpatient in the medical psychiatric unit in a private hospital, continued to be uncooperative with his treatment. An involuntary commitment hearing was held, and Marvin was admitted to the state psychiatric hospital for further treatment. Marvin currently receives many of the same treatments he received at the private facility; however, the state hospital has greater focus on developing insight, improving compliance, and preparing to live back in the community than did the private short-stay inpatient facility.

### State Forensic Psychiatric Hospital Units

The forensic psychiatric unit or state forensic hospital is the most restrictive of all treatment environments. Because of the special care requirements and clear differences in the nurse-patient relationship, forensic units will be described in more detail in Chapter 26.

## COMMUNITY TREATMENT SETTINGS

As hospital-based care becomes less preferable because of the high cost of inpatient stays, community-based alternatives are increasingly being sought. One such alternative was described by a particular hospital as a treatment mall, where the treatment was actually moved from the inpatient unit to an off-grounds building with a menu of treatment activities (Holland et al, 2005). Such approaches to reduce the sense of confinement and increase individual choice tend to have better compliance and participation by patients. Another community-based treatment alternative is the consumer-run drop-in center (Holter and Mowbray, 2005).

The concept of a therapeutic environment has become more applicable to community-based treatment facilities. As the focus of psychiatric care has shifted to the community and away from inpatient and state psychiatric hospitals, community treatment programs have been challenged by applying principles of milieu therapy that were originally intended for inpatient environments. Currently, much psychiatric care takes place in group homes or partial or day hospitals, or through support offered to patients and their family members via home health visits. Once a patient is discharged from the hospital to a community setting, safety remains a priority. For example, a patient preoccupied with internal stimuli (e.g., hallucinations) might be at risk for walking into traffic when leaving a day program. He or she might need an escort home to the family. One study investigating how clients described good community care revealed that the most important attribute is a trusting and stimulating relationship between clients and professionals (van Weeghel, 2005). The rest of this section will focus on the unique aspects of community treatment.

## RESIDENTIAL TREATMENT HOMES

Preparing patients to live in the community requires education on social and independent living skills (Umansky et al, 1999). This was particularly true for patients who spent many years in state psychiatric facilities prior to the deinstitutionalization of the mentally ill. For patients being discharged from state hospitals, intermediary care was required to prepare patients to live independently. This occurred primarily in transitional or group homes, in which there were efforts to assist patients toward independent living and, if this were not possible, to secure the least restrictive residential placement to meet patient needs. Although these types of facilities still exist, some of these residential beds have been made available

to patients residing in the community who need assistance to avoid rehospitalization. In-home treatment by professional staff or coordinated treatment through the corresponding treatment agency is provided to residents throughout the day, either in the home or at an off-site treatment location. Patients generally reported that their greatest sense of being helped occurred with "talking to doctor," followed by "free pass," "medication," "visitors," "non-hospital setting," "making friends with patients," "structure of daily life," "support from team," and "talking to nurses"; the least valued item was "group activities" and verbal therapies (Biancosino et al, 2004).

### How the System Works

Many of these programs are funded by housing and urban development and federal grants. Patients on disability pay rent at these treatment facilities based on their ability to pay. Factored into the calculation of patient cost are considerations for patient care needs, including clothing and personal hygiene. This is highly desirable to some patients as a permanent living solution; for others, it is a transitional stage to prepare them for independent or less supervised living; and for still others, it is most objectionable to consider living in any fashion other than independently, regardless of the cost or other benefits.

Group home staff is usually responsible for getting patients to their appointments and assisting them with their daily care needs, all with the gradual intent, whenever possible, of preparing the resident for independence. Ideally, group home staff secures patient permission for close contact with other members of the treatment team, such as the patient's family, treating psychiatrist, and other mental health care providers. Nursing staff are not always employed in these settings. Salaries of staff who are direct care providers are typically low; thus, an unspoken but obvious conclusion is that the best level of care is not provided to this population. Nurses are ideal care providers and mangers in these homes because of their broad knowledge base, direct experience in patient care delivery, and skill in care coordination. It is encouraging to imagine the outcomes that could be realized with this level of professional staffing; having a nurse available to provide consultation helps improve a group home staff's ability to meet patient care needs.

## PARTIAL HOSPITALIZATION

It is debatable whether partial hospitalization or residential care is more restrictive. In both treatment settings, patients are supervised closely by staff members on a treatment team. In group homes, the place of treatment is the residence; in partial hospitalization, patients usually attend a facility connected with a hospital for intensive treatment and can return home at night. Regulatory agencies and third-party payors require a registered nurse in these facilities to attend, at the minimum, to urgent care matters that might arise and to assist with medication administration and/or management. Treatment is structured in a very similar manner to that in the inpatient environment, but patients are considered safe enough to be able to return to their residence in the evening; in other words, intensive care is required but continued observation is not. After completing a partial hospitalization program, patients might be discharged back to the community mental health center for day treatment or outpatient care, or to a private psychiatrist if they can afford one.

## DAY TREATMENT

Day treatment is similar to the partial hospitalization program described above except that it is less intense. The patient might attend an intensive day treatment program for a prescribed number of hours and specified frequency. Day treatment programs have similar objectives and represent a midpoint between hospitalization and outpatient clinic visits. This varies according to the range of services offered in a community. Supportive treatment programs are often geared more toward maintenance of current function through provision of classes and activities, which support patients' abilities to attend to activities of daily living and social skills development. A meta-analysis on outcomes of psychosocial skills training indicated a moderate to strong relationship to fewer patient symptoms and better functioning (Dilk and Bond, 1996). The importance of such research lies in the demonstration of a positive treatment effect, more than that of medication alone. Consumers and other advocates for patients with chronic mental illness continue to play a significant role in forcing a recovery-oriented approach, instilling a sense of hope; this is in contrast to the approach suggesting that the patient will always be ill, which has been experienced by many patients (consumers) as demoralizing.

## PROGRAMS FOR ASSERTIVE COMMUNITY TREATMENT

Most mental health centers have case management services as part of the continuum of services; however, the level of involvement in patients' daily lives varies. Typically, case managers have as their primary role accessing services for patients. Settings that combine case management with intense programming have been found to be most efficacious. Programs for Assertive Community Treatment (PACT) represent an example of a team of mental health professionals who work intensely with patients to prevent hospitalization. PACT teams have been used widely and are recognized as an important means for delivering psychiatric mental health care in the community (Essock and Kontos, 1995; McFarlane et al, 1996). Such programs involve a team of professionals, including a psychiatrist, an RN, a case manager, and perhaps other mental health professionals. PACT teams take a proactive role and bring the treatment to the patient, if necessary, thereby addressing such frequent problems as follow-up and compliance. Patient consent is required for participation. Such programs are often funded to target particular at-risk populations and are generally well liked by patients. When clients first enter assertive community treatment programs, they often do not trust team members; Leiphart and Barnes (2005) found that trust developed over time, and that those relationships between clients and team members were the most important aspect of the program.

## CONCLUSION

The range of possible services to fill the gaps between state hospital and independent living is often fragmented and inadequate, making the goal of living in the community a difficult one. Some professionals and family believe that institutions (especially long-term care) will always be necessary. On the other hand, human rights advocates continue to argue on behalf of freedom from forced psychiatric treatment. The time for a shift is emerging imminently, but the direction is not yet clear. What is clear is that repeat hospitalizations, routine medication check visits every 3 months (or less often in some facilities), and revolving door short-term admissions to state facilities are not going to accomplish the goal of having patients live independently in the community. National media attention to the increased presence of the mentally ill in jails and prisons highlights that change has not completely taken place for patients with regard to support for living independently; rather, the mental health system is in crisis and, like many crisis situations, responsibility gets shifted. Jails are obviously not the place for the mentally ill, particularly when patients are incarcerated for misdemeanor offenses clearly related to their illness and the limitations so imposed.

Another major change in health care delivery is the ever-increasing use of advanced practice psychiatric nurses to prescribe and evaluate patients' responses to psychotropic drugs (Kaas et al, 1998). Advanced practice psychiatric nurses in community treatment programs can provide quality care with a broad range of skills offered, particularly by the psychiatric nurse who can prescribe medications as well as monitor physical status and provide psychotherapeutic counseling. As in so much of mental health care, even the appropriate role of the advanced practice nurse has not been agreed on.

***Note to Students:*** *These chapters have given an overview of the concept of the treatment environment. Regardless of the clinical setting (e.g., psychiatric, medical, pediatric), the atmosphere and care provided are affected by the variables discussed in this chapter.*

## ▮ Study Notes

1. Milieu therapy was originally designed for the inpatient setting but has increasingly been used in other settings (e.g., mental health clinics), especially in the community.
2. A variety of health care professionals are involved in the treatment milieu of a psychiatric facility, including physicians, nurses, psychologists, social workers, chaplains, and occupational, recreational, and exercise therapists.
3. All members of the treatment team and patients attend therapeutic community meetings to welcome new patients, review milieu rules, and make general announcements about the day's activities. (*Note:* Not all units have therapeutic community meetings.)
4. A variety of treatment activities are used within psychiatric units, such as group therapy, recreational therapy, exercise therapy, spirituality groups, and patient education.
5. The open psychiatric unit is the least restrictive inpatient treatment environment. Generally, patients on the open unit require less close supervision and actively take responsibility for their treatment.
6. Patients in an acute, locked psychiatric unit are often admitted involuntarily and tend to need close supervision and intervention by nursing staff.
7. A special focus of the child-adolescent psychiatric unit is the interpersonal relationships among patients.
8. Medical-psychiatric units are specialty psychiatric environments that address the needs of chronically medically ill patients with coexisting psychiatric problems.
9. Therapeutic activities on a substance abuse unit tend to use confrontation because of the extensive use of denial by this patient population.
10. Patients with both a substance abuse problem and a psychiatric diagnosis can be treated on dual-diagnosis units, which balance confrontational and supportive approaches.
11. Geropsychiatric units address specialized needs of the older adult, including environmental modifications necessary because of sensory losses and other safety factors.
12. The primary differences in the treatment environment of a state hospital setting are the length of stay and the focus on preparing patients for community placement.
13. A forensic psychiatric unit (or hospital) is the most restrictive of all treatment environments.
14. Significant levels of psychiatric care are provided in group homes, partial and day hospitals, and other community settings.
15. Preparing patients to live in the community requires an emphasis on social skills, independent living skills, and prevention of relapse and rehospitalization.

## ▮ References

Ascher-Svanum H, Rochford S, Cisco D, Claveaux A: Patient education about schizophrenia: initial expectations and later satisfaction, *Issues Ment Health Nurs* 22:325, 2001.

Biancosino B, Barbui C, Pera V, et al: Patient opinions on the benefits of treatment programs in residential psychiatric care, *Can J Psychiatry* 49:613, 2004.

Colom F, Vieta E, Sanchez-Moreno J, et al: Psychoeducation in bipolar patients with comorbid personality disorders, *Bipolar Disorder* 6:294, 2004.

Day K, Carreon D, Stump C: The therapeutic design of environments for patients with dementia: a review of the empirical research, *Gerontologist* 40:397, 2000.

Delaney K: Time-out: an overused and misused milieu intervention, *J Child Adolesc Psychiatr Nurs* 12:53, 1999.

Dilk M, Bond G: Meta-analytic evaluation of skills training research for individuals with severe mental illness, *J Consult Clin Psychol* 64:1337, 1996.

Dixon L, Adams C, Lucksted A: Update on family psychoeducation for schizophrenia, *Schizophr Bull* 26:5, 2000.

Donat D, Haverkamp J: Treatment of psychiatric impairment complicated by co-occurring substance use: Impact on rehospitalization, *Psychiatr Rehabil J* 28:78, 2004.

Dowrick C, Dunn G, Ayuso-Mateos JL, et al: Problem-solving treatment and group psychoeducation for depression: multicentre randomized controlled trial. Outcomes of Depression International Network (ODIN) Group, *BMJ* 321:1450, 2000.

Essock SM, Kontos N: Implementing assertive community treatment teams, *Psychiatr Serv* 46:679, 1995.

Geanellos R: The milieu and milieu therapy in adolescent mental health nursing, *Int J Psychiatr Nurs Res* 5:638, 2000.

Gullick K, McDermott B, Stone P, Gibbon P: Seclusion of children and adolescents: psychopathological and family factors, *Int J Ment Health Nurs* 14:37, 2005.

Herz MI, Lamberti JS, Mintz J, et al: A program for relapse prevention in schizophrenia: a controlled study, *Arch Gen Psychiatry* 57:277, 2000.

Holland J, Vidoni-Clark C, Prandoni J, et al: Moving beyond ward-based treatment: a public mental health hospital's transition to a treatment mall, *Psychiatr Rehabil J* 28:295, 2005.

Holter M, Mowbray C: Consumer-run drop-in centers, *Psychiatr Rehabil J* 28:323, 2005.

Inventor B, Henricks J, Rodman L, et al: The impact of medical issues in inpatient geriatric psychiatry, *Issues Ment Health Nurs* 26:23, 2005.

Jackson S, Stevenson C: What do people need psychiatric and mental health nurses for? *J Adv Nurs* 31:378, 2000.

Johansson H, Eklund M: Helping alliance and ward atmosphere in psychiatric in-patient care. *Psychol Psychother* 77:511, 2004.

Kaas MJ, Markley JM: A national perspective on prescriptive authority for advanced practice psychiatric nurses, *J Am Psychiatr Nurs Assoc* 4:190, 1998.

Kathol R: Integrated medicine and psychiatry treatment programs, *Med Psychiatry* 1:10, 1998.

Keatinge D, Scarfe C, Bellchambers H, et al: The manifestation and nursing management of agitation in institutionalized residents with dementia, *Int J Nurs Pract* 6:16, 2000.

Keller MB: Improving the course of illness and promoting continuation of treatment of bipolar disorder, *J Clin Psychiatry* 65(Suppl 15):10, 2004.

Koran LM, Sheline Y, Imai K, et al: Medical disorders among patients admitted to a public-sector psychiatric inpatient unit, *Psychiatr Serv* 53:1623, 2002.

Leiphart L, Barnes M: The client experience of assertive community treatment: a qualitative study, *Psychiatr Rehabil J* 28:395, 2005.

Lloyd GG, Mayou RA: Liaison psychiatry or psychological medicine? *Br J Psychiatry* 183:5, 2003.

McFarlane WR, Dushay RA, Stastny P, et al: A comparison of two levels of family-aide assertive community treatment, *Psychiatr Serv* 47:744, 1996.

Miller TW, Lee LI: Quality assurance: focus on environmental perceptions of psychiatric patients and nursing staff, *J Psychiatr Nurs Ment Health Serv* 18:9, 1980.

Minkoff K: Best practices. Developing standards of care for individuals with co-occurring psychiatric and substance use disorders, *Psychiatr Serv* 52:597, 2001.

Mohr W, Pumariega A: Level systems: inpatient programming whose time has passed, *J Child Adolesc Psychiatr Nurs* 17:113, 2004.

Moos RH: *Evaluating treatment environments: A social ecological approach,* New York, 1974, Wiley.

Motlova L: Psychoeducation as an indispensable complement to pharmacotherapy in schizophrenia, *Pharmacopsychiatry* 33(Suppl 1):47, 2000.

O'Day B, Killeen M, Sutton J, Iezzoni L: Primary care experiences of people with psychiatric disabilities: barriers to care and potential solutions, *Psychiatr Rehabil J* 28:339, 2005.

Pekkala E, Merinder L: Psychoeducation for schizophrenia, *Cochrane Database System Rev* Issue 4, CD002831, 2000.

Prochaska J, Gill P, Hall G: Treatment of tobacco use in an inpatient psychiatric setting, *Psychiatr Serv* 55:1265, 2004.

Riedel-Heller SG, Matschinger H, Angermeyer MC: Mental disorders—who and what might help? Help-seeking and treatment preferences of the lay public, *Soc Psychiatry Psychiatr Epidemiol* 40:167, 2005.

Rossberg JI, Friis S: Patients' and staff's perceptions of the psychiatric ward environment, *Psychiatr Serv* 55:798, 2004.

Sajatovic M, Davies M, Hrouda DR: Enhancement of treatment adherence among patients with bipolar disorder, *Psychiatr Serv* 55:264, 2004.

Schimmel-Spreeuw A, Linssen AC, Heeren TJ: Coping with depression and anxiety: preliminary results of a standardized course for elderly depressed women, *Int Psychogeriatr* 12:77, 2000.

Skodol AE, Plutchik R, Karasu TB: Expectations of hospital treatment: conflicting views of patients and staff, *J Nerv Ment Dis* 168:70, 1980.

Smith M, Specht J, Buckwalter K: Geropsychiatric inpatient care: what is the state of the art? *Issues Ment Health Nurs* 26:11, 2005.

Smith R: Rehab rounds: implementing psychosocial rehabilitation with long-term patients in a public psychiatric hospital, *Psychiatr Serv* 49:593, 1998.

Snyder K, Kymissis P, Kessler K: Anger management for adolescents: efficacy of brief group therapy, *J Am Acad Child Adolesc Psychiatry* 38:1409, 1999.

Teresi J, Holmes D, Ory M: The therapeutic design of environments for people with dementia: further reflections and recent findings from the National Institute on Aging Collaborative Studies of Dementia special care units, *Gerontologist* 40:417, 2000.

Timko C, Moos RH: Outcomes of the treatment climate in psychiatric and substance abuse programs, *J Clin Psychol* 54:1137, 1998.

Umansky R, Telias D, Tzidon E, et al: A school for mental health inpatient preparation for reinsertion in the community, *Int J Psychosoc Rehabil* 3:526, 1999.

U.S. Surgeon General: *Mental health: a report of the Surgeon General,* Washington, DC, 1999, Department of Health and Human Services.

van Weeghel J, Van Audenhove C, Colucci M, et al: The components of good community care for people with severe mental illnesses: views of stakeholders in five European countries, *Psychiatr Rehabil J* 28:274, 2005.

Wancata J, Benda N, Windhaber J, Nowotny M: Does psychiatric co-morbidity increase the length of stay in medical, surgical and gynecological departments? *Gen Hosp Psychiatry* 23:8, 2001.

Zun LS: Evidence-based evaluation of psychiatric patients, *J Emerg Med* 28:35, 2005.

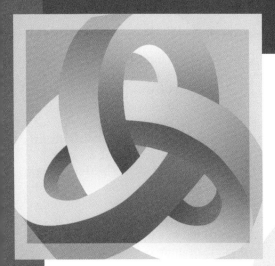

## Chapter 26

# Special Environments: Forensic Psychiatric Treatment Settings

*Beverly K. Hogan and Mona M. Shattell*

### Learning Objectives

*After reading this chapter, you should be able to:*
- Describe the forensic psychiatric care environment.
- Discuss typical nursing care problems unique to the forensic psychiatric setting.
- Discuss the increased significance of limit setting and boundary maintenance in the nurse-patient relationship in a forensic setting.

***Note to Students:*** *All environments in psychiatric nursing are special, and each unit would argue that it has its own has unique features. Although this is certainly true, forensic nursing has emerged as a unique and distinct subspecialty area that requires further detail, highlighting its distinction from mainstream psychiatric nursing practice.*

Forensic nursing is a specialty practice area that has emerged as a distinct specialty and includes many different roles. The International Association of Forensic Nurses (IAFN, 2005) has defined the forensic nurse's role broadly; it deals with legal aspects surrounding various types of trauma and abuse. The IANF recognizes a number of roles of the forensic nurse, including sexual assault nurse examiners (SANEs), legal nurse consultants, forensic psychiatric nurses, and correctional nurses. With so many varied roles under this title, it is easy to see how it would be confusing to a student. This chapter will focus on the forensic psychiatric nurse as a subspecialty area of psychiatric nursing practice involving the management of patients with a mental illness who have been adjudicated to treatment by the criminal courts. Forensic psychiatric facilities have piqued public interest over the last several decades, when the media highlighted such cases as Andrea Yates, the Texas woman who drowned her five children, and Lee Marvo, the teenager who participated in the Washington, DC, sniper shootings with his father figure, John Muhammed. As nurses in forensic settings have developed a unique identity with a particular set of skills, their practice has become distinguished as a specialized area with unique treatment concerns (Love and Morrison, 2002; Sekula et al, 2001). This chapter focuses on the competencies required of the forensic psychiatric nurse in a secure forensic psychiatric facility, particularly the long-term forensic unit.

## STATE FORENSIC PSYCHIATRIC FACILITIES

### INPATIENT FORENSIC FACILITIES AND TYPES OF PATIENTS ADMITTED

The primary difference between an inpatient forensic unit and a regular psychiatric inpatient

**Norm's Notes**

*Speaking frankly, most of you will not be interested in this type of career. Forensic unit staff members care for people who have done something criminal. Sometimes, these crimes have been gruesome and have made national headlines, but I still think reading this chapter will be interesting. It will help you understand our society's attempt to deal with very serious and sometimes very disturbing behaviors. Forensic nurses have an important role to play.*

unit is the requirement of maintaining safety while enforcing the confinement of patients who have a mental illness and have been convicted by a criminal court for a criminal offense.

## Structural Aspects of the Environment

State forensic psychiatric facilities are the most restrictive of all treatment environments. Like prisons, forensic psychiatric facilities are a secure environment with strict rules and regulations to ensure safety and security. Buildings are designed for maximum security to prevent patients from escaping. These individuals have been charged with criminal offenses and are deemed too dangerous to reside in the community. Guard-controlled doors, metal detectors at entry, and strategically placed checkpoints throughout the facility are features shared by forensic psychiatric facilities and prisons. A point of departure in the aims of these institutions is that prisons focus on control, whereas the focus in forensic psychiatric facilities is on treatment (in addition to control).

## TYPES OF PATIENTS ADMITTED TO FORENSIC FACILITIES

The patient in the forensic psychiatric setting is guilty of committing a crime believed to be caused by their mental illness. Alternatively, the forensic psychiatric patient might have committed a crime independently of their mental illness, but is presently too ill to participate in court proceedings. For example, a patient experiencing symptoms of schizophrenia might injure a neighbor because he or she heard voices stating that the neighbor

intended to harm her or him. This is quite different from a patient who injures someone while their illness is stable. A patient judged to have committed a crime in connection with a mental illness might be found not guilty by reason of insanity (NGRI). Unlike a ruling of the courts in which an individual found guilty of a crime is sentenced for a specified period, the NGRI ruling specifies the condition that the patient be confined "until which time it is deemed by the treating facility that the patient is no longer a threat to society." As pointed out in Chapter 5, Legal Issues, usually the person committed to treatment under an insanity plea is actually confined longer than if they were criminally sentenced to prison. Many states stipulate a conditional release for patients committed to forensic psychiatric facilities on an NGRI defense (Parker, 2004). For example, participation in outpatient treatment can be required as a condition of the patient's release. Assertive community treatment (ACT) programs are an example of programs used as a condition of release from a forensic psychiatric facility. Failure to maintain involvement with treatment could result in a return to the criminal justice system (Munetz et al, 2001). Studies have so far suggested promising results in reducing rates of re-arrest and rehospitalization for the forensic psychiatric patient (Parker, 2004). Increasingly, law enforcement officials find themselves in the middle of the crisis in the community care of psychiatric patients (Munetz et al, 2001). Any patient creating a disturbance, but not responded to by the mental health system, invariably comes to the attention of law enforcement. A forensic psychiatric nurse can be of immense service to forensic psychiatric patients and to the community by serving as a liaison between the criminal justice and mental health systems. Because prediction of a patient being dangerous is difficult, close supervision is important to help ensure public safety.

As might be expected, psychiatric disorders such as schizophrenia and bipolar affective disorder are the most common diagnoses of those seeking an insanity defense. It is extremely difficult for other diagnostic categories to use the insanity defense for a crime successfully, although many might attempt this as a plea. Sociopaths have sometimes attempted to claim a propensity for criminal behavior based on biologic evidence;

however, such cases do not meet the conditions for the insanity defense and, as such, these pleas are often halted early in the criminal proceedings. Warren and colleagues (2004) examined more than 5000 sanity evaluations. They determined that the defendants found to be NGRI had psychotic, organic, or affective diagnoses. Defendants with a prior criminal history, drug charges, personality disorder, or intoxication at the time of arrest were unlikely to be found "insane." At their study site (Warren et al, 2004), the State Department of Mental Health required rigorous training of forensic evaluators, which was thought to contribute to the high reliability observed among evaluators. Specifying criteria through such training seems an effective way to ensure consistency in such an important determination as evaluation of sanity and criminal culpability.

Patients might also be admitted to a forensic psychiatric unit for short-term psychiatric assessments done as part of pretrial or sentencing court orders. It is not uncommon for a particular area in a forensic psychiatric setting to be reserved primarily for these short-term assessments and for evaluation of the patient's ability to participate in their own defense. These patients are generally transferred back to the referring facility with a recommendation regarding both their psychiatric illness and their capability to participate in their own defense. If the patient is later found NGRI, confinement and treatment at a forensic psychiatric facility might be ordered by the courts.

## CLINICAL EXAMPLE

Marvin G, a 29-year-old Caucasian man, murdered his mother because he thought she was planning to kill him in his sleep. Marvin heard voices telling him he should kill his mother before she did away with him. Marvin is prescribed Clozaril and had been compliant with this medication regimen; however, he had never told his psychiatrist of these thoughts about his mother. At his trial, expert psychiatric testimony concurred with Marvin's prior diagnosis of paranoid schizophrenia and recommended confinement in a state forensic psychiatric hospital where the patient could be closely monitored and treated. Future discharge is to be reviewed by an expert panel, not before a period of 18 months.

## CRITICAL THINKING QUESTION    1

Should society be investing resources into the treatment of patients who have demonstrated extreme dangerousness? How would one determine when the patient was rehabilitated? What obligation do mental health professionals have to the public's safety?

## CLINICAL EXAMPLE

Mary S, a 22-year-old African-American woman, shot and killed her boyfriend and his sister. During her trial, Mary S stared around the room and giggled for no apparent reason. After being on the stand and pausing for long periods before answering questions, and asking why she was being persecuted by the demons, the judge ordered Mary S to a forensic psychiatric unit for psychiatric evaluation before proceeding further with the trial.

## CRITICAL THINKING QUESTION    2

What type of mental illness would potentially lead someone to injure or murder another person?

## CRITICAL THINKING QUESTION    3

Why are some patients who are violent toward others committed to a local inpatient psychiatric unit or state psychiatric hospital, whereas others end up in a forensic psychiatric unit?

## Rehabilitation and Symptom Stabilization

Obviously, in order for patients in this setting to be eligible for return to the community, both the criminal act and the psychiatric illness must be addressed. To get from point A to point B, activities are structured and closely supervised. Treatment team meetings help maintain the focus on both goals. Although medications are important, programs geared toward many other problems must be offered to give patients an opportunity for improvement. For example, many of these patients have problems with anger, so specific programs targeting anger and aggression management should be offered. Furthermore, a high percentage of this population also has difficult-to-treat substance abuse and/or personality disorders (Ogloff et al, 2004). Creative approaches are required to reach the special interacting and complex needs present in this population. The knowledge base for dealing with the complexity of these multiple, often interacting, problems is not well developed.

## SPECIAL CHALLENGES FOR THE FORENSIC PSYCHIATRIC NURSE

### Dealing With the Potential for Physical Violence

Patients involuntarily admitted to state forensic psychiatric facilities for evaluation and treatment have a history of criminal behavior and thus pose a high risk of violence (Rask and Levander, 2001). Multiple psychiatric diagnoses, especially concomitant personality disorders, substance abuse, and psychoses, also increase the risk of violence. Regulatory agencies recognize violence and behavioral management issues as the primary challenge in forensic psychiatric settings (Love and Morrison, 2002). Security of the staff is an essential concern that must be addressed.

Although acts of violence are not generally caused by staff intentionally, the probability of their occurrence can be influenced by the attitudes and behaviors of the staff. Training in violence prevention and management techniques is essential for forensic psychiatric staff.

Carlsson and colleagues (2004) found that nurses often use knowledge of which they are not always aware, particularly when responding to impending violence in a patient. In this particular study, nurses who were able to acknowledge the threat to their safety reported a decreased intensity of fear. On the other hand, an increased fear level that was not acknowledged often escalated and led to a tendency for nurses to flee, thereby rupturing the caring connection. For example, some nurses forced the issue of controlling behavior as opposed to connecting with the patient and solving problems. Carlsson and colleagues (2004) found subtle ways that nurses made patients feel "wrong, unpleasant, undesired, or disbelieved" just in the nurses' everyday routines or actions. Interactions as benign as handling a patient's request to use personal items can turn into a control battle between patient and nurse. When patients are

dealt with in ways that make them lose their integrity, the probability of acting–out behavior (e.g., verbal or physical aggression) is increased (Carlsson et al, 2004).

In order for forensic units to be therapeutic and thus distinct from prison settings, it is necessary to have balance regarding the issue of behavior control. In Chapter 23, the concept of balance was presented as one essential feature of psychiatric settings. The problem of balancing security needs with treatment needs is even more important in forensic psychiatry. The question that must be answered is, "How can we provide sufficient security to control violence, while maintaining the clinical integrity of treatment?" (Morrison et al, 2002).

Nurses in the forensic setting must address this question while simultaneously operating under the constraints of regulatory agencies that mandate the reduction of restraint and seclusion. Although the efforts to comply with this goal are laudable and can also encourage creativity in the staff, an overzealous zero tolerance policy for restraint and seclusion places undue pressure on the staff and also has the potential for seriously undermining the nurse's ability to maintain control of the unit, particularly with patients with a severe personality disorder (Morrison et al, 2002). Increased violence and staff injuries were addressed in one unit by grouping similar patients together and assuring nurses that restraints could be used in extreme situations. A violence response team was reorganized and, after an initial period of restraint and seclusion use as control of the unit was regained, the use of restraint and seclusion decreased (see Highlighting the Evidence: Current Research box; Morrison et al, 2002). It is imperative in the forensic setting that this type of preplanning occurs, because situations have the potential to get out of control quickly.

Ideally, staff would always be protected from violent assaults, but this is not possible. The aftermath of violent behavior toward health care personnel can have long-term psychological effects on its victims, including feelings of a sense of professional incompetence or failure (Carlsson et al, 2004). When nurses are the target of violence, it is important to offer support and debriefing. Avoiding this topic can result in unhealthy behaviors and attitudes in the nurses. Fortunately, most forensic psychiatric nurses do well at recognizing the patient's behavior as part of their illness.

## Highlighting the Evidence: Current Research

To reduce the occurrence of staff injuries in a forensic psychiatric setting, an expert nurse was employed as a consultant. After meeting, interviewing, and working with staff, the consultant made several recommendations. One of the first was the creation of very specific ward regulations and rules that addressed behavior, dress, and expectations. These rules were clearly written out, explained, and enforced almost immediately. Additionally, units were reorganized so that weaker or sicker patients would be protected from exploitation. Because of the agenda to reduce seclusion and restraints, the staff had been very reluctant to use these interventions and patients could pretty much do what they wanted. An aggression management plan (AMP) was created for each of the known perpetrators of violence. Clear guidelines were written out for

staff, with measurable degrees of behavior indicative of impending violence, including the appropriate clinical interventions for the identified stages of escalation (A = anxiety, B = bold and belligerent, C = crises). A special management team (SMT) was created for the express purpose of restraining at-risk patients, when necessary. This team was outfitted with Kevlar sleeves, helmets with face shields, protective gloves, chest protectors, knee pads, and shin guards to protect them from injury. After an initial increase in the use of restraints and seclusion, the incidence of violence decreased and continued to do so at follow-up (e.g., 1-year, 2-year follow-up). Staff were encouraged to ventilate their feelings about former incidents and received special attention aimed at helping victims of violence.

From Morrison E, Morman G, Bonner G, et al: Reducing staff injuries and violence in a forensic psychiatric setting, *Arch Psychiatr Nurs* 16:108, 2002.

Apart from the prevention and management of potential physical violence, another issue of great importance in the forensic psychiatric setting is verbal abuse.

### Dealing With Verbal Abuse

Just as support and debriefing are important for nursing staff exposed to physical violence, the daily stress of continual verbal abuse of nurses by patients needs to be addressed if staff morale is to be maintained. Repeatedly being called names and being met with hostility from patients that one is trying to help is demoralizing to nursing staff, raising the potential for burnout. Burnout was discussed in the previous chapter (variables affecting the therapeutic environment), with particular emphasis on the effects of secondary traumatization. One might expect this phenomenon to be occur more often in the forensic environment; however, some researchers have actually found forensic psychiatric nurses to be less prone to burnout than their mainstream psychiatric nursing colleagues (Happell et al, 2003). Given the image of forensic psychiatric nursing as dangerous and unpredictable, this finding is somewhat surprising; however, some studies have found morale problems on forensic psychiatric units sur-

prisingly easy to fix. Morrison and colleagues (2002) reported on the use of advanced practice psychiatric nurses to provide staff support and reflective supervision of nurses' clinical practices in a forensic nursing unit with an increased occurrence of violent incidents. The ongoing opportunity to reflect on and discuss reactions to patients was seen by nurses as supportive and helped offset feelings aroused by negative encounters. This type of staff support in an environment where establishing relationships is at best difficult is actively countered by some very negative experiences with patients. The next section will explore how the nurse-patient relationship is affected by the forensic psychiatric setting.

### Difficulties Inherent in the Nurse-Patient Relationship

The nurse-patient relationship in forensic psychiatric settings is much more complex than in nonforensic psychiatric settings. Physical or verbal abuse is sufficiently daunting to interfere with forming a meaningful nurse-patient relationship. Holmes (2005) has noted another potential source of discrepancy for the forensic psychiatric nurse: conflict related to the dual role of caring for patients while also participating in their punishment, by virtue of incarceration (i.e., the forensic environment). Nurses are educated to provide high-quality nursing care; in forensic settings, however, this is not always possible because of the constraints of an environment that is also responsible for enforcing rules related to security and incarceration (Holmes and Federman, 2003). This dual role is difficult for the mental health and legal system to resolve and certainly is not easier for the nurse in this setting who has dual, sometimes conflicting, goals.

Nurses in forensic psychiatric settings are ethically responsible for providing care to mentally ill individuals (patients/inmates), most of whom have committed horrendous criminal acts such as violent murders and rapes. Some studies have suggested that countertransference is a factor interfering with developing a relationship with patients in forensic settings (Encinares et al, 2005). Because of the awful crimes that some patients have committed, nurses might harbor feelings of anger, fear, and hatred toward patients/inmates, which manifests in the nurse-patient relationship in the form of othering. Peternelj-Taylor (2004) has defined *othering* as a judgmental attitude whereby the nurse perceives patients as different, thereby justifying distancing within the context of the nurse-patient relationship. Treating patients/inmates as "monsters" has also been described in the nursing literature as another way that countertransference is manifested in the nurse-patient relationship in this setting (Holmes and Federman, 2003). This type of relating results in distance and misunderstanding and has an enormous impact on the nurse-patient relationship, making it difficult to achieve.

Nurses working in forensic psychiatric settings must be aware of their feelings toward patients/inmates (Encinares et al, 2005). Self-awareness helps counter poor nursing care or maltreatment, which could result from negative conceptions of patients as evil. The nurse, in order to help the patient, must be able to get beyond this reaction to the patient. Just as clinical supervision with an experienced advanced practice nurse can be supportive to staff, an additional benefit is related to assisting staff to maintain an awareness of their feelings, attitudes, and reactions to the patient.

On the other hand, it is noteworthy that the nurse-patient relationship has always been regarded as the cornerstone of psychiatric nursing; however, documentation practices often reflect more of a passive, custodial, observe and report type of approach. One study revealed that nurses were often reluctant to discuss the crime for which the patient was committed, even when the therapeutic relationship is reported to be the focus of nursing intervention (Martin and Street, 2003). Conflict between issues of "care" and "custody," and internal tension arising from caring for patients who might have done incomprehensible horrendous acts, are all notable challenges facing the nurse working in a forensic psychiatric setting (Austin, 2001; Holmes, 2005; Love and Hunter, 1999; Love and Morrison, 2003; Martin, 2001; Martin and Street, 2003; Mason, 2002; Rask and Levander, 2001; Schafer and Peternelj-Taylor, 2003).

One final formidable barrier to effective nurse-patient relationships involves the extreme importance of maintaining professional boundaries with patients (Melia et al, 1999; Peternelj-Taylor, 2002, 2003; Schafer and Peternelj-Taylor, 2003).

## CLINICAL EXAMPLE

James Sean, a 35-year-old Caucasian man, was recently admitted to the forensic psychiatric unit. There are clearly defined markings around several areas of the nursing station, exit doors, restrooms, and certain other areas on the unit. James has been told to remain outside the red line at all times, but walks up and starts trying to ask for an aspirin while inside the red-lined area. The nurse immediately warns the patient and declines to respond to his request until he complies with the stated limit.

## MAINTAINING PROFESSIONAL BOUNDARIES IN THE FORENSIC SETTING

The expertise of forensic psychiatric nursing colleagues such as Colleen Carnes-Love, Eileen Morrison, and several others cited in this chapter (Hunter and Love, 1996; Love and Hunter, 1996, 1999; Love and Morrison, 2003) has provided invaluable information about the extreme importance of close attention to the boundaries of therapeutic relationships, especially among a patient population who experience various mental illnesses, in addition to severe character problems. Manipulation and deviation from prescribed agency boundaries can be particularly dangerous in this situation. Those suffering from substance abuse problems, antisocial personality disorder, and mental illness with a history of violent crime can be a dangerous population, and specific relationship boundaries must be maintained. There are times in most forensic nurses' careers when this boundary is weakened as a result of succumbing to patients' manipulations or charm. Periodic stories in the media attesting to such perilous events as falling in love with a patient, and even assisting a patient in an elopement (escape), underscore the bewildering consequences of inappropriate relationships with patients, particularly in the forensic setting. Again, clinical supervision with an advanced practice nurse is an absolute necessity to assist all staff in remaining clear about the dangers of boundary violations and the insidious manner in which they can occur. It is doubtful that nurses go to work in forensic psychiatric settings to pursue a love interest and yet, it happens, often to the dismay of peers and friends. Certainly, in this environment, where security is the primary concern, boundaries must be maintained with patients/inmates. The balance between establishing a nurse-patient relationship while maintaining adequate boundaries is sometimes hard to achieve. This topic cannot be addressed without discussing those with personality disorders and the skill with which such individuals can manipulate the best-intentioned nurse.

## DEALING WITH SEVERE PERSONALITY DISORDERS

There is little doubt that, of all the diagnoses, personality disorder produces more emotional response in forensic mental health professionals than any other (Woods and Richards, 2005). A high percentage of personality disorder diagnoses can be expected in any forensic setting and represents one of the most challenging aspects of forensic nursing care. Behaviors such as angry outbursts, accusations, manipulation, and exploitation of staff or other patients are so pervasive as to challenge the patience of even the most experienced forensic psychiatric nurses.

For example, as noted previously, a common problem in forensic psychiatric nursing has to do with the extreme importance of maintaining professional boundaries with patients (Love and Morrison, 2002). The repertoire of manipulative behaviors exhibited by the sociopathic personality includes charming the people they target, grandiosity, lying, failing to take responsibility for their own actions (thus blaming others), intimidation,

and violence (verbal or physical). The sociopath is skilled at drawing others in, so it is often easy to forget their predatory nature. When the sociopath is through with the targeted victim, there is generally a shift from charm to harm. We suggest, in addition to ongoing supervision, that a checklist detailing the specific behaviors of the patient should be used. This can serve as an ongoing reminder of the patients' characteristic style of interaction and potentially minimize the ease with which some patients can manipulate others. In other words, if the nurse can see a patient's repertoire of manipulative behaviors in print, the patient's efforts will be less powerful. The Hare Psychopathy Checklist is a tool developed by expert psychologist Robert Hare (1999) as a way to maintain awareness of the hidden mask of sociopathic behaviors. Although Dr. Hare is an expert in the area of the sociopath, he is careful to point out in his books that he can still be manipulated by the sociopath and must find ways to minimize the opportunity for the patient to succeed in their manipulative and deceptive maneuvers.

Responding to a series of unmanageable incidents, including misconduct of a staff nurse at a secure psychiatric facility, Melia and colleagues (1999) suggested that the collusion, victimization, manipulation, anger, and increased emotional intensity generated by dealing with the personality-disordered patient can be minimized by a shift from the traditional one-to-one relationship to a team of nurses. In this approach, two nurses meet with the patient and afterward a third nurse serves as reviewer of the interaction. This approach is said to minimize the staff splitting, frustration, and potential boundary violations that can occur when working one to one with such patients (Melia et al, 1999). Although this might seem counter to mainstream psychiatric nursing, this approach certainly emphasizes the need for staff-to-staff and peer accountability in dealing with severely personality-disordered patients. When relationship boundaries are crossed, it is important to deal with this quickly. Peternelj-Taylor (2002, 2003) has addressed the nurses' difficult decision-making process in finally exposing a colleague who had entered into an inappropriate relationship with a patient. It is worth noting that most aggressive incidents on forensic psychiatric units are perpetrated by patients scoring high on psychopathy scales (Hildebrand et al, 2004). Such patients pose a strong threat to the entire unit if a staff member becomes swayed by the psychopath's charm and skill at manipulation. (See Chapter 33, which discusses personality disorders.) Ignoring such actions is akin to ignoring physical or emotional abuse, alcoholism, addiction, or any other unpleasant behavior—sometimes we pretend these do not exist, even though they might be glaring at us, sometimes from our own mirror.

## MAINTAINING A WORKING RELATIONSHIP WITH UNLICENSED PERSONNEL

It would seem self-evident that relationships among team members on any unit requiring cooperative efforts to deliver care need to be nurtured to maintain this effort. This is especially important in psychiatry, where the treatment environment is greatly affected by the relationships among staff. In the forensic environment, where many patients have personality disorders and thus a propensity for difficulty in managing relationships effectively, staff must actively work at relationships with each other to avoid becoming entangled in the manipulations of character-disordered patients. Unlicensed personnel, under the direction of staff nurses, must be included in treatment planning and offered in-service education and mentoring relationships with professional staff. They are with patients more than any other staff members and, unless creative intervention by nursing staff occurs to keep the relationship of unlicensed personnel focused on the aims of treatment, the potential for their greater identification with patients is higher. Although this might seem obvious, it is easy to become complacent and start to believe that unlicensed staff on the unit with patients are separate from treatment staff. This is a potentially dangerous and certainly countertherapeutic problem, requiring the attention of the forensic psychiatric nurse.

In the next section, the specific interventions used by forensic nurses will be addressed, along with the importance of evidence-based practice in nursing.

## SPECIFIC NURSING INTERVENTIONS USED BY FORENSIC PSYCHIATRIC NURSES

In examining specific skills of forensic psychiatric nurses, most experts agree that there is a need for creativity and further development of evidence-based outcomes for forensic psychiatric nursing. For example, confrontation appears to be a heavily used intervention in forensic settings, although the effectiveness of this approach has not been evaluated (Rask and Levander, 2001). In fact, this intervention might be contrary to the findings of some studies. The confrontational nature of interventions focusing on socially unacceptable behavior has been shown to be a potential source of psychological strain for the patient with schizophrenia (Eklund and Hansson, 1997). Researchers have found that psychotic and nonpsychotic patients require different ward atmospheres. In particular, the presence of a high degree of expressed emotion (EE) has been found to increase the probability of relapse in schizophrenic patients (Eklund and Hansson, 1997; Miura et al, 2004; Rask and Levander, 2001; Woo et al, 2004). With so many complex and interacting variables involved, further research in this area is warranted to delineate specific evidence-based approaches.

A study defining the interventions of forensic nurses revealed that the two main interventions reported by forensic psychiatric nurses were verbal interactions, with a focus on limit setting for problematic behavior, and discussion with patients/inmates about "problems in daily life" (Rask and Levander, 2001). Milieu therapy was the most commonly stated model guiding nursing interventions (Rask and Levander, 2001). The value of research is emphasized when considering the commonly accepted assumption that the nurse-patient relationship is the primary tool in psychiatric nursing, and inferential in forensic psychiatric nursing, but is not actualized in nursing practice (Martin and Street, 2002). If forensic psychiatric nursing is to develop fully as a specialty practice, clearly defined interventions for this unique population must be established and evaluated.

## SUMMARY AND FUTURE DIRECTIONS

Future intervention and patient outcome–based research in forensic nursing are expected to advance this emergent specialty area of nursing. Although forensic psychiatric nursing has been around for some time, it has received minimal attention in the literature. If forensic psychiatric nurses can overcome their professional and physical isolation from other areas of nursing (Love and

Morrison, 2002), and clearly articulate how they affect patients' stabilization and recovery, a new specialty practice will unfold, with new interventions to share with nurses in other areas.

## Study Notes

1. Forensic nursing is a specialty practice area that has emerged as a distinct specialty and includes many different roles such as SANEs, legal nurse consultants, forensic psychiatric nurses, and correctional nurses.

2. The forensic psychiatric nurse is a subspecialty area of psychiatric nursing practice involving the management of patients with a mental illness who have been adjudicated to treatment by the criminal courts.

3. Like prisons, forensic psychiatric facilities are a secure environment with strict rules and regulations to ensure safety and security.

4. The patient in the forensic psychiatric setting is guilty of committing a crime believed to be caused by his or her mental illness.

5. Patients may be admitted to forensic psychiatric settings for short-term psychiatric assessments done as part of pretrial or sentencing court orders.

6. The forensic psychiatric patient may have committed a crime independent of their mental illness but is presently too ill to participate in court proceedings.

7. A patient judged to have committed a crime in connection with a mental illness may be found NGRI.

8. In order for patients in this setting to be eligible for return to the community, *both* the criminal act and the psychiatric illness must be addressed.

9. Patients involuntarily admitted to state forensic psychiatric facilities for evaluation and treatment have a history of criminal behavior and pose a risk of violence.

10. Training in violence prevention and management techniques is essential for forensic psychiatric staff.

11. In order for forensic units to be therapeutic and thus distinct from prison settings, it is necessary to have balance regarding the issue of behavior control.

12. The problem of balancing security needs with treatment needs is important in forensic psychiatry.

13. The nurse-patient relationship in forensic psychiatric settings is much more complex than in nonforensic psychiatric settings.

14. Nurses in forensic psychiatric settings are ethically responsible for providing care to mentally ill individuals (patients/inmates), most of whom have committed horrendous criminal acts.

15. Studies have suggested that countertransference is a factor interfering with developing a relationship with patients in forensic settings.

16. A common problem in forensic psychiatric nursing has to do with the extreme importance of maintaining professional boundaries with patients.

17. In the forensic environment, in which many patients have personality disorders and thus a propensity for difficulty with managing relationships effectively, staff must actively work at relationships with each other to avoid becoming entangled in the manipulations of character-disordered patients.

18. Clinical supervision with an advanced practice nurse is an absolute necessity to assist all staff in remaining clear about the dangers of boundary violations.

19. There is a need for creativity and further development of evidence-based outcomes for forensic psychiatric nursing.

20. Two primary interventions reported by forensic psychiatric nurses are verbal interactions with a focus on limit setting for problematic behavior and discussion with patients/inmates about problems in daily life.

## References

Austin W: Relational ethics in forensic psychiatric settings, *J Psychosoc Nurs* 39:12, 2001.

Carlsson G, Dahlberg K, Lützen K, Nystrom M: Violent encounters in psychiatric care: a phenomenological study of embodied caring knowledge, *Issues Ment Health Nurs* 25:191, 2004.

Eklund M, Hansson L: Relationships between characteristics of the ward atmosphere and treatment outcome in a psychiatric day-care unit based on occupational therapy, *Acta Psychiatr Scand* 95:329, 1997.

Encinares M, McMaster JJ, McNamee J: Risk assessment of forensic patients: nurses' role, *J Psychosoc Nurs Ment Health Serv* 43:30, 2005.

Happell B, Martin T, Pinikahana J: Burnout and job satisfaction: a comparative study of psychiatric nurses from forensic and a mainstream mental health service, *Int J Ment Health Nurs* 12:39, 2003.

Hildebrand M, De Ruiter C, Nijman H: PCL-R psychopathy predicts disruptive behavior among male offenders in a Dutch forensic psychiatric hospital, *J Interpers Viol* 19:139, 2004.

Holmes D: Governing the captives: forensic psychiatric nursing in corrections, *Perspect Psychiatr Care* 41:3, 2005.

Holmes D, Federman C: Constructing monsters: correctional discourse and nursing practice, *Int J Psychiatr Nurs Res* 8:942, 2003.

Hunter ME, Love CC: Total quality management and the reduction of inpatient violence and costs in a forensic psychiatric hospital, *Psychiatr Serv* 47:751, 1996.

International Association of Forensic Nurses: About IAFN. Available at http://www.forensicnurse.org/about/default.html. Accessed July 18, 2005.

Love CC, Hunter M: Engaging patients in violence prevention, *J Psychosoc Nurs Ment Health Serv* 37:32, 1999.

Love CC, Hunter M: Violence in public sector psychiatric hospitals. Benchmarking nursing staff injury rates, *J Psychosoc Nurs Ment Health Serv* 34:30, 1996.

Love C, Morrison E: Forensic psychiatric nursing: struggling to happen, failing to thrive. Available at http://www.forensicnursemag.com/articles/281feat1.html (08/01/02). Accessed July 6, 2005.

Love C, Morrison E, American Academy of Nursing Expert Panel on Violence: American Academy of Nursing Expert Panel on Violence policy recommendations on workplace violence (adopted 2002). *Issues Ment Health Nurs* 24:599, 2003.

Martin T: Something special: forensic psychiatric nursing, *J Psychiatr Ment Health Nurs* 8:25, 2001.

Martin T, Street F: Exploring evidence of the therapeutic relationship in forensic psychiatric nursing, *J Psychiatr Ment Health Nurs* 10:543, 2003.

Mason T: Forensic psychiatric nursing: a literature review and thematic analysis of role tensions, *J Psychiatr Ment Health Nurs* 9:511, 2002.

Melia P, Moran T, Mason T: Triumvirate nursing for personality-disordered patients: crossing the boundaries safely, *J Psychiatr Ment Health Nurs* 6:15, 1999.

Miura Y, Mizuno M, Yamashita C, et al: Expressed emotion and social functioning in chronic schizophrenia, *Compr Psychiatry* 45:469, 2004.

Morrison E, Morman G, Bonner G, et al: Reducing staff injuries and violence in a forensic psychiatric setting, *Arch Psychiatr Nurs* 16:108, 2002.

Munetz MR, Grande TP, Chambers MR: The incarceration of individuals with severe mental disorders, *Community Ment Health J* 37:361, 2001.

Ogloff JR, Lemphers A, Dwyer C: Dual diagnosis in an Australian forensic psychiatric hospital: prevalence and implications for services, *Behav Sci Law* 22:543, 2004.

Parker G: Outcomes of assertive community treatment in an NGRI conditional release program, *J Am Acad Psychiatry Law* 32:291, 2004.

Peternelj-Taylor C: An exploration of othering in forensic psychiatric and correctional nursing, *Can J Nurs Res* 36:130, 2004.

Peternelj-Taylor C: Whistleblowing and boundary violations: exposing a colleague in the forensic milieu, *Nurs Ethics* 10:526, 2003.

Peternelj-Taylor C: Professional boundaries. A matter of therapeutic integrity, *J Psychosoc Nurs Ment Health Serv* 40:22, 2002.

Rask M, Levander S: Interventions in the nurse-patient relationship in forensic psychiatric nursing care: a Swedish survey, *J Psychiatr Ment Health Nurs* 8:323, 2001.

Schafer P, Peternelj-Taylor C: Therapeutic relationships and boundary maintenance: the perspective of forensic patients enrolled in a treatment program for violent offenders, *Issues Ment Health Nurs* 24:605, 2003.

Sekula K, Holmes D, Zoucha R, et al: Forensic psychiatric nursing: discursive practices and the emergence of a specialty, *J Psychosoc Nurs* 39:51, 2001.

Warren JI, Murrie DC, Chauhan P, et al: Opinion formation in evaluating sanity at the time of the offense: an examination of 5175 pre-trial evaluations, *Behav Sci Law* 22:171, 2004.

Woo SM, Goldstein MJ, Nuechterlein KH: Relatives' affective style and the expression of subclinical psychopathology in patients with schizophrenia, *Fam Process* 43:233, 2004.

Woods P, Richards D: Effectiveness of nursing interventions in people with personality disorders, *J Adv Nurs* 44:154, 2003.

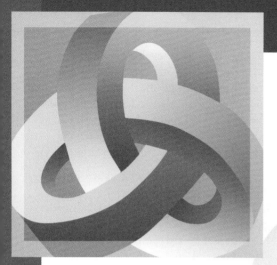

# Chapter 27

# Introduction to Psychopathology

*Norman L. Keltner*

## Learning Objectives

*After reading this chapter, you should be able to:*
- Describe the extent of mental illness in the United States.
- Identify the most common mental disorders in the United States.
- List the three requirements for understanding psychopathology.
- Describe several guidelines applicable to all aspects of psychotherapeutic management.

*Psychoanalysis took a while to conquer the United States, but once it did, after the Second World War, its dominance was unquestioned, and its arrogance breathtaking. Schizophrenia, autism, and numerous other disorders were blamed on the mother, with no evidence, just utter certainty.*

Acocella (2000, p 114)

According to the U.S. Surgeon General's report on mental health (1999), 20% of the U.S. population is affected by mental disorders during a given year. When the full spectrum of mental, emotional, and addictive disorders is included, it is believed that 25% or more of Americans suffer each year (Kessler et al, 2005a); National Institute of Mental Health, 2005; Surgeon General, 1999). As noted in Table 27-1, anxiety disorders are the most prevalent, followed by mood disorders (collectively), alcohol disorders, and major depression. This table, also found in Chapter 1 and in most chapters in this unit, lists prevalence rates for a 12-month period. Lifetime incidence of these disorders is slightly higher (Kessler et al, 2005b). Table 27-2 provides the data for lifetime prevalence rates for the most common mental and chemical abuse disorders. It is important to note that many individuals have a comorbid status—for example, they may be depressed, anxious, and abuse a chemical or have some other combination of disorders. Therefore, psychiatric morbidity is concentrated, with approximately 23% of the population having a history of three or more comorbid disorders (Kessler et al, 2005a). Most of these individuals do not seek professional help, suggesting a great reservoir of unmet mental health needs in the United States.

The incidence of psychopathology is high, and nurses' understanding of psychopathology is basic for effective psychotherapeutic management of mental disorders. Understanding psychopathology requires that knowledge be organized, operational definitions be formed, and criteria for diagnosis be developed. Several diagnostic systems have been developed, but this text presents criteria from the *Diagnostic and Statistical Manual of Mental Disorders* (*DSM*), which is published by the American Psychiatric Association (APA) and is the official diagnostic manual in use in the United States. The current version, *DSM-IV-TR* (fourth revised edition) (American Psychiatric Association [APA], 2000), is the sixth version since the DSM was first published in 1952 (*DSM-I, DSM-II, DSM-III, DSM-III-R, DSM-IV,* and *DSM-IV-TR*). Because diagnostic consistency among clinicians is so important, psychiatric experts are constantly evaluating and updating criteria for this manual. All chapters in this unit are developed around *DSM* criteria that convey important concepts related to each mental disorder discussed. Because people are more than their symptoms, and successful treatment demands an assessment beyond the presenting disorder, the *DSM* involves evaluation on several axes. Five axes have been identified:

*Axis I.* Clinical disorders (e.g., schizophrenia, bipolar disorder, depression)

*Axis II.* Personality or developmental disorders (e.g., paranoid or borderline personality disorders, mental retardation)

*Axis III.* General medical conditions (that are potentially relevant to understanding the mental disorder) (e.g., neoplasms, endocrine disorders)

*Axis IV.* Psychosocial and environmental problems (e.g., divorce, education, housing)

*Axis V.* Global assessment of functioning (e.g., rating of psychological, social, and occupational functioning on a mental health scale [0 to 100])

### Norm's Notes

*This brief chapter provides an overview of some statistics about mental illness and a rationale for the nurse's need to know psychopathologic concepts. A disturbing point that you cannot detect from Table 27-1 is that things are not getting better. I can see it because I've been around a long time and know the older stats. Even though billions and billions of dollars have been spent, just as many people suffer from mental disorders today as they did 20 years ago. I must admit—I'm a little discouraged.*

| Table 27-1 | **12-month Prevalence Rate of Mental Disorders in the United States*** |
|---|---|

| Disorders | Approximate Percentage Over 17 Years of Age | Approximate Number of Persons | Gender Overrepresentation |
|---|---|---|---|
| **Anxiety Disorders** | 18 overall | 36,000,000 | |
| Panic disorder | 3.5 | 7,000,000 | Women |
| Social phobia | 7 | 14,000,000 | Women |
| Specific phobia | 8.7 | 17,000,000 | Women |
| GAD | 3 | 6,000,000 | Women |
| PTSD | 3.5 | 7,000,000 | Women |
| OCD | 1 | 2,000,000 | Equal |
| **Mood Disorders** | 9.5 overall | 19,000,000 | |
| Major depression | 6.7 | | Women |
| Dysthymia | 1.5 | | Women |
| Bipolar I and II | 2.6 | | BD I: Equal BD II: Women? |
| **Impulse Control Disorders** | 9 overall | 18,000,000 | |
| Conduct disorders | 1 | 2,000,000 | Men |
| ADHD | 4 | 8,000,000 | Men |
| **Substance Abuse Disorders** | 3.8 overall | 7,600,000 | |
| Alcohol abuse and dependence | 3.1 | 6,200,000 | Men |
| Drug abuse and dependence | 1.4 | 2,800,000 | Men |
| Schizophrenia | 1.1 | 2,100,000 | Equal |

*Extrapolated from several sources based on current census data.
*ADHD*, attention-deficit/hyperactivity disorder; *BD*, bipolar disorder; *GAD*, general anxiety disorder; *OCD*, obsessive-compulsive disorder; *PTSD*, posttraumatic stress disorder.
From Kessler RC, Chiu WT, Demler O, Walters EE: Prevalence, severity, and comorbidity of 12-month DSM-IV disorders in the national comorbidity survey replication, *Arch Gen Psychiatry* 62:617, 2005; U.S. Surgeon General: *Mental health: a report from the Surgeon General*, Washington, DC, 1999, Department of Health and Human Services: National Institute of Mental Health: *Statistics*. Available at www.nimh.nih.gov/healthinformation/statisticsmenu.cfm. Accessed on April 18, 2005.

| Table 27-2 | Lifetime Prevalence Rates for Mental Disorders in the United States |
| --- | --- |

| Disorder | Lifetime Prevalence Rate (%) |
| --- | --- |
| Anxiety disorders (all) | 28.8 |
| Panic disorder | 4.7 |
| Agoraphobia with panic disorders | 1.4 |
| Social phobia | 12.1 |
| Generalized anxiety disorder | 5.7 |
| Mood disorders (all) | 20.8 |
| Major depressive disorder | 16.6 |
| Bipolar disorder I & II | 3.9 |
| Dysthymia | 2.5 |
| Chemical abuse disorder (all) | 14.6 |
| Alcohol abuse | 13.2 |
| Alcohol dependence | 5.4 |
| Drug abuse | 7.9 |
| Drug dependence | 3 |
| Attention-deficit/hyperactivity disorder | 8.1 |
| Any mental or chemical abuse disorder | 46.4 |

Modified from Kessler RC, Berglund P, Demler O, et al: Lifetime prevalence and age-of-onset distributions of DSM-IV disorders in the national comorbidity survey replication. *Arch Gen Psychiatry* 62:593, 2005.

In addition, each chapter presents a discussion of common behaviors, etiology, and psychotherapeutic management strategies.

## BEHAVIOR

Patients' behaviors are presented to help the student identify behavioral phenomena. Some behaviors can be observed directly (objective assessment, or signs), whereas the patient must report other behaviors (subjective, or symptoms). Knowledge of these signs and symptoms helps the nurse anticipate and plan appropriate interventions.

## ETIOLOGY

For many years, psychiatric clinicians have typically fallen into one of two camps in regard to what causes mental disorders: those who subscribe to the nature argument and believe that mental disorders arise from *nature* (e.g., organic, biologic, genetic) and those who subscribe to the nurture argument and believe that mental disorders arise from *nurture* (e.g., psychodynamic, functional, environmental stressors, early life experiences). In recent years, most clinicians have come to recognize that both views provide valuable insights into the complexities of the human mind. In fact, research has suggested that some life experiences (i.e., nurture) actually change biology (i.e., nature), thus underscoring a more holistic view of mental illness. Threads of the "nature versus nurture" argument (or the "biologic versus psychodynamic" argument) are presented in discussions of etiologies; however, the overriding theme of this unit is the recognition of the unifying symptoms that point to the contributions of each etiologic factor.

## PSYCHOTHERAPEUTIC MANAGEMENT

Sections on psychotherapeutic management in each chapter draw on the general intervention strategies presented in Units II through IV to develop appropriate interventions for each disorder. In addition, a case study and a related nursing care plan are presented for each disorder. A sample nursing care plan is found at the end of this chapter. The following rules provide relevant guidelines for all aspects of psychotherapeutic management:

- Provide support for patients.
- Strengthen patients' self-esteem.
- Treat patients as adults.
- Prevent failure or embarrassment.
- Treat patients as individuals.
- Provide reality testing.
- Handle hostility therapeutically.
- Be calm and matter of fact about norms and limits.

## NURSES NEED TO UNDERSTAND PSYCHOPATHOLOGY

Nurses cannot gain a true understanding of patients with mental disorders until they understand mental disorders. Psychiatric nursing is more than warm, caring feelings about patients. Although being affirming and kind are wonderful attributes in daily life, more is required of the effective psychiatric nurse. This "more" is based on an understanding of psychopathology.

The psychiatric nurse can no more effectively plan and provide psychiatric care without an understanding of psychopathology than can the medical-surgical nurse plan and provide care without an understanding of pathophysiology. In this unit, the authors provide a discussion of psychopathology for each disorder. We have included chapters on the following mental disorders using the language of the *DSM-IV-TR:* schizophrenia, depression, bipolar disorders, anxiety-related disorders, cognitive disorders, personality disorders, sexual disorders, substance-related disorders, dual diagnosis, and eating disorders.

## CRITICAL THINKING QUESTION    1

The biologic versus psychodynamic argument has gone on for a long time. Why is it important to be open to both points of view? Although you might not have used the same words, you probably had a bias one way or the other before you started nursing school. What was your bias?

## ■ Study Notes

1. According to the U.S. Surgeon General, about 25% or more of Americans suffer from some type of mental or addictive disorder in any given 12-month period.

## Care Plan

Name: _____    Admission Date: _____

*DSM-IV-TR* Diagnosis: _____

Assessment    **Areas of strength:** _____
              **Problems:** _____

Diagnoses     _____
              _____

Outcomes      *Short-term goals:*                          *Date met*

              _____            _____
              _____            _____
              _____            _____

              *Long-term goals:*                          *Date met*

              _____            _____
              _____            _____
              _____            _____

Planning/     **Nurse-patient relationship:**
Interventions
              _____
              _____
              _____

              **Psychopharmacology:**

              _____
              _____
              _____

              **Milieu management:**

              _____
              _____
Evaluation    _____
              _____
Referrals     _____
              _____

2. Anxiety disorders are the most common category of mental disorders, followed by mood disorders (collectively), and alcohol disorders.

3. Understanding psychopathology is fundamental for effective psychotherapeutic management; it requires organizing knowledge, defining terms operationally, and developing criteria for diagnosis.

4. The *DSM-IV-TR* (APA, 2000) is the official diagnostic system used in American psychiatry and is emphasized in this textbook.

5. Etiologic explanations of mental disorders can be broadly placed in one of two categories: biologic (natural or organic causes) and psychological (nurturing, psychodynamic, or functional causes).

6. Guidelines appropriate for all aspects of psychiatric care include supportive care, strengthening self-esteem, preventing failure or embarrassment, treating patients as individuals, reinforcing reality, and handling patients' hostility calmly and matter of factly.

## References

Acocella J: The empty couch, *New Yorker,* May 8, 2000, p 112.

American Psychiatric Association: *Diagnostic and statistical manual of mental disorders, text revision,* ed 4, Washington, DC, 2000, APA.

Kessler RC, Chiu WT, Demler O, et al: Prevalence, severity, and comorbidity of 12-month DSM-IV disorders in the national comorbidity survey replication. *Arch Gen Psychiatry* 62:617, 2005a.

Kessler RC, Berglund P, Demler O, et al: Lifetime prevalence and age-of-onset distributions of DSM-IV disorders in the national comorbidity survey replication. *Arch Gen Psychiatry* 62:593, 2005b.

National Institute of Mental Health: *Statistics.* Available at www.nimh.nih.gov/healthinformation/statisticsmenu.cfm. Accessed April 18, 2005.

U.S. Surgeon General: *Mental health: a report from the Surgeon General,* Washington, DC, 1999, Department of Health & Human Services.

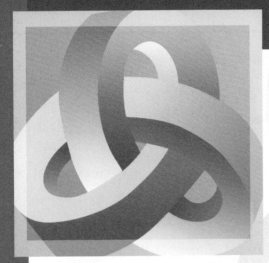

# Chapter 28

# Schizophrenia and Other Psychoses

*Norman L. Keltner*

## Learning Objectives

*After reading this chapter, you should be able to:*

- Define the term *schizophrenia*.
- Describe the major historic figures, events, and theories that have contributed to the current understanding of schizophrenia.
- Identify Bleuler's four A's.
- Recognize the *Diagnostic and Statistical Manual of Mental Disorders,* text revision fourth edition *(DSM-IV-TR)* criteria and terminology for schizophrenia.
- Differentiate and describe *DSM-IV-TR* subtypes, and types I and II subtypes.
- Recognize and describe objective and subjective symptoms of schizophrenia.
- Identify biologic explanations for schizophrenia.
- Describe two theoretical psychodynamic explanations for schizophrenia.
- Develop a nursing care plan for patients with schizophrenia.
- Identify the major drugs used in the treatment of schizophrenia, their mechanisms of action, their target symptoms, and their major side effects.
- Evaluate the effectiveness of nursing interventions for patients with schizophrenia.

There are three inescapable "facts" about schizophrenia (Weinberger, 1987):

1. Age at onset: It is almost always late adolescence or early adulthood.
2. Role of stress: Onset and relapse almost always related to stress.
3. Efficacy of dopamine antagonists: Drugs that block dopamine receptors are therapeutic.

Psychosis is a disruptive mental state in which an individual struggles to distinguish the external world from internally generated perceptions. An impaired ability to relate to others makes it worse. Common symptoms of psychosis include hallucinations, delusions, and difficulty with thought organization. Psychosis can be present in schizophrenia, acute mania, depression, drug intoxication, dementia, and delirium, and can be caused by brain trauma. Schizophrenia is one of the most common causes of psychosis.

## SCHIZOPHRENIA

Although many laypeople are quite sophisticated medically, it is not uncommon to hear the word schizophrenia defined as *split personality*. By split personality, people mean something like a Jekyll and Hyde experience or a multiple personality disorder. This popular depiction does not begin to portray schizophrenia. Schizophrenia is not characterized by a changing personality; it is characterized by a deteriorating personality. Therefore, this popular notion of a dramatic personality change comes far short of capturing the devastat-

**Norm's Notes**

*This might be the most important chapter in this book. Well, not really, but schizophrenia is such a devastating disorder—even though it affects just 1% of the adult population, it has ripple effects that have a disproportionate impact on society. These are people that you might walk by (or around) in our cities, not wanting to interact with them at all. They might scare you at times or offend in other ways. After reading this chapter and having a good clinical experience, I think that your attitude about these individuals will change.*

ing effect that schizophrenia has on the life of a person and the person's family. Simply stated, schizophrenia is one of the most profoundly disabling illnesses, mental or physical, that the nurse will ever encounter.

Schizophrenia is a diagnostic term used to describe a major psychotic disorder characterized by disturbances in:

- Perception (e.g., hallucinations)
- Thought processes (e.g., thought derailment)
- Reality testing (e.g., delusions)
- Feeling (e.g., flat or inappropriate affect)
- Behavior (e.g., social withdrawal)
- Attention (e.g., inability to concentrate)
- Motivation (e.g., cannot initiate or persist in goal-directed activities)

Contributing to the overall deterioration is a decline in psychosocial functioning.

Schizophrenia typically first appears in late adolescence or early adulthood. Schizophrenia affects men and women almost equally; however, gender differences do exist. Box 28-1 highlights a

### 12-Month Prevalence Rate of Mental Disorders in the United States*

| Disorders | Approximate Percentage Over 17 Years of Age | Approximate Number of Persons | Gender Overrepresentation |
|---|---|---|---|
| **Anxiety Disorders** | 18 overall | 36,000,000 | |
| Panic disorder | 3.5 | 7,000,000 | Women |
| Social phobia | 7 | 14,000,000 | Women |
| Specific phobia | 8.7 | 17,000,000 | Women |
| GAD | 3 | 6,000,000 | Women |
| PTSD | 3.5 | 7,000,000 | Women |
| OCD | 1 | 2,000,000 | Equal |
| **Mood Disorders** | 9.5 overall | 19,000,000 | |
| Major depression | 6.7 | | Women |
| Dysthymia | 1.5 | | Women |
| Bipolar I and II | 2.6 | | BD I: Equal BD II: Women? |
| **Impulse Control Disorders** | 9 overall | 18,000,000 | |
| Conduct disorders | 1 | 2,000,000 | Men |
| ADHD | 4 | 8,000,000 | Men |
| **Substance Abuse Disorders** | 3.8 overall | 7,600,000 | |
| Alcohol abuse and dependence | 3.1 | 6,200,000 | Men |
| Drug abuse and dependence | 1.4 | 2,800,000 | Men |
| **Schizophrenia** | 1.1 | 2,100,000 | Equal |

*Extrapolated from several sources based on current census data.
*ADHD*, attention-deficit/hyperactivity disorder; *BD*, bipolar disorder; *GAD*, general anxiety disorder; *OCD*, obsessive-compulsive disorder; *PTSD*, posttraumatic stress disorder.
From Kessler RC, Chiu WT, Demler O, Walters EE: Prevalence, severity, and comorbidity of 12-month DSM-IV disorders in the national comorbidity survey replication, *Arch Gen Psychiatry* 62:617, 2005; U.S. Surgeon General: *Mental health: a report from the Surgeon General*, Washington, DC, 1999, Department of Health and Human Services; and National Institute of Mental Health: *Statistics* www.nimh.nih.gov/healthinformation/statisticsmenu.cfm. Accessed on April 18, 2005.

Box 28-1　**Typical Gender-Based Differences in the Expression of Schizophrenia**

Age of onset in men is typically 4-6 years earlier than it is in women.

Men have a more severe course.

Women have more positive symptoms (see later discussion of positive versus negative symptoms).

Estrogen modulates dopamine function and presumably plays a protective role for women.

Box 28-2　**Prenatal and Perinatal Events Associated With Schizophrenia**

Maternal influenza
Birth during late winter or early spring
Obstetric complications
Prenatal exposure to lead
Maternal starvation
Perinatal exposure to cats (i.e., viral zoonosis)

Data from Bachmann S, Schroder J, Bottmer C, et al: Psychopathology in first-episode schizophrenia and antibodies to *Toxoplasma gondii, Psychopathology* 38:87-90, 2005; Opler MG, Brown AS, Graziano J, et al: Prenatal lead exposure, delta-aminolevulinic acid, and schizophrenia, *Environ Health Perspect* 112:548, 2004; and Sadock BJ, Sadock VA: *Synopsis of psychiatry,* ed 9, Philadelphia, 2003, Lippincott Williams & Wilkins.

Box 28-3　**Epidemiology of Schizophrenia**

1. 1% of the population develops schizophrenia.
2. 95% suffer a lifetime.
3. 33% of all homeless Americans suffer from schizophrenia.
4. 50% experience serious side effects from medications.
5. 10% kill themselves.

Modified from News in mental health nursing, *J Psychosoc Nurs* 35:6, 1997; and American Psychiatric Association: Practice guidelines for the treatment of patients with schizophrenia, *Am J Psychiatry* 154(Suppl 4):1, 1997.

Box 28-4　**Bleuler's Four A's**

**Affective disturbance.** Inappropriate, blunted, or flattened affect
**Autism.** Preoccupation with the self, with little concern for external reality
**Associative looseness.** The stringing together of unrelated topics
**Ambivalence.** Simultaneous opposite feelings

few of those gender differences in expression of this disorder.

Studies have shown that approximately 1% of the population will experience schizophrenia during their lifetime. Although the prevalence rate and symptom presentation for schizophrenia are fairly constant worldwide, inner city residents, those from lower socioeconomic classes, and individuals who experience prenatal difficulties (Box 28-2) (Bachmann et al, 2005; Opler et al, 2004; Sadock and Sadock, 2003) are more likely to be affected (American Psychiatric Association [APA], 2001). Economic costs are in the tens of billions of dollars each year. The cost in human suffering is incalculable. Box 28-3 outlines the statistical epidemiologic realities of schizophrenia.

Morel was the first to name the psychiatric symptoms of schizophrenia. In 1860, while treating an adolescent boy, Morel used the phrase *dementia praecox* (precocious senility) to describe the group of symptoms he observed (Kolb and Brodie, 1982). Kahlbaum (in 1871) and Hecker (in 1874) added to the diagnostic nomenclature with their categories *catatonia* and *hebephrenia* (Kaplan and Saddock, 1995). In 1878, Kraepelin added the term *paranoia* and engaged in a rigorous study of what is now called *schizophrenia*. Kraepelin found commonalities among these three mental disorders (catatonia, hebephrenia, and paranoia) and, in 1899, grouped them under the diagnostic term that Morel had coined 40 years before, dementia praecox (Kaplan and Saddock, 1995). Kraepelin believed that schizophrenia was the result of neuropathologic factors; he envisioned a progressive deteriorating course, resulting in disabling mental impairment with little hope of recovery.

It was left to Bleuler in the early 1900s to coin the term schizophrenia in a book subtitled *The Group of Schizophrenias.* Bleuler believed that schizophrenia does not always follow a course of deterioration (thus, dementia was inappropriate), nor does it always occur early in life (hence, praecox was inappropriate). Bleuler broadened Kraepelin's concept by focusing on symptoms, and identified four primary symptoms that he believed were present in all individuals with schizophrenia. All these classic symptoms begin with the letter "A," which facilitates memorization (Box 28-4).

These two giants of psychiatric history founded two divergent views of schizophrenia. Kraepelin, in using the diagnostic category of dementia praecox, revealed a conceptual alignment between schizophrenia and disorders such as Alzheimer's disease, which have a less optimistic prognosis. Bleuler, on the other hand, developed a school of thought that was much broader and more optimistic than that of Kraepelin. Based on Bleuler's wider grouping, pessimism eased, and some clinicians began to see improvements in their patients. Although Kraepelin based his views on biology, Bleuler, influenced by the master analyst Freud and other psychodynamic theorists, sought psychological explanations for schizophrenia. For most of the twentieth century, Freud's psychoanalytic explanations and, by extension, Bleuler's thinking, dominated the understanding of schizophrenia. However, as the limitations of talking cures became more evident, the psychodynamic approach began to lose its grip on mental health professionals. In the past 20 years or so, a resurgence of interest in biologic research has resulted in renewed respect for Kraepelin's work.

## COURSE OF ILLNESS

Schizophrenia typically first occurs in adolescence or early adulthood, a time during which brain maturation is almost complete. There are three overlapping phases of the disorder:

- *Acute phase.* The patient experiences severe psychotic symptoms.
- *Stabilizing phase.* The patient is getting better.
- *Stable phase.* In this phase, the patient might still experience hallucinations and delusions, but the hallucinations and delusions are not as severe nor as disabling as they were during the acute phase.

Most patients alternate between acute and stable phases.

---

CLINICAL EXAMPLE of *Stable Phase*

Billy is a 39-year-old man living in a psychiatric residential facility who attends a day treatment program Monday through Friday. Although Billy experiences hallucinations frequently, most often visual hallucinations, he is indeed stabilized. All staff members agree that Billy is not a danger to himself or others and that the day treatment program is more appropriate for him than a state hospital would be.

---

CRITICAL THINKING QUESTION    1

Why do you think Kraepelin was so pessimistic about the patients he saw with dementia praecox?

---

**Box 28-5    Evolution of Schizophrenic Subtyping**

| | |
|---|---|
| 1860 | Morel coins the term *dementia praecox.* |
| 1871 | Kahlbaum uses the term *catatonia* to describe patients immobilized by psychological factors. |
| 1874 | Hecker uses the term *hebephrenia* to describe patients with silly, bizarre, and regressed behaviors. |
| 1878 | Kraepelin adds the term *paranoia* to describe highly suspicious patients. He recognizes commonalities among catatonic, hebephrenic, and paranoid individuals. |
| 1899 | Kraepelin groups all three patient categories under the heading *dementia praecox.* |
| 1900s | Bleuler introduces the term *schizophrenia* to describe these mental disorders. He adds the subtype *simple schizophrenia.* |
| 1952 | *DSM-I:* The first attempt to develop a diagnostic manual for nationwide use. *DSM-I* includes nine subtypes. |
| 1968 | *DSM-II:* Developed in an effort to articulate more efficiently a common diagnostic language. *DSM-II* has a total of 11 subtypes. |
| 1980 | *DSM-III:* The authors streamline the diagnostic subtypes to five: disorganized, catatonic, paranoid, undifferentiated, and residual. |
| 1982 | Andreasen and Olsen (1982), Crow (1982), and others suggest a new subtyping approach. They categorize schizophrenia, based on symptoms, into positive (type I) and negative (type II). |
| 1987 | *DSM-III:* Revised; same subtypes. |
| 1994 | *DSM-IV:* Same subtypes as *DSM-III.* |
| 1997 | APA practice guidelines on treating patients with schizophrenia recognize the addition of the subtype "disorganized" to the positive and negative subtyping concept. |
| 2000 | *DSM-IV-TR* is published; same subtypes. |

DSM, *Diagnostic and Statistical Manual of Mental Disorders.*

## *DSM-IV-TR* TERMINOLOGY AND CRITERIA

Since the inception of schizophrenia as a diagnostic entity, attempts have been made to divide it into subtypes. These early attempts resulted in the subtypes catatonic, hebephrenic, and paranoid schizophrenia. As noted in Box 28-5, this early thinking is still reflected in official diagnostic classifications. Currently, the *DSM-IV-TR* identifies five subtypes of schizophrenia: (1) paranoid, (2) disorganized, (3) catatonic, (4) undifferentiated, and (5) residual. Criteria for subtypes, NANDA International nursing diagnoses, and the *DSM-IV-TR* diagnoses related to schizophrenia are found in boxes on pp. 342 and 343.

Although the *DSM-IV-TR* criteria have been thoughtfully deliberated, we find the subtyping approach based on positive versus negative symptoms clinically helpful because it can be predictive of medication response. The student should realize that most patients are not either-or, but have a mixture of positive and negative symptoms.

## POSITIVE VERSUS NEGATIVE SCHIZOPHRENIA

Positive (type I) schizophrenia has a different constellation of symptoms than negative (type II) schizophrenia (Box 28-6). Type I is positive in the sense that symptoms are an embellishment of normal cognition and perception. The symptoms are additional. Positive symptoms are believed to be the result of elevated dopamine levels affecting the limbic areas of the brain.

---

**DSM-IV-TR Criteria   for Schizophrenia**

A. Characteristic symptoms (at least two of the following):
   Delusions
   Hallucinations
   Disorganized speech
   Grossly disorganized or catatonic behavior
   Negative symptoms
B. Social-occupational dysfunction: work, interpersonal, and self-care functioning below the level achieved before onset
C. Duration: continuous signs of the disturbance for at least 6 months
D. Schizoaffective and mood disorders not present and not responsible for the signs and symptoms
E. Not caused by substance abuse or a general medical disorder

Modified from the American Psychiatric Association: *Diagnostic and statistical manual of mental disorders, text revision,* ed 4, Washington, DC, 2000, APA.

---

**DSM-IV-TR Criteria   for Schizophrenia Subtypes**

| | |
|---|---|
| Paranoid | Preoccupation with one or more delusions or frequent auditory hallucinations (content frequently persecutory and/or grandiose) |
| Disorganized | All the following are prominent: disorganized speech, disorganized behavior, flat or inappropriate affect |
| Catatonic | At least two of the following are present:<br>A. Motoric immobility, waxy flexibility, or stupor<br>B. Excessive motor activity (purposeless)<br>C. Extreme negativism or mutism<br>D. Peculiar movements, stereotype of movements, prominent mannerisms, or prominent grimacing<br>E. Echolalia or echopraxia |
| Undifferentiated | Characteristic symptoms (see criteria A) are present, but criteria for paranoid, catatonic, or disorganized subtypes are not met. |
| Residual | A. Characteristic symptoms (see box: *DSM-IV-TR* Criteria for Schizophrenia, criterion A) are no longer present; criteria are unmet for paranoid, catatonic, or disorganized subtypes.<br>B. There is continuing evidence of disturbance, such as the presence of negative symptoms or criteria A symptoms, in an attenuated form (e.g., odd beliefs, unusual perceptual experiences). |

Modified from the American Psychiatric Association: *Diagnostic and statistical manual of mental disorders, text revision,* ed 4, text revision, Washington, DC, 2000, APA.

## DSM-IV-TR and NANDA International Diagnoses Related to Schizophrenia and Other Psychoses

| DSM-IV* | NANDA International† |
|---|---|
| Schizophrenia | Adjustment, impaired |
| Paranoid type | Anxiety |
| Disorganized type | Caregiver role strain |
| Catatonic type | Communication, verbal, impaired |
| Undifferentiated type | Coping, family, compromised |
| Residual type | Coping, family, disabled |
| Schizophreniform disorder | Coping, ineffective |
| Schizoaffective disorder | Identity, personal, disturbed |
| Delusional disorder | Role performance, ineffective |
| Brief psychotic disorder | Self-care deficit, bathing/hygiene |
| Shared psychotic disorder | Self-care deficit, feeding |
| | Self-care deficit, toileting |
| | Self-esteem, situational low |
| | Sensory perception, disturbed (specify) |
| | Social interaction, impaired |
| | Social isolation |
| | Thought processes, disturbed |

*From American Psychiatric Association: *Diagnostic and statistical manual of mental disorders,* ed 4, text revision, Washington, DC, 2000, APA.
†From NANDA International: *NANDA nursing diagnoses: definitions and classifications, 2005-2006,* Philadelphia, 2005, NANDA International.

### CLINICAL EXAMPLE

John is sitting in the dayroom on the psychiatric unit when his eyes begin to dart back and forth, and he becomes increasingly anxious. You ask, "John, are you hearing something that I cannot hear?" "Can't you hear them?" he replies. "They are going to get me." John's auditory hallucination is a positive symptom because it is an exaggeration of a normal perception (he is "hearing" without an auditory stimulus).

Type II is labeled negative because symptoms are essentially an absence or diminution of that which should be—that is, lack of affect, lack of energy, and so on. Type II is related, at least in part, to a hypodopaminergic process. These

### Box 28-6   Positive and Negative Symptoms of Schizophrenia

| Subtype, Prognosis, Onset, and Pathophysiology | Symptoms |
|---|---|
| **Positive or Type I:** | Delusions |
| Prognosis: better | Excitement |
| Onset: acute | Feelings of persecution |
| Pathophysiology: hyperdopaminergia in *mesolimbic* areas | Grandiosity |
| | Hallucinations |
| | Hostility |
| | Ideas of reference |
| | Illusions |
| | Insomnia |
| | Suspiciousness |
| **Negative or Type II:** | Alogia |
| Prognosis: poor | Anergia |
| Onset: chronic | Anhedonia |
| Pathophysiology: hypodopaminergia in *mesocortical* areas | Asocial behavior |
| | Attention deficits |
| | Avolition |
| | Blunted to flattened affect |
| | Communication difficulties |
| | Difficulty with abstractions |
| | Passive social withdrawal |
| | Poor grooming and hygiene |
| | Poverty of speech |

symptoms also can be caused by cortical structural changes. Pathoanatomy consistently mentioned in the literature includes decreased cerebral blood flow (CBF) and increased ventricular brain ratios (VBRs). Decreased frontal blood flow is most pronounced in the dorsolateral prefrontal cortex. Ventricular enlargement can be detected on computed tomography (CT) and magnetic resonance imaging (MRI) with the naked eye. Other pathoanatomic features observed that might contribute to negative symptoms include a modest reduction in brain weight and cerebral atrophy.

### CLINICAL EXAMPLE

Philip Wilson has a long history of mental problems. Mr. Wilson is a patient in the state hospital system. The summary note written by the nursing team leader includes the following observation: "Mr. Wilson is isolative and, for the most part, expressionless. He spends long hours sitting and staring out of the window. Attempts to engage Mr. Wilson in unit activities have not been successful."

An unfortunate side effect of the positive versus negative subtyping approach has been the tendency by a few professionals to be too pessimistic about the prognosis of type II patients. Kopelowicz and Bidder (1992), who cautioned nurses and others against such rash and uninformed thinking, divided negative symptoms into primary and secondary. The secondary symptoms are therapeutically accessible, particularly early in the course of the illness. These symptoms arise from some of the consequences of a schizophrenic diagnosis: medications, hospitalizations, loss of social supports, and a socioeconomic decline. If assessed early, secondary negative symptoms can be arrested.

---

### CLINICAL EXAMPLE

Merritt Burgone is a homeless man with a long history of mental illness. He has not seen his family in many years. Although his family was supportive at one time, they simply grew tired of trying to cope with Mr. Burgone. At this point, even modest improvements in his mental health are compromised by his lack of social support.

---

According to biologic theory, typical antipsychotic drugs (drugs that antagonize primarily dopamine $D_2$ receptors) are likely to be beneficial for positive symptoms because positive schizophrenia is a hyperdopaminergic process. Negative schizophrenia, on the other hand, is thought to be more structurally related and a hypodopaminergic process. Traditional antipsychotics have relatively less effect and might actually cause the negative symptoms to worsen. Accordingly, the more excessive the symptoms are (as in positive schizophrenia), the greater the likelihood of a favorable response to antipsychotics. As was noted in Chapter 18, atypical antipsychotic drugs such as clozapine (Clozaril), risperidone (Risperdal), olanzapine (Zyprexa), quetiapine (Seroquel), ziprasidone (Geodon), and aripiprazole (Abilify) benefit negative symptoms because they affect dopamine receptors and antagonize serotonin 5-HT$_2$ receptors, which liberate dopamine in cortical areas. The latter corrects the hypodopaminergic state. Unfortunately, most of these newer drugs are so expensive that some health maintenance organizations (HMOs) and governments are refusing to pay for them. For example, a 30-day supply of Zyprexa costs $350 or more, whereas the same amount of Haldol costs only a few dollars.

## BEHAVIOR

People who are treated for mental problems come to the attention of mental health professionals in one of two ways. The first is when patients seek help. They do so because they have experienced such troubling subjective symptoms that they want professional intervention. Often, however, professional help is not sought until patients have exhausted self-help aids, friends, and family, leading to the second. The second way in which people come to the attention of the mental health system is by drawing attention to themselves through behaviors that bother, concern, or frighten other people. These indicators of a mental disorder are apparent to others and are called *objective signs*. As discussed in the chapter on legal issues (Chapter 5), help is sometimes resisted, and the person must be treated on an involuntary basis.

Subjective and objective categories are not as discrete as they might appear at first. Hallucinations, for example, are subjective phenomena but might easily cause objective signs that get the attention of others (e.g., a person who talks back to an auditory hallucination). Nonetheless, dividing the expressions of schizophrenia into subjective symptoms and objective signs is a rational and convenient approach for understanding this mental disorder.

Six significant alterations occur in schizophrenia and can be grouped into objective signs or subjective symptoms (Box 28-7). Alterations in personal relationships and alterations of activity are highly visible to others (objective signs), whereas altered perception, alterations of thought, altered consciousness, and alterations of affect are more subjective in nature.

### Objective Signs

#### Alterations in Personal Relationships

Patients with schizophrenia have troubled interpersonal relationships. Often, these problems develop over a long period, well before schizophrenia is diagnosed, and become more pronounced as the illness progresses. It is not uncommon to hear that a person was asocial, a loner, or a social misfit before being diagnosed.

Frequently, patients become less concerned with their appearance and might not bathe without

---

## Box 28-7   Objective and Subjective Behavioral Disorders in Schizophrenia

### Objective Signs

**Alterations in Personal Relationships**
- Decreased attention to appearance and social amenities related to introspection and autism
- Inadequate or inappropriate communication
- Hostility
- Withdrawal

**Alterations of Activity**
- Psychomotor agitation
- Catatonic rigidity
- Echopraxia (repetitive movements)
- Stereotypy (repetitive acts or words)

### Subjective Symptoms

**Altered Perception**
- Hallucinations
- Illusions
- Paranoid thinking

**Alterations of Thought**
- Loose associations
- Retardation
- Blocking
- Autism
- Ambivalence
- Delusions
- Poverty of speech
- Ideas of reference
- Mutism

**Altered Consciousness**
- Confusion
- Incoherent speech
- Clouding
- Sense of "going crazy"

**Alterations of Affect**
- Inappropriate, blunted, flattened, or labile affect
- Apathy
- Ambivalence
- Overreaction
- Anhedonia

---

chomotor agitation); that is, they are unable to sit still and continually pace, or they might be inactive or catatonic. These signs respond to antipsychotic drugs but can also be caused by them. The following example illustrates this point.

### CLINICAL EXAMPLE

The nurse must be careful in assessing alterations in activity. Restlessness might be caused by akathisia (an extrapyramidal side effect [EPSE] of antipsychotic drugs) or might be a manifestation of schizophrenia. Rigidity, on the other hand, might be a warning sign of neuroleptic malignant syndrome (NMS), not catatonia. Both EPSEs and NMS are side effects of antipsychotic drugs. Hence, accurate assessment is critical; although it is appropriate to administer an as-needed (prn) dose of haloperidol for psychomotor agitation or catatonia, it only serves to intensify akathisia and might prove fatal for patients with NMS.

### Subjective Symptoms

Subjective symptoms are, by definition, experienced by patients in a personal way. Patients might hide these symptoms from others. For example, if patients suffer from the delusion that they are a famous person, they might be able to keep it to themselves. In fact, some clinicians advise patients who resist psychiatric care to "keep your symptoms to yourself, and no one will ever know." Presumably, there are individuals in society who are not reporting their subjective symptoms to anyone and thus are avoiding psychiatric intervention. For the most part, however, subjective symptoms of schizophrenia spill over into behavior in public view. Subjective symptoms can be grouped into four categories.

#### Altered Perception

Altered perception includes hallucinations, illusions, and paranoid thinking. Hallucinations are false sensory perceptions and can be auditory, visual, olfactory, tactile, gustatory, or somatic (strange body sensations). Auditory hallucinations are the most common in schizophrenia and often take the form of accusations ("You slut," "Hey, queer") or commands ("Get away from these people"). Visual hallucinations are not as common in schizophrenia as are auditory hallucinations.

persistent prodding. Table manners and other social skills might diminish to the point at which patients are disgusting to others. These behaviors are related to introspection (autism) and apathy. Patients are focused on internal processes to the extent that their external social world collapses. Schizophrenia can cause a diminished energy level (anergia), which also complicates social interactions.

Interpersonal communication becomes inadequate and might be inappropriate. Again, internal processes are at work. Hostility, a somewhat common theme, also distances patients from others. Finally, patients with schizophrenia withdraw, further compromising their ability to engage in meaningful social interactions.

### Alterations of Activity

Patients with schizophrenia also display alterations of activity. Patients might be too active (psy-

(The nurse might suspect a toxic process such as drugs or fever if visual hallucinations are present.) Hallucinations are probably caused by a hyper-dopaminergic state in the limbic areas.

Illusions are misinterpretations of real external stimuli. For example, a tree might be mistaken for a threatening person. Illusions are often associated with physical illness, as well as schizophrenia.

---

CLINICAL EXAMPLE

Delirium: While lying in bed with a low-grade fever, Gladys, a 68-year-old woman, asks, "Are those cobwebs on the wall?" Her son responds, "No, Mama, those are just shadows from your bedside lamp." Gladys laughs and says, "I guess my mind is going."

---

CLINICAL EXAMPLE

Schizophrenia: Tim, a patient in a day treatment program, mistakes a tennis shoe on the porch for a rat.

---

Paranoid thinking is characterized by a persistent interpretation of the actions of others as threatening or demeaning. Paranoid themes can color delusions and hallucinations, as well as the ordinary behavior of others. It is important for the student to differentiate paranoid thinking associated with a paranoid personality disorder from paranoid delusions. Paranoid thinking is less severe than paranoid delusions. Paranoid thinking might be corrected with facts, whereas paranoid delusions cannot.

---

CLINICAL EXAMPLE

Paranoid personality: Bill, a voluntary patient on the adult unit, has sought help because of trouble on the job and at home. His ability to get along with people has deteriorated to the point that he has no friends. Bill's wife has started divorce proceedings, and he has sought treatment, hoping that she will change her mind. Over the last few years, Bill has been obsessed with the thought that his wife is cheating on him. He follows her when she leaves the house, sometimes listens to her telephone calls, and has confronted her with accusations of infidelity. Whenever he finds he is mistaken, he is relieved for a while and apologizes for not trusting her, but soon he begins to have the same paranoid thoughts. His paranoid thinking has caused alterations in his personal relationships.

---

CLINICAL EXAMPLE

Paranoid schizophrenia: Fred is a 28-year-old, unemployed laborer. The police recently brought Fred to the emergency department. Fred had been at the downtown bus station preaching loudly to all who passed. He spoke of a conspiracy of blacks and Jews who plan to take over America. Fred tells the emergency room nurse that he feared for his life. He goes on to explain that he had proof that the FBI was behind President Kennedy's assassination.

---

A final example of altered perception is based on the observation that the ability to adapt perceptually (or attend selectively) is altered in patients with schizophrenia.

---

CLINICAL EXAMPLE

A patient is looking out of a seventh-floor window. The nurse approaches to look and notices activity in the yard below. The nurse assumes that the patient is observing the same activity and comments. The patient, however, is not looking beyond the wire mesh screen in the window. He is unable to filter out what for most people would not be a distraction. The inability to filter out extraneous stimuli (ability to attend selectively) is a perceptual problem for some patients.

---

### Alterations of Thought

Alterations of thought are common in schizophrenia and are disturbing and frightening at times. Antipsychotic drugs are often beneficial. Common thought disorders include thought retardation, blocking, autism, ambivalence, loose associations, delusions, poverty of speech, and concrete thinking.

Thought retardation is a slowing of mental activity. A patient might state, "I just can't think."

Blocking is the interruption of a thought and the inability to recall it. This disorder is very disturbing to patients and, at times, frightening. Blocking might be caused by the intrusion of hallucinations, delusions, or emotional factors. The following is a common example of blocking that could happen to anyone.

## CLINICAL EXAMPLE

Joe, a 49-year-old teacher, is in the middle of a lecture when he loses his "train of thought." He cannot remember what point he is developing or where to go next. He stalls for time, realizing that he is in a potentially embarrassing situation. Finally, he finds his notes and proceeds, a little shaken and distracted but able to continue.

Autism occurs when patients are introspective to the extent that they are distracted from external events. Patients are preoccupied with themselves and might be oblivious to the reality around them, which results in a personalized view of reality.

Ambivalence is a state in which two opposite, strong feelings exist simultaneously. Patients might be both attracted to and repelled by a person, object, or goal. Ambivalence (e.g., love-hate) toward a domineering parent is common. Another common example is the simultaneous need for and fear of people, resulting in immobilization. Schizophrenic patients might be immobilized by their ambivalence regarding a matter as simple as deciding whether to drink orange juice or apple juice for breakfast. In these cases, it is therapeutic for the nurse to make decisions for patients, if patients will allow this. The following clinical example illustrates ambivalence that occurs in some families, and is not meant to depict schizophrenic ambivalence.

## CLINICAL EXAMPLE

Joyce, a 38-year-old librarian, has ambivalent feelings toward her father. He still tells her what to do, and she has a hard time standing up for herself. Joyce realizes that her periodic need for financial assistance is partially responsible for her predicament. Joyce also finds that she avoids calling her father and, because he calls her excessively to find out what she is doing, she cringes when the telephone rings. Although Joyce is not suffering from schizophrenia, she does experience ambivalence. She loves her father but, in her words, "He is driving me crazy."

Loose association is a pattern of speech in which a person's ideas slip off one track onto another that is completely unrelated or only slightly related. An occasional change of topic without obvious connection does not indicate loose associations.

### Example of Loose Associations

The following example of loose associations is based on a conversation with Bill, a 46-year-old patient attending day treatment. Because of the severity of his disorder, he was admitted to a state hospital shortly after this interaction.

Nurse: "How are you doing today, Bill?"

Bill: "Do it. Get it on with monster woman. Do it. Sure Bill sure. Do it. Prevented. There goes the doctor. Kills a woman to have a baby. Fish woman. Purple bologna. That was good. Was that a 38, 25, or 44-45 magnum? White hair. A pig. Ham social security. USDA. USGI grocery store. Paycheck. Money. Funny. Money. Meat. Charles Atlas. Arnold. Hercules. Destroyed Bill. Destroyed Charles Atlas. Charley. Charles Manson. Manchild Part I of Bill. Charley Manson Bill. Helter Skelter. White people. Bride of Frankenstein blood drinkers."

As is readily apparent, Bill's communication pattern at this time is incoherent. With a struggle, one can see some of the underlying connections of these disconnected words and phrases but, overall, Bill's dialogue cannot be followed.

Delusions are fixed, false beliefs and can take many forms. Delusions are described as fixed beliefs because they cannot be changed by logical persuasion. Delusions are described as false because they are not based in reality. Delusional content often relates to life experiences and can include somatic, grandiose, religious, nihilistic, referential, and paranoid content. An example of each type follows:

- *Somatic delusions.* A patient, after medical tests confirm otherwise, still insists, "I have cancer in my stomach."
- *Grandiose delusions.* A patient states, "I am the President."
- *Religious delusions.* A woman attempts to kill her children because she believes the devil wants her to do so: "The devil told me to kill my children."
- *Nihilistic delusions.* A patient states, "I am dead." In response to saying, "If you are dead, how can you talk?" the patient says, "I don't know, but I'm dead."

- *Delusions of reference.* "The TV is talking about me. The guests on *Oprah* are making fun of me."
- *Delusions of influence.* "I can control her with my thoughts."
- *Paranoid delusions.* "They all think that I am a homosexual."

Related phenomena sometimes encountered are the schizophrenic delusions that thoughts can be inserted or withdrawn by others: "Other people can read my mind"; "My thoughts are being broadcast so that everyone can hear."

Poverty of speech is manifested by the inability to formulate and articulate thoughts that are relevant to the discussion at hand. Vocabulary is markedly limited in individuals who experience poverty of speech.

Concrete thinking is the inability to conceptualize the meanings of words and phrases. For example, a concrete response to the proverb "People who live in glass houses should not throw stones" might be construed as "The glass would break." These individuals are likely to misinterpret jokes or similes. For example, the meaning of "a diamond in the rough" or "cool as a cucumber" might be lost completely on a person exhibiting concrete thinking.

### Altered Consciousness

Altered consciousness is perhaps the symptom that is most troubling to patients; fortunately, it is also the most responsive to antipsychotic drugs. Manifestations of altered consciousness include confusion, incoherent speech, clouding, and a sense of going crazy. The last manifestation of altered consciousness, going crazy, deserves special mention. Many students are surprised when they enter a psychiatric facility to find that patients are not crazy. In fact, although psychiatric patients are, by definition, struggling with mental disorders, psychiatric units are not wild, bizarre environments. Patients can readily differentiate between the normal struggle of dealing with a mental disorder and the feeling of going crazy (loss of control). The student will observe that patients on the psychiatric unit define a fellow patient who has become wild or who is loudly talking to himself or herself as crazy. In other words, this behavior is unusual—even on a psychiatric unit. Referring to the discussion of incompetence in Chapter 5,

the student can appreciate why the designation of incompetence is reserved for only a few individuals.

### Alterations of Affect

Alterations of affect are varied and include inappropriate, flattened, blunted, or labile affects; apathy; ambivalence; and overreaction. For example, responding to bad news with laughter is an affective response that does not match the circumstances and is inappropriate. If a patient is unable to generate much affect, and the response to the bad news is weakly appropriate, the affect is blunted or dull. The inability to generate any affective response is referred to as flattened affect. Labile affect is a condition in which emotional tone changes quickly. A patient might be telling a happy story, suddenly begin to cry, and then quickly return to a happy disposition.

Apathy, which can be defined as a lack of concern or interest, is the inability to generate a normal response to people, situations, or the environment.

Another alteration of affect is the tendency to overreact to events. An analogy is the small child who must put so much energy into closing a car door that the door slams shut, offending the ears and nerves of adults nearby. Because of physical limitations, the child has to push as hard as possible to overcome inertia. Because of emotional limitations, schizophrenic patients overreact to normal events to overcome mental and social inertia and, like the child, these patients might offend the sensitivities of those nearby.

## ETIOLOGY

Many authorities suggest that multiple factors must cause schizophrenia, because no single theory satisfactorily explains the disorder. Explanations can be categorized broadly into biologic or psychological (psychodynamic) causes. These two categories parallel the nature versus nurture debate discussed in Chapter 27. Biologic theories and psychodynamic theories are discussed here, followed by a vulnerability-stress model, an eclectic approach that seems to describe the major forces at work in the genesis and outcomes of schizophrenia.

## Biologic Theories: Biochemical, Neurostructural, Genetic, and Perinatal Factors

*People don't cause schizophrenia, they merely blame each other for doing so.*
        E. Fuller Torrey (British Columbia Schizophrenia
                        Society [BCSS], 2006).

Biologic theorists posit that schizophrenia is caused by anatomic or physiologic abnormalities. Biologic explanations include biochemical, neurostructural, genetic, and perinatal risk factors, and other theories. Biologic explanations have driven the development of biologic interventions, such as psychotropic drugs.

Some clinicians have been reluctant to endorse biologic theories because the exclusive use of biologic approaches, such as psychotropic drugs, excludes interpersonal factors. The psychotherapeutic management model, however, recognizes the importance of both biologic and interpersonal interventions.

A positive result of biologic theories has been the minimization of the blaming that is inherent in other explanations. Just as viewing alcoholism as an illness has helped clinicians, families, and patients to get beyond blaming and on to treatment, biologic theories have facilitated the treatment of schizophrenia. To illustrate, just as diabetic patients must learn to cope with illness (e.g., change in lifestyle), psychiatric patients must learn to cope with the limitations of their illness.

### Biochemical Theories

Biochemical theory can be traced to 1952, when Delay and Deniker reported the antipsychotic effects of chlorpromazine. Andreasen and Olsen (1982), Crow (1982), and others have postulated that a biochemical process accounts for the positive symptoms of schizophrenia. The prevailing biochemical explanation is referred to as the *dopamine hypothesis*. According to this hypothesis, excessive dopaminergic activity in limbic areas causes acute positive (type I) symptoms of schizophrenia (hallucinations, delusions, and thought disorders). Excessive dopamine might be a result of increased dopamine synthesis, increased dopamine release, or an increase in the number and activity of dopamine receptors. It is also known that drugs that increase dopamine, such as levodopa and the amphetamines, can cause

a psychotic state (see box: Cigarette Smoking and Schizophrenia). This hypothesis is attractive because it is easy to grasp, and because drugs that block dopamine seem to be extremely effective in the treatment of schizophrenia. However, these drugs take days, weeks, or even months to establish their clinical effectiveness, whereas the central nervous system (CNS) dopamine receptors are blocked within a few minutes. Therefore, it seems that the dopamine hypothesis is too simplistic and that other factors are involved in explaining the effectiveness of antipsychotic drugs.

---

### Cigarette Smoking and Schizophrenia

People with schizophrenia tend to smoke a lot. Although approximately 25% to 30% of the general public smokes, studies have indicated that up to three times as many individuals with schizophrenia smoke (Esterberg and Compton, 2005). The difference in cigarette use between this population and the general population is significant, but there are noticeably fewer attempts at smoking cessation. Some researchers have argued that to deprive the schizophrenic person of the joys of smoking would be unduly cruel—smoking presumably being one of the few pleasures that they have (Dalack et al, 1998).

The question becomes, "Why do people with schizophrenia smoke so much?"

The answer probably lies in the biochemical changes produced by nicotine. All drugs of abuse, for example, cause changes in brain dopamine levels. Dopamine axons from the ventral tegmental area are afferents through the reward pathway, including the putative pleasure nucleus, the nucleus accumbens. Nicotine increases the release of dopamine in the nucleus accumbens (Addington, 1998). This occurs because nicotinic receptors synapse on dopamine afferents in the reward pathway—that is, nicotine modulates dopamine release (Dalack et al, 1998). Nicotine also modulates dopamine afferents to the prefrontal cortex (mesocortical tract). When coupled with the supposition that negative symptoms are related to a hypodopaminergic process, nicotinic stimulation of dopamine in prefrontal areas might produce a therapeutic effect. In other words, the answer to the question, "Why do patients with schizophrenia smoke so much?" is simply this: it makes them feel better.

The dopamine hypothesis, although limited in explanatory power, continues to have great educational value for the following reasons:

1. Drugs that increase dopamine (i.e., dopaminergics such as levodopa and amphetamine) can cause psychotic symptoms.
2. Drugs that block dopamine (i.e., antipsychotics) alleviate psychotic symptoms.

Other proposed neurotransmitter contributors to schizophrenia include serotonin and glutamate. Serotonin inhibits dopamine synthesis and release; therefore, serotonin antagonists potentially increase dopamine levels. This characteristic is one of the neurophysiologic properties presumed to cause atypical antipsychotics to be effective. These agents are now referred to as serotonin-dopamine antagonists (SDAs) by some clinicians and manufacturers.

Reduced levels of glutamate, a product of the Krebs cycle, have been proposed as a causative factor in schizophrenia as well (Kim et al, 1980). Glutamate contributes to the regulation of $N$-methyl-D-aspartate (NMDA) receptors, receptors necessary for cognitive processes. The street drug phencyclidine (PCP) antagonizes NMDA receptors and can cause a psychotic state. Theories suggest that when NMDA receptors are normalized, schizophrenic symptoms are reduced (Ereshefsky and Lacombe, 1993). Treatment with glutamate has not proven particularly promising at this point.

### Neurostructural Theories

The neurostructural theorists have proposed that schizophrenia, particularly negative (type II) schizophrenia, is a result of pathoanatomy. The three specific neurostructural changes mentioned most often are increased VBRs, brain atrophy, and decreased CBF. CT, MRI, positron emission tomography (PET), and single-photon emission computed tomography (SPECT) are techniques used for visualizing the brain. CT and MRI provide images of brain structure (e.g., for VBRs and brain atrophy). PET and SPECT provide information on both brain structure and brain activity (Nasrallah, 1993).

### Ventricular Brain Ratios

The finding that a significant subgroup of individuals with schizophrenia have enlarged ventri-

---

**Selected Structural Brain Imaging Findings in Schizophrenia**

1. Cerebral ventricular enlargement
2. Smaller cerebral and cranial size
3. Hypoplasia of the medial (limbic) temporal structures, especially the hippocampus

From Nasrallah HA: Neurodevelopmental pathogenesis of schizophrenia, *Psychiatr Clin North Am* 16:269, 1993.

---

cles was first reported by Johnstone and colleagues (1976). Individuals with enlarged ventricles have a poor prognosis and exhibit negative symptoms (Andreasen et al, 1982; Andreasen, 1985; Crow, 1982; Rabins et al, 1987).

Although ventricular enlargement is not peculiar to schizophrenia, anatomic findings are substantially different than those for neurodegenerative disorders, such as Alzheimer's disease. Ventricular enlargement in schizophrenia is not associated with a neurodegenerative process (Bogerts et al, 1993; Casanova et al, 1993; Marsh et al, 1994); that is, one would not necessarily expect to find a gradual increase in ventricular volume over time in a patient with schizophrenia. In the patient with Alzheimer's disease, however, ventricles continue to increase in volume as brain cells die. It must be noted that not all patients with schizophrenia have abnormally enlarged ventricles. About 50% of these patients fall within the range of control or normal subjects (Cannon and Marco, 1994). This overlapping effect has led researchers to study monozygotic twins when one twin suffers from schizophrenia. In documented cases in which the affected twin had ventricles falling within the normal range, pathoanatomic deviance can be demonstrated only when contrasted with the ventricles of the unaffected (i.e., nonschizophrenic) twin. Roberts and colleagues (1993) clearly demonstrated that an otherwise normal-appearing ventricle is in actuality enlarged when compared with the perfect control—the ventricles of the monozygotic twin.

### Brain Atrophy

Over 100 years ago, Alzheimer described brain cell loss in schizophrenia. Anatomic pathology in cortical and subcortical areas has been suggested by brain imaging techniques and confirmed by postmortem examinations of individuals with schizophrenia. Limbic, hippocampal, and thalamic structures; temporal lobes; the amygdala; and the substantia nigra are specific lobes and nuclei found to have undergone neuropathologic changes.

### Cerebral Blood Flow

Individuals with atrophic changes also have decreased cortical blood flow, particularly in the prefrontal cortex, with a consequent decrease in metabolic activity (BCSS, 2006; Berman et al, 1987). Cognitive demands, such as organizing, planning, learning from experience, problem solving, introspection, and critical judgment, are compromised (Berman et al, 1987).

### Genetic Theories

Individuals with schizophrenia seem to inherit a predisposition to the disorder because schizophrenia runs in families (Staal et al, 2000). The relatives of individuals with schizophrenia have a greater incidence of the disorder than chance alone would allow (Schultz and Andreasen, 1999). Although an amazing amount of resources have been directed at finding the genetic cause of schizophrenia, the results are far from specific. In fact, almost every chromosome has been linked to schizophrenia (Williams, 2003). Genetic studies hold great promise but much remains to be discovered about this illness.

The genetic risk for schizophrenia is shown in Box 28-8. Of particular interest to clinicians is the risk associated with having a parent afflicted with schizophrenia. Although the risk reaches 35% if both parents have schizophrenia, this higher incidence alone does not adequately address the debate of nature (genetics) versus nurture (upbringing). For instance, a mentally disordered parent might rear children inadequately to the extent that the children are predisposed to schizophrenia based on the parenting skills, not genetics.

To control the nurture variable, researchers have studied twins, both monozygotic (identical) and dizygotic (fraternal) twins. Monozygotic twins have consistently shown a higher concordancy rate (meaning both twins do or do not have symptoms of schizophrenia). Concordancy rates are 50% for monozygotic twins. This rate is 50 times higher than the risk for the general population, and three times higher than the risk for dizygotic twins.

These findings seem to establish the genetic or nature basis of schizophrenia; however, there are still extraneous variables that cannot be explained. For example, many monozygotic twins are dressed alike and often are misidentified; their upbringing might be identical, too. Some argue that it is no wonder that monozygotic twins have a high concordancy rate. Unless researchers can control the environmental variable, the relative impact of nature and nurture cannot be reported with confidence.

To control for the variable of environment, studies have been conducted of monozygotic twins who were separated at birth and reared apart. Monozygotic concordancy rates remained significantly higher in these studies.

---

### CRITICAL THINKING QUESTION    2

Why do people with type I schizophrenia often evolve into type II schizophrenia?

---

### Perinatal Risk Factors

Multiple nongenetic factors influence the development of schizophrenia (McNeil et al, 2000; Rapoport, 2000). Some researchers believe that schizophrenia can be linked to prenatal exposure to influenza, birth during the winter, prenatal exposure to lead, minor malformations developing during early gestation, exposure to viruses from house cats, and complications of pregnancy, particularly during labor and delivery (Andreasen, 1999; McNeil, 1995; Opler et al, 2004; Talan 2001; Torrey and Yolken, 1995). The research about influenza epidemics is far from conclusive,

---

| Box 28-8   Genetic Risk for Schizophrenia | |
|---|---|
| Identical twin affected | 50% |
| Fraternal twin affected | 15% |
| Brother or sister affected | 10% |
| One parent affected | 15% |
| Both parents affected | 35% |
| Second-degree relative affected 2%-3% | |
| No affected relative | 1% |

Modified from Roberts GW, Leigh PN, Weinberger DR: *Neuropsychiatric disorders*, London, 1993, Mosby Europe.

but there is evidence that individuals with schizophrenia are more likely to have been born in the winter months. Research of cohorts conceived during devastating influenza epidemics has revealed a meaningfully higher incidence of schizophrenia in products (i.e., children) of conception during this time. Other researchers have suggested a high incidence of birth trauma and injury among individuals with schizophrenia. These studies suggest a relationship between schizophrenia and birth problems, particularly when adverse events occur during the second trimester of pregnancy (Roberts et al, 1993).

## Psychodynamic Theories

Psychodynamic theories of schizophrenia focus on the individual's responses to life events. The common theme of these theories is the internal reaction to life stressors or conflicts. These explanations include developmental and family theories.

### Developmental Theories of Schizophrenia

During the early part of the twentieth century, two men—Adolph Meyer and Sigmund Freud—held to the significance of developmental psychiatry. They believed that the seeds of mental health and illness are sown in childhood. Freud focused on mental processes, on the unconscious forces that influence individuals. The primary difference between the views of the two men was that Freud focused on fantasy, and Meyer focused on real-life events. An extension of their arguments is that events in early life can cause problems that are as severe as schizophrenia. Freudian concepts are still used meaningfully in discussions of schizophrenia. These include poor ego boundaries, fragile ego, ego disintegration, inadequate ego development, superego dominance, regressed or id behavior, love-hate (ambivalent) relationships, and arrested psychosexual development.

Two later developmental theorists whose work more directly explains schizophrenia are Erikson (1968) and Sullivan (1953). Erikson, who theorized an eight-stage model of human development, saw the first step, trust or mistrust, as crucial to later interpersonal relationships. The child who is deprived of a nurturing, loving environment, who is neglected or rejected, is vulnerable to mental disturbances. Inadequate passage through this stage predisposes the person to mis-

trust, isolative behaviors, and other asocial behaviors—the very behaviors found in schizophrenia. Therapeutic intervention focuses on the reestablishment of trust through consistent, anxiety-free relationships.

Sullivan, using different terms, expressed essentially the same ideas. The absence of warm, nurturing attention during the early years blocks the expression of these same affective responses in later years. Without this capacity, a person exhibits disordered social interactions, as well as other disturbances. These individuals learn to avoid interpersonal interactions because these interactions are painful.

### Family Theories of Schizophrenia

Family theories of schizophrenia are linked naturally to developmental theories. If early life experiences are crucial in development, the argument is made that the family—the environment in which most people grow—is significant to the development of mental health or illness. Lack of a loving and nurturing primary caregiver, inconsistent family behaviors, and faulty communication patterns are thought to be responsible for mental problems in later life.

Outdated and harmful theories specifically tailored to the families of schizophrenic individuals were the schizophrenogenic mother theory and the double-bind theory. The word *schizophrenogenic* literally means to cause schizophrenia. Perhaps this definition has been the greatest single disservice of psychodynamic theories. Essentially, this notion states that the blame for schizophrenia can be placed on the mother. The double-bind theory described family practices in which the child was damned if he did and damned if he didn't. An example often used was the child who was expected to do well in school but was criticized for taking time away from the family to study. Acocella (2000) captured some of the ideology behind these assertions:

> Psychoanalysis took a while to conquer the United States, but once it did, after the Second World War, its dominance was unquestioned, and its arrogance breathtaking. Schizophrenia, autism, and numerous other disorders were blamed on the mother, with no evidence, just utter certainty (p 11).

Geiser and associates (1988) noted that family theories were actually blame theories. Families have been viewed as causative agents, saboteurs of treatment, toxic influences, and as patients themselves. Sometimes, families have been treated with hostility and distrust. Because families bear the brunt of preprofessional and postprofessional care of these patients, it is important to work with families without alienating them.

## CLINICAL EXAMPLE

Many of us think back to our childhood and remember birthday parties and games, such as hide and seek and baseball games. Al thinks back to his past and remembers molestation, cruelty, and punishment. Al has been diagnosed with undifferentiated schizophrenia since the age of 20.

Al is the next to youngest of eight children. According to Al, more than half of his siblings suffer from major mental illness. Al states, "My mama had schizophrenia for 10 years, then God saved her." When asked about his relationship with his mother now, Al states that she left the rest of the family after "daddy" died. When questioned about his father, Al speaks of the way his father used to beat his mother and the children. Al recalls seeing his father beat one brother so severely he thought the boy might die. Al further described a beating he received from his father that left him bleeding. When asked why he thought his father beat him, Al responded, "He got mad a lot. I forgot to get firewood like he asked me to."

In discussing his illness, Al was asked to describe when he first started hearing voices. He replies, "When I was little, after those boys did that to me. I was out fixing my bicycle and I heard the devil talk to me over and over." Al reports numerous incidents of abuse during his life. At one point during the interview, Al states his belief that his schizophrenia is God's punishment for what he had done.

Al's first documented psychiatric episode occurred in the early 1980s. In the psychological evaluation emanating from this experience, the psychiatrist noted the presence of hallucinations and delusions; Al described spaceships, command hallucinations, and stated he had killed Christ. His condition deteriorated further and he was committed to a public hospital. During his hospitalization, Al was diagnosed as having undifferentiated schizophrenia.

Today, Al lives in a residential group home and attends day treatment. He continues to manifest both auditory and visual hallucinations. Although prescribed two atypical antipsychotic drugs, symptom control varies from day to day (Keltner et al, 2001).

## Vulnerability-Stress Model of Schizophrenia

It is generally believed by most clinicians and researchers that schizophrenia has multifactorial causes, many susceptibility genes interacting with numerous environmental factors to yield what is called schizophrenia (Keltner, 2005; Siever and Davis, 2004; Uhl and Grow, 2004). Dr. Thomas Insel (2004), Director of the National Institute of Mental Health, referred to it as a "perfect storm" of events. Suspected environmental influences have been previously discussed.

As previously stated, no single theory adequately answers the questions about the genesis of schizophrenia. The vulnerability-stress model addresses the variety of forces that cause schizophrenia in some cases and, in other cases, that cause the broader schizophrenia spectrum problems of schizoaffective disorders and schizophrenia-related personality disorders. This model recognizes that both biologic (including genetic) and psychodynamic predispositions to schizophrenia, when coupled with stressful life events, can precipitate a schizophrenic process. According to this model, people with a predisposition to schizophrenia might (but not always) avoid serious mental disorder if they are protected from the stresses of life. Individuals with a similar vulnerability might succumb to schizophrenia if exposed to stressors. To illustrate the point, a wealthy person might be spared the brunt of some stressors because of wealth, whereas a poor member of society, struggling to meet basic needs, finds confrontation with stressors a daily event. According to this model, the second person is more likely to display symptoms of schizophrenia.

As noted earlier, schizophrenia is overrepresented among poor people. Individuals with schizophrenia tend to drift downward socioeconomically. This unenviable status enhances their vulnerability by exposing them to constant stressors. Box 28-9 lists some of the daily stressors confronted by poor, mentally ill people (Segal and Vander Voort, 1993).

### Student Example

This situation is easily applied to you and your peers. Students who only need to deal with the stress of nursing school have it hard enough. Students who must deal with the stress of nursing school plus significant financial and family respon-

---

**Box 28-9　Daily Stressors for Seriously Mentally Ill Individuals With Few Resources**

Rising cost of common goods
Loneliness
Troubling thoughts about the future
Too much time on hands
Crime
Filling out forms
Not enough money for entertainment
Regrets over past decisions
Inability to express self
Fear of rejection
Trouble with reading, writing, and spelling

Modified from Segal SP, Vander Voort DJ: Daily hassles of persons with severe mental illness, *Hosp Community Psychiatry* 44:276, 1993.

---

**Box 28-10　Key Objectives for Treating Persons With Schizophrenia**

- Work with the family.
- Treat depression.
- Minimize stressful interactions.
- Treat substance abuse.
- Avoid lengthy, intense verbal interactions.

---

sibilities have a heavier load to manage. When a surprise assignment or change in schedule comes along, the student who already has multiple stressors often has a more difficult time adjusting to school demands.

## SPECIAL ISSUES RELATED TO SCHIZOPHRENIA

A number of special issues need to be clarified to help the student focus on the breadth of concerns involved in the psychiatric nursing care of patients with schizophrenia. Box 28-10 lists key objectives when working with patients and families.

### FAMILIES OF SCHIZOPHRENIC INDIVIDUALS

As noted, families have often been blamed for the problems of individuals with schizophrenia. It is no wonder that some families are suspicious of professionals who might view the family as the villain, nor is it any wonder that many of these families have little desire to be studied.

Although research has substantiated the state of turmoil in these families, many clinicians argue that dysfunctional families are not the cause of schizophrenia but, rather, the result of having a family member with this illness. Nevertheless, once a family becomes destabilized, there is a high probability that the dysfunctional family will have a negative effect on the schizophrenic member.

Individuals with schizophrenia can be a disruptive influence on the family, particularly when they are noncompliant with prescribed medications or when they use mind-altering drugs. Although there is consensus that negative features (e.g., emotionally overinvolved, hostile, critical) are present in many families of schizophrenic patients, it should be noted that these families are studied after schizophrenia has been identified—years after the family might have been disrupted by the illness. This observation leads to the chicken or egg question raised previously: do disruptive families cause individuals to have schizophrenia, or do individuals with schizophrenia cause families to become disruptive?

Although blame might be warranted in some family situations, in most cases it is not. Blaming the family leads to a sense of alienation between the family and treatment team. Nurses should remember that families bear the brunt of care outside the hospital. Most discharged psychiatric patients are sent home to live with their families; therefore, the family's stake in the patient's care is obvious. As time goes on, these families tend to become more and more isolated and feel more and more frustrated, helpless, and hopeless, even though they care very much about the patient.

---

**CLINICAL EXAMPLE**

Pete is 24 years old. At age 19, he began having symptoms that eventually led to a diagnosis of schizophrenia. Through several hospitalizations and outpatient treatment programs, he continued to live at home with his parents. Pete started having delusions that people were watching him. His paranoid thinking reached such levels that his presence in the home completely disrupted family life. Pete would barricade himself in his room, believed that his parents were part of a conspiracy to spy on him, and became physically violent on occasion. Two years earlier, after a fourth hospitalization, Pete's parents informed the treatment team that he was no longer welcome in their home. They verbalized fear of Pete and worried about how he was affecting his younger siblings in the home. Although his parents live within 50 miles of Pete, they seldom visit.

## DEPRESSION AND SUICIDE IN SCHIZOPHRENIA

Depressive symptoms are frequently a part of the psychopathology of schizophrenia, and studies, on average, have suggested that 25% or more of schizophrenic patients experience depression (Keck et al, 2000). These symptoms can occur at any time during the illness, including years after the acute phase, but they do respond to antidepressants. A related phenomenon is the high incidence of suicide (10%) among schizophrenic patients (American Psychiatric Association, 1997). Suicide is the leading cause of premature death in schizophrenia. There are three explanations for the high prevalence of depression (American Psychiatric Association, 1997):

1. Depression is a natural part of schizophrenia.
2. Depression is a reaction to schizophrenia.
3. The biologic nature of the disorder (i.e., schizophrenia is more than a dopamine problem) and the drugs used to treat it produce a depressive syndrome.

## COGNITIVE DYSFUNCTION

That patients with schizophrenia suffer cognitive impairment is well established. For example, memory, attention, and executive function are affected (Andreasen, 1999). Research has shown that cognitive deficits are a better predictor of declining abilities to engage in basic activities of daily living than are positive or negative symptoms (Velligan et al, 2000). Because cognitive ability directly influences so many aspects of successful living, it is important to discuss this aspect of schizophrenia. Traditional antipsychotics do not reduce cognitive symptoms and, in fact, might exacerbate them. For example, extrapyramidal side effects (EPSEs) such as akinesia cause cognitive slowdown. Atypical agents are known to improve performance of some aspects of cognitive ability (Velligan et al, 2000).

---

**Box 28-11    Nursing Interventions to Increase Compliance**

- Observe patients for side effects and intervene accordingly. Akathisia is a troubling side effect that patients cannot tolerate.
- When giving tablets or pills, make sure patients do not "cheek" the medications (hide the medication in cheeks or mouth) to spit them out or hoard them for later.
- Teach patients and their families about drugs, including side effects, potential interactions, and dosage schedules when discharged.
- Depot drugs are effective for patients who do not comply with drug therapy.

---

## RELAPSE

Nonadherence to medications and exposure to significant stressors are the most common causes of relapse. Obviously, psychoeducation aimed at these issues is important. Box 28-11 outlines strategies to help patients adhere to their drug regimen.

## STRESS

One of the three inescapable facts noted in the opening paragraph is the role of stress in onset and relapse. According to the vulnerability-stress model, people with schizophrenia are vulnerable to stress. Common stressors can be categorized as:

1. Biologic (e.g., medical illness)
2. Psychosocial (e.g., loss of a relationship)
3. Sociocultural (e.g., homelessness)
4. Emotional (e.g., persistent criticism)

The therapeutic mandate is to minimize the impact of stress on vulnerable individuals. Two basic strategies are used:

1. Reducing stress and stressor accumulation
2. Developing coping skills

Because of their economic and social status, many individuals face major stressors routinely. Stated another way, some of those most vulnerable to stress have more stress to handle. Helping patients learn to identify and avoid stressful events is an important task for the psychiatric nurse.

## SUBSTANCE ABUSE AMONG PEOPLE WITH SCHIZOPHRENIA

Substance abuse is the most common comorbid psychiatric condition associated with schizophrenia and seems to be increasing. A high percentage of people with schizophrenia abuse alcohol or other drugs or both. Alcohol, marijuana, and cocaine account for most of the drugs abused. Unlike the general population, schizophrenic individuals have little chance of using alcohol in a social manner. This abuse might be related to an underdeveloped reward pathway in the brain (Anonymous, 2003).

Drug abuse has a negative effect on the treatment of these patients and is associated with poor outcomes. Once substance abuse begins, the individual is less likely to take medications and accept other treatments, and more likely to become hostile, violent, and suicidal (Anonymous, 2003). It probably accounts for the overrepresentation of schizophrenic individuals who are jailed. Alcohol, for example, causes disinhibition, aggressiveness, and poor judgment. These symptoms are already present in patients with severe mental illness. Furthermore, these very symptoms and related lack of social skills hinder patients with schizophrenia from fully benefiting from treatment programs such as Alcoholics Anonymous and Narcotics Anonymous.

## CRITICAL THINKING QUESTION   3

Why do you think the rate of substance abuse is so high among individuals with schizophrenia?

## WORK

The lack of work, the inability to work, and the lack of a desire to work are all features of schizophrenia. Because work, or what one does for a living, is a major defining characteristic in this society, the fact that many people with schizophrenia do not work adds to their inability to fit in. The major problem confronting these individuals is not so much a lack of skill but an inability to cope on the job socially. Routine behaviors such as joking, inviting someone out, or having insight into the way one is affecting others are the major obstacles to a productive work life for the schizophrenic population.

## PSYCHOSIS-INDUCED POLYDIPSIA

Psychosis-induced polydipsia, or compulsive water drinking (between 4 and 10 L/day), is seen in 6% to 20% of patients with psychosis (American Psy-

chiatric Association, 1997). The desire to drink probably occurs because of thirst and osmotic dysregulation; it is characterized by a compulsive approach to water ingestion. The major concern associated with polydipsia is hyponatremia. Hyponatremia causes lightheadedness, weakness, lethargy, muscle cramps, nausea and vomiting, confusion, convulsions, and coma. Treatment includes frequent weighings, restricted fluid intake, sodium replacement, and positive reinforcement.

## CONTINUUM OF CARE FOR PEOPLE WITH SCHIZOPHRENIA

*Rather than starting to release patients in a few locales and measuring the outcome, officials implemented the policy in cities and counties across the United States virtually simultaneously, based on widespread hope that the new drugs would cure people and the widespread belief in state legislatures that the policy would save taxpayers money.*
E. Fuller Torrey (1997, p B4)

By "policy," Torrey means deinstitutionalization and, driven by this policy, an array of services, or a continuum of care, has developed. Most clinicians agree that a community setting is good for some patients and an institutional setting is better for others. The continuum of care for people with schizophrenia includes the following (American Psychiatric Association, 1997):

- Hospitalization for acute symptoms
- Long-term hospitalization for patients who are treatment-resistant
- Day treatment for patients needing ongoing supportive care as they stabilize
- Supportive housing for individuals who do not or cannot live with their family, but who need some level of supervision; types of supportive housing include:
  - Foster care
  - Board and care home
  - Nursing home

## PSYCHOTHERAPEUTIC MANAGEMENT

*Most schizophrenics go on for years struggling alone without anyone to help them become stronger than their symptoms.*
P.J. Ruocchio (1989, p 188)

Psychotherapeutic management is aimed at helping patients become stronger than their symptoms.

The nursing interventions used in the treatment of patients with schizophrenia are derived from the appropriate development of the nursing care plan.

## PSYCHOTHERAPEUTIC NURSE-PATIENT RELATIONSHIP

*Pharmacotherapy can improve some of the symptoms of schizophrenia but has limited effect on social impairments that characterize the disorder and limit functioning and quality of life.*

*N.A. Huxley and associates (2000, p 187)*

The objective of the psychotherapeutic nurse-patient relationship is to build a therapeutic alliance with patients. A long-term relationship in which trust has developed is probably more significant and therapeutic than a particular theory of care. It is known that insight therapy has limited usefulness with this population, whereas less invasive modalities such as supportive therapy, problem solving, and social skills training that focus on behavior and not meaning are more helpful. Long-term, trusting relationships yield better compliance with medications and better outcomes with psychological resources.

The objective of this section is to provide basic concepts for working with patients with schizophrenia. General principles for developing a therapeutic nurse-patient relationship are presented. In addition, the Key Nursing Interventions for Developing the Therapentic Nurse-Patient Relationship box lists some of these specific principles, as well as some patient comments that the student might encounter. Examples of therapeutic responses by the nurse are also given.

---

**Patient and Family Education**

**Schizophrenia**

*Illness*

Schizophrenia is a brain disease that disrupts perceptions, thinking, feelings, and behaviors. It can cause distortions of reality, false beliefs, hallucinations, and changes in speech patterns, moods, and behaviors. It disrupts the person's ability to function, socialize, and work.

*Medications*

1. Some of the medicines for schizophrenia might cause temporary, but uncomfortable, side effects. Some of these side effects can be lessened with other medications or nondrug interventions, or both.

2. As a result of these side effects, the person might not want to take the prescribed medicines. The doctor needs to know this immediately.

3. It is crucial for the person to continue taking the medicines, even after the person feels better or the symptoms of illness are no longer evident.

**Other Issues**

Discuss early symptoms with the person, which might indicate a beginning relapse. Make an agreement with the person about the actions that family, friends, or both will take to get the person appropriate help.

---

General principles for developing a therapeutic nurse-patient relationship include the following:

- Be calm when talking to patients. *Rationale:* Anxiety is contagious and counterproductive when working with patients who have schizophrenia.
- Accept patients as they are but do not accept all behaviors. *Rationale:* Everyone wants to be accepted. The focus is on behaviors, which communicates very directly that behaviors can change.
- Keep promises. *Rationale:* Dependability builds trust.
- Be consistent. *Rationale:* Consistency increases trust.
- Be honest. *Rationale:* Honesty increases trust.
- Do not reinforce hallucinations or delusions. *Rationale:* The nurse should simply state his or her perception of reality, voice doubt about the patient's perceptions, and move on to discuss real people or events.
- Orient patients to time, person, and place, if indicated. *Rationale:* Orientation reinforces reality. However, use good judgment. To be continually reminded that you are disoriented takes an emotional toll.
- Do not touch patients without warning them. *Rationale:* Patients who are suspicious might perceive a touch as a threat and retaliate.
- Avoid whispering or laughing when patients are unable to hear all of a conversation. *Rationale:* Have you ever wondered whether you were the subject of discussion when you were around people who whisper or giggle? Suspicious patients will interpret these actions as a personal affront.

## Key Nursing Interventions *for Developing the Therapeutic Nurse-Patient Relationship*

The following are specific interventions and examples for developing a therapeutic nurse-patient relationship, including examples of appropriate responses. These examples are meant to illustrate some of the common situations described in the text. Obviously, each patient is unique, and that uniqueness might necessitate a variation of the response suggested below.

| Intervention | Rationales |
|---|---|
| Do not argue about delusions. | Arguing tends to reinforce delusions and can make patients angry. Reflect reality, and attempt to distract patients in a matter-of-fact manner. |
| | *Patient:* The FBI and the Mafia are both after me. |
| | *Nurse:* I know your thoughts seem real to you; however, it does not seem reasonable to me. I also want you to know that you are safe here. Let's go into the dayroom and talk. |
| | Proceed to talk about occupational therapy efforts (or a similar topic) that focus on the patient's real world. |
| Do not reinforce hallucinations. | *Patient:* The voices are calling me terrible names. |
| | *Nurse:* I do not hear anything but your voice and mine. |
| | *Patient's behavior:* Looks around the room, eyes darting to the corners of the room. |
| | *Nurse:* It looks like you might be listening to something. Are you hearing voices? |
| | This effort might lead to identifying and avoiding triggering events. |
| | *Patient:* Nurse, I started hearing the voices last night right after I went to bed. |
| | *Nurse:* Tell me about your evening last night. There might be a link between something that happened and your hearing voices again. |
| Focus on real people and real events. | This helps patients stay in touch with reality. |
| | *Patient:* I keep hearing the voices. |
| | *Nurse:* I understand, but I want to help you focus away from those voices. Let's go to the dayroom and talk. |
| | Proceed to bring patients closer to reality by talking about daily life. |
| Be diligent in attempting to understand patients. | It is therapeutic to help patients communicate what they want to say; however, use good judgment. Pushing too hard to understand can be frustrating for the patient. |
| | *Patient:* I could have been bitten. It was never a dog's day. |
| | *Nurse:* I am not sure what you are saying, but I want to understand. Are you talking about almost being hurt? |
| Attempt to balance siding with inappropriate behavior and crushing a fragile ego. | Time and effort help the nurse learn to negotiate artfully between these potentially negative outcomes. |
| | *Patient:* I am going to hit that bastard if he says another word to me. |
| | *Nurse:* I know you are upset with him. Let's talk about other ways you can deal with this situation. |
| | If a patient is acting odd and the nurse suspects he or she is hallucinating, the patient should be asked about it. |
| | Help patients identify the stressors that might precipitate hallucinations or delusions. |

- Reinforce positive behaviors. *Rationale:* Appropriate reinforcement can increase positive behaviors.
- Avoid competitive activities with some patients. *Rationale:* Competition is threatening and can lead to decreased self-esteem.

- Do not embarrass patients. *Rationale:* Persons with schizophrenia often avoid contacts because they fear embarrassment.
- For withdrawn patients, start with one-to-one interactions. *Rationale:* Even in group situations, it is probably most therapeutic for inter-

actions to be a series of nurse-patient interactions rather than patient-patient interactions. Nurse-patient interactions are less threatening to patients and can evolve into a wider circle of social interaction.

- Allow and encourage verbalization of feelings. *Rationale:* Patients are helped if they can say what they think without the nurse becoming defensive.

## PSYCHOPHARMACOLOGY

Lieberman (1997) has compared the discovery of antipsychotic drugs to the discovery of insulin. Undoubtedly, the development of this class of medications revolutionized mental health treatment. The student is encouraged to review Chapter 18, which provides a complete discussion of antipsychotic drugs.

Schizophrenic patients need to take their antipsychotic drugs as prescribed, but many do not. Box 28-11 lists some strategies to promote compliance. A review of major side effects is found in Box 28-12. (For a full review of these side effects, see Chapter 18.) Because of racial and ethnic variation, Asians and Hispanics with schizophrenia might need a lower dosage of antipsychotic medi-

cations than Caucasians to achieve the same blood levels (U.S. Surgeon General, 1999).

## MILIEU MANAGEMENT

*Thus, intensely active, highly staffed units might be disruptively intense for schizophrenic patients, who more often benefit from decreased stimulation and a greater measure of solitude and clear role models.*
G. Simpson and P. May (1982, p 148)

Milieu management is an important dimension of the psychiatric nursing care of schizophrenic patients. With the dramatic introduction of psychotropic drugs in the 1950s, other forms of treatment were abandoned. Now that psychopharmacologists have had free reign for many years, it is clear that drugs alone are not enough. A therapeutic treatment approach is best developed with all three components of psychotherapeutic management in place.

Therapeutic manipulation of the environment can occur at both the inpatient and outpatient levels and helps patients function better. General principles that specifically address the environment of schizophrenic patients follow.

### For disruptive patients:
- Set limits on disruptive behavior.
- Decrease environmental stimuli. For example, many nurses find that soft or classical music calms an environment, whereas hard rock or rap music creates agitation.
- Frequently observe escalating patients to intervene. Intervention (e.g., medication) before acting out occurs protects patients and others physically and prevents embarrassment for escalating patients.
- Modify the environment to minimize objects that can be used as weapons. Some units use furniture so heavy that it cannot be lifted by most people.
- Be careful in stating what the staff will do if a patient acts out; however, follow through once a violation occurs (e.g., "If you break the window, we will place you in restraints").
- When using restraints, provide for safety by evaluating the patient's status of hydration, nutrition, elimination, and circulation.

### For withdrawn patients:
- Arrange nonthreatening activities that involve these patients in doing something—for example, a walking tour of a park and painting.

**Box 28-12   Review of Major Side Effects of Antipsychotic Drugs**

Dopamine D$_2$ blockade in nigrostriatal tract, causing *EPSEs:*

    Parkinsonism
    Akathisia
    Dystonias
    Neuroleptic malignant syndrome
    Pisa syndrome

Muscarinic blockade in parasympathetic systems, causing *anticholinergic effects:*

    Dry mouth
    Blurred vision
    Constipation
    Urinary hesitation
    Tachycardia

Hypersensitivity to dopamine in nigrostriatal tract, causing *tardive dyskinesia*

Elevated prolactin related to dopamine blockade in tuberoinfundibular tract, causing *amenorrhea, galactorrhea, impotency, and decreased libido*

Histamine blockade, causing *sedation*

Alpha-1 blockade, causing *orthostatic hypotension*

- Arrange furniture in a semicircle or around a table, which forces patients to sit with someone. Interactions are permitted in this situation, but should not be demanded. Sit in silence with patients who are not ready to respond. Some will move the chair away despite the nurse's efforts.
- Help patients to participate in decision making, as appropriate.
- Reinforce appropriate grooming and hygiene.
- Provide psychosocial rehabilitation—that is, training in community living, social skills, and health care skills.

### For suspicious patients:
- Be matter-of-fact when interacting with these patients.
- Staff members should not laugh or whisper around patients unless the patients can hear what is being said. The nurse should clarify any misperceptions that patients have.
- Do not touch suspicious patients without warning. Avoid close physical contact.
- Be consistent in activities (time, staff, approach).
- Maintain eye contact.

### For patients with impaired communication:
- Be patient and do not pressure patients to make sense.
- Do not place patients in group activities that would frustrate them, damage their self-esteem, or overtax their abilities.
- Provide opportunities for purposeful psycho-motor activity.

### For patients with hallucinations:
- Attempt to provide distracting activities.
- Discourage situations in which patients talk to others about their disordered perceptions.
- Monitor television selections. Some programs seem to cause more perceptual problems than others (e.g., horror movies).
- Monitor for command hallucinations that might increase the potential for patients to become dangerous.
- Have staff members available in the dayroom so that patients can talk to real people about real people or real events.

### For disorganized patients:
- Remove disorganized patients to a less stimulating environment.

- Provide a calm environment; the staff should appear calm.
- Provide safe and relatively simple activities for these patients.

---

**CASE STUDY**

The police bring Bill, a 25-year-old man, to the hospital. He was in a downtown bus station preaching loudly. He states in the emergency room that he had spoken to God and that God had told him to save San Francisco. He admits to hearing both God and Satan arguing and is terrified at times. In talking with his family, staff members discover that Bill was a solid student until about a year ago. He began to struggle in school but continued to pass his course work. He dropped out of school 3 months ago. His family believes his problem started when his girlfriend of 4 years broke off their engagement.

Bill began hearing voices a couple of weeks ago, according to his family, but the family lost contact with him until they were notified of this hospitalization. Bill's family is committed to helping him. On admission to the unit, Bill is oriented to time, place, and person, but states: "God has chosen me to be his special angel. I must save the sinners of San Francisco." Bill then stands up and turns his head rapidly from side to side. When asked why, he says: "God and Satan are arguing about what I should do."

(See the nursing care plan for Bill Wilson on p. 362.)

---

## OTHER PSYCHOTIC DISORDERS

In addition to schizophrenia, several other psychotic disorders are described in the *DSM-IV-TR* with which the student should be familiar. Interventions for these disorders are directed at prominent symptoms and are the same as the interventions used for the symptoms of patients with schizophrenia.

### SCHIZOAFFECTIVE DISORDER

Schizoaffective disorder is a psychosis characterized by both affective (mood disorder) and schizophrenic (thought disorder) symptoms, with substantial loss of occupational and social functioning. Because this disorder is a hybrid of two disorders believed to have different biochemical origins, schizoaffective disorder is somewhat of a puzzle to many clinicians. Affective disorders cause people to be extremely depressed or elated, and schizophrenia is expressed as positive, negative, or even disorganized symptoms. The fact that patients with affective disorders can experience positive and negative symptoms, plus the fact that patients with schizophrenia experience mood changes, partially explains the difficulty in diagnosis. The diagnosis of schizoaffective psychosis helps bridge the gap between the affective disorders and schizophrenia.

In this disorder, schizophrenic symptoms are dominant but are accompanied by major depressive or manic symptoms. Patients with schizoaffective disorder will have experienced delusions or hallucinations in the absence of a prominent mood disturbance, but symptoms of a mood disorder are present for a significant period. The prognosis for schizoaffective disorder is better than that for schizophrenia but significantly less optimistic than the prognosis for mood disorders (American Psychiatric Association, 1997).

## CASE STUDY

A 40-year-old woman with a history of multiple admissions is admitted to the floor. Emma Rice was found wandering downtown incoherent and disheveled. During the assessment interview, Emma is noted to have a flat affect and is withdrawn. She reports not seeing her family for 5 years and cannot remember when she last held a job. There is no history of hallucinatory or delusional thought content in this recent occurrence. The staff knows Emma and knows that, during past admissions, she has responded to the less expensive haloperidol. After admission, Emma says, "Let me go. Go on, onward, backward. (pause) Emma hide, died." When asked where she lives, Emma slowly responds, "Over there, somewhere, anywhere, nowhere." Emma's board and care operator knows her well and has indicated that a bed is being held for Emma.

(See the nursing care plan for Emma Rice on p. 363.)

### CLINICAL EXAMPLE

Patty is a 42-year-old Caucasion woman referred to the county mental health department by her sister after Patty had attempted suicide by combining a large number of benzodiazepines with a six-pack of beer. Patty states that most of her "mental" problems began when she became pregnant at age 18. At the time, she was unmarried and alienated from her parents. Patty raised her young daughter, Billie, alone until she eventually married another man. At

age 25, Patty became pregnant again and gave birth to a son. Her husband, an alcoholic, had abused Patty to some extent, but the abusive behavior became more frequent and more severe as Patty entered her early 30s. There had been suspicion that he had sexually abused Billie, but nothing conclusive was documented. Patty and her husband divorced when the boy was 7 years old. The court awarded the child to the husband. Today, Patty has little contact with her daughter, son, ex-husband, or parents. She frequently has auditory hallucinations telling her to kill herself and has nightmares about killing her son and ex-husband. She attends a day treatment program 5 days a week and lives in a one-bedroom apartment alone. Patty is very sad and always looks at the floor. She is consumed with guilt. She does not initiate conversation with others at the day treatment program. She states that she continues to hear voices and thinks about suicide all the time.

## DELUSIONAL DISORDER

People with delusional disorder display symptoms similar to those seen in patients with schizophrenia. However, substantial differences exist and necessitate a diagnostic differentiation. The following symptoms differentiate delusional disorders from schizophrenic disorders:

- Delusions have a basis in reality.
- The patients have never met the criteria for schizophrenia.
- The behavior of these patients is relatively normal except in relation to their delusions.
- If mood episodes have occurred concurrently with delusions, their total duration has been relatively brief.
- The symptoms are NOT the direct result of a substance-induced or medical condition.

## BRIEF PSYCHOTIC DISORDER

The category of brief psychotic disorder includes all psychotic disturbances that last less than 1 month and are not related to a mood disorder, a general medical condition, or a substance-induced disorder (American Psychiatric Association, 2001). At least one of the following psychotic disturbances must be present: delusions, hallucinations,

## Care Plan

Name: Bill Wilson                                          Admission Date: _____

*DSM-IV-TR* Diagnosis: Schizophrenia: undifferentiated type

| | |
|---|---|
| Assessment | **Areas of strength:** Past accomplishments; past good heterosexual interpersonal relationships (IPRs); alert, oriented to time, place, person; acute symptoms respond to medications; family support. |
| | **Problems:** Religious hallucinations, religious delusions, thought disorder; broken engagement; dropped out of school. |
| Diagnoses | • Disturbed sensory perception (auditory) related to thought disturbance, as evidenced by hallucinations. |
| | • Anxiety related to disturbed perceptions, as evidenced by fear and extraneous movements. |

| Outcomes | | Date met |
|---|---|---|
| | *Short-term goals:* | |
| | • Patient will voice freedom from hallucinations. | _____ |
| | • Patient will report lack of fear of others. | _____ |
| | • Patient will discuss feelings about loss of girlfriend. | _____ |
| | *Long-term goals:* | |
| | • Patient will verbalize need for medication and counseling. | _____ |
| | • Patient will make appointment for outpatient program assessment in mid-July. | _____ |
| | • Patient will return to school in September. | _____ |

| | |
|---|---|
| Planning/ Interventions | **Nurse-patient relationship:** Do not reinforce hallucinations and delusions; voice doubt; encourage identification of strengths and accomplishments; encourage expression of feelings about broken engagement; discuss plans for immediate future. |
| | **Psychopharmacology:** Zyprexa 10 mg qd. |
| | **Milieu management:** Provide distracting activities; monitor television, particularly religious programming and movies with satanic themes; encourage participation in self-esteem and anger management groups. |
| Evaluation | Patient responding to Zyprexa. |
| Referrals | Will see Ms. White, RN, CS, once a week as outpatient. Appointment in 3 weeks with R. Jones for education counseling. |

---

disorganized speech, or grossly disorganized or catatonic behavior. The *DSM-IV-TR* cautions against applying these standards to people from a culture in which they are exhibiting acceptable behavior.

## SCHIZOPHRENIFORM DISORDER

Schizophreniform disorder displays symptoms that are typical of schizophrenia and last at least 1 month but no longer than 6 months. This cautious approach spares the individual the lifelong diagnosis of schizophrenia until professionals are absolutely sure of the diagnosis.

### CRITICAL THINKING QUESTION    4

If a first-degree relative of yours suffered from schizophrenia, what behavior might cause you to refuse to live with that person?

### FUTURE DIRECTIONS

An evolving and interesting area of research focuses on early identification and intervention in schizophrenia. The National Institute of Mental Health, the primary source of funding for neuro-

## Care Plan

Name: Emma Rice                                     Admission Date: _____

*DSM-IV-TR* Diagnosis: Schizophrenia, disorganized type

| | |
|---|---|
| Assessment | **Areas of strength:** Board and care operator knows Emma well and wants her back. Staff knows and understands Emma. |
| | **Problems:** Affective flattening, loose associations, withdrawn, chronic course of illness, no family support. |
| Diagnoses | • Impaired verbal communication related to thought disturbance, as evidenced by impaired articulation and loose association of ideas. |
| | • Bathing and hygiene self-care deficit related to thought disturbance, as evidenced by inability to maintain appearance at satisfactory level. |
| | • Social isolation related to lack of trust, as evidenced by absence of supportive significant other. |

Outcomes

*Short-term goals:*                                                          Date met
• Patient will talk in coherent manner.                    _____
• Patient will carry out ADLs.                                   _____
• Patient will participate in nonthreatening activities.  _____
*Long-term goals:*
• Patient will maintain outpatient program.              _____
• Patient will return to board and care.                     _____
• Patient will comply with medication regimen.        _____

| | |
|---|---|
| Planning/ Interventions | **Nurse-patient relationship:** Be patient; treat as adult; encourage hygiene and appropriate dress; reinforce positive social behaviors; start with one-to-one interactions with nurse, and then encourage independent social behaviors. |
| | **Psychopharmacology:** Haldol 5 mg bid PO (concentrate). Might need long-acting form on discharge. |
| | **Milieu management:** Start patient in occupational therapy by the end of the week; invite patient to sit with staff and other patients; encourage her to make decisions about meals or some other simple tasks; provide resocialization group experience and community living education. |
| Evaluation | Patient stabilized on medications. |
| Referrals | Will see Ms. Brown, RN, CS, once a week and will attend outpatient resocialization group five times a week. Board and care operator will monitor drugs and arrange transportation. |

scientific studies of mental illness, has made this a funding priority. It has long been known that early treatment of schizophrenia symptoms results in better outcomes. Similarly, there is some indication that identifying the prodromal manifestations of schizophrenia might alter the course of illness. The ability to offer screening tests such as blood tests, brain imaging, and checking for simple but often overlooked signs such as impaired smell and eye tracking offers the hope of reducing the disabling effects of schizophrenia. Box 28-13 lists some behavioral early warning signs of schizophrenia. If several of these signs are present in a young person, it behooves the nurse, even if just a neighbor, to suggest professional evaluation. As stated, the earlier the better.

### Box 28-13    Early Warning Signs of Schizophrenia

Deterioration of personal hygiene
Depression
Bizarre behavior
Irrational statements
Sleeping excessively or inability to sleep
Social withdrawal, isolation, and reclusiveness
Shift in basic personality
Unexpected hostility
Deterioration of social relationships
Hyperactivity or inactivity, or alternating between the two
Inability to concentrate or to cope with minor problems
Extreme preoccupation with religion or with the occult
Excessive writing without meaning
Indifference
Dropping out of activities or out of life
Decline in academic or athletic interests
Forgetting things
Losing possessions
Extreme reactions to criticisms

From British Columbia Schizophrenia Society: Schizophrenia: Basic facts about schizophrenia, ed 9. Available at www.mentalhealth.com/book/p40-sc02.html. Accessed February 28, 2006.

### Principles of Psychotherapeutic Management

**Nurse-Patient Relationship Principles**
Focus on behavior, not meaning.
A long-term relationship is most therapeutic.
Accept patient but not all behaviors.
Be consistent.
Do not reinforce hallucinations and delusions.
Avoid whispering or laughing if patient cannot hear all of conversation.

**Psychotropic Drugs**

*Traditional Antipsychotics*
Haloperidol (Haldol)
Fluphenazine (Prolixin)
Chlorpromazine (Thorazine)

*Atypical Antipsychotics*
Clozapine (Clozaril)
Risperidone (Risperdal)
Olanzapine (Zyprexa)
Quetiapine (Seroquel)
Ziprasidone (Geodon)
Aripiprazole (Abilify)

**Milieu Management Principles**
Modify environment to decrease stimulation and for safety.
Staff consistency is crucial.
Arrange environment to reduce withdrawn behavior.
Monitor television watching.
Protect patients' self-esteem.

## Study Notes

1. The concept of schizophrenia has evolved over the last 100 years as a result of the contributions of early theorists, such as Kraepelin and Bleuler, and modern theorists, such as Andreasen, Weinberger, and Torrey.

2. The *DSM-IV-TR* identifies five subtypes of schizophrenia: (1) catatonic, (2) disorganized, (3) paranoid, (4) undifferentiated, and (5) residual.

3. Bleuler identified what he thought to be the four primary symptoms of schizophrenia: (1) affective disturbances, (2) loose associations, (3) ambivalence, and (4) autism (also known as Bleuler's four A's).

4. Andreasen (Andreasen and Olsen, 1982), Crow (1982), and others have conceptualized schizophrenia as having only two subtypes: type I (positive symptoms and usually treatable with traditional antipsychotic drugs) and type II (negative symptoms). More recently, some researchers have added the subtype labeled as disorganized.

5. Objective signs of schizophrenia include alterations in personal relationships and activity.

6. Subjective symptoms of schizophrenia include alterations in perception, thought, consciousness, and affect.

7. Causative theories for schizophrenia are numerous and include both biologic theories (dopamine hypothesis, pathoanatomy, and genetic theories) and psychodynamic theories (developmental and family theories).

8. The dopamine hypothesis—that schizophrenia is a result of increased bioavailability of dopamine in the brain—is a widely held theory of the cause of schizophrenia.

9. Antipsychotic drugs block dopamine receptors and relieve acute symptoms of schizophrenia.

10. Nursing interventions include developing a therapeutic nurse-patient relationship. Several general principles underlie the nurse's interactions with patients who have schizophrenia. These principles include being calm, accepting, dependable, consistent, and honest.

11. In addition to these basic principles, several basic interventions are therapeutic for most patients with schizophrenia. These basic interventions include what *the nurse should not do:* do not reinforce hallucinations and delusions, do not touch patients without warning, do not whisper or laugh when patients cannot hear the conversation, do not compete with patients, and do not embarrass patients; and what *the nurse should do:* provide reality testing, assist with orientation when appropriate, reinforce positive behaviors, and encourage verbalization of feelings.

12. Psychopharmacology is an important part of the nurse's role in caring for patients with schizophrenia. Understanding the importance of adherence to the medication regimen is critical.

13. Nurses are typically responsible for the environment. Strategies for working with disruptive, withdrawn, suspicious, and disorganized patients are crucial for developing a therapeutic environment.

14. Other psychoses listed in the *DSM-IV-TR* include schizoaffective disorder, delusional disorder, brief psychotic disorder, and schizophreniform disorder.

## References

Acocella J: The empty couch, *New Yorker* 8:11, 2000.

Addington J: Group treatment for smoking cessation among persons with schizophrenia, *Psychiatr Serv* 49:925, 1998.

American Psychiatric Association: *Diagnostic and statistical manual of mental disorders, text revision,* ed 4, Washington, DC, 2001, APA.

American Psychiatric Association: Practice guidelines for the treatment of patients with schizophrenia, *Am J Psychiatry* 154(Suppl 4):1, 1997.

Andreasen NC: Understanding the causes of schizophrenia, *N Engl J Med* 340:645, 1999.

Andreasen NC: Positive vs. negative schizophrenia: a critical evaluation, *Schizophr Bull* 11:380, 1985.

Andreasen NC, Olsen S: Negative vs. positive schizophrenia, *Arch Gen Psychiatry* 39:789, 1982.

Andreasen NC, Olsen SA, Dennert JW, Smith MR: Ventricular enlargement in schizophrenia: relationship to positive and negative symptoms, *Am J Psychiatry* 139:297, 1982.

Anonymous: Schizophrenia and drug abuse, *Harvard Ment Health Lett* 20:4, 2003.

Bachmann S, Schroder J, Bottmer C, et al: Psychopathology in first-episode schizophrenia and antibodies to *Toxoplasma gondii, Psychopathology* 38:87-90, 2005.

Becker RE: Depression in schizophrenia, *Hosp Community Psychiatry* 39:1269, 1988.

Berman KF, Weinberger DR, Shelton RC, Zec RF: A relationship between anatomical and physiological brain pathology in schizophrenia: lateral cerebral ventricular size predicts cortical blood flow, *Am J Psychiatry* 144:1277, 1987.

Bogerts B, Lieberman JA, Ashtari M, et al: Hippocampus-amygdala volume and psychopathology in chronic schizophrenia, *Biol Psychiatry* 33:236, 1993.

British Columbia Schizophrenia Society: *Schizophrenia: Basic facts about schizophrenia,* ed 9. Available at www.mentalhealth.com/book/p40-sc02.html. Accessed February 28, 2006.

Cannon TD, Marco E: Structural brain abnormalities as indicators of vulnerability to schizophrenia, *Schizophr Bull* 20:89, 1994.

Casanova MF Carosella NW, Gold JM, et al: A topographical study of senile plaques and neurofibrillary tangles in the hippocampi of patients with Alzheimer's disease and cognitively impaired patients with schizophrenia, *Psychiatry Res* 49:41, 1993.

Crow TJ: Two dimensions of pathology in schizophrenia: dopaminergic and nondopaminergic, *Psychopharmacol Bull* 18:22, 1982.

Dalack GW, Healy DJ, Meador-Woodruff JH: Nicotine dependence in schizophrenia: clinical phenomena and laboratory findings, *Am J Psychiatry* 155:1490, 1998.

Ereshefsky L, Lacombe S: Pharmacological profile of risperidone, *Can J Psychiatry* 38(Suppl 3):S80, 1993.

Erikson E: *Childhood and society,* New York, 1968, WW Norton.

Esterberg ML, Compton MT: Smoking behavior in persons with schizophrenia-spectrum disorder: a qualitative investigation of the transtheoretical model, *Soc Sci Med* 61:293, 2005.

Geiser R, Hoche L, King J: Respite care for the mentally ill patients and their families, *Hosp Community Psychiatry* 39:291, 1988.

Hughes JR, Hatsukami DK, Mitchell JE, Dahlgren LA: Prevalence of smoking among psychiatric outpatients, *Am J Psychiatry* 143:993, 1986.

Huxley NA, Rendall M, Sederer L: Psychosocial treatments in schizophrenia: a review of the past 20 years, *J Nerv Ment Dis* 199:187, 2000.

Insel T: Lecture: Presented at the Summer Genetics Institute, National Institutes of Health, July, 2004.

Johnstone EC, Crow TJ, Frith CD, et al: Cerebral ventricular size and cognitive impairment in chronic schizophrenia, *Lancet* 2:924, 1976.

Kaplan HI, Saddock BJ: *Comprehensive textbook of psychiatry/IV,* ed 6, Baltimore, 1995, Williams & Wilkins.

Keck PE, Strakowski SM, McElroy SL: The efficacy of atypical antipsychotics in the treatment of depressive symptoms, hostility, and suicidality in patients with schizophrenia, *J Clin Psychiatry* 61(Suppl 3):4, 2000.

Keltner NL: Genomic influences on schizophrenia-related neurotransmitter systems, *J Nurs Scholarship* 37:322, 2005.

Keltner NL, James CA, Darling RJ, et al: Nature vs nurture: two brothers with schizophrenia, *Perspect Psychiatr Care* 37:88, 2001.

Kim JS, Kornhuber HH, Schmid-Burgk W, Holzmuller B: Low cerebrospinal fluid glutamate in schizophrenia patients and a new hypothesis on schizophrenia, *Neurosci Lett* 20:379, 1980.

Kolb LC, Brodie HKH: *Modern clinical psychiatry,* Philadelphia, 1982, WB Saunders.

Kopelowicz A, Bidder TG: Dementia praecox: inescapable fate or psychiatric oversight? *Hosp Community Psychiatry* 43:940, 1992.

Lieberman JA: Atypical antipsychotic drugs: the next generation of therapy, *Decade Brain* 8:1, 1997.

Marsh L, Suddath RL, Higgins N, Weinberger DR: Medial temporal lobe structure in schizophrenia: relationship of size to duration of illness, *Schizophr Bull* 11:225, 1994.

McNeil TF: Perinatal risk factors and schizophrenia: selective review and methodological concerns, *Epidemiol Rev* 17:107, 1995.

McNeil TF, Cantor-Graae E, Weinberger DR: Relationship of obstetric complications and differences in size of brain structures in monozygotic twin pairs discordant for schizophrenia, *Am J Psychiatry* 157:203, 2000.

Nasrallah HA: Neurodevelopmental pathogenesis of schizophrenia, *Psychiatr Clin North Am* 16:269, 1993.

NANDA International: *NANDA nursing diagnoses: definitions and classifications, 2005-2006,* Philadelphia, 2005, NANDA.

Opler MG, Brown AS, Graziano J, et al: Prenatal lead exposure, delta-aminolevulinic acid, and schizophrenia, *Environ Health Perspect* 112:548, 2004.

Rabins P, Pearlson G, Jayaram G, et al: Increased ventricle-to-brain ratio in late-onset schizophrenia, *Am J Psychiatry* 144:1216, 1987.

Rapoport JL: The development of neurodevelopmental psychiatry, *Am J Psychiatry* 157:159, 2000.

Roberts GW, Leigh PN, Weinberger DR: *Neuropsychiatric disorders,* London, 1993, Mosby Europe.

Ruocchio PJ: How psychotherapy can help the schizophrenic patient, *Hosp Community Psychiatry* 40:188, 1989.

Sadock BJ, Sadock VA: *Synopsis of psychiatry,* ed 9, Philadelphia, 2003, Lippincott Williams & Wilkins

Schultz SK, Andreasen NC: Schizophrenia, *Lancet* 353:1425, 1999.

Segal SP, Vander Voort DJ: Daily hassles of persons with severe mental illness, *Hosp Community Psychiatry* 44:276, 1993.

Siever LJ, Davis KL: The pathophysiology of schizophrenia disorders: perspectives from the spectrum, *Am J Psychiatry* 161:398, 2004.

Simpson G, Might P: Schizophrenic disorders. In Greist J, Jefferson J, Spitzer R, editors: *Treatment of mental disorders,* New York, 1982, Oxford University Press.

Staal WG, Hulshoff Pol HE, Schnack HG, et al: Structural brain abnormalities in patients with schizophrenia and their healthy siblings, *Am J Psychiatry* 157:416, 2000.

Sullivan HS: *The interpersonal theory of psychiatry,* New York, 1953, WW Norton.

Talan J: Schizophrenia fight leads experts to a retrovirus, *The Brain in the News,* January-May (Special Issue):1, 2001.

Torrey EF: The release of the mentally ill from institutions: a well-intentioned disaster, *Chron High Educ* 43:B4, 1997.

Torrey EF, Yolken RH: Could schizophrenia be a viral zoonosis transmitted from house cats? *Schizophr Bull* 21:167, 1995.

Uhl GR, Grow RW: The burden of complex genetics in brain disorders, *Arch Gen Psychiatry* 61:223, 2004.

U.S. Surgeon General: *Mental health: a report of the Surgeon General,* Washington, DC, 1999, Department of Health and Human Services.

Velligan DI, Bow-Thomas CC, Huntzinger C, et al: Randomized controlled trial of the use of compensatory strategies to enhance adaptive function in outpatients with schizophrenia, *Am J Psychiatry* 157:1317, 2000.

Weinberger DR: Implications of normal brain development for the pathogenesis of schizophrenia, *Arch Gen Psychiatry* 44:660, 1987.

Williams M: Genome-based drug discovery: prioritizing disease-susceptibility/disease-associated genes as novel drug targets for schizophrenia, *Curr Opin Invest Drugs* 41:31, 2003.

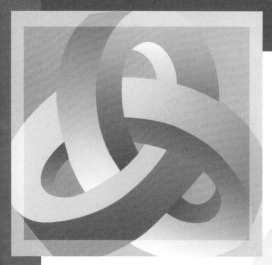

# Chapter 29

# Depression

*Norman L. Keltner*

## Learning Objectives

*After reading this chapter, you should be able to:*

- Recognize the *Diagnostic and Statistical Manual of Mental Disorders,* text revision, fourth edition *(DSM-IV-TR)* criteria and terminology for depressive disorders.
- Compare and contrast major depressive disorder and dysthymic disorder.
- Describe the biologic and psychodynamic explanations for depressive disorders.
- Describe effective nursing interventions for depressed patients.
- Recognize warning signs of suicide.
- Describe interventions to prevent suicide.
- Describe the family issues related to this disorder.

Two major types of depressive disorders are recognized by the American Psychiatric Association (APA): major depressive disorder and dysthymic disorder. However, in reality, it might be more accurate to think in terms of many depressions. The ability to recognize underlying pathologies is growing, and with these advancements come more precise understanding of the variability among depressive disorders. Major depressive disorder and dysthymia are defined as follows.

*Major depressive disorder* is characterized by one or more major depressive episodes, which are defined as at least 2 weeks of depressed mood or loss of interest accompanied by at least four additional symptoms of depression (American Psychiatric Association, 2001). Major depression is a disorder of *severity* and is treatable, with 80% of individuals able to resume normal activities within a few weeks (National Institute of Mental Health, 2001).

*Dysthymic disorder* is characterized by at least 2 years of depressed mood for more days than not (i.e., more than 50% of the time) accompanied by additional depressive symptoms, but that does not meet the criteria for major depression (American Psychiatric Association, 2001). Dysthymia is a disorder of *chronicity.*

*Mood* is a person's state of mind exhibited through feelings and emotions (American Psychiatric Association, 2001). It is normal for all of us to experience different types and levels of moods. Brief periods of highs, lows, and sadness occur for everyone. Mood is considered abnormal when an individual has problems with daily functioning because of the presence of exaggerated feelings and emotions. The *DSM-IV-TR* defines a mood disorder as one in which the predominant feature is the disturbance in a person's mood (American Psychiatric Association, 2001). The *DSM-IV-TR* categorizes mood disorders according to four

## Norm's Notes

*The information here might get personal. Not long ago, I spoke to a woman who was in charge of the student health center at a large university. She said that about 70% of the female students were on an SSRI. I asked that if she were exaggerating to make a point, but she said that she was not. Even if she were fudging a little, what an incredibly high figure. Perhaps most of the women students at this one university felt miserable enough to seek pharmacologic help for depression. I know that most of them would not be described as having major depression, but what a chilling thought. It sounds like an epidemic.*

overarching categories: (1) depressive disorders, (2) bipolar disorders, (3) mood disorder resulting from a general medical condition, and (4) substance-induced mood disorder.

This chapter considers the cause, diagnostic criteria, and treatment of depressive disorders. Chapter 30 addresses these same issues related to bipolar disorders. Box 29-1 summarizes criteria for major depressive disorders. *DSM-IV-TR* and NANDA International diagnoses are listed in the box below.

---

### *DSM-IV-TR* and NANDA International Diagnoses Related to Depression

*DSM-IV**
Dysthymic disorder
Major depressive disorder

NANDA INTERNATIONAL†
Anxiety
Communication, verbal, impaired
Coping, ineffective
Grieving, anticipatory
Grieving, dysfunctional
Hopelessness
Injury, risk for
Nutrition: less than body requirements, imbalanced
Powerlessness, risk for
Self-care deficit, bathing/hygiene
Self-care deficit, dressing/grooming
Self-care deficit, feeding
Self-care deficit, toileting
Self-esteem, chronic low
Sexual dysfunction
Sleep patterns, disturbed
Social isolation
Spiritual distress
Thought processes, disturbed
Violence, self-directed, risk for

*American Psychiatric Association: *Diagnostic and statistical manual of mental disorders, text revision,* ed 4, Washington, DC, 2001, APA.
†NANDA International: *NANDA nursing diagnoses: definitions and classifications, 2005-2006.* Philadelphia, 2005, NANDA International.

---

## DEPRESSIVE DISORDERS

Depression is the oldest and most frequently described psychiatric illness (Belcher and Holdcraft, 2001). The existence of depression has been documented since biblical times. Historically, many important individuals have experienced the devastating symptoms of depression, including King Saul, Job, Elijah, Jeremiah, Mary and Abraham Lincoln, Ernest Hemingway, Eugene O'Neill, and Winston Churchill. More recently, Mrs. Colin Powell, the wife of the nation's former Secretary of State, newscaster Mike Wallace, and actress Brooke Shields are known to have suffered from this disorder. Normal feelings of sadness are appropriate in many situations. In fact, it would be abnormal not to feel sad in certain situations—for example, when a loved one dies or when other losses occur in an individual's life. However, these feelings are usually short-lived and do not completely and permanently alter a person's ability to function.

The *DSM-IV-TR* categorizes depressive disorders into major depressive disorder (MDD), dysthymic disorder, and depressive disorder NOS (not otherwise specified). Depression can manifest itself as a single or recurrent episode and varies somewhat according to age, race, and gender (American Psychiatric Association, 2001). Furthermore, the connection between MDD and suicide is alarming. A discussion of suicide and depression is presented at the end of the chapter. Demographic factors associated with mood disorders are found in Table 29-1.

12-Month Prevalence Rate of Mental Disorders in the United States*

| Disorders | Approximate Percentage Over 17 Years of Age | Approximate Number of Persons | Gender Overrepresentation |
|---|---|---|---|
| **Anxiety Disorders** | 18 overall | 36,000,000 | |
| Panic disorder | 3.5 | 7,000,000 | Women |
| Social phobia | 7 | 14,000,000 | Women |
| Specific phobia | 8.7 | 17,000,000 | Women |
| GAD | 3 | 6,000,000 | Women |
| PTSD | 3.5 | 7,000,000 | Women |
| OCD | 1 | 2,000,000 | Equal |
| **Mood Disorders** | 9.5 overall | 19,000,000 | |
| Major depression | 6.7 | | Women |
| Dysthymia | 1.5 | | Women |
| Bipolar I and II | 2.6 | | BD I: Equal |
| | | | BD II: Women? |
| **Impulse Control Disorders** | 9 overall | 18,000,000 | |
| Conduct disorders | 1 | 2,000,000 | Men |
| ADHD | 4 | 8,000,000 | Men |
| **Substance Abuse Disorders** | 3.8 overall | 7,600,000 | |
| Alcohol abuse and dependence | 3.1 | 6,200,000 | Men |
| Drug abuse and dependence | 1.4 | 2,800,000 | Men |
| **Schizophrenia** | 1.1 | 2,100,000 | Equal |

*Extrapolated from several sources based on current census data.
*ADHD,* Attention-deficit/hyperactivity disorder; *GAD,* generalized anxiety disorder; *OCD,* obsessive-compulsive disorder; *PTSD,* posttraumatic stress disorder.
From Kessler RC, Chiu WT, Demler O, Walters EE: Prevalence, severity, and comorbidity of 12-month DSM-IV disorders in the national comorbidity survey replication. *Arch Gen Psychiatry* 62:617, 2005; U.S. Surgeon General: *Mental health: a report from the Surgeon General,* Washington, DC, 1999, Department of Health and Human Services: National Institute of Mental Health: *Statistics.* Available at: www.nimh.nih.gov/healthinformation/statisticsmenu.cfm. Accessed April 18, 2005.

---

### Box 29-1    Key Features of Major Depressive Disorders

At least a 2-week period of maladaptive functioning is present that is a clear change from previous levels of functioning. At least five of the following symptoms must be present during that 2-week period, one of which must be (1) or (2):

1. Depressed mood
2. Inability to experience pleasure or markedly diminished interest in pleasurable activities
3. Appetite disturbance with weight change (loss or gain of more than 5% of body weight within 1 month)
4. Sleep disturbance
5. Psychomotor disturbance
6. Fatigue or loss of energy
7. Feelings of worthlessness or excessive or inappropriate guilt
8. Diminished ability to concentrate or indecisiveness
9. Recurrent thoughts of death or suicidal ideations

The mood disturbance causes marked distress or significant impairment in social or occupational functioning, or both.

No evidence of a physical or substance-induced cause exists for the patient's symptoms or for the presence of another major mental disorder that accounts for the patient's depressive symptoms.

Modified from the American Psychiatric Association: *Diagnostic and statistical manual of mental disorders,* text revision, ed 4, Washington, DC, 2000, APA.

---

## CRITERIA AND SYMPTOMS OF MAJOR DEPRESSIVE DISORDER

MDD involves psychological, biologic, and social symptoms that impair a person's functioning ability and social interactions. Box 29-2 lists most common and other symptoms of MDD. The *DSM-IV-TR* describes MDD as a mood disorder characterized by symptoms that persist over at minimal 2-week period. A person must have at least five of the nine criteria, one of which must be a depressed mood or anhedonia. The criteria for MDD are:

| Table 29-1 | Demographic Variables Associated With Mood Disorders* | |
| --- | --- | --- |
| **Demographic Variable** | **Most Likely to Be Depressed** | **Least Likely to Be Depressed** |
| Gender | Women | Men |
| Age (yr) | 35-44 | 15-24 |
| Race | Caucasian, Hispanic | African American |
| Income | Low income | High income |
| Education | Less than high school education | High school or more |
| Geography | Urban | Rural |

*In those 15 to 54 years of age.
Modified from Kessler RC, McGonagle KA, Zhou S, et al: Lifetime and 12-month prevalence of DSM-III-R psychiatric disorders in the United States: results from the national comorbidity survey, *Arch Gen Psychiatry* 51:8, 1994.

---

### Box 29-2   Symptoms of Depression

*Most Common Symptoms*
Apathy
Sadness
Sleep disturbances
Hopelessness
Helplessness
Worthlessness
Guilt
Anger

*Other Symptoms*
Fatigue
Thoughts of death
Decreased libido
Ruminations of inadequacy
Psychomotor agitation
Verbal beratings of self
Spontaneous crying
Dependency, passiveness

---

1. Depressed mood
2. Anhedonia (or apathy)
3. Significant change in weight
4. Insomnia or hypersomnia
5. Increased or decreased psychomotor activity
6. Fatigue or energy loss
7. Feelings of worthlessness or guilt
8. Diminished concentration or indecisiveness
9. Recurrent death or suicidal thoughts

Nurses can be instrumental in the assessment of depression. A variety of instruments might be used for assessment purposes. The Hamilton Depression Scale (HAM-D) and the Geriatric Depression Scale (Appendix C) are important examples of these assessment tools.

The *DSM-IV-TR* categorizes MDD into several variants called *specifiers*. These variants include MDD with atypical features, melancholic features, catatonic features, postpartum onset, psychotic features, or seasonal patterns (i.e., seasonal affective disorder). Overarching symptoms are the same across these subgroups, but variances in expression occur. The *DSM-IV-TR* description helps define the population, time frame, and symptoms for these subgroups.

*Atypical depression* is a mood disturbance of depression that generally occurs in younger populations and is more common in women compared with men. This type of depression is expressed by increased appetite or weight gain, hypersomnia, leaden paralysis, and extreme sensitivity to interpersonal rejection. Mood reactivity in which the mood brightens considerably with positive events is another characteristic. Hypersomnia is defined as sleeping 10 hours a day or at least 2 hours more than usual. Leaden paralysis is defined as feeling heavy, leaden, or weighted down in the arms or legs. Feelings of personal rejection tend to be a symptom of long standing and tend to persist after depressive symptoms subside (American Psychiatric Association, 2001). Atypical depression might be the one type of depression in which monoamine oxidase inhibitors (MAOIs) are first-choice drugs (Anonymous, 2005).

*Melancholic depression* is a disturbance of depression occurring most often in older adults that might be misdiagnosed as dementia. This type of depression is characterized by anhedonia and an inability to be cheered up. The mood does not improve, even temporarily. At least three of the following depressive symptoms are found in melancholic patients: depression worse in the morning, early morning awakening, psychomotor retardation or agitation, significant anorexia or weight loss, and excessive or inappropriate guilt. This diagnosis is more likely to be associated with dexamethasone nonsuppression and elevated cortisol levels (see discussion below) (American Psychiatric Association, 2001).

*Catatonic features* are marked by significant psychomotor alterations, including immobility, excessive motor activity, mutism, echolalia (parrot-like repetition of words), and inappropriate posturing. Although this sign is more often associated with schizophrenia, more cases actually occur in patients with mood disorders (American Psychiatric Association, 2001).

*Postpartum depression* is a mood disturbance that occurs during the first 30 days postpartum. Postpartum blues affects approximately 50% to 80% of new mothers (Kennedy and Suttenfeld, 2001). Symptoms include feeling anxious, irritable, or tearful, but also having periods of normalcy. Postpartum depression (about 10% to 15% of new mothers) is more serious compared with postpartum blues (Solomon and Laraia, 2005). Postpartum depression can present with or without psychotic features (fewer than 1% are afflicted with psychosis). Overconcern or even delusional thoughts about the baby's health are not uncommon features of this disorder (American Psychiatric Association, 2001).

In *psychotic depression,* a person has delusions and hallucinations in conjunction with the mood disturbance. These perceptual problems tend to be mood-congruent—that is, delusions of guilt, delusions of deserved punishment, nihilistic delusions (e.g., personal destruction), somatic delusions ("My brain is dying"), and delusions of poverty. Psychotic depression is associated with a poorer prognosis compared with other forms of depression (American Psychiatric Association, 2001). Antidepressants and antipsychotics are usually required for satisfactory treatment (Schwartz, 2005).

*Seasonal affective disorder* (SAD) is a depression occurring in conjunction with a seasonal change most often beginning in fall or winter and remitting in spring (in the Northern Hemisphere). As might be expected, the higher the latitude, the more likely SAD will occur. Women are more likely to be affected by seasonal changes than men (American Psychiatric Association, 2001).

## OCCURRENCE IN SPECIFIC POPULATIONS

### Adults

Depression (all types) is one of the most prevalent mental health problems within the United States, with about 30 million people affected at any given time (Kessler et al, 2003). Depression is predicted to become the leading cause of disability in the future (Venarec, 2000). Women's lifetime risk for depression is 10% to 20% compared with men's lifetime risk of about 5% to 10% (American Psy-

chiatric Association, 2001; Nemeroff, 1998). By later life, this becomes about 50 : 50 (Anonymous, 2003). Although depression can occur at any age, the average age of adult onset is in the mid- to late 20s. Some individuals will have a single episode of clinical depression, recover, and never become depressed again. However, about 80% will eventually have recurrent episodes. Five percent to 10% will experience manic phases in addition to depressive episodes (Nemeroff, 1998). The prevalence rates appear unrelated to ethnicity; however, low-income groups and individuals with a positive family history of depression are at increased risk (up to three times greater risk).

### Children and Adolescents

The occurrence of depression in children and adolescents can be even more devastating than in adults. Children of depressed parents are at greater risk of developing the disorder than are children whose parents are not clinically depressed, and the onset of childhood depression predisposes a child to develop depression as an adult (Depression Guideline Panel [DGP], 1993). Nurses need to be able to assess children and their families for possible symptoms of depression and then develop appropriate interventions for them. Certain events might predispose children and adolescents to develop MDD, including:

1. Loss of parents through divorce, separation, or death
2. Death of other individuals close to the child
3. Death of a pet
4. Move to another neighborhood or town
5. Academic problems or failure
6. Significant physical illness or injury

### Culture, Age, and Gender

It is known that individuals from certain ethnic, racial, or cultural groups might express depressive symptoms differently than European Americans. For example, people from Hispanic, Latino, and Mediterranean groups might describe their sadness or guilt in terms of being nervous or having headaches or stomachaches. Individuals from Asian cultures might describe themselves as being out of balance or feeling weak and nervous. Native-American and Asian-American groups withdraw for meditation and personal growth as part of their culture, so symptoms of depression might be overlooked, ignored, or denied. Chapter 14 presents more specific information on expression of emotional states in different ethnic, racial, and cultural groups.

Nurses and other health care providers can misinterpret symptoms of depression in children, adolescents, women, and older adults. For example, depressive symptoms in children and adolescents might mimic normal developmental changes. On the other hand, women's reports of depression might be dismissed as symptoms of conditions expressed in ways similar to depression. The gender disparity for depression is puzzling. Some research has suggested that the devaluation of women in North America is a primary contributor to the higher incidence of depression among women (Schreiber, 2001). Finally, recognizing symptoms of depression in older adult populations is particularly challenging, because many symptoms of depression are similar to those found in dementia, diabetes, and cardiac conditions (DGP, 1993).

---

### Facts About Depression

1. Slightly fewer than 7% of the adult population of the United States will experience major depression in the next 12 months.
2. Over an entire lifetime, about 16.5% of Americans will suffer from major depression.
3. The first onset of major depression typically occurs between the ages of 25 and 30 years.
4. An episode of depression, on average, lasts about 20 weeks, 12 weeks if treated, and up to 52 weeks if untreated.
5. Most individuals suffering from a first episode of major depression will have another episode (the average is five or six episodes over a lifetime).
6. Some patients never recover from the first episode.
7. Among disabling diseases, depression ranks second in the United States.
8. Stress plays a role in the onset and exacerbation of depression.
9. Early life stress can change brain structure and function, thus lowering the threshold for adult depressive episodes.

Modified from Kessler RC, Chiu WT, Demler O, et al: Prevalence, severity, and comorbidity of 12-month DSM-IV disorders in the National Comorbidity Survey Replication, *Arch Gen Psychiatry* 62:617, 2005; Kessler RC, Berglund P, Demler O, et al: Lifetime prevalence and age of onset distributions of DSM-IV disorders in the National Comorbidity Survey Replication, *Arch Gen Psychiatry* 62:593, 2005; and Sadock BJ, Sadock VA: *Synopsis of psychiatry*, Philadelphia, 2003, Lippincott Williams & Wilkins.

---

### CRITICAL THINKING QUESTION 1

What factors do you think contribute to the high levels of depression in the United States?

---

## DYSTHYMIC DISORDER

Dysthymic disorder is diagnosed when a person has a depressed mood for at least 2 years, for more days than not. The distinction between dysthymia and MDD is subtle, and diagnostic confusion is common. Dysthymic disorder is essentially a disorder of chronicity, whereas severity is the distinguishing factor for MDD. In addition, because a less severe depression might be expected as a patient is recovering from MDD, the *DSM-IV-TR* criteria reduce the possibility of confusing a gradual recovery from MDD with the less severe dysthymic disorder. The *DSM-IV-TR* (American Psychiatric Association, 2001) criteria for dysthymia include:

A. Depressed mood for most of the day, for more days than not
B. Presence of two or more of the following:
   - Poor appetite or overeating
   - Insomnia or hypersomnia
   - Low energy or fatigue
   - Low self-esteem
   - Poor concentration or difficulty making a decision
   - Feelings of hopelessness

---

## BEHAVIOR SYMPTOMATIC OF DEPRESSION

Depression results in both objective and subjective behaviors. Objective signs, such as agitation, can be observed by the nurse. Subjective symptoms, such as hopelessness, are painful but might be hidden by depressed individuals. Objective and subjective symptoms in depression are difficult to differentiate, perhaps more than in schizophrenia. Objective signs are typically extensions of a subjective state. The nurse is encouraged to observe for visible signs of depression and to be aware of, assess for, and expect subjective anguish and anger.

## CLINICAL EXAMPLE

Mrs. Lewis is a 50-year-old woman who presents with dysphoria, tearfulness, suicidal ideation, loss of energy and sexual interest, and insomnia. Although she feels hopeless about the future and worries that she will never get better, she denies that she is really depressed. Mrs. Lewis is an extremely devout woman and believes that someone truly walking with the Lord would not find himself or herself in her situation. Mrs. Lewis believes that she is a burden to her family; she also has fears related to her physical health. Mrs. Lewis also feels guilty for not being able to handle her situation. Her husband, also a religious person, has been dutifully patient throughout all this turmoil but is growing tired of her pessimism, crying, and lack of interest in sex. The nurse fears that a breakup of this 25-year marriage might occur if Mrs. Lewis does not respond to treatment.

## OBJECTIVE SIGNS

Depressed patients often demonstrate behavior that is noticeable to others, but these patients might not want to talk to anyone and might seek to be alone. If someone intrudes into the obsessive thinking of their inner world, depressed patients might become irritable and actually strike out at the intruder. Two general areas of objective signs are alterations of activity and altered social interactions.

### Alterations of Activity

Patients might exhibit psychomotor agitation. They pace, engage in hand-wringing, and might be unable to sit still. These patients might pull or rub their hair, skin, clothing, or other objects. Tying and retying shoes and buttoning and unbuttoning a shirt or blouse are not uncommon behaviors. Psychomotor retardation is marked by a slowing of speech, increased pauses before answering, soft or monotonous speech, decreased frequency of speech (poverty of speech), and muteness. In addition, a general slowing of body movements occurs. Patients might state that they are "tired all the time," even when they are not physically active. For example, a patient might have difficulty getting up from a chair to turn off the television. Even the smallest task might seem unbearable.

Involvement in activities of daily living (ADLs) suffers as well. Depressed individuals often defer carrying out basic personal hygiene measures, such as bathing, shaving, putting on clean clothes, or wiping their mouths after eating. However, these latter objective signs are probably a result of more than a lack of energy. Apathy, a lack of feeling, absence of emotion, or an inability to be motivated, plays an important role in these behaviors as well. An extreme extension of these anergic symptoms is seen in cases in which depressed people lie in bed and become incontinent or constipated because of the inability to muster the energy (both physical and psychological) to walk to the bathroom.

Depressed people usually experience a change in eating behaviors that results in either weight loss or gain. Sleeping patterns change as well. Depressed individuals might experience insomnia (difficulty falling asleep), middle insomnia (difficulty remaining asleep), or terminal insomnia (early morning awakening). Hypersomnia (increased or prolonged sleeping, or both) is an atypical symptom of depression. Depressed people might deny that they are depressed, yet spend hours by themselves. In this case, the nurse should not confuse a request to "go to my room and lie down" with hypersomnia. Many depressed people want to lie down but do not sleep. There, in the solitude of an empty room, these individuals descend into uninterrupted, self-defeating ruminations.

## CLINICAL EXAMPLE

Stan Treback is a 60-year-old Caucasian man who has been successful in business for many years. He recently has become "blue" and does not seem to care about anything. He is cooperative and desires treatment. Stan's symptoms are decreased energy, anxiety, agitation, insomnia, and a weight loss over the past year of 54 pounds. He has many somatic complaints.

### Altered Social Interactions

Depressed individuals often suffer from poor social skills that are linked directly to other symptoms of depression. Underachievement causes a lack of productivity on the job and at home. The self-absorbing nature of depression causes these individuals to be easily distracted and reduces their interest in people, their ideas, or their problems. Depression causes problems with thinking, idea development, and problem solving. In addition, conversations are difficult to maintain, and only with great effort can a depressed person sustain a facial expression of interest and concern. Depressed individuals are also withdrawn and often prefer social isolation over social interaction with others. Hobbies and avocations that were once actively pursued become unimportant and might be abandoned or engaged in half-heartedly. Finally, the body language of depression (e.g., saddened facial expression, drooping posture) serves as a social barrier.

## SUBJECTIVE SYMPTOMS

### Alterations of Affect

Alterations of affect are the symptoms primarily associated with depression, which is reasonable, because these disturbances dominate the internal world of a depressed person. Anxiety, doom and gloom, fear, self-destructive thoughts, and panic attacks are all products of the depressed mind. Because of this anguish, depressed individuals vacillate between sadness and apathy. When the pain becomes too great, patients shut down and become apathetic. Finally, although most laypeople consider sadness to be the universal symptom of distress, apathy actually comes closer to being continually present in depressed individuals.

The overall affective sense is one of low self-esteem. Guilt might include an overreaction to some current failing or might be associated with an indiscretion in the distant past that cannot be forgiven. Guilt can also take the form of accepting responsibility for occurrences in which the person had little impact or take the form of obsessional preoccupation with such thoughts as "What if I had only . . . ?" The person becomes immobilized with should haves and could haves. An even more morbid extension of guilt is the psychotic delusion of guilt for calamities that happened far away, even on the other side of the world.

Anxiety is a companion of depression. Depressed individuals are filled with anxiousness and dread. A ringing telephone holds the potential for catastrophic news. A siren might mean a loved one has been injured; a child at school might not return. Although these terrible things do happen,

most people go on with life somewhat comforted by the knowledge that they will probably not happen if unusual risks are not taken. However, for many depressed individuals, the ringing telephone causes the same anxious reaction each time.

Worthlessness can range from a feeling of inadequacy to total devaluation. Depressed individuals might scan the environment for clues to their inadequacy and, as one person remarked, "I knew I wasn't any good; it just took a while to figure out why."

### Alterations of Cognition

Alterations of cognition include ambivalence and indecision, inability to concentrate, confusion, loss of interest and motivation, memory problems, pessimism, self-blame, self-deprecation, self-destructive thoughts, thoughts of death and dying, and uncertainty. The inability of depressed individuals to make a decision is particularly difficult for others to understand. Faced with even a simple decision, much vacillation is expressed. Once a decision is made, depressed individuals might be obsessed with "what if" questions. Major decisions can be immobilizing.

### Alterations of a Physical Nature

Alterations of a physical nature are common in the depressed individual. Almost all parts of the body can be affected. Common physiologic disorders include abdominal pain, anorexia, chest pain, constipation, dizziness, fatigue, headache, indigestion, insomnia, menstrual changes, nausea and vomiting, and sexual dysfunction. Additionally, as mentioned in the previous section (cultural aspects), some ethnic and racial groups' cultural practices might mimic depressive symptoms, or depression might be expressed somatically.

These subjective symptoms come to the attention of the nurse because of the numerous somatic complaints of depressed individuals. Some people become preoccupied with their bodies to the extent that every twinge, every body change is greeted with great alarm and dread. One recovering depressed patient joked, "I have had a hundred heart attacks." Monitoring of body functions is not uncommon in the general population and is no doubt related to a variety of factors, including perhaps this society's obsession with fitness.

However, overinvestment in self-assessment by depressed individuals is pathologic, and it is the degree of this thinking that sets apart those who are depressed. Chest pain, an unusual spot on the face or abdomen, and stomach pain all can precipitate a panic attack in some people. Panic attacks occur in 15% to 30% of individuals with MDD (American Psychiatric Association, 1993).

### Alterations of Perception

Some depressed individuals suffer from altered perceptions. Delusions and hallucinations are typically congruent with the depressed mood (e.g., a delusion of persecution because of a moral or ethical mistake). Somatic delusions (e.g., "My body is full of cancer") and nihilistic delusions (e.g., "My brain is dying") are not uncommon forms of psychotic delusions in depressed individuals. Hallucinations tend to be less elaborate than those of schizophrenics and tend to focus on personal faults—for example, "You are no good. You don't deserve your family."

## ETIOLOGY OF DEPRESSION

## BIOLOGIC THEORIES OF DEPRESSION

The etiology of depression has been biologically attributed to alterations in neurochemical, genetic, endocrine, and circadian rhythm functions. These alterations produce physical and psychological changes expressed as depression (Warren, 1997).

### Neurochemical Theories

Research findings suggest that a neurochemical depression results when levels of certain neurotransmitters are altered. The biogenic amines norepinephrine and serotonin are most often mentioned, but dopamine, another biogenic amine, is indicated as well. Figure 29-1 illustrates the proposed roles of the three key monoamines. Furthermore, dysregulation of acetylcholine and gamma-aminobutyric acid (GABA) might contribute to the development of biochemical depression as well. More specifically, when the levels of these neurotransmitters are altered at receptor sites, or when receptor sensitivity changes, a neu-

**Proposed Roles for the Three Key Monoamine Systems**

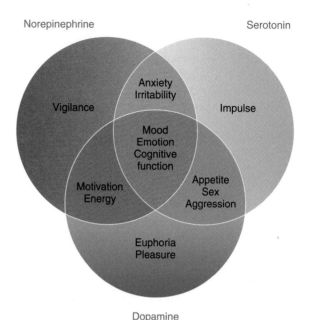

FIGURE 29-1 Proposed roles for the three key monoamine systems. *(From Healy D, McDonagle T: The enhancement of social functioning as a therapeutic principle in the management of depression,* J Psychopharmacology *11(Suppl): S25, 1997.)*

rochemical depression might result. For example, the serotonergic receptors originate in the raphe nuclei of the brainstem and are located near the midline for most of the length of the brainstem. The more rostral neurons (toward the head) project throughout the cortex. Each serotonergic neuron sends over 500,000 terminals to the limbic system and to the cortex, contributing to the regulation of many psychological functions (Dubovsky, 1994). Norepinephrine or noradrenergic pathways originate in the locus ceruleus and innervate all areas of the cortex, the hypothalamus, and the hippocampus (Keltner et al, 2001b). As is the case with serotonin, norepinephrine neurons innervate and contribute to regulation of brain areas with a variety of functions.

It might be appealing to conceptualize depression as a decreased level of serotonin and norepinephrine or to suggest that, by increasing the bioavailability of these amines, depression can be successfully treated. However, doing so oversimplifies both the problem and the solution. A more informed way of looking at depression is to think of it as a monoaminergic dysregulation. It is not so much that monoamines are lacking but that the cells they activate have lost the capacity to respond in a healthy manner; intracellular processes no longer effectively produce the transcription factors necessary for neuronal development. Once the receptor is occupied with serotonin (or norepinephrine), a cascade of intracellular events is initiated (i.e., the second-messenger system). This cascade results in the production of proteins such as enzymes, receptors, and neuroprotective proteins. When some part of this process is dysfunctional, the end products needed for cell sustenance are compromised. Antidepressants probably stabilize this intraneuronal environment.

Other hypotheses include the sensitivity of both presynaptic and postsynaptic receptors and the modulating effects of acetylcholine and GABA on aminergic systems (Keltner et al, 2001a). It is believed, for example, that beta autoreceptors, which normally inhibit the release of norepinephrine, are down-regulated by antidepressants, thus disinhibiting norepinephrine release (i.e., increasing synaptic norepinephrine). Too many norepinephrine or serotonin receptors might be thought of as a positive situation. However, excessive (up-regulation of) receptors indicate insufficient levels of these neurotransmitters. This action is an example of the body compensating for decreased monoamine availability (Nemeroff, 1998). All the up-regulation and down-regulation of receptors, however, might be a result of the intracellular response to antidepressants mentioned earlier. Finally, peptides, dietary practices, and nutritional status are being examined for their biochemical roles in the development of depression, because food intake affects the development of the precursor amino acids required for neurotransmitter synthesis. In summary, there is much to learn about the biochemistry of depression.

## Genetic Theories

Other researchers have contended that depression might be genetically based and that heredity might predispose individuals to develop depression. Several studies have examined the incidence of depression in twins. Research has indicated that up to two thirds of twins are concordant for MDD if one or both of the biologic parents has been diagnosed with MDD (Shuchter et al, 1996).

## Endocrine Theories

Endocrine changes, in relationship to depression, have also been investigated. Normally, the hypothalamic-pituitary-adrenal (HPA) axis is a system that mediates the stress response. However, in some depressed people, this system malfunctions and creates cortisol, thyroid, and hormonal abnormalities. Dysregulation of the HPA axis results in hypercortisolemia (in about 40% to 60% of depressed patients), nonsuppression by dexamethasone, and elevated levels of corticotropin-releasing factor (CRF) (Keltner et al, 2001b). The hypersecretion of cortisol is the result of an overexpression of the CRF gene (leading to increased CRF synthesis) and an increase in CRF-producing neurons in the hypothalamus. This action, in turn, leads to increased pituitary release of adrenocorticotropic hormone (ACTH) and the subsequent hypersecretion of cortisol by the adrenal glands. Nemeroff (1998) has noted that early life exposure to overwhelming trauma literally changes the expression of CRF neurons in the hypothalamus. Events such as early loss of parents, inadequate parenting, or childhood sexual and physical abuse create an adult who is overly responsive to stressors and vulnerable to depression. Essentially, a physical change brought about by childhood stressors causes a long-term or even permanent hyperactivity of central corticotropin-releasing hormones, leaving the adult highly vulnerable to stress. Nemeroff calls this phenomenon the "stress-diathesis model of depression."

The dexamethasone suppression test (DST) fails to suppress cortisol in about 40% of depressed patients. In nondepressed individuals, an elevated serum cortisol level sends a message to the hypothalamus and the anterior pituitary to decrease the release of CRF and ACTH, respectively, slowing cortisol release. Dexamethasone acts only on the anterior pituitary and in nondepressed individuals it suppresses the release of ACTH. In some, but not all, depressed persons, an injection of dexamethasone does not cause cortisol suppression, indicating that the person's stress response mode overrides his or her negative feedback system. This malfunctioning and its results are more pronounced in severely depressed patients (Shuchter et al, 1996). In addition, the presence of endocrine disease, caused by disease in any component of the HPA axis, has also been associated with the development of depressive symptoms (Maes et al, 1994; Shuchter et al, 1996). Controversy exists regarding the role of genetics and hormonal explanations of depression in women; some researchers have contended that women have a predisposition to develop depressive symptoms and MDD because of fluctuations in hormone levels (McGrath et al, 1992). Other researchers have contended that these fluctuations influence the development of MDD through their interaction with neurotransmitters, psychosocial factors, and the stress system (Beeber, 1996; Cockerman, 1992).

### Circadian Rhythm Theories

Individuals experiencing circadian rhythm changes are at increased risk for developing depressive symptoms and MDD. These changes might be caused by medications, nutritional deficiencies, physical or psychological illnesses, hormonal fluctuations associated with a woman's reproductive system, or aging (McEnany, 1995a,b; Warren, 1997). Circadian rhythms are responsible for the daily regulation of wake-sleep cycles, arousal and activity patterns, and hormonal secretions associated with these regulatory mechanisms. In depressed individuals, these regulatory mechanisms are altered, which leads to shortened latency in rapid eye movement (REM) and sleep disturbances such as insomnia, frequent waking, and increasingly intensified dreaming (Shuchter et al, 1996).

### Changes in Brain Anatomy

Evidence exists indicating that depression might result from or cause atrophy of specific brain locations. For example, loss of neurons in the frontal lobes, cerebellum, and basal ganglia has been identified by Soares and Mann (1997a,b). Other findings include a reduction in brain-derived neurotropic factor (BDNF), a protein that helps neurons develop (Duman et al, 1997). Stahl (2000) has suggested that a deficiency in BDNF allows the apoptosis proteins (apoptosis is the cell's self-regulated function of cell extinction) to dominate, leading to premature neuronal death and atrophy in specific brain areas. The hippocampus is particularly susceptible to premature apoptotic processes (Stahl, 2000). Although the notion of identifiable areas of brain atrophy has not been widely embraced, many believe that this hypoth-

esis will become well accepted as diagnostic tools become more advanced.

## PSYCHOLOGICAL THEORIES OF DEPRESSION

The psychological explanations for depression flow from psychoanalytic, cognitive, interpersonal, and behavioral perspectives. In addition, related psychosocial-psychodynamic views explain depression from three general themes: (1) adverse early life experiences, (2) intrapsychic conflicts, or (3) reactions to life events (i.e., stressors), or a combination of all three.

*Psychoanalytic theorists* have contended that depression occurs as a result of an early life loss (Freud, 1957). Freud viewed depression as the aggressive instinct inappropriately directed at the self, often triggered by the loss of a loved person or object (object loss). This loss predisposes the adult to depression when adult losses trigger the memory of the childhood loss. By understanding (i.e., gaining insight into) one's thoughts, feelings, and motives, one can heal. It should be noted that many clinicians believe that this approach is not in the patient's best interest because it focuses on problems in the past and often creates more issues than it solves.

*Cognitive theorists* have contended that depression results when a person perceives all stressful situations as being negative (Beck, 1976; Beck, 1991). In addition, a depressed person reacts to all situations as if they are stressful and sees himself or herself, others, and daily events in a negative light. This reaction to stress is grounded in early childhood losses (e.g., often the loss of the parent through death, leaving the home, or divorce) and serves as the basis for how the depressed person makes decisions and sees himself or herself in relationship to other persons and occurrences. Cognitive therapy aims at symptom removal by identifying and correcting distorted, negative, moment by moment maladaptive thinking and seeks to prevent recurrence by correcting silent assumptions (DGP, 1993). Most clinicians, even those heavily steeped in a biologic framework, believe that medications serve the purpose of preparing the mind to work on faulty thinking. Cognitive approaches are ideal when used in conjunction with antidepressants.

*Interpersonal theorists* believe that when a person has interpersonal difficulties, coping with individuals, life events, and life changes can be inordinately stressful and lead to depression (Klerman, 1989). Role issues, social isolation, prolonged grief reaction, and role transition are major interpersonal themes. Interpersonal difficulties are viewed as causal, concomitant, or exacerbating in maintaining factors for depression (DGP, 1993).

*Behavioral theorists* propose that a person develops depression when he or she develops feelings of helplessness and unworthiness and then learns to use these attitudes to evaluate life outcomes (Abramson et al, 1978).

As noted, psychological or psychodynamic explanations of depression can be categorized under three general themes: (1) debilitating early life experiences, (2) intrapsychic conflicts, or (3) reactions to life events.

### Debilitating Early Life Experiences

According to traditional psychiatric thought, events in early life can lay the foundation for adult depression. Developmental theorists view the early years of life as the foundation of lifelong mental health. Although these theorists use different words to designate life stages, their views of the importance of a solid, nurturing early life environment are similar. Early losses, maternal inconsistency, the giving and withholding of love by the caregiver, and various types of abuse are all given as causative agents for depression.

### Intrapsychic Conflict

Intrapsychic conflict refers to the conflicts people have when they have mixed emotions about a behavior, event, or situation. For instance, an individual who has been brought up to refrain from sexual activity, but who also has strong urges to experience sex, has a conflict. To refrain from sexual activity increases sexual frustration and to engage in sexual activity might cause anxiety, guilt, and fear. People are faced with intrapsychic conflicts all the time. Persistent and unsuccessful resolution of these conflicts can lead to depression.

### Reactions to Life Events (Stress)

Most people view depression as a reaction to life stress. Loss is a major theme: of a loved one, of a job, of self-esteem, of familiar surroundings.

Reacting to loss with grief and sadness is normal; overreacting is abnormal. Probably half of all depressive events are jump-started by stress. However, exactly when normal becomes abnormal is unclear. (See Dysfunctional Grief box.)

---

### CLINICAL EXAMPLE

Elle Jones is a 45-year-old, well-educated, intelligent Caucasian woman who has been in and out of therapy for a long time (15 to 20 years). Elle grew up in northern Mississippi with two brothers and a very physically and emotionally abusive father. Elle reports that, when she was quite young, her mother left home and did not return for several years. Elle left home at age 17 and was married twice and divorced shortly after each marriage. She has a history of depression, and she attempted suicide 20 years ago. After many turbulent years, she started going to bars in hopes "that I might get killed." She refers to this period as her "death hunt days." After emotional and financial collapse, Elle has recently returned to her father's home. He continues to control her life in every way. She has commented that her life is so futile that she would rather be dead.

---

## ASSESSMENT OF DEPRESSION

Assessment of depression might be accomplished through both nonbiologic and biologic assessment methods. The DGP (1993) and Shuchter and colleagues (1996) have recommended that patients be examined—profiled—for an accurate diagnosis of depression. The profile should address *DSM-IV-TR* criteria and biologic findings, including:

1. History of onset of symptoms
2. Presence of comorbid substance, alcohol, and medication use
3. Physical examination to rule out possibility of the presence of medical conditions (Box 29-3 lists medical conditions)
4. Presence of nonmood psychiatric disorders
5. Patient resources and social support systems
6. Interpersonal and coping abilities
7. Level of stressors
8. Presence or level of suicidal ideation

Nurses can be instrumental in collecting all of this information, because they are often the health

## Dysfunctional Grief

If you live long enough you will experience grief—an intense but normal response to loss—typically the loss of someone very close to you. Typically, we think of grief as a reaction to death, but it can also be a reaction to divorce, relocation to another part of the country, terminal illness (e.g., anticipatory grief), or natural disaster (Anonymous, 2002; Zeitlin, 2001). As noted, grief is normal. To lose someone close—for example, a mother, father, brother, sister, wife, husband, or child—and not experience grief is abnormal.

Typically, the grief response lasts about 6 months. People experiencing grief report a choking sensation, emptiness, shortness of breath, weakness, and sighing (Anonymous, 2002). They also use the term *waves* to verbalize how these feelings roll over them. After about 6 months, the grieving person begins to return to normal, but waves of grief can continue to occur for some time (Anonymous, 2002).

During my teenage years (i.e., the early 1960s), I was acquainted with an older woman in my hometown of Manteca, California. She had lost her only son in World War II, and his photograph was displayed on her piano. Not often, but on occasion, she would pick up his photograph and begin to cry. Twenty years later, she still experienced a wave of grief from time to time.

Dysfunctional grief is said to occur when these symptoms extend beyond 6 months. Zeitlin (2001) outlined the risk factors for dysfunctional grieving:

1. History of psychiatric disorders
2. Ambivalent, overly close, or intense relationship with deceased
3. History of multiple, recent losses
4. Loss of a parent or a significant person during childhood
5. Lack of social support
6. Deaths by suicide, AIDS, murder, or other unexpected means

Differentiating grief and depression is not always simple, but the following guidelines can be useful (Anonymous, 2002):

| Grief | Depression |
|---|---|
| Natural response to death | An illness |
| Self-limited and improves with time | Persistent and can worsen |
| Responsive to social contacts | Burdened by social contacts |
| Rarely suicidal | Suicidal ideations common |
| Typically does not need antidepressants | Responsive to antidepressants |

From Anonymous: Coping with grief, *Psychiatr Serv* 53:19, 2002; and Zeitlin SV: Grief and bereavement, *Prim Care* 28:415, 2001.

care professionals who initially assess patients and develop the database for use in the general diagnostic and nursing processes.

## CULTURAL ISSUES AND ASSESSING DEPRESSION

Instrument selection is based on the nurse's clinical knowledge and experience, as well as on the age and mental capability of the person being assessed. Unfortunately, only limited measures have been developed and normed for use in different ethnic, racial, and cultural groups (Jones, 1996). The lack of measurement specificity for these populations can lead to misdiagnosis or underdiagnosis. Because some researchers have contended that culturally competent measures predict relevant criteria more accurately than nonculturally competent measures, this assessment

deficiency should be viewed as clinically significant. Routine review of cultural competence issues will facilitate accurate and valid assessment for all patients.

Culture is the internal and external manifestation of an individual's, group's, or community's beliefs, values, and norms that are used as premises for everyday functioning. Tseng and Streltzer (1997) have recommended that clinicians distinguish between normal cultural behavior and psychopathology by using the following:

1. Cultural competence guidelines, a panel of experts, or both (i.e., someone who understands the culture)
2. *DSM-IV-TR* criteria
3. A functional status measurement
4. The affected person's perception of self and what he or she considers "normal"

## Box 29-3 Medical Conditions Commonly Associated With Depression

**Central Nervous System Disorders**
Alzheimer's disease
Amyotrophic lateral sclerosis (ALS)
Brain tumor
Cerebrovascular accident (stroke)
Chronic subdural hematoma
Multiple sclerosis
Normal-pressure hydrocephalus
Parkinson's disease
Subarachnoid hemorrhage

**Collagen Vascular Diseases**
Polymyalgia rheumatica
Rheumatoid arthritis
Systemic lupus erythematosus
Temporal arteritis

**Toxic-Metabolic Disturbances and Endocrinopathies**
Addison's disease
Cushing's disease
Diabetes mellitus
Electrolyte disorders
Hypoglycemia
Hypothyroidism
Metal intoxication
Parathyroid disorders
Uremia

**Infections**
Acquired immunodeficiency syndrome
Encephalitis
Hepatitis
Infectious mononucleosis
Influenza
Syphilis
Tuberculosis
Viral pneumonia

**Neoplastic Disorders**
Carcinoma of head of pancreas
Chronic myelogenous leukemia
Lymphoma
Other malignant disease
Small cell carcinoma of lung

**Other**
Chronic fatigue syndrome
Chronic obstructive pulmonary disease

Modified from Ford CV, Folks DG: Psychiatric disorders in geriatric medical/surgical patients. II. Review of clinical experience in consultation, *South Med J* 78:397, 1985.

## Box 29-4 Important Points for Administering Antidepressant Drugs

- Most antidepressants have a lag time of 2 to 4 weeks before a full clinical effect occurs.
- Many reports suggest these drugs might provoke suicidal ideation and behavior.
- Suicidal patients may "cheek" these drugs to build up a supply for an overdose. Tricyclic antidepressants (TCAs) have a narrow therapeutic index.
- Monitor vital signs of patients who take TCAs and monoamine oxidase inhibitors (MAOIs):
  1. TCAs can cause orthostatic hypotension, reflex tachycardia, and arrhythmias.
  2. MAOIs have the potential for triggering a hypertensive crisis.
- Monitor sexual side effects of selective serotonin reuptake inhibitors (SSRIs) because they occur fairly frequently and lead to noncompliance.
- Be aware of the drug-drug and food-drug interactions associated with MAOIs.
- Observe for early signs of toxicity:
  1. TCAs: Drowsiness, tachycardia, mydriasis, hypotension, agitation, vomiting, confusion, fever, restlessness, sweating
  2. MAOIs: Dizziness, vertigo, fatigue
  3. SSRIs: Have low probability for causing toxicity

depression increase (U.S. Surgeon General, 1999). Depressive symptoms are relatively common, but because of the overlapping symptoms of physical illness and the depressive side effects of many medications, diagnosis is complex. To acquaint the nurse with potential confounding variables, a list of depression-causing illnesses that share symptoms with depression is presented in Box 29-4. It should be noted that late life depressions (i.e., first depressive episode occurring in later life) are thought to be more likely associated with brain abnormalities rather than genetic or psychological factors.

If the depression is related to a treatable medical illness, elimination of the illness often returns the depressed mood to normal. On the other hand, MDD and medical illness can coexist, and, in these cases, treatment needs to be instituted. The nurse should also be aware that some people who are diagnosed with dementia are, in reality, depressed (referred to as *pseudodementia*). Hence, it is important to differentiate between depression and dementia. Again, depression and dementia can occur comorbidly, in which case both disorders must be treated. Comorbid MDD and dementia

## ASSESSMENT OF DEPRESSION

### In Older Adults

Depression among older adults is a major health concern. The prevalence of MDD declines with age (probably less than 5%), but symptoms of tend to occur early in the course of Alzheimer's disease (DGP, 1993).

Finally, older adults are at increased risk of suicide. Men have a more increased risk than women, with older Caucasian men having the highest risk of suicide in the United States. A discussion of suicide is presented at the end of this chapter.

## Nonbiologic Assessment Measures

Nonbiologic assessments are composed of standardized verbal and written measurement scales. Obtained data can be used in conjunction with the *DSM-IV-TR* criteria and biologic assessments to give a more accurate diagnosis regarding MDD.

## Biologic Assessment Measures

### Dexamethasone Suppression Test

Although not frequently ordered, the DST is a diagnostic test for MDD in adults that measures the function of the HPA axis. Urine and blood samples are collected before the test to determine baseline levels of cortisol. Then, a single injection of the drug dexamethasone is given to the patient. Urine and blood cortisol levels are monitored for 24 hours. A positive result occurs when cortisol levels do not fall (i.e., are not suppressed) or return to 5 mcg/dL or higher within 24 hours. Forty percent of severely depressed patients fail to suppress cortisol. The DST is not specific for depression because individuals suffering from dementia, alcohol withdrawal, and bulimia do not suppress cortisol levels.

### Growth Hormone Assessment

Growth hormone secretion is often used as a biologic assessment measure in childhood depression. Past research has indicated that some depressed children might have decreased secretion of the growth hormone during the day and increased secretion while asleep. This test is not useful in adolescent and adult populations.

### Polysomnographic Measurements

Polysomnographic findings (i.e., examination of sleep patterns) are used to assess depression in adult populations. The REM stage usually begins within 70 to 100 minutes of a person falling asleep and increases in length throughout the night. However, in depressed adults, the REM latency phase is shortened, which results in frequent night and early morning wakening. Antidepressants can restore the normal pattern of REM sleep.

The nurse uses the nursing process to develop appropriate nursing interventions and strategies, expected outcomes, and evaluation of the outcomes for depressed patients. The intervention strategy described in this book, psychotherapeutic management, emphasizes the nurse-patient relationship, psychopharmacology, and milieu management. These concepts are discussed in detail in Units II, III, and IV, respectively. The case study and care plan presented in this section on depression are geared toward the nursing management of the depressed patient who is residing in a psychiatric hospital environment. However, it is important to realize that most psychiatric patients, in the current managed care environment, are hospitalized for short periods or might not be hospitalized at all. Consequently, the nursing management of depressed individuals might occur in medical settings or outpatient clinics. In addition, it is imperative that nurses in any setting be familiar with the *DSM-IV-TR* criteria of MDD and with the information regarding mood disorders presented in this chapter. Finally, it is recommended that the reader refer to Chapter 39 for a detailed explanation of electroconvulsive therapy used in the treatment of depression.

## NURSE-PATIENT RELATIONSHIP

The objective of this section is to provide specific principles of therapeutic communication for nurses who work with depressed patients.

1. Depressed individuals suffer from low self-esteem. The most effective approach to bolster self-esteem is to accept patients as they are (negative attitude and all), help them focus on the positive (accomplishments, good points), provide successful experiences with positive feedback, keep self-help strategies simple, and help patients avoid embarrassing social blunders (e.g., smelly clothes, unkempt appearance).
2. Development of a meaningful relationship in which depressed individuals are valued as human

beings is important to their sense of personal worth. It is important for the nurse to be honest and to work on developing trust. Doing specific things that are in the best interest of each patient develops the trusting relationship. For example, a patient might wish to tell the nurse something of clinical significance but does not want the nurse to share the information with other staff members. The nurse builds trust by telling the patient that significant information will be shared only with staff members who have a need to know. The patient learns to trust the nurse as a professional whose primary concern is the patient's best interest.

3. The nurse who works effectively with depressed patients must have sincere concern for patients and be empathic. The nurse acknowledges the emotional pain and suffering conveyed by patients and offers to help patients work through the pain. Van Os van den Brink, Tiemens, et al (2005) found that empathy, when added to an adequate dosage of antidepressant, bolstered treatment success.

4. It is usually not effective to outline logically why a patient is a worthwhile human being. The nurse can, however, point out even small visible accomplishments and strengths—for example, "I'm glad you combed your hair today." A patient might agree with everything the nurse says but might remain just as depressed. Intellectual understanding does not help severely depressed patients. Cognitive-behavioral therapists, however, have been successful in helping some depressed individuals learn to reprogram negative thoughts—for example, to progress from "I can't do anything right" to "I can learn from my mistakes."

5. Depressed individuals are typically dependent. The nurse might notice that he or she (i.e., the nurse) is taking on responsibility for the depression of patients. The nurse should recognize, but not resent, this tendency in depressed individuals to become dependent. The nurse should reward even small decisions and independent actions.

6. The nurse should not attempt to embarrass patients out of being depressed. For example, pointing out less fortunate people in the hope that such an action might bring depressed individuals to their senses provides,

## Interpersonal Style Continuum

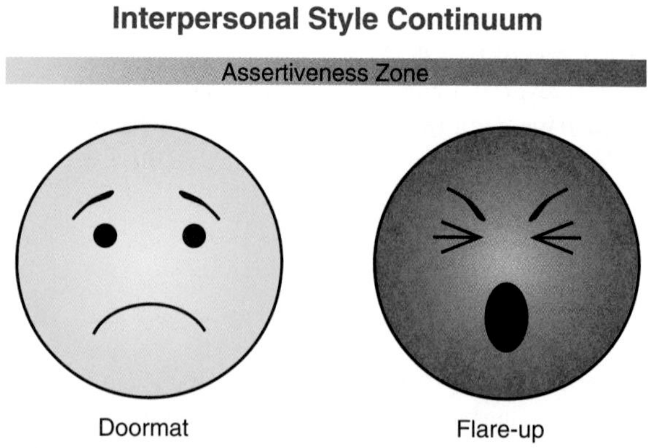

FIGURE 29-2 Depressed individuals often adopt an interpersonal style that causes them to be "doormats"—that is, they allow people to walk all over them. Sometimes the doormat personality will explode when they have had too much. These outbursts are typically followed by even more recrimination and regret. The nurse can help patients learn to avoid these extremes of interpersonal behavior by teaching them to use assertiveness techniques.

at best, short-lived relief based on the misfortune of others.

7. Never reinforce hallucinations, delusions, or irrational beliefs: the nurse cannot agree with the delusions, and arguing seems to reinforce them. The nurse should state his or her perception of reality, voice doubt about the patient's perceptions, and move on to discuss real people and events.

8. Depressed individuals tend to be angry (Figure 29-2). Sometimes, they surprise even themselves with the hateful or hostile things that they say. It is important for the nurse to learn to handle hostility therapeutically by recognizing the anger, not taking it personally and not retaliating in word, deed, or some passive-aggressive form. Encouraging verbal expressions of anger helps release patients' tension.

9. The nurse can help withdrawn patients emerge from their social isolation by spending time with them (even without speaking), providing a nonthreatening one-to-one relationship, practicing assertive interactions, and being accepting.

10. Depressed individuals can have difficulty in making even simple decisions. It is not therapeutic to badger patients into making a decision but it is therapeutic to provide decision-making opportunities as patients are able to comply. Initially, the nurse might need to

## Key Nursing Interventions *for Depressed Patients*

The psychiatric nurse should consider the following intervention principles when working with depressed patients.

| Intervention | Rationale |
|---|---|
| Accept patients where they are and focus on their strengths. | Depressed persons have low self-esteem, and this is the best approach to recapturing some sense of value. |
| Reinforce decision making by patients. | Depressed patients struggle to make even simple decisions. By reinforcing patients' efforts to make simple decisions, the nurse helps patients move toward health. |
| Respond to anger therapeutically. | Depressed persons are typically angry. By understanding that anger is a symptom of depression, the nurse can focus on the issue at hand and help patients move toward a more acceptable style of interaction. |
| Spend time with withdrawn patients. | Withdrawn patients are aware of their surroundings. By spending time (frequent but brief contact) with these patients, the nurse communicates patients' worth and, consequently, might be available during a time when patients feel comfortable with initiating dialogue. |
| Make decisions for patients that they are not ready to make for themselves. | Some patients cannot make a decision. Simply present situations to these patients that do not require decision making (e.g., "It's time to go for a walk"). |
| Involve patients in activities in which they can experience success. | People can feel good about themselves in several ways. One way to develop self-worth is through accomplishment. |

make decisions for patients—for example, "It is time for your bath" or "Here is your apple juice." When possible, the nurse helps guide patients to appropriate decisions by using problem-solving techniques—that is, identifying options, the advantages and disadvantages of each option, and the potential consequences of each decision. (See Key Nursing Interventions for Depressed Patients box.)

## PSYCHOPHARMACOLOGY

To understand the range of information required for effective psychopharmacologic intervention, the student is encouraged to review Chapters 19 and 20, which provides a complete discussion of antidepressant and antimanic drugs. A brief review of critical parameters of antidepressant drug administration is given in Box 29-4 and in Side Effects of Antidepressant Drugs box. Another somatic but nonpharmacologic approach to depression has recently been approved by the U.S. Food and Drug Administration (Splete, 2005). Vagus nerve stimulation (VNS) has demonstrated efficacy in severe, treatment-resistant depression. Specifically, a pacemaker-like device stimulates the vagus nerve and has demonstrated an ability to reduce depression symptoms in more than half the patients studied (Splete, 2005).

### Side Effects of Antidepressant Drugs

**Antidepressants (TCAs, SSRIs)**
Sexual dysfunction (depressed libido, arousal, and/or orgasm)
Dry mouth
Nasal congestion
Urinary hesitancy
Urinary retention
Blurred vision
Constipation
Sedation, ataxia
Confusion
Orthostatic hypotension
Arrhythmias, tachycardia, palpitations
Decreased sweating
**MAOIs**
Overstimulation such as agitation, hypomania
Blurred vision, hypotension, dry mouth, constipation
Hypertensive crisis related to food-drug or drug-drug interactions

*MAOIs,* Monoamine oxidase inhibitors; *SSRIs,* selective serotonin reuptake inhibitors; *TCAs,* tricyclic antidepressants.

## MILIEU MANAGEMENT

Milieu management is an important dimension of the psychiatric nursing care of depressed patients. The student is referred to Unit IV for a complete discussion of milieu management. General principles that specifically address the environment of depressed patients include the following.

### For patients with low self-esteem:

- Encourage patients with low self-esteem to participate in activities, including group activities, in which they will be able to experience accomplishment and receive positive feedback. Most people develop a sense of self-worth through mastery or accomplishment. Simply telling patients that they are okay is not convincing. Provide successful experiences, however small.
- Provide assertiveness training. Many depressed individuals feel like doormats because of their interactional problems; their communication history is typically a lifetime of being taken advantage of, punctuated by periodic outbursts of anger when they become fed up. Assertiveness training helps these patients learn to take care of their needs and to express their feelings along the way; thus, the extremes of "doormat" and "flare-up" are avoided.
- Help patients avoid embarrassing themselves through socially unacceptable appearance or behavior. Many appearance problems are related directly to depressed individuals' preoccupation, apathy, and decreased energy level. For example, food stains on clothes, food in a beard, an unattended runny nose, uncombed hair, urine on trousers, and an unzipped fly might be seen in depressed individuals who cannot pay attention to these hygienic concerns. Help patients shower and dress appropriately. Remind patients to go to the bathroom. In some cases, it is better to encourage patients to walk with the nurse (e.g., to the bathroom area or to the shower).

### For withdrawn patients:

- Keep contacts with withdrawn patients brief but frequent. Depressed patients often do not want anyone around or, at least, anyone to talk to them. Unfortunately, their wishes are not a good indicator of what should be done. Spending time with patients is constructive; allowing patients to isolate themselves is not. Patients might need to increase physical activity before they are able to verbalize issues.
- Many patients are insistent about going to their rooms to lie down. They might stay there all day if the nurse does not intervene. Locking a patient's room during the day might be required to keep the withdrawn or isolative patient from disappearing for hours at a time. Sitting in silence during an activity is better than ruminating in isolation.

### For anorectic patients:

- The nursing staff must take responsibility for ensuring that depressed patients eat. It is irresponsible to set a tray down in front of a depressed person, particularly in his or her room, and then leave. The nurse must encourage patients to eat and might even spoon-feed them, if required.
- Allow patients to participate in selecting preferred foods from the menu.
- Promote a proper diet, adequate fluids, and exercise. Provide small, frequent meals. Record intake.
- Constipation is a side effect not only of antidepressants, but also of depression. A diet with adequate fiber content and sufficient fluids is important. Monitoring and recording bowel elimination is also important.
- If patients will eat food brought from home, permit them to do so.

### For patients with sleep disturbances:

- Depressed individuals want to sleep, but many suffer from insomnia. The tremendous fatigue is real to these patients because the sleep they manage to get is usually not restful. Patients often wake up looking and feeling exhausted. The nursing staff should record the amount and quality of patients' actual sleep. Patients who lie down during the day are not necessarily sleeping but might be isolating themselves. An accurate understanding of the amount of sleep being obtained helps the nurse formulate an intervention strategy.
- People suffering from insomnia often engage in self-defeating behaviors, such as daytime napping and drinking stimulants (e.g., coffee, colas). Eliminating these behaviors increases the likelihood of nighttime sleep.
- Unfortunately, chronic insomnia in a depressed person appears to blunt their response to antidepressants (Jancin, 2005), so successfully

dealing with insomnia offers the possibility of a twofold benefit.

## CRITICAL THINKING QUESTION      2

Do you think physicians have the right to help terminally ill patients end their lives? Should adults in their right mind s be allowed to commit suicide?

## SUICIDE AND DEPRESSION

*Most people who commit suicide die accidentally.*
                                                    *Anonymous*

Suicide is a complex phenomenon influenced by a person's cultural beliefs, values, and norms. Suicide might occur in children, adolescent, and adult populations. Nurses need to assess the following:

*Suicidal ideation level:* Suicidal ideation includes a person's thoughts regarding suicide, as well as suicidal gestures and threats.

*Suicidal gestures:* Suicidal gestures are a person's nonlethal self-injury acts, including cutting or burning of skin areas or ingesting small amounts of drugs. Others often see these gestures as attention-getting measures and do not consider them serious problems that might lead to a suicide attempt or completion.

*Suicidal threats:* Suicidal threats are a person's verbal statements that might declare their intent to commit suicide. Threats often precede an actual suicidal attempt.

*Suicidal attempts:* Suicidal attempts are the actual implementation of a self-injurious act with the express purpose of ending the person's life.

Suicide is a significant cause of death: it is the eleventh leading cause of death in the United States (down from ninth in 1995) and is among the three leading causes of death for people aged 15 to 24 years (Anonymous, 2003a; Mann, 1998). The overall ratio of attempted to complete suicide may be as high as 8 : 1 (Moscicki, 2001). The annual number of suicides in this country is about 11 per 100,000, or roughly 30,000 individuals each year (Centers for Disease Control and Prevention [CDC], 2000).

The prototypical suicide victim is an unemployed male Caucasian, living alone, who has made a serious suicide attempt in the past. Men are four times as likely as women, and Caucasians are twice as likely as African Americans, to complete a suicide attempt successfully (Cugino et al, 1992; Harvard Mental Health Letter, 2003). Over 70% of all suicides are committed by Caucasian men (Pearson, 1998).

The overall suicide rate for the general adult population in the United States is high, but is still considerably lower than for people with psychiatric disorders. Psychiatric diagnosis is the most reliable risk factor for suicide. Approximately 90% of all suicides are committed by individuals with a diagnosable mental or substance abuse disorder. It is estimated that, over a period of 10 to 15 years, 10% to 15% of all patients with depression, schizophrenia, or alcoholism will die by suicide. Table 29-2 compares the suicide rates by diagnostic entity of the general population with those for mentally disordered individuals (Clark et al, 1987). Box 29-5 provides a list of other risk factors that have been related empirically to suicide (USDHHS, 1993).

## CASE STUDY

Bill W. is a 35-year-old African-American man who has been in and out of mental health facilities for several years. Before his formal entrance into the mental health system, he had had several brushes with the law, primarily related to driving under the influence (DUI) of alcohol. It is thought that Bill was actually self-medicating with alcohol and with other substances long before he was able to admit that he had a problem. One year after being diagnosed with major depression, Bill developed hepatitis B through sexual activity. Subsequent to this diagnosis, Bill attempted to kill himself on at least five occasions. During a brief period of his afflic-

tion with depression, he developed auditory hallucinations accusing him of being gay. Although this was a relatively brief episode and did not recur, Bill is very troubled by it, believing that these hallucinations make him "certifiably crazy." Bill now lives with his widowed father who seems to be very pleased to have Bill "back home again." Bill continues to attend an outpatient program 3 days per week. He verbalizes wanting to go back to work, but cannot seem to get moving. A longstanding fear of crowds and people remains. As Bill says, "I'm not out of the woods, but I am a lot better than I was."

## Care Plan

Name: _____    Admission Date: _____

*DSM-IV-TR* Diagnosis: Major depression

| | |
|---|---|
| Assessment | **Areas of strength:** Bill understands his disease, has a good relationship with his father, is financially stable, is willing to acknowledge his problems and work on them, and is motivated to go back to work. |
| | **Problems:** Bill verbalizes motivation but seems "stuck"; he enjoys living with his father, but he is too dependent for a 35-year-old man; he continues to be intimidated by crowds and people and has a suicidal history. |
| Diagnoses | • Risk for self-injury related to depression as evidenced by history of suicide attempts. |
| | • Social isolation related to anxiety, as evidenced by withdrawal from people and uncommunicative behavior. |

| Outcomes | *Short-term goals:* | Date met |
|---|---|---|
| | • Learn and develop coping skills for dealing with other patients at mental health treatment program. | _____ |
| | • Participate in class activities at the mental health center. | _____ |
| | • Develop socialization skills. | _____ |
| | • Continue to comply with medication regimen. | _____ |
| | *Long-term goals:* | |
| | • Seek out information about jobs at his skill level. | _____ |
| | • Practice coping skills learned at mental health center in public areas. | _____ |
| | • Make steps to return to a more independent lifestyle. | _____ |

| | |
|---|---|
| Planning/ Interventions | **Nurse-patient relationship:** Develop a trusting relationship based on honesty and genuine concern for the patient. Spend time with him, and reinforce his strengths and accomplishments. Help patient develop coping skills, and work with him to obtain job information. |
| | **Psychopharmacology:** Risperidone 3 mg qd; sertraline 50 mg qd; alprazolam 1 mg tid. |
| | **Milieu management:** Minimize patient's tendency to isolate himself by encouraging social interaction. As tolerated, draw patient into group situations. Keep environment safe, should patient attempt self-injury. |
| Evaluation | Patient is doing better but still tends to avoid large groups of people. He is compliant with medications, and no psychotic behavior has been observed or reported. |
| Referrals | Patient is a candidate for a mental health system–sponsored apartment in the near future. |

---

**CRITICAL THINKING QUESTION    3**

Why do you think the prevalence of suicide is higher in Caucasians than in other races?

The death by suicide of psychiatric patients is of particular importance to the nurse because of opportunities for assessment and intervention. The psychiatric nurse must continually assess for suicide potential among all patients, but especially among schizophrenic, depressed, and alcoholic patients.

Although there are separate suicide rates for schizophrenics, the depressed, and alcoholics, Hendin (1986) has noted that, when schizophrenic individuals kill themselves, they are typically in a depressed phase, and the act typically is not a product of psychosis. Alcoholics kill themselves usually in response to loss (e.g., divorce, separation, being fired) and when they have been drinking. Hendin made the point that suicide most often is the result of depression, diagnosed or not.

The major themes of suicidal patients are loss, unbearable psychic pain, helplessness, hopelessness, loneliness, and abandonment ("nobody cares").

| Table 29-2 | Clinical Risk Factors for Suicide in the United States |
| --- | --- |
| **Population** | **Suicides per 100,000** |
| Adult general public | <20 |
| Schizophrenic | 140 |
| Depressed | 230 |
| Alcoholic | 270 |

**Box 29-5    Risk Factors of Completed Suicide**

Male
Caucasian or Native American
Age 60 years and older
Hopelessness
General medical illness
Severe anhedonia
Living alone
Prior suicide attempts
Unemployed or financial problems

## Family Issues: Living with the Depressed Person

### Living With a Depressed Mother

Living with a depressed person can be very difficult. The person is often irritable, moody, isolative, and pessimistic. Family members might struggle to get along with the person, co-workers might find the person impossible to please, and children might assume responsibility for their depressed parent's mood. Grunebaum and Cohler (1983) found that children of depressed mothers were more vulnerable to emotional problems than children of mothers with schizophrenia. Schizophrenia, they suggested, is exhibited in such a clearly abnormal fashion that children can recognize the parent as mentally disturbed (i.e., this behavior is abnormal, this behavior is normal). This level of insight affords some degree of emotional insulation from the parent's disruptive behavior. Grunebaum and Cohler (1983) further reasoned that, because the depressed parent is not clearly "abnormal" but rather basically unhappy, moody, sad, and irritable, children are less able to set these boundaries. Hence, living with a depressed parent can trigger emotional insecurity and self-doubt and cause a myriad of intrafamilial communication problems. Two brief clinical examples follow to illustrate the difficulties encountered in families with depressed individuals.

### Living With a Depressed Wife

Joan is a 40-year-old college professor. She has been married for 15 years and has two children, a 13-year-old daughter and an 11-year-old son. Joan admits to a few close friends and to her husband that she is depressed. She has never officially sought help for her depression, but her physician has ordered a tricyclic antidepressant (TCA) at bedtime for sleep. The problems her family faces that are related to her depressed mood are subtle but beginning to take their toll. Joan is never happy nor can she become excited about anything the family does together. She spends much of her time at home, either soaking in the bathtub or in her bedroom reading. She seems to have energy for her research at the university, but for little else. She resents her husband for many things; some are real, others are not. She is often critical of her daughter and then feels remorseful. Joan has great difficulty talking with her family. Her husband, also a professional, realizes that something is wrong, but he is losing patience with his wife. He perceives her lack of interest in sex or even talking with him as signs of a failing marriage. What is not clear is whether the failing marriage precipitated Joan's depressed mood (a reactive depression), whether Joan's depressed mood is causing the marriage to fail (an endogenous depression), or whether there is a synergistic combination of the two.

### Living With a Depressed Husband

Tom is a 60-year-old white man who has been hospitalized numerous times over the years for depression. He has not worked for over 12 years. The past 6 years have been punctuated with threats of suicide and suicidal gestures. He talks about suicide often and has taken out a gun at home on several occasions while talking about killing himself. Tom is the father of four children, three boys and a girl, ages 15 to 32 years. Three children still live at home. Judy, his wife of 35 years, does not know what to do. When Tom's suicide talk becomes serious, she either takes him to the hospital or calls the sheriff's office. The hospital staff, sheriff's deputies, children, Judy, and even Tom are tired of these frequent emergencies. Every time Judy leaves the house and returns, she admits to a fear of finding Tom dead. She is angry with Tom, but she keeps her feelings to herself, for fear of precipitating a suicide attempt. The children living at home become very anxious if they do not see their father as soon as they return from school each day. Judy states that she feels like a prisoner in her own home and cannot take it anymore.

## Patient and Family Education

### Depression

#### Illness

Depression is a life-altering process or state. Depression might be precipitated by overwhelming life stresses including loss (e.g., divorce, death, job), medications, medical illnesses, and specific chemical deficiencies in the brain. These precipitating factors are not mutually exclusive and might interact to produce depression. For example, it is believd that chronic exposure to intense stress can alter brain chemistry. Support for the chemical deficiency view has increased over the last 2 decades because medications known to relieve and correct depressive states correct the chemical deficiencies previously noted. Nine cardinal symptoms define depression: (1) depressed mood, (2) apathy, (3) changes in weight, (4) sleep disturbances, (5) movement disturbances, (6) lack of energy, (7) sense of worthlessness, (8) inability to concentrate, and (9) thoughts of death. An individual with most of these symptoms (depressed mood or apathy must always be present) should be diagnosed as suffering from depression.

#### Medications

1. The most popular antidepressants are the SSRIs. Well-known drugs in this category include Prozac, Zoloft, Paxil, Lexapro, and Celexa. These drugs are effective and have few side effects. However, sexual dysfunction, defined as a loss of interest in sex or the inability to perform sexually, is common and disturbing to many patients. This side effect motivates some patients to stop taking their SSRI. Fortunately, other medications can be added that might restore sexual vitality (e.g., Wellbutrin, Viagra).

2. An older group of medications, referred to as TCAs, is still commonly prescribed (e.g., Elavil, Pamelor, Norpramin). Although they have a higher rate of side effects than the SSRIs, TCAs are as effective and are considerably less expensive. The most common side effects are a decrease in blood pressure when standing, dry mouth, constipation, and a racing heart (at times).

3. A number of newer and very promising agents are now available (e.g., Wellbutrin, Effexor, Remeron). All these drugs seem to be effective and cause fewer side effects for most people.

#### Other Issues

It is easy to be angry with a depressed person—to wonder why that person simply cannot snap out of it. If a family member feels this way, it might help to compare the situation to someone with diabetes. Individuals with diabetes have a reduced level of insulin. They cannot just snap out of it, and nor can a depressed person with changed levels of brain chemicals. On the other hand, just as the person with diabetes is not powerless, neither is the person who is depressed. For example, individuals with diabetes who will not adhere to a diabetic diet or take medications as prescribed can make their condition become worse. So, too, the individual with depression might need to avoid certain substances, associations, and situations.

*SSRIs,* Selective serotonin reuptake inhibitors; *TCAs,* tricyclic antidepressants.

---

These themes complement the common suicidal expressions of a loss of self-esteem, a cry for help, or suicide as a threat. Hendin (1986) underscored that suicidal patients view and use death differently than other people. Suicidal patients tend to use their own death to control others and to maintain control over their own lives. Hence, death is viewed as a means of ensuring control.

## SUICIDE AND OLDER ADULTS

The suicide rate for the general population is 11 per 100,000 (CDC, 1999). The rate for men over age 65 is 28.8 per 100,000. Caucasian men over age 50 account for 10% of the population but 30% of the suicides (CDC, 2000; Anonymous, 2003b). This age group has a high attempt-to-completion ratio that is accounted for probably by the seriousness of the intent and the lethality (guns are used often) of the means (Mellick et al, 1992). Whereas the general attempt-to-completion ratio is 7:1, the ratio is 2:1 in older adults (Gomez and Gomez, 1993). Although the upsurge in recent years of suicide among the young has resulted in much media coverage, the suicide rate among older adults is higher. Young people might use the suicide gesture as a cry for help; older people might just want to die, and they often do.

## ASSESSMENT OF SUICIDAL PATIENTS

It is important for the nurse to assess the suicidal potential of psychiatric patients because these patients are at an increased risk of suicide. Most facilities provide the nurse with a format for evaluating suicidal lethality. The crucial variables are the plan, the method, and the provision for rescue.

### Plan

The more developed is the plan, the high is the risk of suicide. People who have carefully developed a suicidal plan are more serious about suicide and present a higher risk compared with those who have no plan. Although impulsive suicide attempts can result in death, generally they are less often lethal because the lack of planning sometimes foils the effort.

### Method

Some methods of attempting suicide are more lethal than are others. Accessibility of the means to commit suicide is important as well. Having three bottles of pills on hand is more lethal compared with having to make an appointment with a doctor to ask for a prescription. A crucial factor in determining the lethality of a particular method is the amount of time between initiation of the suicide method and delivery of the lethal impact of that method. For instance, the person using a gun has no opportunity to avoid the bullet once the trigger is pulled. On the other hand, sitting in the garage with the motor running affords some time to choose an alternative to self-destruction, as does taking an overdose of certain drugs. Lethal methods of suicide include the use of guns (91%), jumping from high places, drowning (84%), hanging (82%), carbon monoxide poisoning and other gases (64%), and overdose with certain drugs (e.g., barbiturates, alcohol, several central nervous system depressants) (Miller et al, 2004). Methods that are less likely to be lethal include wrist cutting and overdosing on aspirin or Valium.

### Rescue

The person who deliberately attempts to deceive would-be rescuers has an increased lethality potential. For instance, a woman who says she is going to the ocean for the weekend and then drives to the mountains makes it difficult for family and friends to intervene. A person who leaves a note or makes a telephone call before making an attempt is more likely to be rescued.

In summary, the more detailed the plan, the more lethal and accessible the method, and the more effort exerted to block rescue, the greater the likelihood will be of the suicidal effort being successful. However, impulsive efforts of suicidal individuals with rescuers in sight have proved fatal, particularly when a lethal method (e.g., a gun) has been selected.

## SUICIDE INTERVENTIONS

### Face-to-Face

In working face-to-face with suicidal patients, some general guidelines are useful for the nurse.

1. Suspect suicidal ideation in most depressed patients (USDHHS, 1993).
2. Ask patients if they plan to hurt themselves. It is important for the nurse to understand the following:
   a. Talking to patients about their suicidal intentions will not drive them to suicide. Asking patients directly provides useful information and often provides patients with a sense of relief—for example, "Finally, someone hears me."
   b. Many people who have died from suicide did not mean to die; they tragically miscalculated. It can be said accurately that many people who die from suicide do so accidentally. The nurse must take all suicidal threats seriously.
3. If a patient is considering suicide, the nurse should ask about the plan (when and where), method, and how the patient intends to accomplish the suicide. (Is the plan to frustrate rescue attempts?) If the patient wants to use a gun, ask someone at the patient's home to remove the gun. If the patient plans to overdose, ask someone in the home to throw away the pills. Do not offer a weekend pass to this patient. Some clinicians believe that if the method of choice can be blocked, many suicidal patients will not use another method. For example, a woman who might use a drug overdose would not consider jumping off a building.

4. Ask about previous suicide attempts. Ask about the when and the how. How did the patient feel concerning rescue? How was the response to treatment? Previous attempts put individuals at an increased risk.

5. Evaluate patients for depression, recent loss or threat of loss, self-destructive hallucinations, and alcohol or drug use, all of which place individuals at an increased risk for suicide.

6. Once patients are hospitalized, many units protect them by using one of two levels of suicide prevention:

   a. Frequent observation (sometimes referred to as level 1) is used for patients who are not considered to be at immediate risk of suicide. The nursing staff provides periodic observation (every 10 minutes) and monitors drug taking, eating utensils, shaving gear, and other potentially dangerous devices in the environment. The staff communicates concern and control with this close observation of patients and their environment. Patients are asked to sign a contract with the staff stating that they will not harm themselves during hospitalization and will seek out a staff member should they begin to contemplate self-injurious behavior. Clinicians are divided in their view of the efficacy of no-suicide contracts (Valente, 1997).

   b. Continuous observation (sometimes referred to as level 2) is used for patients who present an immediate and serious threat of suicidal behavior. Level 2 also might be initiated for patients who refuse to sign a no-suicide contract. Restraints might be used occasionally, as can neuroleptic drugs. Continuous observation is typically required. This approach is an expensive use of human resources but provides the needed control and human interaction. Patients at serious risk are usually confined to the unit and have restrictions on visitors, where meals are taken, and so on. Harmful objects are removed from the environment.

## Over the Telephone

Former patients frequently call the psychiatric unit or outpatient clinic in which psychiatric nurses work. Helpful guidelines for nurses who work with suicidal individuals over the telephone are as follows (Green and Wilson, 1988):

1. Express genuine concern and a desire to work with callers. ("Let's see what we can do.") Give callers your full attention.

2. Acknowledge how difficult and painful recent losses must be. ("It's been a tough time for you lately.")

3. Assess lethality, especially if the suicidal attempt has begun.

4. Focus on the healthy side of callers. ("You called for help. That tells me you want help, and that's what we want to do.")

5. Ask about alcohol or drug use. If available, these substances increase the lethality level.

6. Ask callers for their ideas about immediate solutions to the current situation. Assess feasibility, appropriateness, and availability. Suggest alternatives if needed.

7. Obtain each caller's name, telephone number, address, and whereabouts during the call. Ask callers how they want to be addressed. ("Your name is Mr. Robert Smith. What would you like me to call you?")

8. If other staff members are available, the nurse might need to direct them to notify the police or send an ambulance. Ask for consent to do so or, at least, inform the caller of the plan.

9. Ask if anyone is with the caller. If someone is present, ask to speak to that person to obtain assistance in planning instructions.

10. If family members can be reached, they should be asked to go to the caller and intervene, if it is safe to do so (ask for caller consent).

11. Refer callers to walk-in crisis services or a regular outpatient counselor.

12. If a caller refuses further help, give the telephone number of a crisis center or a suicide prevention hotline.

## Study Notes

1. Major depression and dysthymia are the most significant depressive disorders.

2. The *DSM-IV-TR* defines major depression as an episode of depression (apathy, weight changes, sleep changes, psychomotor changes,

fatigue, feelings of worthlessness or guilt, decreased cognitive ability, and recurrent thoughts of death) without a history of manic episodes.

3. Dysthymia is characterized by its chronicity.

4. Reacting to a disappointment or loss with sadness, guilt, or depression is normal; however, if any of these reactions persist too long, then a diagnosable condition (either dysthymia or major depression) exists.

5. A high correlation exists between depression and suicide.

6. There are several variants of major depression, including atypical depression, melancholic depression, catatonic depression, postpartum depression, psychotic depression, and seasonal depression.

7. Depression is common in the United States. Women have a lifetime risk of 10% to 20%. Men have a lifetime risk of about 5% to 10%.

8. A number of early life traumas are associated with depression in children.

9. People from different ethnic and cultural groups might experience depression differently.

10. Objective signs of depression include alterations in activity and social interactions.

11. Subjective symptoms of depression include alterations in affect, cognition, physical nature (somatic concerns), and perception.

12. Biologic explanations for depression include neurotransmitter, genetic, endocrine, and circadian rhythm dysfunctions. Psychodynamic explanations concern debilitating early life experiences, intrapsychic conflicts, and reaction to life events.

13. Assessment of depression includes consideration of cultural influences, age (older adults are particularly vulnerable), nonbiologic standardized tests, and biologic indices (DST, growth hormone tests, and polysomnography).

14. Psychotherapeutic management includes developing a therapeutic nurse-patient relationship, administering antidepressant drugs when appropriate, and providing a well-managed milieu with particular emphasis on safety.

15. The psychiatric nurse should suspect suicidal ideation in most depressed patients because suicide is a prevalent theme among this population.

16. The prototypical suicide victim is an unemployed Caucasian man living alone. Over 70% of all suicides are committed by Caucasian men. Elderly men are at particularly high risk.

17. In assessing the lethality of suicide consider the plan, the method, and the prevention of rescue.

18. It is important to ask depressed patients whether they are contemplating suicide. Asking this question will not drive the patient to suicide.

19. Psychiatric inpatient units typically have two levels of suicide contracts. Level 1 usually involves checking on the patient every 10 minutes. Level 2 usually involves continuous direct observation of the patient.

20. Both face-to-face and telephone strategies are important for the nurse to use in working with suicidal patients.

## References

Abramson LY, Seligman ME, Teasdale JD: Learned helplessness in humans: critique and reformulation, *J Abnorm Psychol* 87:48, 1978.

American Psychiatric Association: *Diagnostic and statistical manual of mental disorders, text revision,* ed 4, Washington, DC, 2001, APA.

American Psychiatric Association: Practice guidelines for major depressive disorder in adults, *Am J Psychiatry* 150(Suppl):1, 1993.

Anonymous: Atypical depression. *Harv Ment Health Lett* 22:1, 2005.

Anonymous: Confronting suicide: Part I, *Harv Ment Health Lett* 19:1, 2003a.

Anonymous: Depression in old age. *Harvard Ment Health Lett* 20:5, 2003b.

Beck AT: *Cognitive therapies and the emotional disorders,* New York, 1976, International Universities Press.

Beck AT: *Depression: causes and treatment,* Philadelphia, 1991, University Press.

Beeber LS: Depression in women. In McBride AB, Austin JS, editors: *Psychiatric mental health nursing: integrating the behavioral and biological sciences* (pp. 235-268), Philadelphia, 1996, WB Saunders.

Belcher JVR, Holdcraft C: Web-based information for depression: helpful or hazardous? *J Am Psychiatric Assoc* 7:61, 2001.

Centers for Disease Control and Prevention: *Suicide and suicidal behavior: fact book for year 2001-2002.* Available at http://www.CDCgov/ncipc/fact_book/26_Suicide.htm. Accessed May 3, 2002.

Clark DC, Young MA, Scheftner WA, et al: A field test of Motto's risk estimator for suicide, *Am J Psychiatry* 144:923, 1987.

Cockerman WC: *Sociology of mental disorder,* ed 3, Englewood Cliffs, NJ, 1992, Prentice-Hall.

Cugino A, Markovich EI, Rosenblatt S, et al: Searching for a pattern: repeat suicide attempts, *J Psychosoc Nurs Ment Health Serv* 30:23, 1992.

Depression Guideline Panel: *Depression in primary care. Detection and diagnosis,* vol 1, Washington, DC, 1993, U.S. Government Printing Office (DHHS Publ. No. 93-0550).

Dubovsky SL: Beyond the serotonin reuptake inhibitors: rationales for the development of new serotonergic agents, *J Clin Psychiatry* 55(Suppl 2):34, 1994.

Duman RF, Heninger CR, Nestler EJ: A molecular and cellular theory of depression, *Arch Gen Psychiatry* 54:597, 1997.

Freud S: *Mourning and melancholia,* vol 14, London, 1957, Hogarth Press.

Gomez GE, Gomez EA: Depression in the elderly, *J Psychosoc Nurs Ment Health Serv* 31:28, 1993.

Green LW, Wilson CR: Guidelines for nonprofessionals who receive suicidal phone calls, *Hosp Community Psychiatry* 39:310, 1988.

Grunebaum H, Cohler B: Children of parents hospitalized for mental illness. I. Attentional and interactional studies. In Frank M, editor: *Children of exceptional parents,* New York, 1983, Haworth.

Hendin H: Suicide: a review of new directions in research, *Hosp Community Psychiatry* 37:148, 1986.

Jancin B: Insomnia might blunt response to antidepressants, *Clin Psychiatry News* 33:53, 2005.

Jones RL, editor: *Handbook of tests and measurements for black populations,* vols 1, 2, Hampton, VA, 1996, Cobb & Henry.

Keltner NL, Hogan B, Guy DM: Dopaminergic and serotonergic receptor function in the CNS, *Perspect Psychiatric Care* 37:65, 2001a.

Keltner NL, Hogan B, Knight T, Royals LA: Adrenergic, cholinergic, GABAergic, and glutaminergic receptor function in the CNS, *Perspect Psychiatric Care* 37:140, 2001b.

Kennedy R, Suttenfeld K: Postpartum depression, *Medscape Ment Health* 6:1, 2001. Available at www.medscape.com/viewarticle408688. Accessed April 25, 2006.

Kessler RC, Berglund P, Demler O, et al: The epidemiology of major depressive disorder: results from the National Comorbidity Survey Replication, *JAMA* 289:3095, 2003.

Klerman GL: The interpersonal model. In Mann JJ, editor: *Models of depressive disorders,* New York, 1989, Plenum Press.

Maes M, D'Hondt P, Blockx P, Cosyns P: A further investigation of basal HPT axis function in unipolar depression: effects of diagnosis, hospitalization, and dexamethasone administration, *Psychiatry Res* 51:185, 1994.

Mann JJ: Brain biology influences the risk for suicide, *The decade of the brain,* Arlington, Va, *NAMI* 8:3, 1998.

McEnany GW: *Neuropsychiatric disorders: dementia versus depression versus drug intoxication.* Presented at the Contemporary Forum's Tenth Anniversary Conference on Psychiatric Nursing, Boston, May 1995a.

McEnany GW: *Restless nights: understanding and treating sleep disturbances.* Presented at the Contemporary Forum's Tenth Anniversary Conference on Psychiatric Nursing, Boston, May 1995b.

McGrath E, editor: *Women and depression: risk factors and treatment issues,* Washington, DC, 1992, American Psychological Association.

Mellick E, Buckwalter KC, Stolley JM: Suicide among elderly white men: development of a profile, *J Psychosoc Nurs Ment Health Serv* 30:29, 1992.

Miller M, Azrael D, Hemenway D: The epidemiology of case fatality rates for suicide in the northeast, *Ann Emerg Med* 43:723, 2004.

Moscicki EK: Epidemiology of completed and attempted suicide: toward a framework for prevention, *Clin Neurosci Res,* 2001.

National Institute of Mental Health: Depression information. Available at http:/www.nimh.nih.gov/healthinformation/depressionmenu.cfm. Accessed May 3, 2006.

Nemeroff CB: The neurobiology of depression, *Sci Am* 278:42, 1998.

News and Notes: Cost of depression estimated at nearly $44 billion: time lost from work accounts for largest share, *Hosp Community Psychiatry* 45:85, 1994.

Pearson J: Suicide in the United States, *The decade of the brain,* Arlington, VA, *NAMI* 8:1, 1998.

Schreiber R: Wandering in the dark: women's experiences with depression, *Health Care Women Int* 22:85, 2001.

Schwartz TL: Unipolar, bipolar, and psychotic depression, *Clin Psychiatry News* 33(Suppl):1, 3, 2005.

Shuchter SR, Downs N, Zisook S: *Biologically informed psychotherapy for depression,* New York, 1996, Guilford Press.

Soares JC, Mann JJ: The anatomy of mood disorders: review of structural neuroimaging studies, *Biol Psychiatry* 41:86, 1997a.

Soares JC, Mann JJ: The functional neuroanatomy of mood disorders, *J Psychiatr Res* 31:397, 1997b.

Solomon D, Laraia MT: Pregnancy and postpartum psychiatric disorders. Part I: SSRIs, depression, and anxiety, *APNA News* 17:12, 2005.

Splete H: VNS therapy is approved for severe depression, *Clin Psychiatry News* 33:1, 2005.

Stahl SM: Blue genes and the monoamine hypothesis of depression, *J Clin Psychiatry* 61:77, 2000.

Tseng W, Streltzer J: *Culture and psychopathology: a guide to clinical assessment,* New York, 1997, Brunner/Mazel.

U.S. Department of Health and Human Services: *Depression in primary care, treatment of major depression,* vol 2, Washington DC, 1993, USDHHS.

U.S. Surgeon General: *Mental health: a report of the Surgeon General,* Washington, DC, 1999, Department of Health and Human Services.

Valente SM: Preventing suicide among elderly people, *Am J Nurse Pract* 1:15, 1997.

Venarec E: Depression in the workforce. Part I, *Business Health* 4:48, 2000.

Warren BJ: Depression, stressful life events, social support, and self-esteem in middle class African American women, *Arch Psychiatr Nurs* 11:107, 1997.

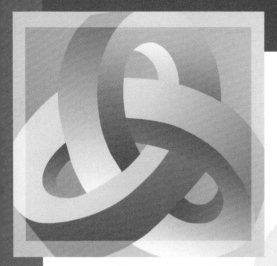

# Chapter 30

# Bipolar Disorders

*Norman L. Keltner*

## Learning Objectives

*After reading this chapter, you should be able to:*
- Recognize the *DSM-IV-TR* criteria and terminology for bipolar disorder.
- Describe the objective and subjective symptoms of bipolar disorder.
- Explain the biologic and psychodynamic hypotheses for bipolar disorder.
- Describe the psychotherapeutic management issues related to bipolar disorder.
- Formulate a nursing care plan for bipolar disorder using the psychotherapeutic management model.

*Nothing is more addictive than the high of a manic euphoria. Once you have tasted that soaring, exhilarating, invincible, phantasmagorical feeling of, "It's great to be me! I can do anything!," once you've experienced the rush of your mind in overdrive, the creativity pouring through it, the connectivity of burgeoning lateral thinking, the ridiculous ease of witty repartee, the unutterable knowledge of your own immensity, your own infinity, then life without another mania is a dreary prospect indeed.*

M. Orum (1996)

## GENERAL DESCRIPTION OF BIPOLAR DISORDER

Bipolar disorders are those in which individuals experience the extremes of mood polarity. Individuals might feel very euphoric or very depressed. It should be noted that a depressive episode is not required for this diagnosis, but a manic episode is required.

Box 30-1 lists the symptoms likely to occur in either a manic episode or a depressive episode. Bipolar disorder can be traced from earliest recorded history to the present day. Thousands of years ago, the Greeks recognized the vacillation between extremes of elation and depression. Other people have also observed and recorded wide mood swings for the historic record. Although the term *bipolar disorder* is the accepted diagnostic terminology, many professionals, and much professional literature, still use the terms *manic-depressive* or *bipolar affective disorder*. Accordingly, the terms are used somewhat interchangeably in this chapter.

Epidemiologic research has indicated that about 5 million women and men in this country will experience bipolar disorders yearly, about 2.6% of the adult population (Kessler et al, 2005a). Of these, a little over 1.2% of the population suffers from the more debilitating bipolar I disorder. Another 2% have what has been referred to as *subthreshold bipolar disorder*. This simply means that a large number of people do not meet the criteria for a diagnosis but nonetheless experience distressing symptoms (Zoler, 2005a). Approximately 3.9% of the population will have bipolar disorders at some point during their lifetime (APA, 2000; Kessler et al, 2005b). (See Box 30-2: Facts About Bipolar Disorder.)

Like schizophrenia, onset tends to be in the early 20s and, for 90% of these individuals, symptoms will be recurrent. The few who have a later onset typically experience a less severe course (Moon, 2005). Bipolar I disorders appear to be equally common among men and women but with evidence of a difference in order of expression. In men, the first episode is more likely to be a manic episode, but for both women and men, depression is more likely to be experienced first (APA, 2002). There is however, evidence to support the belief that pregnancy often causes relapse in women with a history of bipolar disorder (Zoler, 2005b). There are no reports of differential incidence based on ethnic or racial groupings. Some individuals are often misdiagnosed as suffering from schizophrenia when a diagnosis of bipolar disorder would be more appropriate. This misdiagnosis is understandable, because these two disorders share common characteristics (Sherman, 2005). Table 30-1 outlines these similarities.

### Norm's Notes

This is a fascinating subject. Note Ms. Orum's quote at the beginning of the chapter. She is honest—she was addicted to the euphoric highs of manic depression. When you meet persons with this condition, you might be intimidated because they are moving so fast mentally. Their thoughts can fly so quickly that you cannot keep up, but you are there to be therapeutic. Don't feel bad, because this is where your instructor really needs to give you guidance. Talking to a person in a manic state is one of the most challenging situations in psychiatric nursing.

## DSM-IV-TR TERMINOLOGY AND CRITERIA

The *DSM-IV-TR* defines several variations under the category of bipolar disorders, as previously noted. To understand the *DSM-IV-TR* diagnostic categories, the student must be able to distinguish the basic syndromes presented, such as the manic episode and the hypomanic episode.

---

### Box 30-1    Symptoms Occurring During Manic and Depressive Episodes

**Manic Episode**
Elevated mood
Grandiosity, inflated self-esteem
Irritability
Anger
Insomnia
Anorexia
Flamboyant gestures
Flight of ideas, racing thoughts
Distractibility
Hyperactivity
Involvement in pleasurable activities
Loud, rapid speech; talkative
High energy
Increased interest in sex
High rate of suicide
Excessive makeup

***Other Symptoms***
Labile mood
Delusions
Hallucinations
Depressed mood
Low self-esteem

**Depressive Episode**
Withdrawal
Passivity
Insomnia, daytime sleepiness
Anorexia
Sluggish thinking
Difficulty concentrating, distractibility
Inertia
Diminished interest in activities, inappropriate or excessive guilt
Decrease in speech
Fatigue
Decreased interest in sex
High rate of suicide

***Other Symptoms***
Memory loss
Abnormal thoughts about death
Weight loss

## 12-Month Prevalence Rate of Mental Disorders in the United States*

| Disorders | Approximate Percentage Over 17 Years of Age | Approximate Number of Persons | Gender Overrepresentation |
|---|---|---|---|
| **Anxiety Disorders** | 18 overall | 36,000,000 | |
| Panic disorder | 3.5 | 7,000,000 | Women |
| Social phobia | 7 | 14,000,000 | Women |
| Specific phobia | 8.7 | 17,000,000 | Women |
| GAD | 3 | 6,000,000 | Women |
| PTSD | 3.5 | 7,000,000 | Women |
| OCD | 1 | 2,000,000 | Equal |
| **Mood Disorders** | 9.5 overall | 19,000,000 | |
| Major depression | 6.7 | | Women |
| Dysthymia | 1.5 | | Women |
| Bipolar I and II | 2.6 | | BD I: Equal |
| | | | BD II: Women? |
| **Impulse Control Disorders** | 9 overall | 18,000,000 | |
| Conduct disorders | 1 | 2,000,000 | Men |
| ADHD | 4 | 8,000,000 | Men |
| **Substance Abuse Disorders** | 3.8 overall | 7,600,000 | |
| Alcohol abuse and dependence | 3.1 | 6,200,000 | Men |
| Drug abuse and dependence | 1.4 | 2,800,000 | Men |
| **Schizophrenia** | 1.1 | 2,100,000 | Equal |

*Extrapolated from several sources based on current census data.
*ADHD,* Attention-deficit/hyperactivity disorder; *GAD,* generalized anxiety disorder; *OCD,* obsessive-compulsive disorder; *PTSD,* posttraumatic stress disorder.
From Kessler RC, Chiu WT, Demler O, Walters EE: Prevalence, severity, and comorbidity of 12-month DSM-IV disorders in the national comorbidity survey replication, *Arch Gen Psychiatry* 62:617, 2005; U.S. Surgeon General: *Mental health: a report from the Surgeon General,* Washington, DC, 1999, Department of Health and Human Services: National Institute of Mental Health: *Statistics.* Available at: www.nimh.nih.gov/healthinformation/statisticsmenu.cfm. Accessed April 18, 2005.

---

### Box 30-2    Facts About Bipolar Disorder

1. Average age of onset is early 20s for both men and women.
2. Bipolar I disorder occurs equally in men and women.
3. Women might have a higher rate of bipolar II disorder
4. Over 1.2% of the adult population suffers from bipolar I disorder in a given year.
5. Over 2.6% of the adult population suffers from all bipolar disorders in a given year.
6. About 15% of bipolar patients will die at their own hands.
7. About 90% will experience a future episode.
8. Untreated, a person might experience 10 or more episodes over a lifetime.
9. It runs in families.
10. Sixty percent experience chronic interpersonal and occupational difficulties.

Modified from American Psychiatric Association: Practice guidelines for the treatment of patients with bipolar disorder, *Am J Psychiatry* 159(Suppl 4):16, 2002.

---

### Table 30-1    Similarities Between Bipolar I Disorder and Schizophrenia

| | Bipolar I | Schizophrenia |
|---|---|---|
| Gender affected | Equal | Equal |
| Mean age of onset | 20s | 20s |
| Genetic factors | Yes | Yes |
| One affected parent | 25% risk | 15% risk |
| Two parents | 50% risk | 35% risk |
| Identical twin | 40%-70% | 50% |
| Course | Chronic | Chronic |
| Suicide | 15% | 10% |
| Cigarette smoking | Increased | Increased |
| Substance abuse | Increased | Increased |
| Ventricular enlargement | Yes | Yes |
| Hippocampal volume | Reduced | Reduced |
| Very sensitive to stress | Yes | Yes |

Modified from Sherman C: Schizophrenia-bipolar I theory gains traction, *Clin Psychiatry News* 33:27, 2005.

## DSM-IV-TR and NANDA International Diagnoses Related to Mood Disorders

*DSM-IV-TR**
Bipolar I disorder
Bipolar II disorder
Cyclothymic disorder
Dysthymic disorder
Major depressive disorder

NANDA INTERNATIONAL†
Anxiety
Communication, verbal, impaired
Coping, ineffective
Grieving, anticipatory
Grieving, dysfunctional
Hopelessness
Injury, risk for
Nutrition: less than body requirements, imbalanced
Powerlessness
Self-care deficit, bathing/hygiene
Self-care deficit, dressing/grooming
Self-care deficit, feeding
Self-care deficit, toileting
Sexual dysfunction
Sleep patterns, disturbed
Social isolation
Thought processes, disturbed
Violence, self-directed, risk for

*Modified from the American Psychiatric Association: *Diagnostic and statistical manual of mental disorders*, ed 4, *text revision*, Washington, DC, 2000, APA.
†NANDA International: *NANDA nursing diagnoses: definitions and classifications, 2005-2006*, Philadelphia, 2005, NANDA International.

### CRITICAL THINKING QUESTION    1

Can a person fall within the bipolar spectrum but not meet the *DSM-IV-TR* criteria for bipolar disorder?

## MANIC EPISODES

Manic episodes are characterized by an elevated, expansive, or irritable mood and are fundamental to the diagnosis of bipolar I disorder. To meet diagnostic criteria, the symptoms must persist for at least 1 week (or shorter if hospitalization is required). Symptoms are listed in Box 30-1. Manic episodes usually begin suddenly, escalate rapidly, and last from a few days to several months. Judgment is impaired, social blunders occur, and

### Box 30-3    Medical Conditions That Cause Mania

Anoxia
Hyperthyroidism
Hemodialysis
Lyme disease
Hypercalcemia
Acquired immunodeficiency syndrome
Stroke
Brain tumor
Multiple sclerosis
Normal-pressure hydrocephalus
Other neurologic disorders

From Keltner NL, Folks DG: *Psychotropic drugs*, ed 3, St. Louis, 2005, Mosby.

involvement with alcohol and drugs is common. Onset is usually in the early 20s. Individuals experiencing a manic episode have an inflated view of their importance, sometimes reaching grandiosity. ("I'm so important that the President needs my advice on international affairs"). The impairment is sufficiently serious that functioning deteriorates at home, work, school, or in social contexts. Other symptoms include a decreased need for sleep, talkativeness, racing thoughts, and distractibility. The mind seems to go faster and faster. Individuals experiencing a manic episode might engage in risky behavior, such as sexual relationships that are not in keeping with their normal conduct. People might speculate on a risky business venture because they understand the big picture of business. People have lost everything in these periods of manic thinking. Excess is common: spending sprees, sexual indiscretions, loud clothing, and excessive make-up are often seen in individuals in a manic state. Hospitalization is frequently required to prevent harm to the person or to others. Manic episodes can also be part of other mental disorders or a general medical condition (Box 30-3; Keltner and Folks, 2005), or might be substance-induced (Box 30-4).

Fieve (1975), in his highly respected book, *Moodswings*, pointed out that many creative people in this society ride the energy from their manic state to success. Fieve noted that successful producer Joshua Logan (the musical, *South Pacific*) and astronaut Buzz Aldrin (first moon landing) used the tremendous energy from their elevated moods for great accomplishments. Unfortunately, for patients suffering from a manic episode, the climb up the emotional ladder does not stop with elation, and excessive energy moves into psychotic think-

## DSM-IV-TR Criteria for Bipolar Disorders

I. Manic episode:
  A. A distinct period of abnormal and persistent elevated, expansive, or irritable mood that lasts at least 1 week (or less if hospitalization is required).
  B. At least three of the following symptoms must occur during the episode (or four if the patient is only irritable).
    1. Inflated self-esteem or grandiosity
    2. Decreased need for sleep
    3. Very talkative
    4. Flight of ideas or subjective feeling that thoughts are racing
    5. Distractibility
    6. Increase in goal-directed activity (social, occupational, educational, or sexual) or psychomotor agitation
    7. Excessive involvement in pleasurable activities that have a high potential for personal problems (e.g., sexual promiscuity, spending sprees, bad business investments)
  C. Mood disturbance severe enough to cause problems socially, interpersonally, or at work, or the person has to be hospitalized to prevent harm to self or others
  D. Not due to a substance

II. Hypomanic episode: The person experiencing a hypomanic episode meets most of the criteria for manic episode, with two major exceptions: the symptoms must be present "only" 4 days and the person must manifest an unequivocal change in functioning that is observable by others. A hypomanic episode is not severe enough to result in significant impairment or to require hospitalization.

III. Bipolar disorders:
  A. Bipolar episodes are divided into bipolar I and bipolar II. There are six categories of bipolar I. In bipolar I, the patient must have a history of a manic episode.
  B. Bipolar II: The patient has experienced major depression and a hypomanic episode (but not a manic episode)

IV. Cyclothymic disorder: For a period of 2 years, the patient has had numerous periods of hypomanic symptoms and numerous periods of a depressed mood. The patient is never symptom-free for more than 2 months at a time. The patient has never experienced major depression.

Modified from the American Psychiatric Association: *Diagnostic and statistical manual of mental disorders, text revision,* ed 4, Washington, DC, 2000, APA.

---

### Box 30-4    Drugs That Can Cause Mania

Antidepressants
Steroids
Anticholinergics
Stimulants

---

ing and unacceptable behavior. In addition, an equally extreme depression can follow these highs. Both Logan and Aldrin required professional help to restore their moods to normal. Other famous people known to have suffered with bipolar disorder include Kurt Cobain (singer), Patty Duke (actress), Carrie Fisher (actress), Robin Givens (actress), Jimi Hendrix (singer), Margot Kidder (actress), Jane Pauley (television personality), and Ben Stiller (actor) (wikipedia: List of people . . . , 2005).

The following clinical example outlines the success and then the failure of a successful businessman.

## CLINICAL EXAMPLE

Bill Smith is a 50-year-old former chief executive officer of a computer software company. Mr. Smith built the company from scratch into a multimillion dollar-a-year endeavor. In fact, it was Mr. Smith's second time to develop a profitable business from the ground up. In the late 1980s, while in his early 30s, Mr. Smith left a nationally recognized computer company and went into business on his own. Within 3 years, his company was remarkably profitable with what seemed as unlimited potential. Four years later, the business was bankrupt. He started the second business in 1998 and experienced even more success with it. Eventually, the new business became insolvent as well. The reason that both businesses failed is directly linked to Mr. Smith's bipolar disorder. Although he credits the energy and goal-directed drive associated with the illness for helping him achieve great success, grandiose (e.g., unwarranted expansion, excessive spending) and unrealistic (e.g., he believed the government could not function without his computer applications) thinking eventually drove his business into the ground. As he puts it, "I also lost two business, two wives, and three children because of this illness." Both episodes of bipolar disorder required hospitalization.

Mr. Smith has never really recovered from the financial and personal setbacks of his last nervous breakdown. He now lives in a county-operated apartment complex with other people who suffer from persistent mental disorder. Mr. Smith has a limited income and, although significantly improved, continues to display mood lability and other residual symptoms. He volunteers at a community mental health center and acknowledges that he most likely will never be a wheeler-dealer again. He is able to laugh about the good old days, when he would drive into a Cadillac dealership and buy two cars, one for himself and one for his girlfriend of the moment.

## HYPOMANIC EPISODES

*My manias, at least in their early and mild forms, were absolutely intoxicating states that gave rise to great personal pleasure, an incomparable flow of thoughts, and a ceaseless energy that allowed the translation of new ideas into papers and projects.*

Dr. Kay Redfield Jamison (1997, pp 5-6)

The hypomanic episode is similar to the manic episode but denotes a less severe level of impairment. Because patients feel good about themselves and their life, hypomania is perceived as normal. Both bipolar II disorder and cyclothymia diagnoses require evidence of a hypomanic episode. Because the level of severity is somewhat subjective, the *DSM-IV-TR* attempts to differentiate hypomanic from manic episodes with more objective criteria. For a hypomanic episode to be diagnosed, the length of the episode must be at least 4 days in duration, but not severe enough to warrant hospitalization. Additionally, the episode is not severe enough to cause major problems at home, work, school, or in the social milieu, but is observable by others and is distinct from the person's typical behavior. The episode is characterized by an abnormal period of persistent elevated, expansive, or irritable mood. Furthermore,

the individual must experience at least three of the following symptoms:

- Increased self-esteem or grandiosity
- Decreased need for sleep
- Subjective sense that thoughts are racing
- Distractibility
- Increase in goal-directed activity (usually social, occupational, educational, or sexual) or motor agitation
- Excessive involvement in pleasurable activities that have a high potential for painful consequences

At times, it can be difficult to distinguish severe hypomania from mania.

## DEPRESSIVE EPISODES

Bipolar depression differs from unipolar (regular major depression) in some significant ways. First, depressive symptoms tend to be atypical. That is, the patient experiences hypersomnia, not insomnia, hyperphagia, not anorexia, and weight gain, not weight loss. Furthermore, the person might develop an absolute craving for carbohydrates and might experience a leaden paralysis, with little energy to propel himself or herself around (Swann et al, 2005). Bipolar depression typically develops at a younger age than unipolar depression and the patient is more likely to express paranoid thoughts, be irritable, and experience hallucinations (Cassano et al, 2004).

## BIPOLAR DISORDERS

The *DSM-IV-TR* bipolar diagnoses are based on an understanding of manic episodes, hypomanic episodes, and major depression. As noted, the *DSM-IV-TR* divides bipolar diagnoses into bipolar I, bipolar II, cyclothymic disorders, and bipolar disorder NOS. There are six variants of bipolar I disorder, one type of bipolar II disorder, and one type of cyclothymic disorder. Bipolar disorder NOS is not discussed here.

### BIPOLAR DIAGNOSES

#### Bipolar I Disorder

Bipolar I disorder is the most significant of these disorders. In bipolar I, the patient experiences

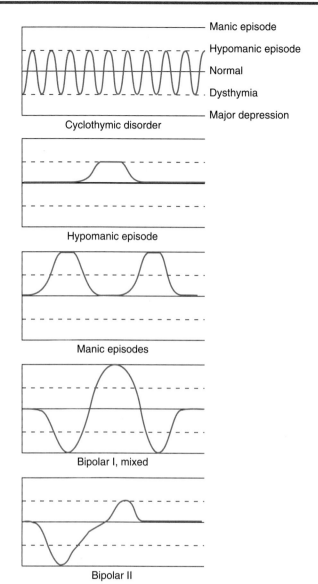

Cyclothymic disorder

Hypomanic episode

Manic episodes

Bipolar I, mixed

Bipolar II

**FIGURE 30-1** Differences in the bipolar disorders on the mood continuum. By understanding this figure, the student will be able to conceptualize the differences among these bipolar disorders.

- Bipolar I disorder, most recent episode mixed (both manic and depressive symptoms)
- Bipolar I disorder, most recent episode depressed
- Bipolar I disorder, most recent episode unspecified

Although it is not important for you as a student to memorize these six variants of bipolar I, take time to contemplate each one and the significance of that level of specificity. Perhaps an additional word is warranted for the bipolar I mixed subtype. This disorder is characterized by both manic and depressive symptoms. In other words, the person is moving 90 miles an hour but is still depressed.

A designation of *rapid cycling* is given if four or more episodes of mania and depression have occurred in 1 year (APA, 2000; Kuyler, 1988).

### Bipolar II Disorder

Bipolar II disorder is similar to bipolar I disorder, with the major exception being that the person has never experienced a manic episode but only a hypomanic episode. In this disorder, the person has experienced major depression but has experienced a hypomanic episode, rather than a full manic episode on the other side of the mood continuum. There might be a higher incidence of this disorder among women. Over the course of a few years, 5% to 15% of these individuals go on to develop a full manic episode (APA, 2000).

---

**CRITICAL THINKING QUESTION**   **2**

What do you think of the following statement? "There are many people in American society who could be diagnosed as hypomanic. Many high-level, workaholic executives are hypomanic and just don't know it."

---

### Cyclothymic Disorder

Cyclothymic disorder is defined as a swing between a hypomanic episode and depressive symptoms. The swings in either direction are not severe enough to warrant the ultimate diagnoses of manic episode and major depression. Using a pendulum as a metaphor, the person experiencing cyclothymic disorder swings from one side to the other but never reaches the extremes of the arc.

swings between manic episodes (defined earlier) and major depression (defined in Chapter 29). Figure 30-1 illustrates the subtle differences in the bipolar disorders. The bipolar I diagnosis can be based on a single manic episode subtype or on several subtypes. The subtypes are:

- Bipolar I disorder, single manic episode
- Bipolar I disorder, most recent event a manic episode
- Bipolar I disorder, most recent event a hypomanic episode

The person is elated and expansive but does not meet the criteria for manic episode. Cyclothymic disorder is characterized by symptoms that have occurred for at least 2 years, without symptom remission for more than 2 months. The person experiences numerous hypomanic episodes and numerous dysthymic level episodes. Cyclothymic disorder is equally distributed between men and women, with a lifetime risk below 1%. About 15% to 50% of these individuals go on to develop full-blown bipolar disorder (St. John, 2005).

## BEHAVIOR

### Objective Behavior

The person experiencing a manic episode appears enthusiastic and euphoric. Other people around that person recognize these behaviors as excessive. Objective behaviors include disturbances of speech; of the individual's social, interpersonal, and occupational relationships; and of activity and appearance. Accordingly, violent behavior, divorce, spousal and child abuse, job loss, and academic failure are relatively common features of this illness.

---

### CLINICAL EXAMPLE

Sue Miller is a 45-year-old Jewish woman who is admitted for bipolar disorder. Police were called to the Greyhound bus station, where they found Ms. Miller annoying customers. She claimed to be a Messianic Jew and was preaching to anyone who would politely listen. She resisted the officers and repeatedly stated that she was the "woman at the well" and had married Christ. On arriving on the unit, it was noted that Ms. Miller had excessive bright red lipstick on, dramatically enhanced eyebrows, and turquoise eye shadow. The rest of her clothing appeared unattended to, and she was dirty and smelly. She is known to the hospital staff and, after her initial physical assessment, was prescribed and received lithium. This particular drug had been quite effective in the past.

---

### Disturbed Speech Patterns

The following are examples of disturbed speech patterns of manic individuals:

- Rapid speech
- Pressured speech
- Loud speech
- Easily distracted

Manic patients might speak loudly in a rapid-fire fashion; they monopolize the dialogue and deflect attempts by others to contribute to the dialogue. Conversations are filled with jokes and puns. Sarcastic and biting remarks are not uncommon. In fact, even though mental health professionals are aware of this tendency, the ability of manic patients to find a weak spot often frustrates, embarrasses, and angers mental health professionals. The tendency to complain often and loudly is also present. Manic patients have the ability to engage staff members in debate and place them on the defensive. Speech is often dramatic, and it is not uncommon for manic individuals to burst into song. Speech is often pressured (i.e., they have a compulsion or strong need to talk).

These patients also are easily distracted. For example, while in the middle of an apparently meaningful discussion, a patient might be distracted by a bird flying outside the window and change the topic of the conversation to flying. This phenomenon, in which patients jump from topic to topic, is referred to as flight of ideas.

### Altered Social, Interpersonal, and Occupational Relationships

Manic individuals often have changes in their relationship patterns, such as:

- Failed relationships
- Job loss and job failure
- Overbearing behavior
- Increased sex drive
- Alienation of family

---

### CLINICAL EXAMPLE

*Demographics:* A young man (Bob, age 30) and a young woman (Mary, age 26), are engaged, with a wedding date planned for the near future.

*Background:* Both are college-educated, with particularly promising careers.

*The setting:* Mary flies into a rage and breaks off the engagement when Bob asks her if she will let the pets out. Mary leaves for 3 weeks, then returns the day before a relative's funeral. Bob attends with her, and she introduces him as her fiancé.

*The crisis:* After the funeral, she tells Bob: "I got married to my old boyfriend while I was gone. It was a mistake. I went to see my doctor. He thinks I have bipolar disorder."

As this clinical example suggests (Shattell and Keltner, 2004), a manic episode can cause chaos in the life of an individual and those close to that person.

It is not surprising that manic patients irritate others with their impulsive behaviors, fault finding, anger, and blaming. This disorder destroys relationships. Listed here are five tendencies that cause social, interpersonal, and occupational problems (Janowsky et al, 1970):

1. Manipulation of the self-esteem of others. Patients use coercive techniques to increase or decrease another's self-esteem. It is easy to fall prey to the manipulation of praise. ("No one here really understands me but you.") It is just as easy to feel the ego-deflating wrath when plans are thwarted. Some insightful nurses have remarked about feeling like "having been played like a yo-yo."
2. Ability to find vulnerability in others. Manic patients can exploit weakness in others or create conflicts among staff members.
3. Ability to shift responsibility. Through the technique mentioned earlier, patients somehow shift personal responsibility (e.g., being late) to someone else. Nurses are particularly vulnerable in this area because they are trained to take responsibility for many concerns of their patients.
4. Limit testing. Manic patients keep pushing the limits established by the treatment setting. If a limit is relaxed, these patients will push it even more.
5. Alienation of family. Manic patients can drive away their families with their behavior (Dore and Romans, 2001). The cyclic nature of the disorder at first inspires hope in the family. After numerous cycles, families often sink into a demoralized state. Divorce related to child and spousal abuse is not uncommon during severe manic episodes.

The same behaviors that drive away family also drive away friends, lovers, bosses, co-workers, ministers, and nonpsychiatric health care providers.

Several trends have been noted among individuals with bipolar disorder:

1. Failed relationships are common for those who do not receive adequate treatment.
2. Most report difficulties maintaining long-term friendships.
3. Job loss and job change are common.
4. A need to engage people, even strangers, in conversation characterizes bipolar disorder. Although at first behavior such as this attracts others, soon the overbearing and intrusive nature of the conversation alienates and even frightens people.
5. Mood lability can cause these individuals to fall in and out of love rapidly, with all the associated problems for themselves and others.

Obviously, the effects of bipolar illness permeate all types of relationships. The expansive mood overflows into excesses as well. The otherwise faithful spouse might become sexually promiscuous, the otherwise thrifty homemaker might go on a shopping or spending spree, and the conservative investor might make a dangerously speculative investment. Divorce rates are two to three times higher than for comparable couples (APA, 2002).

### Alterations in Activity and Appearance

Manic patients are often hyperactive and agitated. Overt manifestations, such as pacing, flamboyant gestures, colorful dress, singing, and excessive use of makeup, are relatively common. Patients also might dress sloppily and omit personal grooming; they might not need sleep, or perhaps need only a few hours per night. Some patients have gone for days without sleep and, at

### Norm's Notes

*Each semester, a number of my students question why a patient's family is distant or even out of the picture altogether. In other words, some students suspect that the family has abandoned the patient. My advice is something you have heard all your life: there are two sides to every story. Some families give up too easily, and others have exhausted all avenues to make things work—and they didn't work. Right or wrong, many tired and demoralized families have flown a white flag and retreated.*

one time, reports of manic patients dropping from exhaustion were common. Many manic patients suffer from poor nutrition because they stop eating; they simply do not have the patience, the ability to sit still long enough, or the desire to eat.

### Subjective Behavior

#### Alterations of Affect

Manic patients experience euphoria and a high regard for self. The inflated self-image can reach levels of grandiosity. Subjectively, the person going through a manic episode experiences an elevated mood, a feeling of joy, and a sense of greatness. A certain sense of invincibility leads to the social, interpersonal, and occupational problems already discussed.

Another significant symptom is a labile or quickly changing affect. Rapid mood swings are exhibited as changing from elation to irritability or from happiness to anger. For example, a 64-year-old woman was laughing and talking about her personal acquaintance with the president. "You know, my husband's name was George." She abruptly began to cry. "He is dead, you know." She quickly returned to the topic of her importance, becoming very excited, with an elevated mood.

#### Alterations of Perception

Delusions and hallucinations occur, and their content is typically consistent with mood. For example, if a patient is grandiose about his or her importance to the government, a mood-congruent delusion might include paranoid thinking related to being pursued by enemy forces.

## ETIOLOGY

### Psychodynamic Theories

At one time, most psychiatric professionals believed that bipolar illness, or manic-depressive illness, was caused by psychological difficulties. Developmental theorists have hypothesized that faulty family dynamics during early life are responsible for manic behaviors in later life. According to this view, the mother (or primary caregiver) enjoys being the giver of life and resents autonomy. As the child grows more independent, the mother becomes unhappy, so to please the mother, the child becomes more dependent; that is, to gain affection, the child at an early age learns to deny his or her own natural tendencies. The unnatural tension between dependence and independence, and the inherent ambivalence in this family environment, can be a causative factor in bipolar illness, according to this view. Others have suggested that the polar events (e.g., approval or disapproval) of childhood are so significant for some people that an adult emotional counterpart to the emotional roller coaster results—for example, receiving approval (elation) and disapproval (depression). Although some psychodynamic explanations seem more credible than others, many professionals believe that family dynamics plays an important role in the genesis of manic-depressive illness.

Another psychodynamic hypothesis explains manic episodes as a defense against or massive denial of depression. According to this view, manic-depressive individuals go through life appearing to be independent and excessive to others (e.g., too pushy, too talkative, and too manipulative), only to be eventually blocked by someone who no longer tolerates being pushed, talked to, or manipulated. When this happens, the manic individual (who is actually overdependent) might become psychotic.

### Neurotransmitter and Structural Hypotheses

Although some professionals still believe in the importance of psychological influences, most are aware of the role of biology. Just as depression seems to be caused by neurotransmitter deficiency, manic episodes also seem to be related to excessive levels of norepinephrine and dopamine, an imbalance between cholinergic and noradrenergic systems, or a deficiency in serotonin. El-Mallakh (1996) proposed that bipolar disorder, including both manic and depressive symptoms, arises from ion dysregulation. Box 30-5 summarizes this interesting hypothesis. If the ion view is correct, the differences between normal depression (or unipolar depression) and the depression associated with bipolar disorder can be more clearly appreciated. Unfortunately, a common diagnostic mistake is incorrectly diagnosing someone as suffering with major depression when they are actually experiencing the depressive aspect of bipolar disorder. Naturally, prescribing an antidepressant

---

## Box 30-5   What Goes Wrong in Bipolar Disorder

What is known about bipolar disorder is that individuals have specific signs and symptoms (e.g., elevated mood, grandiosity, irritability, insomnia, anorexia). What is not known is exactly what causes this disorder to happen. Thus, the question remains, "What goes wrong in bipolar disorder?" El-Mallakh (1996) proposed a convincing model for the pathology of bipolar disorder, suggesting that a disruption in ion regulation is the cause. Ion regulation is important for normal mood. A key part of ion regulation is the sodium (Na) and potassium (K)–activated adenosine triphosphatase (ATPase) pump. As this chapter will explore, bipolar depression and mania are related, and this model proposes a biochemical explanation.

According to this model, both bipolar depression and mania result from a decrease in Na,K-ATPase activity. As activity declines, neuronal membranes become irritable, requiring fewer stimuli to provoke cell firing. Furthermore, as Na accumulates intracellularly because of this faulty pumping action, hyperpolarizing functions of inhibitory neurotransmitters (e.g., gamma-aminobutyric acid [GABA]) are diminished. Additionally, because neurotransmitter release is calcium-dependent, the presynaptic terminals might release more neurotransmitter because of a related deficiency in Na-dependent calcium efflux. All these factors contribute to increased neurotransmitter release and firing—or mania.

However, the very term *bipolar* means two poles—the pole of mania and the pole of depression. These two poles are related. As the Na,K-ATPase pump continues to decrease in activity, neuronal irritability reaches a point at which less stimulation triggers depolarization. The neuron fires more easily, but the action potential loses amplitude. Hence, this loss of amplitude causes calcium channels to decrease their activity and results in a subsequent reduction in neurotransmitter release. Briefly, mania is the first disorder to occur when ion dysregulation occurs but, as the Na,K-ATPase pump becomes more dysfunctional, the depressive side of bipolar disorder develops. Catatonia might be the ultimate expression of ionic dysregulation (El-Mallakh, 1996).

---

would be appropriate for unipolar depression, but such a treatment strategy is not without controversy when the patient has bipolar depression. Giving an antidepressant to a patient with bipolar depression often pushes the individual into a manic state. Nonetheless, treating bipolar depression with antidepressants is not uncommon but usually tried only after several other options have failed.

Perhaps a more compelling view of altered biochemistry in bipolar disorder has been advanced by Manji and Lenox (2000). They outlined the evidence for a breakdown in the complicated second-messenger systems of neurons. In the multistep second-messenger system, once a neurotransmitter binds to a receptor, intracellular processes are triggered. First, a protein (called a G-protein) attaches to the underbelly of the receptor complex, which in turn triggers the attachment of an enzyme. This enzyme stimulates another intracellular entity (often either cyclic adenosine monophosphate [cAMP] or inositol), which causes the activation of protein kinases that turn on transcription factors in the nucleus. At this point, the transcription factors can instruct genes to synthesize such factors as enzymes, receptors, or reuptake proteins or, in other words, the proteins that cause the neuron to function. Manji and Lenox (2000) show that in bipolar disorder there is greater activity than normal with G-proteins and protein kinases and with other steps in the second-messenger system.

Biologic findings also suggest that lesions are more common in this population in areas of the brain such as the right hemisphere or bilateral subcortical and periventricular gray matter (Moore, et al, 2000; Sherman, 2005). Knowing what to make of these structural findings is difficult, but the neurotransmitter hypotheses are consistent with explanations of the putative mechanisms of some antimanic drugs.

### Genetic Considerations

It seems clear that genetics has a role in bipolar disorder (APA, 2002). Monozygotic (identical) twins have a very high concordancy rate, whereas dizygotic (fraternal) twins have a higher rate than normal siblings and other close relatives. Siblings and close relatives have a higher incidence of manic-depressive illness than the general population, and cyclothymic characteristics are common among family members of bipolar patients. The following risks have been established for developing bipolar disorder (Craddock and Jones, 1999):

1. First-degree relative: 5% to 10% chance
2. Identical twin with bipolar disorder: About a 40% to 70% chance

Significant issues arise surrounding family planning counseling for women with bipolar illness, including the heritability of the disease, the stress of parenthood, and the effect an ill parent has on a child. Furthermore, the teratogenicity of lithium, carbamazepine, and valproic acid is a concern when treating a pregnant woman with bipolar disorder. Consequently, pregnant women with bipolar disorder should be prescribed these drugs only when the risk of not doing so is greater than the risk of fetal insult. Because of these teratogenic effects, atypical antipsychotics are more likely to be prescribed to a pregnant woman.

## COMORBIDITY

About 87% of individuals with a manic-hypomanic disorder have a comorbid mental health disorder (Kessler et al, 2005a). Several other mental disorders can be experienced comorbidly in up to 50% of patients with bipolar disorders, including borderline personality disorder, attention-deficit/hyperactivity disorder, generalized anxiety disorder, panic disorder, social phobias, obsessive-compulsive disorder, and posttraumatic stress disorder (St. John, 2005).

Abuse of alcohol and other substances is more common among individuals with bipolar disorder than with any other *DSM-IV-TR* axis I diagnosis (Suppes et al, 2000). Of those diagnosed with bipolar disorder, 60% abuse drugs, according to the landmark National Institute of Mental Health Epidemiologic Catchment Area study (Regier et al, 1993). Additionally, individuals known to abuse drugs are five to eight times more likely to suffer from bipolar disorder than the general public (Kessler et al, 1997; Regier et al, 1993). Some clinicians believe that most first-time diagnoses of bipolar disorder are made in the emergency department related to the consequences of alcohol or other substance abuse. Strakowski and DelBello (2000) have advanced four hypotheses to account for the high rate of substance abuse in bipolar patients:

1. Substance abuse occurs as a symptom of bipolar disorder.
2. Substance abuse is an attempt by bipolar patients to self-medicate.
3. Substance abuse causes bipolar disorders.
4. Substance use and bipolar disorders share a common risk factor.

The use and abuse of alcohol and other substances cause several problems for the bipolar patient: relapse rates increase, response to lithium decreases, remission is delayed, poor treatment compliance occurs, and poor treatment outcomes are common (Suppes et al, 2000). Box 30-6 out-

---

| Box 30-6   Problems With Substance Abuse |
| --- |
| 1. Decreases compliance with antimanic medications |
| 2. Compromises treatment results |
| 3. Increases hospitalizations |

Modified from: Kosten TR, Kosten TA: New medication strategies for comorbid substance use and bipolar affective disorder, *Biol Psychiatry* 56:771, 2004.

---

lines problems with substance abuse in regard to patients with bipolar disorders (Kosten and Kosten, 2004).

## PUTTING IT ALL TOGETHER
### Psychotherapeutic Management

There are three treatment goals when working with bipolar disorder patients:

1. Getting acute mania under control
2. Preventing relapse once remission occurs
3. Returning to the prior level of functioning (i.e., social, occupational, interpersonal)

## NURSE-PATIENT RELATIONSHIP

The Key Nursing Interventions for a Manic Episode box lists specific interventions to be used with patients who experience manic episodes.

- *Matter of fact tone.* A matter of fact tone minimizes the need for the patient to respond defensively and avoids power struggles. By providing emotional support and responding to patients in a matter of fact manner, the nurse conveys both control of the situation and empathy.
- *Clear, concise directions and comments.* Working with hyperactive patients who are highly talkative, easily distracted, experience flight of ideas, and have poor judgment and a labile affect is difficult. When the nurse is confronted with talkative patients, it is not unusual for the nurse to attempt to use familiar skills. For example, most people learn not to interrupt another person until a pause. The pause might never come with manic patients. To be effective, the nurse might need to raise his or her hand and say, "Wait just a minute. I do not want to be rude, but I would like to say something." As a patient starts improving, the nurse might be able to work out a nonverbal signal

## Key Nursing Interventions *for a Manic Episode*

**Patients Too Busy to Eat**

The nurse should use the following interventions to maintain patient's body weight:

1. Provide patients with foods that can be eaten on the run (sometimes referred to as finger foods) because some patients cannot sit long enough to eat.
2. Provide high-protein, high-calorie snacks for patients. A vitamin supplement might be indicated.
3. Weigh patients regularly (sometimes weighing daily is needed).

**Patients Who Cannot Sleep**

Manic patients experience insomnia. The nurse can help patients maximize the opportunity for sleep by doing the following:

1. Provide a quiet place to sleep.
2. Structure patient's days so that there are fewer stimulating activities toward bedtime.
3. Do not allow caffeinated drinks before bedtime.
4. Assess the amount of rest that patients are receiving. Manic patients are not capable of judging the need for rest, and exhaustion and death have resulted from lack of rest.

---

to indicate when the patient needs to stop and let someone else speak. Although manic patients are talkative, there is a tendency for the talk to be superficial. When talking to hyperactive patients, the nurse should keep remarks brief and simple. Many patients literally cannot tolerate a lengthy discussion of any subject.

- *Limit setting.* When the nurse is leading a group, a talkative patient can be disruptive because of these tendencies:
  - Manipulation of the self-esteem of others
  - Ability to find vulnerability of others
  - Ability to shift responsibility to others
  - Limit testing

These patients have the ability to damage the self-esteem of other patients, ridicule the nurse, blame others, pick fights, create problems between patients, and manipulate others. The nurse needs to protect vulnerable patients and keep them from being drawn into the anger that manic patients feel. When the nurse is able to remain calm instead of becoming angry, it helps manic patients and the other patients in the group. This calmness should be based on an understanding of psychopathology; otherwise, it might be simply an unhealthy defense by the nurse. ("You cannot bother me; you are not important enough.") The nurse absolutely does not want to convey that he or she is engaged in an adult version of the childish behavior of plugging the ears and saying, "I can't hear you." It is also important to avoid arguing with patients about unit rules and limits. Do not debate these issues with patients. Simply state the unit policy

and move on. Debating and arguing reinforces the tendencies mentioned earlier.

- *Reinforcement of reality.* Manic patients also experience disturbances in perception. The intervention strategies outlined for other patients with disturbed perceptions are recommended for manic patients as well.
- *Respond to legitimate complaints.* Although many frivolous complaints arise, the nurse must respond to legitimate complaints to defuse irritability and develop trust.
- *Redirect patients into more healthy activity.* The bipolar patient's distractibility serves as an intervention tool when the patient engages in nonproductive behavior.

---

**Patient and Family Education**

**Bipolar Disorder**

*Illness*

Bipolar disorder is a brain disorder that disrupts mood. The patient might experience extreme moods—bouncing from depression to euphoria (or mania) or might primarily exhibit symptoms of mania. A little over 1% of the adult population suffers from bipolar I disorder. Manic episodes are characterized by an elevated mood, irritability, inflated self-esteem, decreased need for sleep, talkativeness, distractibility, and excessive involvement in pleasurable activities. The disorder is typically diagnosed first in the early 20s and occurs

*Continued*

**Patient and Family Education—cont'd**

about equally in men and women. Because of the pursuit of pleasurable activities, many bipolar patients overspend, become sexually involved in situations that they would normally avoid, and invest in unwise business dealings. Both dress and language can become loud and excessive. Involvement with drugs and alcohol is fairly common.

### Medications

Lithium has been the mainstay of treatment for patients with bipolar disorders. It is a naturally occurring element and is located on the periodic table in the same column as sodium and potassium. Lithium is so similar to sodium that the nervous system mistakes it for sodium. However, because lithium reacts more slowly than sodium, it can be given to slow down the nervous system. Lithium works but causes some fairly predictable side effects (e.g., fine tremor, thirst, frequent urination). Although lithium is effective for most patients, it can also cause problems because the difference is slight between a therapeutic dose and a harmful dose (or toxic dose). Because of this concern, patients diagnosed with bipolar disorder must have their blood examined frequently for its lithium content. After chronic and stable use of lithium, blood draws become less frequent.

Antiepileptic drugs are also used to treat bipolar disorder. A number of these agents are used, but the most commonly prescribed are divalproex (Depakote), other valproates, and carbamazepine (Tegretol). These drugs have a wider margin of safety than lithium, but can also produce some significant and serious side effects.

All atypical antipsychotic agents except clozapine have been approved to treat bipolar disorder. These drugs are effective but have been known to cause substantial weight gain.

### Other Issues

Patients with bipolar disorder can be very difficult to live with. Their self-importance, nonstop behavior, talkativeness, style of dress, and irritability can overwhelm a family member. On the other hand, these individuals can be remarkably creative and productive. It is important when living or dealing with individuals with this diagnosis to be matter-of-fact, clear, and concise in communication; set limits; and redirect critical negativism into healthier activities. Although difficult at times, it is important to avoid personalizing negative, sarcastic, and rude comments that these individuals might direct toward you.

## PSYCHOPHARMACOLOGY

The efficacy of lithium in the treatment of bipolar disorder has been recognized for years. Traditionally, lithium has been the most prescribed drug for manic patients. At one time, 80% to 90% of patients responded to lithium, but now only about 50% seem to respond (U.S. Surgeon General, 1999). Checking blood levels of lithium is crucial, because this drug has a narrow therapeutic index. Maintenance blood levels between 0.6 and 1.2 mEq/L are standard and can usually be maintained on a dosage of 900 to 1200 mg/day. There are several alternatives to lithium. Anticonvulsants and atypical antipsychotics are very valuable drugs. The most beneficial anticonvulsants are the valproates, including divalproex (Depakote), carbamazepine (Tegretol), and lamotrigine (Lamictal). The valproic acids seem to be the more effective of these, but lamotrigine does have a special role in treating the depressive phase of bipolar disorder. Newer anticonvulsants such as gabapentin (Neurontin), oxcarbazepine (Trileptal), and topiramate (Topamax) are also used on occasion. Olanzapine and other atypical antipsychotics are also approved for the treatment of acute manic episodes. Overall, these agents have a treatment success rate of about 80%. The use of antidepressants to treat bipolar depression is debatable because these drugs can trigger mania (APA, 2002). A full discussion of these drugs is found in Chapters 19 and 20.

## MILIEU MANAGEMENT

Milieu management is an important dimension of the nursing care of manic patients, because they test the unit or day treatment program perhaps more than any other group of patients.

1. *Safety.* It is important for the nurse to prevent manic patients from hurting themselves or others. Manic patients can become angry when things do not go their way. This pathologic irritability leads to arguments, fights, self-injury (e.g., hitting the wall, not paying attention to the environment), and hurting others. It is reassuring to patients to realize that the staff will not let them harm themselves or others.
2. *Consistency among staff.* Because manic patients tend to create conflict, pick on vulnerable individuals (patients and staff), blame others, test limits, and shift responsibility to others, the

nurse must carefully develop a plan of care. Nursing and other staff members should meet often to defuse conflict and clarify communication. All staff members should be aware of intervention strategies and agree to abide consistently by team decisions. Inexperienced staff members must guard against falling prey to esteem-building statements that tend to split the staff—for example, "You're the only one who understands."

3. *Reduction of environmental stimuli.* Because manic patients are hyperactive, talkative, irritable, and angry, it is important to decrease environmental stimuli. Patients are distractible and respond to all sorts of environmental cues; it is therefore important to modify the environment as much as possible. Helpful environmental modifications include limited activities with others, gross motor activities (e.g., walking, sweeping, aerobics) to discharge some of the need to be active, and a public room free from a television or stereo.

4. *Dealing with patients who are escalating.* Manic patients can become hostile and aggressive. It is important for the staff to deal with this aggressiveness in a calm, confident manner. For patients who are escalating, an antipsychotic drug, such as haloperidol, can be administered to prevent physical aggressiveness, and potential weapons (e.g., chairs, pool cues) can be removed. Limits and the consequences of violating these limits should be reviewed. Do not include limits that are not significant. It is countertherapeutic to defend a poor policy, and it is also countertherapeutic to allow patients to debate a unit issue. It is therapeutic to follow through with appropriate action should a patient violate a unit norm.

5. *Reinforcement of appropriate hygiene and dress.* Bipolar patients often forget hygiene behaviors, thus appearing disheveled and unclean at times. Simple reminders to shower, brush teeth, and wear clean clothes can correct some problems. The nurse should also monitor for flamboyant and suggestive dress that might ultimately embarrass the patient.

6. *Nutrition and sleep issues.* Both inadequate nutrition and inadequate sleep patterns plague bipolar patients. (See the Key Nursing Interventions for a Manic Episode box for appropriate nursing interventions.)

## YOUNG MANIA RATING SCALE (YMRS)

A popular scale for assessing the severity of mania is summarized in Box 30-7 (Shattell and Keltner, 2004). The YMRS is an 11-item scale with a maximum score of 60 possible (Young et al, 1978). Each of the 11 items has a 5-point gradient. For example, item 3, Sexual Interest, can be scored from 0 to 4:

0 = Normal, not increased
1 = Mildly or possibly increased
2 = Definite subjective increase on questioning
3 = Spontaneous sexual content, elaborates on sexual matters, hypersexual by self-report

---

### CASE STUDY

Mr. Casey Tubbs, a 44-year-old electrician, was admitted to the unit with the diagnosis of bipolar I disorder, manic type. The police arrested him after he started a fight with three Hispanic men in a bar. He had been drinking heavily. He was hyperactive, distractible, irritable, talkative, and demanding on admission. He demonstrated flight of ideas and was verbally hostile concerning a Hispanic co-worker, whom he accused of sleeping with his wife. Mr. Tubbs has vowed to get even. He made several comments about Hispanics in general while looking at Mr. Azteca, a Hispanic nurse.

This is Mr. Tubbs' third hospitalization. The first occurred 12 years ago when he contracted a *Candida* infection after having sexual intercourse with his wife. The second hospitalization occurred in 1998. No precipitating event was recorded, nor does Mr. Tubbs recollect anything unusual about the second admission.

Mr. Tubbs has responded well to lithium in the past and, during his last hospitalization, he was also given olanzapine because of his agitation. Between hospitalizations, Mr. Tubbs has functioned well and is considered a good worker. His boss appreciates his perfectionist tendencies. Mrs. Tubbs states that Mr. Tubbs has not slept in 3 days and has not stopped to eat for some time (the actual length of time is not clear). She reports a good marriage until Mr. Tubbs stopped taking his lithium, which he says he will no longer take. She wants him to "get better and come home." The head nurse decides to streamline the admission process because of Mr. Tubbs' agitated state. He is taken to a quiet area and given peanut butter crackers and milk.

4 = Overt sexual acts (toward patients, staff, or interviewer)

The typical minimum score for inclusion in a drug study is 20. Improvement is usually defined as a decrease in a person's YRMS score of 50%. In other studies, improvement might be defined as a specific score, such as 15. It is important to take note of how *success* is being defined on any particular study.

---

**CRITICAL THINKING QUESTION**    `3`

Can a person fall within the bipolar spectrum but not meet the *DSM-IV-TR* criteria for bipolar disorder?

---

## Care Plan

Name: Casey Tubbs                                Admission Date: _____

*DSM-IV-TR* Diagnosis: Bipolar I disorder, most recent episode manic

| | |
|---|---|
| **Assessment** | **Areas of strength:** Patient's marriage is solid between hospitalizations. Patient's boss likes him and is eager for him to return to work. Good adjustment between hospitalizations. He has responded well to lithium in the past. |
| | **Problems:** Patient is threatening and irritating others. Patient has legal problems from bar fight. Patient is threatening to get even with his wife's alleged lover. Patient has not complied with medication regimen recently and states that he will not take lithium. |
| **Diagnoses** | • Violence, high risk for, related to manic dyscontrol and delusions, as evidenced by irritability and verbal hostility. |
| | • Fatigue related to insomnia, as evidenced by lack of sleep for 3 days. |
| | • Nutrition, altered: less than body requirements related to anorexia and hyperactivity, as evidenced by lack of interest in food. |

| **Outcomes** | *Short-term goals:* | *Date met* |
|---|---|---|
| | • Patient will not hurt anyone while in hospital. | _____ |
| | • Patient will comply with medication regimen. | _____ |
| | • Patient will become less agitated. | _____ |
| | • Patient will comply with unit norms and limits. | _____ |
| | *Long-term goals:* | |
| | • Patient will remain free of manic episodes. | _____ |
| | • Patient will continue to take lithium on outpatient basis. | _____ |
| | • Patient will resolve legal problems. | _____ |
| | • Patient will join manic-depressive support group. | _____ |

| | |
|---|---|
| **Planning/ Interventions** | **Nurse–patient relationship:** Talk to patient in matter of fact tone, and clearly indicate that aggressive behaviors are not acceptable. Set firm, clear limits. Do not engage in debates over unit policy or limits. Keep comments brief and simple. Do not respond to sarcastic remarks with anger. Reinforce good behavior and confront (carefully) unacceptable behavior. |
| | **Psychopharmacology:** Lithium carbonate, 600 mg tid, PO (concentrate); olanzapine 15 mg HS. |
| | **Milieu management:** Provide quiet room and decrease stimuli. Do not include in-group activities for a few days. Provide opportunities for rest and monitor sleep. Provide finger foods and weigh daily. Set limits. |
| **Evaluation** | Mr. Tubbs is less agitated and is taking lithium on schedule. Patient is beginning to talk less about his wife's alleged infidelity. Has not lost weight. Patient continues to test limits. |
| **Referrals** | Schedule outpatient appointment and give patient and wife telephone number for manic-depressive support group. |

## Box 30-7   Young Mania Rating Scale (YMRS)

### Guide for Scoring Items

The purpose of each item is to rate the severity of that abnormality in the patient. When several keys are given for a particular grade of severity, the presence of only one is required to qualify for that rating.

The keys provided are guides. One can ignore the keys if that is necessary to indicate severity, although this should be the exception rather than the rule.

Scoring between the points given (whole or half-points) is possible and encouraged after experience with the scale is acquired. This is particularly useful when the severity of a particular item in a patient does not follow the progression indicated by the keys.

#### 1. Elevated Mood
0   Absent
1   Mildly or possibly increased on questioning
2   Definite subjective elevation; optimistic, self-confident; cheerful; appropriate to content
3   Elevated, inappropriate to content; humorous
4   Euphoric; inappropriate laughter; singing

#### 2. Increased Motor Activity/Energy
0   Absent
1   Subjectively increased
2   Animated; gestures increased
3   Excessive energy; hyperactive at times; restless (can be calmed)
4   Motor excitement; continuous hyperactivity (cannot be calmed)

#### 3. Sexual Interest
0   Normal; not increased
1   Mildly or possibly increased
2   Definite subjective increase on questioning
3   Spontaneous sexual content; elaborates on sexual matters; hypersexual by self-report
4   Overt sexual acts (toward patients, staff, or interviewer)

#### 4. Sleep
0   Reports no decrease in sleep
1   Sleeping less than normal amount by up to 1 hour
2   Sleeping less than normal by more than 1 hour
3   Reports decreased need for sleep
4   Denies need for sleep

#### 5. Irritability
0   Absent
2   Subjectively increased
4   Irritable at times during interview; recent episodes of anger or annoyance on ward

6   Frequently irritable during interview; short or curt throughout
8   Hostile, uncooperative; interview impossible

#### 6. Speech (Rate and Amount)
0   No increase
2   Feels talkative
4   Increased rate or amount at times, verbose at times
6   Push; consistently increased rate and amount; difficult to interrupt
8   Pressured; uninterruptible, continuous speech

#### 7. Language/Thought Disorder
0   Absent
2   Circumstantial; mild distractibility; quick thoughts
4   Distractible; loses goal of thought; changes topics frequently; racing thoughts
6   Flight of ideas; tangentiality; difficult to follow; rhyming, echolalia
8   Incoherent; communication impossible

#### 8. Content
0   Normal
2   Questionable plans; new interests
4   Special project(s); hyperreligious
6   Grandiose or paranoid ideas; ideas of reference
8   Delusions; hallucinations

#### 9. Disruptive/Aggressive Behavior
0   Absent, cooperative
2   Sarcastic; loud at times, guarded
4   Demanding; threats on ward
6   Threatens interviewer; shouting; interview difficult
8   Assaultive; destructive; interview impossible

#### 10. Appearance
0   Appropriate dress and grooming
1   Minimally unkempt
2   Poorly groomed; moderately disheveled; overdressed
3   Disheveled; partly clothed; garish makeup
4   Completely unkempt; decorated; bizarre garb

#### 11. Insight
0   Present; admits illness; agrees with need for treatment
1   Possibly ill
2   Admits behavior change, but denies illness
3   Admits possible change in behavior, but denies illness
4   Denies any behavior change

From Young RC, Biggs JT, Ziegler VE, Meyer DA: A rating scale for mania: reliability, validity and sensitivity, *Br J Psychiatry* 133:429-435, 1978. © 1978 The Royal College of Psychiatrists.

## ▌ Study Notes

1. Bipolar disorders (e.g., bipolar disorders I and II) occur in about 2.6% of the adult population in any given 12-month period. About 3.9% of Americans will be affected by this disorder in their lifetime.

2. Manic episodes are characterized by a distinct period (1 week at least or shorter if hospitalized) during which there is an

abnormal and persistent elevated, expansive, or irritable mood. These symptoms tend to occur suddenly and escalate rapidly, lasting from a few days to several months. At least three other symptoms are required (see Box 30-1).

3. Hypomanic episodes are characterized by the set of symptoms that occur in manic episodes, except that the symptoms are not as severe; occur over a 4-day period; do not cause significant social, occupational, or interpersonal problems; and do not require hospitalization.

4. Bipolar I disorder is described as a swing in mood from a manic episode to major depression.

5. Bipolar II disorder is described as a swing in mood from a hypomanic episode to major depression.

6. Cyclothymic disorder is described as a swing in mood from a hypomanic episode to depressive symptoms (but not as severe as those with major depression).

7. Objective signs of bipolar illness include altered speech patterns; altered social, interpersonal, and occupational relationships; and altered activity and appearance.

8. Subjective symptoms of bipolar illness include alterations in affect and perception.

9. Psychodynamic theories of bipolar illness include theories about family dynamics and psychoanalytic explanations that view manic behavior as a defense against overwhelming feelings of depression.

10. Biologic explanations of bipolar disorder include excessive levels of neurotransmitters (norepinephrine, serotonin, and dopamine) and genetics (up to 80% concordancy rates among identical twins in some studies).

11. Lithium is a drug of choice for the treatment of bipolar disorders; however, the valproates (e.g., Depakene, Depakote) are also used extensively. Atypical antipsychotics are the most recently approved agents for bipolar disorder.

## References

American Psychiatric Association: Practice guidelines for the treatment of patients with bipolar disorder, *Am J Psychiatry* 159(Suppl 4):16, 2002.

American Psychiatric Association: *Diagnostic and statistical manual of mental disorders, text revision,* ed 4, Washington, DC, 2000, APA.

Cassano GB, Rucci P, Frank E, et al: The mood spectrum in unipolar and bipolar disorder: arguments for a unitary approach, *Am J Psychiatry* 161:1264, 2004.

Craddock N, Jones I: Genetics of bipolar disorder, *J Med Genet* 36:585, 1999.

Dore G, Romans SE: Impact of bipolar affective disorder on family and partners, *J Affect Disord* 67:147, 2001.

El-Mallakh RS: Lithium: actions and mechanisms. Washington DC, 1996, American Psychiatric Association.

Fieve RR: *Moodswings,* New York, 1975, Bantam.

List of people believed to have been affected by bipolar disorder. Available at http://en.wikipedia.org/wiki/List_of_people_believed_to_have_been_affected_by_bipolar_disorder. Accessed October 6, 2005.

Jamison KR: *An unquiet mind,* Westminster, MD, 1997, Vintage.

Janowsky DS, Leff M, Epstein RS: Playing the manic game, *Arch Gen Psychiatry* 22:252, 1970.

Keltner NL, Folks DG: *Psychotropic drugs,* ed 3, St. Louis, 2005, Mosby.

Kessler RC, Chiu WT, Demler O, et al: Prevalence, severity, and comorbidity of 12-month DSM-IV disorders in the National Comorbidity Survey Replication, *Arch Gen Psychiatry* 62:617, 2005a.

Kessler RC, Berglund P, Demler O, et al: Lifetime and age-of-onset distributions of DSM-IV disorders in the National Comorbidity Survey Replication, *Arch Gen Psychiatry* 62:593, 2005b.

Kessler RC, Crum RM, Warner LA, et al: Lifetime co-occurrence of DSM-III-R alcohol abuse and dependence with other psychiatric disorders in the National Comorbidity Survey, *Arch Gen Psychiatry* 4:313, 1997.

Kosten TR, Kosten TA: New medication strategies for comorbid substance use and bipolar affective disorder, *Biol Psychiatry* 56:771, 2004.

Kuyler PL: Rapid cycling bipolar I illness in three closely related individuals, *Am J Psychiatry* 145:114, 1988.

Manji HK, Lenox RH: The nature of bipolar disorder, *J Clin Psychiatry* 61(Suppl 13):4257, 2000.

Moon AM: Late-onset bipolar patients not as ill as counterparts, *Clin Psychiatry News* 33:48, 2005.

Moore GJ, Bebchuk JM, Wilds IB, et al: Lithium-induced increase in human brain grey matter. *The Lancet* 356:1241, 2000.

Orum M: *Fairytales in reality,* Sydney, Australia, 1996, Seraline.

Regier DA, Farmer ME, Rae DS, et al: Comorbidity of mental disorders with alcohol and other drug abuse: Results from the Epidemiologic Catchment Area (ECA) Study, *JAMA* 264:2511, 1990.

Shattell M, Keltner NL: The case for atypical antipsychotics in bipolar disorder, *Perspect Psychiatr Care* 40:36, 2004.

Sherman C: Schizophrenia-bipolar I theory gains traction, *Clin Psychiatry News* 33:27, 2005.

St. John D: Bipolar affective disorder: diagnosis and current treatment, *Clinician Reviews* 15:44, 2005.

Strakowski SM, DelBello SP: The co-occurrence of bipolar and substance use disorders, *Clin Psychol Rev* 20:191, 2000.

Suppes T, Denehy EB, Gibbons EW: The longitudinal course of bipolar disorder, *J Clin Psychiatry* 61(Suppl 9):23, 2000.

Swann AC, Geller B, Post RM, et al: Practical clues to early recognition of bipolar disorder: a primary care approach, *Prim Care Companion J Clin Psychiatry* 7:15, 2005.

U.S. Surgeon General: *Mental health: a report from the Surgeon General,* Washington, DC, 1999, U.S. Department of Health and Human Services.

Young R, Biggs J, Ziegler VD, Meyer D: A rating scale for mania: reliability, validity, and sensitivity, *Br J Psychiatry* 133:429, 1978.

Zoler ML: High impairment found in subthreshold bipolarity, *Clin Psychiatry News* 33:1, 2005a.

Zoler ML: Pregnancy often triggers bipolar relapse, studies show, *Clin Psychiatry News* 33:42, 2005b.

## ▇ Bibliography

American Psychiatric Association; Practice guidelines for the treatment of patients with bipolar disorder, *Am J Psychiatry* 159(Suppl 4):166, 2002.

Sadock BJ, Sadock VA: *Synopsis of psychiatry,* ed 9, Philadelphia, 2003, Lippincott, Williams & Wilkins.

U.S. Surgeon General *Mental health: a report from the Surgeon General,* Washington, DC, 1999, U.S. Department of Health and Human Services.

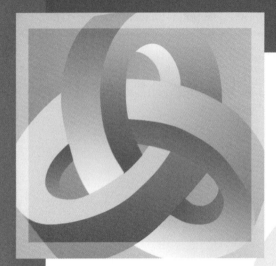

# Chapter 31

# Anxiety-Related, Somatoform, and Dissociative Disorders

*Carol E. Bostrom and Lee H. Schwecke*

## Learning Objectives

*After reading this chapter, you should be able to:*
- Recognize the special terms related to anxiety disorders, somatoform disorders, and dissociative disorders.
- Describe the *Diagnostic and Statistical Manual of Mental Disorders, Text Revision,* Fourth Edition *(DSM-IV-TR)* criteria for these disorders (APA, 2000).
- Describe objective and subjective symptoms of these disorders.
- Develop nursing care plans for individuals with these disorders.
- Evaluate the effectiveness of nursing interventions for individuals with these disorders.
- Recognize issues related to the care of individuals with these disorders.

The disorders discussed in this chapter are classified in the *DSM-IV-TR* as anxiety-related disorders, somatoform disorders, and dissociative disorders. Interventions for each disorder are included. First, to understand anxiety-related disorders, it is crucial to understand *what* anxiety is, *where* it comes from, *why* it is difficult to manage, and *how* individuals normally cope with it. (See Chapter 10 for a conceptualization of the dynamics of anxiety.) To provide effective treatment, it is important to understand the concepts of primary gain and secondary gain. Primary gain refers to the individual's desire to relieve anxiety to feel better and more secure. Secondary gain refers to the attention or support the individual derives from others because of illness. For example, "If I am sick, I cannot leave home to go grocery shopping, so I will call my husband at work and tell him to stop at the

grocery store on his way home to buy the needed items." The assistance from the husband is a secondary gain. Sometimes, the attention or the benefit of the secondary gain becomes more important than reducing the anxiety. This phenomenon complicates the treatment of these patients immeasurably.

## ANXIETY-RELATED DISORDERS

## GENERALIZED ANXIETY DISORDER

In generalized anxiety disorder (GAD), the individual experiences the symptoms of anxiety cognitively and physically. GAD is the most common anxiety disorder and is frequently seen with depression and other anxiety disorders that increase

## 12-Month Prevalence Rate of Mental Disorders in the United States*

| Disorders | Approximate Percentage Over 17 Years of Age | Approximate Number of Persons | Gender Overrepresentation |
|---|---|---|---|
| **Anxiety Disorders** | 18 overall | 36,000,000 | |
| Panic disorder | 3.5 | 7,000,000 | Women |
| Social phobia | 7 | 14,000,000 | Women |
| Specific phobia | 8.7 | 17,000,000 | Women |
| GAD | 3 | 6,000,000 | Women |
| PTSD | 3.5 | 7,000,000 | Women |
| OCD | 1 | 2,000,000 | Equal |
| **Mood Disorders** | 9.5 overall | 19,000,000 | |
| Major depression | 6.7 | | Women |
| Dysthymia | 1.5 | | Women |
| Bipolar I and II | 2.6 | | BD I: Equal |
| | | | BD II: Women? |
| **Impulse Control Disorders** | 9 overall | 18,000,000 | |
| Conduct disorders | 1 | 2,000,000 | Men |
| ADHD | 4 | 8,000,000 | Men |
| **Substance Abuse Disorders** | 3.8 overall | 7,600,000 | |
| Alcohol abuse and dependence | 3.1 | 6,200,000 | Men |
| Drug abuse and dependence | 1.4 | 2,800,000 | Men |
| **Schizophrenia** | 1.1 | 2,100,000 | Equal |

*Extrapolated from several sources based on current census data.
*ADHD,* Attention-deficit/hyperactivity disorder; *GAD,* generalized anxiety disorder; *OCD,* obsessive-compulsive disorder; *PTSD,* posttraumatic stress disorder.
From Kessler RC, Chiu WT, Demler O, Walters EE: Prevalence, severity, and comorbidity of 12-month DSM-IV disorders in the national comorbidity survey replication, *Arch Gen Psychiatry* 62:617, 2005; U.S. Surgeon General: *Mental health: a report from the Surgeon General,* Washington, DC, 1999, Department of Health and Human Services: National Institute of Mental Health: *Statistics.* Available at: www.nimh.nih.gov/healthinformation/statisticsmenu.cfm. Accessed April 18, 2005.

### Norm's Notes

*Anxiety is the most common mental "disorder." There are all types of stressors that just get to us, day in, day out. Some people refer to this phenomenon as life. On top of that, some of us just don't handle life as well as others. Among your classmates you have already identified some people who handle things better than others. Why? Well there are lots of reasons, and this chapter will help you understand them better. It will also look at some types of anxiety that probably go well beyond anything you have experienced. Just as the chapter on depression can hit a little close to home, so can this chapter.*

impairment in functioning (Ballenger et al, 2001). The anxiety or worry is chronic and excessive and might concern everyday events, such as work or school. The debilitating worry can be about nothing in particular or anything at all. The subject of the worry constantly changes (Miller, 2003). These individuals have great difficulty in controlling the anxiety, and worrying becomes a habitual way of coping to prevent a negative occurrence or something bad from happening. Physical symptoms such as dry mouth, and upset stomach are also part of the disorder. The anxiety causes significant distress and impairment in interpersonal, social, or occupational functioning. Because of the sense of helplessness that results from the anxiety, these patients can also experience feelings of depression and possibly pose a danger to self and others (Antai-Ontong, 2003). Frequently, patients have used alcohol or other drugs to the point of abuse in an attempt to feel better. (See the *DSM-IV-TR* Criteria for Generalized Anxiety Disorder box.)

When anxiety is caused by or related to a medical condition, the diagnosis of *anxiety disorder caused by a general medical condition* is used. Presumably, successful treatment of the medical illness will result in a reduced level of anxiety.

## ETIOLOGY

Family and twin studies have suggested a genetic link to the development of GAD (Miller, 2003). In patients with GAD, there might be neurochemical dysregulation in gamma-aminobutyric acid (GABA)–benzodiazepine, norepinephrine, serotonin, neuropeptides, and glutamate (Antai-Ontong, 2003). Some evidence exists that in GAD and panic disorder, patients might have alterations in a number of benzodiazepine receptors. Further research is needed to clearly explain the neurobiologic mechanisms involved in GAD. No one theory fully explains the causes of GAD. Psychosocial and environmental factors also play a role in the development of this disorder, especially for those with heritability for GAD.

---

### DSM-IV-TR Criteria for Generalized Anxiety Disorder

1. Excessive worry and anxiety
2. Difficulty in controlling the worry
3. Anxiety and worry are evident in three or more of the following:
   - Restlessness
   - Fatigue
   - Irritability
   - Decreased ability to concentrate
   - Muscle tension
   - Disturbed sleep

Modified from the American Psychiatric Association: *Diagnostic and statistical manual of mental disorders, text revision,* ed 4, Washington, DC, 2000, APA.

---

### DSM-IV and NANDA International Diagnoses Related to Anxiety-Related Disorders

*DSM-IV\**

*Anxiety Disorders*
Generalized anxiety disorder (GAD)
Panic disorder with or without agoraphobia
Agoraphobia without panic disorder
Specific phobia
Social phobia
Obsessive-compulsive disorder (OCD)
Acute stress disorder (ASD)
Posttraumatic stress disorder (PTSD)
Anxiety disorder due to a general medical condition

*Somatoform Disorders*
Somatization disorder
Pain disorder
Hypochondriasis
Conversion disorder

*Dissociative Disorders*
Dissociative amnesia
Dissociative fugue
Depersonalization disorder
Dissociative identity disorder (multiple personality disorder)

NANDA INTERNATIONAL†
Adjustment, impaired
Anxiety
Body image, disturbed
Breathing pattern, ineffective
Communication, verbal, impaired
Coping, community, ineffective
Coping, ineffective
Fear
Injury, risk for
Pain, chronic
Post-trauma syndrome, risk for
Powerlessness
Role performance, ineffective
Self-esteem, chronic low
Self-esteem, situational low
Self-esteem, situational low, risk for
Sensory perception, disturbed
Sleep patterns, disturbed
Social interaction, impaired
Social isolation
Spiritual distress
Thought processes, disturbed
Violence, other-directed, risk for
Violence, self-directed, risk for

*From the American Psychiatric Association: *Diagnostic and statistical manual of mental disorders, text revision,* ed 4, Washington, DC, 2000, APA.
†From the NANDA International: *NANDA nursing diagnoses: definitions and classifications 2005-2006,* Philadelphia, 2005, NANDA International.

---

### PUTTING IT ALL TOGETHER
Psychotherapeutic Management

## NURSE-PATIENT RELATIONSHIP

The first step in the nurse-patient relationship is for the nurse to assist patients in reducing their level of anxiety. Anxiety must be reduced before problem solving can occur. The nurse's ultimate

## Key Nursing Interventions *to Reduce Anxiety*

1. Provide a calm and quiet environment. *Rationale:* to identify and reduce stimulation, which includes exposure to situations and interactions with other patients that might provoke anxiety.
2. Ask patients to identify what and how they feel. *Rationale:* to help patients increase their recognition of what is happening to them.
3. Encourage patients to describe and discuss their feelings with you. *Rationale:* to help patients increase their awareness of the connection between feelings and behaviors.
4. Help patients identify possible causes of their feelings. *Rationale:* to assist patients in connecting their feelings with earlier experiences.
5. Listen carefully for patients' expressions of helplessness and hopelessness. *Rationale:* to assess for self-harm; patients might be suicidal because they want to escape their pain and do not think that they will ever feel better.
6. Ask patients whether they feel suicidal or have a plan to hurt themselves. *Rationale:* same as above and to initiate suicide precautions, if necessary.
7. Plan and involve patients in activities such as going for walks or playing recreational games. *Rationale:* to help patients release nervous energy and to discourage preoccupation with the self.

goal is to assist patients with developing adaptive coping responses.

Initially, patients need support and reassurance from the nurse. The nurse promotes trust through acceptance of patients' positive and negative feelings and acknowledgment of their discomfort. Conveying empathy tells patients that the nurse is concerned and understanding, and does not minimize the level of distress. For example, the nurse might say, "This must be uncomfortable and painful for you." To help patients manage and reduce their level of anxiety, the nurse should use the interventions found in the Key Nursing Interventions to Reduce Anxiety box.

After the anxiety level has been reduced to a more manageable and comfortable level, the nurse should begin to assist patients in examining their coping behaviors. Through the use of problem-solving methods, adaptive coping skills can increase. The nurse helps the individual to replace the ineffective, maladaptive worrying with effective coping methods for dealing with anxiety. See the Key Nursing Interventions for Problem Solving box.

The process of helping patients learn to use adaptive coping behaviors requires patience and the awareness that individuals learn and change at their own pace. The nurse must also be aware of his or her own verbal and nonverbal behavior when working with these patients, because anxiety is contagious. The nurse should manage his or her own stress and anxiety so that the work between the nurse and the patient is not compromised. The nurse educates the patient about the illness, including the effects of anxiety on the patient's life and on the members of the family.

## PSYCHOPHARMACOLOGY

Antidepressants, such as selective serotonin reuptake inhibitors (SSRIs) and selective serotonin-norepinephrine reuptake inhibitors (SSNRIs), are most effective for treating GAD for anxiety and the presence of comorbid disorders such as depression (Miller, 2003). Because GAD is a chronic disorder, antidepressants are better than benzodiazepines because of the possibility of dependency and tolerance with long-term use of benzodiazepines (Davidson, 2001). Sometimes, benzodiazepines are used on a short-term basis when a quick-acting medication is needed until the antidepressant takes effect. The benzodiazepine is then slowly tapered, if necessary, and discontinued. The tricyclic antidepressants are seldom used because of more serious side effects than with the SSRIs. Buspirone (BuSpar), a nonaddicting non-benzodiazepine, is not as effective as the other medications.

## MILIEU MANAGEMENT

The patient with GAD can benefit from a variety of activities as an inpatient and in the community. Recreational activities help reduce tension and anxiety. The use of relaxation exercises and tapes,

## Key Nursing Interventions    *for Problem Solving*

1. Discuss their present and previous coping mechanisms with patients. *Rationale:* to reinforce effective adaptive behaviors.
2. Discuss with patients the meaning of problems and conflicts. *Rationale:* to help patients appraise stressors, explore their personal values, and define the scope and seriousness of their problems.
3. Use supportive confrontation and teaching. *Rationale:* to increase patients' insight into the negative effects of their maladaptive and dysfunctional coping behaviors.
4. Assist patients with exploring alternative solutions and behaviors. *Rationale:* to increase adaptive coping mechanisms.
5. Encourage patients to test new adaptive coping behaviors through role playing or implementation. *Rationale:* to provide an opportunity for patients to practice new behaviors.
6. Teach patients relaxation exercises. *Rationale:* to reduce the level of anxiety. These techniques help patients manage or control anxiety on their own.
7. Promote the use of hobbies and recreational activities. *Rationale:* to help patients deal with routine feelings of stress and anxiety.

---

### *DSM-IV-TR* Criteria    for Panic Disorder

1. Recurrent, unexpected panic attacks
2. Panic attacks followed by a month or more of worry about having additional attacks, worry about the results of the attacks, and behavior changes related to the attacks
3. Panic disorder possibly accompanied by agoraphobia

Modified from the American Psychiatric Association: *Diagnostic and statistical manual of mental disorders, text revision,* ed 4, Washington, DC, 2000, APA.

meditation, and biofeedback helps decrease tension and promote relaxation and comfort.

Groups that focus on stress management, problem solving, self-esteem, assertiveness, and goal setting are helpful for coping with stress. Cognitive-behavioral therapy (CBT) has been carefully studied and found to be effective in controlling symptoms of anxiety (Antai-Ontong, 2003; Cottraux, 2004; Miller, 2003). Therapeutic touch and acupressure might be useful in reducing anxiety (La Torre, 2001). Depending on the issues and concerns of each patient, various groups can be helpful.

## PANIC DISORDER

Patients with panic disorder experience recurrent panic attacks and are worried about having more attacks. A panic attack develops suddenly, is accompanied by intense fear or discomfort, and peaks within 10 minutes. In addition to somatic symptoms, patients who experience panic attacks fear that they are losing control over themselves, "going crazy," having a heart attack, or dying. Panic attacks can occur during sleep, resulting in exhaustion. (See the *DSM-IV-TR* Criteria for Panic Disorder box.)

According to the *DSM-IV-TR,* panic attacks are (1) unexpected, occur out of the blue, or occur spontaneously, or (2) are situationally bound, meaning that they occur in anticipation of or on exposure to a trigger situation. These patients avoid places where a panic attack has occurred or could occur. Panic attacks that occur in response to a situation or trigger are related to social and specific phobias. Some panic attacks occur later, after exposure to a cue or situation. There is a high comorbidity in those who experience panic attacks in adolescence with the development of other mental illnesses as young adults. Panic attacks are linked to the development of depression, other anxiety disorders, and substance abuse disorders in adults (Goodwin et al, 2004).

Panic disorder can result in agoraphobia because patients fear having a panic attack in a place where embarrassment might occur, where help might not be available, or where escape is impossible. Patients who have panic disorder with agoraphobia use avoidance and restrict their activities outside the home, or require another person to be with them when outside the home. Thus, these patients become agoraphobic as a result of the fear of having an attack outside the home.

# ETIOLOGY

Psychological and biologic factors contribute to the development of panic disorders (Keltner et al, 2003). Susceptibility to panic can be hereditary. Some people might have an increased sensitivity to anxiety and fear and are more susceptible to the effects of trauma, particularly stressful life events such as separation and disrupted attachment in childhood. At the center of the fear mechanism is the amygdala; this includes the hippocampus, thalamus, hypothalamus, locus ceruleus, and other brainstem sites. Life stress and genetic factors can cause panic disorder in adults (Gorman et al, 2000).

According to Gorman and associates (2000) and Keltner and colleagues (2003), three systems work singly or in combination to trigger panic: the sympathetic nervous system, neuroendocrine system, and cognitive processes (Figure 31-1). An individual's catastrophic or "what if" thinking can trigger physiologic (somatic symptoms as in the fight-or-flight response), behavioral (avoidant), and affective (fear) responses. Sensitivity to and vigilance about physiologic symptoms can influence cognitive and neuroendocrine responses. Dysregulation of adrenergic receptors, which results in norepinephrine, serotonin, and GABA receptor impairment, causes decreased regulation of the sympathetic nervous system.

## NURSE-PATIENT RELATIONSHIP

The therapeutic relationship between the nurse and patient with panic disorder is centered on the same issues and interventions discussed for patients with GAD. Interventions specific for patients experiencing a panic attack are described in the Key Nursing Interventions for Panic Attack box. The rationale for the interventions is to help patients manage the panic attack safely, with as little discomfort as possible. With the nurse's assistance, patients' anxiety can be reduced to a more manageable level.

The nurse educates patients about panic disorder to reassure them that they are not losing their minds or dying during an attack. Patients experience relief when given information about the disorder, symptoms that might be experienced, and medications that can relieve symptoms. The nurse should help patients realize that attacks are time-

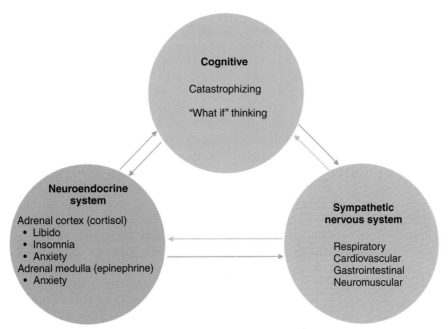

**FIGURE 31-1** Interacting systems of panic attacks. *(From Keltner NL, Perry BA, Williams AR: Panic disorder: a tightening vortex of misery,* Perspect Psychiatr Care *39:41, 2003.)*

## Key Nursing Interventions  *for Panic Attack*

1. Stay with the patient who is having a panic attack and acknowledge the patient's discomfort.
2. Maintain a calm style and demeanor.
3. Speak in short, simple sentences, and give one direction at a time in a calm tone of voice.
4. If the patient is hyperventilating, provide a brown paper bag and focus on breathing with the patient.
5. Allow patients to pace or cry, which enables the release of tension and energy.
6. Communicate to patients that you are in control and will not let anything happen to them.
7. Move or direct patients to a quieter, less stimulating environment. Do not touch these patients; touching can increase feelings of panic.
8. Ask patients to express their perceptions or fears about what is happening to them. *Rationale:* to help patients reduce anxiety to a more manageable and comfortable level.

limited and that symptoms will abate. Cognitive restructuring helps patients reinterpret and reappraise their beliefs regarding the danger of an event or bodily sensations.

## PSYCHOPHARMACOLOGY

SSRIs are most commonly used for the long-term treatment of panic symptoms. Benzodiazepines such as clonazepam (Klonopin) and lorazepam (Ativan) are used for an immediate effect to decrease somatic symptoms until the antidepressant has started working.

Patients with panic disorder might resist drug therapy because it might mean a loss of control at a time when they are struggling to maintain control over themselves and their symptoms. Some patients fear medications and their side effects. A good, simple explanation of the disorder and its biologic components can often convince patients that medication is helpful and that taking it is not a sign of weakness.

The nurse must differentiate symptoms of increased anxiety levels from medication side effects. Anxiety symptoms increase when pertinent issues are addressed or stressors are present. When symptoms of anxiety remain constant, or decrease immediately before the next dose of medication, the symptoms are probably related to the medication. Anxiety reduction strategies (e.g., relaxation exercises) might help patients manage anxiety.

## MILIEU MANAGEMENT

As a patient's anxiety decreases from the panic level to another level of anxiety, gross motor activities, such as walking, jogging, basketball, volleyball, or the use of a stationary bicycle, are appropriate to help decrease tension and anxiety. Other milieu interventions are located in the section on GAD (see earlier). CBT works on thoughts and substitutes rational interpretations for the misinterpretation of bodily responses, as well as helping reappraise beliefs about the danger of an event. Changes in cognition will then lead to decreased avoidant behavior. CBT helps patients control symptoms and improves overall well-being (Miller, 2005c).

## OBSESSIVE-COMPULSIVE DISORDER

According to the *DSM-IV-TR*, obsessions are recurrent and persistent thoughts, ideas, impulses, or images that are experienced as intrusive and senseless. (See the *DSM-IV-TR* Criteria for Obsessive-Compulsive Disorders box.) Individuals with obsessive-compulsive disorder (OCD) recognize that these thoughts are products of their own minds; they know that the thoughts are trivial, ridiculous, or aggressive but they cannot stop, forget, or control them. The thoughts are ego-dystonic and cause distress and anxiety. An example of an aggressive obsession is a woman experiencing an obsession that she has run someone over with her car. An example of a silly obsession is the rhyme, "Sticks and stones may break my bones, but words will never hurt me."

Compulsions can be defined as repetitive behaviors that are performed in a particular manner in

## CASE STUDY

Sandra Johnson, a 41-year-old Caucasian woman, is admitted to the psychiatric unit of a general hospital. She is accompanied by her husband and is coming from the emergency department. Her symptoms in the emergency department were shortness of breath, hyperventilation, palpitations, chest pain, and fear of dying. She stated that these symptoms occurred unexpectedly while she was cooking dinner. She thought she was having a heart attack.

These attacks had happened three times before. The first attack occurred 2 months ago, after which she went to her family physician, who performed electrocardiography and a stress test and conducted a complete physical examination. All results were negative for any physiologic causation of the symptoms. After the second attack, Mrs. Johnson stated that she took 2 weeks off from work because she was worried about having another attack. She had been employed for 5 years as a secretary for a small insurance agency. Just before she was about to return to work, she experienced another attack. After this third attack, she decided not to return to work and to quit her job. She was unable to leave the house to go grocery shopping, drive the children to activities, or go

out socially with her friends. Her husband, who is 42 years old, stated that he and their three daughters, aged 15, 12, and 9 years, were very concerned about her and had been helping her with daily tasks.

After her husband leaves, Mrs. Johnson begins to cry and states that she is letting her family down. They have tried to help her and she cannot do anything at home; she cannot work or even leave the house because she is so afraid of being unable to control the possibility of another attack. She does not understand what is happening to her and wants medication to help her feel better.

On the third day of her hospitalization, Mrs. Johnson tells the nurse that she is upset because her husband has not visited her since her admission. As she continues to talk about her husband, she starts to cry and states that she is afraid of losing him. She reports that 2 or 3 months ago, she noticed a change in her husband. He was less affectionate and was spending more time away from home. Suddenly he had more business trips. She is afraid he is having an affair. She says, "What am I going to do if he leaves? I can't support myself and my children alone. I don't even have a job. I can't go out of the house. I've lost contact with my friends."

## DSM-IV-TR Criteria for Obsessive-Compulsive Disorders

A. Obsessions
  1. Intrusive, inappropriate, recurrent, and persistent thoughts, impulses, or images that are distressful or produce anxiety
  2. Unsuccessful attempts to ignore or neutralize thoughts or impulses by other thoughts or actions
  3. Recognition that obsessions are produced by own thoughts
  4. Not simply excessive worry about real-life problems
B. Compulsions
  1. Repetitive behaviors, such as hand washing, or mental acts, such as counting, performed in response to an obsession
  2. Excessive behaviors or mental acts used to reduce distress or prevent dreaded events
C. Recognition that obsessions or compulsions are unreasonable or excessive
D. Obsessions or compulsions—cause distress, are time-consuming, and interfere with usual daily functioning

Modified from the American Psychiatric Association: *Diagnostic and statistical manual of mental disorders, text revision*, ed 4, Washington, DC, 2000, APA.

response to an obsession. The compulsions are performed to prevent discomfort and to bind or neutralize anxiety. Individuals with OCD experience anxiety if they try to resist the obsessions or compulsions. Some examples of compulsions are repetitive hand washing, checking the locks on doors, counting, and touching. These individuals know or recognize that their actions are absurd, but they are compelled to perform the rituals to avoid an extreme increase in tension and anxiety. They have a great need to control themselves, others, and their environment. Some individuals with OCD find it difficult to express emotions and to be introspective. Depression is a feature associated with this disorder because of its impact on self-esteem and self-worth.

An important feature to remember about OCD is that the obsessions or compulsions can be so severe that they significantly interfere with the patient's normal routine and so time-consuming that they interfere with occupational and social functioning. The obsessions and compulsions also interfere with these patients' interpersonal relationships, because they do not have time to relate to others—they are too busy thinking or doing. People who experience *magical thinking* believe that thinking *equals* doing.

## Care Plan

**Name:** Sandra Johnson                                          Admission Date: _____

*DSM-IV-TR* Diagnosis: Panic disorder with agoraphobia

| | |
|---|---|
| Assessment | **Areas of strength:** Managing her role as mother, homemaker, and secretary; was socially active with her friends; is in relatively good health. |
| | **Problems:** Fear of dying related to fear of heart attack; unable to leave home; fear of losing her husband; feelings of inadequacy. |
| Diagnoses | • Anxiety: panic related to life stress, as evidenced by somatic symptoms and fear of dying. |
| | • Self-esteem disturbance related to feelings of helplessness, as evidenced by inability to function. |
| | • Fear related to avoidance, as evidenced by inability to leave home. |

| Outcomes | *Short-term goals:* | *Date met* |
|---|---|---|
| | • Patient will discuss fears, her sense of inadequacy and helplessness, and anger. | _____ |
| | • Identify relationship between anxiety and physiologic responses. | _____ |
| | • Develop strategies for reducing anxiety, such as relaxation techniques. | _____ |
| | • Use problem-solving techniques for life stresses. | _____ |
| | *Long-term goals:* | |
| | • Patient will meet with husband and social worker to discuss marital issues. | _____ |
| | • Schedule appointment with outpatient therapist for cognitive behavioral therapy, systematic desensitization, or self-exposure training. | _____ |
| | • Identify schedule for attending an agoraphobia support group. | _____ |

| | |
|---|---|
| Planning/ Interventions | **Nurse-patient relationship:** Empathy and supportive-suppressive techniques to keep anxiety at a minimum; encourage ventilation of feelings and issues; help patient to identify relationships among stress, anxiety, and physiologic responses; assist with adaptive coping strategies. |
| | **Psychopharmacology:** Ativan 1 mg q4h prn; Prozac 20 mg q AM. |
| | **Milieu management:** Decrease stimuli and provide quiet, calm atmosphere; monitor anxiety level to prevent escalation; encourage recreational and diversional activities; use quiet room, if necessary; later, encourage problem-solving, assertiveness, communication, problem-centered, self-esteem, and stress management groups. |
| Evaluation | Patient reports being less anxious for the past 2 days. Met with husband and social worker. |
| Referrals | Outpatient appointments for cognitive therapy and self-exposure training. |

---

### CLINICAL EXAMPLE

John is watching a football game on television. As his favorite player prepares to attempt a field goal, John experiences severe anxiety because he thinks the player will miss the field goal. John is afraid that his thinking will cause the player to miss.

Thinking processes in individuals with OCD might also be rigid, and these individuals might be task-oriented. Relaxation is difficult. Patients with OCD are extremely overcontrolled and have a strong sense of right and wrong.

In this society, value is placed on performing well in school and at work. Being responsible and perfectionistic is often rewarded by the boss or by family members. Thus, at times, anyone might be seen as being compulsive. Generally, however, people do not allow their compulsiveness to rule their lives; they are able to maintain a balance between work and play, between role expectations and performance. There is a difference between having characteristics or traits and having an illness. Occasional brooding, rumination, or steadfastness to a task is not usually considered ridiculous or excessively bothersome—these thoughts and feelings do not rule most people's lives.

## CRITICAL THINKING QUESTION 1

A patient with OCD washes her hands after each time she touches anything. Her skin is cracked and bleeding. She states to the nurse, "I can't get my hands free of germs." How is this different from the nurse who washes his or her hands before and after each patient contact on a medical-surgical unit?

## ETIOLOGY

Current views concerning the origin of OCD point to genetic transmission. OCD might run in families. Biologic findings in OCD have identified increased brain activity in the frontal lobe and basal ganglia (Glod and Cawley, 1997). Serotonin dysregulation is involved in the development of OCD, which might account for the effectiveness of clomipramine (Anafranil) and the SSRIs (Wiegartz and Rasminsky, 2005).

## PUTTING IT ALL TOGETHER
### Psychotherapeutic Management

### NURSE-PATIENT RELATIONSHIP

Basic nursing interventions for hospitalized patients with OCD are listed in the Key Nursing Interventions for Obsessive-Compulsive Disorder box.

Therapeutic work involves the nurse helping increase patients' abilities to verbalize feelings, solve problems, and make decisions concerning stressors and problems. The nurse focuses on teaching and helping patients develop adaptive coping behaviors to deal with anxiety. Patients need to learn to substitute positive, anxiety-reducing behaviors for obsessions and rituals. Positive behaviors can include physical exercise, such as walking or using a stationary bicycle. Positive coping behaviors are slowly introduced into each patient's schedule, allowing time for rituals as well as normal activities. The nurse supports patients and positively reinforces nonritualistic behavior. Hobbies and social activities are introduced slowly as patients become more able to handle them.

### PSYCHOPHARMACOLOGY

The antidepressant clomipramine (Anafranil) and the SSRIs, such as fluoxetine (Prozac), sertraline (Zoloft), fluvoxamine (Luvox), and paroxetine (Paxil), are effective in treating OCD. Patients tolerate the SSRIs better than clomipramine (Anafranil) because of a better side effect profile. The treatment of patients with OCD with SSRIs

---

### Key Nursing Interventions for Obsessive-Compulsive Disorder

1. Ensure that basic needs of food, rest, and grooming are met. *Rationale:* patients are too busy to attend to these tasks. Reminders and specific directions are usually necessary.
2. Provide patients with time to perform rituals. *Rationale:* patients need to keep anxiety in check. Later, work to decrease the rituals by setting limits, but never take away a ritual, or panic might ensue.
3. Explain expectations, routines, and changes. *Rationale:* to prevent an increase or escalation of anxiety.
4. Be empathic toward patients and be aware of their need to perform rituals. *Rationale:* to convey acceptance and understanding.
5. Assist patients with connecting behaviors and feelings. *Rationale:* to promote the ability to identify and understand feelings.
6. Structure simple activities, games, or tasks for patients. *Rationale:* to help patients focus on alternatives to their thoughts and actions.
7. Reinforce and recognize positive nonritualistic behaviors. *Rationale:* to increase patients' self-esteem and self-worth.

is unique in that a selective efficacy exists. Other antidepressants are ineffective, a longer therapeutic lag occurs, and higher doses are often required than for treating patients with other disorders (Hollander et al, 2001).

## MILIEU MANAGEMENT

A variety of milieu activities and groups are beneficial to patients. Of particular importance are relaxation exercises and stress management, recreational or social skills, CBT, problem-solving, and communication or assertiveness training groups. Care is always based on the individual needs of patients.

CBT is effective for patients with OCD and can be undertaken on an outpatient basis. This approach encourages patients to contact feared stimuli slowly and then to limit the rituals or number of repetitions (Geffken et al, 2004). Exposure treatment is also effective. (See Chapter 38, Behavior Therapies.) A form of cognitive therapy such as thought stopping can also be used. When an intrusive thought occurs, the patient says "stop" and snaps a rubber band on the wrist or substitutes an adaptive behavior, such as deep breathing, for the ritual. A 7-week group exposure and response prevention therapy was also found to be effective (Himle et al, 2001).

## PHOBIC DISORDERS

Phobic disorders are intense, irrational fear responses to an external object, activity, or situation. Anxiety is experienced if the person comes into contact with the dreaded object or situation. Similar to all anxiety disorders, a phobia is a response to experienced anxiety and is characterized by a persistent fear of *specific* places or things, as opposed to GAD, in which the anxiety is free-floating; thus, anxiety is displaced or externalized to a source outside the body.

Phobias persist even though phobic individuals recognize that they are irrational. People can control the intensity of anxiety simply by avoiding the object or situation they fear.

In the *DSM-IV-TR,* phobias are categorized into three types:

1. *Agoraphobia without history of panic disorder:* a fear of being in public or open spaces, places, or situations in which escape might be difficult or help might not be available—for example, if the person should faint.
2. *Social phobia:* fear of being humiliated, scrutinized, or embarrassed in public—for example, choking while eating in front of others or stumbling while dancing in view of others.
3. *Specific phobia:* fear of a specific object or situation that is not either of the above—for example, fear of animals, flying, or heights.

Exposure to the stimulus results in an anxiety response. It is common to have some fears or phobias about certain objects or situations. Some people are afraid of public speaking, whereas some might be afraid of elevators or heights. However, these fears do not ruin most people's lives to the extent that they can never leave home. Most people are still able to function and fulfill role expectations and responsibilities, and have relationships with others. Phobic symptoms become phobic disorders when they cause severe distress and impair functioning.

## ETIOLOGY

Research has led to theories stating that specific individual, environmental, family, and genetic factors underlie phobic disorders. Types of phobias develop based on the influence of environment and genetic predisposition.

## PUTTING IT ALL TOGETHER
### Psychotherapeutic Management

## NURSE-PATIENT RELATIONSHIP

Patients with phobic disorders are usually treated on an outpatient basis. If the phobia incapacitates a patient to a severe extent, as in panic disorder with agoraphobia, the patient might be hospitalized. Another example in which hospitalization is indicated is the person who has a phobia about germs and might not eat or drink. Some nursing interventions useful for individuals experiencing phobic disorders are the following:

1. Accept patients and their fears with a noncritical attitude.
2. Provide and involve patients in activities that do not increase anxiety but increase involvement, rather than promote avoidance.

3. Help patients with physical safety and comfort needs.
4. Help patients recognize that their behavior is a method of avoiding anxiety.

## PSYCHOPHARMACOLOGY

CBT is the most successful treatment for phobic patients, and medications traditionally have no effect on avoidant behaviors. SSRIs are used to reduce anxiety and depression and block panic attacks, if present.

## MILIEU MANAGEMENT

Assertiveness training and goal-setting groups are beneficial. Social skills groups and other milieu activities help patients redevelop social skills and decrease avoidance.

Behavior therapy, such as systematic desensitization, flooding, exposure, and self-exposure, is most therapeutic for phobic patients. Self-exposure treatment is being used more often to avoid frequent therapy sessions (see Chapter 38).

## ACUTE STRESS DISORDER AND POSTTRAUMATIC STRESS DISORDER

Acute stress disorder (ASD) and posttraumatic stress disorder (PTSD) are somewhat different from the other anxiety disorders. ASD and PTSD are disorders that can develop after exposure to a clearly identifiable traumatic event that threatens the self, others, resources, and/or sense of control or hope. The event overwhelms the individual's usual coping strategies. Some of the traumatic stressors that might precipitate the development of ASD and PTSD are community violence, war, terrorist attack, being a hostage or prisoner of war,

---

### Highlighting the Evidence

| Disorder | Recommended Treatment |
| --- | --- |
| Panic disorder with agoraphobia | Cognitive-behavioral therapy |
| Social phobia | Cognitive-behavioral group therapy |
| Specific phobia | Exposure therapy |
| Obsessive-compulsive disorder | Exposure therapy |
| Generalized anxiety disorder | Cognitive-behavioral therapy |

#### Evidence

In patients with panic disorder with agoraphobia, cognitive-behavioral therapy was found to be superior to relaxation and equally effective to pharmacotherapy in patients with mild to moderate agoraphobia. For patients with severe agoraphobia, treatment was less effective for approximately 60% of those patients at long-term follow-up.

For patients with social phobia, CBTs were found to be encouraging. However, some studies found the benefits of combining cognitive treatment with behavioral approaches to be inconsistent.

Patients with specific phobia received exposure treatment and it was found to be effective in up to 90% of cases, as seen in long-term improvement or complete recovery. Studies on pharmacologic interventions are lacking, probably because of the effectiveness of behavioral treatment.

Exposure response prevention was highly effective for obsessive-compulsive disorder. Cognitive therapy does not appear to be more effective. The use of serotonergic agents is helpful but more research is needed in combining medications and exposure response prevention.

For patients with generalized anxiety disorder, CBT is effective in the research area but, in primary care settings, medications are used most often. Further work is needed to make CBT methods more available.

#### Summary

Numerous research studies have been conducted on the effectiveness of treatments for individuals with the disorders listed. However, the effectiveness of various treatment approaches is not perfect but is encouraging. The treatments themselves need improvement. The addition of medications with these treatments has not been supported and more work in this area is needed.

Modified from Barlow DH, Farchione TJ: Anxiety disorders. In Trafton JA, Gordon WP, editors: *Best practices in the behavioral management of chronic disease*, vol 1: *neuropsychiatric disorders*, Los Altos, CA, 2003-2004, Institute for Disease Management.

torture, disasters, bombings, fatalities in fires or accidents, catastrophic illness, gross injury to self or others, childhood sexual abuse, chronic abuse as a child or adult, rape, assault, and sudden or major personal losses (Solomon and Heide, 2005; Woods and Wineman, 2004). Among American adults, 7.8% to 8% are estimated to have PTSD in their lifetime and women are twice as likely to have PTSD as men (Lombardo and Gray, 2005; Olszewski and Varrasse, 2005). Recent events that have the potential for inducing ASD or PTSD are the London and Spain train bombings and the Afghanistan and Iraq wars.

Anyone experiencing events such as these would be distressed, with intense fear, horror, and a sense of helplessness. (See the *DSM-IV-TR* Criteria for ASD and PTSD box.) To some extent, the type and degree of the initial and later reactions to trauma depend on the individual's preex-isting characteristics and conditions, usual coping style and defense mechanisms, personal and social resources, previous exposure to trauma, and meaning of the event to the individual.

## DIAGNOSTIC CRITERIA

### Dissociative Symptoms and Numbing

The diagnosis of ASD is made when an individual has dissociative symptoms *during or immediately after* the distressing event: amnesia, depersonalization, derealization, decreased awareness of surroundings, numbing, detachment, or lack of emotional response. The diagnosis of PTSD is not made because of any initial reactions at the time of the trauma but is based on characteristic symptoms that occur *1 month or more after* the trauma. It is common for PTSD to be unrecognized for years, sometimes

---

**DSM-IV-TR Criteria** for Acute Stress Disorder and Posttraumatic Stress Disorder

**Acute Stress Disorder (ASD)**
1. Exposure to a traumatic event involving threat of death/injury to self or others, or actual injury to self or others
2. Responses of horror, helplessness, or fear
3. Dissociative symptoms during or immediately after the event:
   - Absence of emotions, numbing, detachment
   - Decreased awareness of surroundings (in a daze)
   - Derealization or depersonalization
   - Amnesia
4. Reexperiencing or reliving the traumatic event: distressing thoughts, dreams, flashbacks, illusions
5. Avoidance of stimuli related to trauma: feelings, thoughts, people, conversations, places, and activities; distress when exposed to reminders of the event
6. Increased arousal or anxiety: sleep disturbance, hypervigilance, startle response, irritability, restlessness, decreased concentration
7. Impairment or distress in functioning—occupational, social, or other important areas
8. Onset: within 4 weeks after the event
9. Duration: 2 days to 4 weeks

**Posttraumatic Stress Disorder (PTSD)**
1. Same criteria as ASD
2. Some criteria as ASD (in children, might be seen as agitated or disorganized behavior)

3. Numbing of responsiveness
   - Restricted affect, such as not being able to love or detachment
   - Sense of foreshortened future (lack of expectations about the future)
   - Inability to recall aspects of the event
4. Same criteria as ASD, *plus*
   - Hallucinations (in children, might be seen as repetitive play, with reenacting aspects of trauma or frightening dreams with no particular theme)
5. Same criteria as ASD, *plus*
   - Decreased participation and interest in activities
   - Estrangement and detachment from others
6. Same criteria as ASD, *plus*
   - Outbursts of anger
7. Same criteria as ASD
8. Onset
   - Acute: within 6 months after the event
   - Delayed: 6 months or more after the event
9. Duration
   - Acute: 1 to 3 months
   - Chronic: 3 months or more

Modified from the American Psychiatric Association: *Diagnostic and statistical manual of mental disorders, text revision*, ed 4, Washington, DC, 2000, APA.

even 10 to 20 years. This is a result, in part, of the major characteristic of both ASD and PTSD—numbing of responsiveness, or reduced involvement with the external world. There is a persistent attempt to avoid situations, activities and, sometimes, even people who might evoke memories of the trauma. These efforts include trying to avoid thoughts and feelings related to the event.

Denial, repression, and suppression are common in both disorders. A constricted or blunted affect, or a limitation in the range of feelings, might occur, such as being unable to show affection. Patients might feel detached or estranged from family and friends. An inability to trust and to love might lead to withdrawal. Interest in activities, even those unrelated to the traumatic event, is often lost. The individual's perceptions about the future might also change, leading to a type of hopelessness—for example, hopelessness about having a family or a career.

## Reexperiencing the Trauma and Intrusive Memories

A second major characteristic of ASD and PTSD is reexperiencing the traumatic event in some way, which might be in the form of intrusive, unwanted memories, upsetting dreams or nightmares, illusions, or suddenly feeling as if the event were recurring (flashbacks). With PTSD, there might be hallucinations related to the traumatic event. It is not known precisely why these unpleasant, frightening experiences begin to break through the denial, repression, or suppression. The triggers for episodes being reexperienced might have obvious connections to the trauma or might not resemble the original situation at all. In the latter case, patients might try to avoid all activities and people in an effort to prevent reexperiencing the flashback.

### CLINICAL EXAMPLE

Three days after a tornado had destroyed her home and seriously injured her son, Joan Marin was found wandering around the hospital in which her son was a patient. She was not injured but complained of nightmares and irritability. She said she could not bear to see her son because he "just wanted to talk about what happened—things I can't remember." Joan has not been to work since the tornado. She was taken to the crisis unit and diagnosed with and treated for ASD.

## Arousal Symptoms

Other criteria of ASD and PTSD include increased arousal, anxiety, restlessness, irritability, disturbances in sleep, and impairment in memory or concentration. Especially with PTSD, there might be occasional outbursts of anger or rage and survivor guilt—guilt about surviving or the actions taken to survive (Kaplan et al, 2001). For example, disaster or terrorist victims and combat soldiers might believe that they survived because of a cowardly act; rape victims might feel guilty for not resisting their attacker.

## Other Symptoms and Problems

Another consequence of ASD and PTSD can be psychological and physiologic symptoms that develop during exposure to situations resembling the original trauma, such as anxiety or panic attacks or psychophysiologic illnesses (e.g., gastrointestinal disorders, headache). Differentiating ASD and PTSD from other disorders is sometimes difficult.

Individuals experiencing posttraumatic symptoms might develop problems with grief, depression, suicidal ideations and attempts, impulsive self-destructive behaviors, anxiety-related disorders, and substance abuse (Foa, Keane, Friedman, 2000; McMillen et al, 2000). Patients might appear avoidant, schizoid, schizophrenic, paranoid, or even manic. These symptoms complicate treatment, especially if the ASD and PTSD are ignored and only the other diagnoses are treated.

Preexisting psychiatric disorders, including personality disorders, can increase the risk of developing ASD and PTSD after a traumatic event (Axelrod et al, 2005). A history of previous traumas, including torture, childhood abuse, rape, and abuse by a partner, leads to an increased risk for PTSD after later traumas. Conversely, events later in life might trigger previously unrecognized PTSD. For example, some World War II and Korean veterans did not show PTSD symptoms until after experiencing retirement, losses, and other processes associated with aging (Snell and Padin-Rivera, 1997). Activation and reactivation of PTSD symptoms have also been reported in veterans following the Gulf War and in people who survived the Oklahoma City bombing (Moyers, 1996), as well as in some who witnessed the events of September 11, 2001—the World Trade Center and Pentagon tragedies.

There might be difficulties such as arrests, unemployment, homelessness, abusiveness, divorce, and paranoia toward authority figures or others whom patients perceive as directly or indirectly responsible for not helping with the original traumatic situation (Amaya-Jackson et al, 1999; Beckham et al, 2000). Mistrust, isolation, abandonment fears, workaholism, focusing on the needs of others, feelings of inadequacy, anger toward God, unresolved grief, and fear of losing control of emotions are common (Bille, 1993).

The family members, friends, and co-workers of individuals with ASD or PTSD might develop problems as well, as "secondary victims." (See Family Issues in Acute Stress Disorders and Posttraumic Stress Disorders box.) In some cases, these individuals experience the same trauma (e.g., accident, fire, disaster) and develop symptoms themselves. The family might or might not be able to help in the treatment of their family member with ASD or PTSD. The whole family or certain members might need treatment.

After a community disaster or a tragedy affecting a nation, many people might experience acute stress or posttraumatic symptoms and initially find it difficult to obtain support from others. When the danger is over, small groups of victims might gather for mutual support and assistance. Fear, concern, uncertainty, frustration, anger, grief, and humor are all to be expected. Disaster personnel often encourage and facilitate debriefing in groups, including groups of emergency personnel. With the 9/11 tragedy and other disasters, the firefighters, emergency medical technicians, disas-

ter workers, and police were not only rescuers, but also victims. They have been found to have higher levels of ASD, PTSD, and depression than those not directly exposed to these situations (Fullerton et al, 2004).

## NEUROCHEMICAL BASIS OF ACUTE STRESS AND POSTTRAUMATIC STRESS DISORDERS

It has been proposed that fear conditioning, a failure of extinction (of the fear-anxiety response), and behavioral sensitization might be important in the development of ASD and PTSD symptomatology following exposure to a traumatic event (Charney, 2004; van der Kolk, 1997). It has been shown that *fear conditioning* to auditory and visual stimuli can last for years and produce relatively indelible emotional and visceral memories. If *extinction* of fear responses does not occur, the responses continue, even when the traumatic event is absent (Beckham et al, 2000; Charney, 2004). Normally, associations leading to the conditioned response would be erased, or new associations would mask the response-producing associations over time. Conditioned fear responses, after being dormant for years, can be reactivated by trauma-associated stimuli. *Sensitization* is the increased magnitude of response to one stimulus, but especially to repeated traumatic stimuli. This behavioral sensitivity produces increased arousal *(hyperarousal)* and stress sensitivity that can endure for a long time (Beckham et al, 2000; Charney, 2004). *Cross-sensitization* can occur, so that there

---

 **Family Issues in Acute Stress Disorder and Posttraumatic Stress Disorder**

Family members, friends, and colleagues of patients with acute stress disorder (ASD) or posttraumatic stress disorder (PTSD) need to be assessed along with patients. Issues to be addressed include the following:

1. Assessing whether any or all members of the family or others have been exposed to the same trauma as the patient and, if so, if family members might be experiencing symptoms of ASD or PTSD as well.
2. Assessing whether any or all of the family members or others are having reactions to the behaviors of the member with ASD or PTSD.

3. Teaching family members and others about the causes, symptoms, and treatment of ASD and PTSD.
4. Educating family members and others about ways to help the patient with ASD or PTSD.
5. Referring family members and others to a support group for families of ASD or PTSD survivors or a related group, if available.
6. Referring members for couple or family counseling, if needed.

is overreaction to other, even minor, stimuli that resemble the original traumatic stimulus (Beckham et al, 2000; Charney, 2004; Friedman, 1997; Solomon and Heide, 2005; van der Kolk, 1997).

Avoidance (behavioral), numbing (emotional), autonomic hyperarousal (somatic), and reexperiencing of the trauma (cognitive, emotional, somatic, and behavioral) are characteristic symptoms of ASD and PTSD. Avoidance and numbing, in response to fear conditioning and behavioral sensitization, are likely to be related to increased endogenous opiate release (Charney, 2004; Friedman, 1997), producing emotional blunting, physical analgesia, and depersonalization. Autonomic hyperarousal, also in response to fear conditioning and behavioral sensitization, is related to increased noradrenergic and dopaminergic system activity and to decreased serotonergic activity, causing fear, anxiety, and fight-or-flight readiness. Reexperiencing the trauma, in response to fear conditioning and failure of extinction, is related to activation of the amygdala, locus ceruleus, hypothalamus, thalamus, and hippocampus (limbic system/hypothalamic-pituitary-adrenal axis), which enhances encoding of traumatic memories and sensory and cognitive memory retrieval (Charney, 2004; Koren et al, 2005; Olszewski and Varrasse, 2005; Solomon and Heide, 2005). Prolonged stress eventually results in down-regulation of corticotropin-releasing hormone (CRH), dehydroepiandrosterone (DHEA), neuropeptide Y, and adrenergic receptors; decreased adrenocorticotropin-releasing hormone (ACTH) release; and increased levels of testosterone and estrogen. The fear-anxiety response can then become blunted and desensitization induced (Charney, 2004; Solomon and Heide, 2005; van der Kolk, 1997). Functional magnetic resonance imaging, magnetic resonance spectroscopy, positron emission tomography, and electroencephalographic findings are beginning to confirm the biochemical evidence (Solomon and Heide, 2005).

Hyperarousal might cause memories to be dissociated, repressed, or stored as bodily sensations that are not available at a conscious level. Fragments of these memories might appear later as physiologic reactions, nightmares, flashbacks, and emotional reenactments of the trauma (van der Kolk, 1997). ASD and PTSD patients typically have more neuromuscular, gastrointestinal, and psychophysiologic symptoms; depression; sleep disturbances; anxiety; maladaptive coping; and altered immune function than individuals who do not have ASD or PTSD (Solomon and Heide, 2005; van der Kolk, 1997). War and terrorism situations might be complicated by exposure to biologic and chemical agents, which can cause many physiologic illnesses as well (Barclay and Vega, 2005; Reeves et al, 2005; Woods, 2005).

The comparatively high incidence of alcohol, opiate, and benzodiazepine abuse in individuals with posttraumatic symptoms might be related to attempts to reduce the symptoms caused by increased noradrenergic and dopaminergic activity. Conversely, addiction to trauma (compulsively exposing oneself to traumatic events) might be explained, in part, by the recurrent increase in endogenous opiates. Individuals with posttraumatic symptoms also have an exaggerated response to amphetamines and cocaine because of their preexisting hyperarousal. After taking these drugs, individuals with posttraumatic symptoms are more vulnerable to paranoia and psychosis (Bremner et al, 1996).

## CRITICAL THINKING QUESTION  2

Ron Jenkins's workplace was severely damaged by an explosion. He was found staring at the cars in the parking lot and repeating that he had to find his car and wife. He was unable to give his address or say where his wife would be at that time of day. He refused to be treated for cuts and bruises until he could find his wife. What interventions would you use at the scene?

## PUTTING IT ALL TOGETHER
### Psychotherapeutic Management

An effective approach with ASD and PTSD is to prevent or minimize the symptoms. Principles of critical incident stress management (CISM) are often applied to disaster situations (including the 9/11 attacks), in which the development of posttraumatic symptoms in some victims is likely. This model provides a wide range of services for primary and secondary victims, including seven core integrated elements: (1) precrisis preparation (including individuals and organizations who will assist in CISM); (2) large-scale demobilization procedures for use after mass disasters; (3) individual acute crisis counseling; (4) brief small group discussions called defusings, designed to assist in acute symptom reduction; (5) longer small group discussions, called critical incident stress debriefings (CISDs), designed to assist in achieving a sense of psychological closure postcrisis and/or facilitate the referral process; (6) family crisis intervention techniques; and (7) follow-up procedures and/or referral for psychological assessment or treatment (Everly et al, 2000). The National Organization of Victims Assistance (NOVA) and the American Red Cross have developed similar models.

The element of CISM related to crisis counseling is similar to the crisis intervention strategies described in Chapter 10, but places more emphasis on mobilizing community resources to assist in crisis management. CISM group work is an organized and structured approach, beginning with a discussion of the goals, rules, and roles of the leaders (who are often both mental health workers and trained peers of the victims). This is followed by a cognitive-oriented discussion of the facts of the incident, beginning with thoughts that group members had when they arrived at the scene. The discussion then moves to an emotional phase, which allows for the expression of the full range of feelings. The final stage focuses on discussion and education about any symptoms of ASD or PTSD that are being experienced, teaching coping strategies to use with any further stress reactions, and ways to prepare for return to work. Ideally, the goal for group debriefing is psychological closure related to the critical event and a return to a precrisis (or an even more functional) level of adaptation. After the group debriefing, the leaders also debrief each other about what they heard and felt while listening to the traumatic experiences being discussed, and about the effectiveness of the group debriefing (Everly et al, 2000). With large-scale disasters, such as at the World Trade Center, closure is much more difficult because of the extended length of time that was required for location and identification of victims and for the final cleanup of the debris.

The treatment of patients who develop ASD or PTSD must be individualized according to age, developmental level, gender, psychiatric history, and family and cultural characteristics (Flouri, 2005); predominant symptoms; and associated problems, such as disorganized behaviors, depression, suicidal ideation, aggression, or substance abuse. (See Chapter 36, on working with dually diagnosed patients and Chapter 41, on survivors of violence, for specific traumas, such as workplace violence, cults, ritual abuse, torture, rape, partner abuse, and childhood sexual abuse, as well as the stages of recovery from trauma.) The goals of treatment are progressive, intensive review of the traumatic experiences (exposure therapy), and then integration of the feelings and memories, often from the least to the most painful. This approach involves moving from a victim status to a survivor status, from "I can't go on because of this" to "I have learned from it and can go on with my life." As with any crisis, there is a potential for growth and the development of improved coping skills, appreciation of the value of life, and enhanced relationships.

## NURSE-PATIENT RELATIONSHIP

The first priority in the relationship with patients experiencing ASD or PTSD is the development of trust. Because these patients have a tendency to be withdrawn, to feel alienated, and to be suspicious of others, developing trust might be difficult. Seeking help or accepting it when offered is also sometimes difficult for patients. When a patient is aware of the current influence of the trauma, there is often a tendency for him or her to believe that "No one can understand what I've been through unless they have been through it too." Therefore, the nurse needs to be nonjudgmental, honest, empathic, and supportive. The nurse can convey the message, "I haven't been through what you have, but the more you tell me, the better I will understand what you have been through and are experiencing." It is important to acknowledge any unfairness or injustices that were part of the trauma. Safety and security are other priorities because of the risk for suicide and aggression.

These patients also need to hear that they are not crazy but are having typical reactions to a serious trauma. Teaching about the dynamics of ASD or PTSD is often appropriate. Depending on the nature of the trauma, the nurse must be prepared to hear horror stories about hideous injuries, unpredicted behaviors, and gross destruction. If the nurse cannot tolerate the stories of atrocities, patients will not feel free to process all the losses and changes that have occurred in their lives as a result of the trauma. Nurses might need help for themselves to avoid vicarious victimization (secondary PTSD), compassion fatigue, or burnout when working with trauma victims in settings such as emergency departments, burn units, accidents, or disaster scenes (Badger, 2001; Boscarino et al, 2004).

It might take time for patients to recognize the relationship between their current problems and the original traumatic event. When patients are not initially aware of the connection between the original trauma and current feelings and problems, the nurse should gently clarify these connections as they emerge.

Patients need to evaluate their past behaviors according to the original context of the situation, not by current values and standards (Figley, 2000). For example, a rape victim who did not resist her knife-wielding attacker needs to judge her behavior in the context of the life-or-death situation, not by someone's comment that she "must have asked for it." Another example is the Afghanistan veteran who must evaluate his experience of killing a woman who was holding an assault weapon within the context of war, not by society's current view of war as immoral. Developing a new perspective on the original trauma, which involves clarifying facts, feelings, and values, is not always easy for patients.

Specific techniques are sometimes used to help patients with ASD and PTSD: exposure therapy (imaginal or in vivo) and systematic desensitization, described in Chapter 38; CBT (multicomponent CBT and multichannel exposure therapy), described in Chapter 4; and eye movement desensitization and reprocessing (EMDR) (Falsetti et al, 2005; Frueh et al, 2004; Lombardo and Gray, 2005; Reeves et al, 2005; Solomon and Heide, 2005).

Patients need significant help in safely verbalizing feelings, particularly anger, that have often been ignored or repressed. This is especially true if there have been destructive outbursts or if patients are trying desperately to remain in control. Writing in a journal is often helpful. Expressive therapy (art, music, and poetry) can facilitate externalizing painful emotions that are difficult to verbalize (Clark, 1997; Hines-Martin and Ising, 1993).

As patients struggle through the sometimes lengthy process of reexperiencing, reintegrating, and processing memories of and feelings about traumatic experiences, they need empathy and reassurance that they will be safe and need to be taught relaxation techniques, so they are not overwhelmed with anxiety (Falsetti et al, 2005). It is also important to take time-outs to focus on emergent problems and potential solutions. These problems, such as finances, housing, and divorce, and their associated feelings, can be as stressful as the original event. Patients need to be involved in problem solving, decision making, and taking specific actions toward overcoming these stresses. Patients' adaptive coping skills and use of relaxation strategies need to be encouraged, whereas dysfunctional activities, especially avoidance of responsibility for one's actions and the abuse of alcohol and drugs, need to be discouraged.

Patients also need to develop interpersonal skills and reestablish relationships that provide support and assistance (Bleiberg and Markowitz, 2005). Couple or family education and counseling might be recommended, if appropriate. Hospitalization of ASD and PTSD patients is normally necessary only if they are suicidal, homicidal, self-mutilating, or unable to function in daily activities. The box, "Key Nursing Interventions for Acute Stress Disorder and Posttraumatic Stress Disorder," lists additional nursing interventions to use for ASD and PTSD.

## PSYCHOPHARMACOLOGY

Medications for patients experiencing ASD or PTSD are used generally for short-term therapy during the acute crisis or for intensive counseling periods to prevent or reverse neurochemical fear conditioning and sensitization. The choice of medications depends on the primary symptoms and the presence of other axis I disorders (Reeves et al, 2005; Schoenfeld et al, 2004).

*Benzodiazepines,* such as clonazepam, might be prescribed to reduce levels of conditioned fear and anxiety symptoms. These medications also might help patients with sleep disturbances and nightmares. There is a risk of dependence, however, especially with patients who are already abusing alcohol or drugs. Other benzodiazepines, such as lorazepam, are usually prescribed on a prn basis for short periods rather than on a fixed dosing schedule. Buspirone (a nonbenzodiazepine) might be an alternative.

## Key Nursing Interventions    *for Acute Stress Disorder and Posttraumatic Stress Disorder*

1. Be nonjudgmental and honest; offer empathy and support; acknowledge any unfairness or injustices related to the trauma. *Rationale:* building trust might be difficult for patients.
2. Assure patients that their feelings and behaviors are typical reactions to serious trauma. *Rationale:* patients often believe that they are going crazy.
3. Help patients recognize the connections between the trauma experience and their current feelings, behaviors, and problems. *Rationale:* patients often are unaware of these connections.
4. Help patients evaluate past behaviors in the context of the trauma, not in the context of current values and standards. *Rationale:* patients often have guilt about past behaviors and are judgmental of themselves.
5. Encourage safe verbalization of feelings, especially anger. *Rationale:* feelings are or have been repressed or suppressed.
6. Encourage adaptive coping strategies, exercise, relaxation techniques, and sleep-promoting strategies. *Rationale:* patients might have been using maladaptive or dysfunctional coping to avoid dealing with feelings and issues.
7. Facilitate progressive review (imaginal or in vivo) of the trauma and its consequences. *Rationale:* review helps patients integrate feelings and memories and begin the grieving process.
8. Encourage patients to establish or reestablish relationships. *Rationale:* relationships (needed for assistance and support) might have been affected by patients' suspiciousness or fear of asking for help.

*Clonidine* and *propranolol* might produce responses similar to those of the benzodiazepines. Both medications can help diminish the peripheral autonomic response associated with fear, anxiety, and nightmares.

*Valproic acid* or *carbamazepine* is sometimes given to patients who are experiencing mood swings, explosive outbursts and intense feelings of being out of control. These medications can help decrease hyperarousal, startle response, and nightmares.

*SSRIs* (especially paroxetine, escitalopram, and sertraline) might reverse continued emergency responses and decrease repetitive behaviors, disturbing images, and somatic states.

*Tricyclic antidepressants* (TCAs) are used occasionally if depression, anhedonia, and sleep disturbances are primary problems. TCAs, especially amitriptyline, are usually given in one dose at bedtime. Trazodone might be used instead of a TCA for sleep.

*Antipsychotics* are used if patients have psychotic thinking. These drugs might be used for hyperarousal and sleep disturbances during acute crisis periods. Low doses of risperidone or quetiapine can help decrease flashbacks and nightmares.

## MILIEU MANAGEMENT

Patients experiencing ASD or PTSD can benefit from many inpatient or outpatient milieu activities. Social activities can help rebuild social skills that have been damaged by suspiciousness and withdrawal. Recreational and exercise programs can help reduce tension and promote relaxation. Groups that might be useful are those that focus on self-esteem, decision making, assertiveness, anger management, stress management, and relaxation techniques. Victims of a variety of traumas might benefit from group meetings that focus on the similarities in their reactions and feelings, such as mistrust, helplessness, fear, guilt, numbing, detachment, nightmares, and flashbacks.

## COMMUNITY RESOURCES

A particularly useful therapeutic aid for patients experiencing ASD and PTSD is group therapy or self-help groups with others who have experienced the same or a similar trauma. A community might have a VA (Veterans Administration) Hospital or veterans' outreach center for war veterans and their spouses, as well as groups for victims of rape, incest, or torture and their family members. A community might hold meetings for victims after a community disaster or national tragedy. There also might be a victim's assistance program for crime victims. Substance abuse programs or groups might also be needed.

## CASE STUDY

Billy Craig was 19 years old when he spent a year in heavy combat in Afghanistan. Although he was upset when his buddies were killed, he was secretly relieved when his wounds got him sent home. He studied forestry and became a ranger in a national forest. He was considered a loner and showed no interest in marriage. He never talked about his experiences in Afghanistan with anyone.

During the television coverage of the latest anniversary of the World Trade Center and Pentagon tragedies, Billy began to have nightmares and flashbacks about killing the enemy and about a friend who was dismembered. Billy became angry more frequently and startled easily. After a month of not seeing him, other rangers found Billy in his cabin, very depressed and surrounded by old guns and grenades. He kept repeating that he should have died in Afghanistan too. He admitted that he was intending to shoot himself. With effort, the rangers convinced him to go with them to the mental health center, where he was admitted, diagnosed with, and treated for delayed posttraumatic stress disorder and major depression.

## ADJUSTMENT DISORDERS

This separate group of adjustment disorders is actually *not* part of the anxiety disorders category but is included here because of its contrasts with ASD and PTSD. The diagnosis of adjustment disorder might be made when symptoms develop within 3 months after an identifiable life event, and the reaction is not severe enough to fit the criteria of ASD or PTSD. Common events or circumstances that might precipitate an adjustment disorder are divorce, moving, marriage, retirement, illness or disability, financial problems, or difficulties in child rearing.

The symptoms of maladaptive reactions to a stressful event or circumstances are not defined as specifically as those for ASD and PTSD, but are still considered more severe than a normal stress response or grief reaction. The acute reaction interferes with functioning but lasts no longer than 6 months *after* the stressor and its consequences have ended. Chronic symptoms might persist more than 6 months if the consequences of the stressor are more enduring, such as a chronic illness or difficulties resulting from a divorce.

The diagnosis of adjustment disorder is based on subcategories according to the predominant feature of the patient's maladaptive stress reaction.

The major feature might be a mood disturbance of *anxiety* or *depression,* or it might be a disturbance with *mixed anxiety and depressed mood.* There might be a *disturbance of conduct*—violation of societal norms or the rights of others. There is a subcategory of *mixed disturbance of emotions and conduct.* The major goals are to recognize the relationship between the stressful situation and current problems and to review and integrate the feelings and memories of the original situation.

## SOMATOFORM DISORDERS

The major characteristic of somatoform disorders is that patients have physical symptoms for which there is *no known organic cause or physiologic mechanism.* Evidence is present or a presumption exists that the physical symptoms are connected to psychological factors or conflicts. These patients are not in control of their symptoms, which are unconscious and involuntary. Patients express conflicts through bodily symptoms and complaints using the defense of somatization. They do not deal with their anxiety or feelings emotionally but displace the anxiety into bodily symptoms. Somatoform disorders are about anxiety that focuses on health matters and will perhaps be classified differently in the *DSM-V* (Mayou et al, 2005).

Patients with somatoform disorders generally see general practitioners and not mental health professionals or psychiatrists. They repeatedly seek medical diagnosis and treatment, even though they have been told that there is no known physiologic or organic evidence to explain their symptoms or disability.

Traditional views concerning somatoform disorders consider repression, denial, and displacement as defense mechanisms used in these disorders. Repression occurs in reference to feelings, conflicts, and unacceptable impulses. Denial of psychological problems is present, even though these patients have been told that there is no physiologic cause or basis for their symptoms.

Current research has suggested that genetic, developmental learning, personality, and sociocultural factors can predispose, precipitate, and maintain somatoform disorders. Emotional and social stress can precipitate these disorders. Individuals with somatoform disorders often appear to be needy and dependent on others.

## Care Plan

**Name:** Billy Craig                                   Admission Date: _____

*DSM-IV-TR* Diagnosis: Posttraumatic stress disorder

| | |
|---|---|
| Assessment | **Areas of strength:** Intelligent, enjoys his work, has supportive co-workers. |
| | **Problems:** Suicidal ideation, flashbacks of and anger about Afghanistan; disturbed sleep; lives in an isolated area. |
| Diagnoses | • Potential for self-directed and other-directed violence related to suicidal ideation and anger, as evidenced by suicidal behavior and statements. |
| | • Sleep pattern disturbance related to nightmares, as evidenced by interrupted sleep, increasing irritability. |
| | • Posttrauma response related to war experiences, as evidenced by reexperiencing of the traumatic events in flashbacks and nightmares. |

| Outcomes | *Short-term goals:* | *Date met* |
|---|---|---|
| | • Patient will agree to talk to staff if he feels suicidal or aggressive toward others. | _____ |
| | • Patient will appropriately verbalize feelings of anger and sadness. | _____ |
| | • Patient will describe his experiences in Afghanistan. | _____ |
| | *Long-term goals:* | |
| | • Patient will schedule outpatient appointments at the veterans' outreach center and at the mental health center. | _____ |

| | |
|---|---|
| Planning/ Interventions | **Nurse–patient relationship:** Assess and monitor suicidal ideations. Assist patient with identification and verbalization of feelings, especially anger. Assist patient in describing Afghanistan experiences. |
| | **Psychopharmacology:** Paroxetine (Paxil) 20 mg 8 AM; quetiapine (Seroquel) 100 mg q hs; lorazepam (Ativan) 1 mg q4h prn. |
| | **Milieu management:** Groups focusing on stress and anger management, relaxation techniques, social skills, and self-esteem. |
| Evaluation | Patient verbalizes that he is no longer suicidal. Patient is beginning to verbalize his anger and sadness about Afghanistan and the loss of his buddies. |
| Referrals | His appointment at the veterans' center is January 12; his appointment at the mental health center is on January 25. |

The somatoform disorders discussed here are somatization disorder, pain disorder, hypochondriasis, and conversion disorder. (See the *DSM-IV-TR* Criteria for Somatoform Disorders box.)

## SOMATIZATION DISORDER

According to the *DSM-IV-TR,* the main characteristic of somatization disorder is that these individuals verbalize recurrent, frequent, and multiple somatic complaints for several years without physiologic cause. This type of disorder usually begins before the age of 30 years. These patients see many physicians over the years and might even have exploratory and unnecessary surgical procedures. Impairment in social and occupational functioning might be present.

According to Brown and associates (2005), chronic emotional abuse might be the major etiology for the development of this disorder. These patients experience a family environment that is emotionally cold and harsh, with insults, rejection, and physical punishment. They experience frightening and intense emotions, which create anxiety and lead to defense mechanisms to cope with the anxiety. Blocking emotions, especially anger, rather than experiencing or verbalizing them is commonly found in patients with somatization disorder (Abbass, 2005). Such patients can

## DSM-IV-TR Criteria for Somatoform Disorders

**Somatization disorder.** Many physical complaints over several years, resulting in treatment being sought or impairment in functioning. It is characterized by four pain, two gastrointestinal, one sexual, and one pseudoneurologic symptom.

**Pain disorder.** Pain in one or more areas of the body that is severe enough to seek treatment; causes impairment in functioning or significant distress.

**Conversion disorder.** One or more symptoms or deficits affecting voluntary motor or sensory function that suggest a neurologic or general medical condition.

**Hypochondriasis.** Preoccupation with fear of having, or the idea that one has, a serious disease; includes misinterpretation of bodily symptoms; preoccupation persists despite medical evaluation and reassurance.

Modified from the American Psychiatric Association: *Diagnostic and statistical manual of mental disorders, text revision,* ed 4, Washington, DC, 2000, APA.

therefore be helped by having them experience and talk about their feelings and conflicts.

## PAIN DISORDER

The chief complaint in pain disorder is severe pain in one or more anatomic sites that causes significant distress or impairment in functioning (APA, 2000). The location or complaint of the pain does not change, unlike the complaints voiced in somatization disorder. Psychological factors play a role in the development and maintenance of pain disorder. No organic basis for this disorder exists.

There might be underlying psychological factors related to pain disorder that patients might not recognize consciously. For example, feelings connected with the loss of a job or status might occur before the development of pain disorder. This type of pain disorder is classified as *pain disorder associated with psychological factors.* In some cases, the pain might allow patients to avoid something that they do not want to do; for example, a woman's chest pain might prevent her from going to work.

Sometimes, there is a physiologic disorder, but the amount of pain or impairment is greatly exaggerated or out of proportion. For example, a patient who has experienced a mild myocardial infarction (MI) is now convinced that he or she can no longer engage in recreational activities such as bicycling or swimming, resulting perhaps from feelings of inadequacy or fear of suffering another MI. This pain disorder would be classified as *pain disorder associated with both psychological factors and a general medical condition.*

Patients with pain disorder are often "doctor shoppers" and might use analgesics excessively without experiencing any relief from their pain. These patients are often anxious about their symptoms and depressed about ever getting better.

## HYPOCHONDRIASIS

Hypochondriacs are worried about having, or believe that they have, a serious disease based on the misinterpretation of bodily signs and sensations (APA, 2000). Medical evaluation and reassurance do not help dispel the fear. These patients displace anxiety onto their bodies and misinterpret bodily symptoms. They are hypersensitive to their symptoms of anxiety and think that they are physically ill, which then increases their anxiety and their physical symptoms (Miller, 2004). This dysfunctional assumption is unique to hypochondriasis (Marcus and Church, 2003). Hypochondriacs check for reassurance from physicians or friends, similar to the compulsive behavior of patients with OCD.

## CONVERSION DISORDER

The major characteristic of conversion disorder is a deficit or alteration in voluntary motor or sensory function that suggests a neurologic or medical condition (APA, 2000). Psychological factors, conflicts, or stressors are associated with or precede the development of this disorder. The most common conversion symptoms suggest neurologic disease such as paralysis, blindness, or seizures. As mentioned earlier, primary gain refers to the alleviation of anxiety that the disorder provides, because conflict is kept out of conscious awareness. Secondary gain is the gratification received as a result of how people in these patients' environment respond to their illness and can prolong conversion symptoms.

## CLINICAL EXAMPLE

Roberta is worried about having an ulcer. She experiences acid indigestion on occasion after dinner. The uncomfortable feeling in her stomach causes her to fear that her stomach acid will burn a hole in the stomach lining. After each episode, Roberta visits her doctor for a physical examination. Based on the negative results from examinations and tests, the doctor has repeatedly told her that she does not have an ulcer.

Another characteristic of this disorder is that the symptom often is determined by the situation that produced it. For example, a soldier suddenly develops paralysis of his or her hand. As a result, he or she can no longer engage in combat because the trigger cannot be pulled on the gun. The symptom is related to the conflict. This soldier can discuss combat, but cannot connect his or her feelings about fighting to the development of the paralysis. This patient also might have an attitude of *la belle indifference,* meaning that he or she expresses little concern or anxiety about the distressing disorder. This lack of concern occurs because the symptom binds the anxiety, so that it is not behaviorally expressed. It might seem as though patients with conversion disorder minimize their illness.

## NURSE-PATIENT RELATIONSHIP

The focus of the nurse–patient relationship is to improve patients' overall levels of functioning by helping them develop adaptive coping behaviors. Patients with somatoform disorders are often unable to identify and express their feelings, needs, and conflicts. Teaching them ways to verbalize feelings appropriately helps eliminate or diminish the need for physical symptoms.

Patients need time to understand their need for physical symptoms. Awareness and insight develop slowly as patients begin to verbalize their needs. For some patients, this awareness and insight take longer to develop. The nurse must convey empathy and reassurance and teach patients about the connection between emotions and physical symptoms.

The physician or psychiatrist orders tests, physical examination, and laboratory workups to assess patients thoroughly for the presence of any physiologic or organic disease or etiology (if this has not been done before admission). The absence of any relevant medical findings strongly suggests that a somatoform disorder is present, especially if stress and conflicts are present in the patient's life.

The nursing interventions used for patients with somatoform disorders are described in the box below.

---

**Key Nursing Interventions** *for Somatoform Disorders*

1. Use a matter-of-fact, caring approach when providing care for physical symptoms. *Rationale:* to decrease secondary gains and to decrease focusing on physical symptoms.
2. Ask patients how they are feeling and ask them to describe their feelings. *Rationale:* to increase verbalization about feelings (especially negative ones), needs, and anxiety rather than about somatization.
3. Assist patients with developing more appropriate ways to verbalize feelings and needs. *Rationale:* to increase adaptive coping through assertiveness.
4. Use positive reinforcement and set limits by withdrawing attention from patients when they focus on physical complaints or make unreasonable demands. *Rationale:* to increase noncomplaining behavior.
5. Be consistent with patients, and have all requests directed to the primary nurse providing care. *Rationale:* to decrease attention-seeking or manipulative behaviors.
6. Use diversion by including patients in milieu activities and recreational games. *Rationale:* to decrease rumination about physical complaints.
7. Do not push awareness of or insight into conflicts or problems. *Rationale:* to prevent an increase in anxiety and the need for physical symptoms.

## CASE STUDY

William Robinson, a 62-year-old white man, was admitted to the psychiatric inpatient unit on June 15 at 10 AM. He walked onto the unit limping and supported by his wife, Harriet. He stated that he was experiencing horrible pain in his left leg and foot. Anger and irritability were evident in his voice.

Mr. Robinson's pain started suddenly about 7 months ago. Since that time, he has seen numerous physicians to obtain treatment and relief from his pain. The last physician told him that his pain was caused by stress, and it was recommended that he be hospitalized to obtain treatment from a physician who has been trained to manage stress-related disorders. The patient stated that he hoped this physician would know what to do, that none of the others did.

Mrs. Robinson brought her husband's medications to the hospital. The nurse found that a number of analgesics had been prescribed, along with sleeping medication. Mr. Robinson said that he took what he wanted, when he wanted, and that it was better than not taking anything at all.

The next day, after visiting her husband, Mrs. Robinson told the nurse that Mr. Robinson needed a lot of help with everything. In fact, she had been so physically tired that she had called their only daughter, Sheila, for assistance. Sheila lives 400 miles away, and they had not seen her for 3 years. Their daughter was so concerned about her parents that she had come to help for 2 weeks last month.

As the conversation continued, Mrs. Robinson told the nurse that her husband had been in good health, except for an occasional cold, until about 8 months ago, when he suddenly started to complain about awful pain in his leg and foot. He had never in all his years working for a cabinetmaker experienced anything like this before. Mrs. Robinson did not know why all this pain was happening now, especially since her husband had retired 9 months earlier. He had been forced to retire early, because the company he worked for had not been doing well and all employees aged 60 and older were forced to retire. She stated that her husband had never said too much about it, and she thought that now they would have time to travel and go on fishing trips, which her husband had always enjoyed. They had gone on many fishing trips as a family while their daughter was growing up and had enjoyed them immensely. Periodically, her husband went fishing with some friends. Since the onset of her husband's pain, however, they had not done anything socially, together or with friends.

From the time he was admitted to the hospital, Mr. Robinson refused to do anything but sit in a lounge chair in the community room. He needed much assistance from staff members to walk to the dining room and to the restroom. At times, his food was brought to him in the community room because he refused to walk to the dining room.

Interactions with the nurse centered on his pain and on requests for pain medication. He described his pain in detail and would talk of little else.

Mr. Robinson was getting Darvon for pain, and an antidepressant as ordered by his physician.

## PSYCHOPHARMACOLOGY

Because patients with somatoform disorders might be using too much medication and taking a variety of drugs, medication for pain should be used temporarily and sparingly. SSRIs are helpful for treating anxiety and depression because of the high incidence of comorbidity of these disorders.

## MILIEU MANAGEMENT

Relaxation exercises, meditation, and CBT are used to treat somatoform disorders. Physical therapy might be indicated to prevent muscle atrophy for an individual with conversion disorder (Miller, 2005a). Assertiveness, decision-making, goal-setting, stress management, and social skills groups often benefit these patients. Family therapy is helpful when family conflict is present.

Because patients with somatoform disorders are usually overusers of medical care, some hospitals and clinics provide group interventions as part of the medical care. These groups focus on underlying psychosocial needs, not on physical needs. The success of this type of treatment approach can result in decreasing hospital costs while providing more appropriate patient care.

## DISSOCIATIVE DISORDERS

Dissociation, which is the removal from conscious awareness of painful feelings, memories, thoughts, or aspects of identity, is an unconscious defense mechanism that protects an individual from the emotional pain of experiences or conflicts that have been repressed. This splitting off helps these individuals endure and survive intense emotion, physical pain, or both.

Dissociation occurs as a result of extreme stress or trauma, such as war or abuse in childhood and adulthood. Individuals might develop PTSD if the trauma is severe and lasting, which can lead to

## Care Plan

Name: William Robinson                                    Admission Date: _____

*DSM-IV-TR* Diagnosis: Pain disorder

| | |
|---|---|
| Assessment | **Areas of strength:** Enjoyed fishing and traveling; had been in good health; wife is very supportive; had worked for many years. |
| | **Problems:** Experiencing pain in his left leg and foot; social functioning has declined; focus with staff is about his pain; secondary gains maintain his sick role. |
| Diagnoses | • Ineffective coping related to anger, as evidenced by complaints of physical pain. |
| | • Chronic pain, related to low self-esteem, as evidenced by inability to verbalize feelings. |
| | • Severe anxiety, related to dependency, as evidenced by inability to care for self. |

Outcomes

*Short-term goals:*                                                                        *Date met*

- Patient will verbalize feelings and needs.                               _____
- Patient will verbalize underlying anger as a result of early            _____
  retirement.
- Patient will verbalize awareness about connecting emotions with         _____
  physical symptoms.
- Patient will develop adaptive coping behaviors.                         _____

*Long-term goals:*

- Patient will assume responsibility for self-care and independent        _____
  functioning.
- Patient will schedule appointments for joint counseling with            _____
  his wife.
- Patient will identify plans to volunteer in his community.              _____
- Patient will plan leisure activities.                                    _____

| | |
|---|---|
| Planning/ Interventions | **Nurse-patient relationship:** Convey interest and support; focus on assisting the patient to verbalize feelings and needs related to anxiety, self-esteem, and anger; give positive feedback when the patient focuses on issues other than pain; set limits on need for attention and medication; teach relaxation exercises. |
| | **Psychopharmacology:** Decrease the use of analgesics. Paxil 20 mg q AM. |
| | **Milieu management:** Encourage participation in assertiveness and communication groups, as well as problem-solving, discharge planning, and social skills groups, and diversional occupational therapy and recreational activities. |
| Evaluation | Patient's focus on pain is decreasing and he is able to assume self-care activities with little assistance. |
| Referrals | Appointments for outpatient group therapy and counseling with wife. |

dissociative identity disorder (Miller, 2005b). Everyone uses dissociation at times. For example, a person might be so engrossed in a book or a movie that they do not hear anything or anyone around them, but this is not pathologic behavior. Everyone forgets things or daydreams, but this does not indicate an illness. Abnormal dissociative states can become dissociative disorders when identity, memory, or consciousness is disturbed or altered. Dissociative disorders in the *DSM-IV-TR* are dissociative amnesia, dissociative fugue, depersonaliza-

tion, and dissociative identity disorder (DID; multiple personality disorder). The *DSM-IV-TR* Criteria for Dissociative Disorders box summarizes the main features of dissociative disorders.

## DISSOCIATIVE AMNESIA

Amnesia is the loss of memory or the inability to recall important personal information. Recent amnesia can occur immediately after a traumatic

## DSM-IV-TR Criteria for Dissociative Disorders

**Dissociative amnesia.** Loss of memory of important personal events that were traumatic or stressful in nature.

**Dissociative fugue.** Sudden, unexpected travel away from home or work with a loss of memory about the past; confusion about identity or assumption of partial or completely new identity is present.

**Depersonalization.** Experiences of feeling detached from, or an outside observer of, one's body or mental processes; reality testing is intact.

**Dissociative identity disorder.** Presence of two or more identities or personalities that take control of the person's behavior; loss of memory for important personal information.

Modified from the American Psychiatric Association: *Diagnostic and statistical manual of mental disorders, text revision,* ed 4, Washington, DC, 2000, APA.

event, such as a car accident. Localized amnesia occurs when the individual cannot remember what occurred during a specific period of time (e.g., not being able to remember what happened for hours after a car accident). The ability to recall some events during a specific period is called *selective amnesia* (APA, 2000). It is important to remember that patients are sometimes found by the police; these patients wander aimlessly and are confused and disoriented. They might be taken to a hospital and might be frightened and perplexed. The precipitant is usually something that causes severe psychosocial stress, such as the threat of physical injury or death.

The *DSM-IV-TR* describes dissociative amnesia as one or more episodes of the inability to recall important personal information that is beyond ordinary forgetfulness. The information is usually stressful or traumatic in nature. The amnesia does not occur only during the course of dissociative identity disorder, nor is it the result of a substance (drug or medication) or a medical condition, such as head trauma (APA, 2000).

## DISSOCIATIVE FUGUE

The major feature of dissociative fugue is sudden, unexpected travel away from home or some other location with the assumption of a new identity (partial or complete) or a confusion about one's identity. The travel and behavior appear normal to casual observers; thus, the person does not seem to be wandering in a confused state.

Fugue states last from a few hours to several days. These episodes are usually accompanied by amnesia; consequently, patients do not remember what happened during the fugue state.

Dissociative fugue is rare and usually follows severe psychosocial stress, such as marital quarrels, personal rejections, military conflict, natural disaster, financial difficulty, and suicidal ideation. Major depression is often present prior to dissociative fugue and there might be a history of childhood trauma (Howley and Ross, 2003). The fugue state then allows escape or flight from an intolerable event or situation.

## DEPERSONALIZATION

According to the *DSM-IV-TR*, depersonalization is included in this group of disorders because the sense of one's reality is changed, but the person is oriented to time, place, and person. In depersonalization, individuals feel detached from parts of their body or from mental processes. Depersonalization involves an altered sense of self, so that individuals feel unreal or strange or believe that danger is not happening to them but to someone else. Therefore, as a response to overwhelming stress, these individuals are protected from overwhelming anxiety. Depersonalization can also involve feeling like a robot or feeling as though one is in a dream; it is often accompanied by symptoms of derealization in which individuals feel that the outside world is changed or unreal. For example, buildings might appear to be leaning, or everything might seem gray and dull.

A diagnosis of depersonalization is made only when the prevalence or intensity of the disorder causes marked distress, interferes with daily functioning, and occurs in the absence of other disorders. An imaging study of depersonalization disorder has suggested abnormalities on limited cortical areas (Simeon et al, 2000). Little research has been done on this disorder to date.

## DISSOCIATIVE IDENTITY DISORDER

The major feature of DID is the existence of two or more identities or personalities that take control of the person's behavior (APA, 2000). The person, or host, is unaware of the other personalities (alters), but the other alters might be aware of each other to varying degrees. Patients can experience memory problems, depersonalization, derealization, identity confusion, time loss, voices conversing with each other, and voices that are persecutory (Dell, 2002).

Traditional views of this disorder consider dissociation to be a defense against extreme anxiety that is aroused in highly painful and emotionally traumatic situations, such as physical, emotional, and sexual abuse. The splitting off of these painful events allows the person to survive the trauma but leaves an impaired personality with disconnected parts, or alters. The alter personalities have feelings and behaviors associated with the trauma.

Each personality is different from the others and from the original personality. Each personality has its own name, behavior traits, memories, emotional characteristics, and social relations. The primary identity might carry the person's name and be depressed, dependent, and guilty, whereas alternate personalities might be hostile, controlling, and self-destructive (APA, 2000).

A shy, quiet woman might have alternate personalities that are promiscuous, flamboyant, childlike, and aggressive. A woman might awaken one morning and find the living room of her apartment littered with toys or strewn with empty alcohol bottles and leftover food. She does not remember what happened because she has amnesia for the span of time when another personality took over, or came out.

Sometimes, a switch to another personality is preceded by a headache, or individuals might cover their face and eyes with their hands. For example, the patient or original personality might state that he or she hears voices talking to one another in his or her head. This might be misdiagnosed as auditory hallucinations, and the disorder misdiagnosed as schizophrenia.

These patients are admitted to inpatient psychiatric units when they are suicidal, meaning that an alter personality is trying to harm or kill one of the other personalities for revelations concerning abuse, for example, or when mutilation or uncontrollable impulses to harm the self are present. Severe anxiety or depression related to the coming out of upsetting alters might also be a reason for admission. The safe structure of a hospital setting provides emotional security for the patient when working with difficult or overwhelming problems.

Some patients experience numerous hospitalizations with different diagnoses before they are finally and accurately diagnosed with DID. The array of symptoms that these patients present might be one reason for inaccurate diagnoses. Another might be that patients do not recognize their symptoms or know what they mean. Patients might think that they are going crazy or losing their mind because they do not understand what their symptoms mean or represent. Thus, these individuals might delay seeking treatment until their disorder severely interrupts their functioning in life. Others around them, such as family members, might not understand what is occurring, might not know how to help, or might want to keep the disorder a secret, especially if the perpetrator of the abuse is a family member.

## PUTTING IT ALL TOGETHER
### Psychotherapeutic Management

## NURSE-PATIENT RELATIONSHIP

The nurse's relationship with individuals experiencing amnesia and fugue includes interventions to establish trust and support. Patients have physiologic and neurologic workups to rule out organic causations. The nurse assists with gathering data regarding feelings, conflicts, or situations that patients experienced before the amnesia or fugue state. Patients also might have sessions under hypnosis to gather data about forgotten material. The nurse should slowly help patients deal with anxiety and conflicts in their lives and improve coping skills.

Patients with depersonalization disorder are not usually found in an inpatient setting unless they have become suicidal, extremely anxious, or depressed. Nurses might work with these patients in outpatient settings.

The treatment goal of DID, ultimately through long-term therapy, is to integrate the personalities or memories, if possible, so that they can survive or coexist in the original personality. The use of hypnosis to retrieve memories is controversial. Some think that this is harmful because it could produce additional alters and false memories (Miller, 2005b).

The nurse provides caring and empathy and works with patients to establish trust because the relationships of these patients with authority figures might have been inconsistent, rigid, and unpredictable. A contract should be initiated for patients' safety and to reduce self-harm and violence. An alter might be homicidal because of revelations concerning abuse. Self-mutilation and suicidal behaviors also might be present when overwhelming anxiety or depression occurs. The nurse needs to remember that, even with the presence of a child alter, the patient is an adult and not a child. Caring and empathy must be balanced with education about the disorder (Shusta-Hochberg, 2004).

The nurse must also be alert to splitting by staff members regarding patients' diagnoses. The staff might divide into groups of believers and nonbelievers regarding the validity of patients' diagnoses. Education about diagnoses, management of feelings, especially anger and rage, and consistency of approach assist the staff in developing a caring, supportive environment for patients so that trust increases and a predictable, positive learning environment is developed.

## PSYCHOPHARMACOLOGY

Medication does not eliminate the dissociative disorder itself. If symptoms of anxiety and depression are present, medications might help. For patients with DID, response to medication might be partial, and an alter's response to medication might be different and inconsistent.

## MILIEU MANAGEMENT

The nurse assumes an important role in the care of patients who are hospitalized in an inpatient psychiatric unit because of suicidal or uncontrollable attempts to harm themselves. Provisions for a safe environment and a trusting relationship are basic for helping these patients, who usually have not had trusting relationships with anyone. Assisting with group sessions; providing emotional security, empathy, acceptance, and support; and helping patients cope with daily living are all involved in nursing care.

For patients with DID, ongoing process-oriented groups, which might be available in some settings, can be nontherapeutic when patients reveal too much and overwhelm the group or

regress. Individual therapy should be in progress and might have been initiated before hospitalization. Task-oriented groups are beneficial. Occupational therapy and art therapy provide patients with a means of nonverbal expression to reveal material that cannot be verbally accessed. Attendance at milieu meetings decreases isolation from the community. For patients with dissociative disorders, cognitive therapy, relaxation, stress management, meditation, and exercise are beneficial. Cognitive therapy can help decrease blame or guilt surrounding issues of physical or sexual abuse.

Before discharge, a safety plan and no-harm contract might be necessary, as well as initiating or continuing a support system for the patient. Self-help groups provide outpatients with the opportunity to practice social skills and problem solving to develop a sense of empowerment and control.

---

### CRITICAL THINKING QUESTION    3

A patient with DID is admitted to the inpatient unit because of a suicide attempt. One of the personalities wants to kill the patient, meaning that the patient is suicidal. The patient refuses to sign a no-harm contract. What issues would you expect to help the patient with, including types of precautions?

---

### Study Notes

1. The concepts of primary and secondary gains are important to understand because primary gain relieves discomfort, whereas secondary gain might encourage patients to maintain their sick role.
2. Understanding the process of anxiety is key to understanding and intervening therapeutically with patients who have these disorders.
3. Patients' anxiety must be reduced to a mild or moderate level before the nurse can work with them on problem solving and adaptive coping.
4. In the category of anxiety-related disorders, patients feel and/or directly express symptoms of anxiety.
5. With ASD, PTSD, and adjustment disorders, the goals are to integrate the traumatic memories and feelings about the original trauma and to move from victim to survivor status.

6. With somatoform disorders, anxiety is expressed through physical symptoms.

7. In DID, anxiety is split off (removed) from conscious awareness, which helps patients survive extreme emotional pain and trauma.

8. Key nursing interventions include helping patients to manage feelings, anxiety, conflicts, and life stressors in an adaptive manner so that they can become independent, functioning adults.

## References

Abbass A: Somatization: diagnosing it soon through emotion-focused interviewing, *J Fam Pract* 54:231, 2005.

Amaya-Jackson L, Davidson JR, Hughes DC, et al: Functional impairment and utilization of services associated with posttraumatic stress in the community, *J Trauma Stress* 12:709, 1999.

American Psychiatric Association: *Diagnostic and statistical manual of mental disorders, text revision,* ed 4, Washington, DC, 2000, APA.

Antai-Ontong D: Current treatment of generalized anxiety disorder, *J Psychosoc Nurs Ment Health Serv* 41:20, 2003.

Axelrod SR, Morgan CA, Southwick SM: Symptoms of posttraumatic stress disorder and borderline personality disorder in veterans of Operation Desert Storm, *Am J Psychiatry* 162:270, 2005.

Badger JM: Understanding secondary traumatic stress, *Am J Nurs* 101:26, 2001.

Ballenger JC, Davidson JR, Lecrubier Y, et al: Consensus statement on generalized anxiety disorder from the international consensus group on depression and anxiety, *J Clin Psychiatry* 62(Suppl 13):47, 2001.

Barclay L, Vega C: Gulf War deployment might have increased the risk of fibromyalgia, chronic fatigue, skin conditions, and dyspepsia. Available at www.medscape.com. Accessed June 6, 2005.

Beckham JC, Moore SD, Reynolds V: Interpersonal hostility and violence in Vietnam combat veterans with chronic posttraumatic stress disorder, *Aggression Violent Behav* 5:451, 2000.

Bille DA: Road to recovery, posttraumatic stress disorder: the hidden victim, *J Psychosoc Nurs Ment Heath Serv* 31:19, 1993.

Bleiberg KL, Markowitz JC: A pilot study of interpersonal psychotherapy for posttraumatic stress disorder, *Am J Psychiatry* 162:181, 2005.

Boscarino JA, Figley CR, Adams RE: Compassion fatigue following the September 11 terrorist attacks: A study of secondary trauma among New York City social workers, *Int J Emerg Ment Health* 6:57, 2004.

Brenner JD, et al: Vietnam vets' PTSD experience, *J Psychosoc Nurs Ment Health Serv* 34(6):148, 1996.

Brown RJ, Schrag A, Trimble MR: Dissociation, childhood interpersonal trauma, and family functioning in patients with somatization disorder, *Am J Psychiatry* 162:899, 2005.

Charney DS: Psychobiological mechanisms of resilience and vulnerability: implications for successful adaptation to extreme stress, *Am J Psychiatry* 161:195, 2004.

Clark C: Posttraumatic stress disorder, *Am J Nurs* 97:27, 1997.

Cottraux J: Recent developments in the research on generalized anxiety disorder, *Curr Opin Psychiatry* 17:49, 2004.

Davidson JR: Pharmacotherapy of generalized anxiety disorder, *J Clin Psychiatry* 62(Suppl 11):46, 2001.

Dell PF: Dissociative phenomenology of dissociative identity disorder, *J Nerv Ment Dis* 190:10, 2002.

Everly GS, Flannery RB, Mitchell JT: Critical incident stress management (CISM): a review of the literature, *Aggression Violent Behav* 5:23, 2000.

Falsetti SA, Resnick HS, Davis J: Multichannel exposure therapy: combining cognitive-behavioral therapies for the treatment of posttraumatic stress disorder with panic attacks, *Behav Modif* 29:70, 2005.

Figley CR: Families coping with trauma, clinical update: posttraumatic stress disorder, *Am Assoc Marriage Family Ther* 2:1, 2000.

Flouri E: Post-traumatic stress disorder (PTSD): what we have learned and what we still have not found out, *J Interpersonal Violence* 20:373, 2005.

Foa EB, Keane TM, Friedman MJ: Guidelines for treatment of PTSD, *J Trauma Stress* 13:539, 2000.

Friedman MJ: Posttraumatic stress disorder, *J Clin Psychiatry* 58:33, 1997.

Frueh B, Buckley TC, Cusack KJ, et al: Cognitive-behavioral treatment for PTSD among people with severe mental illness: a proposed treatment model, *J Psychiatr Pract* 10:26, 2004.

Fullerton CS, Ursano RJ, Wang L: Acute stress disorder, posttraumatic stress disorder, and depression in disaster or rescue workers, *Am J Psychiatry* 161:1370, 2004.

Geffken GR, Storch EA, Gelfand KM, et al: Cognitive behavior therapy for obsessive compulsive disorder, review of treatment techniques, *J Psychosoc Nurs Ment Health Serv* 42:44, 2004.

Glod C, Cawley D: Psychobiology perspectives: the neurobiology of obsessive-compulsive disorders, *J Am Psychiatr Nurs Assoc* 3:120, 1997.

Goodwin RD, Lieb R, Hoefler M, et al: Panic attack as a risk factor for severe psychopathology, *Am J Psychiatry* 161:2207, 2004.

Gorman JM, Kent JM, Sullivan GM, Coplan JD: Neuroanatomical hypothesis of panic disorder, revised, *Am J Psychiatry* 157:493, 2000.

Himle JA, Rassi S, Haghighatgou H, et al: Group behavioral therapy of obsessive-compulsive disorder: seven vs. twelve-week outcomes, *Depress Anxiety* 13:161, 2001.

Hines-Martin VP, Ising M: Use of art therapy with posttraumatic stress disordered veteran clients, *J Psychosoc Nurs Ment Health Serv* 31:29, 1993.

Hollander E, Kaplan A, Allen A, Cartwright C: Pharmacotherapy for obsessive-compulsive disorder, *Psychiatr Clin North Am* 23:643, 2000.

Howley J, Ross CA: The structure of dissociative fugue: a case report, *J Trauma Dissociation* 4:109, 2003.

Kaplan Z, Iancu I, Bodner E: A review of psychological debriefing after extreme stress, *Psychiatr Serv* 52:824, 2001.

Keltner NL, Perry BA, Williams AR: Panic disorder: a tightening vortex of misery, *Perspect Psychiatr Care* 39:38, 2003.

Koren D, Norman D, Cohen A, et al: Increased PTSD risk with combat-related injury: a matched comparison study of injured and uninjured soldiers experiencing the same combat events, *Am J Psychiatry* 162:276, 2005.

La Torre MA: Therapeutic approaches to anxiety—a holistic view, *Perspect Psychiatr Care* 37:28, 2001.

Lombardo TW, Gray MJ: Beyond exposure for posttraumatic stress disorder (PTSD) symptoms: broad-spectrum PTSD treatment strategies, *Behav Modif* 29:3, 2005.

Marcus DK, Church SE: Are dysfunctional beliefs about illness unique to hypochondriasis? *J Psychosom Res* 54(6):543, 2003.

Mayou R, Kirmayer LJ, Simon G, et al: Somatoform disorders: time for a new approach in DSM-V, *Am J Psychiatry* 162:847, 2005.

McMillen JC, North CS, Smith EM: What parts of PTSD are normal: intrusion, avoidance, or arousal? Data from the Northridge, California, earthquake, *J Trauma Stress* 13:57, 2000.

Miller MC: Generalized anxiety disorder: toxic worry, *Harv Ment Health Lett* 19:1, 2003.

Miller MC: Hypochondria, *Harv Ment Health Lett* 21:4, 2004.

Miller MC: Conversion disorder, *Harv Ment Health Lett* 22:1, 2005a.

Miller MC: Falling apart: dissociation and its disorders, *Harv Ment Health Lett* 21:1, 2005b.

Miller MC: Questions and answers, *Harv Ment Health Lett* 21:8, 2005c.

Moyers F: Oklahoma City bombing: exacerbation of symptoms in veterans with PTSD, *Arch Psychiatr Nurs* 10:55, 1996.

Olszewski TM, Varrasse JF: The neurobiology of PTSD: implications for nurses, *J Psychosoc Nurs* 43:41, 2005.

Reeves RR, Parker JD, Konkle-Parker, DJ: War-related mental health of today's veterans, *J Psychosoc Nurs* 43:18, 2005.

Schoenfeld FB, Marmar CR, Neylan TC: Current concepts in pharmacotherapy for posttraumatic stress disorder, *Psychiatr Serv* 55:519, 2004.

Shusta-Hochberg SR: Therapeutic hazards of treating child alters as real children in dissociative identity disorder, *J Trauma Dissociation* 5:13, 2004.

Simeon D, Guralnik O, Hazlett EA, et al: Feeling unreal: a PET study of depersonalization disorder, *Am J Psychiatry* 157:1782, 2000.

Snell FI, Padin-Rivera E: Group treatment for older veterans with post-traumatic stress disorder, *J Psychosoc Nurs Ment Health Serv* 35:10, 1997.

Solomon EP, Heide KM: The biology of trauma: implications for treatment, *J Interpersonal Violence* 20:51, 2005.

van der Kolk BA: The psychobiology of post traumatic stress disorder, *J Clin Psychiatry* 58:16, 1997.

Weigartz PS, Rasminsky S: Treating OCD in patients with psychiatric morbidity: how to keep anxiety, depression, and other disorders from thwarting interventions, *Curr Psychiatry* 4:57, 2005.

Woods SJ: Intimate partner violence and post-traumatic stress disorder symptoms in women: What we know and need to know, *J Interpersonal Violence* 20:394, 2005.

Woods SJ, Wineman, NM: Trauma, posttraumatic stress disorder symptom clusters, and physical health symptoms in post-abused women, *Arch Psychiatr Nurs* 18:26, 2004.

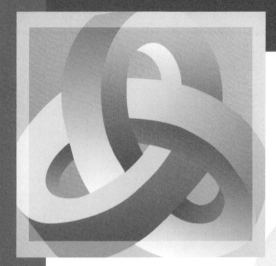

# Chapter 32

# Cognitive Disorders

*Judith A. Wilson*

## Learning Objectives

*After reading this chapter, you should be able to:*

- Describe the biologic and functional changes associated with the most prevalent types of dementia.
- Describe the etiologic aspects and behaviors associated with delirium.
- Be able to use the *Diagnostic and Statistical Manual of Mental Disorders, Text Revision, Fourth Edition (DSM-IV-TR)* to understand the diagnostic criteria used for cognitive disorders.

- Differentiate dementia from delirium.
- Discuss appropriate pharmacologic interventions for patients with dementia.
- Develop a care plan for a patient with dementia.
- Develop effective caregiver interventions.
- Discuss family issues related to cognitive disorders.

## INTRODUCTION

Cognitive disorders comprise a variety of assaults on the human brain. Cognition revolves around learning and memory. Loss of these fundamental abilities is a common thread in all cognitive disorders. In some disorders, these losses might be temporary. However, for most disorders, loss of memory is a harbinger of things to come. This chapter describes the most common cognitive disorders that the nurse might confront.

Other changes in cognition commonly take place. Disorientation, decreased concentration, loss of abstract thinking, and language disturbances might be present. Delusions, hallucinations, and misidentification might frighten the patients. These individuals might not be able to perform routine activities because they have forgotten how to do them in spite of intact motor skills.

Cognitive disorders are divided into reversible and irreversible types. These disorders can span a few hours to many years and might or might not be imminently life-threatening. To cloud the diagnostic picture, patients might have more than one cognitive disorder or a coexisting psychiatric illness. Depression and anxiety are common in these patients.

Patients who exhibit a marked change of mental status often have a cognitive disorder. The *DSM-IV-TR* (American Psychiatric Association [APA], 2000) provides diagnostic criteria for all these disorders. The *DSM-IV-TR* criteria for both delirium and dementia are included in boxes in this chapter. Table 32-1 compares and contrasts dementia and delirium (Wilson and Helton, 2005). Key terms are included, and the student should also consult the glossary in this text. The 12-month prevalence rate of mental disorders in the United States is also

## Norm's Notes

*This chapter is so important. There are more and more of us older people and we are the ones who tend to develop the cognitive disorders discussed in this chapter. Think about it—when you can no longer reason clearly and rationally, the "real" you has been taken. As a kid, I used to wonder if I would rather lose an arm or a leg. Well, kids think about silly stuff. But I know now that I do not want to lose my cognitive functions. Fortunately, our government (run by a bunch of older people) spends a lot of money studying how these conditions can be stopped or reversed. I just want the researchers to hurry.*

included. Pertinent *DSM-IV-TR* diagnoses and current NANDA International diagnoses (NANDA International, 2005), which facilitate care planning, are listed as well.

In dementia research, dozens of diagnostic tools are used, from pen and pencil examinations to sophisticated neuroimaging studies. The Geriatric Depression Scale can be found on the Evolve page. Genetic studies have isolated chromosomes and genes that are related to certain diseases. Since 1993, five different medications for Alzheimer's disease have reached the market.

## OVERVIEW OF NONDEMENTIA COGNITIVE DISORDERS

### MILD COGNITIVE IMPAIRMENT

Mild cognitive impairment (MCI) is a regression in cognition that is not a result of normal

---

**Table 32-1   Dementia and Delirium: Contrast and Comparison**

| Characteristics | Delirium | Dementia |
|---|---|---|
| Onset | Occurs quickly, is obvious | Slow, unnoticeable at first |
| Course | Acute: rapid development, usually hours to days, but can last for months | Chronic: slow development over months and years, with a progressive deterioration spanning 3 to 10 years until death |
| Causes | Usually the result of other physical reasons (e.g., illness, postsurgical problems, toxins) | Usually the primary disorder, but might be related to other illnesses (e.g., AIDS) |
| Memory | Short-term memory is impaired when assessed during an interim lucid or clear moment | Short-term memory is lost initially; long-term memory fails slowly |
| Level of consciousness | Fluctuating level of consciousness; alert at times; sleep is erratic; no pattern | No change; sleep patterns are usually consistent; day-night reversal is common |
| Thought content | Matches level of consciousness | Normal at first; later might be difficult to assess because of confusion or expressive or receptive aphasia and poverty of content |
| Thought process | Logical alternating with illogical, depending on the level of consciousness | Logical at first, then loss of abstraction (e.g., understanding a joke); concrete thinking occurs as the disease progresses |
| Speech | Might have slurred speech | Normal speech |
| Perceptual differences | Hallucinations—*visual:* seeing animals or unusual colors, also picking at the air is a sign; *tactile:* feeling bugs on or under the skin | Misidentification: calling one relative another's name—for example, calling a daughter "mama"; hallucinations might occur in the later stage, usually not at first<br>Delusions: grandiose, paranoid; pathologic jealousy, interfering with belongings and property |
| Mood | Anxiety and fear | Wide range of feelings |
| Affect | Appears bewildered, frightened | Appearance matches feeling |

From Wilson J, Helton B: *PSYCHed: continuing education and consultation, dementia and delirium module,* Birmingham, AL, 2005. (Unpublished.)

12-Month Prevalence Rate of Mental Disorders in the United States*

| Disorders | Approximate Percentage Over 17 Years of Age | Approximate Number of Persons | Gender Overrepresentation |
|---|---|---|---|
| **Anxiety Disorders** | 18 overall | 36,000,000 | |
| Panic disorder | 3.5 | 7,000,000 | Women |
| Social phobia | 7 | 14,000,000 | Women |
| Specific phobia | 8.7 | 17,000,000 | Women |
| GAD | 3 | 6,000,000 | Women |
| PTSD | 3.5 | 7,000,000 | Women |
| OCD | 1 | 2,000,000 | Equal |
| **Mood Disorders** | 9.5 overall | 19,000,000 | |
| Major depression | 6.7 | | Women |
| Dysthymia | 1.5 | | Women |
| Bipolar I and II | 2.6 | | BD I: Equal<br>BD II: Women? |
| **Impulse Control Disorders** | 9 overall | 18,000,000 | |
| Conduct disorders | 1 | 2,000,000 | Men |
| ADHD | 4 | 8,000,000 | Men |
| **Substance Abuse Disorders** | 3.8 overall | 7,600,000 | |
| Alcohol abuse and dependence | 3.1 | 6,200,000 | Men |
| Drug abuse and dependence | 1.4 | 2,800,000 | Men |
| **Schizophrenia** | 1.1 | 2,100,000 | Equal |

*Extrapolated from several sources based on current census data.
*ADHD,* Attention-deficit/hyperactivity disorder; *GAD,* generalized anxiety disorder; *OCD,* obsessive-compulsive disorder; *PTSD,* posttraumatic stress disorder.
From Kessler RC, Chiu WT, Demler O, Walters EE: Prevalence, severity, and comorbidity of 12-month DSM-IV disorders in the national comorbidity survey replication, *Arch Gen Psychiatry* 62:617, 2005; U.S. Surgeon General: *Mental health: a report from the Surgeon General,* Washington, DC, 1999, Department of Health and Human Services: National Institute of Mental Health: *Statistics.* Available at: www.nimh.nih.gov/healthinformation/statisticsmenu.cfm. Accessed April 18, 2005.

aging. Petersen and associates (2005) have referred to MCI as the transitional zone between normal aging and very probable early Alzheimer's disease for those who ultimately develop the disease. Currently, no *DSM-IV-TR* diagnosis exists for MCI. Forgetfulness is the hallmark behavior. Nonmemory areas of function are not impaired enough to lead to a dementia diagnosis. Jack (2003) found that, in the patient with MCI, hippocampal atrophy is predictive of subsequent conversion to Alzheimer's disease. Of 80 patients with MCI, 27 (34%) converted to Alzheimer's disease after 32 months. Other reports have indicated even higher percentages. The National Institute of Aging (NIA) *2000 Progress Report on Alzheimer's Disease* (NIA, 2000) stated that 40% of all patients with MCI develop Alzheimer's disease in 3 years. Morris and colleagues (2001) also concluded that patients with MCI are generally in the early stage of Alzheimer's disease.

No medications are specifically indicated for MCI, but many clinical trials are under way. Anti-oxidants such as vitamins C and E, estrogen, ibuprofen, the statins, and some medications that the U.S. Food and Drug Administration (FDA) has approved for Alzheimer's disease are currently being tested (U.S. Food and Drug Administration, 2005). In a study with 769 subjects, Petersen and co-workers (2005) found that vitamin E offered no benefit but that donepezil slowed the rate of progression to Alzheimer's disease during the first year. These researchers found that 16% of their subjects converted to Alzheimer's disease each year. Although no specific treatments are available, the patient with MCI should stay active, exercise at the appropriate level, eat a well-balanced diet, curb alcohol consumption, and stop tobacco usage. Challenging the brain with mental exercises such as comparing and contrasting is also therapeutic. For example, comparing a book with the movie made about it has been found beneficial: what was the same, what was different? Other ways to stimulate cognition include playing board games, putting together puzzles, and solving word games.

Mr. Hawkins, a 67-year-old retired accountant, had trouble balancing his checkbook. He had forgotten to enter the amounts in the ledger. Mr. Hawkins was aware that he was forgetful and started asking his wife to help him. He did not have any other noticeable change in behavior. Mr. Hawkins enjoyed playing golf with his friends and he could safely drive. However, 3 years later, he was diagnosed with Alzheimer's disease.

## DELIRIUM

The word *delirium* literally means "out of one's furrow," which refers to the dramatic behavioral changes that the person might experience. The hallmark sign of delirium is its acute onset, which is key because the disorder rapidly develops in most cases. Other signs include a fluctuating level of consciousness, slurred speech, nonsensical thoughts, and day-night sleep reversal. The delirious patient might have visual hallucinations—for example, seeing multicolored rats—or have tactile hallucinations, during which the patient might feel bugs under the skin. The patient might pick at the air as if trying to do some routine task, such as opening a prescription bottle. The patient might be able to follow a conversation for a short period, followed by an acute bout of confusion. Emotions are on edge, and the patient might startle easily. The nurse should intervene quickly when delirium is suspected. Assessment and treatment of any underlying physical problem or illness should be addressed, because delirium can be life-threatening. Kirshner (2002) stated that 25% of hospitalized elderly patients who have delirium die within 6 months.

Delirium is the most common complication of the hospitalized older adult patient (Inouye, 2000). *ICU psychosis* is another name for hospital-based delirium. Acute changes in the patient's mental status might serve as a sign that a serious underlying medical illness exists (Inouye et al, 1999). Delirium is associated with many physical illnesses, especially pneumonia, myocardial infarction, and urinary tract infection. Toxic response to medications occurs with prescribed and over-the-counter (OTC) medications. For example, drugs with anticholinergic properties can cause delirium. Such drugs include diphenhydramine (Benadryl), some tricyclic antidepressants, and benztropine (Cogentin). Other drugs, including lithium and divalproex, might become toxic at lower serum levels than the laboratory reference range indicates. Malnourishment, dehydration, constipation, and impactions increase the possibility of developing delirium. The nurse, during the initial medication assessment, should ask the patient or family member about prescription *and* OTC medications. The nurse should also ask about cough syrup, dietary supplements, sleeping pills, and pain medications, in particular.

Dementia is the most consistent risk factor for delirium. Of the patients who have delirium, 30% to 50% have dementia. If the cause of the delirium is the result of a physical illness, treatment should be started to stabilize the patient. Alcohol and drug withdrawal require strict protocols to reduce the likelihood of its occurrence.

If at all possible, delirium prevention is the best medical option. Epling and Taylor (1999) have identified six risk factors for delirium: (1) cognitive impairment, (2) hearing impairment, (3) sleep deprivation, (4) immobility, (5) visual impairment, and (6) dehydration. These researchers developed protocols addressing each risk factor. Most subjects (87%) using these protocols did not develop delirium.

Ms. Helton, a 64-year-old woman, was found crawling around her bedroom. She thought her husband was plotting to kill her. She found his pistol, took it, and was waiting to shoot him when her daughter found her. At that time, she was taking three different OTC preparations that contained diphenhydramine: a sedative, a cough syrup, and a pill for allergies. Discontinuation of the diphenhydramine resulted in a return to the patient's premorbid level of cognitive function. She did not require any further psychiatric care. She and her family were given a list of common OTC and prescribed anticholinergic medications for future reference.

## PSEUDODEMENTIA

Pseudodementia is an inexact term for a cognitive disorder that is almost always associated with depression. Patients might seem as if they have a dementing disorder when they are actually

## DSM-IV-TR Criteria for Delirium

Delirium is characterized by:

1. Disturbances of consciousness (i.e., reduced clarity of awareness of the environment) with reduced ability to focus, sustain, or shift attention.
2. Changes in cognition (e.g., memory deficit, disorientation, language disturbance, perceptual disturbance).
3. Developments over a short period of time (usually hours to days) and with a tendency to fluctuate during the course of the day.

Modified from the American Psychiatric Association: *Diagnostic and statistical manual of mental disorders, text revision,* ed 4, Washington, DC, 2000, APA.

profoundly depressed. These patients are often amotivational and have a lack of energy. When queried, their responses are usually "I don't know" or some other meaningless comment, which makes it seem as though the patient is disoriented and confused.

Some clinicians do not think that this is a real diagnosis. It does not appear in the *DSM-IV-TR.* Is this a separate syndrome or is it always the result of the interaction between depression and dementia (Alexopolos, 2003)? Are there types of depression that are more likely to lead to pseudodementia than others? Does it predict the onset of a dementia?

Treatment is designed for target symptoms such as depression, which might include medications and other modalities—for example psychotherapy, occupational therapy, exercise therapy, and even electroconvulsive treatment.

### CLINICAL EXAMPLE
*of a Patient With Pseudodementia*

Mr. Howell, a 75-year-old man, refused to answer any assessment questions. He said, "I don't know" repeatedly throughout the interview. His wife tried to answer the questions for him. He had stopped taking the antidepressant prescribed for him 2 months before; he could not remember why. Mr. Howell also stopped playing dominoes with his friends. After he was stabilized on the antidepressant medication, Mr. Howell resumed all his usual activities. Two years later, he was diagnosed with Alzheimer's disease.

## DEMENTIA

The word *dementia,* from Latin, literally means "out of one's mind." Dementia is a type of illness with a progressively deteriorating course that ultimately affects cognition, perception, language, behavior, and motor abilities. Over 70 types of dementia have been identified, of which Alzheimer's disease is the most prevalent (Geldmacher, 1997).

A dementia can be either reversible or irreversible. Unfortunately, most dementing illnesses are irreversible, and those that can be reversed might not be completely reversible. Normal pressure hydrocephalus (NPH) and vitamin $B_{12}$ deficiency are two dementias that are potentially reversible. Dementias related to endocrine dysfunction, other metabolic disturbances, and neoplasms might show some improvement after treatment (Perkin, 1998).

### CRITICAL THINKING QUESTION   1
Why is it important to recognize the difference between dementia and delirium?

### CRITICAL THINKING QUESTION   2
Explain why attending a senior center might be therapeutic for a patient with a dementia.

## REVERSIBLE DEMENTIAS

### NORMAL PRESSURE HYDROCEPHALUS

NPH usually presents with a classic triad of symptoms: urinary incontinence, apraxic gait, and dementia. These patients have enlarged lateral and third ventricles, which might be seen on either a computed tomography (CT) or magnetic resonance imaging (MRI) scan of the brain (Moore and Jefferson, 2004). The cause of NPH is impaired return of cerebrospinal fluid to the spinal column from the brain. The cerebrospinal fluid has normal pressure or is slightly elevated when monitored. Urinary urgency or frequency, common signs of a urinary tract infection, might instead be a precursor to incontinence. Gait apraxia might be described as magnetic or as if the patient were walking over a sticky floor.

# *DSM-IV-TR* and NANDA International Diagnoses Related to Cognitive Disorders

*DSM-IV-TR\**

*Delirium Types*
Alcohol

- Induced persisting amnestic disorder
- Intoxication delirium
- Withdrawal delirium

Amphetamine (or amphetamine-like)

- Intoxication delirium

Delirium

- Cannabis intoxication
- Cocaine intoxication
- Inhalant intoxication
- Opioid intoxication
- Phencyclidine (or phencyclidine-like) intoxication delirium
- Sedative, hypnotic, or anxiolytic intoxication delirium

Delirium due to multiple etiologies

Sedative, hypnotic, or anxiolytic withdrawal delirium
Delirium due to [indicate the general medical condition]
Delirium NOS (not otherwise specified)

*Dementia Types*
Dementia

- Substance-induced persisting
- Dementia due to multiple etiologies

Dementia due to Creutzfeldt-Jakob disease
Dementia due to head trauma
Dementia due to HIV (human immunodeficiency virus)
Dementia due to Huntington's disease
Dementia due to Parkinson's disease
Dementia due to Pick's disease
Dementia due to [indicate other general medical condition]
Dementia NOS
Dementia of the Alzheimer's type

- With early onset
- With late onset

Vascular dementia

*Other Disorders*
Amnestic disorder NOS
Amnestic disorder due to [indicate the general medical condition]
Cognitive disorder

Other (or unknown) substance-induced persisting amnestic disorder
Sedative-, hypnotic-, or anxiolytic-persisting amnestic disorder

NANDA INTERNATIONAL†
Anxiety
Anxiety, death
Caregiver role strain, risk for
Comfort, impaired
Communication, verbal, impaired
Confusion, acute
Confusion, chronic
Coping, community, ineffective
Coping, family, compromised
Coping, family, disabled
Coping, family, readiness for enhanced
Coping, ineffective
Denial, ineffective
Diversional activity, deficient
Family processes: alcoholism, dysfunctional
Family processes: interrupted
Fear
Grieving, anticipatory
Grieving, dysfunctional
Hopelessness
Knowledge, deficient
Loneliness, risk for
Memory, impaired
Noncompliance
Powerlessness, risk for
Self-care deficit, bathing/hygiene
Self-care deficit, feeding
Self-care deficit, toileting
Self-esteem, chronic low
Self-esteem, situational low
Sensory perception, disturbed
Sleep patterns, disturbed
Social interaction, impaired
Social isolation
Spiritual distress, risk for
Suicide, risk for
Therapeutic regimen management, community, ineffective
Therapeutic regimen management, effective
Therapeutic regimen management, ineffective
Therapeutic regimen management, family, ineffective
Thought processes, disturbed
Violence, other-directed, risk for
Violence, self-directed, risk for
Wandering

*From the American Psychiatric Association: *Diagnostic and statistical manual of mental disorders, text revision,* ed 4, Washington, DC, 2000, APA.
†From NANDA International: *NANDA-approved nursing diagnoses: definitions and classifications, 2005-2006.* Philadelphia, 2005, NANDA International.

Impairment in activities of daily living is a common presenting problem. Another common early sign is a dulling of personality, with lack of motivation (Perkin, 1998). Judgment and insight might be lacking. Memory loss is the last of three symptoms to appear. If untreated, these symptoms might progress until the patient might be unable to stand or speak, and is ultimately confined to bed.

If caught early, NPH might be reversed. Unfortunately, the patient, family, and clinicians often ignore the initial symptoms. Treatment requires neurosurgery. A ventricular shunt is placed in one of the lateral ventricles in the brain, which then leads to the peritoneum (VP shunt). A small pump is implanted just under the scalp behind the ear. The caregiver activates the pump for the prescribed number of times and frequency each day. The surgery has a 50% success rate (Perkin, 1998). If NPH has progressed and is no longer reversible, the shunting procedure might not arrest further decline.

## CLINICAL EXAMPLE
*of a Patient With Normal Pressure Hydrocephalus*

Mrs. Burkhalter, a 66-year-old woman, was admitted for evaluation. Her husband said that she had been diagnosed with Alzheimer's disease. She was bed-bound, incontinent of urine, and in a fetal position. Mrs. Burkhalter was unable to walk or talk. An MRI scan of her brain was suggestive of NPH. After surgical placement of a VP shunt, the patient was able to have meaningful conversation. She was able to ambulate with assistance. Although the illness was not completely reversed, the patient regained significant function.

## VITAMIN B$_{12}$ DEFICIENCY

Although vitamin B$_{12}$ deficiency is common in older adults, the dementing disorder related to this deficiency is not. If anything interferes with the absorption of vitamin B$_{12}$ in the stomach, inadequate absorption might occur. Pernicious anemia is the most prevalent cause of this deficiency.

In the past, the Schilling test was the preferred diagnostic test for pernicious anemia. Currently, the test for serum antiparietal cell antibodies is usually performed initially. A positive test result

---

### DSM-IV-TR Criteria   for Dementia*

A. The development of multiple cognitive deficits manifested by both
   1. Memory impairment (impaired ability to learn new information or to recall previously learned information).
   2. One (or more) of the following cognitive disturbances:
      a. Aphasia (language disturbance)
      b. Apraxia (impaired ability to carry out motor functions despite intact motor function)
      c. Agnosia (failure to recognize or identify objects despite intact sensory function)
      d. Disturbance of executive functioning (e.g., planning, organizing, sequencing, abstracting)
B. The cognitive deficits in criteria A1 and A2 each cause significant impairment in social or occupational functioning and represent a significant decline from a previous level of functioning.
C. The course is characterized by a gradual onset and continuing cognitive decline.

*These are the common criteria for diagnosing a dementia. Delirium must be ruled out before a dementia can be diagnosed. A dementia related to a general medical condition must first rule out Alzheimer's disease and vascular dementia.
Modified from the American Psychiatric Association: *Diagnostic and statistical manual of mental disorders, text revision,* ed 4, Washington, DC, 2000, APA.

---

indicates that gastric cells are being destroyed and that there is a loss of intrinsic factor.

Dementia related to vitamin B$_{12}$ deficiency is rare. When the deficiency proceeds to this level, demyelinization occurs, leading to axon loss in the brain and in the spinal cord. Paresthesias start in the lower extremities, followed by upper extremity involvement. The person experiencing this form of dementia might also become hyporeflexive or hyperreflexive. Behavioral and mood changes occur. The patient might become psychotic (Moore and Jefferson, 2004).

Vitamin B$_{12}$ replacement should be started immediately and continued throughout the patient's lifetime. Changes take several months to appear. Because vitamin B$_{12}$ supplementation treats the deficiency, the goal is to prevent dementia from developing. The importance of routine health assessments and consumption of a diet rich in vitamin $B_{12}$ are indicated.

### CLINICAL EXAMPLE
*of a Patient With Vitamin $B_{12}$ Deficiency*

Mrs. Washington, an 84-year-old woman, was admitted for cognitive evaluation after the adult protective custody agency found her living in squalor. She was malnourished and dehydrated with a low vitamin $B_{12}$ level. The patient had forgotten to eat. She was also unstable because of weakness in her upper and lower extremities. Vitamin $B_{12}$ replacement therapy was started and continued in the nursing home after discharge.

## IRREVERSIBLE DEMENTIAS

Presently, no cure is available for any of the following dementing disorders, but medications have been developed with FDA indications for Alzheimer's disease. Medications for vascular dementia are in clinical trials. The course of the irreversible dementias might be slowed and plateau, but cognitive decline is inevitable. Through education and support, the nurse can play a pivotal role in assisting both the patient and the family with this devastating diagnosis. Additionally, the nurse can inform patients and family members about the local and national resources available.

Each illness is different in origin and clinical manifestation, but they share some common behaviors. Effective interventions are described in this chapter, as well as important issues faced by patients and their families.

Alzheimer's disease is the most prevalent dementia, representing 50% of all demented patients. Individuals with vascular dementia comprise approximately 20%, and another 25% of patients with dementia have both Alzheimer's disease and vascular dementia. The remaining dementias account for the other 5% (Gruetzner, 2001); this small percentage of dementias includes frontotemporal dementias (e.g., Pick's disease), dementia related to Parkinson's disease (PD), diffuse Lewy body disease (DLBD), acquired immunodeficiency syndrome (AIDS), Huntington's disease (HD), alcoholism, and Creutzfeldt-Jakob disease (CJD). CJD, although rare, sparks interest because of its connection with mad cow disease (Tasman et al, 2000).

### Alzheimer's Disease

Alzheimer's disease, with 4.5 million patients in America, is the most prevalent form of dementia. Alois Alzheimer, a German neurologist, first diagnosed a patient with this disease in 1907. However, the disease did not attract much attention for many years. Biddle and van Sickel, in a 1948 psychiatric nursing text, included only three sentences about Alzheimer's disease. None of the other dementias were mentioned (Biddle and van Sickel, 1948).

Interest in this disease has had a resurgence in the last 20 years (Rosen et al, 2000). Now that Alzheimer's disease has been studied extensively, it is known that the course from onset to death of a patient with Alzheimer's disease might exceed 10 years. The patient having the illness for the shortest duration generally has the most precipitous drop in cognition and function. The patient with a 10- to 20-year course usually has a more gradual and subtle decline. The average life expectancy from onset of disease to death is 8 years (ADEAR, 2006).

Alzheimer's disease, as well as the other types of dementia, is diagnosed after all other disorders have been ruled out. Pseudodementia, MCI, delirium, and other psychiatric illnesses are considered before a dementia diagnosis is made. As previously stated, a patient might have more than one illness, which makes assessment and treatment that much more difficult.

Age is the most significant risk factor for Alzheimer's disease (Gruetzner, 2001). A history of head injury, lower levels of education, and being female are also risk factors (Plassman et al, 2000). Longevity and smaller head size were reasons given for the increased number of women having Alzheimer's disease. However, Snowdon (2001) has asserted that gender alone does not explain this difference.

The three stages of Alzheimer's disease are mild, moderate, and severe. Each stage has typical characteristics, but symptoms might occur outside their expected stage.

Table 32-2 provides information about the stages of Alzheimer's disease (Folstein et al, 1975). When nurses and caregivers understand the

| Table 32-2 | **Stages of Alzheimer's Disease** | |
| --- | --- | --- |
| **Stage** | **Duration (yr)** | **Changes** |
| Mild (MMSE* score = 20-30) | 2-3 | Decreased short-term memory |
| | | Word- and name-finding difficulties |
| | | Decision-making, concentration, reasoning, and judgment problems |
| | | Difficulty performing usual activities |
| | | Denial |
| | | Getting lost |
| | | Repetitive questioning |
| Moderate (MMSE score = 10-19) | 3-4 | Apraxia, agnosia, aphasia with poor comprehension, disorientation, blunting of affect, misidentification, sleep disturbance, delusional, needs assistance with activities of daily living |
| | | Redirectable, extreme emotional lability, self-absorption, supervision with meals, wandering, urinary incontinence, requires supervision |
| Severe (MMSE score = 0-9) | 5-10 | Gait disturbance, unable to feed self, double incontinence, bowel impaction, bed bound, difficulty swallowing, fetal position; requires 24-hour supervision, close observation, or both |

*MMSE*, Mini-mental state examination.
Modified from Folstein MF, Folstein SE, McHugh PR: "Mini-mental state." A practical method for grading the cognitive status of patients for the clinician, *J Psychiatr Res* 12:189, 1975; Wilson J, Helton B: *PSYCHed: continuing education and consultation, dementia module*, Birmingham, AL, 2001. (Unpublished.); and Snowdon D: *Aging with grace*, New York, 2001, Bantam Books.

different stages, they can then plan appropriate interventions.

---

**CRITICAL THINKING QUESTION**    `3`

How do you explain the difference between dementia and Alzheimer's disease?

---

### What Causes Alzheimer's Disease?

Theories abound regarding the causes of Alzheimer's disease. The cholinergic hypothesis is perhaps the most recognized and accepted theory. Simply stated, the level of the neurotransmitter acetylcholine is reduced in the brain. Acetylcholine is the primary neurotransmitter that affects an individual's ability to acquire new information, make simple and complex decisions, and retain memories. Hence, cholinergic dysfunction would contribute to the development of Alzheimer's disease (NIA, 2003).

The nucleus basalis of Meynert in the basal forebrain is the major site of cholinergic cell bodies (90% of cholinergic fibers arise from this site). Axons communicate from this area to the hippo-campus, amygdala, and all layers of the cerebral cortex.

Oxidative stress plays a major part in the destruction of cholinergic cell bodies. Free radicals are produced that can kill these acetylcholine-producing neurons (Stahl, 2000). Tau protein is altered and forms twisted ropelike bundles within the cell, resulting in neurofibrillary tangles. These distorted tubules are then unable to transport molecules through the cell to keep it alive. Consequently, less acetylcholine is available.

Other possible causes of Alzheimer's disease involve deposits of beta amyloid plaque. The patient with Alzheimer's disease is thought to have an abnormality in deoxyribonucleic acid (DNA) that provides the basis for amyloid precursor protein (APP). When the Alzheimer's disease process starts, an inevitable cascade of events follows. The APP moves through the neuronal cell membrane and is cut by an enzyme known as a secretase. If this cut is at the wrong place, APP starts clumping with other similarly cut pieces of APP to form beta amyloid plaque, the sticky protein that attaches to the outside of neurons (NIA, 2003). Cell death results from an overabundance of these plaque formations.

It is unknown whether plaques or neurofibrillary tangles play a more critical role in the development of Alzheimer's disease. In fact, researchers are uncertain whether these tangles and plaques are the cause or result of the disease (Stahl, 2000). Researchers have usually identified themselves as being on one side of the "plaque versus tangle" debate or the other.

Genetics plays a part in Alzheimer's disease development (Bird, 2005). The following chromosomes are paired with these variables: chromosome 21 has the amyloid precursor protein gene, the presenilin 1 gene is found on chromosome 14, and the presenilin 2 gene is found on chromosome 1 (NIA, 2003). These genes are associated with early-onset Alzheimer's disease. Late-onset Alzheimer's disease, the more common form, is associated with chromosomes 9 and 10 (Brookes and Prince, 2005). Additionally, apolipoprotein E4 (Apo-E4) has been linked to the development of amyloid plaque (Cummings et al, 1998). Apo-E4 has been found on chromosome 19 (NIA, 2003). The more amyloid plaque is deposited in the brain, the greater the impairment is thought to be. If one or both parents provide Apo-E4 gene, the recipient is more likely to develop Alzheimer's disease, with the double recipient having the greater risk (Brookes and Prince, 2005). In contrast, however, a person who does not inherit the gene for Apo-E4 might also develop the disease (NIA, 2000; Snowdon, 2001).

The Alzheimer's brain also shrinks, weighing about two thirds the weight of the normal brain. This atrophy begins in the temporal and parietal regions and progresses throughout the entire brain (Snowdon, 2001). Smaller gyri and corresponding larger sulci undergo atrophic changes (Figures 32-1 through 32-4). Atrophy is also occurring in the subcortical areas, which is most apparent in the lateral ventricles. The more the brain shrinks, the larger the ventricles become.

Antioxidants have been found to promote healthy neurons. Free radicals, bits of oxygen fragments that are produced in the dying neuron, start a chain reaction that ends with nerve cell destruction. Vitamins C and E, plus the nonsteroidal anti-inflammatory drugs such as ibuprofen, have some neuroprotective basis (NIA, 2003).

Estrogen replacement therapy for women has produced no improvement in cognition in women who already had Alzheimer's disease (NIA, 2000).

Three years later, the NIA reported these unexpected findings from the Women's Health Initiative Memory Study, which began in 1995. The older women in the study who were given both estrogen and progestin were twice as likely to develop dementia as those taking placebos (NIA, 2003).

An Alzheimer's disease vaccine clinical trial was stopped when some subjects developed brain inflammation. It was thought that the vaccine would interrupt plaque formation. If plaques do not develop, then Alzheimer's disease might either be prevented or slowed. If the disease can be slowed for 10 to 20 years, the patient might die of other causes. In the same way that smallpox vaccine has greatly reduced the worldwide prevalence of that illness, so it is hoped that an Alzheimer's disease vaccine will do the same.

### Environmental Issues

Excessive aluminum from using aluminum cookware or using deodorant with aluminum has not been a proven cause of Alzheimer's disease, according to research on exposure to aluminum (Rondeau, 2002). Instead, the presence of increased levels of aluminum in the brain might be the effect of the dying neurons. Aluminum is a toxin released when the neuron dies. Dental amalgams were also not found to cause Alzheimer's disease (NIA, 2000; Snowdon, 2001). No viral agent that transmits Alzheimer's disease has been identified (Gruetzner, 2001).

### Nontraditional Findings

The traditional roots of Alzheimer's disease development have been discussed, but the cause of Alzheimer's disease is not without controversy. The Nun Study, a longitudinal research study that explored topics related to normal aging and Alzheimer's disease, has generated new questions. David Snowdon, of the Sanders-Brown Center on Aging at the University of Kentucky, began the study in the mid-1980s. In the order of School Sisters of Notre Dame, 678 nuns volunteered to undergo annual assessments and to donate their brains for autopsy after their deaths. This study has been widely covered in both the professional and lay press (Snowdon, 2001).

The Nun Study had some unexpected findings. One sister who lived to be more than 100 years

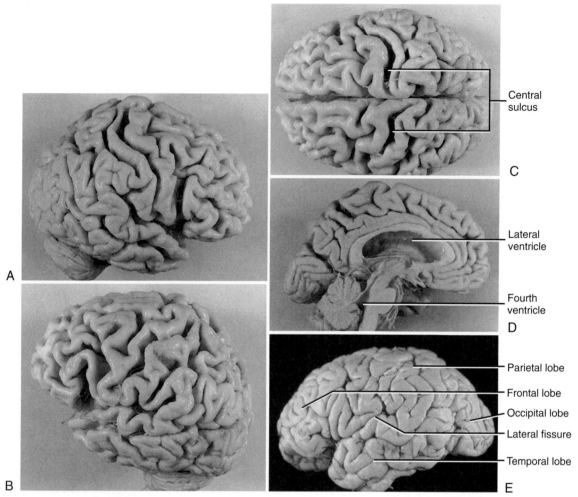

**FIGURE 32-1 A,** Right side of the brain of a patient with Alzheimer's disease. Narrow gyri and larger sulci are demonstrated. **B,** Left side of the same brain demonstrates even narrower gyri and larger sulci. **C,** Superior view. The central sulcus is very wide. **D,** Midsagittal view of the left hemisphere. The greatly enlarged lateral and fourth ventricles are demonstrated. **E,** Normal brain. *(Photographs A to D by Berto Tarin, Western University of Health Science; E courtesy of Dr. Richard E. Powers, University of Alabama at Birmingham Brain Resource Program [UAB-BRP].)*

old showed no signs of cognitive decline, although her brain autopsy showed an abundance of both plaque and tangle formations. Another nun, who died in her 70s, had profound dementia yet had few tangles and plaques. The Nun Study researchers have explored reasons for these unusual findings and concluded (Snowdon, 2003) that the degree of resistance or cognitive reserve has some effect on the clinical manifestations of Alzheimer's disease.

Complex use of language and advanced education were two background issues that were isolated in the nuns who had the highest cognitive ability. Also, nuns with a more positive lifetime attitude were found to be in the highest cognitive group (Snowdon, 2001).

### Classic Behaviors

*Memory loss* is the most noticeable initial problem. Impairment of short-term memory occurs first. The patient and family might think that this loss is a minor problem because the long-term memory remains intact at first. Word-finding difficulty is the easiest problem for the nurse to assess. The patient often describes an object rather than naming it. "The thing you tell time with" for a

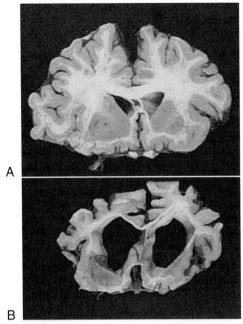

A

B

**FIGURE 32-2 A,** Brain is normal. The sulci and gyri are not atrophied. **B,** Brain shows the effects of Alzheimer's disease. Widened sulci and narrowed gyri are demonstrated. In addition, the lateral ventricles are increased in size because of the decrease in brain mass associated with Alzheimer's disease. *(Courtesy of Dr. Richard E. Powers, UAB-BRP.)*

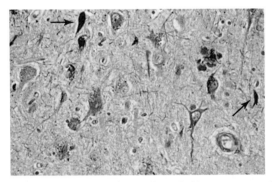

**FIGURE 32-3** The dark, flame-shaped objects are neurofibrillary "tangles," or dead neurons *(arrows).* Tangles are twisted fibrils inside the neuron that disrupt cellular processes and eventually kill the cell. *(Courtesy of Dr. Richard E. Powers, UAB-BRP.)*

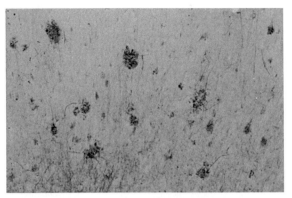

**FIGURE 32-4** The darker objects are plaques, one of two microscopic findings in Alzheimer's disease (the other is the tangles [Figure 32-3]). Because plaques can be found in about 50% of individuals over age 70, it is the quantity of plaques in relation to the person's age that is significant. *(Courtesy of Dr. Richard E. Powers, UAB-BRP.)*

watch is a typical response. Impaired concentration often follows memory problems and word-finding difficulty. Trouble understanding a conversation, comprehending the plot in a book, or following a television program frequently occurs. Withdrawing from a former routine and pleasurable activities because of a lack of interest

and of initiative contributes to further cognitive decline. Box 32-1 outlines what is referred to as the four A's of Alzheimer's disease.

One unusual problem associated with Alzheimer's disease is *misinterpreting the environment.* Visual hallucinations are the most common type of hallucinations seen in Alzheimer's disease. One explanation for these is the Charles Bonnet syndrome. The visual hallucinations usually occur in patients who have visual impairments, most commonly macular degeneration. The patients might report seeing unusual things, such as people and animals. They are often quite vivid and elaborate (Jacob, 2004). One example was a patient who "saw" a Hollywood movie company setting up to film a movie outside in her yard. Of interest, these patients are rarely disturbed by these hallucinations, which confound their caregivers. Patients often have visual hallucinations of dead relatives. One patient was found to be routinely preparing meals for visiting family members, all of whom were deceased. The *voices* or *sounds* typically go along with the visual hallucinations—for example, the perceived deceased relative is *speaking* to the patient. Olfactory, tactile, and gustatory hallucinations are the least common types of hallucinations.

*Delusions* are common. Paranoia about spouses having extramarital affairs, stealing money, and rearranging things in the home and somatic preoccupations are frequent observations that the nurse makes. Whether any of these accusations have any basis in reality must be assessed.

---

**Box 32-1   Four A's of Alzheimer's Disease\* and Adaptive Actions**

**Agnosia.** Impaired ability to recognize or identify familiar objects and people in the absence of a visual or hearing impairment.

- Assess and adapt for visual impairment.
- Do not expect the patient to remember you; introduce yourself.
- Cover mirrors or pictures if they cause distress.
- Name objects and demonstrate their use.
- Keep area free of ingestible hazards (toiletries, chemical cleaning supplies, checkers, buttons, unmonitored medicine).

**Aphasia.** Language disturbances are exhibited in both expressing and understanding spoken words. Expressive aphasia is the inability to express thoughts in words; receptive aphasia is the inability to understand what is said.

- Assess and adapt for hearing loss.
- Observe and use gestures, tone, and facial expressions.
- Provide help with word finding.
- Restate your understanding of behaviors and word fragments.
- Acknowledge feelings expressed verbally and nonverbally.
- Use simple words and phrases; be concise and organized.

- Allow time for response.
- Listen carefully and encourage with nonverbal praise.
- Use pictures, symbols, and signs.

**Amnesia.** Inability to learn new information or to recall previously learned information.

- Do not expect patient to remember you; introduce yourself.
- Do not test the patient's memory unnecessarily.
- Operate in the here and now.
- Provide orientation cues.
- Remember, *you* must adapt when the patient cannot change.
- Compensate for patient's lost judgment or reasoning.

**Apraxia.** Inability to carry out motor activities despite intact motor function.

- Assess and adapt for motor weakness and swallowing difficulties.
- Simplify tasks; give step-by-step instructions and time for response.
- Initiate motion for patient with gentle guidance or touch.

\*Might also be present in other cognitive disorders.

---

Calling a family member or friend by another person's name is known as *misidentification.* Family members are often devastated when the patient cannot remember their name. The nurse can educate the family about misidentification and dispel any idea that it might be a humorous attempt by the patient.

The sundown syndrome is the phrase that describes the period, usually in the afternoon and early evening, during which a patient becomes more agitated and less redirectable. This phenomenon is also called *sundowning,* which is a more accurate term, because the criteria for being a true syndrome are not met (Dewing, 2003). Researchers have yet to find the cause of this behavioral change. The behavior is further confusing to families, because the patient might have good and bad days.

Loss of the ability to care for oneself is particularly difficult for all parties. Over time, the patient forgets how to take care of all personal care needs. Incontinence of bowel and/or bladder and wandering are unmanageable behaviors that make home care no longer possible for many caregivers.

**CLINICAL EXAMPLE**
*of a Patient With Alzheimer's Disease*

Mrs. Jefferson, a 62-year-old woman, has had difficulty recalling the names of people in her church. She had difficulty understanding jokes because she had diminished abstract abilities, instead interpreting them concretely. Mrs. Jefferson had a type of expressive aphasia called *word-finding difficulty.* She described the choir as "those people who sing at church" and her watch as "something you tell time with." At home, she placed her purse in the oven. Each of these occurrences alone is not diagnostic of Alzheimer's disease; however, the cluster of signs should prompt the nurse to consider this diagnosis.

## VASCULAR DEMENTIA

The second most prevalent dementia is vascular dementia, although some researchers now say that DLBD is actually the second most prevalent. However, at present, a separate diagnosis for DLBD is not in the *DSM-IV-TR*. Before the current edition (*DSM-IV*; APA, 1994), vascular dementia was known as multi–infarct dementia. The diagnosis of vascular dementia is made when the brain has multiple vascular lesions in the cortex and subcortical areas (APA, 2000). These affected areas are sometimes called *small strokes*.

Memory loss is the most common presenting complaint. Unlike Alzheimer's disease, the patient with vascular dementia usually maintains the ability to speak without word-finding difficulty. The cognitive changes that occur with vascular dementia are directly related to the location of the lesions. In contrast, the patient with Alzheimer's disease has a more global pattern of deterioration. The time the patient remains at a particular level might be months and years, or vascular changes might occur over a shorter period. If the cognitive levels are plotted on a graph, the decline usually assumes a stepwise pattern of deterioration. Although predictability is impossible, a further decline is likely because the original risk factors are usually still present.

The major risk factors for vascular dementia are hypertension, diabetes mellitus, previous stroke, cardiac arrhythmias, coronary artery disease, tobacco usage, and alcohol and substance abuse. Treatments focus on the patient's medical problems. Although there are no medications with FDA indications for vascular dementia, prescribers are using the Alzheimer's disease medications off label, which means that the medication has not been approved by the FDA for treatment of that particular disease or symptom. Often, aspirin is given to reduce the likelihood of stroke.

### CRITICAL THINKING QUESTION  4
Which risk factors for vascular dementia might be modified by the patient (or the caregiver) for the patient?)

### CRITICAL THINKING QUESTION  5
What does prescribing off label mean and why is it done?

### CLINICAL EXAMPLE
*of a Patient With Vascular Dementia*

Mr. Babb, a 76-year-old man, was hospitalized for depression. During the initial interview, he had difficulty understanding why he was admitted. He did not know the day, date, month, or year; however, he was able to do serial calculations. One week before admission, he had an automobile accident because he pulled out into traffic without looking. Mr. Babb has hypertension and diabetes mellitus. He has had two transient ischemic attacks (TIAs) in the last year.

## FRONTOTEMPORAL LOBE DEMENTIA

Frontotemporal lobe dementia (FLD) is a type of dementia caused by atrophy of the frontal and anterior temporal lobes of the brain. This atrophy might be symmetric or asymmetric. Pick's disease is a subtype of FLD; it features Pick cells and Pick bodies in the brain. Pick cells are swollen and ballooned neurons. This disease is usually diagnosed when patients are over 50 (NINDS, 2005) and the patient might live another 2 to 15 years (Rosen et al, 2000).

The area of the brain affected is responsible for executive functioning. These behaviors include judgment, decision making, impulse control, and abiding by social norms (Litvan et al, 1997). Behavioral changes are usually the first signs that something is wrong. Disinhibition is the most shocking. Disrobing in public, extreme impatience, or openly masturbating typifies FLD behaviors. Difficulties with abstraction, reasoning, lack of initiative, and poor planning might occur. Affective changes, particularly euphoria, acting silly, or insulting behavior, might be present. Also, perseveration of certain behaviors—for example, opening and closing a book repeatedly—might be seen (Jefferson and Moore, 2004). Apraxia, agnosia, and visual-spatial abilities, common signs seen in Alzheimer's disease, are not usually found because of the preservation of the parietal region of the brain. Later in the illness, speech disturbance, memory problems, and gait disturbance occur in a sharp progressive decline (Tasman et al, 1997).

## CLINICAL EXAMPLE
*of a Patient With Frontotemporal Lobe Dementia (Pick's Disease)*

Ms. Brewer, a 66-year-old woman, was found nude in the foyer of her assisted-living facility. She had taken her clothes off three times in a week. Before this occurrence, she had been quite modest. A few days later, she cursed the housekeeper. Ms. Brewer was diagnosed with Pick's disease based on her behavior, her relatively good memory, and neuroimaging that revealed both frontal and anterior temporal lobe atrophy.

## DEMENTIA RELATED TO PARKINSON'S DISEASE

PD is a complex neurologic disorder that affects the extrapyramidal system. All diseases that affect this system have associated aberrant movements. Parkinson's disease is usually diagnosed when patients are in their 50s or 60s, although patients in their 30s, such as the actor Michael J. Fox, have developed the disease. The substantia nigra has approximately a 50% reduction in neurons. Dementia occurs in 15% to 20% of patients with PD (Geldmacher, 1997). Parkinsonian behaviors include muscular rigidity, slow movements (bradykinesia), masklike facies, and stooped posture. Shuffling gait, pill rolling (rubbing the thumb up and down across the tips of the fingers), and drooling are also signs associated with PD (Knopman, 2001). Poor postural reflexes might also be present, which makes these patients prone to falls. Tremor might or might not be present. Freezing refers to the rigid posture that alternates with more fluid movements. Many patients with PD also have depression; this is related to neurologic changes and the grieving process that occurs as these patients become less functional.

Patients with PD might develop cogwheel rigidity, with or without tremor (Young, 1999). One way to assess cogwheel rigidity begins with asking the patient to extend his or her arm. Next, the patient should be asked to flex the arm slowly. At the same time, the nurse tries to extend the patient's arm with one hand. The nurse's other hand should hold the elbow of the extending and flexing arm. Cogwheel rigidity, if present, feels like a ratcheting motion in the patient's elbow. The rate of progression is variable. The majority of patients will be severely debilitated within 15 years.

Pharmaceutical agents that are typically used increase dopamine levels or block acetylcholine (Keltner and Folks, 2005).

## CLINICAL EXAMPLE
*of a Patient With Parkinson's Disease*

Mr. McGreevy, a 72-year-old man, has had PD for 7 years. He has a blunted affect, excessive drooling, and shuffling gait. Last year, the patient was hospitalized for an aspirational pneumonia. Managing his parkinsonian signs was made difficult by frequent visual hallucinations caused by the dopamine component in the levodopa-carbidopa (Sinemet) that he took. He had a prescription for an aypical antipsychotic drug to reduce the hallucinations. The delicate balance of prescribing a dopaminergic for Parkinson's disease (dopamine deficiency in the nigrostriatal tract) and a dopamine blocking antipsychotic medication (excessive dopamine in the mesolimbic tract) to treat hallucinations was a major challenge for his health care providers.

## DIFFUSE LEWY BODY DISEASE

DLBD is the form of dementia that has both cognitive impairment and extrapyramidal signs. (As noted above, many believe that this type of dementia is second only to Alzheimer's disease.) Lewy bodies are intracellular bodies found in neurons. Originally, Lewy bodies were only found in the substantia nigra and therefore were associated only with PD. Now, with better tissue staining methods available, Lewy bodies have been found in the cortex as well. A patient can have Lewy bodies in both places, which makes diagnosis a challenge. Diagnostic questions arise such as the following. "Is DLBD a stand-alone diagnosis?" "Is DLBD a variant of Alzheimer's disease and/or PD." (See comparisons in Tables 32-3 and 32-4 [Stewart, 2003].) Patients with DLBD have what Stewart has called the classic tetrad: Alzheimer's-like dementia, parkinsonian symptoms, prominent psychotic symptoms, and extreme sensitivity to antipsychotic agents. The latter symptom is the one that usually manifests itself, leading clinicians to consider this diagnosis.

DLBD follows a downward course that is much more precipitous than Alzheimer's disease. After the mild stage, the extrapyramidal signs separate the two diseases. The course of DLBD is usually 5 to 8 years (Gomez-Tortosa, 1998).

## Table 32-3 Comparison of Features of Alzheimer's Disease and Diffuse Lewy Body Disease

| Alzheimer's Disease | Diffuse Lewy Body Disease |
|---|---|
| Cortical neuritic plaques, neurofibrillary tangles | Cortical Lewy bodies |
| Accounts for 50% to 60% of all dementias | Accounts for 15% to 20% of all dementias |
| Equally prevalent in men and women | Twice as prevalent in men |
| Often familial | Rarely familial |
| Some daily variability | Prominent daily variability |
| Abrupt deterioration always indicates superimposed illness or drug reaction | Abrupt deterioration common, might be idiopathic ("pseudodelirium") |
| Parkinsonian features very rare, occur late in illness | Parkinsonian features obvious early in illness |
| Autonomic dysfunction rare | Autonomic dysfunction common |
| Incidence of hallucinations 20%, usually in moderately advanced disease | Incidence of hallucinations 80%, usually early in illness |
| Adverse reactions to antipsychotics often seen | Severe or life-threatening adverse reactions to antipsychotics usually occur |

From Stewart J: Defining diffuse Lewy body disease. Tetrad of symptoms distinguishes illness from other dementias, *Postgrad Med* 113:71, 2003 (with permission).

## Table 32-4 Comparison of Features of Parkinson's Disease and Diffuse Lewy Body Disease

| Parkinson's Disease | Diffuse Lewy Body Disease |
|---|---|
| Midbrain Lewy bodies | Cortical Lewy bodies |
| Executive dementia sometimes occurs late in illness | Cortical dementia always occurs early in illness |
| Resting tremor usually present | Resting tremor usually absent |
| Autonomic dysfunction sometimes seen | Autonomic dysfunction very prominent |
| Robust response to levodopa and carbidopa (Sinemet) | Marginal response to levodopa and carbidopa |
| Hallucinations only in response to antiparkinsonian drugs | Hallucinations common in absence of antiparkinsonian drugs |

From Stewart J: Defining diffuse Lewy body disease. Tetrad of symptoms distinguishes illness from other dementias, *Postgrad Med* 113:71, 2003 (with permission).

### CLINICAL EXAMPLE
*of a Patient With Diffuse Lewy Body Disease*

Mr. Hall, a 68-year-old man, started having vivid visual hallucinations. He had fallen twice as a result of his gait disturbance. Mr. Hall slept well at night despite sleeping off and on throughout the day. Some days he seemed like his old self, according to the family. They had a difficult time understanding that this was a hallmark sign of this type of dementia. Instead, they were convinced that he was getting better. He also had been extremely agitated after taking a small dose of an antipsychotic medication.

## CREUTZFELDT-JAKOB DISEASE

Until mad cow disease became headline news, little information appeared in the media about CJD. Now, a variant of CJD has been identified, known as *v-CJD;* it is the human form of mad cow disease. Patients contract this variant after ingesting meat infected with bovine spongiform encephalopathy. Subacute spongiform encephalopathy is a feature of both mad cow disease and CJD.

On microscopic examination, these cells appear like sponges. The cells are stripped of their intracellular material. The infecting agent is the prion, a protein particle, which is unlike either a bacterium or a virus. CJD is one of at least 12 prion-related diseases, all of which are transmissible from one person to another. A genetic component also exists, but this accounts for 10% or less of patients with CJD. When genetics is suspected, the causative agent is a mutation of the tau protein.

Of the individuals who develop this disease, 85% have no known risk factors (NINDS, 2005). CJD is potentially transferable between people when blood and body fluids are present (Moore and Jefferson, 2004; Perkin, 1998). Health care workers who are involved in surgery or autopsy are vulnerable, as are funeral home workers. However, the illness is not contagious by casual contact nor is an airborne pathogen involved.

Dementia is inevitable and occurs early in the disease (NINDS, 2005). Personality changes, seizures, and myoclonic movements might also occur. Impairment of vision and even blindness are not unusual. The course is rapid; on average, most patients die within 6 to 12 months (Perkin, 1998). Only 10% live past a year (NINDS, 2005). The nurse should focus on anticipatory grief for the family and the patient if he or she is cognitively able.

---

### CLINICAL EXAMPLE
*of a Patient With Creutzfeldt-Jakob Disease*

Mrs. Henderson, a 65-year-old woman, became openly hostile to her husband while they were dining out. She had never had outbursts such as this one. In 2 months, her vision was affected and, 3 months later, she was blind. Mrs. Henderson also developed myoclonic jerks that were not controlled with medication. Based on the change in personality, visual impairment, and movement disorder, she was diagnosed with CJD. She died 9 months later. Postmortem examination confirmed the diagnosis.

---

## AIDS DEMENTIA COMPLEX

A dementia related to the late stages of the disease occurs in 20% to 30% of AIDS patients (Hodges, 2001). If it occurs, it might not be expressed until 10 years or so after the infection has started. CT and MRI of the brain might indicate cortical atrophy and enlarged ventricles; however, this tends to be nonspecific (i.e., region-specific neuronal loss is not consistently identified). If the patient does develop dementia, death usually follows within a year. Severe movement problems are usually the first prominent sign. Other symptoms are variable in occurrence and include the following: apathy, lethargy, loss of sex drive, blunted affect, social withdrawal, emotional lability, and problems with abstract thinking. Hallucinations and delusions are not unusual (Jefferson and Moore, 2004).

There is no specific treatment for dementia related to AIDS. Medications for AIDS are to be continued. Other medications might be used to treat the patient symptomatically.

AIDS can occur in all age groups. Behavioral and cognitive changes in the younger patient should alert the nurse to consider ruling out this disease.

---

### CLINICAL EXAMPLE
*of a Patient With AIDS Dementia Complex (ADC)*

Mrs. Browning, a 46-year-old woman, has had AIDS for 8 years. Her family reported that she had been raped 10 years ago. At the time, she did not know that the rapist was HIV-positive. Now, Mrs. Browning is agitated, does not eat, and does not sleep well. In the last 6 months, Mrs. Browning's memory began to fail. Because of the early onset of this cognitive disorder, she had a diagnostic HIV test. She died 11 months after she was diagnosed with ADC.

---

## DEMENTIA ASSOCIATED WITH ALCOHOLISM

This dementia usually occurs decades after the person starts drinking alcohol. Similar to many other dementias, personality changes typically precede memory disturbance. The decline is similar to the course of Alzheimer's disease.

Thiamine deficiency is the main cause of alcohol-related changes. Additionally, the toxic effects of years of drinking alcohol finally take their toll in multiple end-stage organ damage, including the brain. Wernicke's encephalopathy results in motor problems related to alcohol abuse. Most often, the patient develops motor impairments such as ataxia and nystagmus. Korsakoff's syndrome is often associated with Wernicke's encephalopathy. Patients with Korsakoff's syndrome confabulate as they attempt to answer questions (Moore and Jefferson, 2004). This delay is an attempt to cover their severe short-term memory loss. Superficially, these patients seem to know what they are saying. Unless the facts are known, these patients make statements that seem truthful to the nurse.

The brain of a patient with Wernicke-Korsakoff syndrome undergoes several changes. The affected areas of the brain are the medial thalamus and hypothalamus, some of the midbrain gray matter, and the periventricular pons and medulla (Brust, 1998). Other researchers have found that some brain structures (e.g., hippocampus, mammillary bodies) might have reduced volume, whereas the third ventricle is increased in volume (Visser et al, 1999).

With abstinence from alcohol, improvement of cognitive function is possible. However, if dementia is diagnosed, these patients might have an inability to process new information, hindering their rehabilitation and participation in support groups such as Alcoholics Anonymous (AA).

### CLINICAL EXAMPLE
*of a Patient With Dementia Related to Alcoholism*

Mr. Kelly, a 75-year-old man, was admitted to a general hospital for chest pain. Three days later, he was transferred to a geriatric psychiatry unit with altered mental status. Mr. Kelly was unable to speak rationally; he made gestures in the air as if he were having visual hallucinations. His spouse said that he did not have a drinking problem, but he did drink wine each evening. After 3 days of unexpected abstinence, Mr. Kelly was experiencing delirium related to alcohol withdrawal and was placed on an alcohol withdrawal protocol.

Two years later, the patient returned to the hospital with short-term memory loss. He said that he was in Hawaii when asked where he had been before admission. His wife confirmed that Mr. Kelly had not gone to Hawaii. He was confabulating. He had developed Korsakoff's syndrome.

## DEMENTIA RELATED TO HUNTINGTON'S DISEASE

All the dementing illnesses have a sorrowful course. Perhaps none is more tragic than HD. This illness is particularly devastating because it is transmitted only through an autosomal dominant gene that either parent might provide. As such, HD does not skip generations. This illness is not usually diagnosed until patients are in their 30s or 40s, but it can develop sooner or later (Snowdon, 2001). By the time patients are diagnosed with HD, they might have children and even grandchildren. A child has a 50% chance of inheriting the gene and thus the disease.

Personality changes are usually the first signs to appear. A mild-tempered person might develop mood swings or start drinking alcohol. Usually, movement disorders occur after personality changes. These movements, known as choreiform movements, begin with facial twitches or involuntary limb movement and progress to myoclonus (jerking movements) of all extremities (Moore and Jefferson, 2004). The movements place the patient at risk for falling out of a chair or bed. Oddly, many patients do not acknowledge having movement problems, even when severe. Originally, this was thought to be denial, but now there is evidence that these patients might not be aware of this problem (Hodges, 2001).

Chromosome 4 is where the gene associated with HD is located (Snowdon, 2001). Genetic testing involves a simple laboratory serum test; a positive result means that the patient will develop HD. Testing poses an ethical dilemma. For example, should individuals at risk be tested before having children, should they decide not to have children, or should they proceed and take the chance that a child will not have HD? If the patient decides to be tested, the testing should follow strict confidentiality protocols, with extremely limited access to both the testing and results. This protects the patient from personal struggle with this decision, particularly if the test result is positive. Insurance companies and health maintenance organizations could consider a positive test result for Huntington's disease a preexisting condition, even if the disease has not manifested itself. The nurse should be supportive when these issues are raised.

The dementia might develop before or after the choreiform movements begin. Short-term memory is affected first, followed by long-term memory loss. The course is unpredictable because the illness might occur over a short period, or might last decades.

### CLINICAL EXAMPLE
*of a Patient With Dementia Related to Huntington's Disease*

Mrs. Thompson, a 57-year-old woman with HD, was admitted to the psychiatric unit for unmanageable behavior. She had severe myoclonus to the extent that she almost fell out of her wheelchair. She could no longer feed herself and was incontinent of bowel and bladder. She did not know where she was. Based on the previous diagnosis of HD and this recent onset memory loss, Mrs. Thompson was diagnosed with dementia.

CRITICAL THINKING QUESTION     6

Why is genetic counseling essential with a patient who has HD?

## OTHER DEMENTIAS

The most prevalent dementias have been described. Dozens of other types of dementia have been identified. Some dementias are caused by disease—for example neurosyphilis, systemic lupus erythematosus, and Wilson's disease. Still other dementias might be related to metabolic imbalances, such as hypothyroidism and hypocalcemia. Another class of dementias is related to head injuries, toxic effects of medications, heavy metals, or carbon monoxide poisoning (Perkin, 1998).

CRITICAL THINKING QUESTION     7

Is it important to know the type of dementia that a patient has?

## PUTTING IT ALL TOGETHER
### Psychotherapeutic Management

## NURSE-PATIENT RELATIONSHIP

Challenges lie ahead whenever the nurse takes care of patients with dementia. Nothing is more important than getting to know their unique personal qualities. The golden rule is simply this: promote maximum functioning and have patience.

CRITICAL THINKING QUESTION     8

What can the caregiver of a patient with dementia do to reduce stress?

### Communication Strategies

The importance of the nurse-patient relationship cannot be overstated. It is important for the nurse to realize, and to help subordinates realize, that many cognitively impaired individuals live in the moment. They might be incapable of retrieving the past (memory failure) and unable to contemplate the future. Hence, the present is what they have. The nurse must be pleasant, smile, be kind,

use good eye contact and, to repeat, be patient. Here are some tips that will help you be more successful when talking with cognitively impaired individuals.

- If an interaction is going poorly, stop, walk away (providing it is safe to do so), and return in a few minutes with a fresh start.
- Remember, effective communication starts with nonverbal behavior, so use a kind voice and make eye contact.
- Be positive and stay with pleasant subjects.
- Do not use sarcasm, jokes, and metaphors because the patient's loss of abstract thinking makes understanding these language subtleties almost impossible.
- Recognize that patients might not be able to tell the difference between a real argument and an impassioned discussion about a new movie. Observing staff members in such a debate can be frightening and confusing to these patients.
- Use short sentences, not complex ones.
- Give directions slowly, one step at a time.
- Do not finish sentences for patients; give them time to finish their thoughts.
- Approach patients from the front in case they have visual or hearing impairment.
- Lots of chatter can be confusing, because patients struggle to track one conversation when several are going on around them.

### Scheduling Strategies

The way a cognitively impaired patient's day is structured is crucial in the plan of care. The nurse should:

- Develop a schedule that provides structure to the day, because patients adapt better when they have a predictable routine.
- Focus on patient-centered activities.
- Develop singular activities because multiple activities overwhelm the patient. For example, turn off the television while the patient is putting together a puzzle.
- Provide a group experience with one subject approached at a time. Too much stimulation increases anxiety and might lead to agitation.

### Nutritional Strategies

Many patients with cognitive impairment do not want to eat, won't eat, and sometimes can't eat (without great difficulty). Here, again, patience and developing a strategy to meet nutritional needs is important. The nurse should consider the following:

- Make sure that patients are eating properly by tailoring dietary needs to the patient. Serve smaller meals several times per day. If too much food is on the plate, the patient might be overwhelmed.
- Also, finger foods work well for people who will not stay at the table.
- Find out about a patient's favorite foods and provide them as much as possible.
- Remember that beverage supplements can provide nutrition when regular food intake lessens.

### Toileting Strategies

Toileting is a big issue with these patients and often it is this issue that causes families to seek placement outside the home. The nurse should:

- Seek to keep the patient physically comfortable.
- Provide immaculate attention to personal hygiene and toileting needs.
- Take the patient to the bathroom every 2 hours to promote continence (incontinence contributes to the formation of decubitus ulcers, as does immobility).

### Wandering Strategies

Wandering is the second major reason why families choose to place their loved ones in a long-term care facility. Wandering is defined as leaving one's residence, unsupervised, and getting lost. By definition, patients with dementia have cognitive deficits (Algase, 1999a,b), which appear in multiple forms. Visuospatial perceptions might be disturbed. Patients might leave their own residences in search of their "homes" or have day-night reversal and walk at night. To provide a safe place for this activity, some long-term care facilities have wandering paths. The best paths are continuous, without dead ends. Windows, interesting art on the walls, and an unobstructed hallway provide a safe place to wander as well. Furthermore, by making the exit doors to the facility less obvious and painting them with attractive scenes, escapes are reduced.

Photograph the patients and keep the photos updated and on file. Many law enforcement agencies have partnered with the Alzheimer's Association "Safe Return" program. These patients might wear a Safe Return armband that identifies them and provides other personal information. Some families might use global positioning devices, now available from Medic Alert. (This company has provided necklaces and bracelets for patients so emergency medical personnel can obtain information through a toll-free telephone number [1-800-ID ALERT].)

## PSYCHOPHARMACOLOGY

Geriatric patients with cognitive disorder often face the double burden of dealing with a psychiatric diagnosis superimposed on a chronic medical condition. Because of this comorbidity, these individuals are often prescribed many medications. Part of the nurse's role is to ensure that prescribed medications are helping and not harming the patient and to monitor for drug adherence. Because most drugs used in geriatric psychiatry do not have FDA indications specifically for patients with cognitive disorders, nurses must be particularly vigilant in assessing drug effects. Medications for Alzheimer's disease are the exception, however. Some medications have survived the intense scrutiny of FDA approval and are available for use. When nonapproved psychiatric medications are prescribed, the usage is referred to as off label (see earlier discussion). Off-label drugs tend to be used to manage behavior, psychosis, depression, and anxiety associated with Alzheimer's disease. Often, the side effect profile drives the decision on medication choice. For example, some antidepressant medications are activating and some are more sedating. Socially withdrawn depressed patients might benefit from the activating medication, whereas an agitated, depressed patient might benefit from the calming agent. These examples illustrate the need to recognize side effects when choosing a medication for this population.

Unfortunately, many medications might cause or contribute to delirium. Perhaps the most common source of drug-mediated cognitive impairment is those agents that have anticholinergic properties. For example, diphenhydramine (Benadryl) is sold by itself and in combination with many OTC medications (e.g., sinus preparations, cough syrups, and sleeping agents). Two tablets of Tylenol PM, for instance, contain 50 mg of diphenhydramine and can significantly add to the cholinergic deficiency.

MCI and pseudodementia have no medications specifically indicated for them. Treatment is symptomatic; that is, because depression is often the important problem in pseudodementia, antidepressant medications are usually chosen.

## Drugs for Alzheimer's Disease

As previously mentioned, only five medications have FDA approval for Alzheimer's disease and no drugs have been approved for any of the other dementias. An acetylcholine (ACh) deficiency is the neurotransmitter problem most often implicated in Alzheimer's disease. The first drug approved for Alzheimer's disease targeting ACh deficiency was released over 10 years ago. Tacrine (Cognex) was the first in a class of medications called cholinesterase or acetylcholinesterase (AChE) inhibitors. Donepezil (Aricept), rivastigmine (Exelon), and galantamine (Razadyne; formerly known as Reminyl [name changed in 2005]) followed. All four have FDA indications for mild to moderate Alzheimer's disease. These medications in effect boost the level of ACh by preventing its metabolic breakdown. Although these drugs increase the amount of available synaptic acetylcholine, the disease itself continues to progress. In other words, if two patients with equal neurodegeneration were followed clinically for 1 year, one receiving an AChE inhibitor (such as Aricept) and one not receiving any medication at all, they would have approximately equal brain pathology. The Aricept-receiving patient might function better during the year but the underlying disease process would continue in both patients. Obviously, there is much research to be done before treatment of Alzheimer's disease is adequate.

The only agent approved for moderate to severe Alzheimer's disease is memantine (Namenda); it is the only approved medication for Alzheimer's disease that is *not* an AChE inhibitor. Memantine works by blocking abnormal signaling by glutamate at the *N*-methyl-D-aspartate (NMDA) receptor. In so doing, memantine does not affect normal binding of this endogenous neurotransmitter (Keltner and Williams, 2004). Glutamate is the most abundant excitatory neurotransmitter in the brain and is involved with learning and memory; however, overstimulation of these pathways leads to cell death (neuronal excitotoxicity). As opposed to the AChE inhibitors, in which the disease progression continues, memantine is thought to slow the onset of neurodegeneration. The manufacturer has clearly stated that there has been no scientific verification of halting neurodegeneration. Because full NMDA blockade (such as that caused by the street drug PCP [phencyclidine]) can cause psychotic and violent behavior, and full activation can cause excitotoxicity, the makers of memantine walked a fine line during its development.

Memantine can be used by itself or with one of the AChE inhibitors.

***Note to Students:*** *In this chapter, we do not make a distinction between AChE and butyrylcholinesterase. We refer to all cholinesterase (ChE) inhibitors as AChE inhibitors. See Chapter 22 for more detailed information.*

All five of the Alzheimer's disease medications are useful, although to caregivers improvements can be subtle. Prescribers usually start with an AChE inhibitor. Tacrine is rarely used now because of the potential for severe hepatic toxic side effects. Therefore, donepezil, rivastigmine, or galantamine is usually started first. Each of these has FDA approval for mild to moderate Alzheimer's disease. Memantine has FDA approval for moderate to severe Alzheimer's disease. Although memantine can be started first, such a practice is not typical; usually, memantine is added later. One justification for starting a patient on both memantine and an AChE inhibitor is family pressure. Families want everything possible to be done for their loved one and, with Internet and consumer advertising so prevalent, many have more information about what is available. Sometimes, families demand that both the AChE inhibitor and memantine be started at the same time. Although using the two classes of drugs together might be helpful, it does pose problems for clinicians. For example, how does the clinician know if one drug needs to be titrated upward? If the patient improves, how does the clinician know which medication (or both) caused the favorable response? Conversely, if there are any adverse reactions, how can the clinician know which medication caused the effect? Hence, it is usual practice to start an AChE inhibitor and add memantine later.

Convenience in giving medications is always important, but particularly so with these patients

(Table 32-5). Like most people, caregivers prefer simple medication regimens. Extended-release donepezil and galantamine provide once-daily dosing. Rivastigmine and galantamine are given twice daily with meals. Tacrine is given four times daily. Gastrointestinal (GI) adverse effects are the most common, and dosing at mealtime helps lessen this.

Patient and family education about these medications poses a perplexing situation. Most medications are prescribed to produce improvements, but these medications usually level-out the decline. While the disease continues to progress, AChE inhibitors increase the amount of acetylcholine in the areas of the brain most affected, which masks the deterioration of the disease. *Staying the same* for a patient with Alzheimer's disease is actually an improvement because, without the medication, the decline would be evident. Stopping the medications can cause a precipitous increase in the patients' cognitive decline, because they no longer have the artificial boost provided by AChE inhibitors. In the early stage of Alzheimer's disease, cognitive changes are more prominent; however, as the disease progresses, behavioral and functional deficits develop.

Families want to stop these medications for a variety of reasons. Some cannot accept the idea that staying the same is an improvement. On the other hand, some do not want to delay the inevitable. Others have seen the patient go through months and even years of unmanageable behavior. They question the value of the medication. At this point, memantine would be a logical choice of medication, but some families might not want to try anything else.

Expense is another consideration for many families. These drugs are expensive. Some pharmaceutical companies have initiated a variety of cost-saving programs, including medication samples, vouchers for free medications that are attached to written prescriptions, and patient assistance programs, to alleviate financial burdens somewhat.

**CRITICAL THINKING QUESTION** 9

How do you explain that patients taking an AChE inhibitor (e.g., donepezil, rivastigmine, or galantamine) might stay the same over a period of 6 months, and that this is considered an improvement?

**CRITICAL THINKING QUESTION** 10

Should patients take AChE inhibitors for the rest of their lives?

## Other Drugs for Cognitive Disorders

Depression is a real issue in cognitive disorders. Typically, selective serotonin reuptake inhibitors (SSRIs) and venlafaxine (Effexor) are preferred over tricyclic antidepressants (TCAs) and monoamine oxidase inhibitors (MAOIs). TCAs tend to be highly anticholinergic and antiadrenergic, whereas MAOIs have the potential for serious interactions. Psychotic thinking and behavior are also issues for this population. Atypical antipsychotics can be ordered for psychosis but the risk for endocrine changes, such as metabolic syndrome, is becoming more problematic. Mood stabilizers and antianxiety medications are also used when needed in patients with cognitive disorders.

## MILIEU MANAGEMENT

Much is involved in making the patient comfortable. At home, or in a specialized care facility, the room temperature and lighting should be at the patient's preference and not family or staff. Nursing staff should seek to reduce noxious sounds that might offend or frighten patients. Televisions should not be allowed unless there is purposeful viewing. For patients in a specialized care facility, it is important to match roommates' personalities, when possible.

### Memory Aids

A person does not have to have a cognitive disorder to benefit from memory aids. Many patients keep track of appointments on a calendar that has big blocks for each date. Notes are good reminders, but the patient must know to look for them. Directions might be written in large print to instruct patients about how to operate new appliances, such as a new microwave. One patient bought a new television that required three remote controls to operate all the features of the television, cable television box, and DVD player. The three remote controls were consolidated into one universal remote control. The daughter made a

| Table 32-5 | Alternative Formulations of Selected Psychotropic Medications* | | |  |
|---|---|---|---|---|

| Medication (in Usual Class)† | Quick-Dissolving Form | Liquid | Injectable | Miscellaneous |
|---|---|---|---|---|
| **Alzheimer's** | | | | |
| Donepezil (Aricept ODT) | Orally disintegrating tablet (ODT) | | | |
| Galantamine (Razadyne‡) | | Liquid | | |
| Rivastigmine (Exelon) | | Liquid | | |
| **Antianxiety** | | | | |
| Alprazolam (Niravam) | Tablet | | | |
| Clonazepam (Klonopin) | Wafer | | | |
| **Antidepressants§** | | | | |
| Citalopram (Celexa) | | Liquid | | |
| Duloxetine (Cymbalta) | | | | Enteric-coated pellets inside capsule |
| Escitalopram (Lexapro) | | Liquid | | |
| Fluoxetine (Prozac) | | Liquid | | Weekly tablet |
| Mirtazapine (Remeron) | SolTab | | | |
| Paroxetine (Paxil) | | Liquid | | |
| Sertraline (Zoloft) | | Liquid | | |
| **Antipsychotics** | | | | |
| ***Atypical Antipsychotics*** | | | | |
| Aripiprazole (Abilify) | | Liquid | | |
| Olanzapine (Zyprexa) | Zydis | | Short-acting IM | |
| Risperidone (Risperdal) | M-Tabs | Liquid | | |
| Risperidone (Risperdal Consta) | | | Long-acting IM | |
| Ziprasidone (Geodon) | | | Short-acting IM | |
| ***Typical Antipsychotics*** | | | | |
| Fluphenazine (Prolixin) | | Liquid | Short-acting IM | |
| Fluphenazine decanoate | | | Long-acting IM | |
| Halperidol (Haldol) | | Concentrate | Short-acting IM | |
| Haloperidol decanoate | | | Long-acting IM | |
| **Mood Stabilizers** | | | | |
| Carbamazepine (Tegretol) | Chewable tablet | Suspension | | |
| Lamotrigine (Lamictal) | Chewable tablet | | | |
| Lithium | | Liquid | | |
| Divalproex sodium (Depakote) | | | | Sprinkles in a capsule |

*When swallowing pills and capsules is a problem.
†For the most current information, refer to the prescribing information provided by the pharmaceutical company.
‡Formerly known as Reminyl.
§No TCAs, no MAOIs.

photocopy of the new remote control and took it home with her. When the patient had difficulty turning on his television, finding the right channel, or operating the DVD player, he would call his daughter to talk him through it. In another example, a patient's son took digital photographs of each of his mother's pills and then made a daily grid for her with pictures of the real pills according to the time of day that she needed to take them.

Medication administration accuracy and patients' adherence to their medication regimens make a critical combination. A deficit on either side can cause major problems.

Pillboxes for the day, week, or even month help patients keep their medication sorted out. Some

## CASE STUDY

Roberta Evans, an 81-year-old Caucasian female with type 2 diabetes, lived in a retirement community apartment. Since her husband died 5 years ago, this retired high school science teacher had been living independently.

Three weeks before admission to a geropsychiatric unit, she drove her car to a local discount store. While walking to the store, two women approached her in the parking lot. They told Mrs. Evans that they knew a way to invest her money that would double it overnight. Mrs. Evans went to the bank with them, took out $1,000, and gave it to them. Of course, these con artists never returned. Her only child, a son, had moved to Texas about a year ago. He did not call the retirement community director to report what had happened. Instead, when her son heard about the scam, he called a friend who lived locally and had him disable his mother's car battery. Once the patient's car would not start, she started walking out on the busy streets. She never considered that her car could be repaired. Two weeks later, Mrs. Evans wandered away from the retirement community and was found several blocks away. She did not know where she was going and could not remember how to get back to her apartment. A police officer brought her back to the apartment director, who in turn called her son in Texas. He flew in from Texas the next morning.

When he visited his mother in her apartment, he saw plates with dried half-eaten food all over the kitchen and living room. He found the plastic bag with all the diabetes supplies and prescription in it. Dirty clothes were strewn about the apartment. Her bathtub faucet did not work. He did not know how long it had been since she had bathed and his mother could not tell him. She agreed to be evaluated for this change in cognitive status, although she thought nothing was wrong. However, she had connected her son's presence with her driving ban. She said, "I'll do anything to get my car back."

She was admitted to a geriatric psychiatric unit in a university hospital in her town. The multidisciplinary treatment team met the day after Mrs. Evans was admitted to plan her care. Her son did not know what her most recent baseline behavior was, because he had only spoken with her over the telephone during the last year and said he could not detect any changes. The patient was able to take care of her activities of daily living independently once she had prompts, especially for hygiene and grooming. Mrs. Evans attended all the unit activities and enjoyed being with her peers. However, she needed to be reminded to go to each session. She told the music therapist that she was glad that he had started the music group that day. She did not remember participating in music therapy the week before. Mrs. Evans ate well and slept through the night.

She participated in all the diagnostic testing and did not complain. The MRI scan of her brain showed some atrophy. The electroencaphalographic (EEG) results indicated some mild background slowing. The single-photon emission computed tomography (SPECT) scan of her brain indicated lower perfusion in the frontoparietal lobes. Neuropsychological testing showed that the patient had difficulty with short-term memory as well as visuo-spatial difficulties. On admission, she scored 23 out of 30 on the mini-mental state examination. She said, "I don't keep up with these things anymore since I've retired." These findings are consistent with a diagnosis of Alzheimer's disease. She was started on an AChE inhibitor.

Before discharge, the geriatric psychiatrist, nurse, and social worker met with the patient and her son to make treatment recommendations. The results of the diagnostic testing were discussed. The patient had asked the team members while she was still taking the tests to tell her what was wrong. "I'm not crazy, you know!"

The son agreed that it was in his mother's best interest that she be told her diagnosis. The physician told her that she had Alzheimer's disease. She said at first, "I don't believe it." Later, she admitted that she had "memory problems, but I do not have Alzheimer's disease." She reluctantly agreed to move to the assisted living facility in the same retirement community. "I know I need some help with my cooking."

The patient did well in the assisted living facility. She liked the various activities; in addition, her roommate was a woman who had taught in the same high school in which she had taught. Mrs. Evans responded favorably to the AChE inhibitor. She was able to live in the assisted living facility for 3 more years before she had to move to the nursing home.

---

pillboxes even have an alarm in them to remind patients when to take their medications. Sometimes, all a patient needs is a telephone reminder to take the medication. Here are some examples of medication errors that could have been prevented:

1. A patient did not know which medication to take, so he took all his blue pills on one day and all his white pills on another.

2. Another patient took both lorazepam prescribed by one doctor and Ativan prescribed by another. She did not know that they were chemical equivalents.

If there is any doubt about a patient's ability to take medication, ask the patient to demonstrate which medication to take and when.

## Care Plan

Name: Roberta Evans

Admission Date: _____

*DSM-IV-TR* Diagnosis: Dementia of the Alzheimer's type with behavioral disturbance (wandering)

| | |
|---|---|
| Assessment | **Areas of strength:** Willingness to be evaluated, good relationship with fellow residents and staff at the retirement community, strong faith |
| | **Problems:** Short-term memory loss, confusion, poor judgment, wandering |

Diagnoses
- Acute confusion (got lost)
- Memory impairment (forgot that she had been diagnosed with diabetes mellitus, type 2)
- Impaired judgment (being conned out of $1,000)
- Social isolation—relationship with her son: although it is a good one, he lives at a distance
- Self-care deficits—poor personal hygiene and apartment filth
- Wandering

Outcomes

*Short-term goals:*                                                                    Date met
- Patient will have a comprehensive geriatric psychiatric evaluation.          _____
- Patient will be medically stable especially related to new-onset             _____
  diabetes mellitus, type 2.
- Patient will participate in group activities.                                _____
- Patient and son will meet with the multidisciplinary treatment              _____
  team to discuss diagnosis, patient's progress, and plans for
  discharge.

*Long-term goals:*
- Patient will be safe and free of injury (both physical and                   _____
  emotional).
- Patient will be discharged to appropriate level of care.                     _____
- Patient will maintain her independence as long as possible, even             _____
  though she now needs assistance.
- Patient will be introduced to a variety of social activities in which        _____
  she can participate at her new residence.
- Patient will have medical and psychiatric follow up scheduled                _____
  before discharge.
- Patient will have her dignity preserved and her self-esteem                  _____
  enhanced.

Planning/
Interventions

**Nurse-patient relationship:**
- Explain the process of evaluation and treatment by the nursing staff and the rest of the multidisciplinary treatment team.
- Educate the patient about her recent-onset diabetes mellitus, even though she will not be doing the monitoring herself.
- Educate and support the patient regarding this hospitalization, especially the patient's concern that others will think that she is "crazy" (her term).

**Psychopharmacology:**
- Educate the patient and her son about AChE inhibitors and the specific one she is taking.
- Educate the patient and her son about the oral hypoglycemic agent that she is taking for diabetes mellitus type 2.
- Monitor for any adverse reactions.

**Milieu management:**
- Assess and provide the level of care for her activities of daily living associated with bathing, hygiene, and grooming.

## Care Plan—cont'd

Evaluation

- Facilitate interaction between patients who are at her cognitive and functional level in preparation for discharge to a facility where she will have the opportunity to make new acquaintances.
- Patient will meet her short- and long-term goals. She will be prepared to move to the assisted living facility in her retirement community.
- Patient's son has agreed to visit his mother every 3 months and to call her at least once a week. To comply with HIPAA (Health Insurance Portability and Accountability Act) regulations, the patient has signed a release of information so that her son can call the assisted living facility director with any concerns that he might have.

Referrals

- The referral was made to the assisted living facility in her retirement community about her transfer from her apartment.
- The Police Department was notified about the scam artists because this had not been done at the time.

## Study Notes

1. The normal aging process does not include the development of any cognitive disorder.
2. On first glance, delirium and dementia share some commonalities. However, treatment for delirium must be started immediately. Unlike dementia, delirium can be imminently life-threatening.
3. Most types of dementia feature a progressive cognitive deterioration over time. Few types are reversible. NPH, vitamin $B_{12}$ deficiency, and alcohol-related dementia might be reversed in early stages.

   Alzheimer's disease, DLBD, and vascular dementia—the three types of dementia that comprise most of these illnesses—might not be reversed.
4. Alzheimer's disease is not a new disease. Dr. Alois Alzheimer, a German neurologist, first discussed a patient with these signs in 1907. Dr. Frederic Lewy, also a neurologist and a contemporary of Alzheimer's, first described Lewy bodies.
5. Although not a perfect predictor of Alzheimer's disease, a person with MCI is more likely to develop Alzheimer's disease than a person who does not have it.
6. Vascular dementia is caused by little strokes. The progression is unpredictable because it depends on the occurrence of another vascular event. Therefore, the deterioration takes a step-wise progression, meaning that the patient might stay on a plateau for days to years before another ischemic event occurs. Risk factors include hypertension, diabetes mellitus, smoking, and obesity. The reduction of these risk factors might also reduce the likelihood of a subsequent ischemic event. If another little stroke does occur, it might not be as severe as the previous event(s).
7. A pathognomonic (hallmark) sign of DLBD is the hypersensitivity that the patient has with antipsychotic medication. Also, Lewy bodies are found in the neurons of the cerebral cortex.
8. A patient with PD might also have a dementia and/or depression.
9. Patients with dementia who exhibit disruptive behavior might be delirious, confused, or uncomfortable. Many cannot make their needs known.
10. Nursing care must be patient-focused. Dignity must be preserved and safety maintained. Promote as much independence for the patient as possible.
11. Genetics plays a part in some types of dementia (e.g., HD is an autosomal dominant illness). At least six chromosomes have been identified that have some linkage to Alzheimer's disease (chromosomes 1, 9, 10, 14, 19, and 21).
12. Caregiver burden is a significant stressor felt by many caregivers of patients with dementia. The caregivers are at risk for developing physical illnesses or exacerbating current ones (e.g., diabetes mellitus, hypertension) and/or psychiatric disorders (e.g., depression, anxiety).

## References

Algase D: Wandering in dementia, *Am Rev Nurs Res* 17:185, 1999a.

Algase D: Wandering: a dementia–compromised behavior, *J Gerontol Nurs* 25(9):51, 1999b.

Alexopolous G: Clinical and biological interactions in affective and cognitive geriatric syndromes, *Am J Psychiatry* 160:811, 2003.

Alzheimer's Disease Education & Referral Center (ADEAR): *Alzheimer's Disease Fact Sheet.* Available at www.nia.nih.gov/Alzheimers/Publications/adfact.htm. Accessed March 20, 2006.

American Psychiatric Association: *Diagnostic and statistical manual of mental disorders, text revision,* ed 4, Washington, DC, 2000, APA.

American Psychiatric Association: *Diagnostic and statistical manual of mental disorders,* ed 4, Washington, DC, 1994, APA.

Biddle W, van Sickel M: *Introduction to psychiatry,* ed 2, Philadelphia, 1948, WB Saunders.

Bird T: Genetic factors in Alzheimer's disease, *N Engl J Med* 352:862, 2005.

Brookes AJ, Prince JA: Genetic association analysis: lessons from the study of Alzheimer's disease. Mutation research/fundamental and molecular mechanisms of mutagenesis, *Mutat Res* 573:152, 2005.

Brust J: Neurologic emergencies—acute neurologic complications of drug and alcohol abuse, *Neurol Clin* 16:503, 1998.

Cummings J, Vinters HV, Cole GM, Khachaturian ZS: Alzheimer's disease: etiologies, pathophysiology, cognitive reserve, and treatment opportunities, *Neurology* 51(Suppl 1):S2, 1998.

Dewing J: Sundowning in older people with dementia: evidence base, nursing assessment and interventions, *Nursing Older People* 15:8, 24-31, 2003.

Epling J, Taylor H: Preventing delirium in hospitalized older patients, *J Fam Pract* 48:417, 1999.

Folstein MF, Folstein SE, McHugh PR: "Mini-mental state." A practical method for grading the cognitive status of patients for the clinician, *J Psychiatr Res* 12:189, 1975.

Geldmacher D: Differential diagnosis of Alzheimer's disease, *Neurology* 48:PS002, 1997.

Gomez-Tortosa E: Dementia with Lewy bodies, *J Am Geriatr Soc* 46:1449, 1998.

Gruetzner H: *Alzheimer's: a caregiver's guide and sourcebook,* New York, 2001, John Wiley & Sons.

Inouye S: Delirium and other mental status problems in the older patient. In Goldman L, editor: *Cecil textbook of medicine,* ed 21, Baltimore, 2000, WB Saunders.

Inouye S, Bogardus ST Jr, Charpentier PA, et al: A multicomponent intervention to prevent delirium in hospitalized older patients, *N Engl J Med* 340:669, 1999.

Jacob A: Charles Bonnet syndrome—elderly people and visual hallucinations, *BMJ* 328:1552, 2004.

Jack C: Magnetic resonance imaging. In Petersen R, editor: *Mild cognitive impairment,* Oxford, England, 2003, Oxford Unversity Press.

Kay J, Tasman A: *Psychiatry: behavioral science and clinical essentials. Dementia, delirium, and other cognitive disorders,* Baltimore, 2000, WB Saunders.

Keltner N, Folks D: *Psychotropic drugs,* ed 4, St. Louis, 2005, Mosby.

Keltner NL, Williams B: Memantine: a new approach to Alzheimer's disease, *Perspect Psychiatr Care* 40:123, 2004.

Kirshner HS: Delirium and acute confusional state. In Kirshner HS, editor: *Behavioral neurology,* ed 2, Boston, 2002, Butterworth-Heinemann.

Knopman D: An overview of common and non-Alzheimer dementias, *Clin Geriatr Med* 17:281, 2001.

Litvan I, Agid Y, Sastry N, et al: What are the obstacles for an accurate clinical diagnosis of Pick's disease? A clinicopathologic study, *Neurology* 49:62, 1997.

Mace N, Rabins P: *The 36-hour day,* Baltimore, 1991, Johns Hopkins University Press.

Moore P, Jefferson J: *Handbook of medical psychiatry,* ed 2, St. Louis, 2004, Mosby.

Morris J, Storandt M, Miller JP, et al: Mild cognitive impairment represents early-stage Alzheimer's disease, *Arch Neurol* 58:397, 2001.

National Institute of Aging (NIA): *2003 progress report on Alzheimer's disease,* Bethesda, MD, 2003, NIA.

National Institute of Aging (NIA): *2000 progress report on Alzheimer's disease,* Bethesda, MD, 2000, NIA.

National Institute of Neurological Disorders and Stroke (NINDS): *Dementia fact sheet,* Bethesda, MD, 2005, NINDS.

NANDA International: *NANDA-approved nursing diagnoses: definitions and classifications, 2005-2006,* Philadelphia, 2005, NANDA International.

Perkin G: *Mosby's color atlas and text of neurology,* London, 1998, Times Mirror International.

Petersen R, Thomas RG, Grundman N, et al: Vitamin E and donepezil for the treatment of mild cognitive impairment, *N Engl J Med* 352:2379, 2005.

Plassman B, Havlik RJ, Steffens DC, et al: Documented head injury in early adulthood and risk of Alzheimer's disease and other dementias, *Neurology* 55:1158, 2000.

Rondeau V: A review of epidemiologic studies on aluminum and silica in relation to Alzheimer's disease and associated disorders. *Rev Env Hlth* 17(2):107-121, 2002.

Rosen H, Lengenfelder J, Miller B: Frontotemporal dementia, *Neurol Clin* 18:979, 2000.

Snowdon D: Healthy aging and dementia: findings from the Nun Study, *Ann Intern Med* 139(5 Pt 2):450, 2003.

Snowdon D: *Aging with grace: what the Nun Study teaches us about leading longer, healthier, and more meaningful lives,* New York, 2001, Bantam Books.

Stahl S: *Essential psychopharmacology: neuroscientific basis and practical applications,* Cambridge, England, 2000, Cambridge University Press.

Stewart J: Defining diffuse Lewy body disease. Tetrad of symptoms distinguishes illness from other dementias, *Postgrad Med* 113:71, 2003.

Tasman A, Kay J, Lieberman JA, et al: *Psychiatry,* Baltimore, 1997, WB Saunders.

U.S. Food and Drug Administration: *FDA public health advisory: deaths with antipsychotics in elderly patients with behavioral disturbances.* Available at http://www.fda.gov/cder/drug/advisory/antipsychotics.htm Accessed March 20, 2006.

Visser P, Krabbendam L, Verhey FR, et al: Brain correlates of memory dysfunction in alcoholic Korsakoff's syndrome, *J Neurol Neurosurg Psychiatry* 67:774, 1999.

Wilson J, Helton B: *PSYCHed: continuing education and consultation, dementia module,* Birmingham, AL, 2005. (Unpublished.)

Young R: Update on Parkinson's disease, *Am Family Physician* 59:2155, 1999.

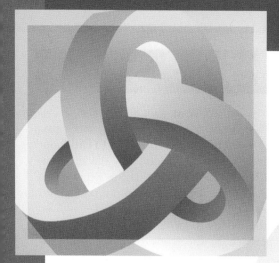

# Chapter 33

# Personality Disorders

*Carol E. Bostrom*

## Learning Objectives

*After reading this chapter, you should be able to:*
- Recognize characteristics of each personality disorder.
- Describe behaviors of individuals with personality disorders.
- Describe nursing interventions for patients with personality disorders.
- Recognize issues related to the care of patients with personality disorders.

This chapter focuses on patients with personality disorders hospitalized in the inpatient psychiatric setting or treated in outpatient programs. Except for the patient with a borderline disorder, these patients are not usually hospitalized because of their personality disorders but because of other mental disorders diagnosed on axis I. The interventions focus primarily on the nurse-patient relationship unique to each personality disorder; however, this chapter does not repeat the general nurse-patient interventions described in Chapter 8. Neither milieu issues nor psychopharmacologic factors will be addressed for each disorder, because unique milieu and pharmacologic interventions are not appropriate for all disorders. Medication might be given if the patient has an axis I diagnosis or a symptom severe enough to interfere with functioning, such as severe anxiety or depression.

All individuals have personality traits and characteristics that make them unique and interesting human beings. Traits are exhibited in the way individuals think about themselves and others and in the way they behave. When traits are inflexible and dysfunctional, individuals generally have problems in functioning and experience subjective distress. Patients with personality disorders suffer lifelong, inflexible, and dysfunctional patterns of relating and behaving. These dysfunctional patterns and behaviors usually cause distress to others. However, individuals with personality disorders might not find their behaviors distressing to themselves; they become distressed because of other people's reactions or behaviors toward them. This reaction affects these individuals by causing immense emotional pain and discomfort. The nurse conveys acceptance of the individual and empathy for emotional pain, regardless of the patient's behavior. Patients with personality disorders are given more psychiatric inpatient, outpatient, and pharmacologic therapy than patients with a major depressive disorder (Bender et al, 2001). Difficulty in managing complicated symptoms and significant impairment in functioning have resulted in increased contact with the mental health system and use of services. Patients do not

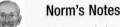

### Norm's Notes

*In my opinion, these disorders are the toughest to treat. For instance, someone with a narcissistic personality disorder can be charming and delightful company but at their center they are always scheming and looking out for number one. They tend to be subversive and undermine authority whenever they can. Note that personality disorders are placed on axis II of the DSM-IV-TR. The other category of disorders placed under axis II is mental retardation. Why are personality disorders placed there? I will answer with another question, "How deep does the yellow go in a banana?" Our personalities go to our core.*

seek treatment to change their personality but want help for depression, anxiety, and alcoholism and for difficulties in work and personal relationships (Grinspoon, 2000c). Personality disorders often coexist with anxiety and mood disorders (Grant et al, 2005).

Personality disorders are listed on axis II. Axis II can also be used to designate developmental disorders, personality traits, or habitual use of particular defense mechanisms. For example, compulsive traits are not the same as obsessive-compulsive personality disorder, which, in turn, is not the same as obsessive-compulsive disorder. Many high-functioning people have compulsive traits, whereas only a few have compulsive personality disorders. Patients benefit from the fact that some nurses might have compulsive traits—for example, rechecking labels, dressings, and drainage tubes.

Criteria for a personality disorder include experiences and behaviors that are very different from those that are usually expected in an individual's culture. The individual must have disturbances in two of the following areas: cognition, affect, interpersonal functioning, and impulse control. The *Diagnostic and Statistical Manual of Mental Disorders,* Text Revision, Fourth Edition *(DSM-IV-TR)* presents general criteria for a personality disorder and criteria specific to each personality disorder (American Psychiatric Association [APA], 2000; see the *DSM-IV-TR* Criteria for Personality Disorders box).

## ETIOLOGY: CONTEMPORARY VIEWS

Between 10 and 15 years ago, the causes of personality disorders were thought to be only psychological in origin based on reactions to childhood experiences and on the reaction of the interpersonal and family environment to the experiences. Child development, family, and environment were key to developing personality disorders.

With the explosion of biologic research, a different approach to the study of factors underlying the development of personality disorders has emerged. Disturbances in cognition, impulsivity and aggression, affective lability, and chronic anxiety in patients with personality disorders are being studied across many personality disorders rather than for a specific personality disorder. This approach will add biologic data and another dimension to psychodynamic theory to increase our understanding of the psychopathology of these disorders (Silk, 2000).

Biologic factors alone are not totally responsible for the occurrence of these disorders. Twin studies have indicated that specific traits, rather than disorders, are inherited.

The social environment, coupled with psychological vulnerability, strongly influences the individual. The effects of societal changes, a stressful environment, and negative childhood experiences, along with biologic factors, are important in the genesis of personality disorders.

## PERSONALITY DISORDER CLUSTERS

According to the *DSM-IV-TR,* the personality disorders are grouped into three clusters based on descriptive features. Cluster A includes the schizoid, schizotypal, and paranoid disorders, characterized by odd or eccentric behaviors. Cluster B includes the narcissistic, histrionic, antisocial, and borderline disorders, characterized by dramatic, emotional, or erratic behaviors. Cluster C includes the dependent, avoidant, and obsessive-compulsive disorders, characterized by anxious or fearful behaviors (APA, 2000).

When a person exhibits features of more than one specific personality disorder or does not meet the full criteria for any one disorder, the classification of "personality disorder not otherwise speci-

## DSM-IV-TR Criteria for Personality Disorders

### Criteria for a Personality Disorder

Disturbances in two or more of the following must be present:

A. Cognition (thinking about self, people, and events)
B. Affectivity (range, intensity, lability, and appropriateness of emotional response)
C. Interpersonal functioning
D. Impulse control

### Cluster A: Odd-Eccentric Behaviors

### Criteria for Paranoid Personality Disorder

A. Suspicious of others
B. Doubts trustworthiness or loyalty of friends and others
C. Fear of confiding in others
D. Suspicious, without justification, of spouse's or sexual partner's fidelity
E. Interprets remarks as demeaning or threatening
F. Holds grudges toward others
G. Becomes angry and threatening when he or she perceives being attacked by others

### Criteria for Schizoid Personality Disorder

A. Lacks desire for close relationships or friends
B. Chooses solitary activities
C. Little interest in sexual experiences
D. Avoids activities
E. Appears cold and detached
F. Lacks close friends
G. Appears indifferent to praise or criticism

### Criteria for Schizotypal Personality Disorder

A. Ideas of reference
B. Magical thinking or odd beliefs
C. Unusual perceptual experiences, including bodily illusions
D. Odd thinking and vague, stereotypical, overelaborate speech
E. Suspicious
F. Blunted or inappropriate affect
G. Odd or eccentric appearance or behavior
H. Few close relationships
I. Excessive social anxiety

### Cluster B: Dramatic, Emotional, Erratic Behaviors

### Criteria for Antisocial Personality Disorder

A. Deceitfulness, as seen in lying or conning others
B. Engages in illegal activities
C. Aggressive behavior
D. Lack of guilt or remorse
E. Irresponsible in work and with finances
F. Impulsiveness
G. Reckless disregard of safety for self or others

### Criteria for Borderline Personality Disorder

A. Frantic avoidance of abandonment, real or imagined
B. Unstable and intense interpersonal relationships
C. Identity disturbances
D. Impulsivity
E. Affective instability
F. Recurrent suicidal behavior or self-mutilating behavior
G. Rapid mood shifts
H. Chronic feelings of emptiness
I. Problems with anger
J. Transient dissociative and paranoid symptoms

### Criteria for Narcissistic Personality Disorder

A. Grandiose self-importance
B. Fantasies of unlimited power, success, or brilliance
C. Believes that he or she is special or unique
D. Needs to be admired
E. Sense of entitlement (i.e., deserves to be favored or given special treatment)
F. Takes advantage of others for own benefit
G. Lacks empathy
H. Envious of others or others are envious of him or her
I. Arrogant or haughty

### Criteria for Histrionic Personality Disorder

A. Needs to be center of attention
B. Displays sexually seductive or provocative behaviors
C. Shallow, rapidly shifting emotions
D. Uses physical appearance to draw attention
E. Uses speech to impress others but is lacking in depth
F. Dramatic expression of emotion
G. Easily influenced by others
H. Exaggerates degree of intimacy with others

### Cluster C: Anxious-Fearful Behaviors

### Criteria for Dependent Personality Disorder

A. Unable to make daily decisions without much advice and reassurance
B. Needs others to be responsible for important areas of life
C. Seldom disagrees with others because of fear of loss of support or approval
D. Problem with initiating projects or doing things on own because of little self-confidence
E. Performs unpleasant tasks to obtain support from others
F. Anxious or helpless when alone because of fear of being unable to care for self
G. Urgently seeks another relationship for support and care after a close relationship ends

*Continued*

## DSM-IV-TR Criteria    for Personality Disorders—cont'd

H. Preoccupied with fear of being alone to care for self

**Criteria for Avoidant Personality Disorder**
A. Avoids occupations involving interpersonal contact because of fears of disapproval or rejection
B. Uninvolved with others unless certain of being liked
C. Fears intimate relationships because of fear of shame or ridicule
D. Preoccupied with being criticized or rejected in social situations
E. Inhibited and feels inadequate in new interpersonal situations
F. Believes self to be socially inept, unappealing, or inferior to others

G. Very reluctant to take risks or engage in new activities because of possibility of being embarrassed

**Criteria for Obsessive-Compulsive Personality Disorder**
A. Preoccupied with details, rules, lists, organization
B. Perfectionism that interferes with task completion
C. Too busy working to have friends or leisure activities
D. Overconscientious and inflexible
E. Unable to discard worthless or worn-out objects
F. Others must do things his or her way in work- or task-related activity
G. Reluctant to spend and hoards money
H. Rigid and stubborn

Modified from the American Psychiatric Association: *Diagnostic and statistical manual of mental disorders, Text Revision,* ed 4, Washington, DC, 2000, APA.

fied" is used. *DSM-IV-TR* diagnoses (APA, 2000) and possible NANDA International nursing diagnoses for personality disorders (NANDA International, 2005) are listed in the box below.

## DSM-IV-TR and NANDA International Diagnoses Related to Personality Disorders

*DSM-IV-TR\**

*Cluster A—Odd, Eccentric Behaviors*
Paranoid personality disorder
Schizoid personality disorder
Schizotypal personality disorder

*Cluster B—Dramatic, Emotional, Erratic Behaviors*
Antisocial personality disorder
Borderline personality disorder
Histrionic personality disorder
Narcissistic personality disorder

*Cluster C—Anxious, Fearful Behaviors*
Avoidant personality disorder
Dependent personality disorder
Obsessive-compulsive disorder

NANDA INTERNATIONAL†
Anxiety
Communication, verbal, impaired
Coping, defensive

Coping, ineffective
Family processes, interrupted
Hopelessness
Loneliness, risk for
Powerlessness
Self-esteem, chronic low
Self-esteem, situational low
Self-esteem, situational low, risk for
Self-mutilation, risk for
Social isolation
Violence, self-directed, risk for
Violence, other-directed, risk for

\*From the American Psychiatric Association: *Diagnostic and statistical manual of mental disorders, text revision,* ed 4, Washington, DC, 2000, APA.
†From NANDA International: *NANDA nursing diagnoses: definitions and classifications, 2005-2006,* Philadelphia, 2005, NANDA International.

## CLUSTER A: ODD-ECCENTRIC

## PARANOID PERSONALITY DISORDER

Suspiciousness and mistrust of people characterize the person with a paranoid personality disorder. These individuals interpret the actions of others as personal threats, which results in an increase in anxiety and the need for vigilance. They are hypersensitive to other people's motives and often act in defense of a fragile self-concept (Bender, 2005). They feel vulnerable because they think others treat them unfairly. Individuals with paranoid personality disorder are unable to laugh at themselves and are often humorless and serious. Speech is logical and goal-directed, although the basis of an argument is false because of their suspiciousness. Other symptoms include prejudice and sometimes ideas of reference. These individuals have a blunted affect, so they might appear to be cold, but they are capable of close relationships with a select few. However, they might be suspicious of people close to them. For example, these individuals might unjustifiably believe that their spouse is having an affair.

Unlike paranoid schizophrenia, people with paranoid personality disorder do not have fixed delusions or hallucinations. Transient psychotic symptoms might be precipitated by extreme stress. People with paranoid personality disorder are hospitalized when their behavior is out of control in response to a threat perceived as overwhelming or immediate. Because they are quick to respond with anger or rage if they feel severely threatened, these individuals might be brought to the hospital because of their loss of control and potential for violence.

## UNIQUE CAUSES

Some evidence has suggested that the paranoid personality disorder tends to occur in biologic relatives of identified patients with schizophrenia and is diagnosed more often in men than in women (APA, 2000).

### CLINICAL EXAMPLE

James Sneed is admitted to the hospital accompanied by a female friend. Mr. Sneed states, "My neighbor is taking my land. He built a fence on my property instead of his." The female friend states that James had barricaded himself in his house, was surrounded by his collection of shotguns, and was threatening to "blow away" his neighbor.

## SCHIZOID PERSONALITY DISORDER

People with schizoid personalities do not want to be involved in interpersonal or social relationships and keep people at an emotional distance. These individuals rarely have close friends and appear uncomfortable interacting with others; they might be thought of as hermits because of their shyness and introversion; they respond with short answers to questions and do not initiate spontaneous conversation; they can function at work successfully, especially if little verbal interaction is required; and, although they are reality-oriented, fantasy and daydreaming might be more gratifying compared with real persons and situations.

If a person with schizoid personality disorder is hospitalized, the nurse-patient relationship will focus initially on building trust, followed by the identification and appropriate verbal expression of feelings. At first, the patient might be able to participate only on the fringe of unit activities because of discomfort and anxiety. Slowly involving the patient in milieu and group activities might help increase social skills.

## SCHIZOTYPAL PERSONALITY DISORDER

Individuals with schizotypal personality disorder appear similar to patients with schizophrenia, with the major exception being that psychotic episodes are infrequent and less severe. These patients have problems in thinking, perceiving, and communicating. Their outward appearance might be eccentric and their behavior odd; they are sensitive to the behaviors of others, especially rejection and anger, and feel that they are different and do not fit in. Paranoid ideation, ideas of reference, and odd beliefs are some of the most prevalent and unchangeable criteria for this disorder (McGlashan et al, 2005). Fantasies about imaginary relationships might be substituted for real relationships. They are uncomfortable around people but are interested in others (Bender, 2005).

When a person with schizotypal personality disorder is hospitalized, interventions offering support, kindness, and gentle suggestions will help the patient become involved in activities with others. It is essential for the nurse to help the patient improve interpersonal relationships, social skills, and appropriate behaviors. Social situations are uncomfortable and cause discomfort and anxiety because of the reactions of others to the patient's appearance and behavior. These patients can benefit from socializing experiences if the interactions are carefully orchestrated. Vocational counseling and assistance with job placement increase the patient's opportunity for success. Low doses of antipsychotic drugs might decrease the severity of symptoms exhibited in the transient psychotic state in relation to thinking, perception, and anxiety.

## UNIQUE CAUSES

Schizotypal personality disorder is more common in the biologic relatives of schizophrenics (APA, 2000). Genetic studies have indicated that patients with this disorder show disturbances (behaviors) similar to those found in people with schizophrenia.

### PUTTING IT ALL TOGETHER
Psychotherapeutic Management

## NURSE-PATIENT RELATIONSHIP

The most important psychotherapeutic task centers on dealing with trust issues. A professional demeanor coupled with honesty and nonintrusiveness will assist in developing some trust. Clear, simple explanations and requests will reduce the patient's feelings of being threatened or controlled. These patients do not tolerate group therapies that expect or involve confrontation or much emotional involvement.

### CLUSTER B: DRAMATIC-ERRATIC

### ANTISOCIAL PERSONALITY DISORDER

The main feature of antisocial personality disorder is a pattern of disregard for the rights of others, which is usually demonstrated by repeated violations of the law. Before the age of 15 years, these behaviors are diagnosed as conduct disorder. Affected individuals engage in unlawful behavior, as evidenced by driving while intoxicated and engaging in spouse or child abuse. They are also promiscuous and feel no guilt about hurting others. Lying, cheating, and stealing are common. Their criminal behavior places them within the judicial and prison systems more than it does the mental health system. Not all criminals, however, have antisocial personality disorder.

The diagnosis of antisocial personality disorder is based on a history of disordered life functioning rather than on mental status. These individuals might experience distress and anxiety because of others' hostility toward them, but they see the problem as being in others and not in themselves. People with antisocial personality disorder might appear to be charming and intellectual; they are smooth talkers and deny and rationalize their behavior. Expected anxiety over their predicament is absent. Guilt, sorrow for offenses, or loyalty is nonexistent, as if they do not have a conscience. These individuals do not behave as responsible, mature, and independent adults.

### CRITICAL THINKING QUESTION   1
A patient with antisocial personality disorder is verbally threatening to the staff when limits are set on his manipulative behaviors. How would the nurse manage the patient's threatening behavior?

## UNIQUE CAUSES

Both genetics and the environment are known to influence the development of antisocial personality disorder. Parents establish an environment in which the parent-child relationship is unstable, resulting in delinquency in their children. Genetic studies of twin or adoptive siblings and family history data have provided significant evidence that suggests a genetic predisposition to this disorder. In other words, children inherit traits that could lead to the development of antisocial personality disorder. Substance abuse and dependency problems are highly correlated with antisocial personality disorder (Grinspoon, 2000a).

A common biologic finding seen in individuals with antisocial personality disorder is a weak response to stress in the autonomic nervous system, as evidenced by a low heart rate and a lack of increase in level of anxiety. They are insensitive to the emotional connotations of language, which might explain their inability to learn from reward and punishment. Brain scans of individuals with antisocial personality disorder have shown lower than average activity in the frontal lobes, which govern judgment and decision making (Grinspoon, 2000b).

## Psychotherapeutic Management

## NURSE-PATIENT RELATIONSHIP

Long-term treatment is necessary for any type of lasting changes to occur. With short-term hospitalization, the nurse can initiate the therapeutic process by setting firm limits. These patients try to manipulate staff and bend rules for their own desires and needs. The nurse must be steadfast and consistent in confronting behaviors and enforcing rules and policies. Consequences of behavior, both for the unit and for the patient's life, are also a point of focus. Helping the patient be aware of consequences is a concrete way to assist the patient in realizing what the results of behaviors are or will be. Pointing out the effects that the patient's behaviors have on others is also part of the therapeutic process. The patient must begin to understand how others feel and react to his or her behaviors, and why they react the way they do. The nurse avoids moralizing and assists the patient in identifying and verbalizing feelings that might reflect anxiety and depression. Membership in a group can help the patient feel accepted as a person, even if the patient's behaviors are not acceptable. Groups of other individuals with this same diagnosis can be effective in confronting inappropriate and manipulative behavior, because these individuals are experts in spotting smooth talking, rationalizing, and lying. Such groups can be effective in helping the antisocial patient. To summarize, the keys to working with the antisocial patient are consistency by the nursing staff and accountability by the patient.

## BORDERLINE PERSONALITY DISORDER

Features of the borderline personality disorder (BPD) include emotional dysregulation, anger, impulsivity, intense psychological pain, impairment in interpersonal or occupational functioning, identity or self-image disturbances, abandonment fears, and self-injurious behavior (Antai-Ontong, 2003; Conklin and Westen, 2005; McGlashan et al, 2005). Of all personality disorders, the borderline personality disorder is the one most commonly treated with high mental health care utilization (Sansone et al, 2005). However, because the full range of symptoms and behaviors is not typically demonstrated during one short-term inpatient hospitalization, it is often difficult to fully appreciate the complexity of these individuals' disorders. These patients usually require hospitalization when they are in a crisis or exhibit self-injurious or suicidal behaviors.

The patient with a BPD has problems with identity, self-image, relationships, thinking, mood, and impulsive behaviors (Lively, 2000). Identity problems are apparent in the patient who is uncertain about his or her self-image, career goals, personal values, and sexual orientation. Interpersonal relationships are chaotic and problems exist in choosing unhealthy relationships and short-term intimate relationships. The patient alternates between overidealization and devaluation of individuals. For example, the patient with BPD "falls in love" with the perfect person and, shortly thereafter, can find no redeeming qualities in the formerly idealized person. The person with BPD cannot appreciate the mixed bag of qualities that most people have.

Manipulation and dependency commonly occur. This patient has great difficulty in being alone and therefore seeks intense but brief relationships. Mood disturbances are exhibited in symptoms of depression, intense anger, and labile mood. Projective identification is used to protect the self. Patients displace their angry feelings onto others to justify their own feelings. Blaming others helps the patient deal with feelings, even though this is dysfunctional and inappropriate. Intense emotional pain contributes to mood shifts, which range from euphoria to crying to acting-out behaviors, such as displays of temper and physical fights, self-mutilation, and suicidal behaviors. Impulsiveness is exhibited in the use of substances and in a tendency toward anorexia-bulimia. Other relatively common impulsive activities include overspending, promiscuity, compulsive overeating, and unhealthy risk taking and decision making. Some behaviors such as self-injury are frantic efforts to avoid abandonment and attempts to cope with affective dysregulation and impulsive aggression (McGlashan et al, 2005).

Research findings have indicated that as many as 75% of individuals with BPD are women and victims of childhood sexual abuse (APA, 2000). This finding is significant because it suggests the possible dynamics of BPD behaviors, which, in turn, determine nursing interventions. The dissociation used by a child sex abuse victim might result in splitting, which is found in the BPD patient. The defense mechanism of splitting is defined as the inability to view both the self and others as having both good and bad qualities. Therefore, the self and others are viewed as either all good or all bad. Splitting helps the individual avoid the pain and feelings associated with past abuse and current situations involving threats of rejection or abandonment. The complexity of behaviors associated with BPD can include severe symptoms of posttraumatic stress disorder and dissociative disorder. See Chapters 31 and 41 for related discussions.

On admission to an inpatient psychiatric unit, the person with a BPD might exhibit a need for attention and affection by contradictory behaviors of manipulation, dependency, or acting out. Frustration on the part of the staff might be seen as rejection. This perception by the patient can lead to increased anger and withdrawal because of fear of abandonment. Shifts between depression, anxiety, euphoria, and anger are seen in the patient's labile mood. Under stress, the patient regresses to immature behaviors and is unable to cope with conflict. The patient vacillates between clinging and disengaged behaviors, as demonstrated by wanting the staff to solve all problems or by the patient viewing the inpatient treatment as unnecessary and meaningless. When progress seems to be occurring, the patient with a BPD might suddenly exhibit opposite behaviors, and it might seem as if the staff will need to start over.

Patients with BPD use self-mutilation or self-injurious behavior for the purpose of self-punishment, tension reduction, improvement in mood, and distraction from intolerable affects (Stanley et al, 2001). Self-injury can be seen in cutting, burning, and severe skin scratching (Muehlenkamp, 2005). After self-mutilating behaviors such as cutting and burning, the patient feels better and appears relieved.

Patients who mutilate themselves are at a serious risk for suicide. Their feelings of hopelessness, despair, and depression contribute to their suicid-ality, and their self-mutilation should never be interpreted as manipulation or as attention-seeking behavior. Patients with BPD are at risk for suicide because of their depression, aggression, impulsivity, underestimation of the lethality of their behavior, and longer and more frequent occurrence of suicidal thoughts. These patients are often unaware of the likelihood of death and misperceive the lethality of their attempts. The lethality of individuals who self-mutilate and attempt suicide is as serious as those who do not self-mutilate and attempt suicide (Stanley et al, 2001). Self-mutilation and suicide attempts should never be minimized or ignored. One in 10 patients with BPD completes suicide and the risk is highest with comorbid substance-related and depressive disorders (Antai-Ontong, 2003).

## UNIQUE CAUSES

The development of BPD might be the result of a combination of temperament, childhood experiences, and neurologic and biochemical dysfunction (Zanarini, 2000). Biologic, environmental, and stress-related factors contribute to the complexity of the disorder. Biologic studies have indicated neurotransmitter dysregulation of the serotonin system, as seen in affective disturbances and impulsive behaviors. Abnormalities of cholinergic and adrenergic systems predispose individuals to dysphoria, emotional lability, and hyperreactivity related to environmental stimuli (Gurvits et al, 2000). An increased norepinephrine level leads to increased reactivity to the environment, which might contribute to affective instability.

Environmental factors include a chaotic home environment, such as emotional discord in the family; neglect of the child's feelings and needs; and verbal, emotional, physical, and sexual abuse.

Stress-related events might trigger the individual's genetically based vulnerable temperament and create misery and frustration. The individual is reminded of earlier stress or trauma, which results in the development of the borderline symptoms and condition (Grinspoon, 2000c). Early trauma and stress affect the hippocampus. Reduced hippocampal volume in adults has been studied through brain imaging. Additionally, the lack of integration of the right and left hemispheres results in abused children using their right hemispheres for frightening memories and left hemispheres when thinking of neutral memories. This might account for the use of splitting by the patient (Gabbard, 2005).

## CRITICAL THINKING QUESTION     2

A 22-year-old woman is admitted to the unit with BPD and self-injurious behaviors. What are the nurse's priorities in caring for this patient?

## PUTTING IT ALL TOGETHER
### Psychotherapeutic Management

## NURSE-PATIENT RELATIONSHIP

The use of empathy by the nurse while maintaining clear boundaries is important in establishing a relationship with the patient diagnosed with BPD. The nurse is not a friend but a health care professional. The nurse acknowledges the reality of the patient's pain, offers support, and empowers and works with the patient to understand, control, and change dysfunctional behaviors. The patient is ultimately in control of his or her own behaviors, even when the behaviors seem out of control (Smith et al, 2001). With the nurse's assistance, the patient can identify and verbalize feelings, control negative behaviors, and slowly begin to replace them with more appropriate actions.

The patient is usually in a crisis situation when hospitalized because of suicidal behavior, self-mutilation, acute personality disorganization, or inability to function. The nurse conducts a suicide assessment and provides a safe environment to decrease self-harm and contain impulses and then works with the patient to find less destructive ways to handle anger, rage, and psychic pain. Alternatives might include ventilation and discussion of feelings, punching pillows, and the use of foam bats. For self-harm behaviors to diminish, the nurse helps the patient identify feelings and verbally express them nonaggressively, which enables the patient to understand that his or her actions are habitual responses to handling emotions. Recognizing behavioral and emotional cues can help the patient decrease impulsive and self-harm behaviors. The nurse then discusses with the patient safe, alternative methods to handle feelings. The use of a behavioral contract to decrease

### CASE STUDY

Sherry Morgan, a 27-year-old woman, is brought to the psychiatric inpatient unit from the emergency department. Both wrists were bandaged after suturing. She vacillates between being angry and crying. Sherry states, "I know I am bad. I should not have done it. I do not want to die, but I am tired of the hassles. You wouldn't understand." During the admission interview, the nurse finds that Sherry has had three previous admissions to this inpatient unit during the past 8 years. Sherry states that she refuses to return to work because her boss accuses her of bothering the other employees instead of doing her own work. She states that her boss is falsely accusing her of using alcohol and drugs and does not accept her reasons for being absent from work. On the morning of admission, she called her outpatient therapist, whom she had not seen in a year and a half; he agreed to see her at 3 PM. When she called the therapist back at noon and found that he was at lunch, she used her scissors to cut her wrists. "I used to think he understood me, but now I know he doesn't care." Her parents are on vacation out of state, and her only close friend is busy with a sick child. She had taken some of her mother's Valium, but it did not calm her down. She has averaged only 3 to 4 hours of sleep each night for the past 5 days and has been unable to eat regular meals. Her attempts to clean her parents' house were not completed. She could not even finish watering her mother's plants. A male acquaintance of 2 weeks was no longer calling her, so she was frequenting several bars and inviting men home. She never heard from these men again, even though she thought that their relationships were sexually satisfying.

Sherry completed 2 years of college and is dressed attractively. She enjoys reading romance novels and has brought five of her favorite books.

self-injurious behaviors in inpatient and outpatient settings provides the patient with clear expectations of behavior. Patients need to recognize that they can choose to harm themselves or choose alternative methods to manage feelings and reduce anxiety (Aviram et al, 2004).

Patients can be helped with understanding themselves and their feelings by having them write in a notebook or journal on a daily basis. In sharing the journal with the nurse, the patient gains an understanding of self and a sense of autonomy and responsibility. This technique can be useful for many patients with BPD.

Patients with BPD who are victims of abuse need to talk about their trauma in a safe environment. The nurse should acknowledge their pain and convey empathy and the appropriateness of their

## Care Plan

Name: Sherry Morgan                                     Admission Date: _____

*DSM-IV-TR* Diagnosis: Axis I—major depression; axis II—borderline personality disorder

| | |
|---|---|
| Assessment | **Areas of strength:** Well-groomed, neat and clean, intelligent, enjoys reading. |
| | **Problems:** Self-mutilating behavior, absence of support system, loss of job, decreased sleeping and eating, irresponsible and impulsive sexual behavior. |
| Diagnoses | • High risk for self-mutilation related to absence of support systems, as evidenced by cutting wrists. |
| | • Defensive coping related to low self-esteem, as evidenced by angry and labile emotions. |

Outcomes    *Short-term goals:*                                    Date met
- Patient will eliminate self-mutilating behavior and appropriately      _____
  verbalize feelings of anger and sadness.
- Patient will use alternative methods of coping with emotions.      _____

*Long-term goals:*
- Patient will schedule outpatient appointment and meeting with      _____
  boss regarding job problems.

| | |
|---|---|
| Planning/ Interventions | **Nurse-patient relationship:** Monitor and set limits on acting-out behaviors. Assist patient with identification and verbalization of feelings. Teach healthy coping behaviors. Discuss fears about accepting responsibility for self and decision making. Discuss behaviors interfering with job performance. |
| | **Psychopharmacology:** Prozac 20 mg q AM, Desyrel 50 mg q HS. |
| | **Milieu management:** Groups focusing on self-esteem, stress and anger management, assertiveness training, social skills, problem-solving skills, discharge planning. |
| Evaluation | Patient has not engaged in self-mutilating behavior. Patient is appropriately verbalizing feelings of anger and sadness. Patient has identified and is using two methods of coping with feelings. Patient has crisis plan when overwhelmed by emotions. |
| Referrals | Appointment weekly after discharge with therapist at outpatient mental health clinic. |

feelings. When patients understand that current behaviors are linked to past trauma, they can learn to recognize and then work toward changing dysfunctional actions toward self and others. See Chapter 41 for more detailed interventions.

The patient with BPD is often manipulative. Consistency, limit setting, and supportive confrontation are necessary interventions to provide clear expectations regarding patient behaviors. These patients are adept at sidestepping rules, avoiding consequences, and pitting staff members against each other, all for the sake of getting what they want. Enforcing unit rules, providing clear structure, and placing the responsibility for appropriate behaviors on the patient, although vigorously resisted, will benefit the person with BPD. The need to help the patient develop

realistic short-term goals must be part of the treatment plan if the patient's responsibility for self is to increase.

The psychiatric nurse is in a perfect position to help the patient with BPD with the daily give and take issues of life that create the many problems for this patient. The nurse should work with the patient on appropriate verbal expression of feelings and assertiveness, even though the nurse's ability to be empathetic, nonjudgmental, and therapeutic is sometimes severely tested by the patient's behaviors. The nurse might feel frustrated and ineffective as a caregiver because of the patient's anger and defenses. Hence, offering superficial solutions to problems, pointing out rules, and interacting superficially might be less frustrating and safer. However, understanding and working with the patient therapeutically can result in a positive experience for the nurse and be of lasting import to the patient.

## PSYCHOPHARMACOLOGY

Psychopharmacology is used for specific symptoms for the patient with BPD. The symptoms are divided into three domains: (1) cognitive-perceptual symptoms, (2) affective or emotional dysregulation, and (3) impulsive-behavioral dyscontrol (Lively, 2000; Soloff, 2000). Medications are only part of the treatment plan and will not solve all the patient's problems. Cognitive-perceptual symptoms might include transitory hallucinations, suspiciousness, paranoid thinking, and delusions. Transient psychotic states resulting from overwhelming stress are treated with low-dose typical and atypical antipsychotics for 3 to 12 weeks to decrease symptoms.

Affective or emotional dysregulation might include depression, labile mood, anger, anxiety, hostility, and mistrust. Selective serotonin reuptake inhibitors (SSRIs) are used to reduce anger, anxiety, chronic emptiness, and temper outbursts. Reducing anxiety facilitates thinking and reduces splitting (Gabbard, 2005). Clonazepam might be useful for anxiety management, if needed (Soloff, 2000). Lithium, valproic acid, and carbamazepine can be used for rapid mood swings.

Impulsive-behavioral dyscontrol symptoms might include suicidal threats and attempts, assaultiveness, impulse-aggression, and binge behaviors involving alcohol, drugs, or sex. SSRIs are used to decrease impulsive behaviors.

---

### CRITICAL THINKING QUESTION   3

Staff members on the unit are frustrated and angry with a patient diagnosed with BPD who is attempting to pit members on the various shifts against each other. They are even beginning to be angry with each other for the inconsistencies occurring with this patient's care. What strategies should the head nurse employ to help the staff and ultimately the treatment of the patient?

---

## MILIEU MANAGEMENT

Interventions mentioned in the nurse-patient relationship discussion regarding firm limits, consistency, and clear structure are basic to the milieu for the BPD patient. The patient's manipulation of other patients must be confronted because the BPD patient can mobilize others against the staff. Consistent communication among staff members is essential to minimize the patient's attempts to divide them.

Group sessions that include dialectical behavior therapy (Dubose and Linehan, 2005; McQuillan et al, 2005), assertiveness training, problem solving, stress management, and anger management are some therapeutic activities that are important for these patients in both inpatient and outpatient settings.

Referral to self-help groups for alcohol and drug problems, eating disorders, and victimization is also important. Substance-related disorders are most likely to interfere with the remission of BPD (Zanarini et al, 2004). Vocational counseling and training are important to foster autonomous and independent functioning. Residential treatment might need to be considered, particularly for patients with chronic self-destructive behavior.

## NARCISSISTIC PERSONALITY DISORDER

The patient with narcissistic personality disorder displays grandiosity about his or her importance and achievements. This grandiosity is unlike the delusions of grandeur found in schizophrenia or bipolar disorders. The grandiosity of the narcissistic personality disorder is based somewhat in reality but is distorted, embellished, or convoluted to meet the patient's needs of self-importance. For example, the male patient might say that he was a star football player in high school and that he could have played for the Indianapolis Colts; he does not tell the nurse that he barely made the second-string football team in high school.

The narcissistic patient overvalues himself or herself; needs to be admired; is arrogant, self-centered, and self-absorbed; and seems indifferent to the criticism of others. This person feels superior and has a sense of entitlement, demanding attention, admiration, and special favors (Miller, 2004).

The patient might appear nonchalant or indifferent to criticism while hiding feelings of anger, rage, or emptiness. Constant reinforcement from others is needed to boost the self-image (Bender,

## Family Issues in Borderline Personality Disorder

### Illness

Borderline personality disorder is caused by multiple factors, including neurotransmitter dysfunction, environmental factors, and stress-related events. The individual has problems with handling feelings and emotions, especially anger and rage. Relationships with others are often intense and the person is afraid of being abandoned by others. Impulsive behaviors can be seen in eating and substance-related problems. Moods can rapidly change and the individual is often overwhelmed by strong emotions, resorting to self-injurious and suicidal behaviors. The individual has difficulty integrating the positive and negative characteristics of others as being part of human nature. Direction or goals in life can quickly change because of not really having a sense of who he or she is or what he or she values and wants to pursue.

### Medication

The individual often benefits from antidepressant medication such as an SSRI—for example, Prozac—or other medications in this category. Medication for anxiety and thinking problems is sometimes prescribed. Medication is used temporarily when symptoms occur; it does not cure or change the personality disorder.

### Issues

Threats to harm oneself in the form of suicide and self-injurious behaviors should be taken seriously. Help should be sought that will enable the individual to receive needed treatment. The individual needs caring, support, and help in dealing with feelings and problems.

---

## Highlighting the Evidence: Balanced Therapy: How to Avoid Conflict and Help Borderline Patients

### Description

Dialectical behavior therapy (DBT) is an evidence-based, comprehensive treatment modality that helps patients with borderline personality disorder (BPD) who have problems regulating emotions and who are suicidal. DBT's outpatient model requires patients to meet weekly in individual psychotherapy and skills training groups. Patients consult with their therapist between sessions by telephone to decrease suicide crisis behaviors, increase behavioral skills, and decrease feelings of conflict and alienation or distance from the therapist.

DBT consists of four stages. In stage 1, patients move from severe behavioral dyscontrol to behavioral control to decrease suicidal and other life-threatening behaviors. Stage 2 consists of moving from desperation to emotional experiencing. In stage 3, patients address problems in living and moving toward happiness/unhappiness. In stage 4, patients move from incompleteness to a capacity for joy and freedom.

### Results

In seven randomized control trials, DBT was shown to be useful to patients with BPD. In the initial trial by DuBose and Linehan (2005), subjects were assessed every 4 months while in treatment for 1 year and for 1 year afterward. DBT was effective in reducing suicide attempts and self-injury, decreasing premature dropout from therapy, reducing emergency room admission and length of psychiatric hospitalization, and reducing drug use, depression, hopelessness, and anger.

### Implications

Nurses trained in DBT can offer patients with BPD an evidence-based effective, comprehensive, and compassionate treatment.

Modified from DuBose AP, Linehan MM: Balanced therapy how to avoid conflict, help 'borderline' patients, *Curr Psychiatry* 4:13, 2005.

2005). Relationships with others seem shallow but might be meaningful if the patient's self-esteem is positively enhanced. The patient cannot empathize with others, and the feelings of others are not understood or considered. These individuals use others selfishly to meet their own needs but do not reciprocate. This type of patient has a sense of entitlement and expects special treatment. The patient uses rationalization to blame others, makes excuses, and provides alibis for self-centered behaviors.

## CLINICAL EXAMPLE

The patient has been admitted to the unit and insists on a private room with a telephone and television because he needs to keep up with the reports on the financial news network.

## UNIQUE CAUSES

Studies of biologic and genetic factors in narcissistic personality disorder have not been conducted. Some theorists believe that the self-centered person is arrested in emotional development because the parents fail to mirror that which is appropriate or inappropriate back to the child (Miller, 2004). Consequently, the child develops without any feedback about his or her behaviors.

## PUTTING IT ALL TOGETHER
### Psychotherapeutic Management

### NURSE-PATIENT RELATIONSHIP

If this patient is hospitalized, the nurse must deal with decreasing the constant recitation of self-importance and grandiosity. The nurse must mirror what the patient sounds like, especially if contradictions exist, and help the patient focus on the identification and verbal expression of feelings. Supportive confrontation is used to point out discrepancies between that which the patient says and that which actually exists to increase responsibility for self. Limit setting and consistency in approach are used to decrease manipulation and entitlement behaviors. Realistic short-term goals focused on the here and now are important to decrease the patient's use of fantasy and rationalization and to increase respon-

sibility for self. The patient needs to be taught that everyone has worth, even if he or she makes mistakes and has imperfections. Group therapy provides the opportunity for the patient to see how his or her behavior affects others and, perhaps for the first time, gives the patient a chance to become involved with the problems of others. Caution must be exercised to not give the patient free rein to talk about himself or herself (Miller, 2004).

## HISTRIONIC PERSONALITY DISORDER

The patient with histrionic personality disorder dramatizes events and draws attention to self. This patient is extroverted and thrives on being the center of attention. Behavior is silly, colorful, frivolous, and seductive. Speech is vague, descriptive, superficial, and overembellished but lacking in detail, insight, and depth. The patient seems to be in a hurry and restless. Temper tantrums and outbursts of anger are seen, as well as overreactions to minor events. This patient might use somatic complaints to avoid responsibility and support dependency. Dissociation is a common defense to avoid feelings. Therefore, this patient cannot deal with his or her true feelings. The patient views relationships with others as special or possessing greater intimacy than is real. Recently met individuals are thought of as being dear friends.

## UNIQUE CAUSES

The causes of histrionic personality disorder are unknown but are probably a result of many factors. In the early mother-child relationship, the mother negates the child's inner feelings. The child then turns to his or her father for nurturance, and the father responds to the child's dramatic emotional behaviors (Gunderson, 1988).

## PUTTING IT ALL TOGETHER
### Psychotherapeutic Management

### NURSE-PATIENT RELATIONSHIP

Positive reinforcement in the form of attention, recognition, or praise is given for unselfish or other-centered behaviors. Because the patient needs much reassurance and feels helpless, the nurse must provide support to facilitate independent problem solving and daily functioning. Because the patient is unaware of and does not deal with feelings, the nurse must help clarify the patient's true feelings and help the patient learn appropriate ways to express them. Working with this type of patient can be frustrating for the nurse because the patient needs time to internalize the meaning of what the nurse is trying to accomplish.

## CLUSTER C: ANXIOUS-FEARFUL

## DEPENDENT PERSONALITY DISORDER

The main characteristic of the dependent personality disorder is a "pervasive and excessive need to be taken care of that leads to submissive and clinging behaviors and fears of separation" (APA, 2000). Dependent individuals want others to make daily decisions for them—for example, the type of clothes to wear and the type of job to seek. They need direction and reassurance. These individuals feel inferior and cling to others excessively because they are afraid that they will be left alone. Avoiding responsibility and expressing helplessness, the patient maintains the need to rely on others. They perceive themselves as being unable to function without the help of others.

Dependent individuals also expect that if they perform good deeds for others, they will be rewarded by someone doing something for them. An intimate relationship with a spouse who is abusive, unfaithful, or an alcoholic is tolerated so as not to disturb the sense of attachment. Passivity and concealing of sexual feelings and anger are a means of avoiding conflict.

### CLINICAL EXAMPLE

The patient has been telling the nurse about her alcoholic, abusive husband. She has been married to him for 16 years. She expresses sadness and frustration about her marriage but states, "How could I leave him? What would I do? Who will take care of me? I could never live alone."

## UNIQUE CAUSES

Biochemical and genetic factors have not been correlated with dependent personality disorder. Psychosocial theories consider culture to be the basis of the development of this disorder. Certain cultures dictate that women should maintain a dependent role. Parents or society might believe that the child should not exhibit certain autonomous behaviors and the child, in turn, might believe that disapproval and loss of attachment are consequences of these behaviors.

### PUTTING IT ALL TOGETHER
Psychotherapeutic Management

## NURSE-PATIENT RELATIONSHIP

The nurse slowly works on decision making with the patient to increase responsibility for self in daily living. The patient needs assistance with managing anxiety because it will increase as the patient assumes more responsibility for self. Assertiveness is an important area of the nurse's teaching which enables the patient to clearly state his or her feelings, needs, and desires. Verbalization of feelings and ways to cope with them are essential.

## AVOIDANT PERSONALITY DISORDER

Patients with the avoidant personality disorder are timid, socially uncomfortable, and withdrawn. They feel inadequate and are hypersensitive to criticism. Although they are fearful and shy, patients with avoidant personality disorder desire relationships but need to be certain of being liked before making social contacts (McGlashan et al, 2005). To keep their anxiety at a minimal level, these individuals avoid situations in which they might be disappointed or rejected. When interacting with someone, this person sounds uncertain and lacks self-confidence and also is afraid to ask questions or speak up in public, withdraws from social support, and conveys helplessness.

## NURSE-PATIENT RELATIONSHIP

Few biologic, genetic, and psychological studies have been conducted. Shyness is common in childhood, but increased shyness and avoidant behavior during adolescence might lead to this disorder. The nurse helps the patient gradually confront his or her fears. Discussing the patient's feelings and fears before and after doing something that he or she is afraid to do is an essential part of the relationship. The nurse supports and directs the patient in accomplishing small goals. Helping the patient be assertive and develop social skills is necessary. The nurse includes the patient in interactions with others and then progresses to small groups as the patient is able to tolerate them. Because of the patient's anxiety, relaxation techniques are taught to enable the person to be successful in interactions. The nurse will give positive feedback to the patient for any real success and for any attempts to engage in interactions with others to promote self-esteem.

## OBSESSIVE-COMPULSIVE PERSONALITY DISORDER

Individuals with obsessive-compulsive personality disorder are perfectionistic and inflexible. These patients are overly strict and often set standards for themselves that are too high; thus, their work is never good enough. They are preoccupied with rules, trivial details, and procedures. They find it difficult to express warmth or tender emotions. There is little give and take in their interactions with others, and they are rigid, controlling, and cold. The patient is serious about all of his or her activities, so having fun or experiencing pleasure is difficult. Because the person is afraid of making mistakes, he or she can be indecisive or will put off decisions until all the facts have been obtained. The person's affect is constricted, and he or she might speak in a monotone.

## UNIQUE CAUSES

Early parent-child relationships around issues of autonomy, control, and authority might predispose a person to this disorder. Recent genetic studies have indicated that this disorder and the more severe obsessive-compulsive disorder might be inherited.

## NURSE-PATIENT RELATIONSHIP

The nurse needs to support the patient in exploring his or her feelings and in attempting new experiences and situations. The nurse helps the patient with decision making and encourages follow-through behavior. At times, a need exists to confront the patient's procrastination and intellectualization. The nurse teaches the patient the importance of leisure activities and exploring interests in this area. Because the patient lacks awareness of the way he or she affects others, the patient needs to look at and understand others' view of him or her. Teaching the patient that he or she is human and that it is all right to make mistakes helps decrease irrational beliefs about the necessity to be perfect.

## Study Notes

1. Personality traits are enduring approaches to the world expressed in the way a person thinks, feels, and behaves.
2. When personality traits become rigid, dysfunctional, and cause distress in self and others, they might be diagnosed as a personality disorder. Personal discomfort arises primarily from others' reactions to or behaviors toward that person.
3. The odd-eccentric cluster of personality disorders includes the following:
   a. Paranoid, characterized by suspiciousness and mistrust
   b. Schizoid, characterized by hermit-like lifestyle, aloneness
   c. Schizotypal, characterized by symptoms similar to but less severe than those of schizophrenia
4. The dramatic-erratic cluster of personality disorders includes the following:
   a. Antisocial, characterized by disregard of others' rights without guilt
   b. Borderline, characterized by problems with self-identity, interpersonal relationships,

emotional dysregulation, and self-injurious behaviors

   c. Narcissistic, characterized by overevaluation of self, arrogance, and indifference to the criticism of others

   d. Histrionic, characterized by dramatic behaviors, attention seeking, and superficiality

5. The anxious-fearful cluster of personality disorders includes the following:

   a. Dependent, characterized by submissiveness, helplessness, fear of responsibility, and reliance on others for decision making

   b. Avoidant, characterized by timidity, socially withdrawn behavior, and hypersensitivity to criticism

   c. Obsessive-compulsive, characterized by indecisiveness, perfectionism, inflexibility, and difficulty expressing feelings

6. Nursing interventions for individuals with personality disorders help the patient recognize specific behaviors distressing to self, others, or both; manage feelings; and develop coping behaviors that are less dysfunctional.

## References

American Psychiatric Association: *Diagnostic and statistical manual of mental disorders, text revision,* ed 4, Washington, DC, 2000, APA.

Antai-Otong D: Treatment considerations for the patient with borderline personality disorder, *Nurs Clin North Am* 38:101, 2003.

Aviram RB, Hellerstein DJ, Gerson J, Stanley B: Adapting supportive psychotherapy for individuals with borderline personality disorder who self-injure or attempt suicide, *J Psychiatr Pract* 10:145, 2004.

Bender DS, Dolan RT, Skodol AE, et al: Treatment utilization by patients with personality disorders, *Am J Psychiatry* 158:295, 2001.

Bender DS: The therapeutic alliance in the treatment of personality disorders, *J Psychiatr Pract* 11:73, 2005.

Conklin CZ, Westen D: Borderline personality disorder in clinical practice, *Am J Psychiatry* 162:867, 2005.

DuBose AP, Linehan MM: Balanced therapy how to avoid conflict, help 'borderline' patients, *Curr Psychiatry* 4:13, 2005.

Gabbard GO: Mind, brain, and personality disorders, *Am J Psychiatry* 162:648, 2005.

Grant BF, Hasin DS, Stinson FS, et al: Co-occurrence of 12-month mood and anxiety disorders and personality disorders in the US: results from the national epidemiologic survey on alcohol and related conditions, *J Psychiatr Res* 39:1, 2005.

Grinspoon L: Antisocial personality—part I, *Harv Ment Health Lett* 17:1, 2000a.

Grinspoon L: Antisocial personality—part II, *Harv Ment Health Lett* 17:1, 2000b.

Grinspoon L: Personality disorders—part II, *Harv Ment Health Lett* 16:1, 2000c.

Gurvits IG, Koenigsberg HW, Siever LJ: Neurotransmitter dysfunction in patients with borderline personality disorder, *Psychiatr Clin North Am* 23:27, 2000.

Livesly WJ: A practical approach to the treatment of patients with borderline personality disorder, *Psychiatr Clin North Am* 23:211, 2000.

McGlashan TH, Grilo CM, Sanislow CA, et al: Two-year prevalence and stability of individual DSM-IV criteria for schizotypal, borderline, avoidant, and obsessive-compulsive personality disorders: toward a hybrid model of axis II disorders, *Am J Psychiatry* 162:883, 2005.

McQuillan A, Nicastro R, Guenot F, et al: Intensive dialectical behavior therapy for outpatients with borderline personality disorder who are in crisis, *Psychiatr Serv* 56:193, 2005.

Miller MC: Narcissism and self-esteem, *Harv Ment Health Lett* 20:1, 2004.

Muehlenkamp JJ: Self-injurious behavior as a separate clinical syndrome, *Am J Orthopsychiatry* 75:324, 2005.

NANDA International: *NANDA nursing diagnoses: definitions and classifications, 2005-2006,* Philadelphia, 2005, NANDA International.

Sansone RA, Songer DA, Miller KA: Childhood abuse, mental healthcare utilization, self-harm behavior, and multiple psychiatric diagnoses among patients with and without a borderline diagnosis, *Compr Psychiatry* 46:117, 2005.

Silk KR: Overview of biologic factors, *Psychiatr Clin North Am* 23:61, 2000.

Smith GW, Ruiz-Sancho AR, Gunderson JG: An intensive outpatient program for patients with borderline personality disorder, *Psychiatr Serv* 52:532, 2001.

Soloff PH: Psychopharmacology of borderline personality disorder, *Psychiatr Clin North Am* 23:169, 2000.

Stanley B, Gameroff MJ, Michalsen V, Mann JJ: Are suicide attempters who self-mutilate a unique population? *Am J Psychiatry* 158:427, 2001.

Zanarini MC: Childhood experiences associated with the development of borderline personality disorder, *Psychiatr Clin North Am* 23:89, 2000.

Zanarini MC, Frankenburg FR, Hennen J, et al: Axis 1 comorbidity in patients with borderline personality disorder: 6-year follow-up and prediction of time to remission, *Am J Psychiatry* 161:2108, 2004.

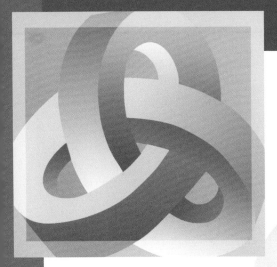

# Chapter 34

# Sexual Disorders

*Carol E. Bostrom*

## Learning Objectives

*After reading this chapter, you should be able to:*

- Recognize the importance of the nurse's role in assessing patients' sexual concerns and problems.
- Describe the categories of sexual dysfunctions, paraphilias, and gender identity disorder.
- Identify the issues related to the care of patients with sexual disorders.
- Demonstrate an understanding of the need for referring patients with sexual disorders for further assessment and treatment.

This chapter presents an overview of sexual disorders and sexual dysfunctions. Normal sexuality and sexual preference issues, such as homosexuality, are not included.

Individuals engage in a wide range of sexual activities, resulting in a wide range of sexual responses. Sexual activity might focus on objects or people; it is unacceptable legally when it involves a nonconsenting individual, a child, or the use of objects in a way that might interfere with healthy relationships. Sexual activity is unacceptable morally when it violates the norms, standards, and values of the culture. Sexual activity should be evaluated according to its effects on the individual and others, such as the level of functioning, self-esteem, and relationships with others.

Considering coercion versus consent between sexual partners is important. An individual's rights and needs should never be violated. Power and control issues affect the definition of consent and the degree of coercion. For example, some clinicians believe that a sexual relationship between a powerful political figure and a young female office worker, although apparently consensual, is actually coercive at its core.

## *DSM-IV-TR* CRITERIA AND TERMINOLOGY

The *Diagnostic and Statistical Manual of Mental Disorders,* Text Revision, Fourth Edition *(DSM-IV-TR,* American Psychiatric Association [APA], 2000) categorizes sexual disorders according to sexual dysfunctions, the paraphilias, and gender identity disorders. Sexual dysfunctions are characterized by the inhibition of sexual appetite or psychophysiologic changes that compromise the sexual response cycle. Paraphilias are characterized by intense sexual urges focused on (1) nonhuman objects, (2) the suffering or humiliation of oneself or one's partner, or (3) children or other nonconsenting individuals. Gender identity disorders are characterized by a discomfort with one's biologic gender or the desire to have the characteristics of the other gender.

**Norm's Notes**

*Well, now we discuss a topic that evokes a kind of morbid curiosity. Sexual disorders come in many varieties, from the inability to participate in healthy sexual activity to behaviors that are illegal, immoral, and sometimes weird. You probably will not run into these individuals during your clinical rotation, but I think you will find this short chapter interesting.*

---

## DSM-IV-TR and NANDA International Diagnoses Related to Sexual Disorders

*DSM-IV*\*
Sexual dysfunction disorders
Paraphilias
Gender identity disorders

NANDA INTERNATIONAL†
Anxiety
Body image, disturbed
Coping, ineffective
Knowledge, deficient
Self-esteem, chronic low
Self-esteem, situational, low
Sexual dysfunction
Sexuality patterns, ineffective
Social interaction, impaired
Spiritual distress

---

\*From the American Psychiatric Association: *Diagnostic and statistical manual of mental disorders, text revision,* ed 4, Washington, DC, 2000, APA.
†From NANDA International: *NANDA nursing diagnoses: definitions and classifications,* 2005-2006, Philadelphia, PA, 2005, NANDA International.

## SEXUAL DYSFUNCTIONS

As part of the admission interview, the nurse assesses each patient for potential or actual problems with sexual functioning. Box 34-1 lists initial questions that the nurse might use to assess the patient's feelings and concerns about sexuality. Potential or actual problems can occur as a result of emotional or physiologic factors, or both. Medications and chemicals can also alter sexual desire and functioning. A thorough assessment or evaluation is necessary for appropriate referral and

---

### Box 34-1    Initial Nursing Assessment of Sexual Concerns

Can you describe any difficulties that you have experienced with sexual performance or satisfaction?

What are your feelings and concerns about sexuality?
How satisfied are you with your sexual relationship?
What type of changes would you like to make in your sexual relationship?
What type of negative sexual experiences have you had?

---

treatment. Treatment is individualized according to the cause or combination of causes. For example, the individual who becomes impotent because of a medical illness or a medication side effect might also have diminished self-esteem and self-confidence that compounds the problem. Therefore, treatment would focus on both the physiologic aspects and emotional needs of the individual.

The phases of human sexual activity have been called the sexual response cycle. There are four phases: the desire phase, the excitement phase, the orgasm phase, and the resolution phase. Sexual dysfunctions are grouped into disorders that compromise one of these phases. Sexual desire disorders effectively stop the sexual response cycle from beginning. Sexual arousal disorders sidetrack the sexual response cycle at the excitement phase. Orgasm disorders arrest the progression of the cycle in the orgasm phase. Finally, sexual pain disorders can abort the sexual response cycle at any phase.

## SEXUAL DESIRE DISORDERS

Individuals with these disorders have little or no sexual desire or have an aversion to sexual contact.

## SEXUAL AROUSAL DISORDERS

Individuals with these disorders cannot maintain the physiologic requirements for sexual intercourse. Women cannot maintain the lubrication-swelling response of sexual excitement, and men cannot maintain an erection.

## ORGASM DISORDERS

Individuals with these disorders cannot complete the sexual response cycle because of the inability to achieve an orgasm. In premature ejaculation, a man reaches orgasm with minimal sexual stimulation, frustrating both himself and his partner.

## SEXUAL PAIN DISORDERS

Individuals with these disorders suffer genital pain (dyspareunia) before, during, or after sexual intercourse. Vaginismus—involuntary spasm of the outer third of the vagina—interferes with sexual intercourse.

---

### CRITICAL THINKING QUESTION   1

A patient with insulin-dependent diabetes states, "After I leave the hospital, I'm going to use only half of the prescribed insulin because I heard insulin might affect my sexual performance." What are your interventions with this patient?

---

## PARAPHILIA

Paraphilia is a condition in which the sexual instinct is expressed in ways that are socially prohibited or unacceptable or are biologically undesirable (APA, 2000).

Individuals with paraphilia might seek inpatient treatment because of a distinct axis I diagnosis that does not reflect a sexual disorder. The nurse on an inpatient unit might encounter individuals admitted with major depression and suicidal ideation who might be trying to avoid criminal prosecution or to be given a lesser sentence by seeking psychiatric treatment. Others might be admitted to inpatient or outpatient care because of axis I disorders and not their paraphilia. Mood disorders, anxiety disorders, and substance disorders might be the reason for seeking treatment. Therefore, the nurse intervenes with behaviors reflective of the axis I diagnosis, rather than specifically addressing the paraphilia.

Individuals with paraphilias do not consider their sexual activities or interests a disorder and do not seek psychiatric treatment for them. Dementia might be associated with the onset of paraphilias, and some professionals consider paraphilias to be part of the obsessive-compulsive spectrum, although the obsessions and compulsions of those with paraphilic disorders consist of pleasurable sexual thoughts and feelings and usually require external intervention to create motivation for change (Krueger and Kaplan, 2001).

Treatment for pedophilia, exhibitionism, and voyeurism generally occurs on an outpatient basis. Information about paraphiliacs comes from individuals who have been arrested and incarcerated, and from their victims. Outpatient treatment programs and programs for incarcerated individuals also provide information about assessment and treatment, with most research being carried out on convicted sex offenders (Cohen and Galynker, 2002).

Paraphiliacs might be men or women, and paraphilic activity might be limited to a period of stress rather than following a chronic or repetitive pattern. Generally, chronic paraphiliacs have a large number of victims. Paraphilias usually begin in adolescence and there is evidence that mood disorders, anxiety and impulse disorders, substance-related disorders, and personality disorders, especially the antisocial and cluster C personality disorders, are frequently comorbid diagnoses. The cause of the paraphilias is unknown. Research studies involving neuropsychological testing, endocrine functioning, brain imaging, and personality characteristics have been conducted. The results are mixed and inconclusive. (See the *DSM-IV-TR* Criteria for Paraphilias box.)

## PEDOPHILIA

Pedophilia involves recurrent intense sexual urges and sexually arousing fantasies involving sexual activity with children. The individual acts on the urges or is distressed by them (APA, 2000). By definition, the victim of pedophilia must be younger than 13 years of age and the pedophile 16 years or older and at least 5 years older than the victim. Pedophilic behavior can be expressed for opposite-sex children, same-sex children, or both. Pedophilia also can be limited to incest. Fondling and oral sex are typical pedophilic behaviors. Vaginal and anal penetration are usually found in incest.

Much controversy exists regarding the personality profiles of sex offenders against minors. Accurately stating the personality characteristics that are present in all sex offenders is impossible. Some of the characteristics reported are shyness, sensitivity, and isolation in social situations; low self-esteem; dependency; depression; low self-confidence; and use of alcohol and drugs. These individuals often have many paraphilias and histories of being abused

## DSM-IV-TR Criteria for Paraphilias

The following paraphilic activities last over a period of 6 months and cause distress or impairment in social, occupational, or other important areas of functioning.

**Exhibitionism**
- Recurrent, intense sexually arousing fantasies, sexual urges, or behaviors involving exposing one's genitals to unsuspecting strangers.

**Fetishism**
- Recurrent, intense sexually arousing fantasies, sexual urges, or behaviors using nonliving objects.

**Frotteurism**
- Recurrent, intense sexually arousing fantasies, sexual urges, or behaviors involving touching and rubbing against a nonconsenting person.

**Pedophilia**
- Recurrent, intense sexually arousing fantasies, sexual urges, or behaviors that involve sexual activity with a child or children generally 13 years of age or younger.
- The person is at least 16 years of age and at least 5 years older than the child or children involved.

**Sexual Masochism**
- Recurrent, intense sexually arousing fantasies, sexual fantasies, urges, or behaviors involving the act of being humiliated, beaten, restrained, or otherwise made to suffer.

**Sexual Sadism**
- Recurrent, intense sexually arousing fantasies, urges, or behaviors involving acts in which the psychological or physical suffering of the victim is sexually exciting to the person.

**Voyeurism**
- Act of observing an unsuspecting person who is naked, in the process of disrobing, or engaging in sexual activity.

Modified from the American Psychiatric Association: *Diagnostic and statistical manual of mental disorders, text revision,* ed 4, Washington, DC, 2000, APA.

## Family Issues in Child Safety

Parents can help keep their children safe by telling them to:

- Not give personal information to or agree to meet someone you met online.
- Not to go near or get inside a stranger's car when someone offers you candy, when someone asks for directions, or when someone asks you to help them find a lost pet.
- Always tell your parents or teacher immediately if someone touches you or asks you to touch them in a way that is confusing, embarrassing, or frightening.

Modified from Miller CM: Pedophilia, *Harv Ment Health Lett* 20:1, 2004.

aggressive; others use aggression in the form of trickery or bribery. The threat of violence might be used to encourage the victim's silence. The use of physical violence might indicate that the offender is a child rapist. The pedophile might seek an occupation that provides easy access to children. Typical occupations are teaching school, working in a day care setting, coaching, or scout leadership. The presence of axis I and axis II disorders in this population is high and, if untreated, plays a role in treatment failure and recidivism of sexual offenders (Raymond et al, 1999). According to Cohen and Galynker (2002), recidivism, dropout, and noncompliance are significant problems in the treatment of pedophilia.

Treatment includes a combination of a variety of cognitive-behavioral methods, antiandrogen medication to lower sexual desires, and selective serotonin reuptake inhibitors (SSRIs). Specialized groups might include victim empathy training, psychoeducation about the illness and medication, coping and social skills training, and relapse prevention (Miller, 2004; Replique, 1999).

## INCEST

Incest is pedophilia with child and adolescent relatives and involves relationships by blood, marriage (step-parents), or live-in partners. Incest is traumatic to children because they are victimized by someone they depend on and trust and are unable to escape their victimization.

and neglected. Witnessing violence in the family is associated with increased risk of abusing others (Wood et al, 1999). To compensate for feelings of powerlessness, the pedophile might need to feel power over the victim through control and domination, and pedophilia provides more control than do relationships with adults (Krueger and Kaplan, 2000; Miller, 2004). Some sex offenders are non-

The characteristics of the perpetrator of incest are as varied as those of the pedophile. Families in which incest occurs might be generally disorganized and exhibit disturbed relationships. Although sex is always involved between the perpetrator and the victim, the perpetrator turns to the child for gratification, intimacy, emotional fulfillment, power, and control. The perpetrator's distorted thinking includes denial of any wrongdoing as well as thinking that he or she is teaching the child about sexuality and giving the child pleasure. Unlike pedophiles, perpetrators of incest do not typically select occupations for access to potential victims because their victims are easily accessible. Treatment is offered to victims and spouses. Some family studies have indicated that victims and spouses do not hate the abuser and do not want others to condemn them (Scheela, 1999).

## EXHIBITIONISM

The primary characteristic of exhibitionism is sexual pleasure derived from exposing one's genitals to an unsuspecting stranger. The stereotypical offender is a young man in a raincoat who flashes women while walking down the street. No other sexual activity is attempted. The exhibitionist is stimulated by the effect of shocking the victim.

## FETISHISM

The primary characteristic of fetishism is the sexual pleasure derived from inanimate objects. Common fetish objects are bras, underpants, stockings, and shoes. Less common fetish objects include urine-soaked and feces-smeared items. The individual with fetishism often masturbates while holding or rubbing these items.

## FROTTEURISM

The primary characteristic of frotteurism is sexual pleasure derived from touching or rubbing one's genitals against a nonconsenting individual's thighs or buttocks. The individual with frotteurism might also attempt to fondle the person's breasts or genitals. Frotteurism usually occurs in a crowded place in which escape into the crowd is possible.

## SEXUAL MASOCHISM

The primary characteristic of sexual masochism is the sexual pleasure derived from being humiliated, beaten, or otherwise made to suffer. Some sexually masochistic individuals enjoy being urinated or defecated on and might pay prostitutes to do so. Hypoxyphilia is the act of enhancing sexual arousal by strangulation or some other oxygen-depleting activity. Apparently, sexual response is heightened by these activities. People have died in their search for enhanced orgasms.

## SEXUAL SADISM

The primary characteristic of sexual sadism is sexual pleasure derived from inflicting psychological or physical suffering on another. Partners can be consenting or masochistic. Sadistic behaviors include spanking, whipping, pinching, beating, burning, and restraining. Some sadistic individuals derive great pleasure from torturing or even killing their victims and might be sadistic rapists. The so-called snuff films, found in the underground of the pornography world, apparently show the actual rape, torture, and murder of women and children for the convenient viewing of sadistic individuals.

## VOYEURISM

The primary characteristic of voyeurism is sexual pleasure derived from observing unsuspecting people who are naked or undressing or who are engaged in sexual activity. The voyeur is commonly referred to as a *peeping Tom*. The voyeur might masturbate during peeping or after returning home.

## GENDER IDENTITY DISORDER

Gender identity disorder in adults involves discomfort with one's gender or the role of that gender. In adults, this disorder can include the desire to live as the other gender or can involve feelings and reactions of the other gender (APA, 2000). See the *DSM-IV-TR* Criteria for Gender Identity Disorder box. Another characteristic is a preoccupation with getting rid of primary and secondary sexual characteristics. These individuals believe that they were born as the wrong gender, experience unhappiness with their own biologic gender, and might desire hormones and surgery to become the opposite gender.

Sexual reassignment surgery is not undertaken immediately on request. The individual must be thoroughly assessed for the presence of other psychiatric disorders that might involve problems with gender identity. The individual desiring sexual reassignment is generally in psychotherapy for 6 to 12 months. Counseling should help the individual clarify issues surrounding their problems and desires. Emotional, medical, surgical, financial, and legal issues are explored, along with the risks involved. Sexual reassignment surgery is not the answer for everyone with gender dissatisfaction (Fee et al, 2003). Some gender identity programs require a written second opinion from another physician or psychologist before proceeding with surgical reassignment. Hormonal treatment and living and relationship changes are slowly made over months while the individual is in therapy. During this time, the individual's attitudes toward sexual reassignment might change and sexual reassignment surgery might not be chosen. People who do choose surgery can be helped to live more comfortable and productive lives.

---

### DSM-IV-TR Criteria for Gender Identity Disorder

A. A strong and persistent cross-gender identification
  1. In children:
     a. Stated desire or insistence that he or she is the other sex
     b. In boys, dressing in female attire; in girls, wearing only masculine clothing
     c. Make believe play or fantasies of being the other sex
     d. Desire to participate in games and pastimes of the other sex
     e. Prefers playmates of the other sex
  2. In adolescents and adults:
     a. Stated desire to be the other sex
     b. Frequently passes as the other sex
     c. Desires to be treated as the other sex
     d. Conviction that he or she has typical feelings and reactions of the other sex
B. Feelings of discomfort with own sex or inappropriateness in gender role of own sex

Modified from the American Psychiatric Association: *Diagnostic and statistical manual of mental disorders, text revision,* ed 4, Washington, DC, 2000, APA.

---

## NURSE-PATIENT RELATIONSHIP

The nurse must have an accepting, empathic, and nonjudgmental attitude if patients are to be comfortable enough to disclose problems with sexuality. This trust comes about only after the nurse has reconciled and accepted his or her own feelings related to sexuality. Patients might interpret the nurse's discomfort with sexual issues and sexuality as disapproval of them and of their sexual issues and concerns. A private area in which to discuss fears or concerns about sexuality and victimization helps patients disclose and discuss their feelings. The nurse discusses options for dealing with sexual issues and problems. Clarification and education might be needed about sexual functioning, effective communication, and healthy relationships. The nurse might also need to intervene with self-esteem issues, anxiety, and guilt.

Helping patients who are perpetrators deal with physical and emotional dimensions is necessary. Physical dimensions might include anorexia, insomnia, and weight loss. Emotional dimensions might include guilt, helplessness, shame, and relief about getting caught. Setting limits on how much information the patient discloses in a group setting, especially if other group members might be victims of sexual assault, must be discussed.

The nurse is involved in the planning of patients' care regarding the specific issues and problems that are addressed during an inpatient stay versus those addressed in outpatient treatment. The nurse also collaborates with social workers and chaplains, if patients so choose, about feelings and religious views. The nurse is legally obligated to report suspected and actual sexual abuse of children to police or appropriate agencies. All states have mandatory child abuse reporting statutes. The nurse discusses possible referrals with patients and family members and refers patients to sex therapists, if necessary. Referrals to outpatient treatment programs or therapy groups for specific disorders might be necessary. Individual, group, and family treatment for incest and support groups for perpetrators and victims might be appropriate.

What approaches would the nurse use while working with patients with sexual problems?

## PSYCHOPHARMACOLOGY

Patients with axis I diagnoses are prescribed psychotherapeutic medication for their specific disorders. The nurse assesses all medications for side effects that affect sexual performance or dysfunction.

Men with paraphilias can be treated with agents to lower testosterone levels, thereby reducing their sex drive. Antiandrogen medications have been proven to suppress pedophilic urges by diminishing sexual desire and fantasy. They can be taken orally or by intramuscular injection for slow release over several months. Medroxyprogesterone (Provera) and leuprolide acetate (LPA, Lupron) inhibit the release of the luteinizing hormone by the pituitary gland, which decreases the production of testosterone by the testes (Miller, 2004). Luteinizing hormone-releasing hormone (LH-RH) agonists inhibit the production of testosterone or produce a pharmacologic castration and reduce sexual drive (Briken, 2002). This medication might become another option in the treatment of paraphilias. In addition to antiandrogens, SSRIs are being used for paraphilias and related disorders (Miller, 2004).

## MILIEU MANAGEMENT

Patients with sexual disorders and dysfunctions benefit from groups dealing with self-esteem, assertiveness, anger management, social and relationship skills, sex education, and stress management. Referrals might be indicated as mentioned previously. Self-help groups such as Sex Addicts Anonymous can benefit some individuals. A multidimensional treatment plan using a combination of education and cognitive-behavioral and family intervention needs to be used to reduce recidivism for sexual offenders. Longitudinal research studies will eventually help determine treatment plans that are effective in reducing recidivism rates.

### CASE STUDY

Bill Wood, 62 years old, has been admitted to the inpatient unit. His wife died 2 years earlier; he has one daughter and three grandchildren. Bill is presently employed but has few friends or hobbies. He visits his daughter and grandchildren approximately once a month. He does not date and does not have any female companions. For the past year, he has noticed an increase in sexual fantasies concerning children. He did not act on the fantasies until a week ago when he was babysitting for his youngest grandchild, 8-year-old Stephanie. He admits to fondling Stephanie's breasts but denies other sexual contact with her. Bill states to the nurse, "I never thought I could be capable of such a horrible thing. I deserve to die. I even thought of killing myself."

### ▇ Study Notes

1. Sexual dysfunctions might occur as the result of psychological, physiologic, and pharmacologic factors.
2. Paraphilias involve sexual activity with objects, children, and consenting or nonconsenting adults that are socially prohibited, unacceptable, or biologically undesirable.

### Highlighting the Evidence: Cognitive-Behavioral Therapies

Various cognitive-behavioral techniques are used to help decrease and/or control sexual urges. These are nonpharmacologic strategies that appear to be the most effective to date.

*Imaginal desensitization:* Sexual situations are described in detail and the individual uses relaxation techniques to tolerate discomfort and to suppress sexual urges.

*Covert sensitization:* The individual verbalizes and associates negative consequences such as imprisonment for their behavior.

*Cognitive restructuring:* The individual's irrational beliefs and rationalizations about their behavior are challenged by group members or therapist.

*Victim empathy training:* Becoming sensitive to victims' feelings is accomplished by watching videotapes of victims' experiences or listening to tapes of victims' experiences.

*Aversive stimulation:* Olfactory aversions, the pairing of noxious odors with the individual's deviant fantasy, interrupts the fantasy and suppresses behavior.

Modified from Krueger RB, Kaplan MS: Behavioral and psychopharmacological treatment of the paraphilic and hypersexual disorders, *J Psychiatr Pract* 8:21, 2002; and Miller MC: Pedophilia, *Harv Ment Health Lett* 20:1, 2004.

## Care Plan

Name: Bill Wood                                          Admission Date: _____

*DSM-IV-TR* Diagnosis: Major depression and pedophilia

| | |
|---|---|
| Assessment | **Areas of strength:** Employed, visits daughter and grandchildren, remorse for contact with child, first offense. |
| | **Problems:** Death of wife, few friends, disturbing sexual fantasies, suicidal ideation. |
| Diagnoses | • Potential for self-directed violence related to guilt, as evidenced by suicidal ideation. |
| | • Sexual dysfunction related to lack of significant other, as evidenced by fondling child. |
| | • Social isolation related to lack of social support, as evidenced by loneliness. |

Outcomes     *Short-term goals:*                                          *Date met*
- Patient will state that he no longer has thoughts of suicide.           _____
- Patient will discuss sexual concerns and needs, and methods            _____
  to satisfy these needs.

*Long-term goals:*
- Patient will contact support groups and senior citizen                 _____
  organizations.
- Patient will attend outpatient appointment, for further assessment     _____
  and treatment of sexual disorder.

| | |
|---|---|
| Planning/ Interventions | **Nurse-patient relationship:** Instruct patient to approach staff when suicidal thoughts occur. Discuss feelings of guilt, remorse, anger, loneliness, and low self-esteem. Discuss the patient's beliefs and values about sexuality with him. Discuss and help the patient to identify sexual concerns, needs, and methods to satisfy needs. |
| | **Psychopharmacology:** Prozac 20 mg q AM. |
| | **Milieu management:** Groups focusing on self-esteem, stress and anger management, assertiveness training, social skills, and discharge planning. |
| Evaluation | Patient reports that he is no longer suicidal. |
| Referrals | He will attend senior citizen activities at his church with a friend. Appointment scheduled at a sexual disorders clinic. |

---

3. Efforts to achieve sexual pleasure do not give individuals the right to violate the rights of others through coercion and control.
4. Currently, cognitive-behavioral techniques and the use of antiandrogen medications are effective treatments for paraphilias.
5. Gender identity disorder in adults involves persistent discomfort with one's biologic gender.
6. The nurse's role in the treatment of sexual disorders is primarily one of referral.

### ▮ References

American Psychiatric Association: *Diagnostic and statistical manual of mental disorders, text revision,* ed 4, Washington, DC, 2000, APA.

Briken P: Pharmacotherapy of paraphilias with luteinizing hormone-releasing hormone agonists, *Arch Gen Psychiatry* 59:469, 2002.

Cohen LJ, Galynker II: Clinical features of pedophilia and implications for treatment, *J Psychiatr Pract* 8:276, 2002.

Fee E, Brown TM, Laylor J: One size does not fit all in the transgender community, *Am J Public Health* 93:899, 2003.

Krueger RB, Kaplan MS: Behavioral and psychopharmacological treatment of the paraphilic and hypersexual disorders, *J Psychiatr Pract* 8:21, 2002.

Krueger RB, Kaplan MS: The paraphilic and hypersexual disorders: an overview, *J Psychiatr Pract* 7:391, 2001.

Miller MC: Pedophilia, *Harv Ment Health Lett* 20:1, 2004.

Raymond NC, Coleman E, Ohlerking F, et al: Psychiatric comorbidity in pedophilic sex offenders, *Am J Psychiatry* 156:786, 1999.

Replique RJ: Assessment and treatment of persons with pedophilia, *J Psychosoc Nurs Ment Health Serv* 37:19, 1999.

Scheela RA: A nurse's experiences, working with sex offenders, *J Psychosoc Nurs Ment Health Serv* 37:25, 1999.

Wood RM, Grossman LS, Kulkarni R, et al: Sexual offenders in custody for control, care and treatment, *Curr Opin Psychiatry* 12:659, 1999.

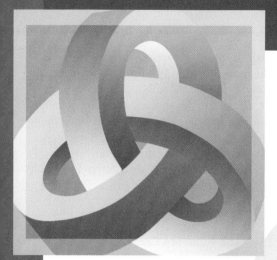

# Chapter 35

# Substance-Related Disorders

*Norman L. Keltner and Gordon I. Pugh\**

## Learning Objectives

*After reading this chapter, you should be able to:*
- Recognize the personal and societal toll of the abuse of alcohol and other drugs.
- Recognize the *Diagnostic and Statistical Manual of Mental Disorders,* Text Revision, Fourth Edition *(DSM-IV-TR)* criteria and terminology for substance-related disorders.
- Recognize and describe objective and subjective symptoms of substance dependence and abuse.
- Describe physiologic, emotional, and interpersonal theoretical explanations for the development of substance-related disorders.
- Develop a nursing care plan for patients with substance-related disorders.
- Evaluate the relative effectiveness of nursing interventions for patients with substance-related disorders.
- Understand the contributions of nonmedical interventions in recovery from substance-related disorders.
- Understand the impact of substance-related disorders on the family.

*Meth cases make mountain of trouble.*
                    *Birmingham News, 2005*

## INTRODUCTION

Drug abuse statistics vary from time to time and from culture to culture. Because of the enormity of these numbers, most people find it difficult to grasp the extent of societal and individual suffering produced by substance abuse and dependence. As Joseph Stalin noted, "A single death is a tragedy; a million deaths is a statistic." Collectively, the statistics of substance-related disorders produce many costs, but even one person's pain is tragic. The stories about real patients in this chapter represent the many individuals who make up these statistics. The effects of their drug and alcohol abuse ripple through our society, touching everyone to some degree.

Humans have used mood-altering substances since at least the beginning of recorded history. Whether using Far Eastern opium, South American cocaine, North American peyote, French wine, or modern pharmaceuticals, humans consistently find ways to alter their mood. Use of mind-altering substances can lead to various complications and problems. Often, however, mind-altering drugs provide therapeutic benefit (e.g., pain relief, decreased anxiety), clouding the

*This chapter is a revision of the text originally written by MaryLou Scavnicky-Mylant and revised by Virginia M. Spaulding.

distinction between therapeutic and abusive use. This chapter concentrates on maladaptive uses of alcohol and other drugs, both legal and illegal, commonly referred to as *drug abuse*. Table 35-1 outlines the extent of drug use in a given month.

As a nurse, you will see patients suffering from the consequences of substance abuse as part of your work. You probably know people personally who suffer from substance-related disorders and who have experienced problems associated with substance abuse; you might suspect that other people suffer from it as well. Your ability to recognize the possibility and to suggest appropriate referrals or interventions might save a home, a family, or a life. Furthermore, as a nurse, friends and acquaintances might turn to you first when they realize that their use has become problematic. Hence, we hope that you take the time to study this information carefully and diligently. The road to recovery begins with the initial assessment.

### Norm's Notes

This is a big problem in the United States and it does not seem to be getting any better. Whenever you hear or read about someone shot dead in a car somewhere, or three young men gunned down in a low-rent motel, or a mom abandoning her kids, it is probably related to drugs. Yes, this is a big problem in our country.

| Table 35-1 | The Numbers Game |
| --- | --- |
| **Substance** | **Current Users** |
| Heroin | 123,000 |
| Cocaine/crack | 1,465,000 |
| Marijuana | ~10,000,000 |
| Alcohol | 109,000,000 |
| Nicotine | 66,500,000 |
| Caffeine | 130,000,000 |

Modified from Nash JM: Addicted: why do people get hooked? *Time* May 5:68, 1997; and Substance Abuse and Mental Health Administration: http://www.oas.samhs.gov/NSduh.htm. Accessed on March 15, 2006.

### 12-Month Prevalence Rate of Mental Disorders in the United States*

| Disorders | Approximate Percentage Over 17 Years of Age | Approximate Number of Persons | Gender Overrepresentation |
| --- | --- | --- | --- |
| **Anxiety Disorders** | 18 overall | 36,000,000 | |
| Panic disorder | 3.5 | 7,000,000 | Women |
| Social phobia | 7 | 14,000,000 | Women |
| Specific phobia | 8.7 | 17,000,000 | Women |
| GAD | 3 | 6,000,000 | Women |
| PTSD | 3.5 | 7,000,000 | Women |
| OCD | 1 | 2,000,000 | Equal |
| **Mood Disorders** | 9.5 overall | 19,000,000 | |
| Major depression | 6.7 | | Women |
| Dysthymia | 1.5 | | Women |
| Bipolar I and II | 2.6 | | BD I: Equal BD II: Women? |
| **Impulse Control Disorders** | 9 overall | 18,000,000 | |
| Conduct disorders | 1 | 2,000,000 | Men |
| ADHD | 4 | 8,000,000 | Men |
| **Substance Abuse Disorders** | 3.8 overall | 7,600,000 | |
| Alcohol abuse and dependence | 3.1 | 6,200,000 | Men |
| Drug abuse and dependence | 1.4 | 2,800,000 | Men |
| **Schizophrenia** | 1.1 | 2,100,000 | Equal |

*Extrapolated from several sources based on current census data.
*ADHD,* Attention-deficit/hyperactivity disorder; *GAD,* generalized anxiety disorder; *OCD,* obsessive-compulsive disorder; *PTSD,* posttraumatic stress disorder.
From Kessler RC, Chiu WT, Demler O, Walters EE: Prevalence, severity, and comorbidity of 12-month DSM-IV disorders in the national comorbidity survey replication, *Arch Gen Psychiatry* 62:617, 2005; U.S. Surgeon General: *Mental health: a report from the Surgeon General,* Washington, DC, 1999, Department of Health and Human Services: National Institute of Mental Health: *Statistics.* Available at: www.nimh.nih.gov/healthinformation/statisticsmenu.cfm. Accessed April 18, 2005.

## CLINICAL EXAMPLE

Robert had an average childhood and made good grades in school. He grew up in a home with both parents and with other siblings. His parents were active in the community. In high school, he was particularly talented in sports and was popular among his peers. Robert was, and is, an immensely likable fellow. He began drinking beer when he was 15 years of age with his baseball teammates. After graduation from high school with honors, he went to college on a baseball scholarship. In college, he was known to smoke some marijuana, but "never let it get in the way" of his sports or his studies. He was good at hiding his drug use. It would never have occurred to him that he "had a problem," not even later when his self-destruction was blatantly apparent to everyone else in his life, except himself. Robert has since learned, however, that he suffers from addiction and has learned how to manage his condition.

At first, he stayed out a little too late one night before a big game, and he had a bad game or two because of his slightly decreased performance. Eventually, he was introduced to cocaine, discovered intravenous (IV) use (mainlining), lost his promising sports career, was divorced by his wife, stole from people, lied to his family, tried to kill himself, and spent time in prison. While he was incarcerated, he realized how self-destructive his drug use had become, and he vowed to do whatever it would take to become and remain drug-free. He reasoned that he had been willing to do a great many things in his search for dope, so he ought to be willing to exert the same amount of energy in his search to break free from its grip on his life. Robert had been hospitalized for detoxification in the past but "wasn't ready." When he attended a small treatment group at the county jail, however, he was ready to listen and learn.

Today, Robert is in his early 30s, has earned his bachelor's degree, has a good job, makes a good salary, is no longer on parole, plays ball with a local community league, is married to a wonderfully supportive spouse, and—most importantly—remains drug-free. Robert's life did not get back together overnight, however. Undoing most of the damage that his drug use caused took several years. Some of the damage he caused can never be repaired, but he is far better off now than he was before he recognized the extent of the problems caused by his drug use.

## ASSESSMENT STRATEGIES FOR CHEMICAL DEPENDENCY

As a component of every assessment, the nurse should inquire about the amount and type of alcohol and other drugs (AOD) used by the patient or the family. The nurse should always ask about the amount of prescription medication the patient actually takes (not simply the amount prescribed, because many people abuse prescription medications as well). The nurse should also question the patient about medical problems associated with AOD use by the patient or family members. Furthermore, because many substance abusers tend to minimize their level of AOD use (as well as the consequences of their use), many facilities routinely use blood or urine drug screens to obtain objective information (Schiller et al, 2000). The importance of this objective data lies in its prevention of AOD minimization. Probably 40% to 60% of AOD users underreport use during their initial interview. Many addicted patients will not readily reveal in an initial interview more than what the nurse can already discover by other means. For example, someone referred to treatment because alcohol use has led to problems with the legal system often does not admit to cocaine or marijuana use until objective testing reveals it. Even then, some patients deny use of the substance detected. Signs and symptoms raising the index of suspicion of a substance-related disorder might include the following:

- Absenteeism, especially after days off
- Frequent accidents or injuries
- Drowsiness
- Slurred speech
- Inattention to appearance
- Increasing isolation
- Frequent secretive disappearances
- Tremors
- Flushed face
- Watery or reddened eyes
- Appearing spaced out
- Odor of alcohol on the breath or strong mouthwash or breath mint smell
- High number of physical complaints

- Disappearing prescriptions (raiding the medicine cabinet)

Denial occurs when the dependent person does not recognize the destructive nature of AOD use, although blatantly obvious to others. Denial prevents the individual from linking his or her problems with AOD use. This inability to see self-destructive behavior and attitudes, or to link life problems with AOD use, defines substance dependence.

Urinalysis often provides the most objective measure of recent drug use (Table 35-2). Blood levels can also detect recent use and trigger treatment protocols. Hair toxicology effectively determines long-term patterns of use but costs more than other methods of detection. Hair samples of Henri Paul, the driver of the car in which Diana, Princess of Wales, died in 1997, were tested in an attempt to find objective evidence about his actual long-term AOD use (Sancton, 1997). Hair toxicology kits available on the retail market enable parents to test the hair of children they suspect of drug abuse. However, blonde hair does not seem to accumulate certain drugs such as cocaine as much as darker hair (Muha, 1997).

| Table 35-2 | Period of Time After Ingestion That Drugs Can Be Detected in the Urine and Blood | | |
|---|---|---|---|
| **Drug** | **Urine** | | **Blood** |
| **Opioids** | | | |
| Heroin | 1-2 days | | 3 days |
| Morphine | 1-2 days | | 3 days |
| Meperidine (Demerol) | 1 day | | 2 days |
| Methadone | 1-7 days | | 1-7 days |
| **Depressants** | | | |
| Barbiturates | 1-7 days | | 7 days |
| Benzodiazepines (Xanax) | 24-36 hours | | 7 days |
| **Stimulants** | | | |
| Amphetamines | 4 hours | | 3 days |
| Cocaine | 2-3 days | | 2-3 days |
| Methamphetamine | 1 day | | 7 days |
| **Hallucinogens** | | | |
| Marijuana | 7-30 days | | Up to 15 weeks |
| LSD | 2-3 days | | 3 days |
| Phencyclidine (PCP) | 7 days | | 7 days |

Modified from Colyar MR: Testing for drugs of abuse. *Adv Nurse Pract* 9:30-31, 2003.

## INTERVIEW APPROACHES

Because underreporting can lead to misdiagnosis, it is important for the nurse to approach the patient in a manner that encourages forthrightness. The nurse should be matter of fact and nonjudgmental while eliciting information that might carry with it some feelings of shame. Most nurses are not prepared for the defensiveness that the person with substance-related problems displays, but some genuine concern for the patient can help overcome this barrier. Furthermore, because drugs and alcohol have personally affected many nurses, it is important for them to be aware of their own feelings and avoid projecting any negative attitudes onto the patient.

Gathering accurate information during the interview claims high priority. As a nurse, you might find it difficult to elicit accurate clinical information from a person such as the woman in Box 35-1. Phrases such as "problem with drinking" or "difficulties with drug use" might be more palatable compared with the labels *addict* or *alcoholic,* but these, too, might not elicit the accurate information sought by the nurse. It might also be helpful initially to focus more on legally or culturally accepted substances such as caffeine and nicotine. The patient's consumption should be evaluated in more detail if the initial assessment data identify the patient as being at higher risk for substance-related problems. We suggest using the terms *problems because of drinking* or *using more than intended* as more accurate and diagnostic, less threatening, and more likely to link patients' AOD use with the problems in their lives. This factor is important both in effective care planning and in providing the patient with positive internal motivation.

Various assessment guides are available to the nurse, including both subjective interview and objective assessment instruments. Early diag-

| Box 35-1 | Defense Mechanisms at Work: Denial |
|---|---|

An intoxicated 60-year-old Madison, Wisconsin, woman, who was dressed as a clown on her way to entertain children at a birthday party, tried to kill her 83-year-old mother-in-law over a beer. "I've had 40 years of hell because of you," she is reported to have told the victim. When asked about her long-standing alcohol problem, she indicated that she has no "problem," except for the mother-in-law.

Modified from *Whad'ya know?* Wisconsin Public Radio, June 4, 1994. The story is from *USA Today,* p 10A, June 3, 1994.

nosis of substance-related disorders is often missed because of misdiagnosing or underdiagnosing related to misunderstandings about AOD disorders or inadequate training or both. Selected instruments are discussed later in this chapter.

Substance abuse is widespread in North America and demands the attention of psychiatric nurses, both as a singular phenomenon and as a variable in other psychiatric disorders. For example, it has been estimated that a third to half of all patients undergoing psychiatric treatment abuse alcohol or drugs or both (U.S. Surgeon General, 1999). Comorbidity or a dual diagnosis is such an important issue that a separate chapter addresses the subject (Chapter 36).

The use and abuse of alcohol and drugs among the general population is one of the most significant social issues of our time. Because of the significance of the problem, this chapter addresses the general issues surrounding substance abuse. To treat the substance-abusing person's condition effectively, the nurse must understand three areas important to effective intervention:

1. The *DSM-IV-TR* criteria used to assess substance-related disorders
2. The nature of the substance being abused
3. The treatment of patients with substance-related disorders

Drugs of abuse fall into several classes: alcohol, barbiturates and other central nervous system (CNS) depressants, opioids, stimulants, and hallucinogens (Table 35-3).

## DSM-IV-TR CRITERIA

The *DSM-IV-TR* specifies criteria for classifications of substance dependence, substance abuse, substance intoxication, and substance withdrawal. Dependence is often marked by physiologic need for the substance, usually in increasing amounts, to gain the same effect; a persistent desire to cut down, which is met with little success; and continued substance use, even though physical, social, and emotional processes are compromised. Regardless of the substance, behavior patterns that meet these criteria indicate a problem. The term *dependence* has generally replaced the term *addiction* for describing compulsive drug use because it more precisely defines the condition. Heroin addiction and alcoholism

are therefore correctly referred to as *drug dependencies.*

### DSM-IV-TR Criteria for Substance-Related Disorders

**Substance Dependence**
A. A maladaptive pattern of substance use as manifested by three or more of the following:
  1. Tolerance
  2. Withdrawal
  3. A need for more of the substance than was intended
  4. Inability to stop using even when wanting to do so
  5. A great deal of time is spent in acquiring the substance or in recovering from its effects
  6. Substance use causes social, occupational, or recreational problems
  7. Continued substance use despite knowledge that the substance is causing physical or psychological problems

**Substance Abuse**
A. A maladaptive pattern of substance use leading to clinically significant impairment or distress as manifested by one or more of the following:
  1. Failure to fulfill major role obligations at work, school, or home
  2. Recurrent substance use in hazardous situations
  3. Recurrent substance-related legal problems
  4. Continued substance use despite problems
B. Has never met the criteria for substance dependence for this class of substance

**Substance Intoxication**
A. The development of a substance-specific syndrome due to a recent ingestion of a substance
B. Clinically significant maladaptive behavioral or psychological changes due to the effect of the substance on the central nervous system
C. Not due to a general medical condition and not better accounted for by another mental disorder

**Substance Withdrawal**
A. The development of a substance-specific syndrome due to the cessation of or reduction in the intake of a substance
B. The substance-specific syndrome causes clinically significant distress or impairment
C. Not due to a general medical condition and not better accounted for by another mental disorder

Modified from the American Psychiatric Association: *Diagnostic and statistical manual of mental disorders, text revision,* ed 4, Washington, DC, 2000, APA.

## Table 35-3  Drug Information

| Class | Examples or Other Names | Withdrawal Syndrome | Withdrawal Treatment | Psychiatric Symptoms During Chronic Use | Overdose Fatal? | Unassisted Withdrawal Fatal? | Overdose Symptoms |
|---|---|---|---|---|---|---|---|
| CNS depressants | Benzodiazepines Barbiturates Other depressants | Tremors, sweats, seizures, anxiety, irritability, hallucinations, death* | Long-acting benzodiazepine, Vistaril | Mood disorder, depression, psychosis, dementia | Yes* | Yes* | Shallow respirations, clammy skin, dilated pupils, weak and rapid pulse, coma, death |
| Opioids | Demerol, heroin, morphine, opium, codeine, Oxycontin | Lacrimations, runny nose, diaphoresis, chills, muscle aches, n/v, diarrhea, leg spasm, goose bumps | Clonidine, supportive medications | Psychosis, mood disorder | Yes | No | Respiratory depression, pulmonary edema, pinpoint pupils, seizures, coma, death |
| Cannabinoids | Marijuana, hash | Craving, irritability | | Psychosis, paranoia | No | No | Hallucinations, paranoia, insomnia, hyperactive |
| Cocaine | Crack, coke, snow | Anhedonia, craving, irritability, fatigue, mood disorder, anxiety | Dopamine agonists, catecholamine precursors | Psychosis | Yes | No | Delirium, psychosis, violence, tachycardia, hypertension, coma, hyperreflexia, myocardial infarction |
| Methamphetamine | Oral: speed, meth Smokable: ice, crystal, crank | Dsyphoria, fatigue, insomnia | Supportive | Psychosis, mood disorder, anxiety disorder | Yes | No | Delirium, psychosis, violence, tachycardia, hypertension, coma, hyperreflexia |
| Inhalants | Gasoline, Freon, paint, and others | Mouth ulcers, gastrointestinal problems, anorexia, confusion, headache | Supportive | Psychosis, panic, memory loss | Yes | No | Seizures, coma |
| Hallucinogens | LSD, psilocybin, PCP | None specific | Supportive | Psychosis, panic | No | No | Seizures, panic, depression |

*CNS*, Central nervous system; *LSD*, lysergic acid diethylamide; *n/v*, nausea and vomiting; *PCP*, phencyclidine.
*For barbiturates.

In 1987, the American Medical Association declared all drug dependencies to be diseases. When chemical dependencies are viewed as diseases, their treatment and understanding are facilitated. This view also reduces the guilt and blame traditionally associated with chemical dependency. Although not all psychiatrists and psychiatric nurses embrace the disease concept of drug dependence, there are convincing arguments for accepting it.

Some professionals use a working definition of chemical dependency that is less rigid compared with the criteria outlined in the *DSM-IV-TR*. These researchers have defined the use of substances as a problem when the effects of such use interfere with and disrupt family, work, and/or social relationships. If these areas of a person's life are being adversely affected, then the person is viewed as having a problem and as being in need of treatment. Still other professionals have simply defined dependence as a state in which "the person feels normal only when the drug is on board."

## ALCOHOL

*Husband Dies After Sherry Enema*
*Lake Jackson, Texas. A woman has been indicted on negligent homicide charges for allegedly giving her husband a sherry enema that killed him. Michael Warner, 58, died last May after the enema caused his blood alcohol level to rise to 0.47 percent. Tammy Warner, 42, was indicted last week. Police said Michael Warner was an alcoholic who could not swallow liquor because of ulcers and heartburn.*
*Birmingham News, 2005*

Alcohol abuse is the primary drug problem in North America and is addressed separately because of the enormity of the problem it poses. The cost to the United States in terms of health problems, lost work hours, family disruption and disintegration, and criminal activity (Box 35-2) has been estimated at more than $185 billion annually (Gordis, 2000). An estimated 4.8% of the adult population in America exhibits symptoms of alcoholism and, along with cardiovascular disease and cancer, it ranks as one of the leading causes of death and disability in the United States (Kessler et al, 2005). Alcoholics have a premature death rate two to four times higher than nonalcoholics. Approximately 100,000 deaths each year are directly related to alcohol. Cirrhosis, other medical problems, homicides (50% alcohol-related),

> **Box 35-2    Alcohol and Crime**
>
> The statistics are striking. Approximately 60% of convicted homicide offenders drank just before committing the offense. Sixty percent of prison inmates drank heavily just before committing the violent crime for which they were incarcerated. The relationship between poverty and homicide is stronger in neighborhoods with higher rates of alcohol consumption than in those with average or below-average rates. Numerous studies have reported a strong association between sexual violence and alcohol, finding that "anywhere between 30% and 90% of convicted rapists are drunk at the time of the offense." Juveniles, especially young men, who drink to the point of drunkenness are more likely than those who do not drink to get into fights, get arrested, commit violent crimes, and recidivate later in life. Alcohol-dependent male factory workers are more than three times as likely to abuse their wives physically than their otherwise comparable non–alcohol-dependent counterparts. The high incidence of drinking among convicted criminals does not necessarily prove that drinking stimulates crime; it might be more accurate to say that criminals who drink are more likely to get caught and convicted than those who do not. However, it is important not to discount or deny the probable, and in some cases patently obvious, connection between alcohol abuse and crime.
>
> From Dilulio JJ Jr: Broken bottles: alcohol, disorder, and crime, *Brookings Review* 14:14, 1996.

and suicides (25% alcohol-related) are directly linked to alcohol use. Accidental deaths such as those from motor vehicle accidents (50% alcohol-related), fires and burns (47% alcohol-related), drownings (34% alcohol-related), and falls (28% alcohol-related) are further examples of the different ways in which alcohol use is lethal (Cherpitel, 1992). In motor vehicle accidents in which pedestrians are killed, 40% of the pedestrians are under the influence of alcohol (Feldman, 1994).

## ETIOLOGY

### *Psychodynamic Theories*

A number of psychological theories have attempted to explain substance dependence. Alcohol-dependent individuals have often been viewed as those who easily succumb to the escape that alcohol provides. More recent theories have described people likely to become dependent on alcohol as more phobic and with greater feelings of inferiority compared with social drinkers. Over time, the search for an alcoholic personality has given way to a multivariate model that incorporates the biopsychosocial components of addiction. Current researchers believe that many of the stereotypical characteristics found in alcohol-dependent people (e.g., dependency, low self-esteem, passivity, introversion) are the result of and not the cause of substance dependence. Psychodynamically oriented treatment tends to emphasize behavioral management techniques and rejects the disease model of substance dependence.

### Biologic Theories

Heredity as an etiology has been studied for many years and continues to provide insight into understanding the genesis of alcoholism. Genetic predisposition is considered to be the single most significant piece of information in identifying alcoholism. Researchers have known for more than 50 years that children of alcoholic parents, even if raised in an alcohol-free environment, are more likely to become alcoholics than children of nonalcoholic parents (Goodwin et al, 1973). Although studies have indicated different degrees of effect, hereditary explanations, at the very least, provide a satisfactory basis for understanding a person's vulnerability to alcohol dependency. However, predisposition suggests neither fatalism nor determinism. Even patients who are genetically predisposed to certain types of cancer, for example, can take steps to minimize their risk. Recognizing their familial predisposition to alcoholism or addiction, individuals can avoid the use of alcohol and drugs.

## PHARMACOKINETICS OF ALCOHOL

### Absorption

Alcohol is absorbed partially from the stomach but mostly from the small intestine. If a person with an empty stomach ingests alcohol, 50% is in the bloodstream within 15 minute with peak levels reached in 40-79 minutes (Colyar, 2003). The form of alcohol consumed affects the rate of absorption. Alcohol in beer and wine is absorbed more slowly compared with alcohol in liquor. This characteristic might be a result, in part, of dilution; beer contains 4% ethanol; wine, 12% ethanol; and whiskey, 40% to 50% ethanol.

| Table 35-4 | The Empty Calories of Booze | |
| --- | --- | --- |

| Beverage | Amount (oz) | Average Calories |
| --- | --- | --- |
| Regular beer | 12 | 150 |
| Light beer | 12 | 110 |
| Gin, rum, vodka | 1 | 65 |
| Liqueurs | 1.5 | 190 |
| Red wine | 4 | 80 |
| White dry wine | 4 | 75 |
| Sweet wine | 4 | 105 |
| Champagne | 4 | 85 |
| Martini | 3.5 | 140 |
| Margarita | 4 | 170 |

From Medline Plus: *Alcohol calorie calculator.* Available at http://www.nlm.nih.gov/medlineplus/substanceabuseproblems. html. Accessed November 18, 2005.

However, dilution of the alcohol in its beverage medium cannot completely account for slower absorption. Food also slows alcohol absorption.

Alcohol also contains what has been referred to as empty calories. Table 35-4 lists the average calorie content of some of the most popular alcoholic drinks.

### Distribution

Ethanol is distributed equally in all body tissue according to water content. Larger individuals (who have greater amounts of body water) can therefore ingest more alcohol than smaller people, who have less body water. Alcohol affects the cerebrum and cerebellum before it affects the spinal cord and the vital centers because the cerebrum and cerebellum contain more water.

### Metabolism

Although the rate of absorption largely determines how quickly a person will become intoxicated, a person's metabolic rate largely determines how long alcohol will affect the body. The healthy body can metabolize 15 ml of alcohol an hour or roughly the alcohol content in a shot of whiskey, can of beer, or glass of wine. Individuals who drink alcohol constantly over a number of years have increased hepatic drug-metabolizing enzymes that hasten alcohol metabolism (metabolic tolerance [pharmacokinetic tolerance]). Hot coffee, sweating it out, and other home remedies do not increase alcohol metabolism, nor do they hasten the sobering up process. Attempts by scientists to develop a pill to prevent or decrease intoxication have been unsuccessful. In late-stage alcoholism, tolerance decreases as the abused liver finally can no longer metabolize the alcohol adequately.

The chemical name for alcohol is ethanol, $CH_3CH_2OH$. Alcohol is primarily metabolized in the liver but 10% is excreted unchanged in the breath, sweat, and urine (Colyar, 2003). The oxidation process can be described chemically as follows:

---

ethanol ($CH_3CH_2OH$) → acetaldehyde ($CH_3CHO$) and hydrogen ($H_2$)

---

- Alcohol = ethanol ($CH_3CH_2OH$); enzyme = alcohol dehydrogenase
- Products = acetaldehyde ($CH_3CHO$) and hydrogen ($H_2$); enzyme = aldehyde dehydrogenase

---

acetaldehyde ($CH_3CHO$) and hydrogen ($H_2$) → acetic acid ($CH_3COOH$)

---

- Product = acetic acid ($CH_3COOH$)

At each step of the metabolic process, an enzyme breaks down the chemical and speeds up the reaction. Alcohol dehydrogenase breaks down $CH_3CH_2OH$ to $CH_3CHO$ and $H_2$. The $H_2$ molecule causes the liver to bypass normal energy sources (the $H_2$ from fat) and to use the $H_2$ from $CH_3CH_2OH$. Fat accumulates because it is not being used as a primary energy source; this leads to fatty liver, hyperlipemia, hepatitis, and, ultimately, cirrhosis. $CH_3CHO$ is toxic to the body; it compromises normal cell function in the liver. If the metabolism of $CH_3CHO$ is impaired, it accumulates in the liver, causing cell death and necrosis. $CH_3CHO$ also interferes with vitamin activation. Aldehyde dehydrogenase breaks down $CH_3CHO$ to $CH_3COOH$, which is a harmless substance. When enzymatic action on $CH_3CHO$ is blocked by the aldehyde dehydrogenase blocker disulfiram (Antabuse), $CH_3CHO$ accumulates, causing severe sickness.

Research confirms the suspicion that women become intoxicated more easily than men, even when studies are controlled for size differences. Frezza and colleagues (1990) discovered that the gastrointestinal tissue of women and of alcohol-dependent men contains little alcohol dehydrogenase. The alcohol dehydrogenase in the gastrointestinal tissue of men who are not dependent on alcohol oxidizes a significant amount of $CH_3CH_2OH$ in the gut before it enters the bloodstream. The inability of women's bodies to undergo this first-pass metabolism accounts for their enhanced vulnerability to alcohol. For example, if a 120-lb man and a 120-lb woman both drink two glasses of alcohol (beer, wine, or liquor), the man's blood alcohol level will be 0.07 and the woman's 0.08 (National Clearinghouse for Alcohol and Drug Information [NCADI], 2005). She is legally drunk and he is not. Furthermore, when a 200-lb man and a 140-lb woman each drink three glasses of alcohol (beer, glass of wine, shot of liquor), their blood alcohol levels will be .06 and 1.0, respectively (NCADI). This is a considerable difference, not only in the eyes of the law but also in behavioral expression.

Another enzyme system, the microsomal ethanol-oxidizing system (MEOS), breaks down some alcohol. This metabolic pathway becomes more important after chronic heavy alcohol consumption (Lieber, 2003). The primary MEOS enzyme is cytochrome P-450 2E1.

### Blood Alcohol Levels

*Alcohol Cited in Oklahoma Student's Death Norman, Oklahoma. A 19-year-old student whose body was found the morning after a party in a fraternity house died from alcohol poisoning, officials said Friday. Blake Adam Hammontree had a blood alcohol level of 0.42 when he died. . . . It was the third death in less than a month at a fraternity house.*

*Birmingham News, 2004*

Blood alcohol levels accurately indicate the amount of ethanol to which the brain is exposed. Behavioral and physiologic effects are predictable for most drinkers. For example, at a 0.05% blood alcohol level, most individuals are predictably feeling good and experience disinhibition (i.e., they might do and say things they would typically just think or think about doing). The box below outlines the typical responses for a given blood alcohol level.

## CLINICAL EFFECTS OF ALCOHOL

| Blood Alcohol Level (%) | Physiologic Effect |
|---|---|
| 0.05 | Euphoria, decreased inhibitions |
| 0.10-0.15 | Labile mood, talkative, impaired judgment |
| 0.15-0.20 | Decreased motor skills, slurred speech, double vision |
| 0.25 | Altered perceptions |
| 0.30 | Altered equilibrium |
| 0.35 | Apathy, inertia |
| 0.40 | Stupor, coma |
| 0.40-0.50 | Severe respiratory depression, death |

Modified from Lehne RA: *Pharmacology for nursing care,* ed 4, Philadelphia, 2004, WB Saunders.

### Tolerance to Alcohol

Tolerance to alcohol is probably related to elevated hepatic enzyme levels (pharmacokinetic tolerance) and to cellular adaptation (pharmacodynamic tolerance). At the point at which the normal drinker might be noticeably drunk after 10 to 12 drinks, the long-term drinker with pharmacodynamic tolerance might seem unaffected by drinking the same amount. However, tolerance to the respiratory depressing effects of alcohol does not develop appreciably. Blood levels just slightly higher than those required to get a buzz on have resulted in the deaths of long-term, pharmacodynamically tolerant drinkers.

## PHYSIOLOGIC EFFECTS

People generally begin consuming alcohol because it causes a reaction they desire. Disinhibition, impaired judgment, and fuzzy thinking are initial responses to alcohol ingestion. These signs represent cerebral intoxication. In many situations, this mental relaxation is pleasant. Alcohol also depresses psychomotor activity. Alcohol has been described as a social lubricant because it relaxes self-imposed barriers that inhibit sociability. Anxiety and tension are relieved, usually for several hours after a drink is taken. Eventually, at least for the alcoholic, drinking becomes defensive; that is, the alcoholic often drinks to avoid the effects of many years of drinking. For example, once the anxiety-reducing effect wears off, more tension and anxiety are produced; thus, the drinker must consume more alcohol to regain the anxiety-free state. Many alcohol-dependent people, even after drinking all they can hold, are not able to quell the rebound psychomotor upheaval caused by years of alcohol-related central nervous system (CNS) irritation. The presenting complaint of many of those who seek treatment for alcohol dependence is nervousness or depression.

### Central Nervous System Effects

The adverse effects of alcohol can be categorized as central or peripheral. CNS effects are related to sedation and toxicity. As the vital centers become affected, a slowed, stuporous to unconscious mental state develops. Large amounts of alcohol can cause sleep, coma, deep anesthesia, or even death. Other common symptoms of intoxication include slurred speech, short retention span, loud talk, and memory deficits. Blackout is the period during which the drinker functions socially but for which the drinker has no memory.

Historically, the brain damage associated with alcoholism was thought to be caused by alcohol-related nutritional deficiencies. Alcohol-dependent people tend to eat poorly, and no doubt this behavior leads to pathologic changes (Lieber, 2003). It is now known, however, that brain damage occurs with drinking, even when a nutritious diet is maintained; neuronal death is probably related to changes in N-methyl-D-aspartate (NDMA) receptor sensitivity heightening the excitotoxicity potential of glutamate (Harper and Matsumoto, 2005). Other neuroregulators are also involved. Brain changes include reduced brain weight, atrophy, reductions in white matter, hippocampal changes, hypothalamic neuronal loss, and cerebellar neuronal loss (Harper and Matsumoto, 2005).

Increased psychomotor activity as a consequence of alcohol is called the *alcohol withdrawal syndrome*. Sedation is the predominant effect of alcohol but, as sedation wears off, psychomotor activity increases. This state is referred to as a *rebound phenomenon*. As the CNS becomes more irritated, the normal drinker feels sick and irritable (a hangover) but lives through it, perhaps vowing never to go through this again. The heavy drinker and the alcoholic have to drink again to resedate the psychomotor system. Eventually, the alcohol-dependent person has to drink larger amounts to feel somewhat normal. Some drinkers reach the

## Table 35-5   Courses of Withdrawal From Addictive Drugs

| Drugs | Length of Acute Detoxification | Common Detoxification Agents | Withdrawal Signs and Symptoms |
|---|---|---|---|
| **CNS Depressants** | | | |
| Alcohol | 3-5 days | Librium, Serax, Valium, Vistaril, alcohol | Anxiety, sweats, tremors, flushed face, irritability, sleeplessness, confusion, seizures, delirium |
| Valium | Slow drug taper, up to 2 wk | Librium, Valium | |
| Phenobarbital | Slow drug taper, 2-4 wk | Librium, phenobarbital | |
| **Opioids** | | | |
| Heroin | 3-5 days | Methadone, other tapering opioid, or nonopioid withdrawal regimen | Yawning, dilated pupils, gooseflesh, vomiting, diarrhea, runny nose and eyes, sleeplessness, anxiety, irritability, elevated blood pressure and pulse, craving for narcotics |
| Morphine | 3-5 days | | |
| Demerol | 3-5 days | | |
| Methadone | 2 wk | | |
| **Stimulants** | | | |
| Amphetamines | 3-5 days | Drug intervention usually not required | General fatigue, apathy, depression, drowsiness, irritability, paranoia |
| Cocaine | 3-5 days | | |
| **Hallucinogen** | | | |
| Marijuana | 2-3 days (metabolites remain in the body up to 2 wk) | Drug intervention usually not required | Few signs of withdrawal, craving for marijuana, general anxiety and restlessness |

From Mueller LA, Ketcham K: *Recovering: how to get and stay sober,* New York, 1987, Bantam Books.

point at which they cannot drink enough alcohol, and CNS irritability is not sedatable. Then, alcoholic tremors, sweating, palpitations, and agitation occur. Although these symptoms usually occur when alcohol ingestion has stopped (Mueller and Ketcham, 1987; Table 35-5), in some cases they occur while the alcohol-dependent person is drinking.

Alcoholic hallucinosis, a state of auditory hallucinations, is a phenomenon that alcohol-dependent people sometimes experience. The brain begins to invent sensory input. Alcoholic hallucinosis usually begins 48 hours or so after drinking has stopped. Usually, within the context of a clear sensorium, frightening voices or sounds are heard.

The ultimate level of CNS irritability is delirium tremens (DTs). In DTs, the body not only invents sensory input, but also has extreme motor agitation. Hallucinations become visual (e.g., the proverbial pink elephants), and the sufferer is tremulous and terrified. Tonic-clonic seizures (grand mal seizures) can occur.

Wernicke-Korsakoff syndrome is a mental disorder characterized by amnesia, clouding of consciousness, confabulation (falsification of memory) and memory loss, and peripheral neuropathy. This disorder results from the poor nutrition of the alcoholic (specifically, inadequate amounts of thiamine and niacin in the diet) and from the neurotoxic nature of alcohol.

### Peripheral Nervous System Effects

Peripheral effects are varied and cause great suffering. For a complete discussion of these various processes, the reader is directed to a medical-surgical textbook. Cirrhosis and peripheral neuritis are the physical health problems most commonly associated with alcohol. As the alcohol-dependent person's liver function becomes impaired, he or she is less able to tolerate alcohol. The person who once boasted of drinking exploits becomes drunk after only a few beers. Physical consequences of cirrhosis include obstructed blood flow (which leads to portal hypertension, ascites, and finally esophageal varices), decreased liver cell function, low serum albumin levels, high ammonia and high bilirubin serum levels, and clotting problems. Peripheral neuritis causes numbness and subsequent injury in the legs, as well as changes in gait.

Alcohol is also an irritant; it burns the mouth and throat and prompts the stomach to secrete more hydrochloric acid. Gastric ulcers develop and then are worsened by alcohol. Alcoholics can experience ulcers, gastritis, bleeding, and hemorrhage in the stomach. Ulcers can eventually perforate, creating a life-threatening situation.

The pancreas is affected by alcohol in many ways. Pancreatitis and diabetes are not uncommon consequences of alcoholism. A malabsorption syndrome is caused by irritation of the intestinal lining. This condition seems to affect B vitamins generally and to lead to a deficiency of vitamin B$_1$ (thiamine) in particular. Thiamine deficiency contributes to peripheral neuritis. Alcohol also has a direct effect on muscle tissue, a condition known as *alcoholic myopathy*. Other organs affected by alcohol include the eyes (loss of peripheral and night vision), the heart (hypertension, enlarged left ventricle), and reproductive organs. As a depressant, alcohol can cause impotence. Furthermore, prolonged drinking shrinks the testicles and decreases testosterone. Sexual potency is further compromised by a failing liver that is unable to detoxify female hormones, thus increasing the level of these hormones and adding to the male's sexual decline. As many men have experienced, alcohol can increase interest in sex but can lead to decreased sexual performance.

CLINICAL EXAMPLE

Anthony is a 36-year-old suffering from alcohol abuse with physiologic dependence. Because alcohol predominates, a primary diagnosis of polysubstance dependence is not appropriate. He has a long history of presentations at the emergency room for suicidal ideations. Alcohol and other drugs are always found in his system. He presents at a local treatment facility, saying, "I just can't keep it up any more. I've been drinking for 23 years and my life is falling apart. Everyone I know hates me. I can't keep a job. No one trusts me. I have to have some help." First, Anthony needed detoxification. He then went through a 28-day treatment program. He attends Alcoholics Anonymous (AA) five times each week and has a sponsor, someone in whom he can confide and from whom he can "learn to live life on life's terms." He also attends an aftercare treatment group three times a week to focus on dealing with his shame. After 108 days of sobriety, Anthony began to think that he was cured and no longer needed his sobriety support system. He drank again. Just before he was pulled over for driving under the influence, he managed to throw away the cocaine he had just bought.

Five months later, the consequences of his past lifestyle are catching up with him. He is considered a habitual offender and has been offered 20 years in prison by the district attorney. The AA program teaches responsibility for one's actions and surrender of self-will to one's "higher power." After getting the alcohol out of his system and reconnecting with AA, Anthony is now, rather than trying to run from his obligations, prepared to go to prison, if necessary. "I did it. I don't want to go to prison, but if that's what God has in mind for me because of my foolish decisions, then so be it. Might be there's somebody out there who needs to hear my story. I can share my experience, strength, and hope, and let them know that God is a way maker." These attitudes of surrender of self-will to one's "higher power" are characteristic of 12-step programs and are considered essential to recovery.

## NURSING ISSUES

### Overdose

People die from overdoses of alcohol because it depresses the CNS. Vital centers become anesthetized, compromising breathing and heart rate and leading to a comatose state or death. Gastrointestinal bleeding or hemorrhage can occur. As a vasodilator, alcohol also leads to heat loss; many people have succumbed to hypothermia in colder climates. People consistently underestimate the potency of alcohol, and deaths have occurred simply because individuals have consumed too much. Almost every year, newspapers report the death of college students by alcohol poisoning (see earlier). Although alcohol alone can kill, most overdose-related deaths are the result of combining alcohol with other CNS depressants.

## Drugs That Affect Drinking

### Disulfiram: Makes Drinking Painful

Disulfiram (Antabuse) inhibits the breakdown of $CH_3CHO$ by the enzyme aldehyde dehydrogenase. Because $CH_3CHO$ is toxic, the person who drinks alcohol while taking disulfiram will become ill (as evidenced by sweating, flushing of the neck and face, tachycardia, hypotension, throbbing headache, nausea and vomiting, palpitations, dyspnea, tremor, weakness, or any combination of these effects). Disulfiram and alcohol can also cause arrhythmias, myocardial infarction, cardiac failure, seizures, coma, and death. The unpleasant response to alcohol is intended to help reinforce the alcoholic's efforts to stop drinking alcohol. Basically, the patient taking disulfiram has to make only one decision a day about drinking: once the pill is taken, the patient dare not drink. Disulfiram is usually started with a single dose of 250 to 500 mg daily. After 1 or 2 weeks, the dose is typically reduced to a maintenance dose of 125 to 250 mg/day. Anecdotal accounts note that some alcoholics will experience an ostensibly spontaneous relapse episode that coincides with their forgetting to take disulfiram for 1 or 2 weeks before their return to alcohol use. Disulfiram is most effective in patients with significant internal motivation for long-term change.

### Naltrexone Hydrochloride: Decreases the Pleasure of Drinking

Naltrexone hydrochloride (ReVia) is an opioid receptor antagonist formerly used to treat narcotic dependence and now approved for the treatment of alcohol dependence. Naltrexone increases abstinence and reduces alcohol craving when used as a part of a comprehensive treatment plan (Sinclair, 2001). Naltrexone interferes with opioid functioning, which probably compromises the pleasurable effects of alcohol. It has been known to cause liver toxicity if taken at higher than recommended levels and is contraindicated for patients who have abused narcotics within 7 to 10 days because it will precipitate opioid withdrawal (Anonymous, 1995). Typically, patients receive 50 mg/day.

### Acamprosate: Restores the Chemical Balance in the Alcoholic Brain

Acamprosate (Campral) was approved in 2004 and was the first new drug for the treatment of alcoholism in 10 years. Although the mechanism of action is not precisely known, it is thought that continuous consumption of alcohol alters the balance between neuronal inhibition and excitation (Forest Laboratories, 2004). Acamprosate is thought to reestablish the prealcoholism balance. This drug can be used once abstinence has begun, but not while the alcohol-dependent person is drinking. It causes neither the aversive effects of disulfiram nor the pleasure-stealing effects of naltrexone. Initial reports have suggested that acomprosate enhances abstaining behaviors. More studies are underway to provide further illumination on this new drug. The recommended dosage of acomprosate is two 333-mg tablets taken three times daily (Forest Laboratories, 2004).

## INTERACTIONS

Alcohol taken with other CNS depressants causes profound CNS depression, often leading to death. For instance, diazepam, which is not lethal when taken alone, has led to death when combined with alcohol. Alcohol should be avoided when a person is taking barbiturates, antipsychotic drugs, antidepressants, benzodiazepines, and other sedatives. Chloral hydrate and lorazepam (Ativan) have been associated with intentional sedating of unsuspecting persons in bars. A chloral hydrate and alcohol combination (the legendary knockout drops) was used years ago to recruit men for ship duty or for robbery. An updated version, with Ativan replacing chloral hydrate, has been used by young women to rob men who picked them up in bars.

## USE BY OLDER ADULTS

Alcoholism in older adults can be roughly divided into two groups:

1. Lifelong users
2. Late-onset users responding to stress

Lifelong users tend to have increased physical, cognitive, and emotional problems associated with their drinking. Late-onset alcoholics include individuals who, as they grow older, tend to cope with the many and persistent losses of later life

**Box 35-3    Older Alcoholics**

Older alcoholics are divided into two groups. About two thirds are early-onset drinkers who have abused alcohol much of their lives and have survived into an unhealthy, unhappy old age. The late-onset group—about one third of all drinkers over age 60—is unlike the general alcoholic population. This group has an excellent chance for recovery. "They are not as impaired physically, emotionally, or cognitively as the early onset drinkers. . . . With abstinence, proper diet, and time, recovery can be complete" (Robertson, 1992).

Heavy drinking in the late-onset group is usually triggered by traumatic loss. The deterioration is rapid, only a 1- to 2-year progression, compared with alcoholics who have been drinking for 20 to 40 years.

From Robertson N: The intimate enemy: will that friendly drink betray you? *Modern Maturity* 35:28, 1992.

by drinking. These individuals, if not effectively treated, can deteriorate rapidly. On the other hand, late-onset alcoholics have a robust response when treated.

Alcohol use in older adults is underreported, frequently unrecognized, and rarely treated (Robertson, 1992; Box 35-3). As the population of older adults has grown, so have the substance-related problems many of these people bring with them. People with impaired liver function do not metabolize alcohol efficiently and can therefore have a low tolerance for alcohol. Decreased liver function is a product of aging and, consequently, many older individuals cannot drink much alcohol without becoming inebriated, confused, and sedated. The nurse should be particularly watchful for combinations of alcohol with other CNS depressants among patients in this age group.

## FETAL ALCOHOL SYNDROME

Pregnant women who drink alcohol run the risk of seriously harming their unborn child. Fetal alcohol syndrome (FAS) is the result of alcohol's inhibiting fetal development during the first trimester. FAS is the third most commonly recognized cause of mental retardation and the only one that is preventable. Characteristic signs of FAS include microcephaly and an associated severe mental retardation. The risk of FAS is directly related to the amount of alcohol that the mother has ingested during pregnancy.

## WITHDRAWAL AND DETOXIFICATION

Withdrawal from alcohol can be painful, scary, and even lethal. As the person abstains from alcohol, he or she begins to reap the consequences of CNS irritation caused by alcohol: tremulousness, nervousness, anxiety, anorexia, nausea and vomiting, insomnia and other sleep disturbances, rapid pulse, high blood pressure, profuse perspiration, diarrhea, fever, unsteady gait, difficulty concentrating, exaggerated startle reflex, and a craving for alcohol or other drugs. As the withdrawal symptoms become increasingly pronounced, hallucinations can occur. The body is undergoing alcohol withdrawal and needs detoxification.

The level of supervision depends on the severity of alcoholism. Mild dependence can be handled on an outpatient basis. Even more heavily dependent cases of alcoholism have been managed by a so-called *cold turkey* method, without medical supervision. In years past, it was not uncommon for former alcoholics to take turns sitting with an individual going through the misery of withdrawal from alcohol. Having gone through this same process, these recovering alcoholics were both sensitive and firm when needed, they understood the pain but knew it was usually survivable, and they knew that individuals had died from withdrawal occasionally when medical assistance was not used.

Because of the misery and risk of death associated with unattended withdrawal, most cases today have medical supervision of some sort. Drugs that have a cross-dependence with alcohol—that is, other CNS depressants—can be used to avoid diminished symptoms of withdrawal. The most commonly used medications are the benzodiazepines, specifically chlordiazepoxide (Librium), lorazepam (Ativan), and diazepam (Valium). These agents minimize symptoms of withdrawal, prevent DTs, and decrease the risk of seizures.

**CASE STUDY**

E.F., a 28-year-old Caucasian man, was brought to treatment by his wife after his third DUI offense in which he ran off the road and into a neighbor's mailbox. He has had a history of alcohol and drug use since age 14. Although neither of his parents drank, he had a grandfather who died from cirrhosis of the liver and bleeding esophageal varices.

E.F. has been in counseling twice before in an effort to salvage his previous marriage. After the breakup of the marriage, he lost his business and became extremely

## CASE STUDY—cont'd

depressed. However, when E.F. drank, he became belligerent and, at one point, threatened his ex-wife and child, forcing her to file for sole custody of their son. During this period, he also began gambling in an effort to make quick money.

E.F. says that he is willing to enter treatment at this time so that he does not lose his wife and because he fears the men to whom he owes gambling debts. He knows that he will be safe in the hospital until he can figure out what to do. He does not believe that he has a problem with alcohol, drugs, or gambling and attributes his misfortunes to the ill will of others. He denies suicidal ideation at this time. Blood alcohol level on admission was 0.02%.

E.F.'s current lifestyle involves hunting and doing things with his wife and two step-children, Ann, 4, and Steve, 6. He misses his 2-year-old son, who lives with his ex-wife.

## CENTRAL NERVOUS SYSTEM DEPRESSANTS

### BARBITURATES

Barbiturates depress the CNS. Barbiturates were first used medicinally as sedatives in the last half of the nineteenth century. It was not until 1950 that researchers were able to confirm their ability to produce physical dependence. CNS depressants decrease the awareness of and response to sensory stimuli.

Barbiturates are used to relieve anxiety or to produce sleep. Common barbiturates include secobarbital (Seconal), pentobarbital (Nembutal), amobarbital (Amytal), and phenobarbital (Luminal). Slang names for these barbiturates include yellow

## Care Plan

Name: E.F.                                                          Admission Date: _____

*DSM-IV-TR* Diagnosis: Alcohol dependence (or alcoholism)

| | |
|---|---|
| Assessment | **Areas of strength:** Has no medical problems and denies suicidal ideation. Has also been in counseling twice and enjoys hunting and doing things with his family. |
| | **Problems:** Has a family history of chemical dependency and long-time use of alcohol and drugs. Denies that alcohol is a problem in his life despite family and occupational problems. |
| Diagnoses | • Ineffective individual coping related to alcohol abuse as evidenced by legal and financial problems. |
| | • Ineffective family coping; disabled related to alcohol abuse, as evidenced by potential marriage separation and financial difficulties. |

Outcomes   *Short-term goals:*                                                 *Date met*
• Patient will state that his marital and occupational problems are          _____
the result of drinking.
*Long-term goals:*
• Patient will remain chemical free on monthly testing, which               _____
will be assessed through urine testing by his probation officer.

Planning/      **Nurse-patient relationship:** Recognize initial need to use denial; discuss the natural
Interventions                          consequences of his drinking and the need for total
                                       abstinence; educate regarding the diagnosis of alcoholism,
                                       offering hope for long-term recovery; encourage attendance
                                       at AA meetings.
               **Psychopharmacology:** No caffeine or sugar; multivitamin daily.
               **Milieu management:** Family treatment; encourage activities of daily living.
Evaluation     According to probation officer, E.F. is sober after 1 month.
Referrals      Refer to AA and make appointment with substance abuse counselor.

jackets, reds, blues, Amy's, and rainbows. These drugs have a narrow therapeutic index, with the lethal dose being only slightly higher than the therapeutic dose. The long-term effects of barbiturate intoxication can be severe because of hypoxia secondary to shallow or absent respirations during intoxication and overdose. Most people recover if treatment is begun early. These drugs produce both physical and psychological dependence. Barbiturates are classified according to their duration of action: ultrashort (30 minutes to 3 hours), short (3 to 4 hours), intermediate (6 to 8 hours), and long (10 to 12 hours). Barbiturates with short to intermediate duration of action have the highest abuse potential. Barbiturates in this category include amobarbital, pentobarbital, and secobarbital.

Barbiturates, usually taken orally, are metabolized by the liver and excreted by the kidneys. When barbiturates are combined with alcohol, dangerous levels of CNS depression can occur.

## PHYSIOLOGIC EFFECTS

Barbiturates cause CNS depression, primarily by increasing gamma-aminobutyric acid (GABA) activity. GABA stimulation decreases awareness of external stimuli, shortens the attention span, and decreases intellectual ability. Barbiturates are used to treat insomnia, to soften withdrawal from heroin, and as anticonvulsants. Drug abusers take barbiturates to maintain a state of relatively anxiety-free living. These drugs are also taken to counteract the effects of amphetamines (to come down) or in place of heroin when it is not available. The acutely intoxicated person will have an unsteady gait, slurred speech, and sustained nystagmus. Chronic users can have mental symptoms that

include confusion, irritability, and insomnia. People who regularly use barbiturates develop a tolerance to the psychological effects but not to the respiratory depression effects. Hence, the user must consume more and more of the barbiturate to achieve a pleasurable effect but eventually increases the dose to the point of depressing respirations.

## NURSING ISSUES

### Overdose

The toxic dose of barbiturates varies but usually an oral dose of 1 g results in serious poisoning, and doses of 2 to 10 g can be fatal. Acute overdose is characterized by CNS and respiratory depression. Coma and death are possible. Treatment is supportive.

### Interactions

Barbiturates interact with many other drugs, but the most significant are those that increase CNS depression. Other CNS depressants such as alcohol, sedatives, tranquilizers, and antihistamines can cause serious CNS depression.

### Use by Older Adults

Barbiturates frequently cause excitement in older adults. Older adults are also more prone to confusion caused by barbiturates.

### Use During Pregnancy

Barbiturates can cause fetal abnormalities. These drugs cross the placental barrier, and fetal serum levels approach maternal blood levels. Infants born

Summary of How Abused Drugs Work

| Abused Substance | Mechanism of Action |
| --- | --- |
| Barbiturates | Increase the effect of GABA |
| Opioids | Mimic endogenous neurotransmitters by stimulating opioid receptors; increase the release of dopamine in the nucleus accumbens |
| Cocaine | Decreases the reuptake of dopamine |
| Amphetamines | Increase the release of norepinephrine; enhance dopamine release; block the reuptake of dopamine; methamphetamine blocks the breakdown of dopamine |
| Ecstasy | Increases the release of serotonin; increases the release of dopamine |
| Marijuana | Stimulates dopamine pathways in the nucleus accumbens |
| LSD | Binds tightly to 5-HT$_2$ receptors, causing a more pronounced effect. |

*GABA,* Gamma-aminobutyric acid; *LSD,* lysergic acid diethylamide.

to mothers who take barbiturates during the last trimester of pregnancy can experience withdrawal symptoms.

## WITHDRAWAL AND DETOXIFICATION

Symptoms of withdrawal from barbiturates are severe and can cause death. Symptoms usually begin 8 to 12 hours after the last dose. Because barbiturates depress the CNS, a rebound effect can occur when a person stops taking them. Minor withdrawal symptoms include anxiety, muscle twitching, tremor, progressive weakness, dizziness, distorted visual perception, nausea and vomiting, insomnia, and orthostatic hypotension. More serious withdrawal symptoms include convulsions and delirium. Untreated, withdrawal symptoms might not decline in intensity for about 1 week (Lehne, 2004). Detoxification requires a cautious and gradual reduction of these drugs. One approach is to reduce the patient's regular dose by 10% each day.

## BENZODIAZEPINES

Benzodiazepines have many legitimate uses and are reviewed in Chapter 21. One benzodiazepine, flunitrazepam (Rohypnol; also known as *roofies, rophies, roche, roaches,* and *ruffies*), is known primarily for its abuse potential (Taylor and Donoghue, 2001). Because of both its sedative and amnesic effects, Rohypnol has been used for date rape. Until relatively recently, Rohypnol was manufactured as a colorless, odorless, and tasteless substance when mixed with liquids. Sexual predators were able to slip it easily into the beverage of an unsuspecting woman and then perpetrate date rape. Again, the amnesia associated with this drug has interfered with prosecution of the perpetrator. Although Rohypnol is not sold in the United States, an active smuggling operation makes it available on the black market.

## GAMMA HYDROXYBUTYRATE

Gamma hydroxybutyrate (GHB) (also known as *G, liquid X, liquid Ecstasy, Georgia homeboy*), is a CNS depressant and is popular among youth as a club drug (Allen, 2001; Taylor and Donoghue,

2001). GHB is taken orally, injected, or snorted. Sexual predators use GHB to incapacitate their victims and render them incapable of remembering the assault. GHB is manufactured from products available in health food stores and has been used as a performance-enhancing drug for athletic competition (Allen, 2001; Whitten, 2001). Interestingly, millions of men and women currently use a number of potential drugs, sold as athletic supplements, despite known deleterious effects (Kanayama et al, 2001). GHB, generally when used with alcohol, has been linked to many deaths. It is now illegal in the United States and is classified as a schedule I drug.

## INHALANTS

Inhalants are inhaled and are commonly used because they are cheap, readily available, and typically legal. Examples include airplane glue, gasoline, rubber cement, polyvinylchloride cement, hair spray, air freshener, spot remover, polish remover, paint remover, and lighter fluid. Inhaled substances can be broken down into three basic groups: hydrocarbon solvents (gasoline and glues), aerosol propellants (propellants in spray cans), and anesthetics and gases (chloroform, nitrous oxide [laughing gas]). Inhalants usually depress the CNS and increase hilarity; they can also cause excitability. Inhalants are particularly dangerous because the amount inhaled cannot be controlled. Deaths from asphyxiation, suffocation, and choking (e.g., on vomit) have been reported. Inhalants cross the blood-brain barrier quickly. Common side effects include mouth ulcers, gastrointestinal problems, anorexia, confusion, headache, and ataxia. Because of their accessibility, children are at a special risk of coming into contact with substances in this category. Some inhalants are highly lipid-soluble to the extent that they become sequestered in fatty tissues, thus having a prolonged effect. Brain damage has been reported with inhalants, including frontal lobe, cerebellar, and hippocampal damage, leading to diminished problem solving, ataxic gait, and memory dysfunction, respectively. Inhalants can be breathed in by sniffing fumes from a container, by bagging (inhaling fumes from a paper bag), and by huffing (inhaling fumes from an inhalant-soaked rag stuffed in the mouth).

## OPIOIDS (NARCOTICS)

Opioids include opium, morphine, codeine, heroin, hydromorphone (Dilaudid), meperidine (Demerol), methadone (Dolophine), hydrocodone (Vicodin), and oxycodone (Oxycontin). Opioids are widely abused. Until what has been called the *cocaine crisis,* the general public viewed heroin as the most prevalent drug of abuse. Although heroin abuse has been relegated to a lower status for some time, it is again becoming a focus of attention, because drug users find it less expensive and less devastating compared with cocaine. Using cocaine and heroin together (called a *speedball*) has grown in popularity. Opioids can be swallowed, smoked, snorted, injected into soft tissue (skin popping), and mainlined (intravenous [IV]).

Parenteral use of heroin, for example, involves the following:

1. Cooking the substance in a spoon or bottle cap
2. Filtering it with a cotton ball
3. Sterilizing a needle with a match
4. Injecting the drug into a vein

Initially, veins in the antecubital space are used but, as vein membranes break down and sclerose (form tracks), they get used up, and other veins are selected for injection. The needle is frequently passed from one user to another. Infections, including acquired immunodeficiency syndrome (AIDS), have been relatively common. Because of AIDS and hepatitis, snorting is increasing in popularity as a route of administration. However, sharing of straws also poses a risk resulting from trauma of the highly vascular mucous membranes in the nasal passages (Gorski, 1996).

### CLINICAL EXAMPLE

Sam Jones is a 32-year-old maintenance man. He has a history of drinking and using marijuana since junior high. He began showing a strong preference for opioids after a visit to the dentist to have a tooth extracted. Since that visit, Sam has had several other teeth extracted and has been to the emergency room several times for various situations requiring treatment for one type of intense pain or another. Sam has lost several jobs because of suspected stealing. Actually, he was only trying to get people's prescriptions that they weren't using anyway and he "would never steal from people." Sam recently started injecting drugs and became obviously impaired fairly quickly. When he was found wandering around the apartment complex with slurred speech and confused thinking, his boss fired him. He left angrily and had a motorcycle accident in which he almost lost his life. He was taken to the trauma unit of the medical center where he began to exhibit narcotic withdrawal the following day. Sam's injuries were so severe that he was "sobered" into agreeing to be evaluated for treatment in the substance abuse treatment program of the medical center. Sam has a long way to go to recover successfully, but exposing him to treatment will at least help him learn more about another way of life, even if he is not ready to fully participate in recovery right now.

## PHYSIOLOGIC EFFECTS

Opioids relieve pain by increasing the pain threshold and by reducing anxiety and fear. These drugs accomplish this by stimulating opioid receptor sites in the brain. The naturally occurring neurotransmitters, the endorphins, produce various responses, including being able to mediate pain and regulate mood by activating opioid receptors. The opioids are endorphin agonists. Drug abusers are attracted by the drug's effect on mood (a feeling of euphoria). Drug abusers frequently refer to the euphoric mood created by morphine and heroin as being better than sex. In fact, IV heroin delivers a rush (lasting less than 1 minute) described as similar to a sexual orgasm. In addition to the euphoria, an overall CNS depression occurs. Drowsiness or nodding and sleep are common effects.

Heroin has a higher abuse potential compared with morphine and other opioids because it more readily passes the blood-brain barrier. Once heroin enters the brain, its chemical structure is changed to that of morphine, so it becomes trapped in the brain, causing a more sustained high. CNS effects of opioids include respiratory depression related to decreased sensitivity to carbon dioxide stimulation by the medullary center for respiration. Respiratory depression is the primary cause of death when opioid-caused death occurs. Peripheral nervous system (PNS) effects include constipation; decreased gastric, biliary, and pancreatic secretions;

urinary retention; hypotension; and reduced pupil size. Pinpoint pupils (miosis) are a sign of opioid overdose. Another opioid, meperidine, is typically the drug of choice for physicians and nurses. Readily available in the health care setting, this drug produces less pupil constriction (hard to detect), is effective if taken orally, and causes less constipation than other opioids (Lehne, 2004).

## NURSING ISSUES

### Overdose

At therapeutic doses prescribed and administered by professionals, morphine and meperidine are helpful and safe analgesics. However, drug abusers who buy these drugs on the street cannot be sure of the amount of opioid they are taking. Street purchases are not standardized, and users occasionally obtain a purer drug form than they anticipated. Inadvertent overdose might thus occur. The primary effect of overdose is respiratory depression. A respiratory rate at or below 12 breaths/minute is cause for concern. A recognizable symptom pattern for overdose is documented:

- The person becomes stuporous and then sleeps.
- The skin is wet and warm.
- Next, a coma develops, accompanied by respiratory depression and hypoxia.
- The skin becomes cold and clammy.
- The pupils dilate.
- Death quickly follows at this point.

Provision of an adequate airway and assisted ventilation, if needed, are treatment priorities. A narcotic antagonist is administered to reverse the effects of opioids.

### Narcotic Antagonists: Antidote to Opioids

The opioids are the only class of commonly abused drugs that have a specific antidote. Naloxone (Narcan), a narcotic antagonist, is the intervention of choice if opioid overdose is suspected. Naloxone blocks the neuroreceptors affected by opioids; thus, the patient responds in a few minutes to an IV injection of naloxone. Respiration improves, and the patient consciously responds. However, because most opioids have a longer lasting effect than naloxone, it is often necessary to repeat the antagonist to maintain adequate respiration. The nurse who administers naloxone must carefully observe the patient to determine whether additional antagonist will be needed. If the dose of the antagonist is proportionately higher than that of the opioids in the system, it is possible to precipitate a state of narcotic withdrawal or abstinence syndrome.

### CLINICAL EXAMPLE

A hospice team member told the following story. The patient was a 70-year-old man suffering from prostate cancer with painful bone metastases. A nursing concern is maintaining a balance between the need for pain management and the risk of respiratory suppression. The patient built up tolerance to his pain medication. His family members were afraid that he was becoming an "addict," so they decided to reduce his medication intake without consulting the physician. Cutting in half and administering a time-release pain pill (a synthetic morphine that lost its time-release properties when broken), they quickly noticed that Dad was not very responsive. He was taken to the hospital, and Narcan was administered. Because it blocks the opioid receptor sites, there was no effective pain relief for this patient. The man was in extreme physical pain because his family was afraid of the legitimate medical uses of pain medication. Additionally, lack of knowledge about how time-release medications work led to an erratic and fatal dose being administered.

### Interactions

The effects of opioids are increased when combined with other CNS depressants. Because the use of multiple drugs is common among drug abusers, the potential for deadly combinations is real. If it is known that heroin was taken and that naloxone does not reverse the CNS depression, it can be safely assumed that other depressants (e.g., barbiturates) were also taken. In cases such as these, supportive nursing care is indicated.

### Use by Older Adults

Some older patients might have chronic medical conditions associated with chronic pain for which long-term narcotic pain medication has been pre-scribed. Older adults are particularly at risk for decreased pulmonary ventilation associated with opioids.

### Use During Pregnancy

Women who abuse opioids give birth to babies who suffer withdrawal symptoms. These drugs can cross the placental barrier and produce respiratory depression in neonates.

### Withdrawal and Detoxification

The unassisted withdrawal from alcohol or barbiturates can be fatal, but unassisted withdrawal from opioids is rarely fatal, although often painful. The term *kicking the habit* comes from the leg spasms associated with the withdrawal from opioids. Withdrawal symptoms are related to the degree of dependence and the abruptness of the discontinuance. Maximal intensity is reached within 36 to 72 hours and subsides in about 1 week. Withdrawal symptoms include yawning, rhinorrhea, sweating, chills, piloerection (goose bumps), tremor, restlessness, irritability, leg spasm, bone pain, diarrhea, and vomiting.

Clonidine has been used successfully for withdrawal by relieving some of the autonomic symptoms (e.g., vomiting and diarrhea). Clonidine does not reduce craving, however. Buprenorphine (Buprenex) and naloxone (Narcan) have been found to be helpful in the detoxification of these individuals (Mathias, 2001). Treatment is primarily symptomatic and supportive.

## SPECIFIC DRUGS

Other opioids include hydromorphone (Dilaudid), a more potent derivative of morphine; levorphanol (Levo-Dromoran), a drug with an action identical to that of morphine but used for less severe pain; meperidine (Demerol), a synthetic narcotic analgesic; pentazocine (Talwin), which has weaker analgesic effects, is less addicting compared with other narcotic drugs, and is not supposed to cause euphoria; and several other related drugs. Fentanyl (Sublimaze), an anesthetic, is similar to but 100 times stronger than morphine and 50 times stronger than heroin. Many deaths have been attributed to fentanyl analogues (Lowinson et al, 1992). These drugs are typically sold as purer heroin.

### Methadone

Methadone (Dolophine), although an opioid similar to morphine, is used specifically to prevent withdrawal symptoms; it is also used as an analgesic in conditions associated with severe pain, such as cancer. Methadone is given orally and is poorly metabolized in the liver. Accordingly, methadone has a much longer half-life (15 to 30 hours) than morphine (about 2 hours). Because of its long half-life, once-daily dosing is effective and useful for outpatient care. When used to help lessen physiologic dependence on opioids, methadone is of great benefit. A longer acting related drug, levomethadyl (Orlaam), can be administered three times weekly instead of every day. This dosing schedule might be preferable for some individuals.

### Heroin

Heroin, which was originally a trade name developed by the Bayer Company in 1898 (Lowinson et al, 1992), was derived from morphine as a cure for morphine addiction, but proved to be more addictive by comparison. It is highly favored by opioid abusers. Heroin is typically taken IV (its effect is felt within 7 to 8 seconds) or smoked or snorted (10 to 15 minutes for effect) (Lehne, 2004). Oral use is less frequent and related to less intensity of the outcome.

### Codeine

Codeine is used primarily as a cough suppressant; its abuse preceded the general drug abuse of the middle to late 1960s because it was easily available in over-the-counter cough syrups. Ease of access was eliminated at about the same time that its drug abuse became recognized as an emerging national problem. Codeine is still a drug of choice for many substance abusers today.

### Oxycodone

Oxycodone (OxyContin), an effective painkiller, has received much attention in the media over the last decade. OxyContin is a time-release form of oxycodone, which has been available in other medications such as Percocet, Percodan, and Tylox for some time. By crushing OxyContin and then swallowing, snorting, or injecting the powder, substance abusers have found another way to achieve a high. Unfortunately, the widespread media coverage of these individuals has made clinicians reluctant to prescribe OxyContin for people suffering from severe pain. Emergency departments located near college campuses have seen a dramatic increase in OxyContin overdoses. Treatment of overdose has become routine because naloxone can quickly reverse the CNS and respiratory depression. The following clinical example, however, details a case in which the obvious was overlooked.

## CLINICAL EXAMPLE

A 32-year-old mother of two was seen in an emergency department in a medium-sized city. She had a history of psychiatric disorders and substance abuse. She admitted to ingesting a large number of OxyContin pills, along with other CNS depressants. She was alert at times but at other times displayed slurred speech and psychomotor retardation. After an initial assessment, it was decided that she should be sent to a free-standing psychiatric facility. Several hours later, she was taken to that facility. Upon admission late in the day, her speech was unintelligible and her respirations were noted to be slowed (12/minute) and irregular. A full assessment was deferred. She died from opioid-induced respiratory depression before morning.

## STIMULANTS

Use of stimulants containing caffeine such as soda, coffee, and tea is widespread. Many people feel sluggish if they do not start their day with a cup of coffee. Other more powerful stimulants, such as amphetamines and cocaine, are widely abused and cause immeasurable harm to society in the United States.

## COCAINE

Coca plants grow high in the Andes Mountains, and the Incas chewed coca leaves long before the Spanish explorers arrived. It should be noted that this plant is not cocoa, from which we get chocolate, but coca. Cocaine is still legitimately used today in some parts of Andean South America. As a mild tea, cocaine can help bring relief for altitude sickness. Cocaine is a fine, white, odorless powder with a bitter taste that was introduced to Western medicine as an anesthetic in 1858. Sigmund Freud was known to use cocaine and believed it to be a remedy for morphine addiction; he reported on the effects of cocaine in his book, *Cocaine Papers*. Cocaine was once used in some cola drinks (e.g., Coca-Cola), and advertisements extolled the ability of cola, as well as of other brain tonics, to refresh. After the Pure Food and Drug Act was passed in 1906, cocaine was eliminated from these beverages. Cocaine (cocaine hydrochloride) and its offspring, crack (freebase cocaine), are now responsible for a major drug problem. Many people have succumbed to this stimulant in their youth. The problems associated with cocaine extend to every level of society.

## PHYSIOLOGIC EFFECTS

Cocaine and its derivatives are addicting stimulants. Cocaine's exhilarating effect is related to its ability to block dopamine reuptake (Castaneda et al, 2000), particularly in the nucleus accumbens pleasure center in the brain (see Chapter 6). Although physical dependence is less severe than with opioid abuse, psychological dependence is intense. Abusers become tongue-tied when attempting to describe the sensations of this drug. Euphoria, increased mental alertness, increased strength, anorexia, and increased sexual stimulation are desired effects of these drugs. Increased motor activity, tachycardia (up to 200 bpm), and high blood pressure are PNS effects. CNS effects include deep respirations (from medullary stimulation), euphoria, increased mental alertness, dilated pupils, anorexia, and increased strength. The cocaine user can be loquacious and stimulated sexually (libido is increased, ejaculation retarded). This latter characteristic undoubtedly adds to the drug's overall appeal. Intense paranoia is common. This paranoia, in combination with other factors such as decreased inhibitions, partly explains why many drug deals go bad and result in someone being murdered.

Less common reactions are specific hallucinations and delusions. Cocaine users report what they think are bugs crawling beneath their skin (formication) and foul smells. Nasal septum perforation has been associated with snorting cocaine and is the result of extreme vasoconstriction, which impedes blood supply to this area and causes nasal necrosis. Death from cocaine is linked to metabolic and respiratory acidosis and hyperthermia associated with prolonged seizures. Tachyarrhythmias and coronary artery spasm have also led to death.

Tolerance to CNS and PNS effects develops quickly because neuronal norepinephrine stores are depleted, causing a need to increase drug amounts to create the desired effect. Tolerance develops to otherwise lethal amounts. Children born to mothers using cocaine are more likely to score lower on tests that measure alertness, attention, and intelligence than children of mothers who do not use cocaine (Zickler, 1999).

## ROUTES OF COCAINE USE

Cocaine hydrochloride is snorted or taken IV, but not smoked. Freebase cocaine (crack) is smoked.

Cocaine passes the blood-brain barrier quickly, causing an instantaneous high. When administered IV (mainlining), cocaine is rapidly metabolized by the liver, thus producing the rush, which, although exhilarating, does not last long. Cocaine exerts both CNS and PNS effects because of its ability to block norepinephrine and dopamine reuptake into presynaptic neurons; it depletes these neurotransmitters. Cocaine can also be swallowed (but is poorly absorbed this way) and snorted. Snorting, in which cocaine is absorbed through the nasal mucosa, was the preferred route of administration especially glamorized in the 1980s. With the discovery of smoking an adulterant-free cocaine crystalline base, freebasing became popular and paved the way for the advent of crack or rock cocaine.

## CRACK

Crack is a less expensive way of using cocaine compared with snorting or mainlining, primarily because it is sold and marketed in smaller packages, most commonly as $10 or $20 rocks. Crack is purported to be the most addictive drug on the streets today. It is produced in a relatively uncomplicated procedure (mixed with baking soda and water, heated, and hardened) and then smoked; it is reported to produce an instantaneous high and almost as instantaneous a crash. An intense desire to smoke again is produced. It is thought that the faster a drug's effect builds and then diminishes, the more

### CASE STUDY

J.R. is a 25-year-old unemployed carpenter who lives with his aunt. One night, he began tearing the house apart, then locked himself in the bathroom, yelling that he was going to kill himself. His aunt called the police, who brought J.R. to the emergency room of the local hospital. The emergency room examiner noted that J.R. was suicidal and having auditory hallucinations, delusions of persecution, disorganized thinking, anorexia, insomnia, anxiety, and agitation. He had been threatening the police and continued to be extremely agitated, threatening the emergency room personnel. Following some history from the aunt, the diagnosis of cocaine intoxication was made.

J.R.'s aunt stated that she had been concerned about possible drug use for the last couple of years but had never pursued the issue with J.R. He was often belligerent and was fired from his job until he was able to get "cleaned up." She had noticed things missing around the house but never questioned J.R. about this.

The emergency room physician decided to keep J.R. in the emergency room until his thinking cleared and to monitor him for tachycardia, cardiac arrhythmia, and seizure activity. The physician ordered 5 mg of diazepam (Valium) IV for 2 to 3 minutes every 10 to 15 minutes if needed for seizures and propranolol (Inderal) IV (0.1 to 0.15 mg/kg at a rate of 0.5 to 0.75 mg every 1 to 2 minutes) should the patient experience cardiac arrhythmias. J.R. was transferred to the psychiatric unit following 4 hours of observation in which there was no seizure activity or cardiac abnormalities.

On arrival at the unit, J.R. was noticeably irritable, agitated, and anxious, and complained of a headache. His responses to questions indicated continuing difficulty in concentration and some disorganized thinking. The care plan on the following page was developed.

addictive it is, thus explaining why crack is considered to be the most addictive drug (Wright, 1999).

Crack is cheap on a per-dose basis, but the user wants more immediately, so it is not an inexpensive drug to use. It is also easy to find. When the user's money is gone, however, the crash often gives way to cocaine-induced depression. This depression is sometimes severe to the point that users attempt suicide.

### CRITICAL THINKING QUESTION    1

Some former cocaine abusers turn to heroin as they grow older. Can you think of a reason why this might be so?

# Care Plan

Name: J.R.

Admission Date: _____

*DSM-IV-TR* Diagnosis: Substance intoxication and dependence

**Assessment**

**Areas of strength:** Young (25 years old); lives with aunt who wants him to return once he begins to feel better; previous employer will rehire him if he gets "clean."

**Problems:** Suicidal ideation, hallucinations (auditory), delusions that someone wants to kill him, thinking disorganized (has difficulty completing thoughts), anorexia, insomnia, anxious (has exaggerated startle reflex), agitated.

**Diagnoses**

- Potential for self-directed violence related to substance abuse or CNS agitation, as evidenced by history of suicide attempt.
- Alterations in perception related to substance abuse or CNS agitation, as evidenced by suicidal ideation, disorganized thinking, hallucinations, and delusions.
- Alteration in nutrition; less than body requirements related to anorexic effect of cocaine, as evidenced by loss of weight.

**Outcomes**

*Short-term goals:*                                                                          *Date met*

- Patient will not experience physical injury during hospitalization.         _____
- Patient will not experience symptoms of cocaine withdrawal.              _____
- Patient will sleep 6 to 8 hours per night.                                          _____
- Patient will admit that cocaine is a problem in his life.                        _____

*Long-term goals:*

- Patient will maintain optimal levels of nutrition and maintain at least 90% of normal weight.                                                           _____
- Patient will attend outpatient Cocaine Anonymous meetings.             _____
- Patient will practice abstinence from psychoactive drugs.                   _____
- Patient will verbalize and show some evidence of developing non–drug-using friends.                                                                     _____

**Planning/ Interventions**

**Nurse-patient relationship:** Develop a contract with patient to report to nurse if suicidal thoughts occur. Establish trusting relationship with patient. Provide reality-based conversation. Accept patient. Set limits on behavior, confront the patient with inconsistencies, and do not allow patient to manipulate. All staff must be consistent. Allow patient to verbalize anxiety and fear. Teach patient the effects of drugs on his body. Encourage independence in self-care, and reinforce examples of self-denial and delayed gratification.

**Psychopharmacology:** Desipramine 50 mg bid for cocaine withdrawal for 2 weeks. Haldol 5 mg PO q4h prn for agitation; Cogentin 2 mg PO with first dose of Haldol on days it is given. Tylenol tabs 2 q4h prn for headache.

**Milieu management:** Provide patient with a quiet room to decrease stimulation and agitation. Provide safe environment, including frequent observation by staff, monitoring of smoking, assessing vital signs prn. Monitor the environment for dangerous objects such as glass, razors, and belts. Provide foods the patient likes to increase interest in food. Provide group setting for patient to explore the issues of substance abuse with other patients and to help the patient get past the notion that no one understands his problems. Orient to surroundings.

**Evaluation**

Patient has not experienced significant cocaine withdrawal; appetite returning. Beginning to sleep better (4 to 6 hours). Patient has not attempted self-injury and denies suicidal intent.

**Referrals**

Outpatient treatment for aftercare, including Cocaine Anonymous meetings and random urine screens for increased accountability.

## CLINICAL EXAMPLE

Gladys is a 32-year-old woman who suffers from cocaine dependence and was referred to outpatient treatment through the legal system because of a possession charge. After her second group therapy session, she requests an individual session with her counselor. There, she reveals that 1 month earlier, other "customers" at the local crack house that she has frequented had raped her. Gladys is frightened and embarrassed; her urge to escape the emotional pain she feels by using is strengthened by her traumatic experience at the crack house. Although Gladys says that she has a supportive family, she is further ashamed and terrified because she thinks that she is pregnant. In her helplessness, Gladys experiences some suicidal ideation and talks about aborting the pregnancy. After she is calm, Gladys agrees to consult with her physician. After she does not return to treatment, no one answers the telephone, and there is no response to letters sent, Gladys is lost to contact. Six months later, Gladys calls her counselor to say that she put aside her shame and talked with her pastor, her mother, and her 12-year-old daughter. She reports that all is going well, although the baby was stillborn. She has not used since that time.

### Table 35-6    Contrasting Methamphetamine and Cocaine

| Methamphetamine | Cocaine |
| --- | --- |
| Synthetic | Plant derived |
| Smoking produces high that lasts 8-24 hours | Smoking produces high lasting 20-30 minutes |
| Half-life, 12 hours | Half-life, 1 hour |
| Limited medical use | Can be used as local anesthetic |

From Medline Plus: *How is methamphetamine different from other stimulants, such as cocaine?* Available at http://www.nida.nih.gov/researchreports/methamph/methamph4.html. Accessed November 18, 2005.

## AMPHETAMINES AND RELATED DRUGS

Amphetamines, which were developed in 1887, have medicinal uses, such as short-term treatment of obesity, attention–deficit/hyperactivity (ADHD) disorders in childhood, and narcolepsy. Amphetamines and some variants referred to as *speed, crystal, meth, ice,* or *crank* are widely abused. Examples of amphetamines include dextroamphetamine (Dexedrine), amphetamine (a 50:50 combination of D-amphetamine and L-amphetamine), methamphetamine (Desoxyn), and an amphetamine mixture (Adderall). Related drugs include methylphenidate (Ritalin), a drug also used in the treatment of ADHD, and 3,4-methylenedioxymethamphetamine (MDMA, Ecstasy).

## METHAMPHETAMINE

This drug is perhaps receiving the most national attention today. Its abuse has been described as an epidemic, and it can be produced quickly and cheaply. The Combat Meth Act of 2005 restricts the sale of some ingredients for methamphetamine (meth) production, such as pseudoephedrine and ephedrine. These drugs now must be kept behind the counter and there is a limitation on the quantity sold. Instructions for home production are readily available on the Internet. Interestingly, one of the main causes of burns significant enough to warrant hospitalization is from explosions experienced by meth cooks.

Methamphetamine (referred to as *speed, meth, crystal, crank,* or *ice*) produces a longer high than cocaine and is typically less expensive by comparison (Table 35-6). It stays in the body 10 times longer than cocaine (Herrick, 2005). Methamphetamine is frequently used as an adulterant of cocaine; it can be snorted, swallowed, injected, or smoked. It causes an immediate intense feeling of pleasure, followed by a lasting high. While high, the meth user doesn't sleep or eat and dental problems develop. Many young women have lost large amounts of weight and users have lost their teeth. When the high wears off, an equally intense crash occurs. Users become paranoid and might hallucinate or even experience violent rages. Long-term use of methamphetamine can cause damage to dopaminergic systems and other brain areas (Zickler, 2000).

Most methamphetamine users never again experience the intense peak of their first high. Many, however, spend their time, money, and health trying to do so. Eventually, methamphetamine abusers use meth to avoid feeling bad.

There are no drugs that effectively help fight methamphetamine addiction. People have to learn to deal with their cravings. Many never do.

## ECSTASY

Ecstasy, 3,4-methylenedioxymethamphetamine (MDMA) (also known as *XTC, E, X, rolls,* or *Adam*) was synthesized in the early 1900s and briefly used at some time later as an adjunct to psychotherapy. The chemical structure of Ecstasy is closely related to that of mescaline and methamphetamine. Ecstasy is a popular club drug, promoted as enhancing closeness to others, affection, and communication abilities (Allen, 2001). At higher doses, an amphetamine-like stimulation occurs, including euphoria, heightened sexuality, diminished self-consciousness, and disinhibition. Ecstasy also produces a psychedelic effect as well. Unpleasant amphetamine-type side effects also occur, such as tachycardia, increased blood pressure, anorexia, dry mouth, and teeth grinding (Taylor and Donoghue, 2001). Ecstasy results in memory impairment and appears to have a profound impact on the serotonin system (Mathias, 1999). Ecstasy has made headlines related to its use at raves, all-night dance parties in which drugs are used to enhance dancing and other activities. Hyperthermia, dehydration, rhabdomyolysis, renal failure, and deaths have been reported. Ecstasy is taken orally, and its effects last up to 6 hours (Taylor and Donoghue, 2001). Some research now indicates an Ecstasy-related loss of serotonin-producing neurons (Hess and DeBoer, 2002). Although the long-term consequences of altered serotonin neurons are not known, decline in memory and mood are likely.

## METABOLISM

Amphetamines are taken orally, well absorbed from the gastrointestinal tract, and excreted basically unchanged by the kidney, and continue to have an effect until cleared. Therapeutic parenteral administration is illegal in the United States, but many speed users self-administer amphetamines IV.

## PHYSIOLOGIC EFFECTS

Amphetamines are indirect-acting sympathomimetics that cause the release of norepinephrine from nerve endings. Amphetamines also block norepinephrine reuptake in presynaptic nerve endings. Similar to cocaine, amphetamines also have a profound effect on the pleasure pathway by enhancing dopamine, sometimes referred to as the pleasure neurotransmitter. Amphetamines block dopamine reuptake but also stimulate excess release of dopamine and retard its enzymatic breakdown. This affect on dopamine and the dopamine system probably accounts for amphetamines' so-called addicting effects. CNS effects range from wakefulness, alertness, heightened concentration, energy, and improved mood to euphoria, insomnia (sometimes desired, sometimes not), and amnesia. The most common side effects of amphetamine use are restlessness, dizziness, agitation, and insomnia. PNS effects are palpitations, tachycardia, and hypertension. Respirations also increase because, similar to cocaine, the amphetamines stimulate the medulla. A psychiatric side effect of amphetamine use is amphetamine-induced psychosis. In the emergency room, this psychotic presentation can be almost indistinguishable from paranoid schizophrenia.

## NURSING ISSUES

### Overdose

Cocaine and amphetamine overdoses have resulted in a number of deaths, resulting primarily from cardiac arrhythmias and respiratory collapse. Smoking cocaine adds to the problem because large amounts reach the system quickly. Toxic levels of amphetamines cause tachycardia, severe hypertension, cardiac ischemia, cerebral hemorrhage, seizures, and coma. Treatment includes induction of vomiting, acidification of the urine, and forced diuresis. In patients with amphetamine psychosis related to toxic levels of these drugs, chlorpromazine or haloperidol given intramuscularly (IM) will antagonize the amphetamine effect.

### Interactions

The effects of cocaine and amphetamines are augmented when combined with other CNS stimulants. Many over-the-counter products such as hay fever medications and decongestants contain stimulants. Urinary alkalinizing agents such as sodium bicarbonate decrease the elimination of amphetamines, whereas urinary acidifying agents increase the elimination of amphetamines.

### Use During Pregnancy

Amphetamines should be used during pregnancy only if clearly needed, because harm to the fetus has been demonstrated. Cocaine-addicted mothers give birth to addicted babies with multiple problems, withdrawal and physical problems of the neonate being only the beginning of a lifetime of resulting effects. About 400,000 infants born each year in the United States are exposed to cocaine in the womb, and are known as *crack babies* when they are born (Anonymous, 1998). As they have reached school age, impaired neurologic development of the exposed fetus has become apparent and is associated with an explosion of children with behavior and learning problems in special education programs.

### Withdrawal and Detoxification

Although cocaine and amphetamines are highly addictive, physical withdrawal is relatively mild. Psychological withdrawal is severe, however, because the drugs are highly pleasurable and because of the depletion of monoamines, which is known to be associated with depression. For individuals withdrawing from amphetamines under medical supervision, the withdrawal process is gradual and safe. Cold turkey withdrawal without medical supervision causes agitation, irritability, and severe depression, frequently with suicidal ideation. As a rule of thumb, the low of withdrawal will be inversely proportional to the high experienced. Withdrawal from cocaine causes intense craving for the drug. A number of approaches are used, all of which aim to restore depleted neurotransmitters. The administration of amino acid catecholamine precursors, such as tyrosine and phenylalanine, tricyclic antidepressants, and the dopamine agonist bromocriptine, is one method used to increase the availability of neurotransmitters.

## HALLUCINOGENS

Hallucinogens, also referred to as psychotomimetics or psychedelics, cause hallucinations. Hallucinogens are divided into two basic groups, natural and synthetic. Natural hallucinogenic substances include mescaline (peyote [from cactus]), psilocybin (psilocin [from mushrooms]), and marijuana (*Cannabis sativa*). Synthetic or semisynthetic substances include lysergic acid diethylamide (LSD) and phencyclidine (PCP). In general, hallucinogens can heighten awareness of reality or can cause a terrifying psychosis-like reaction. Users report distortions in body image and a sense of depersonalization. Particularly frightening is a loss of the sense of reality. Hallucinations depicting grotesque creatures, such as a dog with a snake for a tongue, can be extremely frightening. Emotional consequences of these effects are panic, anxiety, confusion, and paranoid reactions. Some individuals have experienced frank psychotic reactions after minimal use. In the jargon of the hallucinogens, this experience is known as a *bad trip*. The drugs discussed here do not represent an exhaustive accounting of hallucinogens; refer to other sources for a more definitive review of these agents.

## MESCALINE

Mescaline (peyote) is derived from cactus plants found in North America. Native Americans have harvested peyote buttons from cacti and used them in their religious ceremonies. This religious practice was protected by law as part of their worship until 1990, when the U.S. Supreme Court ruled that states can prohibit its use. Mescaline is taken orally, its site of action is probably the norepinephrine synapses, and its effects last up to 12 hours.

### Physiologic Effects

With mescaline, colors are vivid, music is beautiful, and sounds become intense. When users close their eyes, colors and images can be seen. A distorted sense of space and time occurs. A young man who drove his car after taking peyote stated that it seemed to take an eternity to reach a stop sign no more than 50 feet away. The experience is directly related to preingestion expectations. Good experiences include hilarity and joy. The user might feel especially insightful. The answers to questions such as those involving the meaning of life might seem clear. These insights can easily add to the sense of an almost religious experience. If the conversation were recorded and replayed later, however, the users would not be as impressed with their having encountered what they believed to be ultimate truth (this is also true of marijuana). Bad trips are the side effects of concern. Although peyote is less potent than LSD, it still can cause panic, paranoid thinking, and anxiety if the trip is too intense. Dependence does not occur in the strict sense, yet users enjoy the experience and seek to repeat it. Pupil dilation and tremors sometimes occur.

## PSILOCYBIN AND PSILOCIN

Psilocybin is derived from mushrooms *(Psilocybe mexicana)* and converted to psilocin in the stomach.

The effects last up to 8 hours. Hallucinations and time, space, and perceptual alterations are experienced and are the basis of some Native American groups' continued use of psilocybin in religious and other sacred ceremonies to facilitate integration of body, mind, and spirit. Psilocybin dilates the pupils and increases heart rate, blood pressure, and body temperature. Tingling of the skin and involuntary movements can occur. Similar to other hallucinogens, a sense of unreality can be experienced. An inability to concentrate might add to feelings of anxiety and lead to panic and paranoia. Hallucinations and illusions might occur. Although no deaths from psilocybin toxicity have been reported, deaths related to perceptual distortions have occurred.

## MARIJUANA

Cultivation of marijuana (also known as *pot, weed,* and *grass*) has taken place for over 5000 years. Marijuana is the drug most widely used illegally in the United States. Marijuana and other related drugs (hashish and tetrahydrocannabinol [THC]) come from an Indian hemp plant. It is difficult to categorize. Placement with the hallucinogens seems appropriate, but it can also have other categorizations. Marijuana varies significantly in strength depending on the climate and soil conditions in which it is grown.

### Metabolism

The active ingredient in marijuana is delta-9-tetrahydrocannabinol (THC). THC, which is changed to metabolites in the body and stored in fatty tissues, remains in the body for up to 6 weeks after it is smoked and can be detected in blood and urine for 3 days to about 4 weeks, depending

on its level of use. The effects of smoked marijuana last between 2 and 4 hours. If marijuana is ingested, effects might last up to 12 hours.

### Physiologic Effects

Marijuana produces a sense of well-being, is relaxing, and alters perceptions. Euphoria results and is the cause of drug-seeking behaviors. Increased hunger (known as the *munchies*) is an effect that makes marijuana useful for anorexic individuals (e.g., patients with cancer who are undergoing chemotherapy). Marijuana's antiemetic properties make it useful for treating nausea and vomiting associated with chemotherapy. Some states have now legalized its use for this purpose.

Balance and stability are impaired for up to 8 hours after marijuana use. Short-term memory, decision making, and concentration are also impaired. Dry mouth, sore throat, increased heart rate, dilated pupils, conjunctival irritation (i.e., red eyes), and keener sight and hearing are physical responses to marijuana. Marijuana has also been thought to be amotivational, but not all research supports this.

Other effects associated with the use of marijuana include harmful pulmonary effects (bronchitis), weakening of heart contractions, immunosuppression, and reduction of the serum testosterone level and sperm count. Anxiety, impaired judgment, paranoia, and panic are not uncommon reactions to marijuana. Memory is also impaired related to occupation of THC receptors on the hippocampus. These experiences might culminate in some health-compromising behavior. Flashbacks, more commonly associated with LSD, have also been reported. A flashback is a spontaneous reliving of feelings experienced during a high.

| CRITICAL THINKING QUESTION | 2 |
|---|---|

If you believe that marijuana is benign, would you want your neurosurgeon to "take the edge off" by taking a few tokes just before surgery to remove your mother's brain tumor? Yes or no? Explain and justify your answer.

## LYSERGIC ACID DIETHYLAMIDE

Lysergic acid diethylamide (LSD), which stimulates the nervous system by binding tightly to serotonin receptors (i.e., 5-HT$_2$), is taken orally, and the effects are experienced for up to 12 hours. LSD causes a phenomenon known as *synesthesia,* which is the blending of senses (e.g., smelling a color or tasting a sound). Expectations and environment govern the quality of the LSD trip. LSD causes an increase in blood pressure, tachycardia, trembling, and dilated pupils. CNS effects include a sense of unreality, perceptual alterations and distortions, and impaired judgment. Another problem with LSD is flashbacks. Flashbacks are scary and can heighten a sense of going crazy. Bad trips from LSD cause anxiety, paranoia, and acute panic. Some users have suffered psychotic breaks from LSD and have never fully recovered. A number of individuals have killed themselves while under the influence of LSD (Anonymous, 1994; Box 35-4).

## PHENCYCLIDINE AND KETAMINE

Phencyclidine (PCP, angel dust, hog), a synthetic drug, has been traditionally used in veterinary medicine as an anesthetic. Many emergency room nurses are familiar with this drug because PCP-intoxicated individuals are often brought to the emergency room. The unpredictable outbursts of violent behavior of PCP patients are legendary; they literally change from coma to violent behavior and back. Caution must be exercised when providing care to these patients because of their unpredictable behavior. PCP is taken orally, IV, smoked, and snorted. Effects last for 6 to 8 hours.

The PCP user experiences a high. Euphoria and a peaceful, easy feeling can be felt and are sought after. Perceptual distortions are common. Undesired effects of PCP can be serious. Blood pressure and heart rate are elevated. Other PNS effects include ataxia, salivation, and vomiting. A catatonic-type of muscular rigidity alternating with violent outbursts is particularly frightening to bystanders. Psychological symptoms include hostile, bizarre behavior, a blank stare, and agitation.

Ketamine (K, Special K) is a general anesthetic used for minor surgery. It causes a dissociative effect. Bad experiences with ketamine are called a *K-hole.* Because of its amnesic properties, ketamine has also been implicated in date rapes.

### CLINICAL EXAMPLE

Mary Sky is an 18-year-old high school student who has recently become involved with peers who use various hallucinogenic drugs to help them with their spiritual quests. Mary attended a ceremony last night during which she had LSD for the first time. Initially, she experienced anxiety as the sky became a brilliant blue and particular stars seemed to shine brightly, as if they were directly in front of her. Mary soon began smiling a lot and realized the depth of "this process called life" and how we are all "a part of the stars." This heightened experience continued throughout the evening. By the next day, all that remained was memory of bliss and insights, but Mary's actual state of consciousness had returned to its usual state, with all her previously standing inner conflicts.

## NURSING ISSUES

### *Overdose*

High doses of mescaline are not generally toxic. Deaths, however, have occurred. Psilocybin overdose has not been associated with any deaths, and usually a calm environment is all that is needed to assist withdrawal. LSD- and PCP-related deaths are not uncommon. Deaths can be caused by overdose but are more likely to be associated with perceptual disorientation and unresponsiveness to environmental stimuli. Confusion and acute panic can result from an overdose of marijuana, LSD, and other hallucinogens. Diazepam (Valium) can be administered for psilocybin, LSD, and mescaline overdoses and is known to terminate panic attacks caused by these drugs (Hollister et al, 1993). PCP presents greater problems. Diazepam might be given for seizures and agitation and haloperidol (Haldol) for psychotic behavior. Acidifying the urine to a pH of 5.5 accelerates its excretion. Urine screening is the best means of identifying these abused substances.

## Interactions

Mescaline, psilocybin, and LSD can enhance the effects of sympathomimetics. Marijuana should not be used with alcohol, because marijuana masks the nausea and vomiting associated with excessive alcohol consumption. Respiratory depression, coma, and death can occur.

## Use During Pregnancy

A number of birth defects have been associated with these drugs. Obviously, hallucinogenic drugs should not be taken during pregnancy.

## Withdrawal and Detoxification

Hallucinogens do not produce physical dependence, so no withdrawal symptoms occur. Symptoms of withdrawal from marijuana can include extreme irritability, insomnia, restlessness, and hyperactivity. One of the biggest concerns for the nurse is the development of an approach for dealing with the intoxicated person. Basically, the nurse should provide a calm, reassuring environment.

## RELATED ISSUES

## EFFECTS ON FAMILY

Although the substance-dependent person is the designated patient, all family members are affected. The family is usually in need of treatment as well. Family members of addicts and alcoholics are referred to as *co-dependent,* reflecting the process of participating in behaviors that maintain the addiction or allow it to continue without holding the addict or alcoholic accountable for his or her actions. These behaviors become so ingrained that they are difficult to alter when the addict or alcoholic stops using. If the family also gets into recovery via co-dependency treatment or self-help groups such as AA, Narcotics Anonymous, or Co-Dependents Anonymous, they often find many underlying issues of their own that contributed to their selection of a mate with an alcohol or drug problem. For example, many spouses are children of alcoholics or other dysfunctional family systems in which they, out of necessity for survival, had to take on caretaking responsibilities within the family, setting them up to repeat these behaviors in adult relationships. Dealing with these past traumas and learning ways to let others be responsible for themselves are important aspects of family recovery.

In some cases, the family has been affected to the extent that the family member might alternate between rescuing (or enabling) the abuser and blaming the abuser. Examples of rescuing include the following: (1) making excuses for the abuser, (2) lying for the abuser, and (3) doing things that the person with a substance-related problem should have done. Oddly enough, living with a recovering addict or alcoholic can sometimes be more difficult than living with an active user (see Clinical Example that follows). Most units for substance-related disorders have a number of classic stories in which, after abstinence was achieved, the addict or alcoholic was encouraged to start using again, or the spouse separated from the addict or alcoholic. Once drug- and alcohol-free, the person with substance-related problems begins to participate in family functions that have been taken over by other family members. Family roles are difficult to give up, even when they were initially adopted out of necessity. It is sometimes difficult for families and friends to hold the addict or alcoholic accountable; however, on hearing that their loved one is in jail, the family reasons that it is better than hearing the dreaded words from the police, "Your loved one is dead." The clinical example about Bill represents a situation in which a family resists role changes. Sometimes the family gets well, but the addicted person does not. Conversely, sometimes the addicted person gets well and the family does not.

## CLINICAL EXAMPLE

Bill Waters was a 48-year-old house painter. He was an alcoholic and, although he was not as productive as he had been in years past, he still made a good living until recently. In the last 6 months, his alcoholism began to have more and more of an effect on his work. He lost one important job because he was unable to meet the deadlines he had established. His home life had been dysfunctional for years. Weekends were only a blur, because he drank beer continuously and watched television. His wife Wanda made sure that the bills were paid and took care of all the children's needs. Bill never interfered but would occasionally spend money on alcohol before Wanda was able to pay a bill.

In recent years, however, Wanda had caught on to all of Bill's tricks, and he rarely had an opportunity to spend household money. When Bill was too hung over to go to work, Wanda called and made up the excuses. Wanda covered for Bill at church and in other situations in which his heavy drinking would be an embarrassment. Wanda alternated between protecting Bill and blaming him. Her life now revolved around Bill and his problems. After Bill lost an important painting contract, Wanda insisted on treatment. Bill attended a 6-week inpatient treatment program. On his return, Bill was ready to reestablish himself as the husband and father, but Wanda was not ready to trust him. In essence, what had happened, and what happens in many families such as these, is that Wanda had to take over responsibilities of making decisions, and she was not willing to give them up without long-term proof of Bill's sobriety and responsibility. He had promised to stay sober many times before and failed. Bill, on the other hand, had a clear head for a change and wanted to be the "man of the house" again. Although neither Bill nor Wanda was able to articulate the new problems with which they were struggling, they did recognize emotions that they were unable to control. Bill and Wanda soon divorced. A marriage that was able to withstand alcoholism was not able to withstand recovery.

## CHILDREN OF ALCOHOLICS

Several classic roles have been delineated in alcoholic or substance-abusing homes (Wegscheider, 1981; Wegscheider-Cruse, 2000). As the balance in family responsibilities shifts in response to the irresponsible behavior of the alcoholic or addict, children in particular adopt certain roles in an effort to maintain homeostasis. As children of alcoholics grow, they tend to recreate the same dynamics in their relationships to which they became accustomed as children, thus ensuring reenactment of trauma. For example, the hero role is assumed by the child in the alcoholic or addicted family who excels at everything in spite of all the turmoil at home. Table 35-7 describes these roles.

## TREATING THE CHEMICALLY DEPENDENT PERSON

The most common goal of treatment for the chemically dependent person is abstinence from alcohol or drugs. It is believed that the person who is dependent on one substance can easily become dependent on another. The term *cross-dependence* describes this condition. Professionals working with chemically dependent individuals realize their patients' vulnerability and usually refrain from thinking of anyone as being cured. Professionals tend to view treatment as an ongoing, lifelong process in which the person abstaining from formerly abused substances is recovering. The term *recovering* indicates a current and dynamic process but also indicates the ever-present possibility of slipping.

## DIAGNOSTIC TOOLS FOR CHEMICAL DEPENDENCY

Many tools exist for the evaluation of chemical dependency. Criteria set forth in the *DSM-IV-TR* (APA, 2000) are among the most helpful in diagnosing a person with chemical dependence. Early diagnosis can mean a better treatment prognosis. Misdiagnosis can lead to unsuspected withdrawal, drug interactions, or both. Ultimately, an accurate diagnosis might mean the difference between life and death. It is most important that the nurse look for behavioral and physical clues when making diagnostic evaluations with the treatment team.

## TOOLS FOR ALCOHOLISM

Several screening questionnaires have been developed to assist the health care professional in diagnosing alcohol dependency. Among the easiest are the Michigan Alcoholism Screening Test (MAST)

## Table 35-7    Family Roles and Their Features in Alcoholic Families*

| Family Role | Characteristics | Example |
|---|---|---|
| Caretaker | Tends to everyone's needs in the family; makes sure the family looks normal to the outside | Marjorie gets up at 4:30 in the morning so that she can make the kids' lunches, clean up her teenager's room, pay the bills, and clean up the mess her husband made when he ran over the flower bed coming in drunk a few hours earlier. She has to be efficient because she has agreed to do all the carpooling during the month and has to lead the parents' meeting at 7 this morning. |
| Hero | Responsible, wants to be the best; might be the teacher's pet; excels in academics, athletics, or some other area | Jenny gets up early so she can practice for the school play. She hopes to get a scholarship to study drama in Europe. She is an A student and has time for many extracurricular activities including drama, debate, and the school newspaper. She was recently elected class president. |
| Scapegoat | Gets in trouble, breaks rules, defies authority; shifts focus away from the alcoholic or addict | Jimmy is late to school again and was caught smoking in the bathroom. He has been suspended twice this year and is barely passing most of his classes. He slammed the door and ran from the building when the principal was about to call his father. |
| Mascot | Class clown; defuses stress; distracts people from problems with humor and foolishness | Mary has lots of friends and loves to be the life of the party. Whenever anyone is down and out, they can always count on Mary for a good laugh. Last night, when Mary's dad came home drunk, her mom was really upset and Mary had her laughing before it was over with. Mary keeps everyone in the family guessing what she might say or do next. |
| Lost child | Disappears from the activity of the family; does not ever make waves; stays to herself or himself, blends in with the surroundings | Jane is very quiet and unobtrusive. She sits in the back of the class and rarely speaks. She will answer if called, but otherwise no one really notices whether she is there. At home, Jane stays in her room, watches television, and reads and plays alone. She never has friends over and never asks for anything. Jane figures it is best just to try to keep things as calm as possible. |

*These roles were identified by Sharon Wegscheider in her book *Another chance: hope and health for the alcoholic family,* Palo Alto, CA, 1988, Science and Behavior Publishers.

and the CAGE questionnaire. Many other tools are available. The purpose of these tools is to provide an objective assessment for identifying alcoholism or addiction. The health care professional must further assess the potential for a problem of alcoholism or addiction in any patient who answers affirmatively to questions about alcohol or drug use. The problem with most screening tests, particularly for drug abusers, has been their susceptibility to faking and denial on the part of the patient.

### Michigan Alcoholism Screening Test

The MAST is a good screening tool that can help the unconvinced patient gain insight into at least the possibility of a problem if questions are answered honestly. This test can also aid the clinician in diagnostic assessment and can be easily modified to identify other drug problems.

### CAGE Questionnaire

The CAGE questionnaire is another valid instrument. Even easier to administer and possibly perceived as less accusatory compared with the MAST, the following four questions comprise this tool:

1. Have you ever felt you should **C**ut down on your drinking?
2. Have people **A**nnoyed you by criticizing your drinking?
3. Have you ever felt bad or **G**uilty about your drinking?
4. Have you ever had an **E**ye-opener in the morning to steady your nerves or get rid of a hangover?

Two positive responses are suggestive of alcoholism, and three or four positive responses are diagnostic (Whitfield et al, 1986).

## DIAGNOSING DRUG ABUSE

Alcohol abuse and drug abuse have many similarities; however, there are several significant differences: alcohol is typically legal, whereas many drugs of abuse are illegal (or, if legal, taken out of compliance with the law); stages of drug abuse tend to advance more rapidly as compared with alcohol; and drugs can produce their desired effect almost instantly. (See the *DSM-IV-TR* and NANDA International Diagnoses Related to Chemical Dependency box.)

---

### *DSM-IV-TR* and NANDA International Diagnoses Related to Chemical Dependency

*DSM-IV-TR**
Alcohol abuse
Alcohol dependence
Alcohol intoxication
Alcohol intoxication delirium
Alcohol withdrawal
Amphetamine (or related substance) abuse
Amphetamine (or related substance) dependence
Amphetamine (or related substance) intoxication
Amphetamine (or related substance) withdrawal
Caffeine intoxication
Cannabis abuse
Cannabis dependence
Cannabis intoxication
Cocaine abuse
Cocaine dependence
Cocaine intoxication
Cocaine withdrawal
Hallucinogen abuse
Hallucinogen dependence
Hallucinogen intoxication
Hallucinogen persisting perception disorder
Inhalant abuse
Inhalant dependence
Inhalant intoxication
Nicotine dependence
Nicotine withdrawal
Opioid abuse
Opioid dependence
Opioid intoxication
Opioid withdrawal
Phencyclidine (or related substance) abuse
Phencyclidine (or related substance) dependence
Phencyclidine (or related substance) intoxication
Sedative, hypnotic, or anxiolytic abuse
Sedative, hypnotic, or anxiolytic dependence
Sedative, hypnotic, or anxiolytic intoxication
Sedative, hypnotic, or anxiolytic withdrawal
Polysubstance dependence
Other (or unknown) substance abuse

Other (or unknown) substance dependence
Other (or unknown) substance intoxication
Other (or unknown) substance withdrawal

NANDA INTERNATIONAL[†]
Anxiety
Communication, verbal, impaired
Coping, ineffective
Family processes, alcoholism, dysfunctional
Fear
Grieving, dysfunctional
Growth and development, delayed
Hopelessness
Infection, risk for
Injury, risk for
Knowledge, deficient
Noncompliance
Nutrition, less than body requirements, imbalanced
Nutrition, more than body requirements, imbalanced
Nutrition, more than body requirements, risk for imbalanced
Pain, acute
Pain, chronic
Parenting, impaired
Powerlessness
Self-care deficit, bathing/hygiene
Self-care deficit, dressing/grooming
Self-care deficit, feeding
Self-care deficit, toileting
Self-esteem, chronic low
Self-esteem, situational low
Self-esteem, situational low, risk for
Sensory perception, disturbed
Sexual dysfunction
Sleep patterns, disturbed
Social isolation
Spiritual distress
Thought processes, disturbed
Violence, other-directed, risk for
Violence, self-directed, risk for

*From the American Psychiatric Association: *Diagnostic and statistical manual of mental disorders, text revision,* ed 4, Washington, DC, 2000, APA.
[†]From NANDA International: *NANDA nursing diagnoses: definitions and classifications, 2005-2006,* Philadelphia, 2005, NANDA International.

## PSYCHOTHERAPEUTIC MANAGEMENT

Alcoholism is highly treatable. Success of treatment for abuse of other chemical substances varies, but recovery is possible with all chemical dependencies. The success of treatment, however, depends first on the patient's motivation (Box 35-5) and then on the clinician's skill in interpreting data and implementing treatment strategies (Steinberg et al, 1997). The importance of understanding the role of each of the three psychotherapeutic management interventions is crucial. In working with these individuals, the nurse must realize that milieu management has the potential to be more important for this group of patients than for other types of patients. With these ideas in mind, it is important to note that two dominant but divergent general philosophies determine the treatment that most professionals will provide. In the broadest sense, the two umbrella treatment philosophies are (1) the behavioral model and (2) the disease model.

The behavioral model defines addiction as a habit that interferes with work, home, school, health, and relationships, a habit that the addicted individual believes he or she cannot change (Peele and Brodskey, 1991). Adherents of this model point to research that seems to indicate that two brief counseling sessions with the problem drinker's physician can lead to sustained, significantly reduced alcohol consumption (Manissa Communication Group, 1997). One approach of the behavioral model is moderation management—that is, learning to drink in moderation.

The disease model points to physiologic effects and explanations. The goal of treatment is total abstinence. Obviously, when something as significant as alcohol in an alcoholic's life is removed, something must take its place. This can be in the form of counseling groups facilitated by nurses or other professionals or 12-step programs directed by successfully recovering individuals.

The two philosophies vehemently disagree on treatment approaches but do agree that substance dependence frequently shows itself in self-destructive behavior. Most professionals are legitimately concerned about this self-destruction and want to be part of relieving the negative results of AOD use among this population. We see the validity in both perspectives and believe that a proper approach lies somewhere between them. Although a person's initial exposure to AOD use seems to be influenced by both genetic and environmental factors, it also seems that, once ingested, the substance reinforces continued use by its actions on neurons (Roberts and Koob, 1997).

## NURSE-PATIENT RELATIONSHIP

Because most addicted people are experiencing a problem in many areas of their lives when they seek treatment, understanding positive motivators will help in establishing new goals and directions for the patient's life. The patient's ability to function at work, at home, in society, and in many roles has been compromised by alcohol and drugs. Stated another way, almost no one comes to treatment because life is going well. The converse is almost always true: the boss is going to fire him or her, the spouse is going to leave, or the judge is sending the person to jail. Treatment for chemically dependent people is usually initiated out of a crisis. To the degree that treatment can help the patient replace ineffective behaviors with new coping skills, the patient has a better chance of getting and staying sober. Coping skills worthy of

---

### Box 35-5   Motivation

Whether external coercion is a positive influence on treatment outcome is a matter of disagreement. Participants who voluntarily seek treatment are more compliant with their therapists than are those coerced into treatment. Participants who are coerced into treatment might be compliant only while the coercive influence is present and might be compliant only with behaviors specified by the coercive agent. (One example would be the client who does not drive after drinking, but insists on continuing alcohol use, which has proven to contribute to problems in other areas of life.)

In one study (Steinberg et al, 1997), data were contradictory about whether coerced and voluntary participants have different treatment outcomes. "[One measure] found that external motivation was related to a positive treatment outcome only when internal motivation was also present." Internal sources of motivation included spouse/family (28.5%), increasing problems with alcohol, wants to stop but can't (17.1%), and mental health affected by drinking (15.9%). Of the 19 participants with external sources of motivation, 18 (90%) were coerced by their spouses to seek treatment.

From Steinberg ML, Epstein EE, McCrady BS, Hirsch LS: Sources of motivation in a couple's outpatient alcoholism treatment program, *Am J Drug Alcohol Abuse* 23:191, 1997.

nursing effort include work skills and habits, job search skills, homemaking, parenting, financial management, family communication, family role responsibilities, and exploration of leisure activities (Stoffel, 1994).

Establishing a trusting therapeutic relationship with the patient in which the rules for treatment are consistently applied is the benchmark for working with chemically dependent individuals. Genuineness is the single most important quality of this relationship. Expressing empathy and providing a safe environment that minimizes anxiety are also important, especially in the early stages of treatment, while the patient is going through the painful withdrawal process. Engendering feelings of hope for the future is also necessary as the patient begins to establish new life goals. Nurses working with chemically dependent patients must become skilled at confronting denial and managing manipulation.

Because denial is the most predominant defense of the alcoholic, treating it appropriately is important. A group therapy setting seems to provide the best avenue for treatment because groups are especially effective in breaking down the denial process through confrontation, as well as supporting group members who share a common struggle. Confrontation includes telling a patient what is observed through supportive but reflective listening techniques, irrespective of the strength of a patient's denial.

### Confrontation

Here are two common examples of confrontation:

1. "You say you have not been drinking (or using drugs), but I can smell alcohol on your breath (or cocaine was detected in your urine sample)."
2. "I hear you saying that you are in treatment because you believe you need help, so help me understand how you see your need, given your absence from treatment all week without a medical excuse."

What seems to be most effective is when the patient's peers provide appropriate confrontation, as, for example, when Lloyd reported to the group that he had not used alcohol in the last 3 months. Lloyd's peer, Christy, had appropriately used the group for support earlier that session to process her own recent relapse episode. Christy was able to confront Lloyd directly about his lying, because she had happened to see him at the same club where she had been the previous weekend.

### Personal Responsibility

It is important to help the patient learn to foster personal responsibility for recovery. The nurse must cultivate an awareness by the patient that responsibility for change lies within himself or herself. Furthermore, while expressing support and concern for the patient in recovery, the nurse must not shield the patient from the negative consequences of the patient's own addictive behavior.

### Conscience Development

Paradoxically, one of the most effective means for placing responsibility with the patient is in a group that fosters responsibility for another patient in the group. Essentially, patients in these groups are told directly that they have done a poor job of guiding their own lives to the extent that this level of personal responsibility is incomprehensible. However, perhaps they might be able to guide and be responsible for someone else. This idea is novel and intriguing to most patients, until a crisis moment occurs. For example, the program has a rule that no one can drink alcohol on a pass. Joe is responsible for Bill. Bill drinks over the weekend, and Joe is punished. Punishment can range from a loss of coffee privileges to dismissal from the treatment program. Joe, who has perhaps lied, stolen, and connived for years to pursue his dependency, is speechless at the unfairness of the decision. Bill, on the other hand, although feeling some sense of relief at first because he escapes his punishment, soon begins to feel the anger of other group members for causing the innocent Joe to be punished. Bill, who might have perpetrated all types of dastardly events in his life with little remorse (a limited internal conscience), begins to have all sorts of feelings because the group is his conscience now (external conscience). Groups such as these are effective, particularly when occupational or legal consequences are dependent on program completion.

## Lifestyle Issues

The nurse must teach the patient the effects of chemical abuse on the body and provide for the physical and special nutritional needs of the patient. Exercise is crucial to increase mental and physical vitality, as are relaxation, avoidance of stress, and rest. A balanced diet and vitamin and mineral supplements are also essential parts of treatment and recovery. Patients recovering from alcohol or drugs must learn to detach themselves from old playmates and playgrounds that were representative of or involved with their drug use.

## PSYCHOPHARMACOLOGY

Treatment for chemical dependency using medication is becoming increasingly important as knowledge about brain biochemistry increases. Major categories of chemical dependency and pharmacologic approaches to these dependencies are briefly addressed here.

## Medications Used to Treat Alcohol Dependence

Long-acting benzodiazepines such as chlordiazepoxide (Librium), diazepam (Valium), and lorazepam (Ativan) are useful for treatment of alcohol withdrawal. The principle behind this treatment is the rapid substitution of the benzodiazepine for the alcohol to suppress withdrawal symptoms. Benzodiazepines bind to the GABA-benzodiazepine receptor sites, thus explaining their mechanism of action. The next step is a gradual tapering of benzodiazepines over several days. Some clinicians prefer barbiturates for alcohol withdrawal, but respiratory depression and safety concerns dissuade most prescribers.

---

### Patient and Family Education

#### Substance-Related Disorders

##### Illness

There is divided opinion as to whether a substance-related disorder should be described as an illness or disease. To call something a disease implies that symptoms of the disease are beyond the control of the individual. Some professionals find this appealing because it allows the patient and her or his significant others to move beyond blaming and name calling and to focus on treatment. Other professionals disagree; according to them, classifying absenteeism, job loss, frequent accidents and injuries to self and others, inattention to appearance, lying, and sneaking around as symptoms of a disease suggests enabling behavior. Whatever your view, the reality of substance abuse can be seen everywhere. It devastates lives, wrecks homes, kills innocent bystanders, and stifles society and culture. Whatever is said in these pages is too much *and* never enough; too much, because people simply become addicted to substances to blur their reality, and never enough, because it can never capture the enormity, complexity, and gravity of substance-related disorders.

##### Medications

A number of drugs are used in the treatment of substance-related disorders. A brief description of those agents follows.

*Antabuse*—interferes with the metabolic breakdown of alcohol, thus making people extremely sick if they drink while taking this drug.

*ReVia*—reduces the craving for alcohol.

*Benzodiazepines* (e.g., Valium, Ativan)—diminish the symptoms of withdrawal from alcohol.

*Narcan*—used for opioid (e.g., heroin, morphine) overdose.

*Methadone*—used as a substitute for heroin, thus helping ease the person off heroin.

*Orlaam*—same actions as methadone.

##### Other Issues

All family members are affected by substance abuse. Hence, the family is usually also in need of treatment. Families often fluctuate between enabling (e.g., making excuses, lying for, doing things for) and blaming the abuser. An interesting point, verified over and over, is the reality that some families are better at coping with a substance-abusing family member than with dealing with a recovered family member. Awareness of this issue and attempting to think through these dynamics might serve as a preventive mechanism in some situations.

All patients being treated for alcoholism should be given thiamine. Thiamine specifically prevents the development of Wernicke's encephalopathy and its characteristic ataxia, nystagmus, and mental status changes. Disulfiram (Antabuse), an inhibitor of the enzyme aldehyde dehydrogenase, is effective in preventing drinking because of the severe symptoms it causes when combined with alcohol. Naltrexone (ReVia) functions as an opioid-receptor antagonist that is used to reduce alcohol craving.

### Medications Used to Treat Opioid Dependence

Drugs used to treat opioid dependence can be divided into those for opioid overdose and those for long-term treatment. Naloxone (Narcan; see previous discussion) blocks the neuroreceptors affected by opioids. In case of an opioid overdose, naloxone can be given to reverse the opioid-induced CNS depression. Although improvement occurs rapidly in the patient who has taken an overdose, naloxone's effect is short-lived because of its short half-life, and the patient might return to the pre-naloxone state. Maintenance treatment of opioid dependence is accomplished with methadone. Methadone is an opioid with a much longer half-life compared with the prototype opioid morphine and can be given in once-daily doses. Methadone relieves the drug hunger associated with opioid abuse. Typically, no more than 40 mg/day is prescribed. An alternative to methadone is Orlaam, a long-acting methadone cogener with a half-life of 96 hours. Orlaam can be given on a three times/week schedule.

Research has suggested that buprenorphine, a mild narcotic that is used as a pain killer, can be as effective as Orlaam or methadone in heroin treatment (Thomas, 2001). It is an agonist-antagonist opioid, a partial agonist for the mu receptor, and an antagonist for the kappa receptor. This pharmacologic activity seems to reduce the craving for opioids.

Naltrexone (ReVia) prevents euphoria, so it has some therapeutic benefit after the opioids are out of the system.

### Medications Used to Treat Stimulant Dependence

Many medications have been used to treat stimulant dependency. Dopaminergic drugs such as amantadine (Symmetrel) and bromocriptine (Parlodel), anticonvulsants such as carbamazepine (Tegretol), tricyclic antidepressants such as desipramine (Norpramin), and amino acid catecholamine precursors such as tyrosine and phenylalanine have been associated with successful treatment of stimulant dependency (Keltner and Folks, 2005).

### Medications Used to Treat Hallucinogen Dependence

Diazepam has been found to be effective in terminating episodes of panic, violence, and paranoid ideations induced by LSD and other hallucinogens (Hollister et al, 1993).

## MILIEU MANAGEMENT

The six dimensions of milieu management are all important when shaping the milieu of the chemically dependent inpatient. Some of these dimensions are significant for the patient who receives outpatient care as well. Safety issues such as a drug-free environment are critical. Nurses and others must be vigilant to protect the environment from individuals who might bring drugs into the milieu. Psychiatric units are not necessarily drug-free; multiple avenues exist for illicit contraband. Other safety issues such as suicide prevention and thwarting inappropriate sexual behavior continue to be the responsibility of nursing staff. Structural considerations such as an active, meaningful schedule provide for less downtime. Box 35-6 outlines a typical structured day for an inpatient setting. People who abuse alcohol, for example, often structure their day around planning to drink alcohol, drinking alcohol, and being under the influence of alcohol (Stoffel, 1994). Attempts are made to replace the old structure with a new, therapeutic structure. Effective unit structure maximizes what the milieu has to offer the patient. Norms of nonviolent behavior, openness, feedback, and the prohibition of nonprescribed drugs are critical to an effective treatment program. As previously noted, confrontation is a useful technique for working with chemically dependent individuals. Many patients will have never been held accountable; they certainly will rarely have experienced an environment in which direct and sometimes painful comments are expected to be

| Box 35-6 | **Sample Treatment Schedule*** | |
|---|---|---|
| | *Monday through Friday* | *Saturday and Sunday* |
| 7:00 AM | Breakfast | Breakfast |
| 8:00 AM | Morning meditation and spirituality | Community meeting |
| 9:00 AM | Community meeting | Goal setting |
| 11:00 AM | Lecture recovery concepts | Free time |
| 12:00 PM | Lunch | Lunch |
| 1:00 PM | Group therapy | 12-step study |
| 3:00 PM | Goal setting, review of 12-step concepts, journaling | |
| 5:00 PM | Recreation and leisure education | Recreation |
| 6:00 PM | Dinner | Dinner |
| 7:00 PM | Family recovery | Visiting hours |
| 8:00 PM | 12-step meeting | 12-step meeting |

*This is a sample treatment schedule reflecting typical concepts emphasized in most addiction recovery programs. Each program varies but generally includes these basic concepts.

absorbed and digested. Such feedback is necessary to penetrate the strong denial and defensiveness of the addict or alcoholic. Strong norms reinforce the expectation of a reasoned, nonviolent response to such comments.

Limit setting is perhaps the most important and most challenged (i.e., by patients) milieu management technique that the nurse will use. This can be characterized as providing an environment that protects patients from themselves and from other patients. Therefore, the nurse needs to recognize the symptoms of a still actively addicted mind (i.e., mood swings and substance-seeking, stubborn, belligerent, violent, and aggressive behavior) and then set limits on these behaviors. Urine drug screens are also a dimension of limit setting, because these tests reinforce the no-drug policy. If drugs are found, the patient must be confronted and held accountable.

Balance and environmental modification also play significant roles in the well-managed milieu for the chemically dependent patient. Balance is especially important—for example, when using the technique of confrontation. Although confrontation is important and therapeutic, in the hands of some less skilled staff and some patients it can become little more than a heavy-handed counterpart to the abuse patients might have

experienced years ago. The proper technique requires sensitivity to confront without crushing or totally alienating the patient. Skillful confrontation combines knowledge, empathy, and concern with accurate timing.

## INTERVENTION AND TREATMENT PROGRAMS

Many programs exist for the treatment of chemical dependency. The fact that these various programs exist gives testimony to the complexity and seriousness of chemical dependencies in North America.

The best-known intervention programs are AA and Narcotics Anonymous (NA). These programs use a self-help, support group model made up of fellow users in various stages of recovery. Philosophically, AA and NA view psychosocial problems as stemming from substance abuse and generally reject the idea that an underlying psychopathology is responsible for the abuse. AA, with about 1.2 million members in the United States, has established the 12 suggested steps (Box 35-7), which start with a person's admitting personal powerlessness over alcohol and end with the person's being available, night or day, to help another alcoholic in need (Bates, 2005). The popular bumper sticker slogan, "Easy does it," reflects a philosophy of taking life one day at a time and avoiding a frenetic lifestyle. AA and NA subscribe to the belief that only total abstinence can free the chemically dependent person from the bondage of alcohol and drugs, because, they maintain, "A drug is a drug is a drug," meaning that if someone is addicted to one substance, that person is by definition addicted (at least potentially) to all substances. AA's relationship with physicians and mental health professionals has become increasingly cooperative over the last few years.

Although AA in particular has a program that has helped many people, it does not appeal to everyone. Reasons vary, but some professionals believe that the spiritual nature of AA is a deterrent to some who are seeking help. Eight of the 12 steps definitely have a spiritual perspective. Specifically, the concept of a higher power, the expectation that a person tell his or her story publicly, and the notion of making a searching and

## Box 35-7   Twelve Steps of Alcoholics Anonymous

1. Admitted we were powerless over alcohol—that our lives had become unmanageable.
2. Came to believe that a power greater than ourselves could restore us to sanity.
3. Made a decision to turn our will and our lives over to the care of God as we understood Him.
4. Made a searching and fearless moral inventory of ourselves.
5. Admitted to God, to ourselves, and to another human being the exact nature of our wrongs.
6. Were entirely ready to have God remove all these defects of character.
7. Humbly asked Him to remove our shortcomings.
8. Made a list of all persons we had harmed and became willing to make amends to them all.
9. Made direct amends to such people whenever possible, except when to do so would injure them or others.
10. Continued to take personal inventory, and when we were wrong, we promptly admitted it.
11. Sought through prayer and meditation to improve our conscious contact with God as we understood Him, praying only for knowledge of His will and the power to carry that out.
12. Having had a spiritual awakening as the result of these steps, we tried to carry His message to alcoholics, and to practice these principles in all our affairs.

The *Twelve Steps* are reprinted with permission of Alcoholics Anonymous World Services, Inc. Permission to reprint this material does not mean that AA has reviewed or approved the contents of this publication. AA is a program of recovery from alcoholism only—use of the Twelve Steps in connection with programs and activities that are patterned after AA, but that address other problems, does not imply otherwise.

### A Student's Clinical Log*

I went to the substance abuse program on the week of November 2nd. When the two other students and I arrived, we were amazed to see all the teenagers standing in front of the building. As I waited in line to sign in, I heard several of them talking. They were talking about the party they went to last weekend, how they got "messed up," and how they were planning on doing it again the next weekend. They talked about how they hated the substance abuse program and they thought it was a waste of their time. I was bothered by this conversation. If they had that kind of attitude, they did not need to be there. They were wasting their time and money. I should have expected this type of attitude from them. Most of them were there because they had to be there. Some judge thought it was the solution to their problem. I wonder if they were paying for this program or was somebody else "throwing their money away." I think most of them viewed this as a social gathering. I wish I did not think this way. I want to believe that these kids want to "get better," but based on their actions I do not think some of them are ready. They will have to hit rock bottom before they see the error of their ways.

*After an evening at an intensive outpatient program meeting.

### CRITICAL THINKING QUESTION   3

The founders of AA were clear that the recovery process was a spiritual journey. However, we now live in times in which most people are reluctant to speak of spiritual matters for fear of offending others or of imposing their views on others. Do you think that, in our efforts not to "offend" people, we have deemphasized an important part of psychiatric nursing?

## SPECIAL NOTES

## PRESCRIPTION DRUG ABUSE

The traditional stereotype of the addict or alcoholic is the skid row type of individual. One forgets or is shocked to find professionals, especially health care professionals, using drugs. A fairly common form of drug abuse is addiction to

fearless moral inventory and then making amends when needed is incongruent with some people's belief systems. AA continues to be an important treatment alternative for thousands of individuals suffering from alcoholism.

Other programs, developed by more traditionally oriented mental health professionals, might view underlying problems, such as depression or bipolar illness, as the cause of substance abuse. The goal of this therapy is to treat the underlying problem. Proponents of this approach believe that successful treatment of the underlying problem facilitates resolution of the chemical dependency. These programs might use a group format or individual therapy format.

prescription medications, such as pain medications or anxiolytics. People who are addicted to prescriptions have a particularly difficult denial through which to break.

Prescriptions, being legally obtained, are justified as legitimate by the prescription addict. The skills acquired by the prescription addict in maintaining an increasing supply of their drug of choice are accompanied by significant rationalization and sophisticated denial. Because their drugs are acquired legally, prescription drug addicts have a difficult time seeing their use in the same way as a street addict. Awareness and concern about the problem of prescription drug abuse have risen considerably over the last 15 years (Meadows, 2001; Vastag, 2001).

## ADDICTED HEALTH CARE PROFESSIONALS

Addiction and alcoholism among health care professionals are particularly difficult, in that there is a violation of the professional's relationship with the patient. Health care professionals who take drugs from patients are particularly scorned (Bachman, 2001). Many states have adopted non-punitive monitoring programs that allow the nurse an opportunity to work under strict guidelines while actively participating in recovery.

### CLINICAL EXAMPLE

Terry is a 39-year-old opioid-dependent registered nurse whose presentation in treatment is precipitated by the state nursing board. Nursing was Terry's life, and her identity centered on being a nurse. Reporting that it was not uncommon to "share medication" with patients, Terry told of how easy it was at first to document giving the maximum as-needed pain medications in a patient's chart but not always giving them to the actual patient. "I never let one of my patients be in pain, though," Terry reported.

Terry's supervisor did not suspect a problem until medications were unaccounted for. Terry thought that all areas had been covered but was eventually caught, not because of stupidity, but from the kind of impaired judgment that results from drug use.

Terry's nursing license was put on probationary status. Most facilities were unwilling to hire a nurse

on probation; the limitations placed by the board were strict. Terry cannot work the night shift and cannot hold the keys to the medication storage; she must also submit to random drug testing. Without a job, Terry cannot begin to fulfill the conditions of the probation.

Terry was hired as a nurse at a health care facility and has 6 months remaining until another hearing date can be set.

## FINAL THOUGHTS

### EVALUATION

Because abstinence is the overarching goal of most treatments, and because so many people in treatment are referred by the criminal justice system, accurate information is often difficult to acquire. Another complicating factor is deciding exactly which criteria are significant. Unfortunately, there are more questions than answers. Is self-reported abstinence after 6 months, 1 year, or 5 years best? Is self-reporting believable? Should police records be consulted for AOD-related arrests? Outcome evaluations for substance dependence are often among the most confusing of statistics.

### RELAPSE

Not only must the chemically dependent person recover from the dependency or addiction, but also the potential for relapse and readmission to treatment must be addressed. This task can best be accomplished by helping the person see the danger signs of relapse. Rawson and colleagues (1990; quoted in Corrie, 1993) have outlined five warning signs of relapse:

1. Being around other users
2. Severe craving
3. Stopping attendance at AA or NA meetings
4. Not expressing feelings
5. Going through a major emotional crisis

### FOLLOW-UP CARE

Follow-up care is essential for preventing relapse. Patients and nurses need to be aware that recovery has only begun when an inpatient or outpatient program is completed. The few months immediately following completion of a treatment program can be dangerous for the chemically dependent person. Relapse is most common during this period. The nurse should confirm that arrangements for aftercare, outpatient counseling, and self-help support group meetings are made before discharge.

## CRITICAL THINKING QUESTION 4

Is the "Drug War" worth fighting? Justify your answer.

## Study Notes

1. Chemical dependency is a major physical and mental health problem in North America, and most nurses, whether they want to or not, will take care of chemically dependent people.
2. Drugs of abuse can be categorized into basic groups: (1) alcohol, (2) CNS depressants, and (3) opioids, stimulants, and hallucinogens.
3. The *DSM-IV-TR* distinguishes between substance dependence and substance abuse, with substance dependence indicating more severe problems with a substance.
4. Alcohol is the leading drug problem in North America; it exacts a high price economically from our society and is responsible for great suffering and death.
5. Alcohol causes disinhibition and impaired judgment, but is relaxing when first used. The primary concern with respect to alcohol overdose is severe and often fatal CNS depression. Withdrawal causes tremors, nausea, vomiting, tachycardia, diaphoresis, seizures, anxiety, and depression. Withdrawal can be fatal.
6. Other CNS depressants include barbiturates (downers, reds, blues, and rainbows), benzodiazepines such as Librium (green and whites), antipsychotic drugs, and inhalants (gasoline and cement for model airplanes).
7. Depressants cause euphoria, disinhibition, and drowsiness. The primary effect of overdose is respiratory depression. Withdrawal from CNS depressants can be life-threatening.
8. Opioids (narcotics) come from the juice of the opium poppy or are synthetic substances, with opium being the natural product and morphine, codeine, and the semisynthetic heroin

being easily derived from the poppy juice. Synthetic preparations such as meperidine (Demerol), pentazocine (Talwin), propoxyphene (Darvon), and methadone (Dolophine) have been developed in the vain search for a pain reliever with no addicting qualities.

9. Opioids are taken IV, orally, IM, and subcutaneously (skin popping). Overdose can be fatal, with respiratory depression being the most serious side effect. Withdrawal, although unpleasant (influenza-like symptoms), is not particularly life-threatening.
10. Naloxone (Narcan) is an opioid receptor blocker and is given in emergency rooms to treat opioid overdose. Naloxone causes an opioid abstinence syndrome.
11. Stimulants include amphetamines and cocaine. Stimulants cause elation, grandiose thinking, talkativeness, and other less pleasant effects. The primary concerns in the event of overdose are agitation, tachycardia, cardiac arrhythmias, and convulsions. Withdrawal from stimulants, although miserable, is not particularly serious.
12. Hallucinogens include mescaline, marijuana, LSD, and PCP. Hallucinogens cause illusions, hallucinations, diminished ability to perceive time and distance, anxiety, and paranoid thinking. The primary effects of hallucinogenic overdose are intense trips, psychotic reactions, and panic. Withdrawal from hallucinogens can cause anxiety, fear, and panic. However, physical withdrawal has not been found to be particularly serious.
13. Although several treatment approaches are effective, the therapeutic goal for most approaches is abstinence from the substance, although the patient might still be seeking a way to engage in controlled use. (If the patient were able to do that, he or she probably would not qualify as dependent in the first place.)
14. Nursing interventions include group work, education, confrontation, tough love (simply not allowing oneself to be a participant in the patient's self-destruction), providing for physical and nutritional needs, and helping the patient become involved in groups such as AA and NA.
15. Health care professionals have access to medications that can be abused. This has become a significant issue, and hospitals and licensing

boards are making concerted efforts to control this problem.

16. Recovering abusers must be on guard for backsliding to their addictions.

## References

Alcohol cited in Oklahoma student's death. (2004, October 2). *Birmingham News,* p 2A.

Allen LN: Drugs of abuse. In Keltner NL, Folks DG, editors: *Psychotropic drugs,* ed 3, St Louis, 2001, Mosby, pp 366-381.

American Psychiatric Association: *Diagnostic and statistical manual of mental disorders, text revision,* ed 4, Washington, DC, 2000, APA.

Anonymous: Cocaine exposure in utero, *Am J Nurs* 98:9, 1998.

Anonymous: Body of man in 1953 LSD test exhumed. (1994, June 5). *Los Angeles Times,* p A4.

Anonymous: Drug approved to treat alcoholism, *FDA Consumer* 29:2, 1995.

Bachman J: One nurse's story of addiction and recovery, *Colorado Nurse* 101:11, 2001.

Bates F: Study detects some 'heretics' among AA program faithful, *Clin Psychiatry News* 33:50, 2005.

Castaneda R, Levy R, Hardy M, Trujillo M: Long-acting stimulants for the treatment of attention-deficit disorder in cocaine-dependent adults, *Psychiatr Serv* 51:169, 2000.

Cherpitel LJ: The epidemiology of alcohol-related trauma, *Alcohol Health Res World* 16:191, 1992.

Colyar MR: Testing for drugs of abuse, *Adv Nurse Pract* 9:30-31, 2003.

Feldman M: *Whad'ya know?* Wisconsin Public Radio, June 4, 1994. (The story is from *USA Today,* June 3, 1994, p 10A.)

Forest Laboratories: *Campral delayed-release tablets prescribing information,* St. Louis, 2004, Forest Laboratories.

Frezza M, di Padova C, Pozzato G, et al: High blood alcohol levels in women. The role of decreased gastric alcohol dehydrogenase activity and first-pass metabolism, *N Engl J Med* 322:95, 1990.

Goodwin DW, Schulsinger F, Hermansen L, et al: Alcohol problems in adoptees raised apart from alcoholic biological parents, *Arch Gen Psychiatry* 28:238, 1973.

Gordis E: Alcohol and the brain. Neuroscience and neurobehavior. In Armstrong C, Gardner MB, Eckardt M, et al, editors: *Tenth special report to the U.S. Congress on alcohol and health,* Washington, DC, 2000, National Institutes of Health, pp 1-463.

Gorski TT: Alcoholism: disease or addiction? *Professional Counselor* October 15, 1996. Available at http://www2.cdc.gov/ncidod/aip/HepC/HepC.asp. Accessed April 25, 2005.

Gorski TT: *Understanding the twelve steps,* New York, 1992, Simon & Schuster.

Harper C, Matsumoto I: Ethanol and brain damage, *Curr Opin Pharmacol* 5:73, 2005.

Herrick T: The meth epidemic, *Clinician News* 9:21, 2005.

Hess D, DeBoer S: Ecstasy, *Am J Nurs* 102:45, 2002.

Hollister L, Muller-Oerlinghausen B, Rickels K, Shader RI: Clinical uses of benzodiazepines, *J Clin Psychopharmacol* 13:1S, 1993.

Husband dies after sherry enema. (2005, February 4). *Birmingham News,* p 3A.

Kanayama G, Gruber AJ, Pope HG Jr, et al: Over-the-counter drug use in gymnasiums: an underrecognized substance abuse problem? *Psychother Psychosom* 70:137, 2001.

Keltner NL, Folks DG: *Psychotropic drugs,* ed 3, St. Louis, 2005, Mosby.

Kessler RC, Chiu WT, Demler O, Walters EE: Prevalence, severity, and comorbidity of 12-month DSM-IV disorders in the national comorbidity survey replication. *Arch Gen Psychiatry* 62:617, 2005.

Lehne RA: *Pharmacology for nursing care,* ed 4, Philadelphia, 2004, WB Saunders.

Lieber CS: Relationships between nutrition, alcohol use, and liver disease, *Alcohol Res Health* 27:220, 2003.

Lowinson JH, Ruiz P, Millman RB, et al: *Substance abuse: a comprehensive textbook,* ed 3, Baltimore, 1992, Williams & Wilkins.

Manissa Communication Group: U.S. trial confirms value of physician advice to reduce drinking, *Brown Univ Digest Addiction Theory Appl* 16:4, 1997.

Mathias R: NIDA clinical trials network begins first multisite tests of new science-based drug abuse treatment, *NIDA Notes* 15:10, 2001.

Mathias R: "Ecstasy" damages the brain and impairs memory in humans, *NIDA Notes* 14:10, 1999.

Meadows M: Prescription drug use and abuse, *FDA Consumer* 35:18, 2001.

Meth cases make mountain of trouble. (2005, May 1). *Birmingham News,* p 10A.

Mueller LA, Ketcham K: *Recovering: how to get and stay sober,* New York, 1987, Bantam Books.

Muha L: Home drug tests: what concerned parents must know, *Good Housekeeping* July:137, 1997.

Nash JM: Addicted: why do people get hooked? *Time* May 5:68, 1997.

National Clearinghouse for Alcohol and Drug Information, NCADI: *Alcohol.* Available at http://ncadi.samhsa.gov/nongovpubs/bac-chart. Accessed November 18, 2005.

NANDA International: *Nursing diagnoses: definitions and classification, 2005-2006,* Philadelphia, 2005, NANDA International.

Peele S, Brodsky A, Arnold M: *The truth about addiction and recovery,* New York, 1991, Simon and Schuster.

Rawson R, Obert J, McCann M: *The neurobehavioral treatment manual,* Beverly Hills, CA, 1990, Matrix Institute on Addictions; quoted in Corrie D, editor: *CWASAINT trainee notebook,* Atlanta, 1993, Child Welfare Institute.

Roberts A, Koob GF: The neurobiology of addiction, *Alcohol Health Res World* 21:101, 1997.

Robertson N: The intimate enemy: will that friendly drink betray you? *Modern Maturity* 35:28, 1992.

Sancton T: The dossier on Diana's crash, *Time* October 13:50, 1997.

Schiller MJ, Shumway M, Batki SL: Utility of routine drug screening in a psychiatric emergency setting, *Psychiatr Serv* 51:474, 2000.

Sinclair JD: Evidence about the use of naltrexone and for different ways of using it in the treatment of alcoholism, *Alcohol Alcohol* 36:2, 2001.

Steinberg ML, Epstein EE, McCrady BS, Hirsch LS: Sources of motivation in a couple's outpatient alcoholism treatment program, *Am J Drug Alcohol Abuse* 23:191, 1997.

Stoffel VC: Occupational therapists roles in treating substance abuse, *Hosp Community Psychiatry* 45:21, 1994.

Sullivan E, Bissell L, William E: *Chemical dependency in nursing,* Redwood City, CA, 1998, Addison-Wesley.

Taylor B, Donoghue J: Club drugs—its effects on our youth, *Alabama Nurse* 28:20, 2001.

Thomas J: Buprenorphine proves effective, expands options for treatment of heroin addiction, *NIDA Notes* 16:8, 2001.

U.S. Surgeon General, Mental Health: *A report from the surgeon general,* Washington DC, 1999, Department of Health and Human Services.

Vastag B: Mixed message on prescription drug abuse, *JAMA* 285:2183, 2001.

Wegscheider S: *Another chance.* Available at http://www.samhsa.gov/statistics/statistics.html. Accessed November 13, 2005.

Wegscheider-Cruse S: *Another chance: hope and health for the alcoholic,* Palo Alto, CA, 2000, Family Science and Behavior Books.

Whitfield C, Davis J, Barker L: Alcoholism. In Barker LR, Burton JR, Zieve PD, editors: *Principles of ambulatory medicine,* Baltimore, 1986, Williams & Wilkins.

Whitten L: Conference highlights increasing GHB abuse, *NIDA Notes* 16:10, 2001.

Wray J: Psychophysiological aspects of methamphetamine abuse, *J Addictions Nurs* 12:143, 2000.

Wright K: A shot of sanity, *Discover* 9:47, 1999.

Zickler P: Brain imaging studies show long-term damage from methamphetamine abuse, *NIDA Notes* 15:11, 2000.

Zickler P: NIDA studies clarify developmental effects of prenatal cocaine exposure, *NIDA Notes* 14:5, 1999.

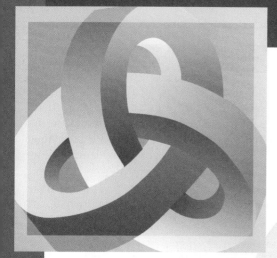

# Chapter 36

# Dual Diagnosis

*Carol E. Bostrom*

## Learning Objectives

*After reading this chapter, you should be able to:*
- Define the term *dual diagnosis*.
- Describe major perspectives related to the etiologies for dual diagnosis.
- Understand issues related to the treatment of dual-diagnosis patients.
- Describe approaches related to treating patients with dual diagnosis.

Traditional psychiatric treatment has divided patients into distinct categories based on the belief that one type of illness or disorder is primary or more urgent than another. Historically, patients were categorized as having either a mental illness or a substance abuse or dependency problem. The mental illness or the substance abuse or dependency problem received separate treatment, without recognition that another diagnosis was appropriate or that there were additional important issues underlying both disorders.

Based on more than 20 years of research, the mental health community has recognized and focused increased attention on dual-diagnosis or co-occurring disorders and their treatment. The complexity of patients' problems with dual diagnosis, resulting in multiple impairments, requires a comprehensive therapeutic treatment approach and individual case management. Part of this effort is to reduce frequent hospitalization, or what has been called the *revolving door syndrome*. Patients with psychiatric illnesses and substance abuse or dependency problems have poor treatment outcomes with high rates of relapse, resulting in high costs in multiple settings.

This chapter discusses issues related to patients with dual diagnoses rather than focusing on specific interventions for this population of patients. Three issues in this area will be addressed: the concept of dual diagnosis, etiology, and treatment.

## DUAL DIAGNOSIS DEFINED

Dual diagnosis refers to the presence of at least one psychiatric disorder in addition to a substance abuse or dependency problem. The psychiatric disorder might be a mental illness or a personality disorder. The psychiatric illness is severe and persistent, causing prolonged disability (Patrick, 2003). An example of a patient with a dual diagnosis is an individual with chronic schizophrenia and alcohol abuse. Another example is a patient with heroin dependency and antisocial personality disorder. Box 36-1 provides examples of dual-diagnosis combinations. Considering the number of axis I and axis II diagnoses, a multitude of combinations is possible. Therefore, patients with dual diagnoses represent a heterogeneous group. Research studies have indicated that about 50% of patients with severe mental illness are affected by substance abuse problems (Drake et al, 2001). Co-occurrence is common and should be expected (Minkoff, 2001).

### Norm's Notes

*Substance abuse is not only a big problem for the population in general, it is a big problem for people with mental disorders. An inordinate number of the homeless have both a mental disorder and a substance abuse problem. People with mental health problems who abuse substances do not help themselves. They might escape their problems momentarily, but these problems don't go away—they usually become worse. This is an important chapter. Make sure you study the causative factors of dual diagnosis.*

## ETIOLOGY

The origins for diagnoses are discussed in the chapters specific to the disorders. One issue that mental health professionals traditionally deal with is which comes first—the mental illness or the substance problem. Because of this dilemma, the treatment of patients has been affected and has followed specific patterns. From the perspective that the mental illness occurred first, many reasons

| Box 36-1 | Examples of Dual Diagnoses |
|---|---|
| Axis | Diagnoses |
| I | Schizophrenia |
|   | Alcohol abuse |
| I | Cocaine abuse |
| II | Antisocial personality disorder |
| I | Major depression |
|   | Anxiolytic dependency |
| I | Major depression |
|   | Marijuana abuse |
| II | Borderline personality disorder |

### 12-Month Prevalence Rate of Mental Disorders in the United States*

| Disorders | Approximate Percentage Over 17 Years of Age | Approximate Number of Persons | Gender Overrepresentation |
|---|---|---|---|
| **Anxiety Disorders** | 18 overall | 36,000,000 | |
| Panic disorder | 3.5 | 7,000,000 | Women |
| Social phobia | 7 | 14,000,000 | Women |
| Specific phobia | 8.7 | 17,000,000 | Women |
| GAD | 3 | 6,000,000 | Women |
| PTSD | 3.5 | 7,000,000 | Women |
| OCD | 1 | 2,000,000 | Equal |
| **Mood Disorders** | 9.5 overall | 19,000,000 | |
| Major depression | 6.7 | | Women |
| Dysthymia | 1.5 | | Women |
| Bipolar I and II | 2.6 | | BD I: Equal |
| | | | BD II: Women? |
| **Impulse Control Disorders** | 9 overall | 18,000,000 | |
| Conduct disorders | 1 | 2,000,000 | Men |
| ADHD | 4 | 8,000,000 | Men |
| **Substance Abuse Disorders** | 3.8 overall | 7,600,000 | |
| Alcohol abuse and dependence | 3.1 | 6,200,000 | Men |
| Drug abuse and dependence | 1.4 | 2,800,000 | Men |
| **Schizophrenia** | 1.1 | 2,100,000 | Equal |

*Extrapolated from several sources based on current census data.
*ADHD,* Attention-deficit/hyperactivity disorder; *GAD,* generalized anxiety disorder; *OCD,* obsessive-compulsive disorder; *PTSD,* posttraumatic stress disorder.
From Kessler RC, Chiu WT, Demler O, Walters EE: Prevalence, severity, and comorbidity of 12-month DSM-IV disorders in the national comorbidity survey replication, *Arch Gen Psychiatry* 62:617, 2005; U.S. Surgeon General: *Mental health: a report from the Surgeon General,* Washington, DC, 1999, Department of Health and Human Services: National Institute of Mental Health: www.nimh.nih.gov/. Accessed April 18, 2005.

might account for the development of a substance problem. As is true for mental illnesses, heredity, impulsivity, and biologic factors might predispose an individual to problems with substances. Some people might be predisposed to develop both a mental illness and a substance abuse problem.

From the perspective that the substance abuse precedes mental illness, it follows that brain chemistry can be altered—that is, neurotransmitter imbalance or depletion. Chemicals can induce acute and chronic psychiatric problems. Substance-induced psychosis, schizophrenia, depression, and mania can occur in vulnerable individuals. Substance abuse can also lead to feelings of guilt, depression, and altered self-esteem. Repeated stimulant use can alter the dopamine system, and alcohol dependence can increase the positive symptoms of schizophrenia (Addington and Addington, 2001; Littrell and Littrell, 1999).

Environmental and psychological factors, such as social networks, drug effects, boredom, dysphoria, unemployment, and poverty, are contributing factors leading to the risk of substance abuse. "There is no evidence that particular substances are used as a function of the biologies of specific mental illnesses" (Drake et al, 2002). However, individuals with mental illness have an increased sensitivity to the effects of drugs and small amounts of exposure can lead to relapse (Ziedonis et al, 2005). Individuals with severe and persistent mental illness such as schizophrenia and bipolar disorder do not need to meet the *Diagnostic and Statistical Manual of Mental Disorders (DSM)* criteria for substance abuse or dependence for such use to provoke problems (Donat and Haverkamp, 2004).

Patients with schizophrenia use substances to feel calmer and as a coping strategy when stressed (Gomez et al, 2000). Others use substances to numb feelings that are too painful to deal with (Kasten, 1999). For patients experiencing psychotic symptoms, self-medicating with alcohol or drugs can help them feel better and less anxious and can decrease the intensity of hallucinations temporarily, but results in a worsening of symptoms after the effects of the alcohol or drug have worn off. Furthermore, using substances does not result in bothersome and uncomfortable side effects as compared with antipsychotics. Patients can also experience some degree of social acceptance when they drink alcohol or use drugs. With the decision to use a substance, the feeling of autonomy or power results in a temporary increase in self-esteem. Problems or issues are avoided, and patients feel better and temporarily in control of themselves. Studies have shown that for individuals with severe mental illness, substance use offers an opportunity to socialize, which can be a prime reason for use (Drake et al, 2002).

Individuals with schizophrenia have reported using alcohol, cannabis, and cocaine to decrease depression, anxiety, and side effects of antipsychotic medication (Addington and Addington, 2001). Individuals with depression sometimes use stimulants to boost their energy so they can work and care for their families. The majority of patients who use substances find only temporary relief, followed by an exacerbation of symptoms (Kasten, 1999). Research generally does not support self-treatment as an explanation for long-term use (Drake et al, 2002). Specific drugs are abused based on market forces, and use begins prior to the development of psychosis.

Substance abuse issues are often present in the population of individuals with personality disorders. Some traits or behaviors of substance abusers are the same as those with personality disorders. Regardless of which disorder or problem came first, the existence of a substance problem, mental illness, or personality disorder complicates diagnosis and treatment, prolongs rehabilitation, increases the incidence of relapse, and is associated with violence, incarceration, homelessness, and human immunodeficiency virus (HIV) and hepatitis infection (Drake et al, 2002). The complexity of these patients' problems requires a holistic, integrated approach.

## TREATMENT ISSUES

Traditional models of treatment have focused on one issue at a time or on the most acute problem first. One model assumed that when mental illness was stabilized, substance use would subside. Another idea suggested that stabilization of the mental illness would enhance patient participation and result in benefit from substance abuse treatment. Some clinicians believed that detoxification from chemical substances must occur before other treatment is possible. All these assumptions were valid for some patients, some of the time. For example, the severely psychotic patient needs antipsychotic medication before being able to participate in treatment groups.

However, many problems exist with these models of treatment. For example, treatment was disrupted when patients had to be transferred from one unit or facility to another. Separate agencies or facilities with different treatment responsibilities did not coordinate and were unable to provide the multiple modalities needed for treatment for patients with dual diagnoses. Continuity of care was difficult to maintain, resulting in gaps in treatment. Consequently, follow-up care was sporadic, and care of patients was not managed effectively or adequately.

Another problem area arises from traditional differences between mental health and substance abuse programs and staff philosophies. A substance abuse program might discourage the use of all psychotropic medications, whereas the psychiatric unit might strongly encourage medication compliance. Confrontational groups on substance abuse units differ greatly from support groups found in psychiatric units. For example, patients with religious delusions, preoccupations, and distortions find it difficult to participate and work in the 12-step recovery program that is part of Alcoholics Anonymous and similar groups.

In the past, education and training for many staff members focused on the type of unit in which they would be working. As a result, staff members were often unprepared to treat patients with other problems. The lack of understanding of dual-diagnosis patients resulted in the staff having unrealistic expectations of what patients might accomplish during a specific time frame. Within the last 25 years, programs integrating treatment for mental illness and substance use have been increasing. Research has shown that integrated treatment programs have positive results—for example, remission of substance use and improvement in mental health (Drake et al, 2001).

## PROBLEMS AFFECTING PROGRAM DEVELOPMENT

Given the heterogeneity of dual-diagnosis patients, many issues have to be considered regarding program development. In working with these patients, the difficulty lies not so much with individual counseling, but with group programming. Treatment programs must identify which issues pertain to the majority of patients and can be managed in large groups and which issues should be addressed in smaller groups. Unique or highly personal issues are more appropriately handled on a one-to-one basis. For example, education about the disease concept of alcoholism or nutrition might be applicable to an entire group of patients. Education about the side effects of specific antidepressants might be appropriate for a select group of patients. A patient might want to discuss his or her feelings about acquired immunodeficiency syndrome (AIDS) on a one-to-one basis before talking in a group. On a given day, changes in a patient's mental status might affect his or her ability to participate in a large group. Therefore, staff members need to be flexible in assigning patients to specific groups.

Patients with dual diagnoses also need flexibility regarding the length of treatment rather than being assigned a fixed number of treatment days, sessions, or appointments. A program that is open-ended, occurs in stages, and provides support and empowerment is necessary for patient compliance with treatment. For patients with severe mental illness, abstinence from a substance is a process and should be a goal of treatment, not a prerequisite.

The staff needs to be aware of and prepared for dealing with issues and conflicts inherent in this population. In groups and in the milieu setting, patients with personality disorders might try to manipulate more regressed members. Depending on the substances abused, conflict might arise around degrees of addiction and drugs of choice ("Cocaine is worse than alcohol" or "My addiction is worse than yours"). Because most patients with dual diagnosis experience difficulties in concentration and memory, educational groups must be structured with concrete concepts, simplified material, and repetition of material. Handouts, role playing, and homework assignments might be helpful to practice and apply key treatment concepts. Often, some patients in this group are perpetrators of violence and others are victims. As a result, victims might find it difficult to participate in or even attend a group with perpetrators.

Another problem exists with program funding. Finances are needed for a system of care with standards for treatment for the diverse populations in managed care systems. The federal government is granting money to states to develop integrated treatment programs for patients with dual diagnosis and to share outcomes (Miller, 2003). Hopefully, additional data will become available on this issue. In dealing with dual-diagnosed patients, it is evident that there are more issues and questions than answers. Continued work and development of models and strategies are necessary for these patients. The hope is that patients will ultimately benefit from more appropriate programming.

---

## CRITICAL THINKING QUESTION   1

What benefits might a patient receive from dual-diagnosis treatment?

---

## PUTTING IT ALL TOGETHER
### Psychotherapeutic Management

Effective treatment for patients with dual diagnoses must be multifaceted and multidisciplinary. Box 36-2 summarizes treatment components. Individual case management for social, medical, and emotional needs requires professional staff members to integrate their knowledge about addictions and mental illness. Education in mental illness and addictions, as well as communication, cooperation, and collaboration among professional staff is required. Integrated treatment is the new standard for evidence-based treatment for dual-diagnosis patients. A combination of mental health and addiction treatment approaches is used to provide seamless care (Ziedonis et al, 2005).

## NURSE-PATIENT RELATIONSHIP

In working with dual-diagnosis patients, the nurse uses a nonjudgmental and individualized approach and considers patients' strengths, deficits, and

---

| Box 36-2 | Treatment Components for Patients With Dual Diagnosis |
|---|---|

Case management
Vocational counseling
Money management
Cognitive-behavioral therapy
Referrals to community resources
Family counseling
Group therapy
Supportive employment
Social skills training
Self-help groups
Psychoeducation groups
Housing

---

ability to use feedback (Patrick, 2003). Interventions are tailored to patients' individual needs, mental illness, and substance problem. The nurse is involved with all these areas simultaneously.

Trust between the nurse and patient develops if the patient believes that the nurse is knowledgeable, skilled, nonjudgmental, and empathic. Trust is especially important with the short length of inpatient hospitalization and outpatient areas along the continuum of care. A supportive relationship, combined with involving the patient in setting achievable, short-term goals, helps the patient build confidence and experience a sense of security. The nurse conveys hope and motivates the patient to participate in treatment.

The nurse needs to ask patients about how substances affect their psychiatric symptoms, moods, and medication effects to assist patients with identifying the short- and long-term effects of using substances. The nurse needs to ask patients about physical or sexual abuse and make referrals for appropriate treatment (Kasten, 1999).

Monitoring patients for exacerbation of symptoms and symptoms of withdrawal is ongoing. (Specific interventions for the relevant mental illness and chemical dependency are found in other chapters.) The nurse is involved in teaching patients about the effects of alcohol and drugs on the mind and body. Patients need education about their mental illness and help in recognizing the signs of relapse regarding their specific mental illness and substance abuse or dependency problem. Strategies for relapse prevention are based on each patient's individual needs.

---

## CRITICAL THINKING QUESTION   2

A young male patient with schizophrenia abuses alcohol. How do the behaviors of this individual's illnesses complicate treatment?

---

## PSYCHOPHARMACOLOGY

Medication is specifically prescribed for patients according to their mental illness. Compliance with prescribed medication is supported by the nurse. Issues related to medication compliance are addressed, such as lack of money or transportation to purchase medications. The nurse teaches patients about side effect management and about potential problems resulting from using alcohol or other substances with medication. (Refer to chapters on psychopharmacology for specific information.) Caution is used in prescribing anxiolytics, which cause dependence (e.g., benzodiazepines). Medications are also used to manage intoxication and withdrawal.

## CASE STUDY

Barbara Abel is a 28-year-old patient who was transferred from CCU because of Prozac (fluoxetine) overdose and alcohol withdrawal. She is weak, shaky, and needs assistance with ambulation. Her diagnoses are major depression and alcohol abuse. Barbara states to the nurse, "I only wanted to sleep, have some peace, and forget my problems. I was so tired and couldn't eat or get out of bed. Ending it all would be better. I'd be happy again and like myself."

Barbara and her husband divorced 3 months ago because "he didn't understand that I needed to have a few drinks to sleep and forget my problems." She is an RN and was employed as a unit manager. She recently lost her job as a result of absenteeism. Barbara moved in with a friend who works as an accountant. Her friend occasionally uses cocaine to "stay on top of things" at work. Two of Barbara's co-workers encouraged her to seek treatment, but she was too tired to make an appointment with her doctor.

## MILIEU MANAGEMENT

Enforcing the rules of the unit or program and setting limits provide structure and clear expectations for patients. Rules and limits help decrease manipulation and conflict among patients on the unit and in group sessions. Treatment groups focus on education about substances, mental illness, relapse prevention, and medication. Modified cognitive-behavioral therapy can be used to improve social skills, problem solving, and information about cravings and triggers of drug use in a highly structured small group setting (Ziedonis et al, 2005). Stress management, including deep breathing and relaxation exercises, assertiveness, and community living skills, is also taught. Teaching communication and social skills by using role playing is used to develop coping skills—that is, how to respond in a situation in which someone is drinking alcohol. The staff must be flexible in assigning patients to groups because of possible changes in mental status resulting from withdrawal

from substances or exacerbation of mental illness symptoms. Supportive, gentle confrontation techniques are more effective than intense confrontation for patients with severe and persistent mental illness.

Attendance at self-help group meetings such as Alcoholics Anonymous and Narcotics Anonymous, and Double Trouble in Recovery and Dual Recovery Anonymous (for dual-diagnosis patients) begins while patients are on the inpatient unit, if possible. Referrals to and involvement with outpatient programs, self-help groups, halfway houses, residential treatment facilities, vocational counseling, and supportive employment are completed before discharge. Supportive employment provides the patient with the opportunity to find a community-based job without prevocational training and lengthy assessment. Employment offers daily structure, finances, self-esteem, and sober co-workers, who help patients develop hope and change their lives (Becker et al, 2005). Sometimes, self-help groups are not attended until later in outpatient treatment, when the patient feels more motivated to attend. Continuity of treatment is necessary to prevent relapse and decrease recidivism.

## CONTINUUM OF CARE

### INTEGRATED TREATMENT FOR DUAL DIAGNOSIS

Integrated treatment programs are effective for patients with dual diagnosis. Treatment that occurs in stages, is open-ended, empowers individuals, and extends beyond weeks or months is beneficial for individuals with a dual diagnosis. Even brief, integrated dual-diagnosis outpatient treatment has been found to reduce inpatient psychiatric hospitalization by 60% 1 year after treatment; for patients with schizophrenia, there was a 74% reduction in hospitalization days (Granholm et al, 2003). With abstinence from alcohol, remission of comorbid axis I disorders occurred during comprehensive long-term alcoholism treatment (Wagner et al, 2004).

The following model from the U.S. Department of Health and Human Services (2005) outlines a program for the treatment of patients with dual diagnosis.

# Care Plan

Name: Barbara Abel                    Admission Date: _____

*DSM-IV-TR* Diagnosis: Alcohol abuse

**Assessment**   **Areas of strength:** RN with nursing and leadership skills. Has basic knowledge about her illnesses from her education. Two co-workers are supportive of her.

**Problems:** Suicide attempt with overdose, alcohol abuse, insomnia, anorexia, recently divorced, no place to stay, unemployed, drug-using friend.

**Diagnoses**
- At risk for violence; self-directed related to depressed mood, as evidenced by suicide attempt.
- Low self-esteem related to divorce and job loss, as evidenced by statement of not liking self.
- At risk for injury related to medication overdose and alcohol withdrawal, as evidenced by weakness and shakiness.
- Altered nutrition; less than body requirements related to depressed mood as evidenced by anorexia.
- Sleep-pattern disturbance related to stress, as evidenced by insomnia.

**Outcomes**   *Short-term goals:*                                            *Date met*
- Patient will verbalize plans for the future.                     _____
- Patient will sleep 6 to 8 hours per night.                       _____
- Patient will eat three balanced meals per day.                   _____
- Patient will recognize and describe problems associated with     _____
  drinking alcohol and depression.
- Patient will make plans to live with a friend who does not use   _____
  drugs or to live at halfway house.

*Long-term goals:*
- Patient will practice abstinence from alcohol.                   _____
- Patient will attend self-help group such as Double Trouble or    _____
  Alcoholics Anonymous.
- Patient will attend outpatient treatment.                        _____
- Patient will be medication-compliant.                            _____
- Patient will live at halfway house or with a friend who does     _____
  not abuse drugs.
- Patient will participate in impaired nurse program through       _____
  the state nurses' association.

**Planning/
Interventions**   **Nurse-patient relationship:** Contract with patient to report to nurse if suicidal thoughts occur. Convey empathy and encourage verbalization of feelings. Reinforce strengths and accomplishments. Teach patient personal signs of relapse and relapse prevention for depression and alcohol abuse. Offer nutritious snacks. Assist patient with ambulation and activities of daily living (ADLs) when necessary and encourage independence when patient is able to perform own ADLs.

**Psychopharmacology:** Sertraline (Zoloft) 50 mg q AM; multivitamin 1 qd.

**Milieu management:** Invite and encourage patient to attend groups on assertiveness, stress management, alcohol, mental illness, medication education, and relapse prevention.

**Evaluation**   Patient denies suicidal ideation. She expresses interest in employment and making alternative living arrangements. She sleeps 6 hours per night and eats three balanced meals per day. The patient identifies some positive characteristics of self and past accomplishments.

**Referrals**   Patient to attend weekly Double Trouble in Recovery meetings and schedule appointments for dual-diagnosis treatment at a mental health clinic.

| Stage | Approach | Stage | Approach |
|-------|----------|-------|----------|
| 1. Precontemplation | Express concern about the patient and the patient's symptoms related to mental illness, substance use, and anxiety. | 4. Action | Encourage and support the client's efforts and adaptive action pertaining to any one disorder. Reinforce the importance of remaining in recovery while acknowledging the discomfort of withdrawal or illness-related symptoms. |
| 2. Contemplation | Discuss positive and negative aspects of substance use, past periods of abstinence, and psychological symptoms. Help the patient consider a trial of abstinence. | 5. Maintenance | Anticipate and discuss difficulties. Continually offer the patient support and motivation to continue working on problems. Reassure the client that relapse or illness-related symptoms will not disrupt the patient-clinician relationship. |
| 3. Preparation | Affirm and discuss the significance of seeking treatment for disorders. Assist the patient with establishing achievable, short-term goals for each disorder. Emphasize that relapse will not disrupt the patient-clinician relationship. | 6. Relapse | Express concern and discuss what can be learned from relapse related to any one disorder. Support the patient and remind the patient that recovery is achievable. |

Modified from U.S. Department of Health and Human Services: *KAP keys for clinicians based on TIP 42 substance abuse treatment for persons with co-occurring disorders,* Washington, DC, 2005, U.S. Department of Health and Human Services, Substance Abuse and Mental Health Services Administration Center for Substance Abuse Treatment.

---

## Highlighting the Evidence: Dual-Diagnosis Disease Management

The following principles underlying dual-diagnosis programs appear to be effective for patients with co-occurring disorders.

1. *Integration of treatment.* Recent studies have supported integrating mental health and substance abuse interventions at the level of clinical interaction or at one site. Multidisciplinary teams include mental health and substance abuse experts who provide interventions tailored to the individual's needs.
2. *Stage-wise interventions.* Stages in treatment consist of establishing trust with the patient, helping the patient develop motivation to engage in recovery, helping the patient acquire skills and supports, and helping the patient develop strategies to prevent relapse.
3. *Assertive outreach.* Difficulty in accessing services necessitates assertive outreach, intensive case management, help with housing, and time to develop trust before formal treatment can begin. Noncompliance and high dropout rates occur without these components.
4. *Motivational interventions.* Effective programs help motivate patients to actively participate in their treatment. Responsibility is placed on the patient to identify and set goals. Not managing one's illness interferes with goal attainment.
5. *Counseling.* Patients need to develop skills to pursue abstinence. Cognitive and behavioral skills along with motivational interventions are used.
6. *Social support interventions.* Social support is a critical component of treatment. It can be obtained from peer groups, social networks, and family interventions.
7. *Long-term perspective.* Recovery occurs in months to years. Effective programs are long-term and community-based. They include rehabilitation activities to prevent relapse and enhance gain.
8. *Comprehensiveness.* Programs provide comprehensive services to help transform aspects of one's life; housing, friends, and stress management are just a few examples to support dual-diagnosis patients.

Current dual-diagnosis outpatient programs involve community mental health services and substance abuse interventions tailored for patients with severe mental illness. Comprehensive integrated interventions are effective in engaging patients in treatment, reducing substance use, and stabilizing mental illness.

Modified from Drake RE: Dual diagnosis. In Trafton JA, Gordon WP, editors: *Best practices in the behavioral management of chronic disease,* vol 1, *Neuropsychiatric disorders,* Los Altos, CA, 2003-2004, Institute for Disease Management.

**Family Issues: Dual Diagnosis**

Families experience much distress in a situation in which a mentally ill relative uses substances. They are angry at their relative for using alcohol or a street drug because an additional problem has been added, often causing the person to be aggressive or violent. The relative might even steal from them to purchase alcohol or drugs.

Family members might feel guilty about thinking that their relative's problem is somehow their fault. It is not. Support and help can be attained from the National Alliance for the Mentally Ill (NAMI), Al-Anon, Alcoholics Anonymous, and Narcotics Anonymous. Some places might even have available a Double Trouble group or another type of self-help group for those with a dual diagnosis.

Enlist the help of members in your family to confront your relative supportively. Ask for behavior change, suggest treatment, limit access to money, provide evidence, and don't argue. Have a plan, including a contact for treatment. Talk to your relative's physician, nurse, treatment team, or clinician.

## Study Notes

1. Dual diagnosis can be defined as the comorbid presence of a substance abuse or dependency disorder and a mental illness or personality disorder.
2. Substance use is a common comorbity for adults with severe mental illness.
3. Patients with dual diagnosis experience higher rates of relapse, hospitalization, victimization, violence, incarceration, homelessness, and HIV and hepatitis infection.
4. The population of dual-diagnosis patients is heterogeneous.
5. Many issues must be addressed in treating dual-diagnosis patients because of their diverse abilities and needs related to their mental illness and substance use.
6. Patients with dual diagnoses benefit from integrated treatment for both substance abuse and mental illness simultaneously.
7. Integrated treatment is based on the patient's needs and occurs in stages.

## References

Addington J, Addington D: Impact of an early psychosis program on substance use, *Psychiatr Rehabil J* 25:60, 2001.

Becker DR, Drake RE, Naughton WJ Jr: Supported employment for people with co-occurring disorders, *Psychiatr Rehabil J* 28:332, 2005.

Donat DC, Haverkamp J: Treatment of psychiatric impairment complicated by co-occurring substance use: impact on rehospitalization, *Psychiatr Rehabil J* 28:78, 2004.

Drake RE: Dual diagnosis. In Trafton JA, Gordon WP, editors: *Best practices in the behavioral management of chronic disease,* vol 1, *Neuropsychiatric disorders,* Los Altos, CA, 2003-2004, Institute for Disease Management.

Drake R, Essock SM, Shaner A, et al: Implementing dual diagnosis services for clients with severe mental illness, *Psychiatr Serv* 52:469, 2001.

Drake RE, Wallach MA, Alverson HA, Mueser KT: Psychosocial aspects of substance abuse by clients with severe mental illness, *J Nerv Ment Dis* 190:100, 2002.

Gomez MB, Primm AB, Tzolova-Iontchev I, et al: A description of precipitants of drug use among dually diagnosed patients with chronic mental illness, *Community Ment Health J* 36:351, 2000.

Granholm E, Anthenelli R, Monteiro R, et al: Brief integrated outpatient dual-diagnosis treatment reduces psychiatric hospitalizations, *Am J Addict* 12:306, 2003.

Kasten BP: Self-medication with alcohol and drugs by persons with severe mental illness, *J Am Psychiatr Nurs Assoc* 5:80, 1999.

Littrell KH, Littrell SH: Schizophrenia and comorbid substance abuse, *J Am Psychiatr Nurs Assoc* 5:S18, 1999.

Miller MC: Dual diagnosis, part II, *Harv Ment Health Lett* 20:1, 2003.

Minkoff K: Developing standards of care for individuals with co-occurring psychiatric and substance use disorders, *Psychiatr Serv* 52:597, 2001.

Patrick DD: Dual diagnosis: substance-related and psychiatric disorders, *Nurs Clin North Am* 38:67, 2003.

U.S. Department of Health and Human Services: *KAP keys for clinicians based on TIP 42 substance abuse treatment for persons with co-occurring disorders,* Washington, DC, 2005, U.S. Department of Health and Human Services, Substance Abuse and Mental Health Services Administration Center for Substance Abuse Treatment.

Wagner T, Krampe H, Stawicki S, et al: Substantial decrease of psychiatric comorbity in chronic alcoholics upon integrated outpatient treatment—results of a prospective study, *J Psychiatr Res* 38:619, 2004.

Ziedonis DM, Smelson D, Rosenthal RN, et al: Improving the care of individuals with schizophrenia and substance use disorders: consensus recommendations, *J Psychiatr Pract* 11:315, 2005.

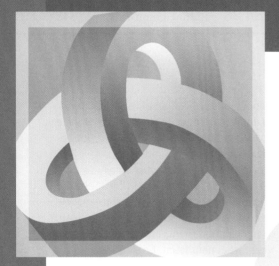

Chapter 37

# Eating Disorders

*Sandra Wood*

## Learning Objectives

*After reading this chapter, you should be able to:*

- Recognize criteria and terminology used in the *Diagnostic and Statistical Manual of Mental Disorders, Text Revision,* Fourth Edition *(DSM-IV-TR)* for eating disorders.
- Recognize and describe objective and subjective symptoms of eating disorders.
- Describe current etiologies for eating disorders.

- Describe treatment issues for professionals who deal with eating-disordered patients.
- Recognize the continuum from dieting to an obvious eating disorder.
- Develop nursing care plans for patients with eating disorders.
- Evaluate the effectiveness of nursing interventions for patients with eating disorders.

American culture has become preoccupied with food, eating, weight, and fitness. Men and women structure their daily schedules around health club and exercise programs in pursuit of increased attractiveness. Books on diets, nutrition, and fitness are sold in greater numbers than ever before. Even so, media reports have indicated that more people are overweight and there is now a greater percentage of American adult and children who qualify as obese (White, 2000). Restaurant portions are larger (Young and Nestle, 2002), and computer graphics technology enables advertisers to make already slender models look even thinner or more enhanced in areas such as the breasts. This presents an inaccurate image of the true size and shape of models and celebrities, and young women and sometimes men chase an unrealistic ideal (Andrist, 2003). Life-threatening eating disorders can be the result.

In this chapter, clinical examples, case studies, and nursing care plans focus on patients with the specific eating disorders of anorexia nervosa and bulimia nervosa, the most common eating disorders. The similarities and differences of these two disorders will be highlighted, as well as the continuum of eating behavior from dieting to anorexia, bulimia, and other eating disorders. Some professionals also consider obesity an eating disorder, but discussing it in detail is beyond the scope of this chapter.

## ANOREXIA NERVOSA

### *DSM-IV-TR* CRITERIA

The *DSM-IV-TR* diagnostic criteria for anorexia nervosa are found in the box to the right.

## Norm's Notes

*When I was a younger psychiatric nurse, it was difficult for me to really believe that eating disorders were legitimate mental health concerns. I just could not grasp that someone could not stop purging, or could start eating, if they really wanted to. I held that uninformed view until I worked with a few young people who could not stop or not start, whatever their particular problem was. I saw how it dominated and, in a few cases, ruined their lives. I can only say this—it is real and it can be devastating.*

Although anorectics limit their intake or refuse to eat, they generally do not lose their appetites. They suppress their appetite in an effort to remain thin or get thinner (Kaye et al, 2000). In fact, they think about food and eating much of the time. Weight or shape is often the most important influence on the eating-disordered person's sense of worth. They might deny that they are dangerously thin, or might acknowledge their underweight status but then deny that their condition is problematic (Halmi, 2005).

| *DSM-IV-TR* Criteria | for Anorexia Nervosa |
|---|---|

A. Refusal to maintain body weight at or above a minimum normal weight for age and height
B. Intense fear of gaining weight or becoming fat, although significantly underweight
C. Disturbance in the way in which one's body weight or shape is experienced, overvaluing of shape or weight, or denial of seriousness of low weight or weight loss
D. In women and female adolescents, the absence of at least three consecutive menstrual cycles
*Restricting type:* During an episode of anorexia nervosa, individuals do *not* engage in recurrent episodes of binge eating or purging.
*Binge-eating or purging type:* During an episode of anorexia nervosa, individuals engage in recurrent episodes of binge eating or purging.

Modified from the American Psychiatric Association: *Diagnostic and statistical manual of mental disorders, text revision,* ed 4, Washington, DC, 2000, APA.

Menstruation might cease early in the illness, before significant weight loss has taken place, or menstruation might continue but be irregular and spotty. If menarche has not been reached, menstruation might not begin. One theory for the cause of amenorrhea suggests that lack of nourishment significantly slows pituitary functioning, fundamental to the menstrual cycle. Women must maintain a body mass index (BMI) of 18 or higher to support menstruation (Muscari, 2002). Levels below this can result in amenorrhea, with accompanying reduction of hormone levels and inadequate development of secondary sexual characteristics. In anorectic men, low sex drive and low testosterone levels might be the equivalent of amenorrhea in female patients (Braun et al, 1999).

Anorexia is less common than bulimia, affecting up to 3.7% of women during their lifetime (Finelli, 2001). Women account for approximately 90% of the reported cases of anorexia nervosa, although anorexia in men appears to be increasing, as noted later in this chapter (Cohane and Pope, 2001). Onset varies from preadolescence to early adulthood, with an increasing incidence at early adolescence (12 to 13 years of age) as well as some new-onset cases in middle and later adulthood (Bulik et al, 2005). These ages correspond with transitional stages in people's lives. Initial morbidity and relapse from adolescent episodes are being seen in adulthood, as well as in adolescence. From 6% to 20% of anorectic patients die as a result of their illness, usually through starvation or suicide, which is a rate higher than in most other psychiatric disorders (Andrist, 2003; Keel et al, 2003; Pompli et al, 2004).

## BEHAVIOR

The onset of anorexia is often insidious because the typical adolescent victim, who is usually female, appears compliant and does not cause problems for others. Because dieting and fad foods are common in adolescence and young adulthood, often no one notices until the young woman has lost a significant amount of weight. A common premorbid personality profile is that of a perfectionistic and introverted girl with self-esteem and peer relationship problems, but victims might also be accomplished and active in school activities (Bulik et al, 2005).

## Objective Signs

The most observable behavior of anorexia nervosa is deliberate weight loss in an effort to control weight through changing eating behaviors. Patients with anorexia nervosa are in two groups: the restricters and the vomiters-purgers. The restricters are more often young people in the normal or slightly above normal weight range for height and build before the eating disorder begins. This group views losing weight as more probable if they simply eat less and avoid social situations in which they are expected to eat. Restricters often withdraw to their rooms and avoid family and friends. It is not uncommon for them to be competitive, compulsive, and obsessive about their activities. They might participate in rigid exercise programs to help reduce their weight (Kaye et al, 2000). Many restricting anorectics become hyperactive to lose weight and because they are highly anxious and unable to relax. They might take early morning walks because of insomnia and a need to burn off calories.

### CLINICAL EXAMPLE

Kristin, age 15, was in the normal weight range when she joined the school volleyball team with her friends. The first time they donned their uniforms, one of Kristin's friends called her "piano legs." Kristin was horrified and began to diet. In addition, she asked her parents to join the local health club so she could exercise to keep in shape for the team. Her entire day revolved around participation on the team to the extent that she forfeited all other social involvement. She did not arrive home until after 9 PM each night because she went to the health club to exercise after a volleyball game or after practice. Kristin lost 21 pounds before anyone noticed.

Compared with restricters, vomiters-purgers are more often overweight before the eating disorder begins, and their weight tends to fluctuate (Kaye et al, 2000). These are usually young women who are prone to dangerous methods of weight reduction, such as induction of vomiting or excessive use of laxatives or diuretics. These anorectic patients commonly deny concerns about weight and typically eat normally in social situations. After the meal, they retreat to the nearest bathroom and purge themselves of the consumed food, although the amount is not excessive, as it is with bulimics. Dental problems frequently occur in these patients because the acidic vomitus decays the enamel on their teeth (Orbanic, 2001). This group also might be susceptible to times when they uncontrollably eat large amounts of food, if unsuccessful in maintaining the severe dietary restriction they impose on themselves. Purgers are more likely to have histories of behavior problems, substance abuse, and open family conflict than restricting anorectics (Kaye et al, 2000).

### CLINICAL EXAMPLE

Tina was always a chubby child. When she was 23 years old, she lost considerable weight by dieting. Shortly thereafter, she began seriously dating and was married. Tina was thrilled with her new look and worked hard to maintain her weight loss, consistently keeping her weight slightly under the ideal for her height. After 2 years of marriage, Tina became pregnant. The thought of gaining weight during her pregnancy upset Tina greatly, and she vowed to herself never to let herself become chubby again. Before long, Tina's doctor noticed that she was not gaining weight at her monthly prenatal checkups and asked what she was eating. When she did a food log for the office nurse, her anorectic behavior was revealed.

Because the intake of nutrients is so low in anorectic patients, their bodies try to adjust by using less energy. Consequently, other physiologic processes are affected. Hypotension, bradycardia, and hypothermia are common. The skin is often dry, and lanugo might appear. Many patients have delayed gastric emptying, causing them to feel full much longer than most people. Thus, these patients do not have the normal desire to eat as often as others. Therefore, they believe they can get by on one small meal a day. Slower abdominal peristalsis combined with decreased intake leads to constipation, fueling the use of laxatives, which leads to dehydration and gives the anorectic a false sense of decreased weight. Dehydration can lead to irreversible renal damage. Refeeding syndrome involving severe shifts in fluid and electrolyte levels from extracellular to intracellular spaces in severely emaciated patients can occur, causing cardiovascular, neurologic, and hematologic complications, and even death (Katzman, 2005). Therefore, refeeding must be done slowly and under very close supervision to prevent serious problems. Pitting edema occurs in some anorectic patients, most often after attempts to gain weight by eating more food during the refeeding process while in treatment. Noticing the swelling, the patient often becomes anxious about the weight gain, immediately stops eating, and might attempt to counteract the perceived weight gain, further complicating the emaciated condition. In addition, osteopenia or osteoporosis might develop as a consequence of prolonged amenorrhea and malnutrition (Muscari, 2002). This bone mass loss might be irreversible if the anorexia goes on long enough. Moreover, studies have found ventricular dilation, decreases in thickness of the left ventricular wall, alterations in the size of the cardiac chambers, and decreased myocardial oxygen uptake, which can lead to life-threatening cardiac arrhythmias (Bulik et al, 2005; Katzman, 2005).

Anorectic patients become preoccupied with food and eating (Bulik et al, 2005). This preoccupation involves all aspects of life. Patients are often found reading many materials on food and dieting and attempting to control family meals because they believe that they are the nutrition authorities in their household. Patients might engage in bizarre behavior regarding food and eating, such as hoarding food or preparing elaborate meals for others but not eating the food they prepare. Elaborate rituals before and during eating might become a compulsion, which adds to the patient's problems and might result in the patient being diagnosed with obsessive-compulsive disorder as well as anorexia (Kaye et al, 2004).

### Subjective Symptoms

An outstanding feature of anorexia nervosa is the conscious fear that these patients have of losing control over the amount of food eaten, resulting in becoming fat. Patients are concerned about being obese, losing weight, or preventing weight gain. Some patients even say that they would rather be dead than fat. This fear motivates them to begin dieting. The fear might be triggered by an event that seems trivial to others, such as an offhand comment by a friend or relative or one or more traumatic events for the patient. These patients might feel abandoned or inadequate, which can precipitate an overall feeling of helplessness. They try to combat helplessness by controlling what they can control—how much food

they eat and, thus, their weight. Much of the patient's energy becomes invested in this effort (Williamson et al, 2004).

In addition to problems with eating behavior and weight concern, anorectic individuals have other psychological symptoms known to be consequences of semistarvation. These patients exhibit depression, irritability, social withdrawal, lessened sex drive, and obsessional symptoms, which are also seen in research studies of starvation. It is believed that some of the anorectic's bizarre behavior might be the result of the starvation (Bruch, 1973; Finnelli, 2001). These symptoms often diminish with weight gain but, if they do not, the patient might be faced with a comorbid condition such as obsessive-compulsive disorder, major depression, substance abuse, or personality disorders (Ro et al, 2005).

## ETIOLOGY

The psychiatrist Hilde Bruch (1973) believed that anorexia was caused by a number of specific disturbances. Today, most experts agree that eating disorders have multifactorial causes, with significant variance among individuals (Kaye et al, 2000). Suggested contributing factors include biologic, sociocultural, family, cognitive, behavioral, and psychodynamic factors.

### Biologic Factors

Earlier in the twentieth century, physiologic disturbances were postulated as causative in anorexia. Currently, researchers believe that the physiologic abnormalities found in anorectic patients are mostly a result of semistarvation and purging behavior rather than the cause of disordered eating. An exception might be increased serotonin levels. Studies have found that, even after long-term weight restoration and recovery, anorectics have increased cerebrospinal fluid (CSF) levels of 5-hydroxyindoleacetic acid (5-HIAA) the major metabolite of serotonin. Serotonin activity is known to have inhibitory effects on a number of areas and might lead to food restriction caused by inhibited appetite, as well as to the rigid, inhibited, anxious, and obsessional behaviors seen in anorectics (Kaye et al, 2005). Unfortunately, the use of selective serotonin reuptake inhibitors (SSRIs), which regulate serotonin levels in depressed patients, has not been as effective in treating anorexia as in treating bulimia. Researchers such as Kaye and associates (2005) have suggested that the malnutrition of anorexia might negate the positive effects of SSRI medication in early treatment; if SSRIs are used to treat anorexia, they should not be started until weight restoration has been achieved.

## Sociocultural Factors

Feminist theorists have highlighted the role of Western philosophical, political, and cultural history in the development of eating disorders. The increased incidence of eating disorders in the twentieth century has been recognized as corresponding to an increasingly and unrealistically thin beauty ideal for women, almost a culture of thinness (Brumberg, 1997; Rand and Wright, 2000). In addition, American culture has advanced the notion that body weight is a matter of personal choice and that shape can be changed at will. Computer imaging technology has resulted in the enhancement of photos on the Internet in response to the current societal standard of beauty. These images encourage dieting, which is a major predisposing factor to both anorexia nervosa and bulimia nervosa (White, 2000).

Another factor is the relational orientation of women, which creates a vulnerability to the opinions of others, particularly during adolescence (Andrist, 2003). American culture stresses the importance of physical attractiveness in obtaining approval and, because of the thin beauty ideal, some girls believe that thinness will lead to approval by others. Lack of approval is interpreted as being caused by a less than ideal body size that causes girls, in particular, to begin dieting.

## Family Factors

Several studies of identical and fraternal twins have suggested a genetic component to the causation of anorexia (Kaye et al, 2000). Family environment might also play a role. Emotional restraint, enmeshed relationships, rigid organization in the family, tight control of child behavior by parents, and avoidance of conflict are other etiologies (Kaye et al, 2000). Odd eating habits and an emphasis on appearance and weight by other family members, especially mothers and sisters, have also been described (Mazzeo et al, 2005). However, the extent to which the observed family problems of anorectics are consequences of the disorder rather than etiologies is still to be determined.

## Cognitive and Behavioral Factors

Behavioral theorists have noted that anorectic behavior develops and is maintained as a function of environmental contingencies. Rejecting food and losing weight, for example, might be reinforced by positive attention from others (Finelli, 2001). The use of behavioral treatments such as assertiveness training and cognitive restructuring is based upon such cognitive factors.

## Psychodynamic Factors

Modern psychoanalytic theorists have stressed the role of sexuality in anorexia nervosa. In addition, some clinicians have suggested that eating disorders might be related to an early history of sexual abuse. Some research indicates that childhood sexual abuse seems to be related to increased body shame, which is a risk factor for eating disorders and self-mutilation (Wonderlich et al, 2001). Sexual abuse might predispose a person to psychiatric disorders in general, rather than to eating disorders in particular.

Some researchers have suggested that anorexia involves a regression to a prepubertal state, so that the adolescent does not mature physically or emotionally. Regression is reinforced when the anorectic adolescent's dependency needs are met. The conscious fear of becoming fat is thought to be the symbolic expression of becoming bigger, or growing up, supposedly the real unconscious fear of the anorectic. Other psychoanalytic theorists have suggested that the drive for thinness might be an attempt to reduce the control of an overcontrolling maternal figure (Stein and Corte, 2003).

Another theory has described anorexia nervosa as an obsession with weight stemming from a fear of being out of control because of the lack of a well-defined self. Patients use reaction formation to organize their lives with a set of rules and regulations for everything they do. They experience a tremendous amount of anxiety if their rules are broken and attempt to regain control by tightening the rules and punishing themselves for their failure (Stein and Corte, 2003).

Experts agree that the causes of anorexia nervosa are multifactorial. Biologic, sociocultural, family, cognitive, behavioral, and psychodynamic factors all might contribute to the disease. Factors contributing to the maintenance of anorexia might be different than those leading to its development.

Today, most research focuses on factors contributing to the onset of dieting (White, 2000). Greater emphasis on factors contributing to the development and maintenance of eating-disordered behavior might result in a better understanding of this disorder and more effective prevention of the disease. Research on adult-onset eating disorders might also prove fruitful, because this phenomenon is being observed more frequently in recent years (Bulik et al, 2005).

## CRITICAL THINKING QUESTION   1

Some theorists contend that adolescent eating disorders are an expression of ambivalence toward becoming an adult. Explain how this might have some validity.

## BULIMIA NERVOSA

### DSM-IV-TR CRITERIA

See the *DSM-IV-TR* Diagnostic Criteria for Bulimia Nervosa box and the NANDA International Diagnoses Related to Eating Disorders box.

| *DSM-IV-TR* Criteria for Bulimia Nervosa |
| --- |
| A. Recurrent episodes of binge eating in a short time period, with intake much greater than average |
| B. A feeling of lack of control over eating behaviors during eating binges |
| C. Recurrent inappropriate compensatory behavior in order to prevent weight gain, such as self-induced vomiting; use of laxatives, enemas, or diuretics; strict dieting or fasting; vigorous exercise; or taking diet pills |
| D. Binge eating and inappropriate compensatory behaviors both occurring, on average, at least twice a week for 3 months |
| E. Self-evaluation unduly influenced by body shape and weight |
| *Purging type:* Regularly engages in self-induced vomiting or the use of laxatives, diuretics, or enemas |
| *Nonpurging type:* Regularly uses strict diet, fasting, or vigorous exercise, but does not regularly engage in purging |

Modified from the American Psychiatric Association: *Diagnostic and statistical manual of mental disorders, text revision,* ed 4, Washington, DC, 2000, APA.

| NANDA International Diagnoses Related to Eating Disorders |
| --- |
| Anxiety (specify level of anxiety) |
| Body image, disturbed |
| Coping, family, compromised |
| Coping, family, disabled |
| Coping, ineffective |
| Denial, ineffective |
| Family processes, interrupted |
| Fluid volume, deficient, risk for |
| Fluid volume, imbalanced, risk for |
| Nutrition: less than body requirements, imbalanced |
| Nutrition: more than body requirements, imbalanced |
| Powerlessness |
| Self-esteem, chronic low |
| Social interaction, impaired |
| Social isolation |

From NANDA International: *NANDA nursing diagnoses: definitions and classifications,* 2005-2006, Philadelphia, NANDA International.

Bulimia nervosa usually begins in adolescence or early adult life, primarily in women, although males have now been diagnosed more often than in the past (Braun et al, 1999). The prevalence of bulimia among adolescents and young adult women is thought to be approximately 1% to 2% of adolescents and 4% of young adults (Orbanic, 2001). The usual course of the disorder is chronic and intermittent over a period of many years. Most commonly, the binge periods alternate with periods of restrictive eating, complicating diagnosis and treatment (Orbanic, 2001).

### BEHAVIOR

The word *bulimia* literally means to have an insatiable appetite. The term is often used to describe massive overeating and is used interchangeably with binge eating or bingeing. Until recently, bulimia nervosa was considered to be part of anorexia nervosa, because almost half of patients diagnosed with anorexia were observed to have binge-eating episodes. Bulimia nervosa is now considered a separate disorder, although there is still much overlap between the disorders (Kaye et al, 2000). The true prevalence of bulimia nervosa is unknown because many patients hide their eating-disordered behaviors. They might be diagnosed with other more familiar psychiatric disorders such as major depression, personality disorders, or posttraumatic stress disorder (Orbanic, 2001). Individuals who seek medical attention (usually for gastrointestinal or menstrual disturbances) could be identified as having bulimia, but the lack of weight loss might blind the treatment provider to the patient's bulimia (Orbanic, 2001).

The onset of the illness is usually between the ages of 15 and 24 years. The disease might develop after anorexia nervosa or following a period of dieting. The dieting predisposes the individual to binge eating, and purging develops as a means of compensating for calories ingested during the binge in an attempt to prevent weight gain. The individual continues restrictive eating during the disorder, which precipitates binge eating and then purging, thus perpetuating the cycle.

---

### CLINICAL EXAMPLE

Mary, age 28, was a young professional with an active social life. Although she was approximately 15 pounds overweight, Mary used her sense of humor to hide any serious concern she had about her appearance. However, Mary worried that her weight might deny her a highly prized job that she wanted. Before applying for the job at a prestigious banking firm, Mary began dieting and ate less food than did her friends at lunch. When she arrived home, however, Mary felt hungry and secretly raided her refrigerator, making several sandwiches before dinner. Despite feeling guilty over her uncontrolled snacking, Mary ate dinner with her roommate. After dinner, feeling uncomfortably full, Mary retreated to the bathroom and vomited until she felt empty. She vowed to try harder to diet the next day, only to have a similar experience.

---

It is important to distinguish overeating from binge eating. To meet *DSM-IV-TR* diagnostic criteria for a binge episode, the eating behavior must qualify as an "objective bulimic episode." That is, the person consumes an unusually large amount of food in a relatively short period (e.g., several thousand calories in less than 2 hours). The amount

of food eaten is considered by others to be atypically large for the particular situation. Additionally, there is a feeling of lack of control over eating during the binge (Orbanic, 2001).

### Objective Signs

Most bulimic patients are secretive about their behavior. A variety of foods might be eaten during a binge, but the most common is high-calorie, high-carbohydrate "snack" food easily ingested in a short period. Some bulimics visit several different fast food restaurants or grocery stores during a binge so that no one knows how much they are eating at one time. Some patients with bulimia have been caught shoplifting food. Most binges occur during the evening or at night. The amount of calories consumed during a binge varies, but is considerably more than the recommended daily allowance (Orbanic, 2001). There is a tendency to eat rapidly during the binge.

Patients report that their bulimic episodes usually end when they begin to induce vomiting, are physically exhausted, suffer from painful abdominal distention, are interrupted by others, or have simply run out of food. After a binge, patients promise themselves to adhere to a strict diet and vow never to binge again, only to return to this behavior because they find themselves addicted to the high they experience when bingeing. Many bulimics resume their usual schedules, as if they had never been interrupted. The frequency of binges varies greatly, depending on the patient. Some patients report having several episodes a day; others report losing control two or three times a week (Orbanic, 2001).

Medical complications in bulimic patients depend on the form and frequency of purging and can include previously described mechanical irritation and dilation of the stomach resulting from binge eating. Fluid and electrolyte abnormalities might result from self-induced vomiting or abuse of laxatives or diuretics; these can include dehydration, hyponatremia, hypochloremia, hypokalemia, and metabolic alkalosis and acidosis. Self-induced vomiting and laxative abuse can cause mechanical irritation and injuries to the gastrointestinal tract. Abuse of laxatives, diuretics, and diet pills can result in addiction. Laxatives can lead to reflex constipation, and both laxatives and diuretics are associated with rebound edema (Orbanic, 2001).

Use of ipecac syrup to induce vomiting is particularly dangerous; it can be toxic and cause fatal cardiomyopathy. Bulimics often have menstrual irregularities or enlarged salivary glands, particularly the parotid glands. Erosion of the dental enamel from chronic vomiting often occurs. Russell's sign, callusing of the knuckles of the fingers used to induce vomiting, is also common. Pancreatitis has also been reported in bulimics (Muscari, 2002).

## SUBJECTIVE SYMPTOMS

Although most bulimic patients have a normal body weight, they are gravely concerned about their body shape and weight. Loss of control over eating causes them great anxiety and shame and, similar to anorectic patients, they express a fear of becoming fat (Orbanic, 2001).

Moods vary considerably among bulimic patients. Some bulimics have reported feeling weak before a binge, followed either by continued anxiety or relief from tension during the binge (Orbanic, 2001). Patients have reported feeling anxious, lonely, or bored, or uncontrollably craving food before the binge. The anxiety present before the binge is replaced with guilt after the binge. If the anxiety is not relieved after the binge, patients feel angry and agitated and might become depressed. Depression appears to be common in bulimic patients. The relationship between bulimia and depression might be one in which one causes the other or there might be independent factors contributing to both disorders. Researchers have found a high rate of mood disorders, particularly depression, in families in which bulimia occurs (Keel et al, 2005). Substance abuse and anxiety disorders also occur at a higher than normal rate among bulimics. It appears that although pharmacotherapy can be helpful, it should be combined with psychotherapy for the most effective long-term outcome.

Most bulimic patients induce vomiting to reduce the fear of becoming fat. Patients might self-induce vomiting by sticking their fingers, a toothbrush, or an eating utensil down their throats; this is a dangerous practice, because patients have swallowed objects used to induce vomiting. Over time, vomiting becomes easier and might require only slight abdominal pressure or no physical manipulation at the end of the binge (Mendell and Logemann, 2001). Some bulimics eat what is known as a *marker* food at the beginning of the binge and then vomit until this food comes back up. This practice is ineffective because food is quickly mixed in the stomach. Furthermore, although bulimics believe that self-induced vomiting rids them of all binge calories, researchers have determined that only a partial amount of calories consumed can be regurgitated. Abuse of laxatives or diuretics primarily causes fluid loss rather than a reduction in absorbed calories (Orbanic, 2001). Other compensatory behavior might include the neglect of insulin requirements by patients with diabetes mellitus (Poirier-Solomon, 2001).

## ETIOLOGY

Similar to anorexia, the causes of bulimia nervosa are thought to be multifactorial, with biologic, sociocultural, family, cognitive, behavioral, and psychodynamic contributing factors. Many of the factors thought to precipitate anorexia are also thought to be involved in bulimia. The focus of this discussion therefore will be on the proposed causes of bulimia that are different than those stated for anorexia.

### Biologic Factors

Brain chemistry has been increasingly implicated in studies relating to the cause of eating disorders, with several neuroendocrine and neurotransmitter abnormalities demonstrated in dieters and in those demonstrating symptoms of eating disorders. Biologic and genetic factors have also been implicated in the causes of bulimia and anorexia. Most researchers believe that illness symptoms are related to the physiologic state of the victims and will lessen when weight is restored. However, serotonin activity appears to be an exception. It has been proposed that, as in depression, there is generally lowered serotonin activity in the brains of bulimics (Kaye et al, 2000). Binge eating is seen by some as a form of self-medication to raise the levels of serotonin. Treatment of bulimia with SSRI antidepressants, particularly fluoxetine (Prozac), appears to be helpful whether or not patients have comorbid depression, so it is not known whether or not the antidepressant has a direct effect on the bulimia (Goldstein et al, 1999).

## Sociocultural Factors

These factors are thought to be the same as those for anorexia nervosa, as noted earlier in this chapter.

## Family Factors

As with anorexia nervosa, a heritable component for bulimia has been proposed. Twin studies have found a higher concordance rate for bulimia in identical than in fraternal twins (Kaye et al, 2000). In addition, mood disorders and substance abuse disorders are found at a higher rate in the families of bulimics (Kaye et al, 2000), which might be a result of both biologic and environmental factors.

Families of bulimics are seen as having a great deal of conflict, being disorganized, lacking in nurturance, and not being cohesive (Kaye et al, 2000). Observations of family interactions have yielded similar data, lending credence to the idea that the bulimia might be a response to chaos in the family.

## Cognitive and Behavioral Factors

Christopher Fairburn and colleagues pioneered work on cognitive-behavioral theory for the maintenance of bulimia nervosa after its onset. According to this theory, bulimia nervosa is maintained by cycles of low self-esteem, extreme concerns about body shape and weight, strict dieting, binge eating, and compensatory behavior, which interact and affect each other. Thus, bulimia is maintained by the behaviors of dieting, bingeing, and purging, which, in turn, are both affected by and contribute to distorted and negative cognitions about the self and the body (Williamson et al, 2004). This theory has led to the development of successful cognitive-behavioral therapy programs for bulimia nervosa that target both eating-disordered behaviors and cognitions (Bakke et al, 2001; O'Dea and Abraham, 2000).

## Psychodynamic Factors

Some psychodynamic theorists have placed particular emphasis on ambivalent feelings of self-esteem in bulimics. The binge eating and purging behavior is thought to express the ambivalence that patients feel toward themselves. On the one hand, patients believe that they are worthy of the nurturing they lack and, because food is a symbolic form of nurturing, they binge. On the other hand, patients feel unworthy of nurturing, so they purge. Bingeing and purging can also be seen as the patient's attempt to numb themselves from the pain in their lives resulting from abuse, neglect, trauma, and strong feelings (Orbanic, 2001).

---

### Comparing Anorexia and Bulimia

**Shared Features**

Restriction of intake at times, especially anorectics

Bingeing or overeating at times, especially bulimics

Purging through vomiting, laxatives, or diuretics

Overexercise

Extreme concern about appearance

Perfectionistic traits—dissatisfaction with appearance and performance in aspects of life such as work or school

Belief that their worth is based solely on appearance

Discomfort in social settings, especially with the opposite gender

Misperception of their size, shape, and level of fat

Low self-esteem

**Differentiation of Behaviors**

| Anorexia | Bulimia |
|---|---|
| Early onset | Later onset |
| Very low weight | More normal weight |
| Amenorrhea for some patients | Menstrual irregularities but not amenorrhea |
| Hormonal imbalance | Fluid and electrolyte imbalance |
| Constipation if not using laxatives | Gastrointestinal problems related to bingeing and purging |

---

## PUTTING IT ALL TOGETHER
### Psychotherapeutic Management

Psychotherapeutic management for anorexia and bulimia shares many characteristics and has some differences. In this section, the commonalities and differences will be highlighted. The psychotherapeutic management of each disorder will vary, depending on the period of treatment being considered and whether the focus is on short- or long-term treatment. For example, when an ano-

## Family Issues: Problems for Children of Mothers Who Have Eating Disorders

Studies have found that mothers with eating disorders are very concerned about their child's well-being, but the child tends to be malnourished because of the mother's concerns about the child's weight and misinterpretation of a normal child's eating behavior. Mothers who have anorexia nervosa tend to overemphasize weight and worry unduly about their children's weight. These concerns can lead mothers to dilute bottles, limit food at mealtimes, keep very little food in the house, and adhere to rigid feeding schedules. Not only do children in such an environment become mal-

nourished, they also learn to eat in the same disordered ways as their mothers. Interventions to help eating-disordered mothers establish healthy eating and exercise habits and promote positive eating environments for their children, as well as resisting external messages promoting thinness, are planned to help prevent eating disorders in the children of mothers who have anorexia nervosa. It is hoped such interventions will have positive effects on the mother's eating disorder as well (Mazzeo et al, 2005).

rectic patient is hospitalized because of extreme weight loss and its life-threatening physical effects, the focus must be on weight restoration before any treatment dealing with changing the patient's perceptions about his or her body or any long-term goals can be addressed.

Management of anorexia is geared toward three primary objectives: (1) increasing weight to at least 90% of the average body weight for the patient's height; (2) helping patients reestablish appropriate eating behavior; and (3) increasing self-esteem, so patients do not need to attain the perfection that they believe thinness provides. The objectives for bulimics are similar but, rather than the need for weight increase, are more likely to focus on stabilizing weight without purging, because bulimics are more likely to be of normal weight.

When patients are in the starvation phase of anorexia and malnutrition has become a serious medical problem, treatment occurs in a medical environment in which appropriate supplies and equipment, such as intravenous lines and feeding tubes, are readily available for feeding the patient if he or she will not do so voluntarily. Refeeding and weight restoration in anorexia must be done slowly and carefully, with close monitoring by experts to avoid life-threatening physical complications and possible death. As for the treatment of anorexia nervosa, medical stabilization of the bulimic patient is the initial treatment goal. After medical stabilization, psychotherapy is the treatment of choice (Castro et al, 2004). When medical crises are resolved, patients are transferred to a psychiatric unit or are seen in an outpatient

program, in which effective psychotherapeutic intervention can occur.

Cognitive-behavioral therapy has the greatest research support, although limited evidence exists suggesting that interpersonal psychotherapy might have similar effectiveness (McIntosh et al, 2000). Pharmacotherapy is used as an adjunct to psychotherapy for bulimics, when indicated (Nakash-Eisikovits et al, 2002).

Nurses might encounter anorectic or bulimic patients on an inpatient basis in a medical or psychiatric unit or on an outpatient basis in a physician's office, clinic, or school. Bulimics are less likely to be encountered in inpatient settings unless their purging has led to medical complications, but should be hospitalized in the following circumstances: (1) to treat a psychiatric or medical crisis; (2) when respite is needed from a chaotic home life so that the bulimic can examine his or her living situation more objectively; and (3) if the patient cannot obtain treatment in their home community. In any setting, a multidisciplinary treatment approach is crucial. Members of the treatment team should include a physician, nurse, dietitian, and psychotherapist specializing in the treatment of eating disorders. These patients need thorough medical and psychiatric assessment, medical monitoring, nutritional education and counseling, and psychotherapy (Stewart and Williamson, 2004). Assessment should include use of instruments from self-reporting to more structured interview tools, as well as differential diagnosis of other psychiatric conditions, including affective disorders, personality disorders, anxiety disorders such as obsessive-compulsive

## Highlighting the Evidence

### Comparison of Family Therapy and Family Group Psychoeducation in Adolescents With Anorexia Nervosa

*Description:* This late 1990s study at an eating disorders program in Toronto, Canada, compared 4 months of family therapy with a psychiatrist and two social workers to 4 months of family psychoeducation with an occupational therapist, dietitian, and registered nurse. A group of 25 adolescent girls meeting the *DSM-IV-TR* criteria for anorexia and admitted to the hospital needing treatment for weight restoration met the criteria for the study and were randomly placed in the family therapy or family psychoeducation group. The study was undertaken to determine which of the two treatment methods was more effective.

*Results:* In both groups, weight restoration (from 77% to 96% of ideal body weight) was achieved for a majority of patients. Hospital length of stay was also similar for both groups. Both groups acknowledged more family pathology at the end of treatment than at the beginning. There appeared to be no significant difference between the treatment modalities, although family group psychoeducation was less expensive than family therapy.

*Implications:* Because family group psychoeducation is a less expensive and more easily administered treatment due, in part, to the type of personnel needed to present the program, it might be a more effective treatment in situations in which costs of care are severely constrained.

Modified from Geist R, Heinmaa M, Stephens D, et al: Comparison of family therapy and family group psychoeducation in adolescents with anorexia nervosa, *Can J Psychiatry* 45:173, 2000.

disorders, and substance abuse or dependence (Pike, 2005).

Treatment for comorbid diagnoses with psychotherapy and medication will enhance the success of treatment for the eating disorder. Premorbid physical conditions that should be ruled out include thyroid conditions, bowel disease or other gastrointestinal conditions, pancreatitis, cancer, or the effects of medications. If eating behaviors are caused by one of these conditions, therapeutic effectiveness involves different treatments than if the eating behaviors were solely the result of an eating disorder. Patients with diabetes might also develop eating disorders, thus increasing their risk of serious medical complications of diabetes in the future and the risk of ketoacidosis in the present (Poirier-Solomon, 2001).

Working with anorectic or bulimic patients presents a challenge to the psychotherapeutic team as patients continue their struggle to maintain control. When the treatment team requires weight gain or an end to bingeing and purging, patients perceive themselves as losing control, which triggers unconscious feelings of helplessness and resistance to treatment goals and interventions. Consciously, patients again experience the fear of becoming fat. This fear underlies the need to gain more control, restarting the vicious cycle of disordered eating. Nurses need to confront this fear openly and help patients to find ways to deal with it (Cummings et al, 2001). See the Tips for Professionals From Persons Recovering From Eating Disorders box. NANDA International nursing diagnoses for eating disorders are listed in the box noted earlier in this chapter. Also see the Key Nursing Interventions for Patients With Eating Disorders box.

## NURSE-PATIENT RELATIONSHIP

Because most anorectic patients have been forced into treatment by concerned family or friends, developing a therapeutic alliance is a challenge. Patients might believe that the nurse's purpose is simply to make them gain weight, so the nurse is perceived as an enemy, not an ally. Bulimic patients differ from anorectic patients in that bulimics are more likely to want help. They are more likely to enter therapy of their own volition, are eager to please, and so behave in a manner that will lead therapists to like them. However, in trying to please, bulimic patients have a tendency to become manipulative and might conceal the full extent of their problem. The desire to be helped is the greatest strength of bulimic patients.

See Chapters 7 and 8 for general information about communicating with patients and developing rapport and trust with patients. Specific thera-

## Tips for Professionals and Families From Persons Recovering From Eating Disorders*

Be wary of rigidly applying *DSM-IV-TR* criteria in the detection of eating disorders.

- Some patients never binge or purge but control weight with exercise and restriction of intake.
- Some patients do not stop menstruating, although there might be changes in their cycles.
- Depression, anxiety, neglect, and domestic violence might predispose patients to eating disorders or be seen comorbidly with them. If only these disorders are treated without treating the eating disorder, efforts will likely fail.
- Patients' concentration on exactness and perfection might lead them to deny their illness by rationalizing that, if they do not exhibit *all* the criteria of the disorder, they do not have the disorder.
- Patients might recognize that their body image is distorted but might be unable to stop their destructive behavior.
- Not all eating-disordered patients have rituals about eating. They might simply avoid being in situations in which they have to eat in front of others.

When educating adolescents about eating disorders, avoid using films or other graphic materials that might teach the teens more ways to beat the system regarding eating and maintaining healthy weight.

Dishonesty (lying to self and others) is a hallmark of patients with eating disorders. Honesty toward self and others is the key to recovery and relapse prevention.

Watch for the onset of eating disorders at times of major life transition with increased pressure on an individual to fit in or adjust. These times include the move to middle school from elementary school, to high school from junior high or middle school, and graduation from high school with the move to college or a job.

Patients with eating disorders believe that calories are everywhere and go to great lengths to avoid them, including not smelling food or licking stamps for fear calories will be absorbed.

Media images of very thin models and celebrities might be viewed by very young girls as an ideal to be achieved, but most patients use media images of thinness to justify their behavior after becoming eating-disordered rather than motivation to begin their disordered eating.

*I wish to acknowledge the sharing of a local chapter of the Anorexia and Associated Disorders Association of Indianapolis support group in 2000, whose members offered their experience and information to help professionals deal with individuals such as themselves.

## Key Nursing Interventions   *for Patients with Eating Disorders*

- Monitor daily caloric intake and electrolyte status while in the hospital; patients should not gain too much weight too quickly.
- Observe patients for signs of purging or other compensation for food consumed.
- Monitor activity level and encourage appropriate levels of activity for patient.
- Weigh daily while in hospital, but encourage patient to diminish focus on weight after refeeding.
- Plan for a dietitian to meet with patients and families to (1) provide accurate information on nutrition, (2) discuss a realistic and healthy diet, and (3) assist the nurses in monitoring the nutritional intake of the patient (particularly crucial for patients who are diabetic or pregnant).
- Encourage use of therapies or support groups to attain healthy weight and prevent relapse.
- Promote patient decision making concerning issues other than food.
- Promote positive self-concept and perceptions of body, as well as interactions with others.

peutic communication techniques helpful for eating-disordered patients include the following:

- Convey warmth and sincerity. Patients must believe that the nurse genuinely understands and cares about their concerns and efforts to

overcome their ambivalence about treatment (Sloan, 1999).

- Listen empathically. Although anorectic patients will likely deny that weight is a problem, they do admit being lonely and tired of compulsively striving to meet unreachable goals. Bulimics are more likely to admit their problems with weight, but still feel helpless in addressing them (Muscari, 2002; Sloan, 1999).

- Be honest. Patients enter treatment distrustful of everyone. Honesty is essential to developing a trusting relationship with any eating-disordered patient.
- Set appropriate behavioral limits. Because of control needs, patients are likely to attempt to manipulate the nurse. A clear contract between the nurse and patient will help establish trust and minimize power struggles.
- Assist patients in identifying their positive qualities. Because self-esteem is low, patients need to see concrete evidence of their positive qualities. Improving the patients' self-worth is a primary objective in recovery (Sloan, 1999).
- Collaborate with patients. To elicit cooperation, engage patients in planning to foster trust and a sense of control that will diminish their need to maintain control through disordered eating (Sloan, 1999).
- Teach patients about their disorders. Providing accurate information about eating disorders should decrease denial and help patients understand the disease's effects on their bodies and minds (Sloan, 1999).
- Determine the anorectic's ability to be weighed in the early stages of treatment. Often, anorectics need to be weighed with their backs to the scale to help patients reduce their focus on body weight.
- Initiate a behavior modification program with patient input that rewards weight gain or lack of purging with meaningful privileges or rewards. Although the idea of gaining weight is stressful to patients, it is crucial to recovery. When a safe weight is attained, allow patients more control of their own progress and program as long as they do not backslide. Patients must eventually take control of maintaining a safe weight.
- Model and teach appropriate social skills. Acquiring social skills, particularly expressing emotions assertively, is crucial for patients with eating disorders. Encourage patients to examine their interpersonal relationships and work to decrease their loneliness.
- Help patients identify and express bodily sensations and feelings related to their disorders. Anorectic patients have little bodily awareness other than a distorted perception of their size (Sloan, 1999).
- Identify non–weight-related interests of the patient. Involvement with these interests can reduce anxiety as patients invest their energies in areas not related to eating. Encourage the development of new hobbies and interests that are not food-related.

## PSYCHOPHARMACOLOGY

Currently, no psychopharmacologic agent is approved specifically for anorexia nervosa. Medication management of anxiety, depression, somatic disturbances, or other comorbid conditions is appropriate and might assist in treatment of the patient's anorexia. Small amounts of anxiolytics might help patients with eating if given just before meals when refeeding is occurring. Anxiolytics can also be used to decrease the anxiety that fuels a bulimic's bingeing and purging, although antidepressants are a safer, more effective way to achieve that end. Long-term use of anxiolytics can lead to medication dependence, adding to the patient's woes. The atypical antipsychotic olanzapine (Zyprexa) has been tried to promote weight gain, with some success, but it is unclear whether the weight gain is a result of the medication's tendency to cause weight gain or its effect on disturbed thought content and process, such as that experienced by anorectic patients (Attia and Schroeder, 2005).

Treatment with antidepressants, especially the SSRI antidepressants, has proved helpful in reducing bingeing, purging, and depression in bulimic patients (Nakash-Eisikovits et al, 2002). These drugs have been shown to have a positive effect on associated mood disturbances and preoccupation with shape and weight. Interestingly, antidepressants appear to be equally effective in both depressed and nondepressed patients with bulimia nervosa. These results suggest that the mechanism of the drug action might not be antidepressant, but might have direct central effects on neurotransmitter systems, particularly serotonin and norepinephrine. It should be noted, however, that although antidepressants have beneficial effects in the short term, this improvement does not appear to be maintained over the long term (Nakash-Eisikovits et al, 2002). Generally, psychotherapy is recommended before a trial of an antidepressant. Antidepressants are considered when the patient has failed to respond adequately to psychotherapy alone or when there is comorbidity with severe clinical depression.

## MILIEU MANAGEMENT

- Provide an orientation to the setting to prepare the patient for inpatient or outpatient treatment so that fears will be reduced.
- Provide a warm, nurturing atmosphere. It is important for patients to feel support to reduce anxiety and increase trust.
- Closely observe patients. Avoidance behaviors should be identified to plan appropriate interventions. Common behaviors include hiding food in a paper napkin to be discarded later, leaving bread crusts on the plate and discarding the rest, discarding food into plants or out the window, spilling food while eating so it cannot be determined how much the patient really ate, and holding food in the mouth to be discarded when the patient brushes his or her teeth. Respond to such behaviors with nonjudgmental confrontation, conveying understanding of weight gain fears.
- Encourage the patient to approach a team member if feeling the need to purge. Expression of feelings reduces anxiety and helps patients discover alternatives to restricting food or vomiting.
- Involve the patient's family in treatment, when appropriate. If the family denies the problem or is not supportive of treatment, the family might need to be temporarily excluded from the treatment team. If parents, particularly of minors, provide emotional support, treatment efforts have a greater chance of success. Families must understand the disorder and its treatment. Family therapy and family education are crucial components for helping eating-disordered adolescents in both short- and long-term treatment (Geist et al, 2000; Melrose, 2000).
- Respond with consistency. The behavioral program or treatment regimen implemented must be constantly adhered to by the entire staff to diminish patient manipulation and avoid sabotage of treatment.
- Encourage participation in art, recreation, and other types of therapy. These modalities teach patients alternative ways to express their feelings and provide activities other than focusing on food and dieting.
- Involve a dietitian in the treatment plan who can teach proper nutrition while providing patients with an opportunity to select menus. Increase caloric intake gradually to increase patient cooperation in the weight gain program, maintain patient safety, and avoid the medical risks in adding weight too quickly. Encourage compliance with planned schedules for meals and snacks. Regularization of eating prevents the precipitation of binge eating resulting from dieting or restrictive eating practices. Encourage all patients to follow the advice of dietitians regarding normalization of eating (Stewart and Williamson, 2004).
- Encourage patient attendance at group therapy sessions. Providing an opportunity for patients to participate in a group with peers helps them see that they are not alone in having difficulty expressing feelings and dealing with developmental issues. Nurse-led support groups encourage patients to share issues, feelings, and fears (Muscari, 2002).
- Recommend follow-up psychotherapeutic groups and support groups for patients and their families and individual psychotherapy for patients with a qualified therapist. These sessions are particularly beneficial following significant weight gain and after discharge from a treatment program (Castro et al, 2004). Patients might relapse or even die because of lack of appropriate outpatient follow-up, or might even attempt suicide (Pompli et al, 2004). A comprehensive continuum of care provides the best option for relapse prevention in view of the chronic nature of the disease (Cummings et al, 2001).

Treatment in various settings from outpatient to day treatment and finally inpatient treatment for the most physically compromised patients has been attempted, but research has not shown any clear difference in results related to the treatment setting (Fairburn, 2005). A stepped care approach might be useful, in which patients first participate in a simple treatment, such as guided self-help or a psychoeducational group with their families and then, if they do not respond, are referred for cognitive-behavior therapy. Patients who do not improve with therapy can then be referred for a more intensive form of treatment, such as interpersonal psychotherapy, partial or full hospitalization, and possibly antidepressant medication.

## CASE STUDY

Sarah, a 17-year-old girl, was brought to the hospital by her parents and outpatient therapist, whom she had been seeing weekly for 1 month. Sarah and the therapist had a contract of a 2-pound weight gain every week, but Sarah had continued to lose weight. On admission, she was 5 feet 5 inches tall and weighed 86 pounds. Sarah strongly opposed her hospitalization and denied she had a problem.

Sarah is the youngest of three daughters, ages 27, 24, and 17, a late addition to her middle-class family. Sarah's parents admitted that she had been steadily losing weight for the last 6 months. At first, Sarah's parents believed that she was just dieting but, when they began to see her ribs and vertebrae through her nightgown, they became gravely concerned.

Sarah was recently named recipient of a college scholarship. She has been active in school activities and was well liked by her teachers because of her hard work. Although she appeared to have many friends, Sarah claimed that she only had one real friend, another anorectic.

Sarah said her obsession with weight began approximately 6 months ago, when the family went to visit the oldest daughter, whom Sarah idolized. One afternoon, the three sisters went berry picking, and the oldest told Sarah, "Don't eat all the berries, or you'll grow into a real chub!" Sarah interpreted this to mean that her sister thought she was fat. She became obsessed with food and became a vegetarian. She adopted the role of planning menus and educating the family on proper nutrition.

When her mother attempted to intervene, Sarah screamed that she knew what she was doing and was tired of being treated like a baby. If her mother attempted further control over Sarah's eating behavior, Sara refused to eat at all. The situation at home deteriorated until there was little communication between family members and Sarah. She engaged in irrational rituals and lost 30 pounds. When Sara began to look very thin, they persuaded her to seek help, although she continued to lose weight during outpatient therapy.

Sarah is a likable young lady. The other adolescents in the hospital were attracted to her and wanted to be her friend. However, they noticed Sarah's odd eating habits, such as mixing cornflakes in vanilla pudding and pouring cranberry juice over cereals. At first, she resisted eating meals and snacks, but complied when faced with tube feeding to replace what she refused to eat. Sarah always dressed in baggy overalls and wore oversized sweaters. When other patients asked Sarah if she felt cold, she quietly told them that she did not want them to stare at her fat body, a comment that tended to put off her peers.

During break times, Sarah was found writing morbid poetry, which contained subtle suicidal messages. She preferred to be alone and became irritable and rude when asked to participate in group therapy sessions. Sarah tried to be as compliant as she thought others wanted her to be; however, the lack of control she experienced in the hospital added to her anxiety and discomfort and fueled her denial that she had a problem.

## EATING DISORDERS IN MALES

The incidence of eating disorders among males is currently 10% to 15% of the eating-disordered population, with speculation that this figure might increase as men become more comfortable seeking treatment (Ray, 2004). Identification of partial and full syndrome eating-disordered males has increased the numbers of males with eating disorders. Although diagnosis, etiologies, and treatment of males and females with eating disorders are similar, there appear to be differences in onset, presentation, and assessment. For example, males are more likely than females with eating disorders to have a history of obesity before the onset of symptoms of an eating disorder and to have a later onset and higher initial BMI before becoming eating-disordered. Males also tend to feel less guilt than in females about episodes of bingeing and purging. Comorbidity with other psychiatric disorders is higher in males than in females with eating disorders (Woodside et al, 2001). Dieting or bingeing is more often related to a desire to build a lean body for participation in sports, such as competing in a lower weight class in wrestling (Ray, 2004).

Although controversial, some research has shown that male patients with eating disorders exhibit a higher frequency of concerns about gender or sexual identity, homosexual orientation, and asexuality (Meyer et al, 2001; Ray, 2004). It should be noted, however, that although some eating-disordered males have a homosexual orientation, this is still a minority of cases. Sexual orientation might represent a risk factor for eating disorders, because homosexual males might place particular emphasis on physical attractiveness (Ray, 2004).

Treatment for males with eating disorders is similar to that for females. From a psychotherapeutic management standpoint, the following three areas need particular focus with males:

## Care Plan

Name: Sarah H                                              Admission Date: _____

*DSM-IV-TR* Diagnosis: Anorexia nervosa

| | |
|---|---|
| Assessment | **Areas of strength:** Intelligence; past achievements; likableness; past healthy interpersonal relationships; good personal hygiene; some insight into reasons for hospitalization; family support. |
| | **Problems:** Low weight, disturbed body image, low self-esteem, depression, lack of accurate knowledge regarding nutrition, manipulativeness. |
| Diagnoses | • Alteration in nutrition; less than body requirements, related to not eating enough nutrients, as evidenced by continued weight loss and inappropriate eating habits. |
| | • Disturbance in body image, related to feeling fat when actually underweight, as evidenced by inappropriate dress and comments about how fat she is. |
| | • Disturbance in self-esteem, related to fear of becoming fat and repulsive, as evidenced by suicidal messages in poetry and by social withdrawal. |
| | • Knowledge deficit in proper nutrition, related to fear of being fat, as evidenced by odd eating habits and refusal to eat certain foods. |

| | | |
|---|---|---|
| Outcomes | *Short-term goals:* | Date met |
| | • Patient will gain 1 pound per week. | _____ |
| | • Patient will identify two positive qualities about herself. | _____ |
| | • Patient will discuss fears of losing control. | _____ |
| | *Long-term goals:* | |
| | • Patient will gain at least 20 pounds within 6 months. | _____ |
| | • Patient will verbalize knowledge of illness and proper nutrition. | _____ |
| | • Patient will identify at least three alternative coping mechanisms to use when feeling out of control. | _____ |
| | • Patient will verbalize increased comfort in relating to peers. | _____ |

| | |
|---|---|
| Planning/ Interventions | **Nurse-patient relationship:** Establish a contract to meet with the patient daily to discuss feelings; express concern for the patient; encourage verbalization of feelings about depression and/or lack of control; encourage patient to identify positive qualities about herself. |
| | **Milieu management:** Encourage patient to attend meals and sit with peers; encourage participation in group therapy to discuss feelings with peers; encourage patient to share positive qualities of herself with peers; maintain consistency of unit rules and make certain that patient is adhering to them. |
| Evaluation | Patient gained 2 pounds in the first 10 days of hospitalization; attended all unit activities; attended individual therapy with Ms. M, RN, and stated one positive thing about herself. |
| Referrals | Patient has been given information about an eating disorder support group in her community and a person to contact regarding group attendance after discharge. |

1. The excessive attention that adolescent boys can place on attaining a masculine physique and its effect on their body image
2. Dietary habits to promote health, fitness, and muscle mass without using disordered eating patterns
3. The expression of feelings and the exploration of any underlying sexual identity concerns

Although most adolescents with eating disorders have difficulty expressing their feelings, boys seem to have more difficulty than girls. A therapeutic relationship can be especially instrumental in the recovery of these young men (Ray, 2004).

CRITICAL THINKING QUESTION   2

A 17-year-old boy remarks to you that he feels too fat and is afraid that he will not be able to "make weight" for wrestling. You do not observe that the patient is overweight. How do you begin to assess whether the patient is suffering from an eating disorder?

## BINGE-EATING DISORDER

The *DSM-IV-TR* lists binge-eating disorder (BED) as a condition that has not met diagnostic criteria for inclusion in the *DSM-IV-TR* manual, but might warrant further research and study. BED shares many criteria of bulimia nervosa (lack of control over intake, patient distress, and guilt over bingeing) but without the regular compensation for excess intake through purging, laxatives, fasting, or overexercise. As a consequence, individuals with BED tend to be overweight to a moderate or greater degree and their weight tends to fluctuate more compared with those with anorexia or bulimia. As with bulimia, the onset of this disorder tends to be later than that of anorexia, generally beginning in late adolescence to early adulthood. These patients are diagnosed as eating disorder not otherwise specified (NOS), with the notation that the patient's symptoms meet the research criteria for BED.

Other examples of NOS disorders include the patient who meets all criteria for anorexia nervosa except amenorrhea or who has a regular pattern of vomiting for weight control after normal eating.

### Web Resources

- These sites represent a small sampling of available resources for professionals, patients, and families. Nurses should evaluate the appropriateness of web resources as with all other resources before giving them to patients and families.
- There is a disturbing phenomenon on the Internet known as *pro anorexia* (pro ana) and *pro bulimia* (pro mia) web sites, bulletin boards, and chat rooms hosted by those suffering from eating disorders and proclaiming anorexia and bulimia as lifestyle choices rather than life-threatening illnesses. These sites offer tips on how to be the "best anorectic" or "best bulimic" and often feature alarming pictures of those with the disorders in a macabre competition of thinness. The web addresses of these sites are often passed from patient to patient, making them very difficult to track and control (Andrist, 2003).

**National Association of Anorexia and Associated Disorders (ANAD)**
http://www.anad.org
This site is sponsored and maintained by ANAD, the oldest national nonprofit organization devoted to helping eating-disordered patients and their families through providing networking, support groups, and advocacy for patients and their families. Current efforts are directed at monitoring and advocating against media references that portray eating disorders as funny and that the organization believes are dangerous and demeaning.

**Eating Disorders Referral and Information Center (EDRIC)**
http://www.edreferral.com
This site is sponsored and maintained by the International Eating Disorders Referral Organization, a nonprofit organization. The web site contains much information and many links to other resources, as well as referrals worldwide to caregivers experienced in treating eating disorders.

**Anorexia and Related Disorders, Inc. (ANRED)**
http://www.anred.com
This site is sponsored and maintained by a group of mental health professionals (including a nurse) with many years of experience treating eating-disordered patients. This group is nonprofit, provides links to other resources, and exists primarily as an educational resource. The web site cautions patients that direct professional care is needed to overcome their illness.

**Something Fishy Web Site on Eating Disorders**
http://www.something-fishy.org/edaso.html
This site serves as a clearinghouse for eating disorder resources and information. It provides discussion forums for those experiencing eating disorders and another forum for loved ones of those with eating disorders and proclaims itself as pro recovery.

These individuals might not be underweight or demonstrate binge eating and so are not identified as having an eating disorder. Clinicians should recognize the importance of early detection and treatment before the NOS illness becomes more severe (American Psychiatric Association, 2000).

for the patient's height or if medical complications related to the patient's condition are present.

## Study Notes

1. Anorexia nervosa is characterized by a refusal to maintain body weight at or above a minimally normal weight for age and height, an intense fear of becoming fat, a distorted body image, and amenorrhea or irregular menstrual cycles in women and low testosterone levels in men.

2. Anorectic dieters might begin their illness in a normal weight range but then isolate themselves socially from others, become competitive concerning weight loss, and exercise excessively.

3. Bulimia is characterized by episodes of binge eating, a feeling of lack of control over eating, use of compensatory behavior, and an overconcern with body shape and weight. Depression commonly coexists with bulimia.

4. Anorectic and bulimic patients suffer a variety of physiologic problems that can cause death. Personality and emotional changes are also evident in these patients, which might result from the eating disorder or might be a contributing factor in its genesis.

5. The causes of eating disorders are thought to be multifactorial, including biologic, sociocultural, familial, cognitive, behavioral, and psychodynamic factors.

6. Cognitive-behavioral therapy has the most research support in the treatment of eating disorders.

7. The incidence of eating disorders in males is increasing, with similarities in presentation and treatment to eating-disordered females, although eating disorders in males seem to appear at a later age than in females.

8. Nursing interventions with eating-disordered patients require caring, supportive relationships, limit setting, a behavior modification program, and a consistent milieu. Family involvement, individual psychotherapy, and group therapy are also essential.

9. Hospitalization with a structured milieu and antidepressant medications might be needed if weight decreases below what is appropriate

## References

American Psychiatric Association: *Diagnostic and statistical manual of mental disorders, text revision,* ed 4, Washington, DC, 2000, APA.

Andrist L: Media images, body dissatisfaction and disordered eating in adolescent women, *Am J Maternal/Child Nurs* 28:119, 2003.

Attia E, Schroeder L: Pharmacologic treatment of anorexia nervosa: where do we go from here? *Int J Eat Disord* 37:S60, 2005.

Bakke B, Mitchell J, Wonderlich S, Erickson R: Administering cognitive-behavioral therapy for bulimia nervosa via telemedicine in rural settings, *Int J Eat Disord* 30:454, 2001.

Braun D, Sunday S, Huang A, Halmi K: More males seek treatment for eating disorders, *Int J Eat Disord* 25:415, 1999.

Bruch H: *Eating disorders,* New York, 1973, Basic Books.

Brumberg JJ: *The body project: an intimate history of American girls,* New York, 1997, Random House.

Bulik CM, Reba L, Siega-Riz AM, Reichborn-Kjennerud T: Anorexia nervosa: definition, epidemiology, and cycle of risk, *Int J Eat Disord* 37:S2, 2005.

Castro J, Gila A, Puig J, et al: Predictors of rehospitalization after total weight recovery in adolescents with anorexia nervosa, *Int J Eat Disord* 36:22, 2004.

Cohane GH, Pope HG: Body image in boys: a review of the literature, *Int J Eat Disord* 29:373, 2001.

Cummings MM, Waller D, Johnson C, et al: Developing and implementing a comprehensive program for children and adolescents with eating disorders, *J Child Adolesc Psychiatr Nurs* 14:167, 2001.

Fairburn CG: Evidence-based treatment of anorexia nervosa, *Int J Eat Disord* 37:S26, 2005.

Finelli L: Revisiting the identity issue in anorexia, *J Psychosoc Nurs* 39:23, 2001.

Geist R, Heinmaa M, Stephens D, et al: Comparison of family therapy and family group psychoeducation in adolescents with anorexia nervosa, *Can J Psychiatry* 45:173, 2000.

Goldstein DJ, Wilson MG, Ascroft RC, Al-Banna M: Effectiveness of fluoxetine therapy in bulimia nervosa regardless of comorbid depression, *Int J Eat Disord* 25:19, 1999.

Halmi K: Psychopathology of anorexia nervosa, *Int J Eat Disord* 37:S20, 2005.

Katzman DK: Medical complications in adolescents with anorexia nervosa: a review of the literature, *Int J Eat Disord* 37:S52, 2005.

Kaye WH, Bulik CM, Thornton L, et al: Comorbidity of anxiety disorders with anorexia and bulimia nervosa, *Am J Psychiatry* 161:2215, 2004.

Kaye WH, Frank GK, Bailer UF, Henry SE: Neurobiology of anorexia nervosa: clinical implications of alterations of the function of serotonin and other neuronal systems, *Int J Eat Disord* 37:S15, 2005.

Kaye WH, Klump KL, Frank GKW, Strober M: Anorexia and bulimia nervosa, *Annu Rev Med* 51:299, 2000.

Keel PK, Dorer DJ, Eddy KT, et al: Predictors of mortality in eating disorders, *Arch Gen Psychiatry* 60:179, 2003.

Mazzeo SE, Zucker NL, Gerke CK, et al: Parenting concerns of women with histories of eating disorders, *Int J Eat Disord* 37:S77, 2005.

McIntosh WV, Bulik CM, McKenzie JM, et al: Interpersonal psychotherapy for anorexia nervosa, *Int J Eat Disord* 27:125, 2000.

Melrose C: Facilitating a multidisciplinary parent support and education group guided by Allen's developmental health nursing model, *J Psychosoc Nurs* 38:19, 2000.

Mendell DA, Logemann JA: Bulimia and swallowing: cause for concern, *Int J Eat Disord* 30:252, 2001.

Meyer C, Blisset J, Oldfield C: Sexual orientation and eating psychopathology: the role of masculinity and femininity, *Int J Eat Disord* 29:314, 2001.

Muscari M: Effective management of adolescents with anorexia and bulimia, *J Psychosoc Nurs* 40:23, 2002.

Nakash-Eisikovits O, Dierberger A, Westen D: A multidisciplinary meta-analysis of pharmacotherapy for bulimia nervosa: summarizing the range of outcomes in controlled clinical trials, *Harv Rev Psychiatry* 10:193, 2002.

NANDA International: *Nursing diagnoses: definitions and classification, 2005-2006,* Philadelphia, 2005, NANDA International.

O'Dea JA, Abraham S: Improving the body image, eating attitudes and behaviors of young male and female adolescents: a new educational approach that focuses on self-esteem, *Int J Eat Disord* 28:43, 2000.

Orbanic S: Understanding bulimia, *Am J Nurs* 101:35, 2001.

Pike K: Assessment of anorexia nervosa, *Int J Eat Disord* 37:S22, 2005.

Poirier-Solomon L: Eating disorders and diabetes, *Diabetes Forecast* 11:43, 2001.

Pompli M, Mancinelli I, Girardi P, et al: Suicide in anorexia nervosa: a meta-analysis, *Int J Eat Disord* 36:99, 2004.

Rand CSW, Wright BA: Continuity and change in the evaluation of ideal and acceptable body sizes across a wide age span, *Int J Eat Disord* 28:90, 2000.

Ray SL: Eating disorders in adolescent males, *Prof School Counseling* 8:98, 2004.

Ro O, Martinson EW, Hoffart A, Rosenvinge J: Two-year prospective study of personality disorders in adults with long-standing eating disorders, *Int J Eat Disord* 37:112, 2005.

Sloan G: Anorexia nervosa: a cognitive behavioural approach, *Nurs Standard* 13:43, 1999.

Stein KF, Corte C: Reconceptualizing causative factors and intervention strategies in the eating disorders: a shift from body image to self-concept impairments, *Arch Psychiatr Nurs* 17:57, 2003.

Stewart TM, Williamson DA: Multidisciplinary treatment of eating disorders—part 2, *Behav Mod* 28:831, 2004.

White JH: The prevention of eating disorders: a review of the research on risk factors with implications for practice, *J Child Adolesc Nurs* 13:76, 2000.

Williamson DA, White MA, York-Crowe E, Stewart TM: Cognitive-behavioral theories of eating disorders, *Behav Mod* 28:711-738, 2004.

Wonderlich SA, Crosby RD, Mitchell JE, et al: Eating disturbance and sexual trauma in childhood and adulthood, *Int J Eat Disord* 30:401, 2001.

Woodside DB, Garfinkel PE, Lin E, et al: Comparisons of men with full or partial eating disorders, men without eating disorders, and women with eating disorders in the community, *Am J Psychiatry* 158:570, 2001.

Young L, Nestle M: The contribution of expanding portion size to the U.S. obesity epidemic, *Am J Publ Health* 92:246, 2002.

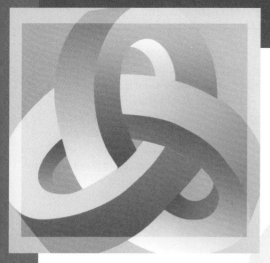

# Chapter 38

# Behavior Therapies

*Lee H. Schwecke*

## Learning Objectives

*After reading this chapter, you should be able to:*

- Identify three techniques for increasing a behavior.
- Describe two schedules of reinforcement.
- Identify four techniques for decreasing a behavior.
- Understand the principles of a token economy program.
- Discuss three techniques for helping patients deal with disturbing stimuli.
- Explain the nursing process using behavior modification principles.

## FOUNDATIONS OF BEHAVIOR THERAPIES

Behavior therapy is a distinctive approach to influencing interactions among individuals and between individuals and their environment. The principles used in behavior therapy were derived from research in conditioned reflex and operant conditioning. Applications of behavior therapy principles are common and effective in psychiatric nursing, especially in helping patients deal with anxiety and change their behaviors. Behavior therapy is typically combined with cognitive therapy and psychotropic medications to address the entire scope of problematic thoughts, feelings, and behaviors (Falsetti et al, 2005).

### CLASSICAL CONDITIONING

The origin of classical conditioning is credited to Pavlov (1927) and his research on stimulus and response in laboratory animals. Pavlov was involved in studying reflexes and the various aspects of the secretion of gastric juices in dogs when he discovered that the dogs began salivating before they were presented with food. *Respondent conditioning* is the process of pairing a neutral stimulus with an eliciting stimulus; thus, ultimately, the neutral stimulus alone elicits the response.

### OPERANT CONDITIONING

The basis of the operant learning theory was derived from numerous controlled experiments with animals and was reported originally by B. F. Skinner (1938, 1953, 1956). Attention is directed to the events that immediately precede and follow a person's specific behavior. Theoretical inner causes of behavior, such as psychological, neurologic, or conceptual states, are not denied; however, they are *not* viewed as relevant to the analysis of behavior.

A response is any movement or observable behavior. The operant response (the behavior being analyzed) can be described and measured (frequency, duration, magnitude). A stimulus is an

### Norm's Notes

*When I was in graduate school, I had a professor who was a pure behaviorist. In fact, his weight loss method was totally behavioral—he had people smear something disgusting on their favorite food and then eat it. Well, that put a distaste in my mouth (pun intended) for behavior therapy. Fortunately, I have learned about other behavioral approaches that make sense and that are effective. This chapter reviews information you probably had in a psychology course but does it in a way that illustrates its application to nursing practice.*

event that immediately precedes or follows a behavior.

Primary reinforcers for behaviors are events of biologic importance (e.g., food, water, sexual contact, coat on a cold day, bed for sleeping). Secondary or generalized reinforcers are events that have been paired repeatedly with a primary reinforcer (e.g., money, tickets, diplomas, attention of others).

## APPLICATION OF BEHAVIOR THERAPY IN PSYCHIATRIC NURSING PRACTICE

Behavior therapy is used with children, adolescents, groups, couples, and families. Behavior modification has been used in inpatient and outpatient settings and in skills-training programs. The most common uses are with posttraumatic stress disorder (PTSD), anxiety disorders, traumatic memories, addictions, and social and general anxiety, especially when one or more of these are concomitant or are in combination with other psychiatric disorders. Additionally, behavioral principles form the basis of self-control treatment programs, such as those used for changes in behaviors (e.g., eating, exercise, assertive communication).

## BEHAVIOR MODIFICATION: HELPING PATIENTS CHANGE BEHAVIOR

When patients' problem behaviors are reinforced or maintained by consequences of the behavior, operant conditioning (commonly called behavior modification) is the model used. Functional analysis involves a behavioral and reinforcement history. It is important to include the patient in this process of behavioral contracting, which is often put into writing. The contract includes unacceptable and acceptable behaviors, as well as rewards and consequences. Contingencies that can be controlled by the therapist, patient, or family are altered to create a change in the problematic behaviors.

### Increasing the Probability That a Behavior Will Recur

#### Conditioning

Conditioning is the strengthening of a response by reinforcement. Positive reinforcement follows a behavior with a reinforcing stimulus that increases the probability that the behavior will recur. For example, asking for help in an assertive way occurs more frequently when followed by attention and suggestions (reinforcement) in a communication skills group. Negative reinforcement is the process of removing a stimulus from a situation immediately after a behavior occurs, which increases the probability of the behavior occurring. For example, when a person steps into an uncomfortably hot shower and turns the dial to reduce the water temperature, the behavior (turning the dial) is reinforced. The stimulus (uncomfortably hot water) is removed.

The timing of reinforcement is important. When reinforcers are presented according to a time schedule (rather than being contingent on a particular response), any behavior immediately preceding the reinforcer is strengthened.

#### Premack Principle

When a person is observed often enjoying a particular activity, the opportunity to engage in that activity can be used as a reinforcer for other behaviors that occur less frequently (Premack, 1962). For example, the opportunity to watch television might be used as a reinforcer for cleaning the living area.

#### Shaping

Shaping is a process of reinforcing successive approximations of responses to increase the probability of a behavior. For example, to increase the probability of a patient saying "no" in an assertive way, each time the patient makes a response that approximates the target response (or gets closer to the target response), reinforcement is presented until that response occurs at a high frequency. Then, reinforcement is withheld until the next response more closely approximates the target behavior, and so on, until the target behavior is performed. The selective reinforcement of each behavior that more closely approximates the target response is called *differential reinforcement*.

## Schedules of Reinforcement

### Continuous Reinforcement

Continuous reinforcement is the presentation of reinforcing stimuli following each occurrence of the selected response. Continuous reinforcement is used primarily during the initial phases of conditioning or shaping a behavior and results in a high rate of behavior, such as when a professional provides reinforcement each time a patient uses appropriate comments during role playing of conflict management skills.

### Intermittent Reinforcement

Intermittent reinforcement is the presentation of the reinforcer following the target response according to a selected number of responses (ratio schedule). An example would be after every fifth target response or according to a selected time period (interval schedule) of 10 minutes after every target response. Schedules might vary as well.

## Decreasing the Probability That a Behavior Will Recur

### Differential Reinforcement of Other Behavior

Differential reinforcement is a technique used to decrease the frequency of a behavior. When the goal of treatment is to decrease a behavior, another behavior, incompatible with the target behavior, can be reinforced. Target behavior, if emitted, is not reinforced. To decrease the soft speaking of a patient in a group, attention of the group is available only when the patient speaks in a normal, audible voice. The soft speaking voice, incompatible with a normal voice, is ignored.

### Extinction

Extinction is the gradual decrease in the rate of responses when the reinforcement is no longer available. The rate of responses might increase for a short time and then begin to decrease gra-dually. Emotional responses characteristically occur during extinction. A familiar example is the behavior that occurs when the button to start an elevator is pushed. When the elevator door fails to close, repeated and sometimes rapid button-pushing behavior occurs for a short period, and then stops. Banging or pulling on the elevator door (an emotional response) might occur during this time. Use of a behavior technique called *social extinction* involves the withdrawal of attention from a patient when he or she acts inappropriately in the setting.

### Negative Consequence

Negative consequence is the presentation of an event immediately following a response that decreases the probability of that response recurring—for example, putting a child in his or her room immediately after seeing the child playing in the street. Another example is having a patient apologize to other patients and mop the floor after throwing food. Negative consequences usually result in the immediate suppression of the particular response. For inpatients, a common form of this technique is to withdraw privileges as a consequence of acting-out behaviors. Unfortunately, a negative consequence can result in an increase in emotional behavior or aggressive responses, so it is used when other techniques are not effective in decreasing the frequency of a particular response.

### Time-Out

Time-out is a negative consequence technique in which the person is removed from a setting in which ongoing reinforcers are available. When a patient is exhibiting aggressive behavior that is followed by social reinforcement from other patients, the patient might be moved to another room in which no social reinforcement is available.

## Skills Training

When behavioral responses are not appropriate for a person's age and life situation, new behaviors are acquired through teaching anger management skills, social skills, and problem-solving procedures. Instruction, modeling, behavior rehearsal, corrective feedback, positive reinforcement, programmed practice, and flexibility exercises are used for these programs (Turner et al, 2005). Imitation and shaping are also used. Nurses often make individual assessments of the social skills of patients and form small groups to conduct training of skills that are appropriate for the patients but have not been seen in the hospital situation. An example is assertiveness training in which assertiveness is defined, described, and compared with passive and aggressive responses. Assertive responses are modeled. The patients then practice these responses and use them in role-playing and homework assignments (Mishra et al, 2000). Reinforcement is given when assertiveness is appropriately demonstrated.

### Contingency Contracting

Contingency contracting is the arrangement of conditions that enable patients to participate in setting target behaviors and selecting reinforcers. The therapist and patients jointly specify what, how, when, and where behavioral change will occur. Criteria for the delivery of reinforcement are defined. The type, amount, and schedule of reinforcement are specified. For example, a contract specifies that, if the patient approaches the nurse to ask for his or her medications at the scheduled time, he or she can join a reward walk with the nurse and other patients after dinner.

### Self-Control

The direct management of behavioral contingencies by a therapist is usually impractical for adult patients in an outpatient treatment setting. A more frequently used approach is the development of a self-control program with contingency contracting in which patients do the assessment, change their behaviors, provide their own reinforcement, and evaluate the results. This approach can be used with thought stopping, when patients have automatic negative thoughts. Patients are taught to say to themselves "stop," and to substitute a positive thought (Lyon, 2001).

---

**CRITICAL THINKING QUESTION**    `1`

Jennifer O'Conner inflicts superficial cuts on her wrists when she receives negative consequences for seductive behavior with male patients. Positive reinforcement for opposing behaviors, social extinction, and time-out have not been successful. What behavioral approaches would you plan instead?

---

| | S | M | T | W | T | F | S |
|---|---|---|---|---|---|---|---|
| Get up on time | X | X | X | | | | |
| Make bed | | X | | | | | |
| Complete ADLs | X | X | X | | | | |
| Go to group on time | X | X | X | | | | |
| Participate in group | | | X | | | | |
| Do own laundry | X | | | | | | |
| Take medicines on time | | X | X | | | | |
| Assertively approach staff | X | | X | | | | |

FIGURE 38-1 Expected outcomes for patient. *ADLs,* Activities of daily living.

### Token Economy

*Token economy* was originally the term used to describe the use of operant principles in the management of behavior with groups of patients in inpatient or outpatient partial hospital programs (Ayllon and Azrin, 1968). It is now used more often with individual patients who, because of the severity of their illness, have trouble with daily functioning. Tokens (tangible conditioned reinforcers) are presented to patients when they exhibit specific target behaviors. A simple example is presented in Figure 38-1. Tokens can be exchanged for positive reinforcers, such as privileges and favorite foods or activities.

## RESPONDENT CONDITIONING: HELPING PATIENTS COPE WITH DISTURBING STIMULI

When patients' problem behaviors are related to particular stimuli situations, such as those related to pain, phobias, and PTSD, respondent conditioning is the model used. Treatment might involve making changes in stimulus situations or in control of problematic behaviors.

### Reciprocal Inhibition

The process of strengthening alternative responses to fear or anxiety associated with a stimulus is called *reciprocal inhibition* or *counterconditioning* (Yates, 1970). Relaxation techniques, for instance, can be taught to highly anxious patients or those in pain. A person cannot be relaxed and anxious simultaneously. Techniques often taught are positive and affirming self-talk, yoga, deep breathing, meditation, progressive muscle relaxation, and positive or pleasant imagery (Mishra et al, 2000; Nakao et al, 2001). For example, the patient is instructed to tense and relax specific muscle groups, in a sequence, until relaxation is achieved. Several sessions of practice are usually carried out with the therapist, audiotape prompts, written instructions, or any combination of these.

## Exposure Models

### Systematic Desensitization—In vivo

Originally developed by Wolpe (1958) for the treatment of anxiety, systematic desensitization is the planned progressive or graduated exposure to stimuli in real life (in vivo) that elicit fear or anxiety while the anxiety or fear response is suppressed with relaxation techniques. A biofeedback program might also be used to reach and maintain a state of relaxation or pain control (Mishra et al, 2000). Exposure models are now used more often in combination with other therapies such as education, supportive therapy, cognitive-behavioral therapy, and skills training (described earlier), especially for patients with complicated problems such as PTSD or multiple *Diagnostic Statistical Manual of Mental Disorders*, Text Revision, Fourth Edition (*DSM-IV-TR*) diagnoses (Freuh et al, 2004; Turner et al, 2005).

Hierarchies of the fear-eliciting stimuli are constructed through a detailed assessment (Freuh et al, 2004). For example, a patient with a fear of being in open and crowded places that limits appropriate shopping behavior might report a hierarchy of fear-eliciting situations as follows: standing in the doorway of the house; standing outside several feet from the house, then two blocks away, then several blocks away; being in a small, empty store; being in an empty department store; being in an empty shopping center; being in a small, crowded store, a crowded department store, and then a crowded shopping center. The stimulus least likely to evoke fear or anxiety is introduced initially, followed by gradual exposure to more fearful stimuli.

Hierarchies related to traumatic events could include conditioned external and internal cues (Falsetti et al, 2005):

Examples of external cues include places, situations, objects, smells, and sounds associated with the trauma. Internal cues include emotions, such as fear and disgust, the physiological arousal experienced during traumatic events, and conditions experienced during the event, such as thoughts of dying or going crazy (p. 73).

Patients need to be aware that exposure initially increases their emotional and physical distress, so they are prepared to engage in the process. However, prolonged, repeated exposure, along with relaxation, eventually decreases the fear and anxiety (Geffken et al, 2004; Turner et al, 2005).

In the presence of the therapist, patients actually place themselves, systematically, in the least to the most fearful situations. Patients carry out this self-exposure while using incompatible competing responses to fear and anxiety. In using exposure techniques, the therapist carefully helps patients experience a gradual decrease of the fear or anxiety response in the presence of the eliciting stimulus. Later in the therapy process, patients might practice exposure independently, as homework, especially if a patient is in outpatient therapy.

### Systematic Desensitization—Imaginal

Systematic desensitization might also be practiced with the imagining of traumatic events, beginning with the least traumatic aspects of the trauma. Patients might be asked to write about or write and then talk about each aspect with the therapist. Writing assignments and journaling might be give as homework between sessions (Lombardo and Gray, 2005). Relaxation techniques are still used as in imaginal desensitization.

### Flooding or Implosion

Flooding or implosion is a process in which patients imagine or place themselves in the fearful situation; that is, they immerse themselves in the feared stimuli (Freuh et al, 2005). For example, an individual with a fear of elevators would stand in an elevator until his or her anxiety subsides. This is normally done when accompanied by the therapist.

## EXAMPLE OF BEHAVIORAL INTERVENTIONS

The behavioral nursing process consists of an assessment of behavior and related contingencies, a behavioral nursing diagnosis, outcome identification and planning, implementing an intervention program, and an evaluation of the results of the intervention. Occasions for conducting this process occur in daily interactions with patients. The interactions focus on providing a well-structured therapeutic environment, assisting patients with here and now living problems, and helping them learn behavioral patterns related to emotional health. The following example illustrates the use of a behavioral approach for skills training in a group of patients with chronic psychiatric disorders who were participating in a structured outpatient day program that used a modified token economy system. Skills desired included assertiveness (patients asking for a staff talk), communication (starting and continuing a conversation in appropriate ways), reporting improvements to staff, making a plan for specific methods of self-care, and contracting with staff about treatment events or outcomes.

As part of the treatment program, each patient carried a behavioral rating card that listed specific expected behaviors (e.g., self-care activities, management of personal items and living area, attendance at prescribed treatment events). When the patients demonstrated these behaviors, a staff member rated the behavior and initialed the card. At the end of each day, each patient's ratings on the behavior cards were tallied and reinforcement was presented contingent on the score for the day. Examples of the reinforcements were opportunities to engage in the purchase of items at the snack bar and/or participation in recreation activities. The skills training groups consisted of four to six patients who met daily during the week. The sessions began with a brief orientation period and an introduction of specific skills relevant to that session. Next, there was a demonstration and role playing using the skills, followed by discussion and homework suggestions. Specific techniques that the nurse used were positive reinforcement (social reinforcement by the nurse and/or initialing the rating card) contingent on appropriate behavior, modeling and imitation, contingency contracting, homework, self-control, and extinction (withholding of reinforcement) following undesired behaviors.

Each group member's progress was evaluated with the use of a recording form that listed target behaviors. Seven patients showed consistent increases in target behaviors over the period of the group session. One patient demonstrated a relatively high rate of target behaviors during the

initial group session and continued this rate. Demonstration of target behaviors by two of the patients was variable and consistently low throughout the sessions. For these two patients, the group intervention program was not effective in changing target behaviors during the period that they were involved in the group.

---

### CRITICAL THINKING QUESTION    2

What phobias, in addition to the ones mentioned in this text, might systematic desensitization be successful in overcoming?

---

## ▇ Study Notes

1. Classical conditioning is based on the involuntary stimulus-response reaction. After repeated pairing of eliciting and neutral stimuli, the neutral stimulus alone produces the expected response.
2. Operant conditioning focuses on the external variables that precede and follow the response to learn which variables control behaviors. Reinforcers are particularly important.
3. Behavior therapy begins with a functional analysis of behavior and environmental contingencies as the basis for developing a treatment program.
4. Behavior modification programs can be used for various problematic behaviors in a variety of settings.
5. Increasing the probability of a desired behavior can occur with conditioning, reinforcement, or shaping.
6. Decreasing the probability of an undesirable behavior can occur with reinforcement of an incompatible behavior, extinction, time-out, and/or negative consequence.
7. New behaviors might be acquired in skills training through the use of modeling and imitation techniques, as well as through reinforcement and shaping.
8. Self-control and token economy programs are varieties of reinforcement approaches.
9. Respondent conditioning is useful in altering an unpleasant response to a specific stimulus. Reciprocal inhibition, systematic desensitization (in vivo or imaginal exposure), and flooding are varieties of this approach.
10. Behavioral nursing interventions involve baseline observations, analysis of behaviors,

problem specification, outcome identification, formulation of treatment plans, intervention, and evaluation.

## References

Ayllon T, Azrin N: *The token economy,* New York, 1968, Appleton-Century-Crofts.

Falsetti SA, Resnick HS, Davis J: Multichannel exposure therapy: combining cognitive-behavioral therapies for the treatment of posttraumatic stress disorder with panic attacks, *Behav Modif* 29:70, 2005.

Freuh BC, Buckley TC, Cusack KJ, et al: Cognitive-behavioral treatment for PTSD among people with severe mental illness: a proposed treatment model, *J Psychiatr Pract* 10:26, 2004.

Geffken GR, Storch EA, Gelfand KM, et al: Cognitive-behavioral therapy for obsessive-compulsive disorder: review of treatment techniques, *J Psychosoc Nurs Ment Health Serv* 42:44, 2004.

Lombardo TW, Gray MJ: Beyond exposure for posttraumatic stress disorder (PTSD) symptoms, *Behav Modif* 29:3, 2005.

Lyon BL: Strategies to enhance positive situational focusing skills, *Reflections on Nursing Leadership,* Third quarter:5, 2001.

Mishra KD, Gatchel RJ, Gardea MA: The relative efficacy of three cognitive-behavioral treatment approaches to temporomandibular disorders, *J Behav Med* 23:293, 2000.

Nakao M, Myers P, Fricchione G, et al: Somatization and symptom reduction through a behavioral medicine intervention in a mind/body medicine clinic, *Behav Med* 26:169, 2001.

Pavlov IP: *Conditioned reflexes* (trans. by GV Anrep), London, 1927, Oxford University Press.

Premack K: Reversibility of the reinforcement relation, *Science* 136:255, 1962.

Skinner BF: A case history in scientific method, *Am J Psychol* 11:211, 1956.

Skinner BF: *Science and human behavior,* New York, 1953, Free Press.

Skinner BF: *The behavior of organisms,* New York, 1938, Appleton-Century-Crofts.

Turner SM, Beidel DC, Freuh, BC: Multicomponent behavioral treatment for chronic combat-related posttraumatic stress disorder, *Behav Modif* 29:39, 2005.

Wolpe J: *Psychotherapy by reciprocal inhibition,* Stanford, CT, 1958, Stanford University Press.

Yates AJ: *Behavior therapy,* New York, 1970, Wiley.

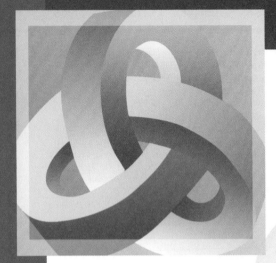

# Chapter 39

# Somatic Therapies

*Norman L. Keltner*

## Learning Objectives

*After reading this chapter, you should be able to:*

- Identify the major indications for electroconvulsive therapy (ECT).
- Compare modern ECT with traditional ECT depicted in some movies.
- Name and understand the purpose of the drugs used in conjunction with ECT.
- Describe the nurse's role in caring for patients before and after ECT.
- Describe and discuss the ethical, legal, social, and biologic concerns related to psychosurgery.

*Electroshock has undergone fundamental changes since its introduction 65 years ago. It is no longer the bone-breaking, memory-modifying, fearsome treatment featured in films. Anesthesia, controlled oxygenation, and muscle relaxation make the procedure so safe that the risks are less than those which accompany the use of psychotropic drugs. Indeed, for the elderly, the systemically ill, and pregnant women, electroshock is a safer treatment for mental illnesses than any alternative.*

Max Fink (1999, p. ix)

Somatic therapies are treatment approaches that use physiologic or physical interventions to effect behavioral change. The most common form of somatic therapy is electroconvulsive therapy (ECT), which will be discussed at length. Box 39-1 outlines early efforts in somatic therapy, summarizing the history of insulin-coma therapy and initial convulsive therapies. A brief review of psychosurgery, a highly controversial and rarely used therapy, follows the ECT discussion. Psychosurgery's inclusion traces its relevance to historical, ethical, and legal issues profoundly affecting psychiatric care. A brief discussion of other somatic therapies, such as transcranial magnetic stimulation and phototherapy, concludes the chapter.

ECT and psychosurgery emerged as treatment forms in the 1930s. The roots of ECT lie in the misconception of early twentieth-century psychiatrists that epilepsy and schizophrenia were incompatible (Abrams, 1997). Advocates of ECT and psychosurgery envisioned and promised dramatic relief from the curse of mental illness. Over time, inappropriate use and disappointing results, coupled with the development of psychotropic drugs and a growing general distrust of psychiatric hospitals, created a climate of hostility toward these therapies and their practitioners. In the 1960s and early 1970s, the use of both therapies came to a virtual standstill. In about the last 20 years, however, ECT has emerged once again as a useful treatment alternative when more traditional approaches have failed. Psychosurgery, on the other hand, remains a treatment of last resort and is infrequently per-

## Norm's Notes

*Somatic therapies, especially electroconvulsive therapy, are terribly misunderstood. If antidepressants are not working for someone with a severe depression, electroconvulsive therapy will usually help them. If you know someone who just cannot seem to improve with the various antidepressant medications available, particularly if that person has entertained thoughts of suicide, please talk to someone in his or her family about this option. The kind of procedure you see in older movies has not been used in most hospitals (in industrialized countries) since the 1960s. It is safe and it is effective. And it saves lives.*

formed. With rigid treatment criteria and careful pretreatment evaluation, many psychiatric patients respond to these somatic therapies.

## ELECTROCONVULSIVE THERAPY

Ugo Cerletti and Luciano Bini (Cerletti's assistant), two Italian psychiatrists, introduced ECT in 1938. The first patient suffered from schizophrenia and, after 11 treatments, experienced a full recovery. The first ECT treatment in the United States was in 1940.

ECT was once commonly referred to as *electroshock therapy* (EST) or simply *shock therapy*. Both terms are considered pejorative today.

During ECT, an electric current is passed through the brain, causing a seizure. Historically, this seizure resulted in a full grand mal convulsion accompanied by the various complications of these convulsions—that is, muscle soreness, fractures, dislocations, sprains, and tongue lacerations. These seizures and the resulting grotesque facial grimaces have been dramatically captured on film and graphically detailed in literature. In films and novels, ECT has been portrayed as a devious tool used by psychiatrists and psychiatric nurses, who are themselves demented. The late Ken Kesey's book, *One Flew Over the Cuckoo's Nest,* and the 1975 movie of the same name created a firestorm of hostility against the use of ECT. In his book, Kesey portrayed ECT as an agent used to maintain

---

### Box 39-1   Early Somatic Therapies

**Insulin-Coma Therapy: 1933**

Insulin-coma therapy was introduced in 1933 by the Viennese physician Manfred Sakel after he accidentally discovered that giving too much insulin to a psychotic diabetic patient produced a reduction in the patient's symptoms. Insulin shock therapy gained a wide following for some time in hopes of alleviating the debilitating symptoms of psychosis (Colaizzi, 1996; Dorman, 1995).

**First Convulsive Therapies: 1934**

Ladislas Meduna, a Hungarian, was the originator of convulsive therapy. In 1934, Meduna introduced camphor oil–induced and then Metrazol-induced convulsion therapy based on his pathologic observation that the glial cells of patients with schizophrenia were different than those of individuals with epilepsy. Meduna erroneously concluded that schizophrenia and epilepsy were mutually exclusive disorders (Abrams, 1997). Fink (1999) has chronicled one of Meduna's first patients, a 33-year-old man who had been psychotic, mute, and withdrawn for 4 years:

> Two days after the fifth (camphor oil) injection, on February 10 in the morning, for the first time in four years, he got out of his bed, began to talk, requested breakfast, dressed himself without help, was interested in everything around him, and asked about his disease and how long he had been in the hospital. When the patient was told he had been in the hospital for 4 years he did not believe it! (p. 88)

---

control over sane but highly individualistic patients. This public attack on ECT, linked with reports of inappropriate use, virtually stopped the use of ECT in this country. Inappropriate use of ECT included administering ECT for almost all conditions and, from the accounts of former patients, using it as punishment for noncompliant behavior.

ECT was used most often during the early 1950s, when it was given to almost every patient who did not respond to other treatment forms (Swartz, 1993a). In large state hospitals, ECT was given to as many as 20 or more patients on a psychiatric ward, typically without written consent. One patient after another, some under their own power, others literally manhandled and restrained, would take their place on the bed to be given ECT. Nursing staff would hold the patient in place (to decrease fractures and dislocations), insert the mouth guard (to prevent tongue bites), put paste on the electrodes, and hold the electrodes in place on each side of the head (usually the temple area). A nurse would then hold the chin and jaw in proper alignment, and the physician in the background would push a button to deliver the shock. A full grand mal seizure would occur—a tonic seizure followed by a significantly longer clonic seizure. After convulsion activity ended, the patient was turned on his or her side and tied in place (to prevent aspiration) while a staff member or helper patient stayed at the bedside until consciousness returned. The ECT team then moved on to the next patient. This unforgettable scene, depicted in novels and films and reported by former patients, contributed to a growing public fear of ECT.

Despite the negative perceptions, however, ECT remains a viable treatment approach because many mental health professionals know it to be an effective treatment. Unfortunately, in the process of waiting to evaluate the efficacy of other treatments, many patients have suffered needlessly. Many clinicians now argue that ECT should be considered as a treatment choice earlier in the treatment process. About 100,000 patients receive ECT treatments annually in the United States (Smith, 2001).

## MODERN ELECTROCONVULSIVE THERAPY

During ECT, an electric current is passed through the brain for 0.2 to 8.0 seconds, causing a seizure (Fink, 1999). Induction of a seizure is necessary for a therapeutic outcome (Krystal et al, 2000). The seizure resulting from ECT must be of sufficient quality to produce the best effect. Seizures are timed and subdivided into motor convulsions (at least 20 seconds required), increased heart rate (for 30 to 50 seconds), and a brain seizure as monitored by an electroencephalogram (EEG) (for 30 to 150 seconds) (Fink, 1999). The patient is given an oximeter-monitored anesthetic to ensure optimal oxygenation. The events leading up to, during, and after treatment, including nursing responsibilities, are presented here.

### Preparation for Electroconvulsive Therapy

- The patient must have a pretreatment evaluation, including physical examination, laboratory work (blood count, blood chemistries, urinalysis), and baseline memory abilities.
- A consent form must be signed. Because ECT is often given as a treatment of last resort, some

patients are profoundly depressed to the extent that, by the time ECT is ordered, a truly informed consent is almost a contradiction in terms (Rose et al, 2005). In these cases, family members and facility legal staff should be involved.
- If possible, the routine use of benzodiazepines or barbiturates for nighttime sedation should be eliminated because of their ability to raise the seizure threshold (i.e., make it more difficult to stimulate a seizure).
- A trained electrotherapist and an anesthesiologist should be available.

### Nursing Responsibilities Before Electroconvulsive Therapy

- The patient should not be given anything by mouth for approximately 6 to 8 hours before ECT, except for cardiac, antihypertensive, and a few other medications.
- Atropine (or glycopyrrolate [Robinul]) should be given as ordered. Atropine can be given 1 hour before treatment or intravenously immediately preceding treatment (Box 39-2). Atropine reduces secretions and subsequent risk of aspiration and counteracts the ECT-induced vagal stimulation.
- The patient should be asked to urinate before the treatment (seizure-induced incontinence is common).
- The patient's hairpins, contact lenses, hearing aid, and dentures should be removed.
- Vital signs should be taken.
- The nurse should be positive about the treatment and attempt to reduce the patient's anxiety.

### Procedures During Electroconvulsive Therapy

- An intravenous line is inserted.
- Electrodes are attached to the proper place on the head. Electrodes are typically held in place with a rubber strap.
- The bite block is inserted.
- Methohexital (Brevital) or another short-acting barbiturate is given intravenously. The barbiturate causes immediate anesthesia, preempting the anxiety associated with waiting for the jolt to hit and the anxiety caused by succinylcholine (see next).
- Succinylcholine (Anectine) is a neuromuscular blocking agent and is given intravenously. Suc-

## Box 39-2   Drugs Used for Electroconvulsive Therapy

**Atropine**

**Class:** Anticholinergic

**Actions:** Atropine is used before ECT for several reasons:

1. Inhibition of salivation and respiratory tract secretions to minimize aspiration
2. Decreases the potential for cardiovascular depression resulting from ECT, succinylcholine, methohexital, or any combination

*Pharmacokinetics*
   *Onset:* Orally, 30 minutes; intramuscularly, 15 minutes; IV, 1 minute
   *Dose:* 0.4 to 0.6 mg

**Side Effects:** Typical anticholinergic effects

**Succinylcholine (Anectine)**

**Class:** Ultrashort-acting neuromuscular blocker

**Actions:** Prevents the musculoskeletal complications from induced convulsions

*Pharmacokinetics*
   *Onset:* 30 to 60 seconds; duration of action, 5 minutes
   *Dose:* 0.6 mg/kg IV

**Side Effects:** Prolonged apnea, respiratory depression, fasciculations

**Methohexital (Brevital)**

**Class:** Ultrashort-acting barbiturate

**Actions:** Induces a light coma preceding delivery of ECT

*Pharmacokinetics*
   *Onset:* 10 to 15 seconds; duration of action, 5 to 7 minutes
   *Dose:* 1.5 mg/kg (typically 50 to 120 mg)

**Side Effects:** Respiratory depression, hypotension, myocardial depression, decreased cardiac output

---

cinylcholine causes paralysis but not sedation (it does not cross the blood-brain barrier), thereby leaving the patient conscious but unable to breathe.

- Succinylcholine prevents the external manifestations of a grand mal seizure, thus minimizing fractures or dislocations, but it does not affect the brain seizure.
- The anesthesiologist mechanically ventilates the patient with 100% oxygen immediately before the treatment.
- The electrical impulse is typically given for 0.2 to 8.0 seconds.
- The seizure should last a certain length of time to be of therapeutic value (see previous point).

If the seizure lasts less than this amount of time, the physician must decide whether to stimulate another seizure. Seizure duration longer than 180 seconds is associated with a less favorable outcome and can be terminated with diazepam or another benzodiazepine.

- Monitoring devices include those for heart rate and rhythm, blood pressure, and electroencephalography (EEG).
- Ventilation and monitoring continue until the patient recovers.

### Nursing Responsibilities After Electroconvulsive Therapy

- The nurse or anesthesiologist mechanically ventilates the patient with 100% oxygen until the patient can breathe unassisted.
- The nurse monitors for respiratory problems.
- ECT causes confusion and disorientation; thus, it is important to help with reorientation (time, place, person) as the patient emerges from this groggy state.
- Because approximately 5% to 10% of these patients awake in an agitated state, the nurse might need to administer a benzodiazepine, as needed (Fitzsimons, 1995).
- Observation is necessary until the patient is oriented and steady, particularly when the patient first attempts to stand.
- All aspects of the treatment should be carefully documented for the patient's record.

An EEG recording monitors seizure activity. Blood pressure, oxygen saturation, and heart rate are also monitored. Oxygen is administered immediately before and after treatment because of interruption of breathing caused by the succinylcholine and the electrically induced seizure.

### CRITICAL THINKING QUESTION   1

ECT has been considered a political issue. Do you think that opponents of ECT tend to be more on the left or the right of the political spectrum?

ECT is more effective than antidepressants in the treatment of severe depression. Nonetheless, there is reluctance to use ECT. If you or a member of your family were severely depressed, which of these two treatment forms would you want? Carefully consider the stigma of ECT, as well as the effects of anesthesia and memory loss.

# HOW DOES ELECTROCONVULSIVE THERAPY WORK?

The short answer is that no one knows for sure, although over 100 theories have been advanced to explain ECT (Sackiem, 1993). Four of these theories seem most promising (Bezchlibnyk-Butler and Jeffries, 2004; Fink, 1999; Kellner and McCall, 1997).

1. ECT alters the endocrine system in ways that promote an antidepressant effect. For example, levels of corticotropin-releasing hormone (CRH), adrenocorticotropic hormone (ACTH), thyrotropin-releasing hormone (TRH), prolactin, vasopressin, and various peptides are altered as well.
2. ECT alters neurotransmitter systems that contribute to mental disorders (e.g., acetylcholine, dopamine, gamma-aminobutyric acid [GABA], norepinephrine, serotonin).
3. ECT alters (raises) the seizure threshold, which, in turn, causes an antidepressant effect.
4. ECT alters (increases) the permeability of the blood-brain barrier.

# NUMBER OF TREATMENTS

Typically, patients are given ECT two to three times a week, up to a total of 6 to 12 treatments (or until the patient improves or is obviously not going to improve). Patients often experience relief after two or three treatments, but occasionally up to 20 are needed. If improvement is not observed after about 12 treatments, then continuing ECT is usually not helpful. Although ECT is generally effective, relapse occurs frequently. Many patients require continuation or maintenance ECT treatments to function at their best (see later discussion).

# INDICATIONS FOR ELECTROCONVULSIVE THERAPY: MAJOR DEPRESSION

Although ECT was originally developed for schizophrenia, its primary indication soon shifted to patients who were severely depressed, particularly those manifesting delusions and psychomotor retardation (Box 39-3). Severely depressed patients account for about 85% to 90% of all patients receiving ECT. These patients respond better and

---

**Box 39-3    Indications for Electroconvulsive Therapy**

- *Major depression:* ECT is appropriate treatment when associated with:
  1. Nonresponse to an adequate trial of antidepressants
  2. High suicide potential
  3. Dehydration
  4. Depressive stupor
  5. Catatonia
  6. Delusions
- Prophylaxis of recurrent major depression (i.e., maintenance ECT)
- Severe mania not controlled by medications
- Postpartum psychosis after nonresponse to antidepressants
- Schizophrenia (catatonic type) when nonresponsive to medications
- Movement disorders refractory to treatment (e.g., Parkinson's disease, neuroleptic malignant syndrome, tardive dyskinesia, myasthenia gravis)

Modified from Bezchlibyk-Butler KZ, Jeffries JJ: *Clinical handbook of psychotropic drugs,* Seattle, 2004, Hogrefe & Huber; Calarge CA, Crowe RR, Electroconvulsive therapy and myasthenia gravis, *Ann Clin Psychiatry* 16:225, 2004; Husain SS, Kevan IM, Linnell R, Scott AI: Electroconvulsive therapy in depressive illness that has not responded to drug treatment, *J Affect Disord* 82:121, 2004; Sadock BJ, Sadock VA: *Synopsis of psychiatry,* ed 9, Philadelphia, 2003, JB Lippincott.

---

more rapidly to ECT than to antidepressants (Bowden, 1985; Coffey and Weiner, 1990). Potter and Rudorfer (1993) have suggested a hierarchy of patients who should receive ECT:

1. Patients who require a rapid response (e.g., suicidal or catatonic patients)
2. Patients who cannot tolerate or be exposed to pharmacotherapy (e.g., pregnant women)
3. Patients who are depressed but have not responded to multiple and adequate trials of medication

## CLINICAL EXAMPLE

Penny Jones is a 48-year-old woman who worked for the postal service until 3 weeks ago. She was admitted to an acute psychiatric facility accompanied by her daughter, who indicated that her mother had lost 30 pounds during the last 4 months. The daughter further described her mother as having a poor appetite, being isolative, awakening early in the morning with the inability to fall back to sleep, and verbalizing thoughts with suicidal overtones. The daughter stated that her mother's actions scare her.

Ms. Jones states that life is intolerable, and she does not want to live anymore without Jerry. The daughter explains that Jerry was the patient's husband, who died 5 months ago.

Ms. Jones sought psychiatric help immediately and was prescribed sertraline 25 mg per day for 1 week, then 50 mg qd. She improved slightly but has relapsed into a deeper depression and has lately begun to verbalize suicidal thoughts. Based on her poor response to antidepressants and her suicidal thoughts, a course of six ECT treatments was prescribed. Ms. Jones tolerated the procedures well. Her suicidal ideations ceased, she began interacting with others spontaneously, and regained her appetite. She was discharged during the third week of her hospitalization.

Disorders, depressive symptoms, and conditions that respond to ECT are found in Table 39-1 (Swartz, 1993b). Box 39-4 lists conditions that do not respond to ECT.

---

**Box 39-4  Conditions Nonresponsive to Electroconvulsive Therapy**

Anxiety disorders
Behavioral disorders
Mild depressions
Personality disorders
Phobic disorders
Somatoform disorders

---

# CONTRAINDICATIONS TO ELECTROCONVULSIVE THERAPY

Ziring (1993) has suggested that ECT should be viewed similarly to many lifesaving surgeries; that is, although there might be conditions that place an ECT recipient at risk, the risk might be warranted if the patient's condition is serious enough (e.g., severe depression, active suicidal ideations). Most clinicians believe that the conditions listed in Box 39-5 create some level of risk for a patient who receives ECT.

---

**Box 39-5  Conditions Causing Increased Risk for Patients Receiving Electroconvulsive Therapy**

**Very High Risk**
Recent myocardial infarction
Recent cerebrovascular accident
Intracranial mass
Increased intracranial pressure

**High Risk**
Angina pectoris
Congestive heart failure
Extremely loose teeth (aspiration)
Severe pulmonary disease
Severe osteoporosis
Major bone fractures
Glaucoma
Retinal detachment
Thrombophlebitis
High-risk pregnancy
Use of monoamine oxidase inhibitors (MAOIs) (severe hypertension)*
Use of clozapine (seizures, delirium)

*Some studies indicate that MAOIs given in conjunction with ECT do not cause a serious interaction.
Modified from Ziring B: Issues in the perioperative care of the patient with psychiatric illness, *Med Clin North Am* 77:443, 1993; Bezchlibnyk-Butler KZ, Jeffries JJ: *Clinical handbook of psychotropic drugs*, Seattle, 2004, Hogrefe & Huber.

---

**Table 39-1  Disorders, Depressive Symptoms, and Conditions That Respond to Electroconvulsive Therapy**

| Disorders | Depressive Symptoms | Conditions |
|---|---|---|
| Severe depression | Anhedonia | Tardive dystonia |
| Refractory depression | Anorexia | Tardive dyskinesia |
| Catatonia | Delusions | Akathisia |
| Mania | Insomnia | Parkinsonian symptoms |
| Some types of schizophrenia | Muteness | Neuroleptic malignant syndrome |
| | Psychomotor retardation | |
| | Suicidal ideations | |

From Swartz CM: Seizure benefit: grand mal or grand bene? *Neurol Clin* 11:151, 1993b.

# ADVANTAGES OF ELECTROCONVULSIVE THERAPY

Historically, ECT has been viewed as providing the fastest relief for depression (Roose and Nobler, 2001).

ECT is a safe procedure; only a few ECT-related deaths have been reported (Nuttall et al, 2004; Sackeim et al, 1993). ECT has about the same risk as that associated with general anesthesia, one death per 50,000 patients (Gitlin et al, 1993), and is safer compared with tricyclic antidepressants (i.e., fewer cardiotoxic effects, cannot be used to attempt suicide). Furthermore, ECT is not only safe, but it is also more effective than antidepressants for certain groups of patients. Potter and Rudorfer (1993) stated that up to 90% of severely depressed patients respond to ECT. Finally, ECT can be used safely and effectively in older patients, even those regarded as the old-old (older than 85 years), and in adolescents (Cohen et al, 2000; Tomac et al, 1997).

# DISADVANTAGES OF ELECTROCONVULSIVE THERAPY

## Provision of Only Temporary Relief

The major disadvantage of ECT is that treatment provides only temporary relief; it does not provide a permanent cure. Certainly, many patients are able to remain free of depression for long periods, and others might never need treatment again. However, some patients receiving ECT might need another series of treatments within a few months. Some psychiatrists order maintenance or continuation ECT (about once a month for 6 to 12 months or longer); however, there is still much to learn about the benefits of this approach. Studies have suggested that continued periodic treatments of ECT plus an antidepressant significantly reduce relapse rates (Gagne et al, 2000).

## Memory Loss

Memory impairment, both retrograde (memory before treatment) and anterograde (memory and the ability to learn new things after treatment), has been frequently cited as a side effect of ECT. Events closest in time to ECT are most frequently affected. Although it is true that memory is impaired for events both before and after each treatment, and that confusion occurs immediately after each treatment, there does not seem to be any substantial loss of mental function for most patients once the treatment series has been completed. Furthermore, because depression can cause memory loss as well, it is not always clear whether memory impairment is related to ECT or to depression. Unilateral placement of the electrodes—that is, both electrodes placed on the nondominant side of the head (for right-handed individuals, this would be the right side)—minimizes treatment impact on memory and learning but might not be as effective (Bailine et al, 2000). Bifrontal placement (placed a few inches apart on the front of the head) also causes fewer problems with memory and learning (Abrams, 1997; Bailine et al, 2000).

## Adverse Physiologic Effects

Adverse physiologic effects of ECT include cardiac effects such as hypertension, arrhythmias, alterations of cardiac output, and changes in cerebrovascular dynamics. Hemodynamic changes, in combination with increased muscle tone, have been postulated to result in a generalized increase in oxygen consumption. Increases in myocardial oxygen consumption might result in ischemia (Ziring, 1993). Other problems that have been reported include hyponatremia (Greer and Stewart, 1993) and migraine headaches (Weinstein, 1993). ECT does not cause brain damage (Abrams, 1997).

# OTHER SOMATIC THERAPIES

# PSYCHOSURGERY (LOBOTOMY)

This brief introduction to psychosurgery discusses an important historical period in psychiatric care. To appreciate today's advances in psychiatric care and patient advocacy, one must understand issues and debates that shaped today's mental health environment.

It is difficult to find an area of psychiatry surrounded by more controversy than psychosurgery. Psychosurgery destroys brain tissue for the purpose of relieving intractable mental disorders not amenable to other therapies. A review of the literature suggests that medical scientists have strongly held views on both the efficacy and ethics of this procedure. Obviously, clinicians should eliminate all other options before using this drastic approach.

Dorman (1995) has suggested that this radical treatment was adopted because of the convergence of four existing conditions in psychiatric care:

1. The persistent appalling conditions in state hospitals
2. The rivalry between neurology and psychiatry
3. The use of other radical treatments (e.g., ECT)
4. New theories regarding frontal lobe brain function

### Historical Overview of Lobotomies

The man considered the modern-day pioneer in psychosurgery was Antonio Egas Moniz, a Portuguese neurologist. In 1935, Moniz, with the assistance of Lima, performed a series of psychosurgical operations on 20 severely ill institutionalized patients. These researchers reported that 14 members of this cohort showed improvement (Cosgrove and Rauch, 1995) and coined the term *psychosurgery*. In 1949, Moniz received the Nobel Prize in Medicine and Physiology for his work.

Walter Freeman, a neurologist, and his neurosurgeon colleague, James Watts, were impressed with the work of Moniz and began performing these surgeries in the United States in 1936. Although a neurologist, Freeman treated many psychiatric patients and sought treatment approaches that were more efficient compared with standard treatment modalities. Psychosurgery was the procedure he was looking for. Before his retirement, Freeman (1971) performed over 3500 psychosurgeries. In addition, Freeman toured the country, stopping at large state mental institutions to demonstrate his technique. In Freeman's wake, local practitioners began performing psychosurgery. Colaizzi (1996) has vividly described Freeman's visit to a hospital in 1950.

Freeman's reputation has been sullied somewhat by what appears to be high-handed or pejorative language. Dorman (1995) has retrieved some of Freeman's remarks, which detract from his work:

> Some patients come to operation at the end of a long and exasperating series of medical treatments, hospital treatments, shock treatments, including endocrines and vitamins mixed with their physiotherapy and psychotherapy. They are still desperate, and will go to any length to get rid of their distress.

Other patients can't be dragged into the hospital and have to be held down on a bed in a hotel room until sufficient shock treatment can be given to render them manageable. We like both types. (p. 60)

Freeman also recorded a conversation with a 24-year-old laborer who was awake during the surgery (Dorman, 1995):

*Freeman:* Are you scared?
*Patient:* Yeah.
*(2 minutes later)*
*Freeman:* How do you feel?
*Patient:* I don't feel anything, but they're cutting me now.
*Freeman:* You wanted it?
*Patient:* Yes, but I didn't think you'd do it awake. Oh, gee whiz, I'm dying. Oh, doctor. Please stop. Oh, God. I'm goin' again. Oh, oh, oh. Ow *(chisel on skull),* oh, this is awful. Ow *(grabs Freeman's hand and sinks nails into it).* Oh, God, I'm goin', please stop.
*(After cuts have been made)*
*Freeman:* What's happened to your fear?
*Patient:* Gone.
*Freeman:* Why were you afraid?
*Patient:* I don't know.
*Freeman:* Feel okay?
*Patient:* Yes. I feel pretty good right now. (p. 58)

Moreover, in response to critics of his surgical technique, Freeman referred to concerns about sterile procedure as "all that germ crap" (Dorman, 1995).

Psychosurgical intervention was widely used in the 1940s and 1950s, but a sharp decline occurred after the introduction of psychotropic drugs to state hospitals in the early to mid-1950s (Figure 39-1). As previously mentioned, psychosurgery suffered some of the same public rejection as ECT. Again, the popular novel *One Flew Over the Cuckoo's Nest* depicted the defiant hero as the victim of a treacherous state hospital staff. The patient's defiance eventually resulted in the ultimate punishment—a lobotomy—and he emerged from the lobotomy room a vegetable, his defiant character finally conquered. This depiction of psychosurgery helped shape public opinion about this procedure. Most professionals soon abandoned psychosurgery treatment.

### Ethical Concerns

As might be expected, many concerns have been voiced regarding the ethics of psychosurgery. To

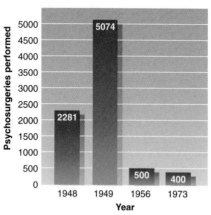

**FIGURE 39-1** Psychosurgery performed in the years before and after the discovery and introduction of antipsychotic drugs. *(From Valenstein ES: The psychosurgery debate, San Francisco, 1980, WH Freeman.)*

destroy brain tissue constitutes an extreme and irreversible tactic. Without room for error, most clinicians believe that psychosurgery should be abandoned.

### Indications for Psychosurgery

Although extremely rare, when psychosurgery is indicated it most likely is used for obsessive-compulsive disorder or aggressiveness related to a mental disorder.

## BRIGHT LIGHT THERAPY

Bright light therapy (BLT), formerly called *phototherapy*, exposes patients to intense light (5000 lux-hours) each day. The rationale for this treatment comes from several studies plus anecdotal reports indicating that environmental factors play a role in mood disorders. Seasonal affective disorder (SAD), for example, results from decreased exposure to sunlight and usually occurs in and around the winter season. BLT used for SAD sufferers relieves symptoms of depression. Apparently, morning administration is most beneficial.

BLT works in just a few days. The precise mechanism of action of how exposure to intense light produces an antidepressant effect remains unclear; however, it is believed that its therapeutic effect is mediated by the eyes, not the skin. Other conditions thought to respond to light therapy include bulimia, sleep maintenance insomnia, and nonseasonal depression. Because phototherapy produces few if any significant adverse effects

(e.g., nausea, eye irritation), the risk-benefit ratio favors its use. Contraindications include glaucoma, catatracts, and use of photosensitizing medications.

**CRITICAL THINKING QUESTION    2**

Does it make common sense that a bright light could improve a person's mental health?  Does a sunny day help your mood?

## REPETITIVE TRANSCRANIAL MAGNETIC STIMULATION

Transcranial magnetic stimulation (TMS) or repetitive transcranial magnetic stimulation (rTMS) produces a magnetic field over the brain, influencing brain activity. Apparently, TMS increases the release of neurotransmitters and/or down-regulates beta-adrenergic receptors, thus ameliorating depressive symptoms and possibly other disorders. Because TMS does not require anesthesia, it is an attractive alternative to ECT if conclusive evidence of its efficacy can be demonstrated. Some studies have suggested that it is as effective as ECT in nonpsychotic patients (Fitzgerald, 2004). Adverse effects include seizures in previously seizure-free individuals, headache, and transient hearing loss. Patients with metal implanted in their bodies (e.g., plates), pacemakers, heart disease, or increased intracranial pressure should be carefully evaluated before receiving TMS.

**CRITICAL THINKING QUESTION    3**

What are some of the potential abuses of psychosurgery in a society in which physicians are held in high esteem?

### ▌ Study Notes

1. Somatic therapies are treatment approaches that use physiologic or physical interventions to effect behavioral change.
2. The most common form of somatic therapy is ECT.
3. During ECT, an electric current is passed through the brain, causing a grand mal seizure.
4. Modern ECT uses anesthesia and muscle relaxants to prevent convulsive jerks that once caused

broken bones; oxygen is given to guard against brain damage.

5. ECT is indicated for the treatment of severe depression, depression that is unresponsive to other treatments, mania, catatonia, and some types of schizophrenia.

6. Psychosurgery (lobotomy), a controversial brain surgery, is performed to provide relief from mental disorders that have been resistant to other treatment forms.

7. Some individuals suffer depressive symptoms (SAD) in response to decreased sunlight availability (i.e., during the winter months). Bright light therapy, the exposure to intense artificial light, reduces these symptoms.

8. Symptoms of depression can be reduced by rTMS of the brain, perhaps by increasing levels of neurotransmitters.

## References

Abrams R: *Electroconvulsive therapy,* New York, 1997, Oxford University Press.

Bailine SH, Rifkin A, Kayne E, et al: Comparison of bifrontal and bitemporal ECT for major depression, *Am J Psychiatry* 157:121, 2000.

Bezchlibnyk-Butler KZ, Jeffries JJ: *Clinical handbook of psychotropic drugs,* Seattle, 2004, Hogrefe & Huber.

Bowden CL: Current treatment of depression, *Hosp Community Psychiatry* 36:1192, 1985.

Calarge CA, Crowe RR: Electroconvulsive therapy and myasthenia gravis, *Ann Clin Psychiatry* 16:225, 2004.

Coffey CE, Weiner RD: Electroconvulsive therapy: an update, *Hosp Community Psychiatry* 41:515, 1990.

Cohen D, Taieb O, Flament M, et al: Absence of cognitive impairment at long-term follow-up in adolescents treated with ECT for severe mood disorder, *Am J Psychiatry* 157:460, 2000.

Colaizzi J: Transorbital lobotomy at Eastern State Hospital (1951-1954), *J Psychosoc Nurs Ment Health Serv* 34:16, 1996.

Cosgrove CR, Rauch SL: Psychosurgery, *Nurs Clin North Am* 6:167, 1995.

Dorman J: The history of psychosurgery, *Tex Med* 91:54, 1995.

Fink M: *Electroshock,* New York, 1999, Oxford University Press.

Fitzgerald P: Repetitive transcranial magnetic stimulation and electroconvulsive therapy; complementary or competitive therapeutic options in depression? *Australas Psychiatry* 12:234, 2004.

Fitzsimons L: Electroconvulsive therapy: what nurses need to know, *J Psychosoc Nurs Ment Health Serv* 33:14, 1995.

Freeman W: Frontal lobotomy in early schizophrenia: long-term follow-up in 415 cases, *Br J Psychiatry* 119:621, 1971.

Gagne GG Jr, Furman MJ, Carpenter LL, Price L: Efficacy of continuation ECT and antidepressant drugs compared to long-term antidepressants alone in depressed patients, *Am J Psychiatry* 157:1960, 2000.

Gitlin MC, O'Neill PT, Barber MJ, Jahr JS: Splenic rupture after electroconvulsive therapy, *Anesth Analg* 76:1363, 1993.

Greer R, Stewart R: Hyponatremia and ECT, *Am J Psychiatry* 150:1272, 1993.

Husain SS, Kevan IM, Linnell R, Scott AI: Electroconvulsive therapy in depressive illness that has not responded to drug treatment, *J Affect Disord* 83:121, 2004.

Kellner C, McCall W: Novel electrode placements: time to reassess, *J ECT* 15:115, 1999.

Krystal AD, Dean MD, Weiner RD, et al: ECT stimulus intensity: are present ECT devices too limited? *Am J Psychiatry* 157:963, 2000.

Nuttall GA, Bowersox MR, Douglass SB, et al: Morbidity and mortality in the use of electroconvulsive therapy, *J ECT* 20:237, 2004.

Potter W, Rudorfer M: Electroconvulsive therapy: a modern medical procedure, *N Engl J Med* 328:12, 1993.

Roose SP, Nobler M: ECT and onset of action, *J Clin Psychiatry* 62(Suppl 4):24, 2001.

Rose DS, Wykes TH, Bindman JP, Fleischmann PS: Information, consent and perceived coercion: patients' perspectives on electroconvulsive therapy, *Br J Psychiatry* 186:54, 2005.

Sadock BJ, Sadock VA: *Synopsis of psychiatry,* ed 9, Philadelphia, 2003, JB Lippincott.

Sackeim HA, Prudic J, Devanand DP, et al: Effects of stimulus intensity and electrode placement on the efficacy and cognitive effects of electroconvulsive therapy, *N Engl J Med* 328:839, 1993.

Smith D: Shock and disbelief, *Atlantic Monthly* February:79, 2001.

Swartz CM: ECT or programmed seizures? *Am J Psychiatry* 150:1274, 1993a.

Swartz CM: Seizure benefit: grand mal or grand bene? *Neurol Clin* 11:151, 1993b.

Tomac TA, Rummans TA, Pileggi TS: Safety and efficacy of electroconvulsive therapy in patients over age 85, *Am J Geriatr Psychiatry* 5:126, 1997.

Valenstein ES: *The psychosurgery debate,* San Francisco, 1980, WH Freeman.

Weinstein MD: Migraine occurring as sequela of electroconvulsive therapy, *Headache* 33:45, 1993.

Ziring B: Issues in the perioperative care of the patient with psychiatric illness, *Med Clin North Am* 77:443, 1993.

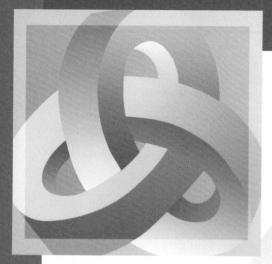

# Chapter 40

# Alternative and Complementary Therapies

*Beverly K. Hogan*

---

## Learning Objectives

*After reading this chapter, you should be able to:*

- Define alternative therapy.
- Trace the historical use of alternative therapies to their current state of use.
- Define complementary therapy and give an example to illustrate what is meant by complementary versus alternative therapy.
- Name common alternative and complementary therapies used for psychiatric symptoms and discuss current research conclusions regarding their efficacy.

- Describe how various alternative and complementary therapies are regulated.
- Name three dangerous interactions with herbal therapies.
- Explain the role of the nurse in assessment and intervention with clients using alternative or complementary therapies.

---

A 1998 comprehensive survey on Americans' use of alternative and complementary therapies has continued to provide data from which other studies have emerged (Barnes et al, 2004) (Table 40-1). Each year, nearly $1 trillion is spent on health care in the United States, of which $22 billion is spent on alternative therapies. This figure is remarkable, considering that most of this money is an out of pocket expense, not usually reimbursed by health insurance (Eisenberg et al, 1998; Snyder and Lindquist, 2001). Eighty percent of the world's population relies on therapies called *alternative* in the United States (Folks and Gabel, 2001), but that are mainstream in other countries (Yarnell and Abascal, 2004). Estimates have suggested that one of three consumers in the United States uses alternative therapies in one form or another. Eisenberg and colleagues (1998) found an almost 50% increase in alternative care visits from a previous survey (in 1990). Clearly, the American health care consumer is willing to consider treatments offered outside conventional medicine (Bridevauxa and Salesa, 2004).

Among people using alternative therapies along with traditional medicine, fewer than half disclose this use to their health care provider (Eisenberg et al, 1998; Robinson and McGrail, 2004). Because alternative therapies might interact with traditional therapies and might also have their own side effects, it is important to know whether the patient is using these therapies. Robinson and McGrail (2004) found that the primary reasons people give for nondisclosure of their use of alternative therapies are related to a:

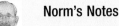

### Norm's Notes

*This is a hot topic, and presents a moving target. It is almost impossible to keep up with the various claims being made on late night or early morning television. Some of these agents or remedies really work and as for the others—well, you can hardly tell what works. Maybe they work for some people and not for others. I think the author of this chapter has done a good job of selecting those therapies that have some support. The average nurse should know something about them.*

1. Belief that health care professionals will have a negative reaction
2. Belief that health care practitioners cannot or do not understand these therapies, or
3. Desire to have some control over their health care

Nurses need to know about these therapies to provide culturally competent care and obtain essential information (Snyder and Lindquist, 2001; McDowell and Burman, 2004).

Mental health service consumers are also seeking alternative treatments (Parslow and Jorm, 2004; Simon et al, 2004). In fact, the most commonly used herbs are for mental health–related symptoms (Beaubrun and Gray, 2000). The majority of people in the United States with self-defined anxiety attacks or severe depression use some form of alternative or complementary therapy to treat these conditions. Most users of complementary and alternative medicine (CAM) do not report their use, suggesting that herbals are being used to augment prescribed psychotropic medicine (Kessler et al, 2001; Parslow and Jorm, 2004). The importance of this issue is reflected by the inclusion of this chapter in a psychiatric nursing textbook; hopefully, other nursing textbooks are doing the same.

The issue of alternative medicine demands our attention as health care professionals. The statistical data show a high probability of use and a low probability of disclosure. Regardless of whether the health care professional endorses or recommends the use of alternative therapies, they affect the treatment provided by conventional practitioners. This chapter will use the term *alternative* to refer to therapies that are not generally accepted by conventional Western medicine. Complementary therapy

| Table 40-1 | Summary of Studies Cited in Chapter |  |
| --- | --- | --- |

**Herbals**

***St. John's Wort***

Beaubrun and Gray, 2000; Knuppel and Linde, 2004; Linde and Knuppel, 2005

***Kava-Kava***

Anke and Ramzan, 2004a; Thompson et al, 2004; Wong et al, 1998

***Valerian***

Agins and Lehne, 2004; Glass et al, 2003; Hallam et al, 2003; Malva et al, 2004

***Gingko***

Abascal, 2005b; Beaubrun and Gray, 2000; Wong et al, 1998

**Omega-3 Fatty Acids**

Cronin, 2004; Fenton et al, 2004; Hallahan and Garland, 2004; Harris et al, 2004; Joy et al, 2000; Meletis and Barker, 2004; Silvers et al, 2005; Stoll, 2001; Stoll et al, 1999

**Acupuncture**

Acupuncture: NIH Consensus Conference Statement [ANCCS], 1997; Ernst, 1998; Luo et al, 1998; Macpherson et al, 2004; Shwartz et al, 1999; Vickers and Zollman, 1999

**Massage Therapy**

Ernst, 1998; Moyer et al, 2004; Reader et al, 2005; Schlossberg, 2005a,b

**Meditative Practices**

Infante et al, 2001; Kabat-Zinn et al, 1992; Lavey et al, 2005; Miller et al, 1995; Shannahoff-Khalsa, 2004; Shannahoff-Khalsa and Beckett, 1996; Tooley et al, 2000

will be used to refer to treatments used in conjunction with conventional Western medicine. Thus, complementary and alternative medicine therapies will be referred to together as CAM therapies.

A historical perspective of CAM therapy will be presented to provide a context for this topic. It will be followed by a review of therapies with some scientific support with regard to psychiatric patients. Finally, the implications of this information and the consequent controversies will be examined within the context of nursing care.

***Note to Students:*** *Coverage of the entire field of CAM therapies is beyond the scope of this text. See Box 40-1 for additional resources on CAM therapies.*

**Box 40-1    Resources for Learning More About Alternative and Complementary Medicine**

- American Botanical Council: www.herbalgram.org or www.herbs.org
- U.S. Food and Drug Administration: www.fda.gov
- National Center for Complementary and Alternative Medicine, National Institutes of Health: www.nccam.nih.gov
- Kush RD, Bleicher P, Raymond S, et al: *Physician's Desk Reference of Herbal Medicine,* ed 3, Montvale, NJ, 2004, Thomson Healthcare.
- Linda Skidmore-Roth: *Mosby's Handbook of Herbs and Natural Supplements,* ed 3, St. Louis, 2004, Mosby.

## HISTORICAL PERSPECTIVE

In ancient times, belief held that fate, evil spirits, or gods caused illness. Hippocrates, the father of modern medicine, is credited with introducing beliefs suggesting that illness resulted from an interaction between the mind-body and the environment. Care of the whole person was considered central to the practice of medicine and, well into the 1800s, alternative therapies and conventional medicine peacefully coexisted. However, as surgical techniques improved and microbes came to be understood as disease-causing agents, a preference for more scientifically based therapies developed. By the 1900s, alternative therapy was dismissed as quackery. Medical advances continued throughout the twentieth century but, as early as the 1960s, a growing dissatisfaction with health care was becoming apparent. Not only had conventional medicine failed to live up to its promise, but it had also created a cadre of chronic diseases and toxic medications. Many consumers began the search for more palatable alternatives. Furthermore, conventional medicine, with its reliance on scientific methodologies and single-agent causation, had created a dual system of care (i.e., not holistic), in which psychological and spiritual issues were left to other disciplines. Although acute care medicine became effective in keeping people from dying, it did little to enhance quality of life (Gaydos, 2001; Snyder and Lindquist, 2001). This growing dissatisfaction, coupled with other events (see later discussion), formed the groundswell for this emerging field.

One event that gave credence to the alternative health movement arose from concerns about the effects of stress on health. A proliferation of research and the development of the new field of psychoneuroimmunology resulted. These scientifically based findings brought about a renewed interest in mind-body interactions. Ironically, this holistic approach to medicine was similar to what Hippocrates had envisioned. Modalities that had remained in mainstream medicine in the East were becoming popularized as alternative therapy in the West. A dissatisfied yet receptive consumer waited.

The growing popularity of alternative treatments attracted the attention of many special-interest groups and eventually resulted in the federal government's creation of the Office of Alternative Medicine (OAM). The OAM's mission was to provide the public with information regarding the safety and efficacy of these therapies. The U.S. Food and Drug Administration (FDA) was unable to regulate herbals because herbs were classified as dietary and nutritional supplements. In 1994, the FDA, as a result of the Dietary Supplement and Health Education Act (DSHEA), was able to require labeling on herbals, stating that there was "no proof of efficacy, safety, or standards for quality control" (Dietary Supplement Health and Education Act of 1994, 2005). In Germany, France, the United Kingdom, and Canada, the quality and safety of herbs are enforced by the federal government (Keltner and Folks, 2005). As herbals and other alternative therapies continued to gain popularity in the United States, the OAM, as a division of the National Institutes of Health (NIH), broadened its scope to include research as an objective and was renamed the National Center for Complementary and Alternative Medicine (NCCAM). One directive of the NCCAM is to fund research into the efficacy and safety of alternative treatments. The remainder of this chapter will focus on biologically based therapies, mind-body–based therapies, whole medical systems, and general concerns related to CAM.

## BIOLOGICALLY BASED THERAPIES

The biologically based therapies include such subcategories as herbals and vitamins, minerals, and nutritional supplements.

## Highlighting the Evidence

It is often assumed that people from other cultural backgrounds use alternative and complementary therapies in large quantities. The Hispanic population, in particular, is often said to have a number of healers within their community to whom they turn when ill; it is also assumed that their theories of hot and cold are highly relevant to their beliefs about health care. These practices among people with a Hispanic background can easily become assumptions and represent another stereotype, as opposed to knowing what is true for a particular patient. A study done on Hispanics has called this assumption into question and warns against stereotyping based on someone's cultural background (Mikhail et al, 2004).

A cross-sectional survey of 179 urban Hispanics from northern and southern California was conducted to establish the use and prevalence patterns for alternative and complementary medicine. Of those studied, 63%, most whom were women (75%), reported using some form of alternative therapy, mainly herbal remedies.

The highest users were more likely to have a low income and educational level, and to lack proficiency in the English language.

Even among those using herbal remedies, only 5% believed that herbal remedies were superior to conventional Western medicine. Of the alternative therapy users, 61% had more confidence in their Western medical provider than in their own healers. At least 45% of the users of herbal therapy thought Western medicines were safer than herbal remedies. In contrast to the assumption that patients with Hispanic backgrounds are high users of alternative therapy and place great confidence in their healers, most people in this study had a higher regard for Western conventional medicine.

Although it is helpful know about health care practices in other cultures, it is important to avoid assumptions and stereotypes when providing nursing care. Treating all patients as individuals takes precedence over one's cultural knowledge.

From Mikhail N, Wali S, Ziment I: Use of alternative medicine among Hispanics, *J Altern Complem Med* 10:851, 2004.

## HERBAL THERAPIES (HERBACEUTICALS)

Herbs include plant roots, tree barks, berries, leaves, resins, and flowers. Herbal therapy has been used for centuries and was referred to in the writings of Hippocrates. Although 30% of all modern drugs are derived from plants, only 1% of plants have been analyzed for their potential medicinal uses. Other cultures have known the value of various herbs for treating particular conditions and some have developed a wide knowledge base, although it would not be considered scientific by our standards (Mikhail et al, 2004). Even so, herbal medicine use, scientifically proven or not, is an important part of the health beliefs of many people.

In the United States, 20% of people use herbs for chronic conditions. Most herbs are generally not recommended for use in pregnancy, and some are known abortifacients (Folks and Gabel, 2001). A common misconception associated with

herbals is that natural equals not harmful. There are numerous reports in medical and scientific journals of severe reactions to herbs, including liver failure, renal failure, gastrointestinal (GI) tract obstruction, cardiac arrhythmias, seizure exacerbation, development of psychiatric symptoms, and even fatalities (Anke and Razman, 2004a,b; Clough et al 2004; Ernst et al, 2004). The variability of herbal preparations and their impurities make adverse reactions possible, although not predictable. Even though many people in other parts of the world have used herbals safely for thousands of years, commercial preparations in the United States might not be equivalent. Some have suggested that the time has come for a new way to report reactions, such as reliable online information and a feedback system (Peters et al, 2003). In particular, reports and investigations should focus on the responses of sensitive subpopulations, such as pregnant women, the young, and the elderly (NTP Fact Sheet, 2003).

## Table 40-2  Common Herbs Used to Treat Psychiatric Symptoms

| Herbal Product (Dosage) | Contraindications | Adverse Side Effects | Drug Interactions |
|---|---|---|---|
| Angelica (1-2 g twice daily; whole herb) | Diabetes<br>Peptic ulcer disease<br>Bleeding disorders<br>Pregnancy<br>Breast-feeding | CV: Decreased BP<br>GI: Anorexia, flatulence, spasms, dyspepsia<br>Integumentary: photosensitivity, phototoxicity, dermatitis | Increased PTT with anticoagulants |
| Chamomile (300-400 mg, up to six times/day) | Known abortifacient<br>Cross-sensitivity to sunflowers, ragweed, and members of aster family (echinacea) | Hypersensitivity-allergic reactions<br>Burning of face, mouth, eyes, and mucous membranes | Anticoagulants<br>Increases effects of CNS drugs |
| Gingko biloba (120 mg/day) | Pregnancy<br>Breast-feeding<br>Peptic ulcer disease and other bleeding problems | Headache, anxiety, and restlessness | Trazodone |
| Kava-kava (100-200 mg/day) | Liver disease (?) | Scaling of skin<br>Overdose | Antiparkinsonian agents, benzodiazepines, CNS depressants |
| Melatonin | | | More data needed |
| St. John's wort (900 mg/day) | Pregnancy<br>Breast-feeding | Dizziness, insomnia, restlessness, constipation, abdominal cramps, photosensitivity | Protease inhibitors<br>Olanzapine (Zyprexa)<br>Oral contraceptives |
| *Valeriana officinalis* (400-900 mg/day) | Pregnancy<br>Breast-feeding | Dependence | MAOIs, warfarin, phenytoin |

*BP,* Blood pressure; *CNS,* central nervous system; *CV,* cardiovascular; *GI,* gastrointestinal; *MAOIs,* monoamine oxidase inhibitors; *PTT,* prothrombin time.
From Drugs used in alternative and complementary medicine. In Keltner N, Folks D, editors: *Psychotropic drugs,* ed 4, St. Louis, 2005, Mosby.

Four of the 12 most common herbs are used to treat or prevent psychiatric symptoms (Beaubrun and Gray, 2000). For example, herbals are among the most frequently tried alternative therapies for depression (Ernst, 1998; Linde et al, 2005; Parskow and Jorm, 2004). Table 40-2 provides a summary of herbals used for psychiatric symptoms. The use of herbal preparations for mental health–related symptoms is apparently so common that it has been called part of the hidden mental health network (Simon et al, 2004).

A noteworthy caveat from a study examining the lay public's preference for treatment of mental health–related symptoms did *not* identify treatment with psychotropic medication nor visiting a psychiatrist as the first choice (except in the case of schizophrenia). Instead, alternative therapies or psychotherapy were more likely to be recommended (Riedel-Heller et al, 2005). Clearly, this is a topic of importance in a psychiatric nursing course.

## HERBALS TO TREAT ANXIETY AND DEPRESSION

### St. John's Wort

This herb is a popular treatment for mild to moderate depression; it is also used to treat anxiety, seasonal affective disorder, and sleep disorders. The herb is available in capsule, tea, or tincture form. St. John's wort is among the top-selling botanical products in the United States. If efficacy is firmly established, St John's wort is expected to be in even greater demand because of having fewer and less severe side effects compared with traditional antidepressant drugs (Linde et al, 2005; NCCAM, 2001).

Although no consensus exists regarding the mechanism of action for St. John's wort, it is thought to have an affinity for a number of neurotransmitters (Keltner and Folks, 2005). Several mechanisms of action of St. John's wort have been proposed, including the following:

- Inhibition of monoamine (serotonin, dopamine, and norepinephrine) reuptake
- Modulation of interleukin-6 (IL-6) activity

Increases in the levels of IL-6, a protein involved in intercellular communication in the immune system, might lead to increases in adrenal regulatory hormones such as cortisol (elevated cortisol is associated with depression; see Chapter 29) (Folks and Gable, 2001).

An analysis of 23 European clinical studies of St. John's wort concluded that it has antidepressive effects in cases of mild to moderate depression (the dose varied considerably among the studies [Linde and Knuppel, 2005]). These studies compared St. John's wort with tricyclic antidepressants (TCAs) but not the newer antidepressants. More recent studies have shown inconsistent and mixed results with regard to the effectiveness of St. John's wort (Hicks et al, 2005; Knuppel and Linde, 2004; Linde and Knuppel, 2005). Studies are beginning to compare St. John's wort with selective serotonin reuptake inhibitors (SSRIs), showing similarity in effectiveness (Szegedi et al, 2005; vanGurp et al, 2002). Given the number of prescriptions written annually for SSRIs, St. John's wort is a potential contender for treating less severe forms of depression.

St. John's wort is generally safe, with most side effects emerging at dose ranges exceeding those recommended for depression. There have been case reports of St. John's wort exacerbating mania. It might increase the risk for serotonin syndrome and should not be taken with other antidepressants, particularly SSRIs (Beaubrun and Gray, 2000; Zhou et al, 2004). St. John's wort is thought to induce an increase in cytochrome P450 3A4 levels, thus potentially speeding the metabolism of many drugs. For example, St. John's wort decreases blood levels of protease inhibitors, such as those used in treatment of human immunodeficiency virus (HIV) infection (Folks and Gabel, 2001; Skidmore-Roth, 2001). The mechanisms for a number of other interactions have not been clearly elucidated, thus intensifying the need for health care workers to be aware of patients taking this herbal (Zhou et al, 2004; Hobblyn and Brooks, 2005). Some reports have suggested that St. John's wort might reduce the effectiveness of oral contraceptives, thereby increasing the risk of pregnancy (Ayd, 2000; Zhou et al, 2004). In summary, St. John's wort appears to be efficacious in the treatment of mild to moderate depression; its use in severe depression *cannot* be recommended (Beaubrun and Gray, 2000; Knuppel and Linde, 2004; Linde and Knuppel, 2005); and the high potential for interactions with conventional and herbal medicines must be noted.

## CLINICAL EXAMPLE

Sam S. is a 47-year-old male Caucasian who has been treated for depression on several occasions in the past. Sam has had several recurrences of depression because he does not like taking "psychiatric drugs." Sam began taking St. John's wort, made by Nature's Source, at a dose of 750 mg/day. Sam believes that his depression is improved and feels better about taking a "natural" herb. Because Sam has never had an episode of severe depression and has never been suicidal, Sam's psychiatrist agrees with Sam's plan to continue St. John's wort and asks Sam to come in for psychiatric evaluation of his depression every 6 months.

## S-Adenosylmethionine (SAM-e)

SAM-e has been shown to be effective for depression associated with HIV infection (Shippy et al, 2004). Although SAM-e is widely used in Europe, it is only beginning to be popular in the United States. A number of studies have suggested SAM-e to be useful as an adjunct or sole therapy for depression (Brown et al, 1999). One study from Harvard University found that SAM-e augmented antidepressant response in conventional antidepressant nonresponders (Alpert et al, 2004).

## Kava-Kava

Kava-kava is part of traditional religious and social ceremonies in Polynesia and other Pacific islands. Kava-kava is prized for its ability to soothe the worried mind. The active ingredients are kava-kava pyrones, which are thought to inhibit monoamine oxidase B (Uebelhack et al, 1998). Kava-kava has also been assumed to have an affinity for benzodiazepine receptors (Folks and Gabel, 2001), thus explaining its effectiveness in reducing anxiety. There appear to be few side effects associated with kava lactories when taken in the recommended dose range (100 to 200 mg/day) (Beaubrun and Gray, 2000). Kava-kava does not appear to affect cognitive functioning, mental acuity, or coordination at regular doses (Cairney et al, 2003). At higher than recommended doses, elevated liver enzyme levels and impaired motor coordination have been reported (Cairney, 2003). Kava-kava has been reported to produce electroencephalographic (EEG) changes similar to those seen with benzodiazepines, thus reinforcing comparisons with those agents (Wong et al, 1998). Unlike benzodiazepines, which impair cognitive performance and produce subjective feelings of dysphoria, kava-kava is a potent anxiolytic agent capable of facilitating cognitive functioning and improving mood, sometimes to the point of exhilaration (Thompson et al, 2004).

Kava-kava interacts with antiparkinson drugs, benzodiazepines, and other drugs that act on the central nervous system (CNS) (Skidmore-Roth, 2001). Long-term use can cause scaling of the skin (Keltner and Folks, 2005; McEnany, 2001a). There was widespread panic when reports of kava-kava causing liver failure were publicized in the media, but these reports have not resulted in fewer sales (Mills et al, 2004). As a result of concern regarding hepatoxicity, sales of kava-kava have been banned in Germany, Canada, Switzerland, and France, but not in the United States (Agins and Lehne, 2003). There are some indications that hepatotoxicity was secondary to kava-kava's potent inhibition of the cytochrome P-450 systems, increasing the likelihood of interactions with other herbals or conventional medications, which were the real culprits (Anke and Ramzan, 2004a,b; Clouatre, 2004; Hobblyn and Brooks, 2005). Other reports have indicated that liver problems are rare when kava-kava is used alone and that liver enzyme levels return to baseline after discontinuation of kava-kava (Clough et al, 2003). Even so, reports of both sudden death (Clough et al, 2004) and acute hepatotoxicity clearly indicate the need for caution (Estes et al, 2003).

In summary, kava-kava has been used for centuries by people around the world with apparent safety. Recently, concerns of liver failure have caused a reassessment of its use. Whether adverse reactions are related directly to kava-kava or have more to do with the inconsistency in purity, labeling, or manufacturing is not known at this time.

### CLINICAL EXAMPLE

Sherry S., a 26-year-old African-American woman, was admitted to the psychiatric unit for depression with psychotic features. Sherry received a 1-mg injection of lorazepam (Ativan) in the emergency room. On admission to the unit, Sherry was noted to have slurred speech, poor coordination, and slow responses. Sherry has not been on any scheduled or prescribed medications, but the nurse found a bottle of kava-kava among Sherry's belongings. Sherry's excessive response to the lorazepam (Ativan) was most likely a result of her concomitant use of the herbal preparation kava-kava.

### Valerian

Over 250 different species of valerian are native to Europe and Asia. The variety used for anxiety comes from the plant *Valeriana officinalis.* Considerable difference exists in the potency of valerian, depending on the manufacturing process. The general dose range of 400 to 900 mg/day has been shown to be effective in decreasing sleep latency, nocturnal awakening, and a subjective sense of good sleep (Beaubrun and Gray, 2000). There is some indication that the sedative effect develops slowly over a period of weeks (Agins and Lehne, 2004). Valerian has an affinity for gamma-aminobutyric acid (GABA) A and serotonin 1a receptors (Keltner and Folks, 2005). Valerian has been extensively studied for its effectiveness in relieving anxiety. In a direct comparison with triazolam (Halcion), temazepam (Restoril), and diphenhydramine (Benadryl), valerian provided equivalent anxiolytic benefit with a slightly better side effect profile (Glass et al, 2003; Hallam et al, 2003). There are also preliminary reports of a possible neuroprotective function for valerian (Malva et al, 2004; Taibi et al, 2004).

Possible adverse effects of valerian include enhancing the effects of other CNS-acting drugs and negating the effects of other drugs, including monoamine oxidase inhibitors (MAOIs), warfarin, and phenytoin (Skidmore-Roth, 2001). There have been some indications that the valepotriate content of valerian has possible carcinogenic effects. *Valeriana officinalis,* the most commonly purchased form of valerian, has the lowest concentration of valepotriate (Taibi et al, 2004). Valerian must be protected from light and moisture or its effectiveness is altered (Keltner and Folks, 2005).

In summary, *Valeriana officinalis* appears to be useful for anxiety and insomnia; however, some clinicians caution regarding potential dependence and withdrawal. Based on the notion that valerian effects are mediated by GABA, caution should be taken with regard to preanesthetic use as well (Yuan et al, 2004).

## ANXIOLYTIC HERBALS WITHOUT SUFFICIENT EVIDENCE OF EFFICACY AND SAFETY

### Chamomile

Like other herbals that are calmative, chamomile has an affinity for benzodiazepine receptors and might also interact with the histamine system (Keltner and Folks, 2005). Multiple studies have demonstrated the herb's ability to promote relaxation and sleep and decrease anxiety (Skidmore-Roth, 2001). In a study of the effect of 300 mg/kg of chamomile administered to laboratory rats, a decreased sleep latency was observed (Shinomiya et al, 2005), suggesting that the reported effects of chamomile as a hypnotic are probably valid.

### Angelica

Several studies have shown angelica to cause significant muscle relaxation without changes in level of consciousness. At present, studies on the use of angelica for specific psychiatric disorders are insufficient, but it remains a promising herb for treating anxiety because of its potential to facilitate relaxation without also impairing cognition and motor behavior. In laboratory testing, angelica essential oils decreased aggressive behavior and increased social interaction in mice (Min et al, 2005).

### Other Herbals for Anxiety

The search for the perfect mood-altering drug, devoid of negative effects, remains elusive but some herbals for anxiety have shown preliminary promise. Lavender, linseed, passion flower, lemon balm, oat seed, and California poppy are all known to herbalists as potentially useful for treating anxiety. Abascal and Yarnell (2004c) have suggested continued testing of these herbals as an alternative to the benzodiazepines.

## HERBALS FOR MEMORY AND DEMENTIA

### Ginkgo

As one of the top-selling herbs in the United States, gingko has demonstrated improvement in memory, concentration, and mood in patients with dementia. A 52-week double-blind, placebo-controlled study of participants who were given 120 mg/day of gingko showed an overall improvement on cognitive subscales of the Alzheimer rating scale (Beaubrun and Gray, 2000). Ginkgo has also proven useful in brain trauma and cerebral insufficiency. One to 3 months is required to achieve the full effect. Multicenter controlled studies have demonstrated the ability of ginkgo to improve memory and attention (Folks and Gabel, 2001). Studies have also been undertaken to evaluate a possible neuroprotective function in healthy adults, but there have not been enough studies to replicate findings and further testing is indicated to assess for an effect of gingko in increasing alertness and sensory function (Mattes and Pawlik, 2004). The proposed improvement in cognitive functioning is thought to occur by the antioxidant effect of gingko, an effect that might protect against the tissue and cell damage of oxygen free radicals (Keltner and Folks, 2005). Research has shown that medicines that act by curtailing beta amyloid have potentially negative effects (Abascal, 2005a). (See Chapter 32 for a discussion of the role of beta amyloid in Alzheimer's disease.)

Current recommendations suggest that research in Alzheimer's should focus on antioxidants that might slow down or perhaps prevent disease progression. Gingko is part of a botanical treatment plan consisting of several other herbals (lemon balm, tumeric, sage, rosemary) and other dietary modifications recommended by herbalists to slow or delay the progression of Alzheimer's disease (Abascal, 2005b). Random controlled trials of gingko and four standard cholinesterase inhibitors showed no difference in therapeutic effects (McEnany, 2001b).

At least one trial has demonstrated improvement in depression when gingko was used to augment antidepressant therapy in medication-refractory patients (Wong et al, 1998). Ginkgo has also been used as an antidote to treat erectile dysfunction caused by antidepressants. Ginkgo helps modulate vascular tone and decreases thrombosis by antagonizing the platelet-activating factor; it might increase the effects of anticoagulants and should be used with caution in patients with potential bleeding problems, such as peptic ulcer disease (Folks and Gabel, 2001; Skidmore-Roth, 2001). Of particular concern with regard to inter-actions is the fact that elderly patients are often on multiple drugs, raising the risk of an interaction if they are also taking gingko. For example, gingko interacts with several psychotropic drugs, aspirin, ibuprofen, some antihypertensives, and cardiovas-cular drugs (Bressler, 2005). Pharmacologic side effects, caused by an increased release of catechol-amines, include headache, anxiety, and restlessness (Skidmore-Roth, 2001).

In summary, gingko has shown promise in treat-ing dementia and in improving memory, circula-tory impairment, and a number of other conditions. However, the results are inconclusive and close monitoring is required for patients on other medi-cations because of the potential for interaction.

## HERBALS THAT MIGHT CAUSE PROBLEMS FOR PSYCHIATRIC PATIENTS

- Ginseng can exacerbate mania and precipitate acute anxiety and insomnia.
- Evening primrose can exacerbate mania.
- Ephedra can cause nervousness, irritability, and insomnia.
- Yohimbine (often taken for its ability to stimu-late sexual excitation) can cause nervousness, irritability, and insomnia.
- Reports have suggested that severe extrapyra-midal symptoms have been seen after heavy betel nut consumption in patients on neuro-leptics (Ayd, 2000).
- Herbals are known to interact with certain drugs and raise a concern for patients taking drugs with a narrow therapeutic window, such as TCAs and lithium (Hatcher, 2001).

### CLINICAL EXAMPLE

Thomas J. is a 76-year-old African-American man who has been on maintenance doses of Coumadin after open heart surgery 6 months ago. Thomas was admitted to the general medical unit with an abnormal prothrombin time. When assessing his medication adherence practices, Thomas tells the nurse practitioner that he takes gingko for his memory. The treatment team was able to make appropriate dose adjustments for the Coumadin and further evaluated his complaints about his memory.

## VITAMINS, MINERALS, AND NUTRITIONAL SUPPLEMENT THERAPIES

### Melatonin

Several studies have demonstrated the efficacy of melatonin in reducing sleep onset latency and the number of nocturnal awakenings. Some promising studies have been conducted on the use of mela-tonin in resynchronizing the biological clock and preventing what has been called *ICU syndrome* (i.e., delirium, psychosis) (Arendt, 2005; McEnany, 2001a).

Some have attributed many problems to an excessive, almost phobic, avoidance of the sun, an extreme no more helpful than overexposure (Horowitz, 2004). Sunlight is essential for the body's production of vitamin D and also affects levels of melatonin, which are important for regu-lating circadian rhythms. Seasonal affective disor-der (SAD), thought to be related to altered sunlight and melatonin levels, has been effectively treated by sunlight or full-spectrum lighting. Melatonin might have some role in the treatment of SAD as well as sleep disorders (Arendt, 2005).

### Vitamin E

A meta-analaysis published in 2005 concluded that there was little evidence of benefit and even some suggestion of harm for patients using vitamin E for protective effects (Miller et al, 2005). This led many concerned consumers to wonder whether they should discontinue this practice. Proponents of vitamin E argue that the meta-analysis failed to distinguish between natural and synthetic forms of vitamin E and also failed to control for medica-tions and chronic diseases (Yale, 2005). Such con-fusing mixed results exemplify one way in which consumers have come to mistrust the health care system. It appears that this particular study received premature publicity in the absence of planned counseling and interpretation of results for consumers. Vitamin E is frequently recommended for patients with tardive dyskinesia and is often recommended for allaying the development of dementia.

## Vitamin C

Although neither vitamin C nor E alone shows a protective benefit in preventing Alzheimer's disease, there might be a synergistic effect if the two are taken together (Zandi and Anthony, 2004).

## Folate, Niacin, Pyridoxine, and Zinc

A number of psychiatric disorders have been associated with vitamin and mineral deficiencies. For example, folic acid deficiency is commonly found in patients with mood disorders, vitamin B deficiency (particularly niacin and pyroxidine) has been associated with anxiety, and zinc deficiency is linked to attention-deficit/hyperactivity disorder (Coppen and Bolander-Gouaille, 2005; Meletis and Barker, 2004; Sachdev et al, 2005; Tiemeier et al, 2003).

## Omega-3 Fatty Acids

The interest in essential fatty acids (EFAs) began when the observation was made that people living in areas where fish constitutes a large portion of their diet have a lower incidence of disease. Omega-3 and omega-6 EFAs have now been well established as essential for normal functioning of the nervous system. Research has shown that the ratio of these EFAs is important for proper neurotransmitter function and other brain neuronal activity. Although the exact ratio has not been agreed on, it is generally accepted that a typical Western diet contains far greater amounts of omega-6 EFAs and smaller amounts of omega-3 EFAs, thus disrupting the balance considered optimal for neuronal and brain function. Apparently, omega-6 EFAs, in the absence of at least an equivalent amount of omega-3 EFAs, can promote an inflammatory response, with oxidative damage to cell membranes, thereby increasing the likelihood of several diseases. The FDA has already endorsed fish oil supplementation, a source of omega-3 EFAs, for its cardiovascular benefits (U.S. Food and Drug Administration, 2004).

Problems with lipid metabolism have been suggested in both bipolar disorder and schizophrenia (Cronin, 2004). Clinical studies with psychiatric patients have shown decreased levels of omega-3 EFAs and some improvement in symptoms with supplementation (Harris et al, 2004). Early results from a few trials have also suggested a positive effect of omega-3 fatty acids over placebo for clinical outcomes in patients with schizophrenia (Fenton et al, 2001; Joy et al, 2000, 2003). The benefit of this type of supplementation in patients with schizophrenia continues to be promising (Meletis and Barker, 2004). Patients with subacute mania treated with omega-3 fatty acids had significantly longer periods of remission compared with a placebo group (Stoll et al, 1999). Beneficial effects for depression and schizophrenia have also been observed (Stoll, 2001). Some studies failed to find a significant improvement with supplemental fish oil compared with antidepressant therapy alone (Silvers et al, 2005).

The psychiatric conditions of attention-deficit/hyperactivity disorder and borderline personality disorder, as well as the phenomena of deliberate self-harm and violence, have been ameliorated by the supplementation of EFAs in a number of recent clinical trials (Hallahan and Garland, 2004). Also, what these disorders share in common is impulsivity, a behavior known to be associated with low cerebrospinal levels of serotonin. Supplementation with fish oil, which is high in omega-3 fatty acids, is thought to increase available serotonin and reduce impulsivity, particularly aggression (Hallahan and Garland, 2004).

## MIND-BODY-BASED THERAPIES

Mind-body medicine is another category of CAM therapies that focuses on the relationship between mind and body and the many ways in which emotions, thoughts, and beliefs influence the endocrine and immune system to affect health directly (NCCAM, 2005). Some examples of mind-body therapies are meditation, yoga, spiritual practices, and massage therapy.

Research has shown some support for mind-body therapies for specific physical problems, stress-related conditions, and anxiety (Wolsko et al, 2004). Central to the concept of mind-body therapies is healing intention. According to this view, the health care practitioner must possess a compassionate, warm, and accepting attitude to elicit the healing process. Mindfulness requires the ability to experience the moment with complete presence. Some would refer to this as being in the moment, or the now. Such presence and focus are essential for treatment (Schmidt, 2004). Meditation, yoga, and spiritual practices and guided imagery and visualization have proven effective.

## MEDITATION, YOGA, AND SPIRITUAL PRACTICES

Several studies have been conducted over the last several decades on the beneficial effects of meditation for psychiatric conditions. One apparent effect is a modulation of sympathetic tone, suggesting increased resilience to daily stresses (Infante et al, 2001). In a study of practitioners of transcendental meditation, catecholamine levels were found to be significantly lower compared with those in control groups. Normally, catecholamine levels follow a circadian rhythm, with increased levels during the morning followed by gradual decrease through the day. Infante and colleagues have suggested that a lack of rhythmic changes in catecholamine levels in these practitioners represents a lowered hormonal response to daily stress. They also demonstrated significantly higher levels of melatonin following meditation. Numerous positive health benefits have been attributed to melatonin's functions, such as maintenance of biologic rhythms, augmentation of the immune system, and antiaging, anticancer, and antistress effects (Tooley et al, 2000). Other studies have found a potential use of meditation for anxiety disorders (Kabat-Zinn et al, 1992; Miller et al, 1995).

Yoga is a particular type of meditative practice that includes controlled breathing, and positioning of the body into various poses. Yoga comes from Hindu and Buddhist traditions and emphasizes both meditation and relaxation. One small pilot study ($N = 5$) showed a 71% reduction in obsessive-compulsive disorder (OCD) symptoms for subjects practicing yoga (Shannahoff-Khalsa and Beckett, 1996). Five patients were well stabilized on fluoxetine (Prozac) before the study, three stopped medication after 7 months or less, and two experienced significantly reduced symp-

### CASE STUDY

Herbie Plant is a 29-year-old Caucasian male who presents for help with severe anxiety. Herbie says that he cannot concentrate at work and has been late on several occasions. Car travel to work has become a problem since Herbie had a panic attack while driving on a crowded freeway. He reports being so anxious around co-workers that they end up distancing themselves from him. Herbie reports having had mild problems with anxiety off and on through his school-age years but reports it usually dissipated. He is particularly concerned because his relationship with his girlfriend has been affected due to his constant worry that he is "losing his mind."

Herbie looks mildly anxious. Although he reports being despondent at times because of his problems, he does not believe that he is depressed. Herbie requests reassurance frequently, and although he is taking an antianxiety medication, he prefers not to take any medication. Screening lab studies were within normal limits as were thyroid function studies. A baseline electrocardiogram was also within normal limits, and the physical exam was unremarkable except as noted above. The urine drug screen was negative for cocaine, amphetamines, opioids, marijuana, barbiturates, and benzodiazepines. The *DSM-IV-TR* diagnosis is Panic Disorder Without Agoraphobia. His current treatment plan includes lorazepam as needed and cognitive behavioral therapy. Though Herbie admits to some improvement, he is seeking complementary strategies to achieve greater symptom relief.

toms. A follow-up randomized control trial was conducted on a larger number of subjects ($N = 22$) comparing a particular type of yoga (Kundalini) to meditation with a relaxation focus (Shannahoff-Khalsa, 2004). Those using the Kundalini technique showed significantly more improvement. The technique (described in detail in the report) is said to be specific for patients with OCD (Shannahoff-Khalsa, 2004). Yoga is also effective for general anxiety and for improving mood in a group of psychiatric inpatients, according to some researchers (Lavey et al, 2005). It is important that research studies explain the particular technique because there are a number of different forms of yoga.

Similar to meditative practices are spiritual therapies. The primary spiritual therapy used as an alternative or complementary health care practice is prayer. When used for health concerns, prayer is considered an alternative health practice. Studies suggest that African Americans and women, in

# Care Plan

**Name:** Herbie Plant

**Admission Date:** _____

*DSM-IV-TR* Diagnosis: Panic disorder without agoraphobia

| | |
|---|---|
| Assessment | **Areas of strength:** Highly motivated to try anything perceived as helpful; has a supportive girlfriend; lives near a church that offers meditation and yoga classes for a nominal fee. |
| | **Problems:** Extremely high anxiety level; prone to impulsiveness; trouble driving to work; very dependent on girlfriend to take over tasks and errands when he is extremely anxious. |
| Diagnoses | • Ineffective coping related to high anxiety level and impulsivity |
| | • Strained relationship with girlfriend related to dependency |
| | • Anticipatory fear related to panic attacks while driving |

Outcomes

*Short-term goals:*                                                                     *Date met*

• Patient will attend yoga and meditation classes three times
per week.                                                                             _____

• Patient will work with cognitive-behavioral nurse therapist three
times per week for six weeks. Patient will complete homework          _____
assignments in self-help workbooks selected by patient from
therapist's library.

*Long-term goals:*

• Patient will be able to drive self to work.                                  _____

• Patient will maintain an anxiety self-care plan with yoga and
meditation or self-help exercises.                                             _____

• Patient will be able to manage his own personal tasks and
errands.                                                                              _____

| | |
|---|---|
| Planning/ Interventions | **Nurse-patient relationship:** Encourage independent behaviors; assist patient to a lower level of anxiety and encourage anxiety reduction activities; discuss impact of anxiety and dependency on relationship with girlfriend; assist in developing a plan for returning to driving; provide teaching on anxiety, panic, and different treatment approaches shown to be effective, such as meditation, cognitive-behavioral therapy, and alternative and complementary therapies. |
| | **Psychopharmacology:** Patient will consider a selective serotonin reuptake inhibitor if medication supplementation is necessary. |
| | **Milieu management:** Provide soft relaxation music in the waiting area; arrange waiting room so that patient can have privacy if desired. |
| Evaluation | Patient will have remission of panic attacks. |
| Referrals | Patient will see B. Kalm, APRN, BC, three times per week; patient and girlfriend will see RN in physician's office for teaching session and monitoring of progress; patient to attend yoga and meditation sessions at church. |

particular, are more likely to rely on community supports, particularly the church (Seniors Use Prayer to Cope with Stress, 2000). Studies have indicated that although only 10% of people using prayer discuss it with their physicians, the majority would like to do so, especially if going through end-of-life care (McCaffrey et al, 2004). There is some indication that physicians make an effort to respect the patient's religious views but admit great difficulty when their belief system differs fundamentally from the patient's belief system (Curlin et al, 2005).

## MASSAGE THERAPY

Massage therapy is defined as manual manipulation of soft tissue, with the intent to promote well-being (Moyer et al, 2004). Studies have revealed an immediate positive effect on the subjective sense of well-being after a single session of massage therapy (Moyer et al, 2004). Although research has been confounded with methodologic problems, particularly in terms of being able to replicate them, studies have begun to appear in the literature about the effect of massage therapy on mental health–related problems. One study documented improvement in mood after a treatment period of 5 days in adolescents with adjustment disorder and depression. The treatment duration and sample size were insufficient to draw conclusions beyond this limited period (Ernst, 2004). A meta-analysis of massage therapy studies revealed the greatest effect to be an overall increase in mood and decrease in anxiety with a course of several sessions. Benefits of massage for depression and anxiety were similar to the benefits revealed in meta-analysis studies of psychotherapy sessions (Moyer et al, 2004). Research has documented a measurable reduction in elevated stress hormones (e.g., epinephrine, norepinephrine, and cortisol) as well as an increase in dopamine and serotonin, all of which are thought to enhance mood. Overall, significant findings have emerged to suggest massage therapy as an effective intervention for patients with depressive or anxiety disorders (Moyer et al, 2004).

There has even been some indication that massage used adjunctively with alcohol detoxification medication protocols shows promise in reducing some of the sympathetic nervous system overactivity associated with alcohol withdrawal (Reader et al, 2005). Hospitals with integrative medicine departments are starting to incorporate massage therapy into these programs (Schlossberg, 2005a,b).

Understandably, there might be a concern about the effect of touching patients' bodies, particularly in a psychiatric setting; however, this is an issue that is part of a massage therapist's training and education, which includes clear guidelines regarding boundaries and professional ethics. It should be noted that the massage that one might get in a massage parlor or even at some spa resorts might not be therapeutic massage. Therapeutic massage therapists generally have graduated from an accredited school and carry credentials such as RMT and have a license or evidence of certification or registration (Anonymous, 2005).

## GUIDED IMAGERY AND VISUALIZATION

Guided imagery and visualization are also important aspects of mind-body medicine and go hand in hand with meditative practices. These techniques, whereby patients are assisted in using imagery and their imagination to visualize desired results, have been successfully used as part of cognitive-behavioral interventions to alter negative thought processes, as well as to improve immune response. Health care practitioners in oncology are generally well aware of how these types of mind-based therapies can influence the patient's treatment response.

## WHOLE MEDICAL SYSTEMS

Medical systems of care that are more than single therapies and involve a system of beliefs that are alternative to those of conventional medicine are called *whole medical systems*. The particular therapies used are part of an overall system of care. Examples of whole systems of care in the United States include traditional Chinese medicine (TCM), homeopathic medicine, and naturopathy. By no means is this a comprehensive list of all the whole medical systems that are alternatives to conventional Western medicine.

## TRADITIONAL CHINESE MEDICINE

TCM is a completely different way of approaching health and illness than that used in Western medicine. The TCM approach with the most scientific support is acupuncture. It is important to note that acupuncture is only one element of a larger system known as TCM.

### CRITICAL THINKING QUESTION    1

If asked to make recommendations about alternative therapies, what criteria should be used in making any recommendations or giving advice? What would you tell someone about alternative therapies? What cautions would you advise about alternative therapies?

## ACUPUNCTURE

Acupuncture is one of the most thoroughly researched and documented alternative practices. Many conventional therapies have not been as thoroughly studied as acupuncture. In its original form, acupuncture was based on the principle that the workings of the human body are controlled by a vital force or energy called Qi (pronounced "chee"), which circulates between the organs along channels called meridians. Acupuncture points are located along meridians and fine needles are inserted through the skin and left in position briefly, sometimes with manual or electrical stimulation. Acupuncture is only one means of altering the flow of Qi in TCM. Acupuncture needles are extremely fine and do not hurt in the same way as, for example, the needles used for an injection (Acupuncture: NIH Consensus Conference Statement [ANCCS], 1997).

Acupuncture has been used successfully for a variety of conditions (Vickers and Zollman, 1999). Several studies have demonstrated the effectiveness of acupuncture for major depression.

Clinical research suggests acupuncture to be equivalent to amitriptyline (Elavil) when measuring treatment effects and rates of recurrence of depression (Ernst, 1998; Luo et al, 1998). Acupuncture might be especially useful for patients who are unable to tolerate the anticholinergic side effects of TCAs. Patients with mild to moderate depression respond well to acupuncture, and efforts are underway to develop a specific acupuncture protocol for treating depression (Macpherson et al, 2004).

Acupuncture is also useful as a complementary therapy in the treatment of substance abuse. Outpatient acupuncture patients were less likely to be readmitted for relapse when compared with those in residential detoxification programs 6 months after treatment (Shwartz et al, 1999). A 1997 consensus panel for the NIH composed of 25 expert presenters and 12 panel members evaluated the available literature on the efficacy of acupuncture for various conditions. The panel concluded that sufficient evidence existed to support its endorsement as a complementary therapy for drug addiction (ANCCS, 1997). Treatment success is apparently dependent on correct needle placement. The correct method of needle placement is referred to in TCM as the *five-point system* and has been carefully outlined by the National Acupuncture Detoxification Association (D'Alberto, 2004).

Although there have been reports of serious adverse events associated with acupuncture, such as pneumothorax, hepatitis, and other infections, these side effects are believed to be a result of poor technique by untrained acupuncturists. Side effects and risks associated with acupuncture are rare but might include contact dermatitis, pain in the puncture region, ecchymosis with or without pain, malaise, transient hypotension, forgotten needles, minor hemorrhage, or aggravation of the initial complaint (Yamashita et al, 1998).

Not surprisingly, Western medicine is not satisfied with the explanation of acupuncture's mechanism of action (i.e., restoring Qi). The search for more scientific explanations does suggest an alteration in neurotransmitters, neurohormonal mechanisms, and blood flow. Additional evidence substantiates an alteration of the sensory pathways affecting functions in the brain and the periphery (ANCCS, 1997). Acupuncturists are willing and interested in participating in research, particularly if they are permitted to have input into the research or if the research question is one that is particularly relevant to public opinion (Fitter and Thomas, 2005). Overall, as one part of the system of TCM, acupuncture has been accepted by many consumers and by conventional medical practitioners as a viable alternative or complementary therapy for a number of conditions.

| CRITICAL THINKING QUESTION | 2 |
|---|---|

Acupuncture, which has traditionally been considered an alternative therapy, is now widely used by many people; several studies have supported its use for certain conditions. At what point does an alternative therapy become a conventional therapy?

## NATUROPATHIC AND HOMEOPATHIC REMEDIES FOR AFFECTIVE AND ANXIETY DISORDERS

Naturopathy encompasses many natural healing practices, including herbal and homeopathic preparations, nutritional counseling, and light therapy. Naturopathy falls under the NCAAM alternative therapy category of whole medical systems. A naturopathic doctor (ND) is licensed to practice naturopathic healing methods, including the prescribing of homeopathic remedies.

Homeopathy is a system of care that attempts to stimulate the body to heal itself. Symptoms are believed to represent the body's attempt to restore itself to health; thus, a homeopath will use a remedy to stimulate the body to move in the direction it is already going. For example, instead of trying to stop a cough with suppressants, as conventional medicine does, a homeopath will give a remedy that would cause a cough in a healthy person and thus stimulate the ill body to restore itself.

In conventional therapy, the goal is control of the illness through regular use of medical substances. Homeopathy's aim is the complete restoration of health. Symptoms are not seen as something wrong that must be corrected but rather as signs of the way in which the body is attempting to help itself. Although Hippocrates first postulated this principle of "likes curing like," Samuel Hahnemann established the first practical application in 1796 (National Center for Homeopathy, 2001).

The exact nature of symptoms is important because even slightly different symptoms require different homeopathic treatments. Any substance might be considered a homeopathic medicine if it has known effects that mimic the symptoms, syndromes, or conditions that it is administered to treat and is manufactured according to the specifications of the *Homeopathic Pharmacopoeia of the United States* (HPUS; National Center for Homeopathy [NCH], 2001). In some sense, it is like giving an immunization; a minute amount of a virus is used to encourage the body's immune system to respond. In the case of homeopathic medicine, the medicine is given to encourage the body's response, most often to an existing problem.

The HPUS is a standard reference text detailing the sources, composition, and preparation of the homeopathic drugs, which are prescribed on the basis of the "law of similars." An example of a homeopathic drug is aconite or wolf's bane, prescribed when symptoms come on suddenly, especially if exposure to cold might be a causative factor (NCH, 2001).

Few studies on homeopathic remedies for psychiatric symptoms have been done. One small study ($N = 12$) suggested the possible usefulness of homeopathy in the treatment of affective and anxiety disorders in patients with mild to severe symptomatic conditions (Davidson et al, 1997). A reduction in test anxiety has been reported with a homeopathic solution known as *Argentum nitricum;* however, the result could not be replicated in a subsequent trial by other researchers (Baker et al, 2003).

In general, research on homeopathic remedies has been difficult because of problems of replication. Of all the alternative therapies, Western medicine reserves its greatest skepticism for homeopathy. Although homeopathy has little support in the literature, it has an extremely strong following and is fiercely defended by those who believe in its capacity to heal (Bauer, 2005).

## GENERAL CONCERNS REGARDING CAM THERAPIES

## ISSUES OF SAFETY AND EFFICACY OF HERBALS

The method of manufacture of herbals determines the potency of an herb. Herbal concentration and dose potency are highly dependent on several factors, for which there can be great variability (St. John's Wort and the Treatment of Depression). Although the American Herbal Association and the American Botanical Council have attempted to regulate safety, there is currently no guarantee of purity or standardization of herbal products. A *Los Angeles Times* survey indicated that three of ten herbal products contained only half the potency listed on the product label (Beaubrun and Gray, 2000; Hatcher, 2001; Snyder and Lindquist, 2001).

Although safety and purity of herbal preparations should certainly be standardized for consistency, one has only to watch television or see biilboards along the highway advertising FDA-approved medicines that have been recalled, removed from the market, or studied with excess industry bias. Some clearly believe that there are inconsistent standards applied to herbals (Kirsch, 2003). Strong feelings abound regarding the need for conventional medicine to have control of herbal medicines; for example, Agins and Lehne (2004) have emphatically stated,

> It's time for the scientific community to stop giving alternative therapy a free ride. There cannot be two kinds of medicine—conventional and alternative.

There is only medicine that has been adequately tested and medicine that may or may not work . . . If it is found to be reasonably safe and effective, it will be accepted. (p. 1139)

It might be useful to remember that it was the medical community that rejected these remedies in the first place and, whether or not medical practitioners believe them useful, people will take them anyway. Apparently, the solution to this threat is regulation. Ironically, a lack of control and a feeling of powerlessness is what led many consumers to look outside conventional medicine in the first place. Previously grandfathered in the DSHEA, the use of herbs is now threatened by efforts to restrict the sale of herbs as part of consumer safety. Referred to as the CODEX rules, these rules represent an international effort to restrict health claims for herbals and would require a physician's prescription, thus defeating one of the primary reasons why people turn to herbals. Interestingly, there is no recommendation that the prescribing of herbals be left to certified herbalists or NDs. There is a fine line between the rights of individuals and responsibilities of the government. Since herbs have become popular and profitable, some regulation may be necessary for consumer safety. Standardization of doses enables greater consistency by people self-administering herbals.

Another potential problem includes findings that many people using alternative remedies are doing so without any type of supervision (Eisenberg et al, 1998). Potentially, this self-medicating might lead to a dangerous delay in seeking more efficacious care. For example, if the treatment does not work, the patient might become more symptomatic during the trial of herbals and become less able to seek other medical care. Anxiety is a good example. Overreliance on herbals can present some of the same problems as benzodiazepine dependence and/or abuse. Delaying more effective treatments such as cognitive-behavioral psychotherapy might make it more difficult to achieve the maximum benefit offered by this approach. Patients using both conventional and alternative medicines without informing their physician place themselves at risk for herb-drug interaction, over- or undermedication, and difficulty in appropriate management of their health. Nondisclosure, as opposed to talking about one's values and beliefs with their health care provider, interferes with a collaborative relationship between patient and health care provider. Box 40-2 pro-

## Box 40-2  General Precautions for Consumers and Health Care Professionals Regarding Herbals

- Avoid products with multiple herbs. Check the active and inactive ingredients for possible combinations and additives.
- Avoid imported herbs because of differences in dose effects.
- Buy only from reputable, established companies and with the *United States Pharmacopoeia* (USP) seal of approval.
- Always inform health care provider of any use of herbal products, including topicals.
- Discontinue if any unusual side effects occur and report adverse reactions to Medwatch at 1-800-332-1088.
- Avoid herbals during pregnancy, when attempting to get pregnant, and during breast-feeding.
- Avoid self-medicating with herbals before a medical illness has been ruled out.

vides a summary of general precautions regarding herbals.

## CRITICAL THINKING QUESTION  3

What are the implications of patients self-medicating with alternative therapies? Are there any dangers? What are the possible benefits?

## COMPETENCE OF PRACTITIONERS

Training and credentialing of practitioners are important. There are opportunities, without regulation, for tremendous variation in the preparation and expertise of practitioners. Regulatory requirements vary from state to state and not all states require licensure or even certification. Most states, but not all, require the practitioner to register their practice with the government. Box 40-3 lists helpful questions to ask alternative care practitioners. The best-regulated alternative therapies are acupuncture and naturopathy.

## CRITICAL THINKING QUESTION  4

If alternative care practitioners cannot practice medicine, how is it that medical doctors can practice alternative care?

## ACUPUNCTURE

Acupuncture is regulated by practice acts in 26 states. States not having practice acts limit the practice of acupuncture to designated medical providers or require medical supervision. Acupuncturists are held to the same standard of care as licensed physicians (Sale, 2001). Professional acupuncturists train for up to 4 years full time and might acquire university degrees on completion of their training. Some acupuncturists have also completed training in the principles and practice of Chinese herbalism. Accredited acupuncture courses include conventional anatomy, physiology, pathology, and diagnosis. A national credentialing agency, the National Commission for Certification of Acupuncturists, provides examinations for entry-level practice. This agency also serves as a disciplinary and grievance board, giving consumers an avenue for holding practitioners accountable.

## NATUROPATHY

Great variation also exists among naturopathic practitioners (Boon et al, 2004). Most definitions of what constitutes naturopathic practice place emphasis on the use of natural substances or methods that stimulate the body's natural capacity for healing. Naturopathic practice might include a variety of therapies, and naturopaths often prescribe homeopathic and herbal remedies. Wide arrays of natural therapies are usually included under the scope of practice for naturopathy. In the United States, several universities offer the naturopathic doctorate. One of the first was Bastyr University in Seattle. In 1994, Bastyr University achieved recognition when a research center for HIV/AIDS was established there. A government-funded clinic for the underserved marked one of several other areas in which NDs were gaining the respect of government agencies (Pizzorno, 2005). It should be noted that several correspondence schools also offer the naturopathic doctorate. Many health care professionals do not view university and correspondence programs as equivalent.

NDs are licensed to practice in 12 states. States without licensing might still have practitioners that practice under another professional license. Some states prohibit the practice of naturopathy, except by physicians (Sale, 2001). Legally, practitioners are accountable under the law and could be sued for practicing outside the scope of their practice.

## HOMEOPATHY

Practice acts exist in some states, requiring licensure to practice homeopathy (Sale, 2001). The legal system expects a practitioner to make and document referrals for serious conditions. Practitioners might encourage patients to inform their health care provider of their homeopathic therapy.

In some other countries, physicians are trained in the methods considered mainstream in that country but, when they emigrate to the United States, they are not legally permitted to practice their native medicine. Some foreign-trained practitioners have concerns with the way in which their therapies are integrated into Western medical practice, recognizing a risk of losing time-honored traditions (Mason, 2004).

In the United Kingdom, the Health Professions Council regulates more than 13 independent professions and it is expected that more will join these ranks, including a Complementary Alternative Therapy Council (Stone, 2005). Washington was the first state to require the integration of a full range of CAM providers, including chiropractors, naturopathic physicians, acupuncturists, and massage practitioners, into commercial health insurance coverage (Watts et al, 2004). Although some hospitals have begun the process of integrating CAM therapies into their menu of services for patients, the regulatory requirements, credentialing, and scope of practice are not by any means uniform, suggesting that a number of issues still need to be resolved (Cohen et al, 2005a). It is recommended that greater uniformity in definitions, standardization of licensure requirements and practices, and more centers for interdisciplinary training will enhance the research and development of an integrated health care system (Cohen et al, 2005a,b).

## NURSES AND ALTERNATIVE THERAPIES

Many nurses have pursued education, specialized training, or additional certification to enable them to administer alternative therapies (Frisch, 2001a, b; Snyder and Lindquist, 2001). The American Holistic Nurses Association (AHNA) offers certification in holistic nursing, whereby a nurse can become a certified holistic nurse (HNC). The HNC designation implies that the registered nurse meets competency standards for integrating the CAM into their own self-care and the care of their patients. The AHNA requires completion of an examination and adherence to standards of practice. The AHNA admits that the HNC designation has more to do with the attitude of the practitioner than with specific techniques (American Holistic Nurses Association, 2002). Similar to all certifications, the HNC designation is recognition of excellence in a particular area. Many HNC nurses use CAM therapies in their daily practice. It is generally recommended that nurses using CAM therapies in practice adhere to agency policy, pursue a nursing outcome, and document within a nursing context (Frisch, 2001).

## FUTURE DIRECTIONS OF INTEGRATIVE HEALTH CARE

As conventional health care has advanced technologically and diagnostically, it makes sense that a focus be shifted to the biologic aspects of health. Western medicine has been called "broken" by some and amazingly "miraculous" by others. One thing is clear: the public wants the opportunity to be empowered in their health care. Three decades of research have revealed that the mind-body connection is a powerful one. There is a call for all health care practitioners to incorporate the core concepts of CAM therapies into the care of patients. The health care practitioner in a newly evolving health care system must have interpersonal competencies that promote respect, empathy, and concern for the patient they are treating (Gilbert, 2003).

The term *integrative health care* connotes blending the best practices from both conventional and alternative medicine. Health care practitioners are entering the health care environment at one of the most opportune moments in the history of medicine. Conventional health care has become a comprehensive science, with the capability to diagnose all types of disease states of the body and mind. Barrett and colleagues (2003) have noted that the definition of health adopted by the World Health Organization, "a state of complete physical, mental and social well-being," is not easily reconciled with the general disease-treating framework of conventional medicine. At the same time, some alternative health care practitioners can provide such an excellent healing environment that a treatment effect occurs, independent of the curative method used. The move toward alternative therapies is a natural occurrence in a system of health care that has become fragmented and focused on cost, disease, and overreliance on medication. A combined approach offers the patient the absolute best in world health care.

The direction of alternative, complementary, or integrative medicine depends greatly on economic and political powers (Barrett et al, 2003). Some health care practitioners are vehemently opposed to the alternative and complementary health movement. Ernst and colleagues (2004) have called for an open mind in regard to CAM therapies, pointing out that dissenters often are using circular reasoning—that is, alternative therapies are considered a waste of research funds because there is no scientific proof of their efficacy. Consumer empowerment and choice can be a threatening concept for health care practitioners used to a more authoritative approach.

The alternative health care movement has implications for psychiatry. Whereas once little was known about biologic markers for mental illness, much is now known. Research has revealed a plethora of knowledge about neurotransmitters, hormonal influences, and structural abnormalities of the brain. Intrapsychic and environmental influences on this system were ignored along the way to our current state of focusing almost exclusively on the biologic aspects of mental illness (Riedel-Heller et al, 2005).

### Norm's Notes

*The use of alternative and complementary therapies is widespread and still growing. Traditional medicine has not been able to meet the needs of a public that believes good health is a right. The statistical table of mental disorder prevalence in Chapter 1 and in all psychopathology chapters reflects data that have not changed much for about 30 years. However, during that time, many new and supposedly wonderful medications have been discovered. The conventional psychotropic drug industry is a multibillion dollar concern, but the actual number of people with a drug-treatable disorder has increased. Consequently, many Americans now look outside the traditional psychiatric drug manufacturing complex to see whether they can "fix" themselves. In brief, the alternative and complementary approach to mental health care derives, in part, from this disillusionment and disappointment.*

The values of alternative and naturopathic medicine run the risk of falling prey to the same ills afflicting conventional medicine if conflict over its use becomes too intense. When considering alternative therapies, it is important to keep an open mind—remember that some are helpful, some cause harm, and some, although harmless, probably offer no more than a placebo effect. The alternative therapy movement holds a valuable lesson if we can learn it: patients want to be treated holistically. If, instead of learning this lesson, medicine (and nursing) determines how to profit from controlling a patient's access to alternative treatments, the opportunity to defragment the health care system will be lost. Many consider integrative medicine both an opportunity to transform medicine and a sign that the next major transformation is unfolding before us. Hopefully, we will listen to this message and respond.

***Note to students:*** *One thing that has likely been crossing your mind as you read this chapter is that the very definition of what is alternative is itself quite controversial. By the strictest definition, anything that is not considered mainstream medicine with approved indications would be considered alternative. Whether something is considered alternative or complementary depends* on the purpose of the treatment and who is recommending the treatment. Furthermore, what is alternative at the moment might be mainstream in the near future (Astin, 1998; Frisch, 2001).

| CRITICAL THINKING QUESTION | 5 |
|---|---|

What do you think about patients taking health into their own hands and engaging in practices that have not been proven by the scientific method and endorsed by the medical community?

### Study Notes

1. Alternative therapies are therapies that are used instead of mainstream medicine; complementary therapies are those outside mainstream medicine that are used along with traditional medical therapies.
2. Increasing numbers of patients are using alternative or complementary therapies. The public is clearly becoming more receptive to alternative treatments.
3. Alternative health practices have been around for centuries but lost favor with the disease-based scientific model of care. A renewed interest in alternative health practices has emerged as dissatisfaction with our current system of care has grown.
4. The NIH has created an office of complementary and alternative medicine, initially called the OAM and recently renamed as NCCAM.
5. The FDA does not regulate herbal products but does require labeling that indicates lack of proven efficacy and quality control standards.
6. St. John's wort is the most widely used herbal for depression. Studies have generally demonstrated the effectiveness of St. John's wort for mild to moderate depression. It should not be taken with other antidepressants, especially SSRIs, and generally has a high potential for interaction with other drugs. In particular, it might interfere with the protease inhibitors often used for HIV-positive patients.
7. Kava-kava is an herbal anxiolytic without the problems of altered coordination and alertness associated with normal doses of the benzodiazepines. Problems can occur if taken with CNS-acting drugs, and overdose is possi-

ble. Concerns about liver toxicity have decreased but have not eliminated sales in the United States. It is unclear what mechanism is involved in altering liver function in certain individuals.

8. Valerian is an herbal anxiolytic useful for anxiety and insomnia. Withdrawal syndromes similar to benzodiazepine discontinuation can occur. Valerian might increase the effects of other centrally acting drugs and might reduce the effectiveness of anticoagulants and antiseizure drugs.

9. Chamomile and angelica have also been used for anxiety but have fewer supporting studies compared with kava-kava and valerian.

10. Gingko is one of the top selling herbals in the United States and is effective for brain trauma, memory impairment, and cerebral insufficiency. Gingko should not be taken by anyone with a history of bleeding problems.

11. Melatonin has been suggested as possibly useful for ICU syndrome and for sleep.

12. Acupuncture is one of the most thoroughly researched alternative therapies and shows evidence of effectiveness in the treatment of substance abuse when used in conjunction with traditional therapies.

13. Meditation, yoga, and spiritual practices have been found useful for regulating anxiety levels.

14. Omega-3 fatty acids, found in fish oils, have promise for improving clinical outcomes in many conditions, including mania and schizophrenia.

15. Homeopathy, which is a system and philosophy of care using natural remedies to stimulate the body to heal itself, is based on the law of similars, or "like cures like." Approved homeopathic remedies can be found in the HPUS. Scientific studies have been difficult to replicate.

16. Some herbals are known to be problematic for psychiatric patients, particularly evening primrose, ephedra, yohimbine, ginseng, chaste tree, and betel nut.

17. One concern about patients taking herbals without supervision is that patients might delay seeking essential treatment.

18. Health care professionals should routinely question patients about the use of herbals or other alternative therapies. It is essential to examine one's own attitude and manner so that patients feel comfortable disclosing their use.

19. The alternative therapies that are best regulated include acupuncture and homeopathy. States vary greatly in their individual regulation of alternative health care practitioners. The direction that legal and regulatory statutes take will depend on many political and economic factors.

20. Nurses demonstrating the ability to integrate CAM into their clinical practice can be certified through examination and adherence to standards of practice by the American Holistic Nurses Association, with the designation of HNC. Nurses possessing HNC credentials might also have been trained in alternative therapies through special education or credentialing.

21. Nurse and physician education can be expected to include alternative and complementary medicine as part of their core curriculum in the future. The NCCAM offers training grants that as yet have not been fully used by schools, as had originally been hoped.

22. The concept of alternative versus complementary therapy, by definition, changes as the therapy becomes incorporated into mainstream medicine.

23. One way of conceptualizing the alternative and complementary medicine movement is as a paradigm shift, calling for a change in the currently dichotomized and increasingly impersonal system of care in the United States.

## References

Abascal K, Yarnell E: Alzheimer's disease, part 1: biology and botanicals, *J Altern Complem Med* 10:18, 2004a.

Abascal K, Yarnell E: Alzheimer's disease, part 2: a botanical treatment plan, *J Altern Complem Med* 10:67, 2004b.

Abascal K, Yarnell E: Nervine drugs for treating anxiety, *J Altern Complem Med* 10:309, 2004c.

Acupuncture: NIH Consensus Conference Statement [ANCCS], November 3-5, 1997. Available at http://consensus.nih.gov/1997/1997Acupuncture107html.htm. Accessed May 28, 2006.

Agins A, Lehne R: Herbal supplements. In Lehne R: *Pharmacology for nursing care* (pp. 1171-1174), St. Louis, 2003, WB Saunders.

Alpert JE, Papakostas G, Mischoulon D, et al: S-Adenosyl-L-methionine (SAMe) as an adjunct for resistant major depressive disorder: an open trial following partial or nonresponse to selective serotonin reuptake inhibitors or venlafaxine, *Clin Psychopharmacol* 24:661, 2004.

American Holistic Nurses Association: *Certification*. Available at http:www.ahna.org/edu/education.html, 2002; http://www.ahncc.org/pages/1/index.htm. Accessed May 28, 2006.

Anke J, Ramzan I: Kava hepatotoxicity: are we any closer to the truth? *Planta Med* 70:193, 2004a.

Anke J, Ramzan I: Pharmacokinetic and pharmacodynamic drug interactions with kava (*Piper methysticum* Forst. f.), *J Ethnopharmacol* 93:153, 2004b.

Anonymous: Laws and regulations: legislation news, *Massage* July-August (Issue 116):164, 2005.

Arendt J: Melatonin: characteristics, concerns, prospects, *J Biol Rhythms* 20:291, 2005.

Astin JA: Why patients use alternative medicine: results of a national study, *JAMA* 279:1548, 1998.

Ayd F: Evaluating interactions between herbal and psychoactive medications, *Psychiatr Times* 17:45, 2000.

Baker D, Myers SP, Howden I, Brooks L: The effects of homeopathic *Argentum nitricum* on test anxiety, *Complem Ther Med* 11:65, 2003.

Barnes P, Powell-Griner E, McFann K, Nahin R: Complementary and alternative medicine use among adults: United States, 2002, *Adv Data* 343:1, 2004.

Barrett B, Marchand L, Scheder J, et al: Themes of holism, empowerment, access, and legitimacy define complementary, alternative, and integrative medicine in relation to conventional biomedicine, *J Altern Complem Med* 9:937, 2003.

Bauer L: Homeopathy: a view from the outside, *J Altern Complem Med* 11:1, 2005.

Beaubrun G, Gray G: A review of herbal medicines for psychiatric disorders, *Psychiatr Serv* 51:1130, 2000.

Boon H, Cherkin D, Erro J, et al: Practice patterns of naturopathic physicians: results from a random survey of licensed practitioners in two U.S. states, *BMC Complem Altern Med* 4:14, 2004.

Bressler R: Herb-drug interactions: interactions between Ginkgo biloba and prescription medications, *Geriatrics* 60:30, 2005.

Bridevauxa I, Salesa A: Erratum to a survey of patients' out-of-pocket payments for complementary and alternative medicine therapies, *Complem Ther Med* 12:144, 2004.

Brown R, Bottiglieri T, Colman C: *Stop depression now: SAM-e: the breakthrough supplement that works as well as prescription drugs in half the time with no side effects,* New York, 1999, GP Putnam Sons.

Cairney S, Maruffi P, Clough A, et al: Saccade and cognitive impairment associated with kava intoxication, *Hum Psychopharmacol Clin Exp* 18:525, 2003.

Clough AR, Bailie RS, Currie B: Liver function test abnormalities in users of aqueous kava extracts, *J Toxicol Clin Toxicol* 41:821, 2003.

Clough AR, Rowley K, O'Dea K: Kava use, dyslipidaemia and biomarkers of dietary quality in aboriginal people in Arnhem Land in the Northern Territory (NT), Australia, *Eur J Clin Nutr* 58:1090, 2004.

Clouatre DL: Kava kava: examining new reports of toxicity, *Toxicol Lett* 150:85, 2004.

Cohen M, Davis R, Schachter S, Eisenberg D: Emerging credentialing practices, malpractice liability policies, and guidelines governing complementary and alternative medical practices and dietary supplement recommendations, *Arch Intern Med* 165:289, 2005a.

Cohen M, Sandler L, Hrbek A, et al: Policies pertaining to complementary and alternative medical therapies in a random sample of 39 academic health centers, *Altern Ther Health Med* 11:36, 2005b.

Commission E Monographs: Introduction. Available at http://www.herbalgram.org/default.asp?c=comission_e. Accessed September 22, 2001.

Coppen A, Bolander-Gouaille C: Treatment of depression: time to consider folic acid and vitamin $B_{12}$, *J Psychopharmacol* 19:59, 2005.

Cronin D: Supporting mental health with polyunsaturated fatty acids, *J Altern Complem Med* 10:95, 2004.

Curlin F, Roach C, Gorawara-Bhat R, et al: When patients choose faith over medicine: physician perspectives on religiously related conflict in the medical encounter, *Arch Intern Med* 165:88, 2005.

Davidson JR Morrison RM, Shore J, et al: Homeopathic treatment of depression and anxiety, *Altern Ther Health Med* 3:46, 1997.

D'Alberto A: Auricular acupuncture in the treatment of crack-cocaine abuse: review of the efficacy, the use of national acupuncture detoxification association protocol and the selection of sham points, *J Altern Complem Med* 10:985, 2004.

*Dietary Supplement Health and Education Act of 1994,* 2005, Available at http://www.cfsan.fda.gov/~dms/dietsup.html. Retrieved June 14, 2006.

Eisenberg D, Davis RB, Ettner SL, et al: Trends in alternative medicine use in the United States, 1990-1997: results of a follow-up national survey, *JAMA* 280:1569, 1998.

Ernst E: The "improbability" of complementary and alternative medicine, *Arch Intern Med* 164:914, 2004.

Ernst E: Harmless herbs? A review of the recent literature, *Am J Med* 104:170, 1998.

Estes JD, Stolpman D, Olyaei A, et al: High prevalence of potentially hepatotoxic herbal supplement use in patients with fulminant hepatic failure. *Arch Surg* 138:852, 2003.

Fenton WS, Dicerson F, Boronow J, et al: A placebo-controlled trial of omega-3 fatty acid (ethyl eicosapentaenoic acid) supplementation for residual symptoms and cognitive impairment in schizophrenia, *Am J Psychiatry* 158:2071, 2001.

Fitter M, Thomas K: Duty, curiosity, and enlightened self-interest: what makes acupuncture practitioners participate in national research studies? Guest editorial/commentary, *J Altern Complem Med* 11:227, 2005.

Folks D, Gabel T: Herbaceuticals in psychiatry. In Keltner N, Folks D, editors: *Psychotropic drugs,* ed 3 (pp. 513-539), St. Louis, 2001, Mosby.

Frisch N: Nursing as a context for alternative/complementary modalities, May 31, 2001, *Online J Issues Nurs* 6(2):Manuscript 2, 2001a. Available at http://www.nursingworld.org/ojin/topic15/tpc15_2.htm. Accessed 2001.

Frisch N: Standards for holistic nursing practice: a way to think about our care that includes complementary and alternative modalities, May 31, 2001, *Online J Issues Nurs* 6:Manuscript 4, 2001b. Available at http://www.nursingworld.org/ojin/topic15/tpc15_4.htm. Accessed 2001.

Gaydos HL: Complementary and alternative therapies in nursing education: trends and issues, May 31, 2001, *Online J Issues Nurs* 6:Manuscript 5, 2001. Available at http://www.nursingworld.org/ojin/topic15/tpc15_5.htm. Accessed 2001.

Gilbert M: Weaving medicine back together: mind-body medicine in the twenty-first century, *J Altern Complem Med* 9:563, 2003.

Glass JR, Sproule BA, Herrmann N, et al: Acute pharmacological effects of temazepam, diphenhydramine, and valerian in healthy elderly subjects, *J Clin Psychopharmacol* 23:260, 2003.

Hallahan B, Garland M: Essential fatty acids and their role in the treatment of impulsivity disorders, *Prostaglandins, Leukotrienes & Essential Fatty Acids* 71:211, 2004.

Hallam KT, Olver JS, McGrath C, Norman TR: Comparative cognitive and psychomotor effects of single doses of *Valeriana officianalis* and triazolam in healthy volunteers, *Hum Psychopharmacology* 18:619, 2003.

Harris J, Hibbeln J, Mackey R, Muldoon M: Statin treatment alters serum n-3 and n-6 fatty acids in hypercholesterolemia patients. *Prostaglandins, Leukotrienes & Essential Fatty Acids* 71:263, 2004.

Hatcher T: The proverbial herb, *Am J Nurs* 101:36, 2001.

Hicks S, Walker A, Gallagher J, et al: The significance of non-significance in randomized controlled studies: a discussion inspired by a double-blinded study on St. John's wort for premenstrual symptoms, *J Altern Complem Med* 10:925, 2004.

Hoblyn JC, Brooks JO: Herbal supplements in older adults. Consider interactions and adverse events that may result from supplement use, *Geriatrics* 60(2):18, 22-23, 2005.

Horowitz S: The brighter aspects of ultraviolet light, *J Altern Complem Med* 10:304, 2004.

Infante JR, Torres-Avisbal M, Pinel P, et al: Catecholamine levels in practitioners of the transcendental meditation technique, *Physiol Behav* 72:141, 2001.

Joy CB, Mumby-Croft R, Joy LA: Polyunsaturated fatty acid supplementation for schizophrenia, *Cochrane Database System Rev* Issue 2:update of CD001257, 2003.

Joy CB, Mumby-Croft R, Joy LA: Polyunsaturated fatty acid (fish or evening primrose oil) for schizophrenia, *Cochrane Database System Rev* Issue 2:CD001257, 2000.

Kabat-Zinn J, Massion AO, Kristeller J, et al: Effectiveness of a meditation-based stress reduction program in the treatment of anxiety disorders, *Am J Psychiatry* 149:936, 1992.

Keiko Honda K, Jacobson J: Use of complementary and alternative medicine among United States adults: the influences of personality, coping strategies, and social support, *Prev Med* 40:46, 2005.

Keltner N, Folks D: Drugs used in alternative and complementary medicine In Keltner N, Folks D, editors: *Psychotropic drugs,* ed 4 (pp. 513-546), St. Louis, 2005, Mosby.

Kessler R, Soukup J, Davis RB, et al: The use of complementary and alternative therapies to treat anxiety and depression in the United States, *Am J Psychiatry* 158:289, 2001.

Kirsch I: St John's wort, conventional medication, and placebo: an egregious double standard, *Complem Ther Med* 11:193, 2003.

Knuppel L, Linde K: Adverse effects of St. John's Wort: a systematic review, *J Clin Psychiatry* 65:1470, 2004.

Lavey R, Sherman T, Mueser K, et al: The effects of yoga on mood in psychiatric inpatients, *Psychiatr Rehabil J* 28:399, 2005.

Linde K, Knuppel L: Large-scale observational studies of hypericum extracts in patients with depressive disorders—a systematic review, *Phytomedicine* 12:148, 2005.

Linde K, Mulrow CD, Berner M, Egger M: St John's wort for depression, *Cochrane Database System Rev* 18(2):CD000448, 2005.

Luo H, Meng F, Jia Y, Zhao X: Clinical research on the therapeutic effect of the electro-acupuncture treatment in patients with depression, *Psychiatry Clin Neurosci* 52(Suppl):S338, 1998.

Macpherson H, Thorpe L, Thomas K, Geddes D: Acupuncture for depression: first steps toward a clinical evaluation, *J Altern Complem Med* 10:1083, 2004.

Malva JO, Santos S, Macedo T: Neuroprotective properties of *Valeriana officinalis* extracts. *Neurotox Res* 6:131, 2004.

Mason R: Naturalizing ACM and its practitioners: an interview with Nathan Waxman, M.A., J.D., *J Altern Complem Ther* 10:271, 2004.

Mattes R, Pawlik M: Effects of Ginkgo biloba on alertness and chemosensory function in healthy adults, *Hum Psychopharmacol Clin Exp* 19:81, 2004.

McCaffrey A, Eisenberg D, Legedza A, et al: Prayer for health concerns: results of a national survey on prevalence and patterns of use, *Arch Intern Med* 164:858, 2004.

McDowell J, Burman M: Complementary and alternative medicine: a qualitative study of beliefs of a small sample of Rocky Mountain area nurses, *Med Surg Nurs* 13:383, 2004.

McEnany G: Herbal psychotropics, part 3: focus on kava, valerian, and melatonin, *J Am Psychiatr Nurs Assoc* 6:126, 2001a.

McEnany G: Herbal psychotropics, part 4: focus on ginkgo biloba, L-carnitine, lactobacillus, acidophilus, and ginger root, *J Am Psychiatr Nurs Assoc* 7:22, 2001b.

Meletis C, Barker J: Mental health not all in the mind—really a matter of cellular biochemistry, *J Altern Complem Med* 10:28, 2004.

Mikhail N, Wali S, Ziment I: Use of alternative medicine among Hispanics, *J Altern Complem Med* 10:851, 2004.

Miller E, Pastor-Barriuso B, Dalal D, et al: Meta-analysis: high-dosage vitamin E supplementation might increase all-cause mortality, *Ann Intern Med* 142:37, 2005.

Miller JJ, Fletcher K, Kabat-Zinn J: Three-year follow-up and clinical implications of a mindfulness meditation-based stress reduction intervention in the treatment of anxiety disorders, *Gen Hosp Psychiatry* 17:192, 1995.

Mills E, Singh R, Ross C, et al: Impact of federal safety advisories on health food store advice, *J Gen Intern Med* 19:269, 2004.

Min L, Chen SW, Li WJ, et al: The effects of angelica essential oil in social interaction and hole-board tests. *Pharmacol Biochem Behav* 81:838, 2005.

Moyer C, Rounds J, Hannum W: A meta-analysis of massage therapy research, *Psychol Bull* 130:3, 2004.

National Center for Complementary and Alternative (NCCAM): Mind-body medicine: an overview. Available at http://nccam.nih.gov/health/backgrounds/mindbody.htm. Accessed August 2, 2005.

National Center for Complementary and Alternative Medicine Fact Sheets: St. John's wort, 2001. Available at http://nccam.nih.gov/fcp/factsheets/stjohnswort/stjohnswort.htm. Accessed September 22, 2001.

National Center for Homeopathy: *Introduction to homeopathy: natural medicine for the twenty-first century.* Available at http://www.homeopathic.org/introduction.htm. Accessed August 20, 2005.

NTP Herbal Medicine Fact Sheet, 2003. Available at http://ntp.niehs.nih.gov/ntp/htdocs/liason/factsheets/HerbMedFacts.pdf. Accessed September 16, 2005.

Parslow R, Jorm A: Individuals prescribed antidepressants or anxiolytics might replace or augment such medications with complementary and alternative medicines (CAMs), *J Affect Disord* 82:77, 2004.

Peters D, Donaldson J, Chaussalet T, et al: Time for a new approach for reporting herbal medicine adverse events? *J Altern Complem Med* 9:607, 2003.

Pizzorno J: Naturopathic medicine—a 10-year perspective (from a 35-year view), *Altern Ther* 11:24, 2005.

Reader M, Young R, Connor J: Massage therapy improves the management of alcohol withdrawal syndrome, *J Altern Complem Med* 11:311, 2005.

Riedel-Heller S, Matschinger H, Angermeyer M: Mental disorders—who and what might help? Help-seeking and treatment preferences of the lay public, *Soc Psychiatry Psychiatr Epidemiol* 40:167, 2005.

Robinson A, McGrail M: Disclosure of CAM use to medical practitioners: a review of qualitative and quantitative studies, *Complem Ther Med* 12:90, 2004.

Sachdev PS, Parslow RA, Lux O, et al: Relationship of homocysteine, folic acid and vitamin B$_{12}$ with depression in a middle-aged community sample, *Psychol Med* 35:529, 2005.

St. John's Wort and the Treatment of Depression, NCCAM Publication No. D005. Available at http://nccam.nih.gov/health/stjohnswort/index.htm. Accessed March 15, 2006.

Sale DM: Overview of legislative development concerning alternative health care in the United States, 2001. Available at http://www.healthy.net/public/legal-lg/regulations/fetzer.htm. Accessed October 20, 2001.

Schlossberg B: Michigan Hospital integrates massage, *Massage* July-August:28, 2005a.

Schlossberg B: Massage boosts mental health services, *Massage* July-August:31, 2005b.

Schmidt S: Mindfulness and healing intention: concepts, practice, and research evaluation, *J Altern Complem Med* 10:S7, 2004.

Seniors use prayer to cope with stress; prayer no. 1 alternative remedy, December 28, 2000. *University of Florida News.* Available at http://www.napa.ufl.edu/2000news/prayer.htm. Accessed August 2, 2005.

Shannahoff-Khalsa D: An introduction to Kundalini yoga meditation techniques that are specific for the treatment of psychiatric disorders, *J Altern Complem Med* 10:91, 2004.

Shannahoff-Khalsa DS, Beckett LR: Clinical case report: efficacy of yogic techniques in the treatment of obsessive compulsive disorders, *Int J Neurosci* 85:1, 1996.

Shinomiya K, Inoue T, Utsu Y, et al: Hypnotic activities of chamomile and passiflora extracts in sleep-disturbed rats, *Biol Pharm Bull* 28:808, 2005.

Shippy RA, Mendez D, Jones K, et al: *S*-Adenosylmethionine (SAM-e) for the treatment of depression in people living with HIV/AIDS, *BMC Psychiatry* 4:38, 2004.

Shwartz M, Saitz R, Mulvey K, Brannigan P: The value of acupuncture detoxification programs in a substance abuse treatment system, *J Subst Abuse Treat* 17:305, 1999.

Silvers K, Woolley C, Hamilton F, et al: Randomised double-blind placebo-controlled trial of fish oil in the treatment of depression, *Prostaglandins, Leukotrienes & Essential Fatty Acids* 72:211, 2005.

Simon G, Cherkin D, Sherman K, et al: Mental health visits to complementary and alternative medicine providers, *Gen Hosp Psychiatry* 26:171, 2004.

Skidmore-Roth L: *Handbook of herbs and natural supplements,* St. Louis, 2001, Mosby.

Snyder M, Lindquist R: Issues in complementary therapies: how we got to where we are, May 31, 2001. *Online J Issues Nurs* 6:Manuscript 1, 2001. Available http://www.nursingworld.org/ojin/topic15/tpc15_1.htm. Accessed October 20, 2001.

Stoll AL, Severus WE, Freeman MP, et al: Omega-3 fatty acids in bipolar disorder: a preliminary double-blind, placebo-controlled trial, *Arch Gen Psychiatry* 56:407, 1999.

Stoll AL: *The omega-3 connection: the groundbreaking anti-depression diet and brain program,* New York, 2001, Simon and Schuster.

Stone J: Regulation of CAM practitioners: reflecting on the last 10 years, *Complem Ther Clin Pract* 11:5, 2005.

Szegedi A, Kohnen R, Dienel A, Kieser M: Acute treatment of moderate to severe depression with hypericum extract WS5570 (St. John's wort): randomised controlled double-blind non-inferiority trial versus paroxetine, *BMJ* 330:503, 2005.

Taibi D, Bourguignon ZC, Taylor A: Valerian use for sleep disorders related to rheumatoid arthritis, *Holistic Nurs Pract* 18:120, 2004.

Thompson R, Ruch W, Hasenohrl RU: Enhanced cognitive performance and cheerful mood by standardized extracts of *Piper methysticum* (Kava-kava), *Hum Psychopharmacol* 19:243, 2004.

Tiemeier H, van Tuijl H, Hoffman A, et al: Plasma fatty acid composition and depression are associated in the elderly: the Rotterdam study, *Am J Clin Nutr* 78:40, 2003.

Tooley GA, Armstrong SM, Norman TR, Sali A: Acute increases in night-time plasma melatonin levels following a period of meditation, *Biol Psychol* 53:69, 2000.

Uebelhack R, Franke L, Schewe HJ: Inhibition of platelet MAO-B by kava pyrone-enriched extract from *Piper methysticum* Forster (kava-kava), *Pharmacopsychiatry* 31:187, 1998.

U.S. Food and Drug Administration: FDA announces qualified health claims for omega-3 fatty acids, September 8, 2004. Available at http://www.fda.gov/bbs/topics/news/2004/NEW01115.html. Accessed October 20, 2005.

vanGurp G, Meterissian G, Haiek L, et al: St John's wort or sertraline? Randomized controlled trial in primary care, *Can Fam Physician* 48:905, 2002.

Vickers A, Zollman C: ABC of complementary medicine. Acupuncture, *BMJ* 319:973, 1999.

Watts C, Lafferty W, Baden A: The effect of mandating complementary and alternative medicine services on insurance benefits in Washington state, *J Altern Complem Med* 10:1001, 2004.

Wolsko P, Eisenberg D, Davis R, Phillips R: Use of mind-body medical therapies: results of a national survey, *J Gen Intern Med* 19:43, 2004.

Wong A, Smith M, Boon H: Herbal remedies in psychiatric practice, *Arch Gen Psychiatry* 55:1033, 1998.

Yale S: The vitamin E metaanalysis: cause for concern? *Altern Complem Ther* 11:7, 2005.

Yamashita H, Tsukayama H, Tanno Y, Nishijo K: Adverse events related to acupuncture, *JAMA* 280:1563, 1998.

Yarnell E, Abascal K: Herbal medicine in Korea: alternative is mainstream, *Altern Complem Ther* 10:161, 2004.

Yuan CS, Mehendale S, Xiao Y, et al: The gamma-aminobutyric acidergic effects of valerian and valerenic acid on rat brainstem neuronal activity, *Anesth Analg* 98:353, 2004.

Zandi P, Anthony J: Reduced risk of Alzheimer disease in users of antioxidant vitamin supplements: the Cache County Study, *Arch Neurol* 61:82, 2004.

Zhou S, Chan E, Pan SQ, et al: Pharmacokinetic interactions of drugs with St John's wort, *J Psychopharmacol* 18:262, 2004.

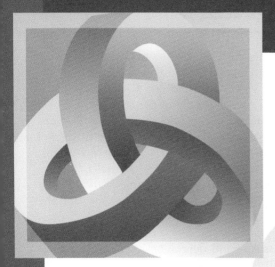

# Chapter 41

# Survivors of Violence and Trauma

*Lee H. Schwecke*

## Learning Objectives

*After reading this chapter, you should be able to:*
- Recognize the seriousness of violence and trauma in the United States.
- Describe the emotional reactions of adult victims of crime, workplace violence, terrorism, torture, ritual abuse, mind control, rape and sexual assault, childhood sexual abuse, and partner abuse.
- Recognize the dynamics involved in interpersonal violence crimes.

- Analyze the way in which the cycle of violence inhibits individuals from leaving abusive relationships.
- Identify the needs of victims of violence and trauma.
- Describe strategies for facilitating the transition from victim to survivor of violence or trauma.
- Develop a nursing care plan for survivors of violence and trauma.

The victimization of any individual by another creates serious mental health, social, community, and legal problems. Violence in all forms is prevalent in this society. Nurses, regardless of their areas of practice, will come into contact with the victims—as inpatients, outpatients, home care patients, emergency care patients, parents of patients, friends, and relatives. Although the victims are typically seen initially for physical injuries, their psychological needs require attention if long-term mental health problems are to be prevented.

Forensic nursing is emerging as a vital aspect of the holistic care of victims and perpetrators of violent crimes and their families (Peternelj-Taylor, 2001). This care includes obtaining clinical histories, documenting evidence, including photographs of injuries, and carrying out quality nursing interventions in a holistic care framework, which

includes consideration of all the medical-legal aspects of the patient's problems (Hammer, 2000). The rights of the alleged perpetrators of crime, suspects, and victims must be protected so that the legal case will not be jeopardized (Piercy and Greenwood, 2002).

This chapter focuses on victims of violence and trauma, beginning with a brief overview of general reactions to any crime, workplace violence, terrorism, torture, and ritual abuse, followed by a more in-depth look at rape, adult survivors of childhood sexual abuse, and individuals abused by their partners. A small number of perpetrators of rape, sexual abuse, and partner abuse are female, but the more common pattern of this victimization is males against females. The short- and long-term reactions of victims described in this chapter are generally true for both male and female victims; however, men sometimes have a more

**Norm's Notes**

*If ever there was a timely topic, this is it. I read just this morning in my local paper about a husband and wife who were arrested on child pornography charges. The national evening news yesterday centered on a report about a sophisticated ring of child pornographers who committed deeds so barbaric that the newscaster refused to describe them on the air. The victims, when they survive such abuse, are potentially scarred for life. How in the world do they ever learn to trust again? Lee Schwecke has had a lot of experience with survivors of violence and trauma, and has a lot to share in this chapter.*

difficult time admitting to and dealing with their emotional victimization than women. The added impact on males of sexual violation by other males, both as children and as adults, is a result, in part, of their fears about homosexuality (Ray, 2001).

Beyond the scope of this chapter are the issues of peer victimization and crime and violence by children and adolescents, despite national attention to gangs, school shootings, date violence (verbal, physical, and sexual), bullying, hate crimes against certain populations, property damage, and fighting (with or without weapons). Also beyond the scope of the chapter is the issue of elder abuse. Unfortunately, older adults can be the victims of all the crimes discussed in this chapter, as well as the particular crimes in the category of elder abuse, such as emotional and financial abuse, neglect, and abandonment, despite their inability to provide for their own self-care.

## VIOLATION BY CRIME

### EFFECTS OF CRIMES

Not all crimes involve physical violence, injury, and threat to life; however, all crimes involve emotional violation and trauma. The victim's identity is affected, even with the loss or destruction of possessions and property, because these are a representation of an individual's identity and have personal significance. Crime undermines

foundations formed in the first two stages of human development, regardless of the victim's age when the crime occurred (see Chapter 4). There is a loss of *trust,* not only in the criminal, but also to some degree in all other individuals. Victims also lose self-esteem, a sense of ability to control their own lives and themselves (*autonomy* issues), as well as having *identity* issues (Rowell, 2005).

Emotional reactions to crime vary greatly according to the individual, the situation, and the meaning of the crime to that person. However, typical reactions are denial, fear, anxiety, anger, powerlessness, and depression. A sense of failure and guilt is common; victims wonder what they did to cause the crime and how they might have prevented or stopped it. Victims usually feel ashamed and unworthy, as well as contaminated or dirty, whether or not they were physically touched by the perpetrator. Fantasies of revenge or a wish for legal retribution are typical. The relationships of victims to family and friends can be disturbed, in part, because of the loss of trust, but also because of the response of others. Caring individuals often imply that the victim was responsible for the crime, with questions such as, "Why were you there alone at night? Why were you carrying so much cash? Why didn't you install that burglar alarm?" The victim might feel alienated and isolated. Hospital personnel, the police, and the legal system might also unwittingly convey what could be called a *blame the victim* attitude in their manner of questioning and in focusing only on the facts, without any emotional support or empathy.

Workplace violence is a particular crime that is getting increased employer and media attention recently and is included here because nurses, in nonpsychiatric and psychiatric settings, are two or three times more likely to be victims than other professionals (Gates, 2004; Morrison and Love, 2003). This type of crime includes verbal abuse, sexual harassment, stalking, assault and battery, rape, and murder perpetrated by patients or their visitors, other employees, former or current partners of employees, and intruders from the outside looking for specific items, such as money or drugs (Gilmore-Hall, 2001; Institute for Safe Medication Practices, 2004). A 1999 study on workplace violence done by the National Institute for Occupational Safety and Health found that 38% of reported assaults took place in health care facilities and fewer than half of these assaults were committed by patients (Worthington and Franklin, 2000).

*Verbal abuse* by other employees includes intimidation, condescending language or tone, reluctance or refusal to answer questions, negative or threatening language, rude gestures, threats to or actual reporting of the nurse to a manager, ostracism, offensive notes or e-mail, criticism, humiliation, screaming, and sabotage (Institute for Safe Medication Practices, 2004; Leiper, 2005). In a 1999 survey, 94% of the nurses reported verbal abuse, with an average of five or six incidents per month (Stringer, 2001). Verbal abuse, especially when the abusers are physicians, nurse managers, or supervisors, has been linked to the high turnover of nursing staff and, indirectly, to the nursing shortage (Gates, 2004; Leiper, 2005; Parks, 2001; Stringer, 2001).

Sexual harassment is defined (Farella, 2001) as

an unwelcomed sexual advance or conduct on the job that creates an intimidating, hostile, or offensive working environment . . . [ranging from] . . . repeated offensive or belittling jokes to pornography or outright sexual assault. (p. 14)

According to a 1988 survey of the federal workforce, 42% of all women and 15% of all men have experienced some form of harassment (Farella, 2001).

Stalking is a crime that can occur anywhere but often follows victims to their workplace. Stalking is obsessional pursuit, harassment, and intimidation by a person who has or believes that he or she has a significant personal relationship with the object of his or her unwanted attention. Stalkers might send letters, packages, or e-mails; make harassing phone calls; or follow and/or appear repeatedly at the victim's home or workplace. Sometimes they kill pets, vandalize or destroy property, and physically or sexually assault, or even murder, their victims (Muscari, 2005). One survey indicated that 2% of all men and 8% of all women have been stalked at least once in their lifetimes. Men account for 87% of the stalkers, and women are their victims in 60% of cases. However, some cases involve female-male, male-male, or female-female stalking (Muscari, 2005).

The media tends to focus on the stalking of celebrities and public officials by strangers. The stalkers in these cases tend to be psychotic or have delusions about their victims and the supposed love relationship. However, most cases of stalking occur as the victim is trying to end a casual, dating, or marital relationship (Mawson, 2005). This pattern is more likely than celebrity stalking to involve physical violence (80%) and sexual assault (30%) and to be carried out by nondelusional individuals.

The Occupational Safety and Health Administration (OSHA) encourages voluntary compliance by employers with their workplace violence guidelines, published in 1998. Briefly, these guidelines suggest the following: (1) systematic education of all employees about verbal abuse, sexual harassment, and other forms of violence, along with ways to prevent and deal with them; (2) development of corporate policies and procedures related to workplace violence and reporting procedures; (3) definition of roles for supervisors, employee health staff, and security personnel; and (4) provision for treatment and counseling for employee victims (Farella, 2001; Gilmore-Hall, 2001; Monarch, 2000; Morrison and Love, 2005; Trossman, 2001). Counseling is most often provided by Employee Assistance Programs (EAPs; Paul and Blum, 2005).

## RECOVERY FROM VIOLENCE AND TRAUMA

Many models have been formulated about the process of recovery from traumas such as crimes and disasters. Most researchers agree that the duration and severity of the trauma, the victim's resources, and the nature of help available during and immediately after the crime, trauma, or disaster influence recovery. Typically, three stages of recovery are defined: (1) initial disorganization (impact), (2) a struggle to adapt (recoil), and (3) reconstruction (reorganization). The brief summary here is derived from the views of Foa (2005), Lacy and Benedek (2003), Pasquali (2003), and Tynhurst (1951). The stages are not clearly separated, and the readjustment process is not smooth. Vacillation among the stages might occur, and recovery might take months or years.

### Impact

The initial reaction to a single-event trauma usually lasts from a few minutes to a few days. Common responses are shock, denial, disbelief, and confusion. There might be paralyzing fear, hysteria, horror, anger, rage, shame, guilt, a sense of helplessness and vulnerability, physiologic responses, and disturbed sleeping and eating. These reactions might occur for a longer time when the trauma is ongoing, such as harassment, stalking, or disaster. Some victims react less visibly or in a delayed manner; they look calm, organized, and rational, and take all the necessary actions initially needed. Later, the other reactions might occur. Occasionally, the victim's reaction might include dissociative symptoms (amnesia, depersonalization, numbing, detachment), intrusive memories (nightmares, flashbacks), and severe anxiety. These symptoms might indicate that the victim is experiencing acute stress disorder (ASD) (see Chapter 31).

### Recoil

In the recoil stage, victims begin the struggle to adapt. The immediate danger might be over, but a great deal of emotional stress remains. In the beginning of this phase, there are periods in which victims look and act normal and are able to carry out daily routines at home and at work. Activity helps suppress fears, anger, and sadness. Later in this phase, there is a desire to talk about all the details of and feelings about the trauma ("What happened?"). Victims often feel a need for support and to be temporarily dependent. Fantasies of revenge for the crime are natural during this stage. In the weeks and months following trauma, victims gradually become aware of the full impact that the event has had on their lives.

### Reorganization

Reorganization might take months or years to accomplish. Although the trauma is not forgotten, the anxiety, fear, and anger diminish, and victims reconstruct their lives. The beginning of this phase includes reviewing and organizing what happened and why ("Why me?"); attributing blame to self, others, or both; justifying one's own actions at the time and later ("Why did I act the way I did then and since then?"); and regaining a sense of control and self-protection. Grief over losses resolves slowly. Lingering nightmares, frustrations, and disillusionment might occur; however, these subside as victims become reengaged in life and activities. If reorganization is not effective, victims might experience degrees of symptoms that, in some cases, are clinically diagnosable (e.g.,

posttraumatic stress disorder [PTSD]) and need appropriate treatment (Lacy and Benedek, 2003). See Chapter 31.

Even with satisfactory recovery, victims sense that they and their lives are, and always will be, different as a result of the crime ("What if it happens again?"). Moving from victim to survivor or victor status is the goal for those experiencing trauma (Rowell, 2005), which can be accomplished by integrating the memories of the trauma and moving on in life with restored functioning, a reasonable sense of safety and security, healthy relationships, and improved self-esteem.

## PUTTING IT ALL TOGETHER
### Psychotherapeutic Management

## NURSE-PATIENT RELATIONSHIP

Although trust, empathy, emotional support, and a willingness to listen are important in all stages of recovery, specialized care is needed in each stage. During the *impact stage,* the focus is on the survivor's need for physical safety and emotional security (see Chapter 10 for these crisis intervention strategies). Reassurance, protection from further harm, and sometimes medical care are needed. Survivors might need clear, simple directions on what to do, where to go, and what to avoid. It is crucial that nurses avoid accusations (blaming), intimidations, unnecessary intrusions, and invasion of privacy. In most instances, crisis intervention occurs face to face at the scene of the trauma or in the emergency room. For survivors who are superficially calm and in control, the crisis intervention might be needed a few hours or days later, when the trauma reality hits. Phone numbers for crisis telephone or walk-in services can be given to survivors before they leave the police interview at the scene or the emergency room.

During the *recoil stage,* survivors need validation of their worth and rights as victims. Referrals can be made to a victim's assistance program and for legal, insurance, or financial assistance, if needed. If family and friends are not fully available during the episodes of emotional turmoil in the recoil phase, then short-term counseling might be beneficial. During the struggle to adjust, support groups with other survivors can be useful. Whether the group is of short duration (6 to 8 weeks) or ongoing, and whether the group is professionally led or self-led, there is value in receiving information, encouragement, and companionship from others "who have been there."

During the *reorganization stage,* most survivors are able to recover and grow with minimal assistance. Appropriate humor might play a role in decreasing aggression and stress (Pasquali, 2003). Long-term counseling is sometimes needed to overcome anxiety, phobias, depression, suicidal ideation, or other posttraumatic symptoms. It is uncommon for survivors to need hospitalization beyond initial medical care. Exceptions include survivors who are unable to function or meet their basic needs, or those who become suicidal.

## PSYCHOPHARMACOLOGY

Survivors of crime do not generally need medications. Antianxiety agents (benzodiazepines) are prescribed occasionally for short-term use to decrease anxiety and facilitate sleep.

## MILIEU MANAGEMENT

Many communities have temporary or ongoing groups for survivors of disasters, divorce, death of a loved one, sudden infant death syndrome (SIDS), rape, incest, and physical and emotional abuse, as well as for those affected by suicide, mass murders, torture, and abduction of children.

## TERRORISM

### NATURE OF THE PROBLEM

September 11, 2001 is the day that awakened the United States to the realities of terrorism—its unpredictability and devastation. Before this day, terrorism was a news story about terrible acts in foreign countries. Terrorism can be perpetrated under the justification of various military, political, social, cultural, or religious reasons. Acts of terrorism can involve plane crashes, bombings, military warfare, biologic and chemical agents, trained or programmed assassins, and suicide or homicide bombers. Terrorism rarely affects only a single individual; victimization can involve thousands who have been injured or killed in a single event. The victims of terrorism include those who were injured or killed; police, fire, and rescue personnel; businesses and their employees; the friends and families of all the victims; and potentially anyone who witnessed the tragedy (directly or through the media).

## EFFECTS

Terrorism can have more devastating results than natural disasters or major accidents because terrorism is not only perpetrated by humans, but it is also not accidental. The purpose of terrorism is to terrorize, kill, or injure targeted groups and to generate fear that it can or will happen again (Foa, 2005; Pasquali, 2003). The trauma of terrorism is more pervasive, long-lasting, and severe than other violent crimes. Survivors typically experience some degree of grief and mourning and acute or posttraumatic stress symptoms, which are expected reactions to an abnormal and horrifying event. See Box 41-1 (p. 608) for a list of typical reactions to terrorism. The event might also retrigger memories of previous traumatic experiences or lead to new or exacerbation of preexisting disorders (Ai et al, 2005).

## RECOVERY

Most individuals will recover with the support of loved ones, co-workers, and friends; memorial or religious services and community meetings; sleep, stress management techniques, relaxation techniques, physical activities; and a return to normal activities (Foa, 2005; Miller, 2005). Critical incident stress management strategies (described with PTSD in Chapter 31) can also facilitate recovery and prevent other untoward consequences (Lacy and Benedek, 2003; New York Academy of Medicine, 2005; Pasquali, 2003).

A major goal of recovery is to regain some sense of trust, safety, and security while acknowledging that future terrorist attacks are possible. In general, recovery will parallel the stages of recovery described earlier (*impact, recoil,* and *reorganization*) but might be lengthier and more complicated, depending on the severity and duration of the trauma. On a larger scale, most cities and hospitals are reviewing their disaster plans for the capability to respond to terrorist attacks, biologic and chemical warfare, and large-scale bombings. For many cities, an effort has been made to improve citywide, coordinated plans among police, fire, and rescue agencies, as well as hospitals, mental health

---

### Box 41-1    Specific Responses Resulting From Terrorism, Torture, Serial Ritual Abuse, Mind Control

Shock, disbelief, fear, anxiety, powerlessness
Insecurity, guilt, shame, spiritual distress
Unresponsiveness, dissociation, numbness
Decreased concentration, confusion
Panic, terror, sense of violation, anger, rage
Aggression, fantasies of revenge, impulsiveness
Helplessness, hopelessness, despair
Suicidal or homicidal ideation, self-mutilation
Mistrust, suspiciousness, paranoia, alienation
Estrangement, withdrawal, isolation
Fatigue, insomnia, nightmares, flashbacks
Memory disturbances, amnesia
Hyperarousal, stress sensitivity, startle response
Denial, repression, suppression, intellectualization
Body kinesthetic memories, psychosomatic
   symptoms
Extreme passivity, loss of self-esteem
Depression, prolonged grieving, substance abuse
Sexual dysfunctions, eating disorder, anxiety
   disorder
Labile emotions, personality changes

Modified from van der Kolk B, McFarlane AC, Weissaeth L: *Traumatic stress: the effects of overwhelming experience on mind, body, and society,* New York, 1996, Guilford Press; Turkus JA: The treatment challenge, *Many Voices* 12:6, 2000; Anorexia Nervosa and Associated Disorders (Indianapolis Chapter of ANAD): Personal interviews: Indianapolis, 2002, ANAD; Valente S: Controversies and challenges of ritual abuse, *J Psychosoc Nurs* 38:8, 2000; Miller MC: Disaster and trauma, *Harv Ment Health Lett* 18:1, 2002; Lacy TJ, Benedek DM: Terrorism and weapons of mass destruction: managing the behavioral reaction in primary care, *South Med J* 96:394, 2003.

---

facilities, and local, state, and federal emergency management administrations. Psychiatric nurses and mental health personnel with mental health disaster management skills are included in the planning.

## TORTURE, RITUAL ABUSE, AND MIND CONTROL

## NATURE OF THE PROBLEM

Public and professional attention to the effects of torture, serial ritual abuse (SRA), and mind control (MC) on mental health has waned in recent years, although the crimes have not, according to the victims. These crimes might be perpetrated by individuals, relatives, gangs, cults (satanic or nonsatanic), hate groups, or military-political organizations (e.g., Al Qaeda, Sadam Hussein's regime, Abu Ghraib Prison). Gangs are responsible for an increased number of homicides, other physical violence, and intimidation, according to the FBI (Ragavan and Guttman, 2004). The actions of Muslim gangs in France in November 2005 are another example of the destruction that can occur in a country. The effect is more severe because they involve multiple, calculated, and organized crimes against each victim or group of victims. This type of crime is used to create fear, humiliation, and submission in individuals, communities, and societies.

Statistics on the prevalence of torture, SRA, and MC are not readily available because of the problems in acknowledging, reporting, and proving occurrences, but the rates might be similar to those of family child abuse (Valente, 2000). The threat of further harm to the self, pets, or family tends to keep victims silent. Especially in SRA and MC, perpetrators might use triggers to maintain victims' silence or to control their actions, such as special words, hand signals, or greeting cards (Anorexia Nervosa and Associated Disorders [Indianapolis], 2002). Drug and MC experiments began before the 1970s (e.g., LSD experiments and covert military-political operation [MK-ULTRA] programming that trained or programmed assassins for U.S. security forces) (Katchen, 2005; McGonigle, 1999). MK-ULTRA operations (noted in movies—*Conspiracy Theory, The Bourne Identity, The Bourne Supremacy*) are becoming more widely known, because the Freedom of Information Act has resulted in the declassification of military and political documents.

### Tactics

According to survivors, torture involves physical, psychological, pharmacologic, MC, or sexual manipulation, or any combination of these aimed at damaging the victim's identity, personality, emotional stability, spirit, and physical integrity. Torture, SRA, and MC can begin with abduction and detention and end with execution, or can be ongoing over time. It might also include human trafficking, sex trade operations, and prolonged interrogation. Tactics can include using hot irons, electric shock, submersion, suffocation, large doses of drugs, beatings, physical restraint, confinement in cramped and buried containers, watching or forced participation in others' torture, gang rape, sexual and physical mutilation, being tied or hung in the air (or both), being photographed during the abuse, starvation, sensory and sleep deprivation, brainwashing, indoctrination, programming, threats to or lies about the safety of loved ones and pets, over-stimulation, mock executions, electronic harassment (microchip implants, as in the movie *Manchurian Candidate*), and threats with weapons (ANAD, 2002; Dowbecko, 2005; McCollough-Zander and Larson, 2004; Sarson and MacDonald, 2004; Tolces, 2005; Valente, 2000).

## EFFECTS

Common outcomes of torture, SRA, and MC are injuries to the head, teeth, and genitals, as well as bone fractures, dislocations, scars, burns, pain, and chronic headaches. The emotional effects are more severe and longer lasting than those caused by other crimes; they include a sense of violation, dehumanization, humiliation, guilt about harming others or animals, identity and personality changes, and damaged social and family relationships. Trauma-specific fears (e.g., small dark spaces or nudity), hypersexuality, and obsessions with rituals, magic, or devils are common. Victims might have been forced or programmed to commit crimes against others. They might talk about topics that might not make sense to professionals, such as the Greek alphabet, sex trade, white slavery, drinking blood, satanic rituals and holidays, and the *Satanic Bible* (written by Anton LaVey) (ANAD, 2002; Valente, 2000). Other specific responses resulting from torture, SRA, and MC are listed in Box 41-1.

There is much controversy about assigning psychiatric diagnoses (e.g., PTSD, adjustment disorder, major depression, dysthymia, anxiety disorder, dissociative identity disorder, or other dissociative disorders) to victims who are having *typical* reactions to *horrific* crimes (Torem, 2000). The major concern is that diagnosis is another form of victimization, stigmatization, and discounting of the validity of reports of these crimes. Blaming the victim draws attention away from the individual, social, cultural, and political variables creating and fostering torture, SRA, and MC and from research on strategies for prevention. Some professionals even view PTSD as insufficient for acknowledging the catastrophic effects experienced by victims and their families.

## RECOVERY

Because torture, SRA, and MC tend to be ongoing, the *impact* stage of recovery persists but might wax and wane over the years. In the *recoil* stage, adaptation is difficult because of the severity of the emotional stress remaining after these crimes end. Although supportive, cognitive-behavioral, psychodynamic, and pharmacologic approaches (Lacy and Benedek, 2003; McCollough-Zander and Larson, 2004) are useful in helping these survivors *reorganize* their lives, this stage is likely to be prolonged, with more relapses during other life crises. Admission to a specialized program or psychiatric unit might be needed during intense therapy periods, when the risk of self-mutilation, suicide, or increased substance abuse is present. The major goals for recovery (Howe, 2003; Lacy and Benedek, 2003; McCollough-Zander and Larson, 2004; Valente, 2000) include the following:

1. Decreasing, and eventually eliminating, self-destructive behaviors (self-mutilation, suicide attempts, substance abuse, and manipulation)
2. Developing emotion management skills and acknowledging the thoughts, feelings, and behaviors as "normal reactions to abnormal situations"
3. Expressing and dealing appropriately and safely with the intense emotions, especially anxiety, guilt, anger, rage, and desire for revenge
4. Becoming aware of suppressed or repressed thoughts and feelings, positive emotions, and body memories and reactions
5. Allowing oneself to grieve for the variety of losses experienced
6. Processing and integrating the memories of the experiences, often from the least to the most bizarre experiences (as in the recovery from PTSD and the integration of multiple personalities)
7. Developing or reestablishing healthy relationships with family, friends, and the community
8. Developing boundaries, a sense of privacy, self-integrity, and empathy
9. Using complementary or alternative medicine and spiritual practices that are helpful
10. Becoming aware of new perspectives in life and reasons to live, in spite of the past

11. Regaining a sense of hope, personal power, and control over oneself and one's life

## NURSE-PATIENT RELATIONSHIP

Conveying acceptance, caring, and support; ensuring confidentiality; and believing what is being described are crucial if survivors are going to trust someone enough to discuss their experiences (McCollough-Zander and Larson, 2004). Survivors must have time and space to process the issues at their own pace and within their own cultural framework. Survivors might need prompting, which also conveys understanding, such as, "It sounds as if you have been traumatized in some way" or "I wonder if you have experienced activities using rituals." Strategies used with patients experiencing PTSD are particularly useful for survivors of torture, SRA, and MC (see Chapter 31). Depending on the origin of the torture, SRA, or MC (individuals, relatives, gangs, hate groups, cults, military-political organizations), it might be crucial to understand the survivor's family, religious, cultural, and political background. Referrals for treatment or correction of physical injuries might be appropriate, such as dentists, plastic surgeons, gynecologists, neurologists, or gastroenterologists (Turkus, 2000).

## PSYCHOPHARMACOLOGY

Using medication for treating survivors of torture, SRA, and MC is highly controversial, especially because drugs were often a part of the abuse as it occurred. Sometimes the medications used in treating PTSD, anxiety disorders, depression (especially selective serotonin reuptake inhibitors, SSRIs), sleep disturbances, and psychosis are effective (Lacy and Benedek, 2003; McCollough-Zander and Larson, 2004).

## MILIEU MANAGEMENT

Specialized treatment centers, such as the Center for Victims of Torture in Minnesota (McCollough-Zander and Larson, 2004) and The Center: Post-Traumatic Disorders Program in Washington, DC, use a multidisciplinary approach in providing treatment and rehabilitation for survivors and their families. Some of the 30 centers and programs use bicultural counselors to facilitate counseling with immigrants and former gang members. Self-help and therapy groups might be useful for survivors with similar experiences and needs, such as political refugees; rape, childhood sexual abuse, and partner abuse survivors; and former cult and gang members.

## NATURE OF THE PROBLEM

Statistics indicate that rape is an underreported crime in the United States; probably only 16% of rapes are reported (Jordan, 2004). Valid statistics are not available for sexual assault and rape because of this lack of reporting. It is estimated that one in four adult women have been raped in their lifetime (Campbell and Wasco, 2005). In one school system, in 2003, 8.5% of the female students reported having been raped (Cerdorian, 2005). The elderly are vulnerable at home and in extended care facilities, especially if they have medical conditions, a physical or mental disability, or dementia (any of which might result in their reports being discounted by caregivers, family, and officials) (Burgess et al, 2005). Rape of men by men is increasing, but is rarely reported. Of the reported sexual assaults and rapes, probably 90% involve a male perpetrator and a female victim (Brown, 2001).

One major problem in reporting rape is that laws and attitudes vary in different states and communities. In general, rape is considered forcible penetration of the victim's body by the perpetrator's penis, fingers, or object without consent (Martin et al, 2000). Any other form of forced sexual contact (from touch to mutilation) is considered sexual assault. Despite sexual contact, it is generally acknowledged that rape is not sexually motivated, but involves a desire for power and control, a wish to humiliate the victim, and the playing out of a (sexual) fantasy (Brown, 2001). Some police and prosecutors still do not pursue rape as a charge if the two individuals know each other (Jordan, 2004), despite the fact that, in 90% of reported rapes, the victim knows the offender at least casually (Brown, 2001). Date or acquaintance rape might be complicated by the use of amnesiacs (date rape drugs), other drugs, and alcohol, which interfere with remembering the rape (Osterman et al, 2001). Some states lack marital rape statutes, or prosecutors are reluctant to charge husbands with raping their wives. Unfortunately, many in our society ignore rape or convey the message that anyone who is raped asked for it (blaming the victim).

## EFFECTS

Similar to all crime victims, the rape victim experiences a severe violation and all the possible emotions of the *impact* stage. In addition to internal and external bodily injuries, there might be a threat to life with weapons, to return and rape again, or to kill the victim if the rape is reported, or the perpetrator might kill the victim during or after the rape (Brown, 2001). Victims usually live but wish they had died. The traumatic memories of the rape usually include tastes, smells, sounds, and sights, as well tactile sensations and physical pain (Brown, 2001). These memories and the powerlessness, loss of control, fear, shame, guilt, humiliation, rage, and feelings of being contaminated or dirty might be overwhelming. A typical reaction of the victim is the wish to regain a sense of control and retreat to a safe place, take a thorough shower, and destroy any damaged belongings. To do this, however, would destroy most of the evidence that is required if the victim decides to report the rape and prosecute. Avoiding medical attention also places victims at risk for acquired immunodeficiency syndrome (AIDS), hepatitis B infection, sexually transmitted diseases (STDs), pregnancy, and improper healing of any physical injuries (Campbell and Wasco, 2005; Piercy and Greenwood, 2002).

## RECOVERY

Despite an outward appearance of calm composure and a denial at times of the need for help (as in silent or delayed reactions), the rape survivor needs assistance, information, and support. It might not be until the survivor begins the up and down struggle of the *recoil* stage that the losses, anger, and needs are recognized. In an emergency department, collecting evidence and taking away clothes might be a priority for staff but, for the survivor, it is perceived as further intrusion and violation. To staff, survivors might seem resistant

---

### Box 41-2   Needs and Rights of Rape Survivors

1. Crisis intervention: information, counseling, and referrals
2. Help with basic needs: housing, transportation, child care, safety
3. Medical information and care: information about pregnancy prevention, testing for sexually transmitted diseases, follow-up care, and counseling
4. Advocacy for whatever choices are made about reporting or prosecuting
5. Protection of rights: to privacy, confidentiality, gentleness, sensitivity, and explanations of procedures and tests
6. Protection of rights: to refuse collection of evidence, to determine who will and will not be present during examinations, to get copies of all medical and legal reports, and to apply for reimbursement through victim's compensation
7. Fairness, information, and protection of legal rights during investigations, hearings, and trial, including not being asked about prior sexual experiences with anyone other than the suspect or defendant
8. Reasonable protection against further harm: escorts to court, restraining order, additional patrols, even relocation, if necessary

---

and uncooperative, whereas survivors are trying to protect themselves and regain a sense of control (Brown, 2001). Box 41-2 lists some of the needs and rights of rape survivors.

Many communities have developed specialized services for rape survivors (e.g., Centers for Hope) within clinics or hospitals (as part of the emergency departments). Sexual assault nurse examiners (SANE) have skills in collecting forensic evidence while providing empathy, support, and information (Campbell and Wasco, 2005). Nurses also can encourage the beginning of the recovery process by challenging any myths stated by the survivors, such as, "I should have fought him off" or "I shouldn't have been drinking" (Brown, 2001; Girardin, 2001; Piercy and Greenwood, 2002).

Specialized rape services have information packets prepared for rape survivors and staff in hospitals, counseling centers, and other crisis areas. Survivors can be encouraged to keep the information sheets, as well as phone numbers of resources, for later use. The temporarily composed and calm victim who denies the need for help should be especially encouraged to take materials home. A

SANE might also call a sexual assault advocate, an advocate from a victim's assistance program, or a rape crisis counselor to initiate contact with the survivor and make periodic follow-up contact days, weeks, and even months later, when emotional, physical, or legal issues and concerns might arise (Brown, 2001; Campbell and Wasco, 2005).

In the *recoil* stage, most survivors begin to react to the significant effect that rape has had on their lives; they might alternately deny and admit to experiencing turmoil. Fear and mistrust are major issues and might be directed toward individuals resembling the perpetrator or toward everyone around them, especially if others convey any hint of blaming the victim. Survivors might be afraid to leave the one place they designate as safe. They might be able to go out with family and friends, but they more often avoid strangers, places similar to the rape scene, and intimacy, especially sexual relationships. If the rapes occurred in their residence, survivors might move or at least make safety-related changes to prevent recurrence, or they might ask for someone to stay with them at night for a while. Being alone and unprotected is usually frightening, especially when nightmares and traumatic memories occur. Survivors need help in reaffirming that they are worthwhile individuals, with dignity and rights, who did not cause and did not deserve the rape. They need to know that their anger is natural, especially about the violation of person and privacy, the humiliation, and the sense of powerlessness. Survivors often question whether they might have fought off the attacker. Survival is most important; if the victim survived the rape, then he or she did exactly what was necessary to stay alive.

## RAPE TRAUMA SYMPTOMS

One way to monitor and evaluate the rape survivor's responses to the trauma and recovery process through the recoil and reorganization stages is to assess periodically for improvements in the rape trauma symptoms (DiVasto, 1985):

- Sleep disturbances, nightmares
- Loss of appetite, somatic symptoms
- Fears, anxiety, phobias, suspicion
- Decrease in activities and motivation
- Disruptions in relationships with partner, family, friends
- Self-blame, guilt, shame
- Lowered self-esteem, feelings of worthlessness

It is important to remember that survivors vacillate in the recoil stage between repression or suppression and dealing with the trauma. Even progress in the reorganization stage is not smooth; backslides occur at times, especially if new situations trigger memories of the rape. Survivors might avoid future routine gynecologic and rectal examinations to avoid reexperiencing the trauma (Osterman et al, 2001). The use of restraints during an inpatient stay might also reactivate the trauma symptoms. The goals of recovery from rape and sexual assault are the same as those for all survivors of crime. In addition, rape survivors might need to develop or regain healthy sexual functioning and relationships (Osterman et al, 2001). Victims need to transfer traumatic memories to narrative or past memories by processing the sensory memories and decreasing their strength and influence, enabling them to move from victim to survivor status (Brown, 2001).

## PUTTING IT ALL TOGETHER
### Psychotherapeutic Management

## NURSE-PATIENT RELATIONSHIP

The rape or sexual assault survivor needs continual empathy, support, and an opportunity to process the events and intense feelings, as well as to regain a sense of psychological and physical safety (Osterman et al, 2001). Although it is more time- and energy-consuming, the best approach in collecting evidence and providing nursing care is to move slowly and supportively at the individual survivor's pace and to give rationales for and descriptions of procedures and referrals. Nurses can be particularly helpful to rape survivors. Male and especially female survivors tend to feel safer with a woman and might refuse to talk to a man, especially alone. The presence of a SANE or sexual assault advocate during examinations and interrogations can be reassuring. Survivors might or might not choose to have a friend or family member stay with them for additional support or help them get home. A sense of shame or guilt might interfere with reaching out for support (Osterman et al, 2001).

Crisis intervention is the most appropriate approach during the impact stage. Short-term counseling and a rape support group can be beneficial during the recoil stage. Long-term counseling might be needed during the reorganization stage, especially if the survivor decides to prosecute the perpetrator. A lengthy legal process can seriously delay recovery because of having to relive the events and emotions. In many trial situations, the survivor is still treated as a criminal during cross-examinations. On the other hand, conviction and imprisonment of the perpetrator can help survivors feel vindicated, compensated, and safer in their environments.

If the symptoms of rape trauma do not gradually diminish and if reorganization of lifestyle does not seem to occur, the survivor needs to be assessed for and helped with any new problems, such as posttraumatic stress, anxiety, excessive anger and guilt, depression, acting out, isolation, suicidal thoughts, self-destructive behaviors, eating and sexual disorders, substance abuse, phobias, and/or negative or destructive relationships with others, as well as reactivation of childhood sexual abuse memories (Campbell and Wasco, 2004; Faravelli et al, 2004). With any of these behaviors, longer term counseling might be a necessity and hospitalization for safety becomes essential.

## PSYCHOPHARMACOLOGY

Although rarely prescribed to rape survivors, benzodiazepines to reduce anxiety and provide for sleep might be used on a temporary basis. Alternatively, an antidepressant taken at bedtime (especially trazodone [Desyrel]), might be ordered if symptoms of depression exist with a sleep disturbance. If nightmares or traumatic memories are severe, a low dose of an atypical antipsychotic such as risperidone (Risperdal) or quetiapine (Seroquel) might be indicated.

## MILIEU MANAGEMENT

Referral can be made to a rape support group or center, which encourages expressing anger safely, overcoming guilt and shame, building self-esteem and trust, and assisting in regaining control of the survivor's life and a sense of safety. Support groups are sometimes available for relatives, especially partners, of rape survivors to help them deal with the trauma, stereotyping and myths, and changes

occurring in the survivors, themselves, and their relationship with the survivors.

### CLINICAL EXAMPLE

A 24-year-old woman called a rape crisis line complaining of anxiety at work, not sleeping, fear of being out at night, overwhelming anger, and feeling dirty and ashamed. For several weeks she thought that a co-worker was watching her. Last Friday, as she was leaving work late, the co-worker pushed her into her car and raped her. She did not report the rape and hid in her apartment all weekend. She forced herself to go to work on Monday. The man acted friendly toward her, as if nothing had happened.

# ADULT SURVIVORS OF CHILDHOOD SEXUAL ABUSE

## NATURE OF THE PROBLEM

The crimes of child pornography and childhood sexual abuse (by nonrelatives) and incest (by relatives) are especially destructive for two major reasons: the crimes are not one-time occurrences, and the perpetrators might be known and trusted. Unfortunately, these crimes are common. Studies have indicated that 15% to 30% of all girls and 4% to 16% of all boys have experienced childhood sexual abuse (Cook, 2005; Valente, 2005). The incidence of sexual abuse of boys might actually be much higher. It is sometimes harder for men to reveal the abuse because of the fear of being seen as unable to protect themselves, weak, or gay (Cook, 2005; Ray, 2001; Valente, 2005). However, the number of children who have been sexually abused and never reported it, even when they became adults, is not actually known.

Sexual abuse and incest include voyeurism and exhibitionism, which can lead to intercourse and mutilation, but always involve a younger victim who is not capable of giving consent to the older, more powerful individual. For 75% of the adult female survivors in one study, the abuse began before the age of 7 years and 62% had multiple perpetrators (Jonzon and Lindblad, 2005; Valente, 2005). Male perpetrators are commonly fathers, uncles, stepfathers, older brothers, cousins, grandfathers, neighbors, scout leaders, camp counselors, coaches, and religious leaders. Less frequently, the perpetrators are females—mothers, older sisters, other relatives, day care workers, teachers, coaches, neighbors, and babysitters. Perpetrators tend to choose either male or female victims, so there can be male to male, male to female, female to male, and female to female abuse. However, 92% of the females were victimized by male perpetrators and 38% of the males were victimized by female perpetrators (Lie and Barclay, 2005a). Victims are from every social, cultural, ethnic, and economic group (Cook, 2005).

Although sexual abuse can be violent, it often is not. Coercion is possible because of the victim's dependent, trusting, or loving relationship with the perpetrator. The victim is urged to maintain the secret with various threats, such as the following: the victim will be taken away from the family; the perpetrator will be put in a mental hospital or jail; the parents will divorce; the other parent will get sick; there will be no abuse of siblings if the victim is compliant; love will be withdrawn; no one would believe the victim anyway; or there will be physical abuse if the victim does not comply. Even when no physical violence takes place, victims usually fear that it will occur if they resist the perpetrator. Factors such as family conflicts or disorganization, witnessing violence, parental loss, parental mental illness, economic instability, secrecy and communication difficulties, substance abuse, and other forms of abuse (emotional, verbal, physical) and neglect seem to correlate with sexual abuse (Davis and Petretic-Jackson, 2000; Gladstone et al, 2004; Goodwin, 2005).

Even if the young victims want to disclose the abuse, it is difficult for them because they lack the words and concepts to describe the event. An emotional reaction of fear and confusion usually occurs, and some physical pain, but not a moral, ethical, or legal concept of right or wrong. Most victims who, as children, tried to tell a parent or other adult were often met with disbelief, denial, or pressure to retract their accusations. It is difficult for a parent to believe that the partner they love or a respected member of the community is capable of sexual abuse. Police, prosecutors, judges, mental health professionals, and the general public might discount a child's report as unreliable, a fantasy, distorted, or faked at the urging of a parent, especially if there is a custody dispute in progress (Davis and Petretic-Jackson, 2000). There

are also potential benefits from the sexual relationship; the child is made to feel special, with extra attention from and time with the perpetrator that other children do not enjoy. A certain power comes from pleasing the adult and receiving a degree of (distorted) affection (Davis and Petretic-Jackson, 2000). At times, the child might even have the physical experience of sensual pleasure (Valente, 2005). However, the emotional pleasure and concept of adult sexual love are absent. (It should be noted that all children make bids for attention and affection. Even if they are cute, coy, or flirtatious, these desires should not be viewed as seduction. Perpetrators of sexual abuse choose to misinterpret the child's behavior to meet their own needs and should still be held responsible for the crime.)

# EFFECTS OF CHILDHOOD SEXUAL ABUSE

## On the Child

For the victim, the prolonged stress of the abuse might lead to changes in his or her neurobiology, as in the stress response described in Chapter 10. Another result is disturbed growth and development (beginning with trust and autonomy issues), ambivalence about the experience (both the benefits and the pain), and denial of what is happening to protect the whole family or the community. The young child is fulfilling the roles of child and lover to the perpetrator, and roles of child and protector to the rest of the family or community (protecting them from the horrible secret). As a result, the child begins a long-term process of taking care of others to the exclusion of personal needs. Basically, the child wishes for love, not sex, but eventually feels guilty, exploited, betrayed, angry, dirty, helpless, and responsible. Denial, repression, suppression, rationalization, and dissociation are mechanisms used by young victims to cope with this no-win situation. Sleep and eating disturbances, enuresis, anxiety, depression, aggression, an active fantasy life, masturbation, sexualized play, sexual aggression, poor impulse control, cruelty to animals, spiritual distress, somatization, alienation, fear, shame, self-blame, self-destructive behaviors, running away, and truancy are common (Cook, 2005; Davis and Petretic-Jackson, 2000; Valente, 2005). The more severe the abuse, the more likely that repression will begin near puberty.

If the sexual abuse continues throughout adolescence, repression is less likely. Repression normally lasts until victims are in their 20s or 30s and are having trouble with intimate relationships and/or parenting.

---

### CLINICAL EXAMPLE

Children who were examined following ritual abuse in a day care center reported being locked in a cage, put in a coffin, held underwater, injected with needles, tied and hung from hooks, sexually assaulted, and threatened with guns and knives. The children were told that if they told anyone about the abuse, their parents, siblings, or pets would be killed.

---

## On the Adolescent

As adolescents, sexual abuse victims show mostly overt methods of dysfunctional coping, such as impulsive acting out, violence toward or abuse of others, cruelty to animals, self-destructive behaviors, sleeping and eating disorders, suicide attempts, running away, truancy, delinquency, substance abuse, spiritual distress, sexual acting out, prostitution, early pregnancy, and early marriage (Cook, 2005; Davis and Petretic-Jackson, 2000; Valente, 2005). For victims who cope through self-mutilation, these behaviors tend to begin between the ages of 12 and 14 years (Cerdorian, 2005).

Adolescents might have fantasies of revenge and wish for the perpetrator's death. The anger toward the perpetrator and other adults (for not protecting them) approaches rage but is not directly expressed. Victims might not even be aware of the reason for their rage, shame, guilt, confusion, sense of alienation, and isolation and might not realize that their acting-out behaviors are related to the abuse. Regression, depression, depersonalization, dissociation, manipulation, low self-esteem, impaired social skills, spiritual distress, thought and memory disturbances, self-neglect, aimlessness, and withdrawal are common. Sexual abuse survivors are also more likely than the general population to be raped and battered by partners in adolescence and later in life (Davis and Petretic-Jackson, 2000; Gladstone et al, 2004; Kreidler et al, 2000; Valente, 2005).

## On the Adult

For many victims of childhood sexual abuse, the process of surviving childhood and adolescence and becoming an adult is similar to delayed PTSD responses: repression of memories (even nonsexual ones), followed by a breakthrough of unwanted, intrusive memories. The memories might begin as nightmares, kinesthetic sensations (such as flinching or vaginal pain when touched by a partner in the same way as the perpetrator), or flashbacks. The memories might return gradually, in pieces, or in a sudden, overwhelming flood. Victims cannot be rushed to remember the abuse before they are ready to cope with it.

On the surface, adult victims might look relatively uninjured because of denial, dissociation, amnesia, emotional deadening, or repression. They enter counseling for manifestations of the abuse rather than for the incest or sexual abuse itself. The list of typical reactions in Box 41-3 can be used as a checklist to identify the issues to be addressed in counseling. Victims who see this list typically express amazement (that so much has resulted from the sexual abuse) and relief (that there is finally an explanation for all their "craziness"). Up to this point, victims might tend to deny or minimize the relationship of the sexual abuse to any of their current problems. It then becomes evident to victims that the event has disturbed their entire growth and development process and their self-esteem, and has set them up for other abusive relationships. Only one third of victims ever receive counseling specifically focusing on the childhood sexual abuse (Gladstone et al, 2004). Until counseling finally focuses on the anger and underlying cause of their reactions, victims tend to seek treatment repeatedly, without relief.

The inability to handle the memories of abuse and the painful emotions, especially anger, often induces thoughts of suicide to escape the pain and depression, to die with the secret, to avoid conflict with the family or perpetrator, to stop feeling "crazy," and to end the nightmares and flashbacks that are so frightening. Self-harm or mutilation, without even feeling the pain, is a common way of dealing with the emotional pain, loss, rage, and abandonment. Dissociation during the mutilation is common. Victims describe various patterns of their mutilation (ANAD, 2002; Cerdorian, 2005; Starr, 2004):

## Box 41-3    Adult Manifestations of Childhood Sexual Abuse

**Memory Disturbances**
Amnesia about the abuse
Memory gaps about childhood
Inability to think straight

**Keeping Unnecessary Secrets**

*Relationship Issues*
Trouble connecting with others
Running away from others
Fear of men or fear of women
Trouble trusting others and their motives
Fear of intimacy
Fear of abandonment and rejection
Unable to maintain intimacy
Trouble giving and receiving affection
Feeling alienated from others
Fear of being used/abused
Trouble saying "no"
Taking care of others
Trouble with parenting
Entering abusive relationships
Poor choices of partners

*Body Symptoms*
Vague and transient pains
Memories of physical pain
Chronic pain or migraine headaches
Gagging, nausea, vomiting
Unpleasant sensation when touched
Negative, distorted body image
Self-conscious about body
Overly conscious of appearance

*Anger Issues*
Fear of expressing anger
Holding anger in
Crying instead of being angry
Fantasies of revenge
Feeling violent, full of rage
Fear of violence
Homicidal thoughts

*Anxiety Issues*
Easily startled
Inability to relax
Fear of being attacked, exposed
Hypervigilance
Feeling like a frightened child
Fear of the dark
Panic attacks
Phobias, agoraphobia

*Addiction Issues*
Alcohol/drug abuse or dependence
Compulsive spending

*Intrusive Thoughts and Memories*
Intense nightmares, unwanted thoughts
Flashbacks: feeling, seeing, smelling, tasting, hearing

*Detachment Issues*
Feeling numb, unreal
Disconnected from feelings from body
Feeling as if there are "personalities" inside
"Out-of-body" experiences

*Control Issues*
Fear of authority, rules
Need to be in control, feeling out of control
Pretending to be out of control (or helpless)
Fear of being vulnerable
Ambivalent about being taken care of
Letting others be in control
Trying to control others
Allowing children to be abused

*Identity Issues*
Confusion about identity or roles
Negative self-image
Need to be perfect or perfectly bad
Underachievement or overachievement
Need to be totally competent

*Sexual Issues*
Concealing sexual feelings
Discomfort with sexual touching
Feeling nonsexual
Lack of orgasms, sexual dysfunctions
Confusion about sexuality/sexual identity
Feeling "dirty"
Trading sex for favors
Promiscuity, prostitution
Wondering if one is gay

*Self-Punishment*
Suicidal thoughts, attempts
Wanting to die or to be dead
Self-mutilation
Compulsive eating or dieting
Bingeing, purging

*Other Feelings*
Low self-esteem, guilt, shame
Fear of feelings
Feeling stuck
Feeling like a failure
Chronic dissatisfaction
Frozen emotions
Lack of a sense of humor
Feeling inadequate
Feeling walled in
Feeling "crazy"

1. When feeling overwhelmed, they inflict harm as a cry for help when they believe that no one is listening or cares.
2. When emotions build up, they go numb or dissociate and have to inflict pain to make sure that they can still feel.
3. When they are feeling unreal (depersonalization), they draw blood to make sure that they are alive.
4. They cause physical pain so that they do not have to focus on the emotional pain.
5. They punish themselves when they are feeling self-loathing, guilt, shame, or fear.
6. They use the mutilation as a way of avoiding suicide.
7. They use the mutilation to relieve the anger or rage toward self and others.
8. They might use the mutilation as an attempt to manipulate others.
9. The mutilation might become chronic and addictive, especially if it produces a high (related to endogenous opiates/endorphines).

Some evidence has suggested that suicide attempts might have share similar, as well as unique, dynamics as self-mutilation and also might become a chronic pattern or addiction (Mynatt, 2000).

Alcohol and drugs are often used to avoid or numb the pain and memories and to bring fleeting pleasure that is otherwise elusive (Davis and Petretic-Jackson, 2000; Gladstone et al, 2004). Food might also provide brief pleasure or fill an emptiness inside (bingeing), but leads to feeling bloated and guilty and a need to purge. Although sex is not usually enjoyable, it can bring relief from loneliness, temporary attention, affection, and approval. On the other hand, sexual encounters might trigger traumatic flashbacks, anxiety, fear, shame, disgust, or a sense of helplessness. Healthy adult relationships and sexual intimacy are difficult because of problems in trusting anyone and the history of linking abuse and love. Victims have boundary issues, trouble setting limits with others, and difficulty with asking for what they really need (Davis and Petretic-Jackson, 2000). Victims also tend to be caretakers, rescuers, and codependents.

Victims' reactions to the trauma (see Box 41-3) are often labeled as clinical symptoms. When an Axis I diagnosis is given to patients, it is commonly depression (atypical type), PTSD, substance abuse disorder, eating disorder, anxiety disorder, somatoform disorder, dissociative disorder (including dissociative identity disorder), or impulse-control disorder. Axis II personality disorder diagnoses are commonly borderline, narcissistic, histrionic, avoidant, dependent, atypical, or mixed disorders (Davis and Petretic-Jackson, 2000; Kreidler et al, 2000).

Receiving a diagnosis is a major problem, not only because of the stigma and blaming the victim, but also because the diagnosis often becomes the focus of treatment rather than the underlying issues. Lack of appropriate treatment carries a major risk, not only for adult survivors but also for their children, especially if the survivors are still in a stage of repression. Evidence has suggested that untreated or improperly treated victims occasionally set up dysfunctional, disorganized families, in which there is incestuous abuse of the children. With their own denial, repression, amnesia, or other mechanisms, survivors have trouble relating to their partners and are unable to see the partners' involvement with their children. Perpetrators (and occasionally victims) might sexually abuse their younger siblings, children, grandchildren, nieces, nephews, and others. Examples of incest have surfaced within three and four generations of a family. Breaking this cycle is of crucial importance.

## CLINICAL EXAMPLE

Jan Lester, 30 years of age, was admitted to a psychiatric unit as a result of suicidal ideations and 12 superficial cuts on her wrists. Nine months ago, she began having nightmares about being awakened at night as a child with someone on top of her. During the nightmares, she would wake up crying with strange body sensations, gagging, pressure on her chest, and vaginal pain. As the nightmares and memories became more complete and vivid, she realized her father had frequently had sex with her while her mother was asleep. As her father's fiftieth birthday approached, she felt as if she could not tolerate going to his party. She wanted to be dead but was unable to force herself to cut her wrists more deeply. She wanted help.

## RECOVERY

In some ways, recovery from childhood sexual abuse or incest is similar to recovery from all crimes and/or from PTSD, but it tends to be more complex, difficult, and lengthy by comparison, especially if emotional abuse by the family is ongoing or if the survivor still lives with the abuser. The memories and emotions are strong, painful, and confusing. The intense anger and ambivalence toward the perpetrator (because the victim is still seeking approval and love from the perpetrator) are hard for both the survivors and nurse to handle. Survivors need to know in the beginning that the symptoms and emotional pain will probably worsen before they improve as the experiences are reviewed. Therefore, survivors need to learn emotion management to tolerate the distress and use safety measures prior to using imaginal exposure techniques (Dunbar, 2004; Goodwin, 2005). (See the discussion of dialectical behavioral therapy [DBT] in Chapter 4 and systematic desensitization in Chapter 38.)

Although outpatient counseling often takes 2 years or longer, survivors tend to engage in treatment sporadically. It is common for survivors to initially disclose, discuss, vent, and feel cured. Then, as new crises or relationship problems emerge, survivors return to counseling to deal with each issue and its possible connection to the original trauma. Getting a patient to commit to continuous, long-term counseling is sometimes difficult, but the nurse can emphasize the desirability and value of at least sporadic counseling.

The overall goals of recovery are safety and security, rebuilding trust, improved self-esteem and self-acceptance, forgiveness of self, adaptive coping with life and its stresses, assertiveness skills, the capacity for intimate relationships and genuine sexual pleasure, improvements in affect, and reduced anxiety, anger, shame, guilt, fear, and dissociation, as well as the prevention of suicide and sexual abuse of future generations (Davis and Petretic-Jackson, 2000; Kreidler et al, 2000).

## PUTTING IT ALL TOGETHER
### Psychotherapeutic Management

## NURSE-PATIENT RELATIONSHIP

Much depends on the nurse's ability to develop a trusting relationship with the survivor quickly. Empathy, active support, compassion, warmth, and being nonjudgmental are crucial. Survivors need to be calmly and matter of factly asked about childhood sexual abuse, because they are not likely to reveal it spontaneously. The old and perhaps current coercions to keep the secret remain strong in the minds of survivors; they need to feel safe about confidentiality and the nurse's acceptance before disclosure can occur. How much detail is revealed and how soon depends, in part, on the nurse's ability to be receptive to the experiences without being critical of the perpetrator, of other adults in the family, or of the survivor's loyalty to them. The survivor needs to be reassured that all the experiences and emotions (positive, negative, and ambivalent) are valid and that exploring them is the beginning of the process of working through recovery (Davis and Petretic-Jackson, 2000). It is usually helpful for survivors to be reminded periodically that they were not responsible for and did not deserve the sexual abuse, are not to be blamed, were not in control of the situation, and that the way they coped in the past was the best they could do at the time. Cognitive-behavioral approaches and education about the dynamics of sexual abuse and reassurances about recovery can be useful in correcting faulty perceptions about the abuse, decreasing self-blame and guilt, and instilling hope for the future despite the inability to change the past. (See Key Nursing Interventions for Survivors of Childhood Abuse box.)

Mentally and emotionally reexperiencing traumatic events (see discussion of imaginal exposure in Chapter 38) is disturbing; only periodic, small doses might be tolerable. It is helpful to remind survivors that they went through the abuse alone, but do not have to remember it alone. If traumatic flashbacks or dissociation occur, it is important to bring the survivors back to the present by reminding them where they are and that the nurse is with them now. The nurse and survivors can monitor their safety and tolerance of the process to prevent becoming overwhelmed, retreating, attempting suicide, or self-mutilating. Anger release strategies, such as using a foam bat (batacca) while talking to a chair that represents the perpetrator or nonprotective adult, often help the survivor express thoughts and feelings that could not be expressed in childhood. Play therapy, therapeutic stories, and art therapy can be especially useful in helping children process their abuse (Bennett, 1997; Hinds, 1997). Writing memories and painful feelings in an ongoing journal and writing "letters," which will not be sent, to the perpetrator and nonprotectors can be useful (Cerdorian, 2005).

## Key Nursing Interventions *for Survivors of Childhood Abuse*

- Contract for safety and control of impulses to harm self or others.
- Set limits on self-destructive or self-harm patterns.
- Establish a trusting and supportive environment.
- Accept all feelings and reactions as normal responses.
- Ask permission before touching survivors.
- Reinforce that recovery is possible, even if it is difficult.
- Educate about the dynamics of abuse and recovery processes.
- Assist survivors in understanding current behaviors as reflections of survival strategies used in childhood.
- Facilitate reevaluation of the sexual abuse, its circumstances, and its effects, but without pressuring.
- Encourage coping choices that are in survivors' best interests.
- Discuss safeguarding other children if the perpetrator still poses a risk.
- Support choices about future disclosures, confrontation, or reporting.
- Be aware that family members and others might feel split loyalty and engage in dysfunctional roles and interaction patterns.
- Decrease feelings of isolation, shame, and stigma.
- Encourage self-acceptance.
- Facilitate acknowledgment, forgiveness, and love for the child within.
- Teach and encourage stress management and anger reduction.
- Facilitate the transfer of responsibility and anger to the perpetrator but set limits on acting out fantasies of revenge.
- Foster separation and individuation from the family and its patterns.
- Help to find meaning in the experience and mourning of all the losses (grieving is a very painful experience).
- Facilitate the change from victim to survivor status (reexperiencing and integrating the positive, negative, and ambivalent feelings and memories).
- Facilitate reexperiencing and reworking of maturational tasks that were missed or experienced prematurely.
- Educate about life skills, communication skills, coping skills, assertiveness, decision making, conflict resolution, boundary setting, friendship, intimacy, sexuality, and parenting.
- Refer to outpatient counseling and appropriate support groups.

Confrontation of the family or perpetrator by the survivor is not necessarily a desired outcome or safe option. Confrontation might be done symbolically or verbally with the nurse and/or in the letters, rather than directly with the perpetrator and other family members. If survivors choose to confront directly, much preparation is needed before this can happen. Survivors need to consider, plan for, and rehearse their reactions to all the typical responses of family members, such as denial, rationalization, and blaming the victim. Confessions and apologies are unlikely. (See the family issues box.) Survivors can be helped to debate the benefits and risks of confrontation, as well as the degree and type of contact they want to have with the family, even if they do not confront them or if the survivors need to protect their own children. An important consideration for the nurse and survivor to discuss is the mandatory reporting of child abuse if younger children are currently victims of abuse. This type of reporting is understandably difficult for both the nurse and the survivor, but needs to be carefully and directly addressed.

When survivors are in outpatient counseling, it is important to consider priorities in each counseling session. Current crises and problems need to be addressed (instead of the sexual abuse) as they arise. For example, gynecologic and physical examinations might be distressing and trigger flashbacks (Roberts, 2000). This aspect is also critical for self-destructive behaviors that are increased because of counseling, such as suicidal ideation, self-mutilation, and substance abuse. Hospitalization might be necessary if the crisis is severe. Although survivors view recovery as frightening and painful, they also experience relief that they are making progress.

## PSYCHOPHARMACOLOGY

Medications are not always needed or desirable for adult survivors of childhood sexual abuse, especially if substance abuse is a problem or potential problem. For the small number of survivors with serious psychopathology, medications should be given according to the Axis I diagnosis, such as depression. An antidepressant such as trazodone (Desyrel) might be used if the depressive symptoms are interfering with sleep. Benzodiazepines or clonidine might be given on a short-term basis to help control the emotional or autonomic arousal that occurs during the reexperiencing of traumatic memories. Occasionally, low doses of risperidone (Risperdal) or quetiapine (Seroquel) are given for persistent and severely disturbing nightmares, flashbacks, and/or agitation.

## MILIEU MANAGEMENT

On an outpatient basis and during any brief hospitalizations, cognitive-behavioral and affect management groups can be a useful adjunct to nursing care (Kreidler et al, 2000). If available, a short-term or ongoing sexual abuse or incest recovery group is beneficial. Some self-help groups include Incest Survivors Anonymous, Survivors of Sexual Abuse, and Daughters and Sons United. Parents United (for the nonperpetrator parent) can be suggested, if appropriate. The perpetrator might also be referred to counseling. Family therapy is sometimes appropriate.

Other groups that might be recommended, depending on the symptoms and needs of the survivor, are Co-dependency Anonymous, Adult Children of Alcoholics, Alcoholics or Narcotics Anonymous, and Emotions Anonymous. Survivors might also be directed to classes or short-term groups that address issues such as decision making, problem solving, communication or relationship skills, conflict resolution, anger management, parenting skills, and human sexuality.

### CRITICAL THINKING QUESTION    1

You are working with a patient who was sexually abused as a child by her father. The father insists on visiting his daughter and telling you about her history of emotional problems and lying about the family. What is your approach in working with the father?

## PARTNER ABUSE

## NATURE OF THE PROBLEM

Estimates are that more than 25% to 50% of men and women worldwide (from adolescents to the elderly) have suffered physical assault by a partner at least once in their lifetime (Daniels, 2005; Dutton and Nicholls, 2005; Miller, 2004; Tilley and Brackley, 2004). The number is even higher when psychological abuse and other violations of rights are considered (Figure 41-1; Daniels, 2005; Dutton and Nicholls, 2005). It is difficult to collect statistics on female to female, female to male, and male to male abuse because of the lack of reporting (Dutton and Nicholls, 2005). Women are abused, raped, tortured, or beaten by their husband, boyfriend or girlfriend, male or female lover, former partner, or estranged partner (Daniels, 2005), and most of this abuse goes unreported, even when injuries are severe enough to require treatment. Prior partner abuse increases the risk of it occurring during pregnancy (Tilley and Brackley, 2004). In primary care practice, it has been estimated that 34% to 46% of the female patients are victims of partner abuse (Lie and Barclay, 2005b).

Dating violence in the adolescent population is estimated to be 10% to 35%, and there is a trend for this to occur in younger age groups than in past years. Even middle school children (grades 6 through 8) are being affected as they get into emotional and sexual dating relationships. Contributing factors for these children include witnessing parental violence, prior victimization or abuse, earlier puberty, typical stresses and issues of early adolescence, earlier use of drugs and alcohol, and exposure to media violence (Close, 2005; Miller, 2004).

Partner abuse victims tend to conceal their victimization. They are acutely aware that disclosure of their plight will be met with denial or be minimized by the partner, friends, and relatives and by increased abuse by their partners (Merrell, 2001). As abused women become more independent (both emotionally and financially), the incidence of violence by their partners increases as well. The fact that 30% to 50% of all women killed in the United States are killed by a partner as they tried to leave or had left supports women's fears (Gerard, 2000; Jordan, 2004; Logan and Walker, 2004).

## Family Issues: False Memories? False Allegations?

Some families, including members of the False Memory Syndrome Foundation, claim that they have been wrongly accused of sexual abuse by their children or adult children. These families and some professionals especially challenge the validity of the processes of repression and delayed recovery of memories of abuse. They warn that those who interview children, those who counsel children and adults, and members of support groups can implant false memories and provide support for false allegations. These families and professionals question the credentials and training of many who counsel children and adults who claim that they were abused. They cite studies of recent and long-term memory to support their views about distorted and false memories. They sometimes question the claims of serious emotional damage to victims as a result of actual sexual abuse. They support the premise that false memories and false allegations are destroying the families of these children.

Other professionals and adult survivors of childhood sexual abuse maintain that the graphic details of children's traumatic memories and the use of sexual descriptions, very advanced for their age at the time, support the credibility of the abuse charges. These professionals and survivors claim that denial, repression, amnesia, and dissociation are real and are used by children, adolescents, and adults to protect themselves emotionally from the abuse as it was happening and from the later realization of its moral, legal, ethical, and emotional significance. These individuals maintain that 75% or more of survivors are able to collect strong corroborating evidence of their abuse and recovered memories. They cite recent neurochemical studies of traumatic memory processes, stress, and PTSD (see Chapter 31) to support their view of the validity of repression, dissociation, and recovered memories. They acknowledge that 2% to

10% of claims of sexual abuse by children and divorcing parents might be false, but report that perhaps 75% to 90% of valid child abuse is never reported by children, agencies, and professionals. They point out that the False Memory Syndrome Foundation admits that it collects only information on denials of charges of abuse but has no way of knowing if these denials are true or false. Survivors and professionals contend that those who molest children typically threaten the victims to "keep the secret" and use denial, minimization, and rationalization when charged with abuse. They also express concern that claims of false memories and false allegations are efforts to disconfirm and "blame the victim," protect abusers (and society), and minimize the severity of the short- and long-term effects of abuse. They contend that families are being destroyed by interfamilial violence (not the reports of abuse) and that abused children suffer emotional pain and a wide variety of problems throughout childhood, adolescence, and adulthood.

As a result of this controversy, it is recommended that those working with possible survivors of childhood sexual abuse do the following:

1. Allow patients' memories to emerge without pressure and leading questions.
2. Avoid specific sexual abuse explanations for patients' symptoms.
3. Follow established guidelines for interviewing child victims and others to assess the credibility of memories and testimony.
4. Interview anyone who might provide corroboration or disconfirming evidence.
5. Use established therapeutic techniques rather than nonestablished methods.
6. Avoid using hypnosis and sodium amytal injections as a way of recovering repressed memories.

Modified from Gardner RA: *True and false accusations of child sex abuse,* New York, 1992; Leavitt F: Iatrogenic memory change: examining the empirical evidence, *Forensic Psychology* 19:21, 2001; Loftus EF, Potage DC: Repressed memories: when are they real? *Psychiatr Clin North Am* 22:61, 1999; Valente S: Controversies and challenges of ritual abuse, *J Psychosoc Nurs* 38:8, 2000; Satel SL: Who needs trauma initiatives? *Psychiatr Serv* 52:815, 2001; van der Kolk B, McFarlane AC, Weissaeth L: *Traumatic stress: the effects of overwhelming experience on mind, body, and society,* New York, 1996, Guilford Press; Anorexia Nervosa and Associated Disorders (Indianapolis Chapter of National ANAD): Personal interviews, Indianapolis, 2002, ANAD; Katchen MH: Ritual abuse vs religious abuse: the development of an artificial distinction, *MKzine* 3:9, 2005.

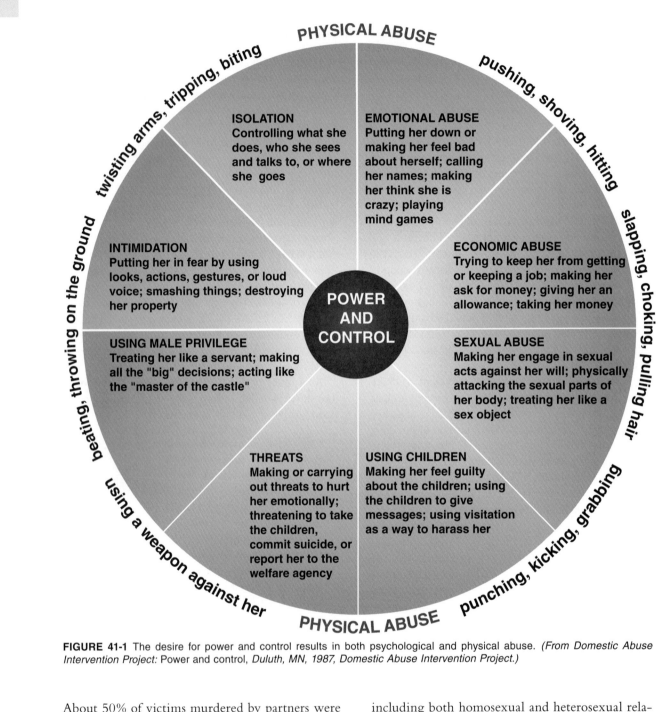

**FIGURE 41-1** The desire for power and control results in both psychological and physical abuse. *(From Domestic Abuse Intervention Project: Power and control, Duluth, MN, 1987, Domestic Abuse Intervention Project.)*

About 50% of victims murdered by partners were seen in the emergency departments for injuries at other times before they died (Gerard, 2000). Men are also killed by their partners (4% of all male homicides; Daniels, 2005). Homicide occurs, sometimes in self-defense during the abuse or after a history of beatings.

Studies have shown that partner abuse crosses all social, racial, cultural, and economic classes,

including both homosexual and heterosexual relationships, but is more often reported by individuals on welfare. This tendency is because the victims are more likely to be in contact with reporting agencies, such as public health nurses, welfare offices, public clinics, and emergency rooms. Individuals with higher incomes are likely to obtain private services that do not report the abuse (Poirier, 2000). Nurses in any setting need to screen patients for any past or current abuse (Lewis-O'Connor, 2004).

The relationship of alcohol and drug abuse to violent behavior has been the subject of many studies on partner abuse. Some abusers are abstainers, but more are substance abusers (Murphy et al, 2005). The victim's view is that the abuser uses alcohol and drugs as an excuse for their violence and drink when they are about to become violent. Victims have also reported a correlation between increased intake of alcohol and the severity of violence (Murphy et al, 2005). The combination of substance abuse and violence encourages victims to blame the substance rather than hold the batterers accountable for their violent behaviors. Women often describe their abusers as *Dr. Jekyll and Mr. Hyde,* with changing personalities—gentle, loving, and kind at times; rude, uncaring, and violent at other times. This change is explained, in part, by the cycle of violence described later.

In some relationships, violence is mutual (Dutton and Nicholls, 2005) and is the result of efforts to resolve negative communications and escalating conflicts. These couples are often motivated to change and can be taught more effective skills for handling conflict and anger. This mutual violence pattern differs from, but can become, the more common pattern of using violence to exploit and control a partner, often arising out of anger, fear of abandonment, and jealousy (McClellan and Killeen, 2000). This second pattern almost always involves a man abusing a woman, and the man has little motivation to change. Separate interventions and therapy with the man might interrupt the cycle of violence (Merrell, 2001). Other studies have reported that men and women use violence almost equally in the nonmutual abuse pattern and those with Axis II personality disorders have somewhat higher rates of violence with their partners (Dutton and Nicholls, 2005).

The nature of modern society is a factor to be considered in partner abuse. The portrayal of physical and sexual violence in the media (e.g., the Internet, television, music videos, and films) continues to increase in frequency and severity. Women are still portrayed by the media as second-class citizens at times. However, women younger than 30 are more aggressive in their intimate relationships than women older than 30 (Dutton and Nicholls, 2005). In addition, it is well documented that witnesses of family violence and victims of child abuse and neglect tend to become perpetrators of other violence or the abusers and partners of abusers (Smith et al, 2004; Woods and Wineman, 2004).

## EFFECTS

Most experts acknowledge the development of learned helplessness, hopelessness, isolation, and resignation in response to ongoing emotional and physical abuse. Abused women report that they fear and hate the abuse, but have a tendency to believe their partner's view that they deserve the abuse. Box 41-4 presents common reasons why women endure long-term abuse. Another accepted

---

**Box 41-4   Why Women Stay as Long as They Do**

**Situational Factors**
- Economic dependence; lack of job skills
- Fear of greater physical danger to themselves and their children if they attempt to leave or have partner arrested
- Fear of emotional damage to children because of being without a father
- Fear of losing custody of children
- Lack of alternative housing
- Social isolation; lack of support from family or friends
- Lack of information regarding alternatives
- Fear of involvement in court processes
- Fear of retaliation from partner or partner's family

**Emotional Factors**
- Poor self-image; fear of being alone
- Being in a state of denial and living a secret
- Personal embarrassment and protecting the image of husband and family
- Insecurity over potential independence and lack of emotional support
- Guilt about failure of marriage or relationship
- Fear that partner is not able to survive alone
- Belief that partner is sick and needs her help
- Belief that partner will change
- Ambivalence and fear about making formidable life changes and having increased responsibility

**Cultural Factors**
- Knowing that batterers are not held accountable for their violent actions
- Believing that the abuse is her fault
- Being raised to be passive and submissive
- Developing survival skills instead of escape skills
- Recognizing that the legal system is a male-dominated system

**Plus: She Still Loves Him**

Modified from Julian Center Shelter, Indianapolis, and Task Force on Families in Crisis, Nashville, TN.

view of why women endure abuse is the cycle of violence (Box 41-5). During the honeymoon stage, the good side of the man is evident, and the woman is reminded of their love and the happy potential of the relationship (Farella, 2000; Gerard, 2000; Walker, 1979). Women report thinking that they can help their partners overcome their problems and violent behaviors. There is still a shortage of safe places to go, as well as a shortage of services to help victims become independent. Many states still have ineffective or outdated laws that indirectly perpetuate abuse rather than foster

arrest of the abuser for assault and battery. Arrest is a way that batterers get the message that their violence is a crime and not their right (Jordan, 2004; Williams, 2005).

Battered woman syndrome has been suggested as a subclassification of PTSD because repetitive abuse is a serious threat to the victim's health and life. Victims often report nightmares, flashbacks, recurrent fears of more violence, emotional detachment, numbness, startle response, sleep problems, guilt, impaired concentration, and hypervigilance. However, there are other symptoms, such as

---

**Box 41-5 Cycle of Violence**

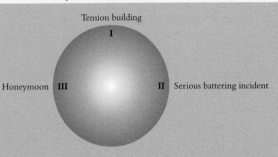

Tension building

I

Honeymoon III    II Serious battering incident

**Man**

*I. Tension building*
He has excessively high expectations of her.
He blames her for anything that goes wrong.
He does not try to control his behaviors.
He is aware of his inappropriate behaviors but does not admit it.
Verbal and minor physical abuse increase.
Afraid that she will leave, he gets more possessive to keep her captive.
He gets frantic and more controlling.
He misinterprets her withdrawal as rejection.

*II. Serious battering incident*
The trigger event is an internal or external event or substance.
The battering usually occurs in private.
He will threaten more harm if she tries to get help (police, medical).
He tries to justify his behaviors but does not understand what happens.
He minimizes the severity of the abuse.
His stress is relieved.

*III. Honeymoon*
He is loving, charming, begging for forgiveness, making promises.
He truly believes that he will never abuse again.

He feels that he taught her a lesson and she will not act up again.
He preys on her guilt to keep her trapped.

**Woman**

*I. Tension building*
She is nurturing, compliant, and tries to please him.
She denies the seriousness of their problems.
She feels she can control his behaviors.
She tries to alter his behavior to stay safe.
She tries to prevent his anger.
She blames external factors: alcohol, work.
She takes minor abuse, but does not feel she deserves it.
She gets scared and tries to hide (withdrawal).
She might call for help as the tension becomes unbearable.

*II. Serious battering incident*
In cases of long-term battering, she might provoke it just to get it over with.
She might call for help if she is afraid of being killed.
Her initial reaction is shock, disbelief, and denial.
Fearing more abuse if police come, she might plead for them not to arrest him.
She is anxious, ashamed, humiliated, sleepless, fatigued, depressed.
She does not seek help for injuries for a day or more and lies about the cause of injuries.

*III. Honeymoon*
She sees his loving behaviors as the real person and tries to make up.
She wants to believe that the abuse will never happen again.
She feels that if she stays, he will get help; the thought of leaving makes her feel guilty.
She believes in the permanency of the relationship and gets trapped.

Modified from Walker L: *The battered woman,* New York, 1979, Harper & Row; Gerard M: Domestic violence: how to screen and intervene, *RN* 63:52, 2000; McFarlane J, Malecha A, Gist J, et al: Increasing the safety promoting behaviors of abused women, *Am J Nurs* 104:40, 2004.

depression, hostility, low self-esteem, self-blame, relative passivity, impaired decision making, psychosomatic complaints, fatalism, social isolation, and an unwillingness to seek help (ANAD, 2002; Logan and Walker, 2004). As with PTSD, battered women show typical reactions to a chronic trauma, not symptoms of psychopathology. Labeling and blaming the victims again shifts responsibility away from the perpetrators.

According to victims, it is unlikely that abused women will leave their partners until they realize that the cycle is not going to stop and they have the emotional support to leave and a safe place to go. Fearing that the next beating might be fatal, finding that their partners are physically or sexually abusing their children, and realizing that their children are learning to be abusive are incentives for leaving permanently (ANAD, 2002; Miller, 2004).

## RECOVERY

Immediately preceding or at the beginning of a serious battering incident, victims are frightened, amenable to crisis intervention, and more likely to call the police or a crisis service agency for help. Getting victims and their children to a shelter or other safe place, if they will go, is desirable when immediate danger of injury is present. If injuries have occurred, victims should be encouraged to go to an emergency department. In any case, crisis workers, shelter workers, or nurses can begin the important process of assessment and providing information that can make a dent in the cycle of abuse. Even if the survivors are not yet ready to leave their partners, they can be given an easily concealed card with telephone numbers of police, prosecutors, crisis services, victims' assistance, shelters, and support groups, and perhaps a short message about the inevitability of the cycle of violence and the fact that no one deserves to be abused. If contact is only by phone or if they are worried that the abusers will find the card, they can be asked to write down the phone numbers on the back of a picture in their wallets or be told to call 911. (In some cities, such as Indianapolis, dialing 211 provides a direct connection to the Domestic Violence Network.) Survivors can also be given ideas for developing a safety or escape plan (Daniels, 2005), such as packing a bag with medicines and clothes for them and their children, house and car keys,

money and change for the pay telephone (if they don't have a cell phone), and important phone numbers and papers (e.g., bank account numbers, birth certificates, social security numbers, medical insurance cards, no contact orders). They should also be informed of the protections afforded by legal statutes, protective orders, and more recent antistalking laws. Long-term goals for survivors of partner abuse are to develop self-confidence, self-respect, independence, healthy support systems, and a sense of freedom, safety, and empowerment.

## PUTTING IT ALL TOGETHER
### Psychotherapeutic Management

## NURSE-PATIENT RELATIONSHIP

Because most abused women seek help for their injuries and somatic symptoms at least once, nurses can be instrumental in offering information and assistance. Nurses in emergency departments, clinics, physicians' offices, and community health agencies need to know how to recognize a survivor, make an assessment, and make a referral to available services. Some common cues to abuse are listed in Box 41-6. The assessment process is often difficult because survivors fear disclosure, are embarrassed about the situation, desire to be treated quickly and leave, and sometimes the abusers are present. It is important to interview the victim privately and with sensitivity, empathy, and compassion. Box 41-7 describes other responses that survivors consider helpful.

The most crucial information to document in an initial contact is the following:

1. Identity and current location of the abuser
2. Location and safety of any children
3. Length and frequency of abuse
4. Types of abuse (physical, psychological, sexual, financial) and use of weapons
5. Types and locations of injuries (photographs and body maps are preferred)
6. Availability of weapons at the place of residence
7. Use and abuse of substances and medications by victim and abuser
8. Active and passive suicidal ideations (with or without a plan or a wish to be dead)

### Box 41-6 Common Cues to Partner Abuse

- Repeated, vague symptoms or illnesses that are not confirmed by tests, such as backache, abdominal pain, indigestion, headaches, hyperventilation, anxiety, insomnia, fatigue, anorexia, heart palpitations
- Unexplained injuries or ones with unlikely explanations and embarrassment about them
- Hidden injuries such as those in areas concealed by clothes or visible on physical or x-ray examination only—for example, head and neck injuries, internal injuries, genital injuries, scars, burns, joint pain or dislocations, numbness, hearing problems, or bald spots
- Injuries with recognizable marks such as those from a belt, iron, raised ring, teeth, fingertips, cigarette, gun, or knife
- Multiple fractures or bruises in various stages of healing
- Jumpiness or flinching in the presence of the abuser
- Substance abuse and suicidal thoughts or attempts
- Attempts to conceal fear of the partner
- Continual efforts to keep partner from getting angry
- Denial of any problems in the relationship
- Lack of relationships with family or friends
- Isolation or confinement to home
- Guilt, depression, anxiety, low self-esteem, sense of failure, concealed anger
- Continual justification of own actions and whereabouts to partner
- Continual justification of the abuser's actions in public; excusing or rationalizing the behaviors
- Believing in family unity at all costs and in traditional stereotypes
- Believing in managing alone, even when help is offered
- An oversolicitous partner who does not want to leave the victim alone with hospital or agency staff or even with family and friends

Modified from Constantine RE, Bricker PL: Social support, stress, and depression among battered women in the judicial setting, *J Am Psychiatr Nurses Assoc* 3:81, 1997; Merrell J: Social support for victims of domestic violence, *J Psychosoc Nurs* 39:31, 2001; Miller MC: Countering domestic violence, *Harv Ment Health Lett* 20:1, 2004.

### Box 41-7 Helpful Responses to Partner Abuse

- Be nonjudgmental, objective, and nonthreatening.
- Ask directly if abuse is occurring.
- Identify the abuser's behavior as abusive.
- Acknowledge the seriousness of the abuse.
- Assist the victim in assessing internal strengths.
- Encourage the use of personal resources.
- Give the victim a list of resources: shelters, financial aid, police, and legal assistance.
- Allow victim to choose own options.
- Offer names of relevant support groups.
- Help victim to develop a safety or escape plan.
- Tell the abuser to stop the abuse and get help.
- Do not disbelieve or blame the victim.
- Do not get angry with the victim.
- Do not refuse to help if the victim is not ready to leave the abuser.
- Do not align with the abuser against the victim.
- Do not push the victim to leave the abuser before ready.

9. Types of service desired (police, legal, shelter, crisis counseling, knowledgeable clergy, social service agencies, and transportation)
10. Referrals made

Even if the initial contact is brief, it is important to convey to survivors that they are not alone in their abuse and that there are those who are willing and able to help when they are ready. Survivors also need to be told more than once that they do not deserve the abuse. The nurse must convey to survivors that they are important and have dignity and worth. They need acknowledgment of their mental and physical exhaustion, fears, and ambivalence about the abuser, leaving, and their wish to help the abuser, as well as themselves. It is difficult for nurses and all professionals to accept that survivors cannot be pushed, rushed, or coerced into leaving the abuser before they are ready. In fact, survivors might want to try couples' counseling and even personal counseling (when the abuser refuses counseling) more than once before giving up hope of saving the relationship and of helping the ones they love. It is important to recognize and to acknowledge that it is common for survivors to leave and return several times. Survivors need not feel guilty or ashamed for trying to improve the relationship. In fact, the guilt of leaving will be lessened if they believe they have tried everything and are finally able to acknowledge that nothing will change, because the abusers are the only ones who can control the violence and stop the abuse.

When an abused woman does leave her partner, the problems are not over. Box 41-8 describes some of the common reactions the abuser might have and ways in which he might behave. Psychological and physical abuse might continue after

## Box 41-8   If You Have Left an Abusive Man . . .

1. Your problems are not over.
2. Your abuser will try to locate you through family and friends. He will play on their sympathy or intimidate them.
3. He will repeatedly apologize, make promises about changing, and give gifts.
4. Next, he will threaten or intimidate you, your children, family, and/or friends.
5. He might threaten to kill himself because of you.
6. He often threatens to take your children away.
7. In another step, he will enter counseling and/or will express religious fervor.
8. He might try to find a counselor or religious leader to try to convince you to return to him.
9. Next, he might harass and stalk (begging, crying, phone calls, written or verbal threats, legal actions, or following you from location to location).

Regardless of his tactics, take advantage of legal, community, and personal resources to protect yourself and your children.

Modified from the Salvation Army Domestic Violence Program, Indianapolis.

12. Decreasing co-dependency behaviors
13. Building a new, improved support system
14. Setting goals and specific plans for immediate future
15. Resolving grief

Referrals might also be needed for job counseling or training, legal assistance, financial aid, child care, and permanent housing. At any stage during working with survivors, brief hospitalization might be needed because of injuries, suicide attempts, self-mutilation, or substance abuse and for treatment of serious problems such as depression, anxiety, or panic attacks.

### CRITICAL THINKING QUESTION   2

Your co-worker is sharing with you that she is thinking about leaving her husband because of his drinking and long-term emotional abuse of her. She expresses a fear that he might try to kill her and a fear of raising her two children alone. What information would you offer her?

separation (Logan and Walker, 2004). Survivors frequently need longer term counseling and social services to recover and become independent, especially if the abuser is unwilling to participate in couples' counseling or an abusers' program (often a court-ordered program of group education and counseling lasting 26 weeks or longer). Nursing interventions for survivors (individually or in groups, using cognitive-behavioral techniques) generally focus on the following:

1. Monitoring safety from partner abuse and preventing suicide
2. Reiterating information about abuse, the cycle of violence, and the abuser's accountability
3. Building self-esteem, confidence, independence, and sense of hope
4. Sharing of feelings, especially anger, frustration, fear, and anxiety
5. Decreasing shame, guilt, embarrassment, manipulation, and isolation
6. Confirming personal rights, as well as legal rights
7. Teaching stress management techniques
8. Teaching communication techniques
9. Teaching conflict resolution techniques
10. Teaching assertiveness training
11. Teaching parenting techniques

## PSYCHOPHARMACOLOGY

Medications normally are not needed but are commonly given to survivors. Often misprescribed medications are antidepressants, benzodiazepines, and hypnotics. These same medications might be used appropriately if the survivor's symptoms of depression, anxiety, sleeplessness, or nightmares or flashbacks are severe. Continual assessment is needed to determine when medications are no longer needed to prevent abuse and addiction.

## MILIEU MANAGEMENT

Groups in inpatient or outpatient settings that might be relevant for survivors are those focusing on self-esteem, problem solving, assertiveness, relationship issues, stress management, and codependency. Substance abuse groups should be recommended, if necessary. In the community, a group for abused women is desirable. A newer form of intervention is a telephone support program that focuses on safety-promoting behaviors. Six calls over 8 weeks have encouraged increased use of these behaviors, which were more likely to be practiced even 18 months later (McFarlane et al, 2004).

## CRITICAL THINKING QUESTION    3

As an emergency room nurse, you are treating a 19-year-old male victim who was tortured and raped by a local gang. The victim refuses to give any details or to identify members of the gang. Describe what information you would give him about being a victim and the benefits of follow-up counseling.

## ■ Study Notes

1. Not all crimes involve physical violence and injury; however, all crimes involve emotional violation and injury. Victims lose a sense of the ability to control their own lives, as well as losing trust in others.
2. Progression through the stages of recovery from a crime might take years. Crisis intervention and group meetings with other survivors can facilitate recovery.
3. In assisting survivors, sensitivity to their needs is crucial to build trust and to avoid blaming the victim.
4. Information about counseling resources and support groups can be given to the survivors of rape and partner abuse for later use, even if there is an initial denial of the need for help.
5. The reexperiencing and working through of any traumatic crime, especially torture, SRA, MC, and childhood sexual abuse memories, is a painful, lengthy, and sometimes sporadic process that requires intense support and empathy.
6. Adult survivors of childhood sexual abuse might repress memories for years as a result of the emotional turmoil and sense of being betrayed by the abuser and others.
7. Adult survivors of childhood sexual abuse typically enter counseling for a variety of overt problems, unaware of how these are related to childhood trauma.

## CASE STUDY

Rachael Benton, a 26-year-old survivor of incest by her father, is married to Richard. She has an 8-year-old child, Matthew; Richard has three boys, Robert, James, and Daniel, ages 11, 8, and 7, who live with them. Angela, age 5, was born after Rachael and Richard were married. Matthew was removed from the home after being abused by Robert. Rachael sought help by attending a battered women's group.

Rachael's situation was difficult to resolve. Because of heavy drinking, Richard was missing work and changing jobs. His income declined and was sporadic but expenses did not decline. Without insurance, Rachael's repeated treatment of menstrual irregularities, back pain, chronic and severe headaches, and diarrhea were not paid for. She avoided treatment for bruises, a superficial knife wound, head cuts, and contusions. Richard repeatedly punched her stomach during a pregnancy, causing a miscarriage.

It was when Richard raped her that Rachael realized that there was no hope for change and that she had to leave. As Rachael became more assertive and independent, Richard demanded that she stay home, bought a shotgun to convince her to stay, and took the starter off the car. He rode to work with co-workers. Rachael had not adopted Richard's boys, so she could not take them with her. She was afraid that his verbal abuse of them would turn to physical violence when she left. Richard knew about all the places she thought of going.

It took 4 months to develop, coordinate, and implement arrangements so that Rachael and Angela were safe in leaving Richard. Neighbors, friends, and teachers were warned of the potential abuse of the boys and given the phone number for anonymously reporting child abuse. Rachael's mother rented her a small trailer in a rural town and obtained forms for Aid to Families with Dependent Children. Rachael secretly and gradually packed clothes and important documents in the trunk of a group member's car.

One night (14 months after the group began) Richard got drunk, beat Rachael, and tried to rape her again. She fought him off and waited until he passed out. The group member with the packed car drove her to the new trailer. As expected, Richard got his shotgun and went to every friend of Rachael's, but none knew where she was. He drove to Rachael's mother's home, and she called the sheriff when his car pulled into the driveway. Richard was escorted out of the county and warned not to return. Within a week, Daniel's teacher filed a child abuse report about bruises found on him. Within 2 weeks, the boys were removed from the home and returned to their natural mother.

Rachael has received proper medical treatment and feels healthier. She is now divorced, going through a job training program, and maintaining her secret location. She feels safe but is still in counseling once a month to complete her emotional recovery. She attends a support group for battered women once a week.

## Care Plan

Name: Rachael Benton

Admission Date:_____

*DSM-IV-TR* Diagnosis: Physical abuse of an adult by partner

| | |
|---|---|
| Assessment | **Areas of strength:** Bright, articulate, and capable of problem solving; mother and one friend willing to help; developing trust in group and beginning to process her feelings and rights. |
| | **Problems:** Lack of safe housing and employment; inability to remove husband's children from the house and fear he will abuse them; fear of increased abuse of her, even death, if she tries to leave; severe headaches. |
| Diagnoses | • Decisional conflict related to dysfunctional marriage, as evidenced by attendance in a battered women's support group. |
| | • Posttrauma syndrome related to previous sexual abuse and physical, emotional, and economic abuse, as evidenced by physical wounds, fear, and emotional trauma. |
| | • Fear (of leaving husband) related to potential abuse of sons, as evidenced by reluctance to leave without stepsons. |

Outcomes  *Short-term goals:*                                                      *Date met*

• Patient will remove bullets from gun; design an escape plan.          _____

• Patient will verbalize ability to survive on her own; confirm         _____
  housing in rural county.

*Long-term goals:*

• Patient will enroll in job training program.                          _____

• Patient will obtain legal assistance for divorce.                     _____

• Patient will seek medical treatment for chronic problems.             _____

| | |
|---|---|
| Planning/ Interventions | **Nurse-patient relationship:** Listen nonjudgmentally and empathically; accept strange behaviors related to secrecy and self-protection; avoid disparaging spouse and pressuring to leave; locate resources for training, finances, counseling, and medical care in rural county. |
| | **Psychopharmacology:** Desyrel, 50 mg at bedtime, to alleviate moderate depression and improve sleep; Tylenol No. 3 prn for severe headaches. |
| | **Milieu management:** Encourage continuing in local support group; locate support group in rural county; continue assessment of safety of patient and children. |
| Evaluation | Patient has moved to rural county and joined support group; is receiving counseling and medical care. Husband's children were removed and placed with natural mother. |
| Referrals | Has an appointment with a job training program in the rural county. |

8. The concepts of learned helplessness, the cycle of violence, and other situational, emotional, and cultural factors help explain why survivors often remain with their abusive partners.

9. Immediately preceding or at the beginning of a serious battering incident is when abuse victims are most amenable to crisis intervention and referrals for needed services.

10. Patience, support, and information are critical aspects of nursing interventions with all survivors.

## References

Ai AL, Cascio T, Santangelo LK, Evans-Campbell T: Hope, meaning, and growth following the September 11, 2001, terrorist attacks, *J Interpers Violence* 20:523, 2005.

Anorexia Nervosa and Associated Disorders (Indianapolis Chapter of ANAD): Personal interviews, Indianapolis, 2002, ANAD.

Bennett L: Projective methods in caring for sexually abused young people, *J Psychosoc Nurs Ment Health Serv* 35:18, 1997.

Brown K: Rape and sexual assault: the nursing role, *Nurs Spectrum (Metro Edition)* 29, August:29, 2001.

Burgess AW, Brown K, Bell K, et al: Sexual abuse of older adults, *Am J Nurs* 105:66, 2005.

Campbell R, Wasco SM: Understanding rape and sexual assault, *J Interpers Violence* 20:127, 2005.

Cerdorian K: The needs of adolescent girls who self-harm, *J Psychosoc Nurs Mental Health Serv* 43:40, 2005.

Close SM: Dating violence in middle school and high school youth, *J Child Adolesc Psychiatr Nurs* 18:2, 2005.

Cook LJ: The ultimate deception: childhood sexual abuse in the church, *J Psychosoc Nurs* 43:19, 2005.

Daniels K: Violence and depression: a deadly comorbidity, *J Psychosoc Nurs* 43:45, 2005.

Davis JL, Petretic-Jackson PA: The impact of child sexual abuse on adult interpersonal function: a review and synthesis of the empirical literature, *Aggression Violent Behav* 5:291, 2000.

Dowbecko U: "The Manchurian Candidate": all-American conspiracy, *MKzine* 3:5, 2005.

Dunbar B: Anger management: a holistic approach, *J Am Psychiatr Nurses Assoc* 10:16, 2004.

Dutton DG, Nicholls TL: The gender paradigm in domestic violence research and theory: part I—the conflict of theory and data, *Aggression Violent Behav* 10:680, 2005.

DiVasto P: Measuring the aftermath of rape, *J Psychosoc Nurs Ment Health Serv* 23:33, 1985.

Farella C: Hot and bothering: sexual harassment in the workplace is no joke, *Nurs Spectrum (Metro Edition)* September:14, 2001.

Farella C: Love shouldn't hurt: understanding domestic violence, *Nurs Spectrum (Metro Edition)* November:14, 2000.

Faravelli C, Giugni A, Salvatori S, Ricca V: Psychopathology after rape, *Am J Psychiatry* 161:1483, 2004.

Foa EB: The psychological aftermath of Hurricane Katrina, *Medscape Psychiatry Ment Health* 8:1, 2005.

Gates D: Burgers or bruises? Being assaulted shouldn't be part of a nurse's aide's job, *Am J Nurs* 104:13, 2004.

Gerard M: Domestic violence: how to screen and intervene, *RN* 63:52, 2000.

Gilmore-Hall A: Violence in the workplace: are you prepared? *Am J Nurs* 101:55, 2001.

Girardin B: Is this forensic specialty for you? *RN* 64:37, 2001.

Gladstone GL, Parker GB, Mitchell PB, et al: Implications of childhood trauma for depressed women, *Am J Psychiatry* 161:1417, 2004.

Goodwin JM: Redefining borderline syndromes as posttraumatic and rediscovering emotional containment as a first stage in treatment, *J Interpers Violence* 20:20, 2005.

Hammer R: Caring in forensic nursing: expanding the holistic model, *J Psychosoc Nurs* 38:18, 2000.

Hinds J: Once upon a time: therapeutic stories as a psychiatric nursing intervention, *J Psychosoc Nurs Ment Health Serv* 35:46, 1997.

Howe EG: Treating torture victims and enhancing human rights, *Psychiatry* 66:65, 2003.

Institute for Safe Medication Practices: For most nurses, intimidation is commonplace, *RN* 67:17, 2004.

Jonzon E, Lindblad F: Adult female victims of sexual abuse, *J Interpers Violence* 20:651, 2005.

Jordan CE: Intimate partner violence and the justice system, *J Interpers Violence* 19:1412, 2004.

Katchen MH: Ritual abuse vs. religious abuse: the development of an artificial distinction, *MKzine* 3:9, 2005.

Kreidler MC, Zupancic MK, Bell C, Longo MB: Trauma and dissociation: treatment perspectives, *Perspect Psychiatr Care* 36:77, 2000.

Lacy TJ, Benedek DM: Terrorism and weapons of mass destruction: managing the behavioral reaction in primary care, *South Med J* 96:394, 2003.

Leiper J: Nurse against nurse: how to stop horizontal violence, *Nursing 2005* 35:44, 2005.

Lewis-O'Conner A: "Dying to tell?" Do mandatory reporting laws benefit victims of domestic violence? *Am J Nurs* 104:75, 2004.

Lie D, Barclay L: Consequence of childhood sexual abuse similar for both sexes, *Medscape CME* Retrieved from www.medscape.com. Accessed July 11, 2005a.

Lie D, Barclay L: Patients might prefer that physicians ask about family conflict, *Medscape CME* Retrieved from www.medscape.com. Accessed June 3, 2005b.

Logan TK, Walker R: Separation as a risk factor for victims of intimate partner violence: beyond lethality and injury, *J Interpers Violence* 19:1478, 2004.

Martin L, Rosen LN, Durand DB, et al: Psychological and physical health effects of sexual assaults and nonsexual traumas among male and female United States Army soldiers, *Behav Med* 26:23, 2000.

Mawson AR: Intentional injury and the behavioral syndrome, *Aggression Viol Behav* 10:375, 2005.

McClellan AC, Killeen MR: Attachment theory and violence toward women by male intimate partners, *J Nurs Scholarship* Fourth Quarter:353, 2000.

McCollough-Zander K, Sarson S: "The fear is still in me": caring for survivors of torture, *Am J Nurs* 104:54, 2004.

McFarlane J, Malecha A, Gist J, et al: Increasing the safety-promoting behaviors of abused women, *Am J Nurs* 104:40, 2004.

McGonigle HL: The law and mind control, *S.M.A.R.T. News,* August 15, 1999.

Merrell J: Social support for victims of domestic violence, *J Psychosoc Nurs* 39:30, 2001.

Miller MC: The biology of child maltreatment, *Harv Ment Health Lett* 21:1, 2005.

Miller MC: Countering domestic violence, *Harv Ment Health Lett* 20:1, 2004.

Monarch K: Protect yourself from sexual harassment, *Am J Nurs* 100:75, 2000.

Morrison EF, Love CC: An evaluation of four programs for the management of aggression in psychiatric settings, *Arch Psychiatr Nurs* 17:146, 2003.

Murphy CM, Winters J, O'Farrell TJ, et al: Alcohol consumption and intimate partner violence by alcoholic men: comparing violent and nonviolent conflicts, *Psychol Addictive Behav* 19:35, 2005.

Muscari ME: What should I do when a client is being stalked? *Medscape Nurses* 7:1, 2005. Retrieved from www.medscape.com. Accessed July 11, 2005.

Mynatt S: Repeated suicide attempts, *J Psychosoc Nurs* 38:24, 2000.

New York Academy of Medicine: Worksite crisis intervention helped New Yorkers curb level of mental distress for up to two years after the World Trade Center disaster, *LifeNet* 16:1, Fall 2004/Winter 2005.

Osterman JE, Barbiaz J, Johnson P: Emergency interventions for rape victims, *Psychiatr Serv* 52:733, 2001.

Parks S: Silence verbal abuse, *Nurs Spectrum (Metro Edition)* August:20, 2001.

Paul J, Blum D: Workplace disaster preparedness and response: the employee assistance program continuum of services, *Int J Emerg Ment Health* 7:169, 2005.

Pasquali EA: Humor: an antidote for terrorism, *J Holistic Nurs* 21:398, 2003.

Peternelj-Taylor C: Forensic psychiatric nursing: a work in progress, *J Psychosoc Nurs* 39:8, 2001.

Piercy D, Greenwood M: DOVE program takes flight, *Nurs Spectrum (Metro Edition)* January:18, 2002.

Poirier N: Psychosocial characteristics discriminating between battered women and other women psychiatric inpatients, *J Am Psychiatr Nurs Assoc* 6:144, 2000.

Ragavan C, Guttman M: Terror on the streets, *U.S. News and World Report,* December 13, 2004, p. 21.

Ray SL: Male survivors' perspectives of incest/sexual abuse, *Perspect Psychiatr Care* 37:49, 2001.

Roberts SJ: Primary health care of survivors of childhood sexual abuse: how can psychiatric nurses be helpful? *J Am Psychiatr Nurses Assoc* 6:191, 2000.

Rothschild B: *The body remembers: the psychophysiology of trauma and trauma treatment,* New York, 2000, WW Norton.

Rowell PA: The victor(y) over interpersonal trauma, *J Am Psychiatric Nurses Assoc* 11:103, 2005.

Sarson J, MacDonald L: Human trafficking and ritual abuse-torture From Persons against Ritual Abuse-Torture. Available at http://www.ritualabusetorture.org. Accessed August 5, 2004.

Starr DL: Clients who self-mutilate, *J Psychosoc Nursing* 42:33, 2004.

Stith SM, Smith DB, Penn CE, et al: Intimate partner physical abuse perpetration and victimization risk factors: a meta-analytic review, *Aggression Violent Behav* 10:65, 2004.

Stringer H: Raging bullies, *Nurse Week* February 12:10, 2001.

Tilley DS, Brackley M: Violent lives of women: critical points for intervention—phase I, focus groups, *Perspect Psychiatr Care* 40:157, 2004.

Tolces R: Electronic harassment, *MKzine* 3:5, 2005.

Torem MS: The role of medication in treatment of dissociative disorders, *Many Voices* 12:6, 2000.

Trossman S: Illinois RNs win workplace safety measures, *Am Nurse* January/February:1, 2001.

Turkus JA: The treatment challenge, *Many Voices* 12:6, 2000.

Tynhurst JS: Individual reactions to community disaster, *Am J Psychiatry* 107:764, 1951.

Valente SM: Controversies and challenges of ritual abuse, *J Psychosoc Nurs* 38:8, 2000.

Valente SM: Sexual abuse of boys, *J Child Adolesc Psychiatr Nurs* 18:10, 2005.

van der Kolk B, McFarlane AC, Weissaeth L: *Traumatic stress: the effects of overwhelming experience on mind, body, and society,* New York, 1996, Guilford Press.

Walker L: *The battered woman,* New York, 1979, Harper & Row.

Williams KR: Arrest and intimate partner violence: toward a more complete application of deterrence theory, *Aggression Violent Behav* 10:660, 2005.

Woods SJ, Wineman NM: Trauma, posttraumatic stress disorder symptom clusters, and physical health symptoms in post-abused women, *Arch Psychiatr Nurs* 18:26, 2004.

Worthington K, Franklin P: Workplace violence, *Am J Nurs* 100:73, 2000.

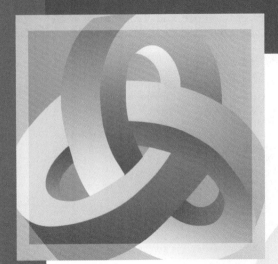

# Chapter 42

# Child and Adolescent Psychiatric Nursing

*Lawrence Scahill and Maryellen Pachler*

## Learning Objectives

*After reading this chapter, you should be able to:*

- Describe the major categories of child psychiatric disorders.
- Describe the frequency of serious psychiatric disorders in children and adolescents.
- Identify genetic and environmental factors that can elevate the risk of developing a psychiatric disorder.
- Describe the symptoms of the selected child and adolescent psychiatric disorders.
- Identify principles of nursing intervention with children and adolescents.

Recent contributions from several disciplines have increased our understanding of psychiatric disorders that occur in childhood. Through the field of epidemiology, appreciation for the frequency and distribution of child psychiatric disorders has increased. Dramatic developments in neuroscience have deepened our grasp of the biologic underpinnings of some psychiatric disorders, such as attention-deficit/hyperactivity disorder (ADHD), autism, and Tourette's syndrome. Studies in behavioral genetics have shown that several psychiatric disorders of childhood have a strong genetic contribution, although environmental contributions should always be considered. Recent investigations in molecular genetics suggest that specific genes are associated with some psychiatric disorders. Clinical research has provided information to guide both pharmacologic and behavioral approaches to treatment. Despite these advances, however, the etiologic factors of most childhood psychiatric disorders remain unknown, and many treatments lack empirical support.

This chapter reviews the major categories and frequency of child psychiatric disorders, as well as the factors that influence the probability of developing a psychiatric disorder. The clinical features of selected child psychiatric disorders are also described. The chapter concludes with a brief discussion of treatment issues, including psychopharmacologic and behavior therapy, as well as a description of the treatment settings in child and adolescent psychiatry.

## SCOPE OF THE PROBLEM

A report from the U.S. Surgeon General (U.S. Public Health Service, 2000) has estimated that 10% of school-age children have serious mental health problems. Another 10% has milder problems that might pose some interference with

### Norm's Notes

*In my opinion, Larry Scahill is the foremost authority on child and adolescent psychiatric nursing in this country. Whenever he speaks, or writes, I listen. Just this morning, in my local paper, a front page article discussed the overuse of antipsychotic medications by children. This chapter provides a balanced view of what can be done for young people with mental health problems. There is absolutely no doubt that the number of people in these diagnostic categories is increasing rapidly, such as those with autism or ADHD. This chapter will give you a better understanding of these disorders, which are all around us.*

interpersonal relationships and adjustment to school. This percentage translates into an estimated 8 to 12 million youngsters with significant mental health problems in the United States. Despite the documented frequency of psychiatric disorders in children and adolescents, as few as one in five are using specialized mental health services (Burns et al, 2004; U.S. Public Health Service, 2000). In lieu of obtaining mental health services in child psychiatric clinics, children might receive mental health services in primary care settings and public schools (Briggs-Gowan et al, 2000; U.S. Public Health Service, 2000).

## EPIDEMIOLOGY OF CHILD PSYCHIATRIC DISORDERS

Epidemiology is the study of the frequency and distribution of disease conditions in a population. The primary concerns in epidemiology are how common a disorder is in a given population and whether particular subgroups are at increased risk for developing a specific disorder. For example, men are more likely to have a myocardial infarction than women, although women are at higher risk than men for osteoporosis. Recently, methods of epidemiology have been applied to child psychiatry, resulting in a better understanding of both the frequency and the distribution of these disorders in the population. This effort has profited from improvements in the operational criteria of psychiatric disorders and diagnostic interview methods built on these criteria.

Any number of genetic or environmental characteristics might influence the likelihood of developing a psychiatric disorder. Characteristics that increase the probability of having a psychiatric disorder are called *risk factors*. Although often described as separate, genetic influences and environmental conditions might interact to elevate the risk of a child psychiatric disorder. Thus, risk factors for a psychiatric disorder can be additive. Examples of biologic risk factors include the inherited genetic abnormality seen in fragile X syndrome, which is among the most common genetic forms of mental retardation. Poverty, child abuse, overcrowded living conditions, and exposure to alcohol in utero are examples of environmental risk factors.

## GENETIC FACTORS

Several psychiatric disorders are presumed to have an important genetic component. Indeed, for depression, anxiety disorders, tic disorders, and ADHD, having a close family member with that specific disorder might be the single largest risk factor for that same disorder in a child. Various methods are used to study the role of genetics in the cause of psychiatric disorders, including twin, family, and adoption studies, as well as studies of affected siblings. More recently, powerful new techniques developed in the field of molecular biology are being applied to the study of psychiatric disorders (Abelson et al, 2005). Among the first questions to ask when considering the genetic contribution for a given disorder is whether the disorder recurs more frequently in families compared with the general population. However, simply showing that a disorder such as depression is more common in children who have a depressed parent does not prove that depression is inherited. For example, the developmental impact of having a depressed parent might increase the risk of depression in a child through environmental influences.

To establish that genetic inheritance confers vulnerability for a psychiatric disorder, researchers have carried out twin and adoption studies. Twin studies exploit the fact that identical (monozygotic) twins have 100% of their genes in common, whereas dizygotic twins share an average of 50% of their genes. Thus, if a disorder is truly genetic, it should be present in both identical twins, whereas the expected *concordance* in dizygotic twins would be significantly lower. On the other hand, disorders caused by environmental influences exert similar impact on development, regardless of whether the twins are genetically identical. Thus, if a disorder were primarily the result of environmental influences, there would be no difference in the concordance between monozygotic and dizygotic twins. Twin studies have demonstrated a strong genetic contribution in ADHD (Levy et al, 1997; Hudziak et al, 2005), obsessive-compulsive disorder (OCD) (Carey and Gottesman, 1981), Tourette's syndrome (TS) (Price et al, 1985), and autism (Rutter et al, 1999). Although none of these disorders shows 100% concordance in monozygotic twins, the percentage of mutually affected monozygotic twins is significantly higher than in dizygotic twins for each of these disorders.

Although twins can provide strong support for a genetic factor, these methods do not elucidate the mode of inheritance (Box 42-1). If a disorder runs in families and is genetically inherited, it would be expected to recur in specific patterns within families. The formal method for evaluating the pattern of inheritance in families is called *segregation analysis*. Through segregation analysis, known models of inheritance can be compared with the observed pattern.

If a disorder is genetically inherited, it implies that the action of one or more genes is abnormal. Recently developed techniques in molecular biology might lead to the identification of a gene or genes that cause psychiatric disorders of childhood. The primary function of genes is to encode for proteins in a series of carefully engineered steps, from deoxyribonucleic acid (DNA) to ribonucleic acid (RNA) to a specific protein. Thus, a genetically determined disorder is ultimately caused by a disruption in function of these molecular procedures, resulting in impaired function of the protein product (State et al, 2000). In fragile X syndrome, for example, the gene that regulates an early step in the process of protein manufacture (i.e., transcription of the DNA message to RNA) appears to be defective. The precise mechanism whereby this disruption in the molecular biology produces the physical characteristics and symptoms of fragile X syndrome remains unclear.

## ENVIRONMENTAL FACTORS

Broadly speaking, environmental factors are any and all nongenetic exposures, including intrauterine insults, adverse family conditions, poverty, unsupportive community circumstances, natural disasters, traumatic events, and toxic substances (e.g., ingesting lead paint). Ideally, genetic and environmental influences can be distinguished. In actuality, however, genetic and environmental factors interact in complex ways, making it difficult to attribute exclusive causality. For example, phenylketonuria (PKU) is a metabolic defect inherited in an autosomal recessive fashion that results in a toxic accumulation of phenylalanine in the brain. However, if PKU is detected, a low-phenylalanine diet will limit the negative impact of the inherited metabolic defect.

## PSYCHOSOCIAL ADVERSITY

Several studies have shown that conditions marked by psychosocial adversity, such as poverty, family discord, overcrowded living conditions, sexual abuse, physical abuse, and a parent with a history

---

### Box 42-1  Types of Inheritance

**Autosomal Dominant**
One parent is affected with the disorder and passes on a single copy of the disease-causing gene to the affected offspring. Huntington's chorea is an example of a neuropsychiatric disorder that is inherited as an autosomal dominant condition.

**Autosomal Recessive**
To be affected, the child must have two copies of the disease-causing gene. Each unaffected parent passes on one disease-causing gene to the affected offspring. Phenylketonuria is the result of autosomal recessive inheritance.

**Sex-Linked Inheritance**
Recalling that women have an XX karyotype and men have an XY karyotype, it is possible for a mother to carry a trait on one X chromosome without being affected. Although the gene is not expressed in the mother, the male offspring is affected. Some forms of hemophilia follow a sex-linked inheritance pattern.

**Polygenetic Inheritance**
Some disorders recur in higher than expected rates in families but follow more complex patterns than autosomal dominant or autosomal recessive inheritance. These disorders are presumed to be caused by several genes acting in combination. Schizophrenia, Tourette's syndrome, autism, and some forms of learning disability are believed to follow a polygenetic pattern.

of substance abuse or a psychiatric disorder, are associated with psychiatric disorders in children and adolescents (Biederman et al, 1995; Scahill et al, 1999). Moreover, these risk factors appear to be additive. In a clinical sample of children with ADHD, Biederman and colleagues (1995) found that, as the number of these adverse elements increases, the likelihood of ADHD also increases. As previously suggested, however, the association of these adverse psychosocial conditions with child psychiatric disorders does not preclude a genetic contribution.

On the other hand, it is clear that not all children who are exposed to psychosocial disadvantage develop a psychiatric disorder. Indeed, some children seem to grow and mature into well-adjusted individuals despite the presence of multiple environmental risk factors. The environmental and constitutional elements that account for these resilient children are poorly understood and deserve further investigation. It might be that a supportive relationship with a member of the extended family or community protects the child from the adverse effects of psychosocial conditions. Resilience can also be fostered within the environment so that the ill effects of a genetic vulnerability can be mitigated. For example, a child with an inherited vulnerability for ADHD is more likely to achieve an optimal outcome if reared in a predictable family environment than would a child with a similar vulnerability reared in a more chaotic family circumstance.

### Family Systems

Families develop in a manner that is analogous to child development. Although families come in several sizes and compositions, families typically begin with the formation of a couple. When the couple comes together, each individual makes a transition from single life to family life. This transition to family life takes a major step forward with conception and birth (or adoption) of a child. Each subsequent phase of the child's development—infancy, toddler, school age, adolescence, and young adulthood—calls for an adjustment by the family unit. The rules, rituals, and communication patterns that define the family system have an impact on the child's development. Similarly, the child's development influences the family system.

## DIAGNOSTIC CATEGORIES OF CHILD PSYCHIATRIC DISORDERS

The introduction of the *Diagnostic and Statistical Manual of Mental Disorders,* third edition *(DSM-III)* in 1980 (American Psychiatric Association [APA], 1980) represented an important milestone in the definition of mental illness. For the first time, psychiatric diagnoses were described in operational terms with clearly stated (although not necessarily empirically verified) criteria. The *DSM-III* also introduced a multiaxial diagnostic system that not only included the primary mental illness (axis I), but also noted the presence of mental retardation (axis II), medical illness (axis III), psychosocial stressors (axis IV), and assessment of functioning (axis V). The *DSM-IV-TR* (APA, 2000) contains several changes from *DSM-III* and *DSM-IV* but retains the same essential features.

Childhood psychiatric disorders can be divided into several broad categories, such as developmental disorders, disruptive behavior disorders, internalizing disorders, tic disorders, psychotic disorders, and elimination disorders.

## DEVELOPMENTAL DISORDERS

### MENTAL RETARDATION

Mental retardation is defined by subaverage intelligence (intelligence quotient [IQ] below 70) accompanied by impairments in performing age-expected activities in daily living. Intelligence is measured by a standardized test and can be used to define the degree of mental retardation (Table 42-1). Impaired adaptive functioning is often a clinical judgment, but standardized assessments such as the Vineland Adaptive Behavior Scales (Sparrow et al, 1984) are available.

| Table 42-1 | *DSM-IV* Classification of Mental Retardation |
|---|---|
| **Severity** | **IQ Range** |
| Mild | 55-69 |
| Moderate | 40-54 |
| Severe | 25-39 |
| Profound | Below 25 |

| Table 42-2 | Selected Pervasive Developmental Disorders in *DSM-IV-TR* |
|---|---|
| **Disorder** | **Prevalence** |
| Autistic disorder | 15 to 20/10,000 |
| Asperger's disorder | 2 to 10/10,000* |
| PDD—not otherwise specified | 20 to 40/10,000* |

*Accuracy of estimate is hampered by changes in definition.
*PDD,* Pervasive developmental disorder.

The prevalence of mental retardation is estimated at 2.0%, with a range from 1.0% to 2.5%. Most of the mentally retarded (nearly 90%) are in the mildly retarded range. The causes of mental retardation vary from specific genetic abnormalities such as fragile X syndrome, trisomy 21 (Down syndrome), and phenylketonuria to multifactorial causes, in which several genes are presumed to interact with environmental factors. In addition to intellectual handicap, mentally retarded children might also have a psychiatric disorder.

## PERVASIVE DEVELOPMENTAL DISORDERS

The pervasive developmental disorders (PDDs) are a group of disorders characterized by impairments across multiple domains of development. Although not a defining feature of PDDs, many of these children demonstrate varying degrees of mental retardation. Table 42-2 presents the more common forms of PDD described in *DSM-IV.*

These PDDs share several common features, including delayed socialization and stereotypical behaviors such as rocking, hand flapping, and peculiar preoccupations. These children are rigid and often intolerant of change in routines. They also tend to perseverate on themes of idiosyncratic interest and are prone to behavioral outbursts in response to modest environmental demands.

### Autistic Disorder

Since the first description of autism by Leo Kanner over 50 years ago, several theories have been advanced concerning its cause. For example, in the 1950s and 1960s, serious consideration was given to the notion that detached professional parents might be the cause of autism (Volkmar, 2005). This explanation is no longer accepted and suggests a bias of ascertainment, in that professional families were more likely to seek treatment from medical centers that evaluated children with profound developmental delays. In addition, this conceptualization fails to recognize that the parental indifference might have been rooted in the child's incapacity for reciprocal communication. More recently, measles, mumps, and rubella (MMR) vaccine has been blamed for an apparent increase in the prevalence of autism, although the evidence to support this claim is not compelling (Acosta and Pearl, 2003).

A recent epidemiologic study reported a prevalence of 2 per 1000 for autistic disorder in children (Chakrabarti and Fombonne, 2005). This estimate, which is two to four times higher than previous estimates, might not reflect an increase in the prevalence of autistic disorder; rather, it probably reflects improved classification of children with developmental disorders. For example, a substantial percentage of children with autistic disorder are mentally retarded and about 25% have seizure disorders. Prior studies might have classified these children as mentally retarded rather than as children with autism. Family genetic and twin data suggest a strong genetic contribution to autism, but the specific cause remains unknown. Several studies have observed higher serum levels of serotonin in children with autism, resulting in considerable research interest in the serotonin system. However, the failure to replicate this finding in other studies suggests that hyperserotonemia might be true only for some autistic patients. Further evidence implicating the serotonin system comes from a study that observed an association between autism and the structure of the serotonin receptor (Acosta and Pearl, 2003). If this finding is replicated, it might have important implications for pharmacotherapy in autism.

Autism can be differentiated from the other forms of PDD because it has an early age of onset (before 30 months of age), social relatedness is profoundly disturbed, communication is delayed and deviant, and the delayed developmental profile is relatively constant (e.g., in Rett syndrome, a rare developmental disorder, previously acquired skills rapidly decline). Children with autism appear aloof and indifferent to others and seem to prefer inanimate objects to human contact. Language, if present, is characterized by abnormal intonation, pronoun reversals, and echolalia (repetition of words or phrases spoken by others). Other common features of autism, which might also be present in other variants of PDD, are stereotypical behaviors such as rocking and hand flapping, extraordinary insistence on sameness, and preoccupation with peculiar interests (e.g., fans, air conditioners, train schedules).

### Asperger's Disorder

Asperger's disorder was also described about 50 years ago, but it was not included in *DSM-III* or *DSM-III-R* (revised version). Compared with children with autism, children with Asperger's disorder are less likely to be mentally retarded, and their linguistic handicap is less severe. Indeed, these children often have normal intelligence, and verbal intelligence is typically higher than performance intelligence. The social deficits in Asperger's disorder include inept initiation of social interactions, impaired reading of social cues, and a tendency toward concrete interpretation of language. Speech tends to be stilted and intonation is abnormal. These children tend to be clumsy, have difficulty managing transitions, and are preoccupied with matters of private interest.

The prevalence of Asperger's disorder is estimated at 1 per 1000 (Chakrabarti and Fombonne, 2005). Asperger's syndrome appears to be more common in boys than in girls. Although no genetic marker has been identified, the disorder often runs in families, with high recurrence in fathers.

### Pervasive Developmental Disorder— Not Otherwise Specified

The classification of pervasive developmental disorder—not otherwise specified (PDD-NOS) is a residual category reserved for children who do not meet criteria for a more specific type of PDD, such as autism or Asperger's syndrome. The prevalence is difficult to estimate with accuracy because of changes in the definition. For example, *DSM-III* and *DSM-III-R* do not include this category. Given the heterogeneity of PDD-NOS, it is unlikely that a single etiologic factor will ever be identified. Both genetic and environmental causes, particularly perinatal exposures, probably play a role in the cause of PDD-NOS.

Children with PDD-NOS exhibit traits that are similar to those described for autism and Asperger's disorder. Differential diagnosis is determined by age of onset, severity of speech and language deficit, degree of social impairment, and level of interest in interpersonal relationships (Koenig and Scahill, 2001). In general, these features are less severe in PDD-NOS than in autism.

## SPECIFIC DEVELOPMENTAL DISORDERS

Specific developmental disorders are characterized by a delay in a discrete domain of development. This section focuses on learning disorders and communication disorders.

### Learning Disorders

Learning disorder (also called learning disability) is characterized by a significant discrepancy between aptitude (IQ) and achievement in a particular area, such as reading or mathematics. The specificity of the delay is what differentiates learning disorders from the more global deficits observed in mental retardation and PDD.

The most common type of learning disorder is reading disability (also called *dyslexia*). Estimates range from 3% to 17% of school-age children, with boys being affected more often than girls in most studies (Liederman et al, 2005). However, in a large community survey, no gender difference in reading disability was present (Shaywitz and Shaywitz, 2005). In clinical samples, reading disability is associated with a range of psychiatric disorders, but whether this apparent association is caused by characteristics that are related to seeking treatment is unclear. Less is known about the prevalence of nonverbal learning disorder (mathematics disorder), with estimates ranging from 0.1% to 1.0% and no apparent difference between boys and girls.

## COMMUNICATION DISORDERS

Communication disorders involve speech (the motor aspects of speaking) or language, which refers to the formulation and comprehension of verbal communication. The prevalence of speech and language disorders has been reported in two estimate studies (Law et al, 2000; Shriberg et al, 1999). Data indicate that 25% of 5-year-old children and 2% of 8-year-old children (the median prevalence estimate across these studies falls in the range of 8% to 9%) present with speech and language disorders. Communication deficits present early in childhood do resolve in some children. In a longitudinal study, speech and language disorders were shown to be strongly associated with psychiatric disorders (Clegg et al, 2005). Whether the psychiatric disorder and the communication disorder share an underlying cause or whether the prior presence of a communication disorder is a predisposing factor for development of a psychiatric disorder is unclear.

Theories suggest that language delay and reading disability might share the same underlying phonologic defect (Shaywitz and Shaywitz, 2005). Both reading disability and a speech or language handicap can exert a negative impact on socialization and education. For example, peers might tease a child with an articulation defect or stuttering, causing withdrawal and a poor self-image. Because reading is a cornerstone of learning, children with reading disability might fall behind their peers in school—especially if the reading disability is undetected.

## ATTENTION-DEFICIT AND DISRUPTIVE BEHAVIOR DISORDERS

This group includes three relatively common child psychiatric disorders: ADHD, oppositional defiant disorder (ODD), and conduct disorder (Table 42-3). These disorders are more common in boys than girls and are associated with low socioeconomic status, urban living, single parenthood, family dysfunction, learning disabilities, language delay, and a positive family history of a disruptive behavior disorder (Biederman et al, 1995; Pauls, 2005; Scahill et al, 1999).

## ATTENTION-DEFICIT/ HYPERACTIVITY DISORDER

ADHD is characterized by inattention, impulsiveness, and overactivity. *DSM-IV* represents another

| Table 42-3 | **Types and Prevalence of Disruptive Behavior Disorders** |

| Disorder | Range of Estimates (%) |
| --- | --- |
| Attention-deficit/hyperactivity disorder | 2-11 |
| Oppositional defiant disorder | 5-10 |
| Conduct disorder | 4-10 |

conceptualization of ADHD and allows the description of a primarily hyperactive-impulsive type, a primarily inattentive type, or a combined type (see the *DSM-IV-TR* Criteria for Attention-

| *DSM-IV-TR* Criteria | for Attention-Deficit/Hyperactivity Disorder |

A. Either 1 or 2:
  1. Inattention: At least six of the following symptoms of inattention have persisted for at least 6 months and are maladaptive:
     a. Inattentive to details or makes careless mistakes in schoolwork.
     b. Difficulty sustaining attention in tasks or play.
     c. Does not seem to listen to what is being said.
     d. Poor follow-through on instructions and fails to finish schoolwork and chores.
     e. Difficulties with organizing tasks.
     f. Avoids or strongly dislikes sustained mental effort.
     g. Often loses things necessary for tasks or activities.
     h. Is often easily distracted by extraneous stimuli.
     i. Is often forgetful in daily activities.
  2. Hyperactivity-impulsivity: At least six symptoms of hyperactivity-impulsivity that are maladaptive and have persisted for at least 6 months:
     a. Hyperactivity
        i. Fidgety
        ii. Inappropriately leaves seat (in classroom)
        iii. Inappropriate running or climbing
        iv. Difficulty in playing or engaging in leisure activities quietly
        v. Often on the go
        vi. Talks excessively
     b. Impulsivity
        i. Blurts out answers to questions
        ii. Often has difficulty waiting in lines or awaiting turn
        iii. Often interrupts or intrudes on others
B. Onset no later than 7 years of age:
  1. Other criteria concern context of behavior, level of impairment, and the need to rule out other diagnoses.

Modified from the American Psychiatric Association: *Diagnostic and statistical manual of mental disorders, text revision,* ed 4, Washington, DC, 2000, APA.

Deficit/Hyperactivity Disorder box). Typically, children with ADHD are restless, overactive, distractible, reckless, and disruptive. ADHD is a relatively common disorder in school-age children, affecting an estimated 2% to 11% (Costello et al, 1996; Wolraich et al, 1996). ADHD is a frequent presenting complaint in child mental health clinics, and long-term disability is not uncommon (Barkley, 1998). Thus, ADHD is of significant public health importance.

Several environmental exposures have been proposed as potential causes of ADHD, including perinatal insults, head injury, psychosocial adversity, lead poisoning, and diet (e.g., food allergies, sensitivity to food additives). These hypotheses might explain some cases of ADHD; it is unlikely, however, that any one of these exposures alone will explain a significant portion of children with ADHD. Large community-based studies have confirmed that psychosocial adversity is highly associated with ADHD (Scahill et al, 1999). Whether these adverse psychosocial conditions are causal or contributing factors to other undetermined factors is unclear. The claim that food additives or allergies cause ADHD is supported largely by case reports, because most controlled studies have failed to support a causative role for diet in ADHD (Eigenmann and Haenggeli, 2004).

Based on evidence from twin and family studies, genetic endowment clearly plays a role in the cause of ADHD. Although identical twins are not fully concordant for ADHD, monozygotic twins are far more likely to be mutually affected than dizygotic twins (Hudziak et al, 2005; Levy et al, 1997). Family genetic studies have also shown that biologic relatives of children with ADHD are more likely to be affected by ADHD than biologic relatives of pediatric controls (Pauls, 2005).

The cause of ADHD remains unknown, but a growing body of evidence has suggested that subtle dysfunction in the frontal lobe and functionally related subcortical structures plays an essential role in the core symptoms of ADHD (Barkley, 1998). The frontal lobe, which is responsible for planning, attention, and regulation of motor activity, has been shown on volumetric magnetic resonance imaging (MRI) to be slightly smaller in boys with ADHD than in controls (Castellanos et al, 1996). Positron emission tomography (PET) has also shown that adults with a history of ADHD have reduced meta-

bolic activity (hypoperfusion) in the frontal lobe (Swanson and Volkow, 2001). Although not a consistent finding, structural MRI studies have also found small volumetric differences in the basal ganglia (Castellanos et al, 1996). These subcortical structures are highly connected to the frontal lobe and play a role in cognition and motor activity.

## OPPOSITIONAL DEFIANT DISORDER

ODD is defined by an enduring pattern of disobedience, argumentativeness, explosive angry outbursts, low frustration tolerance, and a tendency to blame others for quarrels or accidents. This pattern of behavior might begin early in development. Indeed, ODD is the most common psychiatric diagnosis of preschool children. As a child progresses through development, ODD tends to be associated with comorbid diagnoses of anxiety and mood disorders and either a single or comorbid diagnosis of ADHD (Lavigne et al, 2001).

By definition, children with ODD are frequently in conflict with adults. They might also have trouble maintaining friendships. In both clinical populations and community samples, substantial overlap with ADHD exists, although the two disorders do not always occur together.

## CONDUCT DISORDER

Conduct disorder is distinguishable from ODD because it is characterized by more serious violations of social standards, such as aggression, vandalism, cruelty to animals, stealing, lying, and truancy.

As with the other disruptive behavior disorders, comorbidity is common in conduct disorder, with higher than expected rates of ADHD, depression, and learning disorders. The relationship between ADHD and conduct disorder is intriguing and points out the potential contribution of family genetic studies. Faraone and colleagues (1991) have shown that children with ADHD plus conduct disorder were more likely to have conduct disorder in their families than were children with ADHD alone. The rate of ADHD in the families of both subgroups was similar, whether or not conduct disorder was present in the index child. As pointed out by the authors, these findings suggest that ADHD plus conduct disorder might represent a particular form of ADHD that is distinguishable from ADHD alone.

## INTERNALIZING DISORDERS

### ANXIETY DISORDERS

*DSM-IV* defines several anxiety disorders, including generalized anxiety disorder, separation anxiety, agoraphobia, panic disorder, posttraumatic stress disorder, and obsessive-compulsive disorder. This section focuses on separation anxiety and obsessive-compulsive disorder. Generalized anxiety disorder, agoraphobia, panic disorder, and posttraumatic stress disorder are described in Chapter 31.

#### Separation Anxiety Disorder

Many children experience some discomfort on separation from their mother or major attachment figure. For children with separation anxiety disorder, profound distress on entry to school might occur, and some children might refuse to go to school. In some cases, the child might "shadow" the mother around the house and not let the mother out of sight. When asked, most children with separation anxiety disorder will express worry about harm or permanent loss of the mother or major attachment figure.

The prevalence of separation anxiety disorder is estimated at 4% of school-age children. The diagnosis of separation anxiety disorder in *DSM-IV-TR* is based on childhood onset of excessive anxiety on separation from home or a major attachment figure. The manifestations typically include acute distress accompanied by reluctance or refusal on separation and frequent nightmares about separation. The excessive anxiety must be present for at least a month and be the source of significant impairment at home, at school, or with friends.

Anxiety disorders recur in families at a much higher than expected rate, and it is likely that both environmental and genetic factors play a causative role in separation anxiety disorder. Life events, such as a family move, a change to a new school, or a death in the family, might predate the onset of separation anxiety. Additional evidence suggests that extreme shyness (fearfulness in new situations) is a heritable trait, and that the presence of this trait in a child elevates the risk of an anxiety disorder (Biederman et al, 2001). Additional research is needed to determine the relative contribution of genetic and environmental factors in separation anxiety disorder.

### OBSESSIVE-COMPULSIVE DISORDER

OCD is a heterogenous disorder affecting 2% to 3% of adolescents and adults (Karno et al, 1988; Valleni-Basile et al, 1994). Although the prevalence is probably lower in the prepubertal age group (Costello et al, 1996), OCD can be identified in children as young as 5 years of age (Scahill et al, 2003).

Obsessions are recurring thoughts or images that are disturbing and difficult to push out of the mind. Compulsions are repetitive behaviors that the person feels obliged to complete. Attempts to resist these ritualized behaviors typically increase anxiety and intensify the urge to perform the compulsion. In many cases, the reported purpose of the ritual is to prevent some dreaded event, whereas other patients state that the ritual is done to achieve a sense of completion. In either case, the performance of the compulsion achieves a momentary decrease in anxiety. This reduction in anxiety, albeit brief, reinforces the compulsive habit.

Common obsessions in children and adolescents, such as contamination, fear of harm coming to self or family members, worry about acting on unwanted aggressive impulses, and concern about order and symmetry, are similar to those reported by adults. Common compulsions include hand washing, cleaning rituals, requesting reassurance about matters of health and well-being, ordering and arranging objects, complex touching habits, checking, counting, and repetition of routine activities to achieve a sense of completion. To warrant a diagnosis of OCD, obsessional worries, compulsive habits, or both must waste time (at least an hour per day), cause distress, and interfere with daily activities.

Data from several lines of research have converged over the last 25 years to clarify the neurobiologic factors of OCD. These data, derived primarily from neuroimaging studies, suggest that OCD is caused by dysregulation of brain circuits that connect the cortex, basal ganglia, and thalamus (Rauch et al, 2001). Another source of evidence is the replicated finding in both children and adults that antidepressant drugs that block serotonin at presynaptic reuptake sites are effective for most patients with OCD (Chiu and Leonard, 2003). By contrast, drugs that block the presynaptic reuptake of norepinephrine are not effective in OCD.

# MOOD DISORDERS

*DSM-IV-TR* defines several mood disorders, including major depressive disorder, dysthymic disorder, bipolar I and bipolar II disorders, and cyclothymic disorder. Although these disorders can occur in children and adolescents, they are more common in adults (see Chapters 29 and 30). This section provides a brief discussion of major depressive disorder and bipolar disorder in children and adolescents.

## Major Depressive Disorder

Depression is characterized by sadness, feelings of worthlessness, loss of interest in usual activities, sleep or appetite disturbance, loss of energy, diminished activity, decreased capacity to concentrate, and recurrent thoughts of death or suicide. At least five of these symptoms must be present on a daily basis and persist for at least 2 weeks (APA, 2000). The manifestations of depression in children are similar to those observed in adults. However, children might be less able to verbalize their feelings and irritability might be a predominant feature in children and adolescents. The prevalence of depression in children and adolescents ranges from 1% to 8%, with important differences by age and gender. Overall, depression is less common in prepubertal children, with boys at slightly higher risk than girls in the younger age group. During adolescence, depression is more common in girls.

As with other psychiatric disorders of childhood, comorbid mental disorders are common in children with major depressive disorder (MDD). The most frequent comorbid disorders in both children and adolescents include dysthymia, anxiety disorders, and disruptive behavior disorders. In adolescents, personality disorders such as borderline personality and substance abuse are of particular concern.

A large body of data shows that depression involves the hypothalamic-pituitary-adrenal axis, as well as the norepinephrine and serotonin systems in the brain, but the precise mechanism is not well understood. Family studies provide evidence that the risk for depression is substantially higher if a history of depression exists in an immediate family member (Birmaher and Brent, 2003; Klein et al, 2001; Zubenko et al, 2001).

---

**CRITICAL THINKING QUESTION**  [1]

A child with separation anxiety expresses recurring worry about a parent's safety. How is this different from OCD?

---

## Bipolar Disorder

*DSM-IV-TR* defines two major types of bipolar disorder, bipolar I and bipolar II. Bipolar I disorder is defined by mania with or without a history of depression. Bipolar II disorder is characterized by a history of major depression and hypomania, but not a full manic episode (Box 42-2) (APA, 2000).

The existence of bipolar illness in young children is a matter of controversy. Some investigators have suggested that bipolar illness is rare in prepubertal children, whereas others have contended that it is simply underdiagnosed. This debate is further complicated by disagreement concerning whether bipolar illness in children has the same clinical features as those seen in adults (Carlson, 2003; Giedd, 2000). In its classic form, adult bipolar disorder is an episodic condition characterized by clear-cut manic episodes, including decreased need for sleep, elated mood, grandiose thinking, increased goal-directed behavior, racing thoughts, and excessive output of speech. Between manic episodes, adults with bipolar disorder show variable functioning—some patients might be quite productive. By contrast, children who exhibit manic symptoms are often significantly impaired between manic episodes. The chronic symptoms observed in these patients include mood instability,

---

**Box 42-2    Manic Episode**

Persistent period (at least 1 week) of expansive or irritable mood accompanied by three or more of the following:

- Inflated self-esteem
- Decreased need for sleep
- Pressure of speech
- Racing thoughts
- Highly distractible
- Increase in goal-directed activity (or agitation)
- Unrestrained involvement in pleasurable activities

impulsive behavior, and hyperactivity, symptoms that clearly overlap with bipolar disorder. Whether children who show this chronic symptom picture should be diagnosed with bipolar illness is the center of the debate about bipolar disorder in children. Data from a large-scale community survey have suggested that the core symptoms of bipolar illness are relatively common, affecting 4 to 6% of adolescents (Lewinsohn et al, 1995). The combined prevalence of bipolar I and bipolar II in this sample was approximately 1%. A subsequent follow-up assessment of this same community sample showed that the presence of core symptoms in the first study did not predict the subsequent onset of bipolar illness (Lewinsohn et al., 2000). These results suggest that core symptoms are relatively common, but more clearly defined bipolar disorders are less common. The frequency of core bipolar symptoms that fall below the diagnostic threshold indicates the potential for false-positive case results. In the clinical setting, therefore, clinicians should beware of the over-diagnosis of bipolar disorders in children and adolescents.

## TIC DISORDERS

Tic disorder is a general term used to describe several disorders that are characterized by motor or phonic tics, or both. Motor tics are typically rapid, jerky movements of the eyes, face, neck, and shoulders, but other muscle groups might also be involved. Motor tics might also take the form of slower and more purposeful movements. The most common phonic tics are throat clearing, grunting, or other repetitive noises. More complex sounds such as words, parts of words, and obscenities are expressed by a minority of patients. Table 42-4 presents a list of tic disorders and their defining features.

As shown in Table 42-4, TS is a chronic movement disorder that is defined by the presence of multiple motor and phonic tics. The prevalence of TS is estimated to be between 1 and 10 cases per 1000, with several studies falling in a narrower range of 3 to 6 cases per 1000 (Scahill et al, 2005). The prevalence of TS is three to six times higher in boys than in girls (Kurlan et al, 2001).

The observation in the 1970s that the potent dopamine postsynaptic blocker haloperidol reduced tics prompted speculation about the role of central dopamine systems in TS. Since then, several other neurochemical systems have been implicated in TS, including norepinephrine, endogenous opioids, serotonin, and androgens. Several family genetic studies reported data consistent with autosomal dominant inheritance. These studies also showed that the range of expression is variable and probably includes TS, chronic motor or chronic vocal tic disorder, and OCD as well (Pauls, 2003). Further support for a genetic hypothesis came from twin studies indicating that monozygotic twins are far more likely to be concordant for TS than dizygotic twins. In many cases, however, concordant monozygotic twins were not equally affected, suggesting that environmental factors also have an impact on the expression of the gene. Other family genetic studies have suggested that the inheritance of TS might involve more than a single gene rather than a straightforward autosomal dominant pattern (Walkup et al, 1996).

Although the cause of TS is unknown, several lines of evidence point to dysregulation of circuits that travel from the cortex through the basal ganglia and back (Peterson et al, 2003). The basal ganglia are a group of subcortical structures that play an important role in planning and executing movement, as well as higher cognitive functions. These circuits are organized into five parallel, minimally overlapping pathways, each of which appears to serve separate functions. Dysregulation of one or more of these circuits has been implicated in the pathophysiologic nature of several disorders, including OCD, schizophrenia, TS,

| Table 42-4 | Types and Features of Tic Disorders in *DSM-IV-TR* |
|---|---|
| **Tic Disorder** | **Clinical Features** |
| Transient tic disorder | Motor *and/or* phonic tics for at least 2 weeks, but less than 1 year |
| Chronic tic disorder | Either motor *or* phonic tics for more than 1 year |
| Tourette's disorder* | Both motor *and* phonic tics for more than 1 year |

*In *DSM-IV*, Tourette's disorder is also called Tourette syndrome.

Huntington's chorea, and Parkinson's disease (Mink, 2001; Peterson et al, 2003).

## PSYCHOTIC DISORDERS

Psychotic symptoms might occur in the context of several disorders, such as bipolar illness, depression, and PDD. Psychotic disorders such as schizophrenia are defined using the same criteria as those for adults and are rare in children. For example, childhood-onset schizophrenia is estimated at 2 cases per 100,000, compared with 2 to 10 cases per 1000 in the late teens. The precise cause of schizophrenia is unknown but, as previously suggested, genetic influence is strongly implied. Neuroimaging data suggest a loss of inhibitory control in pathways connecting the frontal lobe to subcortical structures, including the basal ganglia and thalamus (Nicolson and Rapoport, 2003).

## ELIMINATION DISORDERS

### ENURESIS

Enuresis usually refers to bed-wetting (nocturnal enuresis). However, enuresis can also be characterized by repeated urination on clothing during waking hours (diurnal enuresis). For nocturnal enuresis, *DSM-IV-TR* specifies that bed-wetting occur at least twice per week for a duration of 3 months and that the child be at least 5 years of age. Boys are more often affected than girls and the prevalence goes down with age. An estimated 6.7% of 5-year-old boys, 3% of boys ages 9 to 11, and 1% of 14-year-old boys have nocturnal enuresis.

### ENCOPRESIS

Encopresis is defined as soiling clothing with feces or depositing feces in inappropriate places by a child 4 years of age or older. Additional diagnostic criteria require that the soiling occur at least once per month and that it not be the result of a medical disorder, such as aganglionic megacolon (Hirschsprung's disease). The most common cause of encopresis is leakage of stool around a fecal impaction. Fecal impaction might start because the child withholds in response to the urge to defecate. Over time, a loss of muscle tone might occur in the lower bowel, and the child loses the normal urge to defecate and might not even be aware of the leakage. Encopresis affects an estimated 1.5% of school-age children and is three to four times more common in boys than in girls. As with enuresis, the frequency of the condition decreases with age.

### CLINICAL EXAMPLE

Alan, a 9-year-old fourth grader, was referred by his pediatrician to the outpatient clinic for an evaluation of his overactivity, impulsiveness, poor concentration, and disruptive behavior in school. At the time of referral, he lived with his mother and younger sister in a small apartment after having moved from a neighboring town. His mother works part time as a waitress. The history revealed that he had been treated with methylphenidate (Ritalin) in the second grade with uncertain benefit. However, his mother was unable to recall the dose or the duration of treatment.

The developmental history was remarkable for significant marital discord during the pregnancy, resulting in the couple's first separation. This marital discord was characterized by the father's alcohol abuse, parental arguments, and occasional physical fights. The couple finally divorced 3 years later, just before the birth of Alan's younger sister. Alan achieved motor milestones early, but was late in speech and language acquisition. He had only a few words by 2 years of age and, when he entered preschool at the age of 3 years, his speech was poorly understood by nonfamily members.

Overactivity and inability to play with other children without fighting led to Alan's dismissal from the first preschool. His mother reported that Alan did better in the second preschool, which had a more structured program. He remained in this program until the first grade, when he entered the public school. In the first and second grades, Alan's teachers reported that he was hard to manage because of overactivity, calling out without permission, and interfering with the affairs of other children. Although generally good-natured, Alan's intrusive style and occasional aggressive behavior caused him to be rejected by his classmates. He was highly distractible and unable to stay on task. Not surprisingly, he fell behind academically and was barely able to read at the end of second grade.

CLINICAL EXAMPLE—cont'd

In his current school setting, Alan has been frequently ejected from the classroom for disruptive behavior. After instigating a fight in the schoolyard, he had been admonished to stay away from older boys during recess.

Alan was a healthy boy with no history of serious injuries or illnesses or hospitalizations. He had multiple middle ear infections during the first 3 years of life, but had not had any since the age of 5 years. Review of body systems revealed a recent history of intermittent constipation and soiling. According to Alan's mother, this problem had occurred in second grade, but resolved without intervention after 1 or 2 months. He had no known allergies to foods or medication; his last physical examination was before the start of fourth grade.

## Treatment

### Treatment Settings

Traditionally, there were two treatment settings for children and adolescents with psychiatric disorders: specialized inpatient units and outpatient services. Driven in part by the high cost of inpatient care, and by the recognition that the level of care should be congruent with symptom severity, a wider range of mental health services has emerged in recent years. It is now possible in some communities to receive mental health services in the home, school-based clinics, after-school programs, specialized educational programs, day hospitals, therapeutic foster homes, and residential treatment centers, as well as the traditional outpatient and inpatient settings. In all likelihood, this range of mental health services will expand.

## PSYCHOPHARMACOLOGY

Several different classes of medications are used in the treatment of children and adolescents with psychiatric disorders (Scahill and Rains, 2004). Many of the drugs used in the treatment of children and adolescents with serious psychiatric symptoms were developed for other purposes (Table 42-5). In addition, the same drug might be prescribed for any one of several problems. Unfortunately, many of these medications have entered clinical practice without the benefit of carefully controlled studies to guide their use. For example, clonidine was developed as an antihypertensive medication and is used in the treatment of ADHD and tics. Although studies have been conducted in both children and adults with tics, the data supporting its use in ADHD have been limited until rather recently (Tourette's Syndrome Study Group, 2002).

An important guiding principle in pediatric psychopharmacology is that children are physiologically different from adults. These differences can have an impact on dose, clinical response, and side effects. For example, children often require larger doses of psychotropic drugs, on a milligram-per-kilogram basis, than adults to obtain beneficial effects. Although it is not completely clear why this is true, it might be because children have more efficient liver metabolism and glomerular filtration systems than adults (Vinks and Walson, 2003). Because of developmental differences in neural pathways, drug effects (pharmacodynamics) might be different in children compared with adults. For example, norepinephrine, dopamine, and serotonin systems all undergo developmental changes in childhood (Vinks and Walson, 2003). These developmental differences might explain the inconsistent effects of tricyclic antidepressants (TCAs) in children with depression compared with adults and the more frequently observed activating side effects of selective serotonin reuptake inhibitors (SSRIs) in children (Chiu and Leonard, 2003; Gundersen and Geller, 2003).

## STIMULANTS

The most frequently used stimulants are methylphenidate (Ritalin), dextroamphetamine (Dexedrine), and the mixed amphetamine compound (D,L-amphetamine) Adderall. Of these various preparations, methylphenidate is by far the most common, being used by approximately 3% of school-age children. The preference for methylphenidate over the other stimulants is probably because of its familiarity (Ford et al, 2003). Another less commonly used stimulant is pemoline (Cylert). Because of concern about the risk of hepatic failure, this medication is falling out of use and in September 1999 was withdrawn from the market in Canada.

One federally funded multisite study enrolled 576 children and randomly assigned them to one

| Table 42-5 | Level of Evidence for Medications Used in the Treatment of Children and Adolescents With Psychiatric Disorders | |
| --- | --- | --- |

| Class | Purpose(s) | Empirical Support* |
| --- | --- | --- |
| Stimulants | ADHD | Excellent |
| Tricyclic antidepressants | 1. Depression | Fair |
| | 2. ADHD | Good |
| | 3. Enuresis | Good |
| | 4. Separation anxiety | Fair |
| | 5. OCD (clomipramine) | Excellent |
| Serotonin reuptake inhibitors | 1. OCD | Excellent |
| | 2. Depression | Good |
| | 3. Anxiety | Good |
| Traditional antipsychotics | 1. Psychosis | Excellent |
| | 2. Tics (haloperidol and pimozide) | Excellent |
| | 3. Severe impulsiveness in ADHD | Good |
| | 4. Agitation in PDD | Good |
| Atypical antipsychotics (risperidone best studied to date) | 1. Psychosis | Good |
| | 2. Aggression in PDD | Excellent |
| | 3. Tics | Excellent |
| | 4. Severe disruptive behavior in ODD and CD | Excellent |
| Alpha-2 agonists | 1. Tics (clonidine) | Good |
| | 2. ADHD (clonidine and guanfacine) | Good |
| Mood stabilizers | 1. Mania (lithium) | Good |
| | 2. Mania (valproate) | Fair |

*Poor, No controlled studies in pediatric populations; support from open-label studies only; *fair*, at least one controlled study in pediatric populations, might be concern about side effects; *good*, some data from controlled studies, but findings are inconsistent; *excellent*, consistent body of efficacy and safety data from more than one controlled study (see text for details).
*ADHD*, Attention-deficit/hyperactivity disorder; *CD*, conduct disorder; *OCD*, obsessive-compulsive disorder; *ODD*, oppositional defiant disorder; *PDD*, pervasive developmental disorder.

of four groups: (1) expert medication management (from one of the research centers), (2) expert medication management with behavioral treatment, (3) behavioral treatment alone, or (4) treatment in the community. In this design, treatment in the community was the control condition. The behavior-therapy program in the behavior treatment–only group and the combined treatment group was the same and was delivered in structured fashion to ensure consistency across sites. Important questions for the study included whether expert medication management would be superior to treatment obtained in the community, and whether behavior therapy would show additive benefit when combined with medication treatment. Subjects were reassessed at 14 months. Compared with the community controls and the behavior therapy–only groups, the groups who received expert medication management alone or expert medication management with behavior therapy did significantly better on ratings from teachers and parents. No difference occurred

between the behavior treatment–only and community controls (MTA Cooperative Group, 1999). In both the expertly managed medication groups and the community control group, methylphenidate was the most commonly used drug. The medication management at the research centers tended to involve higher doses on average and to use three doses per day rather than two, which was the norm in the community sample.

The follow-up study of 520 children conducted by the same research group (MTA Cooperative Group, 2004) examined the long-term benefits and impact of stimulant medication on growth at 24 months. All four treatment groups showed some loss of benefit from the 14- to 24-month assessment. The children who remained on medication showed the least amount of deterioration compared with those who had not taken medication. In contrast to these beneficial effects, children who remained on medication showed slightly slower growth rates than children who were never treated with stimulant medication.

Methylphenidate was also studied in a group of 66 children (age range, 5 to 14 years) with PDD accompanied by hyperactivity and impulsive behavior (Research Units on Pediatric Psychopharmacology Autism Network, 2005a). For each of 4 weeks in the study, children received a different dose of methylphenidate (low, medium, or high) or placebo. Parents, teachers, and the research team were blinded to dose level or placebo. Overall, methylphenidate was superior to placebo, but the magnitude of effect was smaller than the large effects observed in typically developing children with ADHD. Seven of 66 subjects exited the study because of adverse effects. These side effects, which included insomnia, decreased appetite, irritability, and increased self-injury, were most likely to occur during the highest dose week (0.5 to 0.6 mg/kg for the morning dose). Although methylphenidate appears useful in children with PDD and hyperactivity, the magnitude of benefit is modest and this population appears more susceptible to adverse effects than typically developing children with ADHD.

The optimal daily dosage of methylphenidate ranges between 0.6 and 1.5 mg/kg of body weight per day in three divided doses. This level translates into roughly 10 mg twice daily (breakfast and lunch) and 5 mg at 4 PM for a 45-pound (20-kg) child. Slightly higher doses might be tried in cases showing equivocal response, but doses above 60 mg per day are not recommended. The usual dose of dextroamphetamine (or D,L-amphetamine) is lower than that of methylphenidate and is typically given twice daily. The total daily dosage is typically in the range of 10 to 20 mg/day for younger children and 30 to 40 mg/day for older children (i.e., for a total dosage of 0.3 mg and 1 mg/kg per day).

Immediate-release methylphenidate and the amphetamines are given just before or with meals to prevent loss of appetite. Other adverse effects of the stimulants include insomnia, irritability, tics and abnormal movements, a tendency to become overfocused on details and, rarely, agitation and psychotic symptoms. In the usual short-acting form, methylphenidate and the amphetamines have a duration of action of about 4 and 6 hours, respectively. As the medication effects wear off, a behavioral rebound can occur. To soften the rebound effect later in the day, the third dose of methylphenidate or the second dose of amphetamine is typically lower than the previous dose. Additionally, long-acting preparations of methylphenidate (Concerta, Metadate CD or ER, Ritalin LA) and D,L-amphetamine (Adderall XR) are available (Rains and Scahill, 2004). These long-acting preparations facilitate dosing by eliminating the need for a second or third daily dose. Because the release is sustained throughout the day, dosing flexibility is limited.

## TRICYCLIC ANTIDEPRESSANTS

TCAs, including imipramine, desipramine, nortriptyline, and clomipramine, are a group of chemically related compounds that have been used in children and adolescents for over 30 years. As suggested in Table 42-5, these agents have been used in the treatment of depression, enuresis, separation anxiety, ADHD, and OCD with mixed results, depending on the specific agent and the disorder in question.

To date, the efficacy of the TCAs in the treatment of children with depression has not been demonstrated (Gundersen and Geller, 2003). Placebo-controlled studies have demonstrated the effectiveness of desipramine in the treatment of ADHD (Spencer et al, 2002). However, concern about alterations in cardiac conduction has decreased enthusiasm for the use of desipramine in pediatric populations. Imipramine has been studied in controlled trials for separation anxiety, with inconsistent results (Klein et al, 1992). Imipramine has demonstrated efficacy in the treatment of enuresis. However, since the introduction of the synthetic antidiuretic hormone desmopressin (DDAVP), the use of imipramine for enuresis has declined.

Clomipramine is unique in that, in addition to the norepinephrine reuptake properties common to the other TCAs, it also has potent serotonin reuptake properties (Gundersen and Geller, 2003). This mechanism is believed to be the explanation for its effectiveness in the treatment of OCD. In a multicenter trial, clomipramine was superior to placebo in adolescents with OCD (DeVeaugh-Geiss et al, 1992). The typical dose of clomipramine ranges from 75 to 200 mg, depending on the age of the child, with younger children on the lower end of the range.

The side effects of the TCAs include dry mouth, fatigue, dizziness, sweating, weight gain, urinary retention, tremor, tachycardia, and agitation. These adverse effects can often be managed by lowering the dose or changing the dosage schedule (e.g., splitting into two doses per day). All TCAs can affect cardiac conduction. Therefore, children and adolescents treated with any TCA should receive a cardiogram at baseline and periodically during treatment. Resting heart rate over 120 bpm is cause for concern, warranting consultation with the clinical team. The TCAs are also vulnerable to drug-drug interaction. For example, commonly used drugs such as erythromycin can interfere with the metabolism of the TCA, resulting in a rapid and dramatic increase in the level of the TCA. Given that the risk of adverse effects of the TCAs increases at higher drug levels, drug-drug interactions should be avoided.

## SELECTIVE SEROTONIN REUPTAKE INHIBITORS

SSRIs are a group of chemically unrelated compounds that were developed as antidepressants. The success of clomipramine in the treatment of OCD prompted great interest in these drugs for the treatment of OCD, as well as depression. Currently, six SSRIs are marketed in the United States, including fluoxetine (Prozac), sertraline (Zoloft), paroxetine (Paxil), fluvoxamine (Luvox), citalopram (Celexa), and escitalopram (Lexapro). Each has shown efficacy in the treatment of depression in adults. Fluoxetine, sertraline, and fluvoxamine have also demonstrated efficacy for OCD in controlled trials in both children and adults (Chiu and Leonard, 2003). Fluoxetine, sertraline, paroxetine, and citalopram have been examined in placebo-controlled trials in children and adolescents with depression. Results of these studies are mixed and only fluoxetine has been shown to be superior to placebo in more than two trials (Hamrin and Scahill, 2005). Currently, sertraline, fluvoxamine, and fluoxetine are approved for use in children with OCD; fluoxetine is approved for MDD.

The precise mechanism of the SSRIs is not completely understood. It is known that SSRIs block the return of serotonin into the presynaptic neuron—hence, the term *reuptake inhibitors.* All six of the SSRIs have relatively long half-lives, permitting single daily dosing, with the exception of fluvoxamine, which is often given twice daily (Box 42-3).

### Box 42-3    Selective Serotonin Reuptake Inhibitors

**Fluoxetine**
Fluoxetine (Prozac) comes in a 10- or 20-mg capsule, a liquid form, and a weekly dosage formulation. Because of its long half-life (fluoxetine also has an active metabolite with an even longer half-life), the dose is typically increased slowly to avoid overshooting the optimal dose. The typical starting dosage is 5 to 10 mg/day, and the dosage range for most children and adolescents is between 10 and 40 mg/day. Fluoxetine has been shown to be effective in the treatment of depression and OCD in pediatric studies.

**Sertraline**
Sertraline (Zoloft) has shown superiority to placebo in large-scale studies in OCD and is available in 50- and 100-mg tablets that can easily be broken in half. The starting dosage might be 25 mg/day, with gradual increases to 25 to 150 mg in children. Adolescents might receive slightly higher doses. Some patients respond at lower doses, so dosing should be individualized.

**Fluvoxamine**
Fluvoxamine (Luvox) has been evaluated in a large multicenter study in children and adolescents with OCD and now has approval from the FDA for use in pediatric populations. The medication comes in 25-, 50-, and 100-mg tablets, each of which can be broken in half. Treatment might begin with 12.5 to 25 mg/day and might be increased by 25 mg every 5 to 7 days, as tolerated. The typical dosage range is 50 to 200 mg/day in children. It is often administered in two divided doses.

**Paroxetine**
Paroxetine (Paxil) comes in 20- and 30-mg tablets that can be broken in half. To date, paroxetine has been studied in depression and OCD in pediatric populations. A reasonable starting dosage would be 10 mg/day to a total of 10 to 40 mg in a single daily dose.

### Side Effects of the Selective Serotonin Reuptake Inhibitors

The most common side effect of the SSRIs in children and adolescents is *behavioral activation,* which might be characterized by motor restlessness, insomnia, hypomania, and disinhibition. The risk of behavioral activation is greatest early in treatment, but it might also be seen with dose increases (Chiu and Leonard, 2003). In some cases, what appears to be activation becomes a manic episode. Either activation or a true manic episode requires intervention. Other side effects include abdominal pain, heartburn, diarrhea, and decreased appetite.

In October 2004, the FDA issued a warning about the use of SSRIs in pediatric patients because of increased concerns regarding behavioral activation. Based on pooled analyses of 24 placebo-controlled trials involving over 4000 pediatric patients, the FDA expressed concern about the possibility of worsening depression, emergence of suicidal thoughts and behaviors, hyperactivity, irritability, and impulsiveness following the initiation of SSRI treatment. A carefully conducted multisite study involved four treatment groups: (1) fluoxetine alone, (2) fluoxetine with cognitive-behavioral treatment (CBT), (3) CBT alone, and (4) placebo (see below for more details). Fluoxetine was superior to placebo and CBT alone (Treatment of Adolescents with Depression Study, 2004). The fluoxetine group also showed a slightly higher rate of suicidal thought and self-harming behavior (e.g., cutting behavior) than the placebo group. Thus, although SSRI medication—especially fluoxetine—has been shown to be effective in treating depression, children treated with an SSRI should be monitored for suicidal thoughts and planning, even as their depression improves (Hamrin and Scahill, 2005).

When a child is placed on an SSRI for OCD or depression and has a positive response, parents frequently inquire about the duration of treatment. In the absence of clear evidence to guide the decision, most clinicians suggest discontinuation after a symptom-free period of 8 to 12 months (Birmaher et al, 1998). Parents should be discouraged from abrupt withdrawal because of reports of emotional instability, dizziness, nausea, nervousness, and confusion on abrupt withdrawal of sertraline and paroxetine (Rosenbaum et al, 1998). Fluoxetine, which has a longer half-life, was not associated with these complaints. Fluvoxamine, citalopram, and escitalopram were not evaluated in this study. However, because fluvoxamine is also relatively short-acting compared with fluoxetine, abrupt withdrawal of fluvoxamine should be avoided. Similarly, although citalopram and escitalopram have longer half-lives than fluvoxamine, they also should probably not be stopped abruptly. Children and parents should also be informed that symptoms of OCD or depression might return after planned discontinuation of an SSRI.

A multisite study conducted by the Research Unit on Pediatric Psychopharmacology Anxiety Group evaluated the efficacy and safety of fluvoxamine in childhood-onset anxiety disorders (Anonymous, 2001). The study included 128 children and adolescents (age range, 6 to 17 years) with generalized anxiety disorder, separation anxiety disorder, social phobia, or any combination. Before randomization, eligible subjects were given 4 weeks of cognitive psychotherapy. Subjects who remained symptomatic after the 4-week psychotherapy were randomized to fluvoxamine or a placebo for 8 weeks under double-blind conditions. After 8 weeks of treatment at an average dose of $4.4 \pm 2.2$ mg/kg, a 52% improvement was noted on the Pediatric Anxiety Rating Scale (PARS) in the fluvoxamine group compared with a 16% improvement in the placebo group. The side effects observed in this study were similar to those reported in pediatric samples with OCD. The most common adverse effects included abdominal discomfort, behavioral activation, headache, and drowsiness (higher than 20% for each).

As noted above, fluoxetine was studied in a National Institute of Mental Health–funded, multisite trial of 439 patients ages 12 to 17 years with major depression (Treatment of Adolescents with Depression Study, 2004). Subjects were randomly assigned to fluoxetine alone, CBT alone, fluoxetine plus CBT, or placebo. Fluoxetine alone or in combination with CBT was superior to placebo on a clinician measure of depression. Although fluoxetine plus CBT was better than fluoxetine alone, the difference was not statistically significant. Of all patients receiving an SSRI ($N = 216$), 7% expressed suicidal ideation compared with 4% of the 223 children in the non–drug-treated groups (i.e., CBT-only and placebo groups). Six of the 216 (3%) fluoxetine-treated subjects exhibited mania, hypomania, or elevated mood symptoms compared with 1% (2 of 223) subjects in the non–drug-treated groups.

Sertraline was studied in a multisite trial of 112 subjects ages 7 to 17 years by the Pediatric OCD Treatment Study Team (2004). Participants were randomized to receive CBT alone, CBT combined with sertraline, sertraline alone, or placebo for 12 weeks. All three treatments were superior to placebo alone and no subjects experienced self-harm, suicidal ideation, or intent. Furthermore, combined treatment was superior to CBT alone or sertraline alone. This was the first study in child psychiatry to show that the combination of medication and CBT is superior to medication alone. However, the interpretation of this finding is complicated by the observation that CBT appeared to be more successful in one of the study sites than in the others.

## TRADITIONAL ANTIPSYCHOTICS

Traditional antipsychotics, such as the phenothiazines and haloperidol, primarily block $D_2$ dopamine receptors. These medications have been used for a range of problems, including psychosis, tics, and aggression. The newer atypical antipsychotics such as olanzapine and risperidone not only block dopamine receptors, but are potent antagonists of specific serotonin receptors as well. This pharmacologic property appears to be protective against neurologic side effects.

### Side Effects of the Traditional Antipsychotics

Low-potency antipsychotics are associated with sedation and orthostatic hypotension. By contrast, the higher potency agents are associated with extrapyramidal side effects (EPSEs), such as dystonia, dyskinesia, akathisia (subjective feeling of restlessness), and parkinsonism. In some cases, the dystonia is acute and severe, characterized by torticollis and rolling of the eyes upward (i.e., oculogyric crisis). Treatment of acute dystonia includes immediate injection of an anticholinergic medication such as benztropine (Cogentin) and slowing down the rate of increase of the antipsychotic. Other side effects of the traditional antipsychotics include cognitive blunting, irritability, depressed mood, blurred vision, dry mouth, and weight gain. Finally, long-term treatment with an antipsychotic places the patient at increased risk for tardive dyskinesia (Campbell et al, 1997), a chronic neurologic condition involving abnormal movements of the face, mouth, and sometimes the arms. These potential short- and long-term side effects should be discussed with the child and family before and during treatment with this group of medications.

## ATYPICAL ANTIPSYCHOTICS

Concerns about the potential long- and short-term adverse effects of the traditional antipsychotics have prompted the development of a new class of antipsychotics. The first medication of this new class was clozapine, which was introduced in the 1960s. Although early results were encouraging, clozapine was nearly withdrawn from use because of concerns about agranulocytosis. Currently, clozapine is reserved for cases of treatment-refractory schizophrenia. The atypical antipsychotics block both serotonin and, to some extent, dopamine receptors. Over the last few years, several agents with this dual action have been introduced, such as risperidone (Risperdal), olanzapine (Zyprexa), quetiapine (Seroquel), ziprasidone (Geodon), and aripiprazole (Abilify). In addition to the treatment of psychosis, these medications are used to treat other target symptoms, including aggression, tantrums and self-injury in autism, severe disruptive behavior, and tics in TS (Aman et al, 2002; Research Units on Pediatric Psychopharmacology, 2002; Research Units on Pediatric Psychopharmacology Autism Network, 2005b; Scahill et al, 2003) (Box 42-4). Perhaps because it was the first of the new atypical antipsychotics to enter the marketplace, risperidone is the best studied of this class of medications (Findling et al, 2003).

Risperidone came on the market in early 1994. Since then, risperidone has been evaluated in several open-label studies in children and adolescents with a wide range of problems, including tic disorders, PDD, schizophrenia, and severe disruptive behavior. The usual daily dosage ranges from 0.5 to 2.5 mg. Neurologic side effects associated with the traditional antipsychotics are rare. The most common adverse effects across these studies include sedation, increased appetite, and weight gain. Children who are placed on this drug should be weighed at baseline; diet, appetite, and weight should be monitored during treatment. One case of dramatically elevated liver function tests accompanied by fatty infiltration has been reported (Kumra et al, 1997).

The Research Units on Pediatric Psychopharmacology (RUPP) Autism Network (McCracken et al, 2002) evaluated the efficacy and safety of risperidone in children and adolescents with autism accompanied by tantrums, aggression, and self-injury. This placebo-controlled study in 101 children with autism showed that risperidone at an average dosage of 1.8 mg/day was superior to placebo for reducing aggression, tantrums, and self-injury (McCracken et al, 2002). These gains were stable over a 6-month follow-up period without having to increase the dosage of medication. In the last phase of the study, children were randomized to gradual withdrawal to placebo or

## Box 42-4 Traditional Antipsychotics

### Thioridazine
Thioridazine (Mellaril) is a low-potency antipsychotic in the phenothiazine chemical family. It has been used for the treatment of severe hyperactivity and/or agitation. The introduction of the atypical antipsychotics and concern about the potential for inducing cardiac arrhythmias have contributed to the decline in the use of thioridazine.

### Thiothixene
Thiothixene (Navane) is an antipsychotic of intermediate potency that is used primarily for psychosis or severe agitation. In children, treatment typically begins with 2 mg two or three times daily, with gradual increases to 5 mg two or three times daily. This schedule might be more aggressive, and higher dosage levels might be used in acute psychotic states.

### Haloperidol
Haloperidol (Haldol) is a high-potency antipsychotic that is unrelated to the phenothiazines. It has been studied in pediatric populations for the treatment of psychosis, PDD, conduct disorder, and tic disorders. The typical dosage ranges from 1 to 2 mg/day for the treatment of tics to 10 mg/day for the management of acute psychosis.

### Pimozide
Pimozide (Orap) is another high-potency antipsychotic that is used specifically for the treatment of tics. It comes in 1- and 2-mg tablets; the typical dosage range is 1 to 4 mg/day.

### Risperidone
Risperidone (Risperdal) is a newer atypical antipsychotic medication that has potent dopamine- and serotonin-blocking properties. Risperidone is effective for the treatment of tics, as well as aggression, agitation, and self-injury in children with autism and severe disruptive behavior.

continued treatment with risperidone under double-blind conditions. The group of children who gradually switched to placebo showed a significantly higher rate of relapse (i.e., return of tantrums, aggression, or self-injury) than the group who continued treatment with risperidone (Anonymous, 2005).

## NONSTIMULANT MEDICATIONS FOR ATTENTION-DEFICIT/HYPERACTIVITY DISORDER

### ALPHA-2 AGONISTS

The alpha-2 agonists, clonidine (Catapres) and guanfacine (Tenex), were developed as antihypertensive agents. These drugs reduce norepinephrine activity in the brain. Clonidine can be useful for the treatment of tics, as shown in a double-blind study (Leckman et al, 1991). Support for the use of clonidine in the treatment of ADHD is less consistent, although one placebo-controlled study showed that it was superior to placebo in a sample of children with tic disorders and ADHD. In addition, the combination of clonidine and methylphenidate provided additional benefits (Tourette's Syndrome Study Group, 2002). The typical daily dosage of clonidine ranges from 0.15 to 0.25 mg divided into three or four doses. The most common side effect of clonidine is sedation. Dry mouth, headache, irritability, and sleep disturbance might also occur. Although rarely a problem, blood pressure should be monitored during treatment, especially when starting the medication. Abrupt discontinuation can cause a rebound in blood pressure and should be avoided.

In dosages ranging from 1 to 4 mg/day in three divided doses, guanfacine has been evaluated in two placebo-controlled trials. In one study, 17 children with ADHD and a tic disorder were randomly assigned to receive guanfacine and 17 received placebo. After 8 weeks of treatment, the guanfacine group showed improvements in ADHD symptoms and tics compared with the placebo group (Scahill et al, 2001). Adverse effects are similar to those of clonidine, although guanfacine is less sedating than clonidine. Guanfacine is of increasing interest for the treatment of ADHD, but more studies are needed.

## ATOMOXETINE

Atomoxetine (Strattera) is a nonstimulant medication that was originally developed as an antidepressant. Similar to the older TCA desipramine, atomoxetine is a potent norepinephrine reuptake inhibitor. Unlike desipramine, it does not appear to affect cardiac conduction. Atomoxetine has been evaluated in several studies, showing that it is safe and effective for the treatment of children with ADHD (Michelson et al, 2001, 2002). Based on these results, atomoxetine is now FDA-approved for the treatment of ADHD. The magnitude of benefit for atomoxetine in these trials is about 30% over baseline, which is clearly lower than the expected level of benefit associated with the stimulants (MTA Cooperative Group, 1999).

Studies of atomoxetine in children and adolescents with ADHD have used once-daily or twice-daily dosing strategies. Comparing results across these studies, it is clear that both dosing regimens are superior to placebo for reducing ADHD symptoms (Michelson et al, 2001, 2002). Thus, whether atomoxetine is given once or twice daily might be a case-by-case decision. Compliance might be better with once-daily dosing, but adverse effects might be slightly lower with twice-daily dosing.

Common side effects of atomoxetine include headache, upper abdominal pain, decreased appetite, nausea, weight loss, irritability, dizziness, and somnolence (Wernicke and Kratochvil, 2002). Decreased appetite and weight loss are most common early in treatment and might be attenuated by slow upward adjustment. Atomoxetine is available in 10-, 18-, 25-, 40-, and 60-mg tablets.

## COGNITIVE-BEHAVIORAL THERAPY

Currently, treatment of children and adolescents often involves a multimodal approach, which might include medication, family treatment, group therapy, and individual therapy for the child. CBT is a form of individual therapy that has been successfully used for children with disruptive behavior disorders, anxiety disorders, and depression. Other psychotherapeutic interventions such as interpersonal therapy (IPT) have been shown to be effective in adults and adolescents (Mufson et al, 1999). This section focuses on cognitive-behavioral techniques used in the treatment of ADHD and OCD.

### ATTENTION-DEFICIT/HYPERACTIVITY DISORDER

Recalling that the hallmark features of ADHD are inattention, overactivity, and impulsiveness, the goal of CBT in ADHD is to improve the child's ability to stop, look, and listen before acting. Several approaches have been developed to accomplish this.

### Social Skills Training

Social skills training teaches the child to recognize the impact of his or her behavior on others.

Because impulsive children and adolescents often fail to recognize the adverse effects of their verbal and nonverbal behavior, social skills training uses instruction, role playing, and positive reinforcement to improve interpersonal relationships and enhance social outcomes.

### Problem-Solving Skills Training

Problem-solving skills training focuses on defective cognitive processes such as assessment of situations, as well as interpretation of events and expectations of others. Children with disruptive behavior problems often misinterpret the intentions of others—for example, perceiving hostility when none was intended. Through instruction and role playing, problem-solving skills training teaches the child to generate alternative interpretations for the behavior of others and options for a response. These options are then evaluated for their likely consequences on the situation and on interpersonal relationships.

### Parent Training

The reckless and impulsive behavior of children with ADHD and other disruptive behavior disorders often elicits punitive responses from their parents. Parent training attempts to provide parents with a more complete understanding of their child's behavior and new ways of responding to it. These programs emphasize the importance of clear limits concerning unwanted behavior and positive reinforcement (positive attention, praise, and tangible rewards) for desired behaviors. The use of point systems and mild punishments such as time-out is also presented. Parent training programs might be offered in a group format or in a family therapy setting (Barkley, 1998).

### OBSESSIVE-COMPULSIVE DISORDER

CBT for OCD is based on exposure and response prevention. Exposure refers to deliberate confrontation of a situation or event that triggers anxiety or the urge to perform the ritual. Response prevention consists of blocking the compulsive behavior despite the presence of the urge to complete it. For example, if the patient feared contamination and felt the need to wash after touching sticky materials, the patient might be encouraged to touch a sticky counter and then refrain from washing. These techniques have clearly demonstrated their usefulness in the treatment of adults with OCD and recently have been applied to children (POTS, 2004).

The theory behind exposure and response prevention is that rising anxiety occurs in response to external events (a trigger). Second, the anxiety associated with the triggering event or situation is exaggerated. Third, because the performance of the ritual results in a rapid decline in anxiety, it reinforces the idea that the compulsive behavior is a useful strategy for managing anxiety. Unfortunately, the success of the ritualized behavior is typically short-lived. Finally, systematic confrontation of the triggering event or situation results in decreased anxiety, even if the ritual is not performed. Box 42-5 presents a traditional treatment plan for the case presented earlier in this section.

## CRITICAL THINKING QUESTION    2

When working with a parent of a child with ADHD, how might a nurse explain the child's need for structure in the home without seeming to blame the parent for the child's problem behavior?

## ■ Study Notes

1. Current prevalence estimates of psychiatric disorders in children indicate that they are relatively common, but only a small percentage of children are receiving appropriate treatment.
2. Risk factors for childhood psychiatric disorders include genetic factors and adverse environmental influences, such as perinatal complications, and psychosocial adversities, such as poverty, single-parent family, family conflict, and a parent with a mental illness.
3. The presence of a risk factor increases the likelihood of developing a mental illness.

---

### Box 42-5    Treatment Plan: Alan

**Diagnosis**

| | |
|---|---|
| Axis I | ADHD: combined type |
| | Encopresis |
| | Reading disorder |
| Axis II | None |
| Axis III | None |
| Axis IV | Academic problems |
| | Inadequate finances |
| | Family dysfunction |
| Axis V | Global assessment of functioning: 50 |

**Goals**
1. Reduce overactivity and impulsive behavior.
2. Improve social judgment.
3. Remediate delayed reading skills.
4. Restore normal bowel function.

**Placement**
The treatment plan includes placement in a day treatment program beause of the degree of impulsiveness and tendency to provoke retaliation from others. This placement will also permit the application of multiple treatments, including social skills training, parent training for Alan's mother, and close monitoring of pharmacotherapy. The day hospital program will also include a psychoeducational evaluation to clarify his reading disability and generate remediation strategies.

**Medication**
After a 2-week observation period, a trial of methylphenidate will be initiated. Despite report of a previous unsuccessful trial, available evidence suggests that the trial was inadequate. Therefore, before moving on to another stimulant or to a nonstimulant alternative, response to methylphenidate in a carefully monitored trial is appropriate. The medication will be started at 5 mg/day and increased to 5 mg tid (8 AM, 12 noon, and 4 PM) after 4 days. If well tolerated, the dosage will be increased 4 days later to 10 mg in the morning, 10 mg at noon, and 5 mg at 4 PM. Thereafter, the dose will be increased depending on response, with a maximum dosage of 30 to 40 mg/day in three divided doses with the third dose roughly half of the morning and noon doses.

**Bowel Retraining Program**
In collaboration with his primary care providers, a bowel retraining program will be initiated. Step 1 is educating the mother and Alan about normal bowel function and the vicious cycle of fecal impaction and leakage of stool around the hardened mass of stool. This educational effort should help decrease the mother's anger at Alan for this problem and will help motivate Alan to engage in solving the problem. Step 2 is to clean out the bowel (e.g., with a laxative and mineral oil). Step 3 is the behavioral treatment program, which typically involves daily sitting on the toilet after each meal for 10 minutes. Rewards in the form of stickers or points will be given at school and at home for participating in the program. Special bonuses can be awarded for successful defecation. The stickers or points can be cashed in for small prizes at the end of each week.

4. Children can be motivated by their peers. Psychotherapeutic management of children in the psychiatric inpatient setting is most effective when the nurse-patient relationship and milieu issues are considered jointly.

5. Resilience is the ability of a child to maintain an optimal development course despite exposure to undesirable environmental conditions.

6. ADHD is the most common pediatric behavioral disorder. Central nervous system stimulants are the drugs most frequently used to treat children with ADHD.

7. Symptoms of autism include significant delays in socialization and communication, as well as repetitive behavior and restricted patterns of behavior.

8. Depression is uncommon in young children, but the prevalence increases in adolescents. Until recently, no antidepressant had been shown to be superior to a placebo in children and adolescents.

## References

Abelson JF, Kwan KY, O'Roak BJ, et al: Sequence variants in SLITRK1 are associated with Tourette's syndrome, *Science* 310:317, 2005.

Acosta MT, Pearl PL: The neurobiology of autism: new pieces of the puzzle, *Curr Neurol Neurosci Rep* 3:149, 2003.

Aman MG, De Smedt G, Derivan A, et al: Risperidone Disruptive Behavior Study Group: Double-blind, placebo-controlled study of risperidone for the treatment of disruptive behaviors in children with subaverage intelligence, *Am J Psychiatry* 159:1337, 2002.

American Psychiatric Association: *Diagnostic and statistical manual of mental disorders, text revision,* ed 4, Washington, DC, 2000, APA.

American Psychiatric Association: *Diagnostic and statistical manual of mental disorders,* ed 4, Washington, DC, 1994, APA.

American Psychiatric Association: *Diagnostic and statistical manual of mental disorders,* ed 3, Washington, DC, 1980, APA.

Anonymous: Randomized, controlled, crossover trial of methylphenidate in pervasive developmental disorders with hyperactivity, *Arch Gen Psychiatry* 62:1266, 2005.

Anonymous: Fluvoxamine in the treatment of children and adolescents with anxiety disorders. The Research Unit on Pediatric Psychopharmacology Anxiety Study Group, *N Engl J Med* 344:1279, 2001.

Barkley RA: *Attention deficit hyperactivity disorder: a handbook for diagnosis and treatment,* New York, 1998, Guilford Press.

Biederman J, Hirshfeld-Becker DR, Rosenbaum JF, et al: Further evidence of association between behavioral inhibition and social anxiety in children, *Am J Psychiatry* 158:1673, 2001.

Biederman J, Milberger S, Faraone SV, et al: Family-environmental risk factors for attention-deficit hyperactivity disorder. A test of Rutter's indicators of adversity, *Arch Gen Psychiatry* 52:464, 1995.

Birmaher B, Brent DA: Depressive disorders. In Martin A, Scahill L, Charney D, Leckman J, editors: *Pediatric psychopharmacology* (pp. 466-483), New York, 2003, Oxford University Press.

Briggs-Gowan MJ, Horwitz SM, Schwab-Stone ME, et al: Mental health in pediatric settings: distribution of disorders and factors related to service use, *J Am Acad Child Psychiatry* 39:841, 2000.

Burns BJ, Phillips SD, Wagner HR, et al: Mental health need and access to mental health services by youths involved with child welfare: a national survey, *J Am Acad Child Adolesc Psychiatry* 43:960, 2004.

Campbell M, Armenteros JL, Malone RP, et al: Neuroleptic-related dyskinesias in autistic children: a prospective, longitudinal study, *J Am Acad Child Adolesc Psychiatry* 36:835, 1997.

Carey G, Gottesman II: Twin and family studies of anxiety, phobic, and obsessive-compulsive disorders. In Klein DF, Rabkin J, editors: *Anxiety: new research and changing concepts,* New York, 1981, Raven.

Carlson GA: Bipolar disorder. In Martin A, Scahill L, Charney D, Leckman J, editors: *Pediatric psychopharmacology,* New York, 2003, Oxford University Press, pp 484-496.

Castellanos FX, Giedd JN, Marsh WL, et al: Quantitative brain magnetic resonance imaging in attention-deficit hyperactivity disorder, *Arch Gen Psychiatry* 53:607, 1996.

Chakrabarti S, Fombonne E: Pervasive developmental disorders in preschool children: confirmation of high prevalence, *Am J Psychiatry* 162:1133, 2005.

Chiu S, Leonard H: Antidepressants I: selective serotonin reuptake inhibitors. In Martin A, Scahill L, Charney D, Leckman J, editors: *Pediatric psychopharmacology,* New York, 2003, Oxford University Press, pp 274-283.

Clegg J, Hollis C, Mawhood L, Rutter M: Developmental language disorders—a follow-up in later adult life. Cognitive, language and psychosocial outcomes, *J Child Psychol Psychiatry* 46:128, 2005.

Costello EJ, Angold A, Burns BJ, et al: The Great Smoky Mountains study of youth: goals, design, methods, and the prevalence of DSM-III-R disorders, *Arch Gen Psychiatry* 53:1129, 1996.

DeVeaugh-Geiss J, Moroz G, Biederman J, et al: Clomipramine hydrochloride in childhood and adolescent obsessive-compulsive disorder: a multicenter trial, *J Am Acad Child Adolesc Psychiatry* 31:45, 1992.

Eigenmann PA. Haenggeli CA: Food colourings and preservatives—allergy and hyperactivity. *Lancet* 364:823, 2004.

Faraone SV, Biederman J, Keenan K, Tsuang MT: Separation of DSM-III attention deficit disorder and conduct disorder: evidence from a family-genetic study of American child psychiatric patients, *Psychol Med* 21:109, 1991.

Findling RL, McNamara NK, Gracious BL: Antipsychotic agents: traditional and atypical. In Martin A, Scahill L, Charney D, Leckman J, editors: *Pediatric psychopharmacology: principles and practice,* New York, 2003, Oxford University, pp 328-340.

Ford RE, Greenhill LL, Posner K: Stimulants. In Martin A, Scahill L, Charney DS, Leckman JF, editors: *Pediatric psychopharmacology,* New York, 2003, Oxford University Press, pp 255-263.

Giedd JN: Bipolar disorder attention-deficit/hyperactivity disorder in children and adolescents, *J Clin Psychiatry* 61:31, 2000.

Gundersen K, Geller B: Antidepressants II: tricyclic agents. In Martin A, Scahill L, Charney D, Leckman J, editors: *Pediatric psychopharmacology* (pp. 284-294), New York, 2003, Oxford University Press.

Hamrin V, Scahill L: Selective serotonin reuptake inhibitors in children and adolescents with major depression: current controversies and recommendations, *Issues Ment Health Nurs* 26: 433, 2005.

Hudziak JJ, Derks EM, Althoff RR, et al: The genetic and environmental contributions to attention deficit hyperactivity disorder as measured by the Conners' rating scales—revised, *Am J Psychiatry* 162:1614, 2005.

Karno M, Golding JM, Sorenson SB, Burnam MA: The epidemiology of obsessive-compulsive disorder in five U.S. communities, *Arch Gen Psychiatry* 45:1094, 1988.

Klein DN, Lewinsohn PM, Seeley JR, Rohde P: A family study of major depressive disorder in a community sample of adolescents, *Arch Gen Psychiatry* 58:13, 2001.

Klein RG, Koplewicz HS, Kanner A: Imipramine treatment of children with separation anxiety, *J Am Acad Child Adolesc Psychiatry* 31:21, 1992.

Koenig K, Scahill L: Assessment of children with pervasive developmental disorders, *J Child Adolesc Psychiatr Nurs* 14:159, 2001.

Kumra S, Herion D, Jacobsen LK, et al: Case study: risperidone-induced hepatoxicity in pediatric patients, *J Am Acad Child Adolesc Psychiatry* 36:701, 1997.

Kurlan R, McDermott MP, Deeley C, et al: Prevalence of tics in schoolchildren and association with placement in special education, *Neurology* 57:1383, 2001.

Lavigne JV, Cicchetti C, Gibbons RD, et al: Oppositional defiant disorder with onset in preschool years: longitudinal stability and pathways to other disorders, *J Am Acad Child Adolesc Psychiatry* 40:1393, 2001.

Law J, Boyle J, Harris F, et al: Prevalence and natural history of primary speech and language delay: findings from a systematic review of the literature. *Int J Lang Commun Disord* 35:165, 2000.

Leckman JF, Hardin MT, Riddle MA, et al: Clonidine treatment of Gilles de la Tourette's syndrome, *Arch Gen Psychiatry* 48:324, 1991.

Levy F, Hay DA, McStephen M, et al: Attention-deficit hyperactivity disorder: a category or a continuum? Genetic analysis of a large-scale twin study, *J Am Acad Child Adolesc Psychiatry* 36:737, 1997.

Lewinsohn PM, Klein DN, Seeley JR: Bipolar disorder during adolescence and young adulthood in a community sample, *Bipolar Disord* 2:281, 2000.

Lewinsohn PM, Klein DN, Seeley JR: Bipolar disorders in a community sample of older adolescents: prevalence, phenomenology, co-morbidity, and course, *J Am Acad Child Adolesc Psychiatry* 34:454, 1995.

Liederman J, Kantrowitz L, Flannery K: Male vulnerability to reading disability is not likely to be a myth: a call for new data, *J Learn Disabil* 38:109, 2005.

Michelson D, Allen AJ, Busner J, et al: Once-daily atomoxetine treatment for children and adolescents with attention deficit hyperactivity disorder: a randomized, placebo-controlled study, *Am J Psychiatry* 159:1896, 2002.

Michelson D, Faries D, Wernicke J, et al: Atomoxetine in the treatment of children and adolescents with attention-deficit/hyperactivity disorder: a randomized, placebo-controlled, dose-response study, *Pediatrics* 108:E83, 2001.

Mink JW: Neurobiology of basal ganglia circuits in Tourette syndrome: faulty inhibition of unwanted motor patterns? *Adv Neurol* 85:113, 2001.

MTA Cooperative Group: National Institute of Mental Health Multimodal Treatment Study of ADHD follow-up: changes in effectiveness and growth after the end of treatment, *Pediatrics* 113:762, 2004.

MTA Cooperative Group: A 14-month randomized clinical trial of treatment strategies for attention-deficit/hyperactivity disorder. The Multimodal Treatment Study of Children with ADHD, *Arch Gen Psychiatry* 56:1073, 1999.

Mufson L, Weissman MM, Moreau D, Garfinkel R: Efficacy of interpersonal psychotherapy for depressed adolescents, *Arch Gen Psychiatry* 56:573, 1999.

Nicolson R, Rapoport J: Neurobiology of childhood schizophrenia and other related disorders. In Martin A, Scahill L, Charney D, Leckman J, editors: *Pediatric psychopharmacology* (pp. 184-194), New York, 2003, Oxford University Press.

Pauls DL: The genetics of attention-deficit/hyperactivity disorder, *Biol Psychiatry* 57:1310, 2005.

Pauls DL: An update on the genetics of Gilles de la Tourette syndrome, *J Psychosom Res* 55:7, 2003.

Pediatric OCD Treatment Study (POTS) Team: Cognitive-behavior therapy, sertraline, and their combination for children and adolescents with obsessive-compulsive disorder: the pediatric OCD Treatment Study (POTS) randomized controlled trial, *JAMA* 292:1969, 2004.

Peterson BS, Thomas P, Kane MJ, et al: Basal ganglia volumes in patients with Gilles de la Tourette syndrome, *Arch Gen Psychiatry* 60:415, 2003.

Price RA, Kidd KK, Cohen DJ, et al: A twin study of Tourette syndrome, *Arch Gen Psychiatry* 42:815, 1985.

Rains A, Scahill L: New long-acting stimulants in children with ADHD, *J Child Adolesc Psychiatr Nurs* 17:177, 2004.

Rauch SL, Whalen PJ, Curran T, et al: Probing striato-thalamic function in obsessive-compulsive disorder and Tourette syndrome using neuroimaging methods, *Adv Neurol* 85:207, 2001.

Rosenbaum JF, Fava M, Hoog SL, et al: Selective serotonin reuptake inhibitor discontinuation syndrome: a randomized clinical trial, *Biol Psychiatry* 44:77, 1998.

Research Units on Pediatric Psychopharmacology Autism Network: Risperidone in children with autism for serious behavioral problems, *N Engl J Med* 347(5):314, 2002.

Research Units on Pediatric Psychopharmacology Autism Network: A randomized controlled crossover trial of methylphenidate in pervasive developmental disorders with hyperactivity, *Arch Gen Psychiatry* 62:1266, 2005a.

Research Units on Pediatric Psychopharmacology Autism Network: Risperidone treatment of autistic disorder: longer term benefits and blinded discontinuation after 6 months, *Am J Psychiatry* 162:1361, 2005b.

Rutter M, Silberg J, O'Connor T, Simonoff E: Genetics and child psychiatry: II. empirical research findings, *J Child Psychol Psychiatry* 40:19, 1999.

Scahill L, Rains A: Psychopharmacology for children. In Keltner NL, Folks DG, editors: *Psychotropic drugs,* ed 3 (pp. 468-495), St. Louis, 2005, Mosby.

Scahill L, Sukhodolsky D, Williams S, Leckman JF: The public health importance of tics and tic disorders, *Adv Neurol* 96:240, 2005.

Scahill L, Leckman JF, Schultz RT, et al: A placebo-controlled trial of risperidone in Tourette syndrome, *Neurology* 60:1130, 2003.

Scahill L, Chappell PB, Kim YS, et al: A placebo-controlled study of guanfacine in the treatment of children with tic disorders and attention deficit hyperactivity disorder, *Am J Psychiatry* 158:1067, 2001.

Scahill L, Schwab-Stone M, Merikangas KR, et al: Psychosocial and clinical correlates of ADHD in a community sample of young children, *J Am Acad Child Adolesc Psychiatry* 38:976, 1999.

Shaywitz SE, Shaywitz BE: Dyslexia (specific reading disability), *Biol Psychiatry* 57:1301, 2005.

Shriberg LD, Tomblin JB, McSweeny JL: Prevalence of speech delay in 6-year-old children and comorbidity with language impairment, *J Speech Lang Hear Res* 42:1461, 1999.

Sparrow SS, Balla DA, Cicchetti DV: *Vineland adaptive behavior scales,* Circle Pines, MN, 1984, American Guidance Clinic.

Spencer T, Biederman J, Coffey B, et al: A double-blind comparison of desipramine and placebo in children and adolescents with chronic tic disorder and comorbid attention-deficit/hyperactivity disorder, *Arch Gen Psychiatry* 59:649, 2002.

State MW, Lombroso PJ, Pauls DL, Leckman JF: The genetics of childhood psychiatric disorders: a decade of progress, *J Am Acad Child Adolesc Psychiatry* 39:946, 2000.

Swanson J, Volkow N: Pharmacokinetic and pharmacodynamic properties of methylphenidate in humans. In Solanto MV, Arnsten AFT, Castellanos FX, editors: *Stimulant drugs and ADHD. Basic and clinical neuroscience* (pp. 259-282), New York, 2001, Oxford University Press.

Tourette's Syndrome Study Group: Treatment of ADHD in children with tics: a randomized controlled trial, *Neurology* 58:527, 2002.

Treatment for Adolescents With Depression Study (TADS) Team: Fluoxetine, cognitive-behavioral therapy, and their combination for adolescents with depression: treatment for Adolescents With Depression Study (TADS) randomized controlled trial, *JAMA* 292:807, 2004.

U.S. Food and Drug Adminstration. (2004). *Questions and answers on antidepressant use in children, adolescents and adults.* Available at http://www.fda.gov/cder/drug/antidepressants/Q&A_antidepressants.htm. Accessed November 30, 2004.

U.S. Public Health Service: *Report of the Surgeon General's conference on children's mental health: a national action agenda,* Washington, DC, 2000, Department of Health and Human Services.

Valleni-Basile LA, Garrison CZ, Jackson KL, et al: Frequency of obsessive-compulsive disorder in a community sample of young adolescents, *J Am Acad Child Adolesc Psychiatry* 33:782, 1994.

Vinks AA, Walson PD: Pharmacokinetics I: Developmental principles. In Martin A, Scahill L, Charney D, Leckman J, editors: *Pediatric psychopharmacology,* New York, 2003, Oxford University Press, pp 44-53.

Volkmar FR: *Handbook of autism and pervasive developmental disorders,* ed 3, New York, 2005, Wiley.

Walkup JT, LaBuda MC, Singer HS, et al: Family study and segregation analysis of Tourette syndrome: evidence for a mixed model of inheritance, *Am J Hum Genet* 59:684, 1996.

Wernicke JF, Kratochvil CJ: Safety profile of atomoxetine in the treatment of children and adolescents with ADHD, *J Clin Psychiatry* 63(Suppl 12):50, 2002.

Wolraich M, Hannah JN, Pinnock TY, et al: Comparison of diagnostic criteria for attention-deficit hyperactivity disorder, *J Am Acad Child Adolesc Psychiatry* 35:319, 1996.

Zubenko GS, Zubenko WN, Spiker DG, et al: Malignancy of recurrent, early-onset major depression: a family study, *Am J Med Genet* 105:690, 2001.

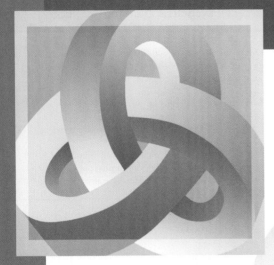

# Chapter 43

# Mental Disorders in Older Adults

*Norman L. Keltner*

## Learning Objectives

*After reading this chapter, you should be able to:*

- Describe the barriers to mental health care that exist for older adults.
- Describe the various treatment options and care settings available to older Americans.
- Identify the unique variations in symptoms of mental disorders evidenced by older adults.

- Identify major substance abuse issues in older adults.
- Recognize pharmacokinetic and pharmacodynamic changes in older adults that affect pharmacotherapy.
- Describe the psychological assessment of older adults.
- Identify therapeutic goals for older adults.

## INTRODUCTION

Currently, approximately 3.6 million older Americans (aobut 20%) suffer from mental disorders, and the National Institute of Mental Health (NIMH) projects that 15 million older adults will need mental health services by the year 2030 (Administration on Aging [AoA], 2005; NIMH, 1999a; U.S. Department of Health and Human Services [USDHHS], 1999). This number includes individuals who experience mental disorders for the first time in late life and those whose early-onset psychiatric disorders persist as chronic or recurrent conditions. Mental disorders in older adults might have a clear biochemical basis or might be a reaction to stressors commonly occurring in late adulthood. Regardless of cause, mental illness exacts a high toll in excess disability and disproportionate use of health care services.

Rapid growth in the older population (36.3 million strong) is fueling interest in issues surrounding mental health and aging. In 2000, 12.4% of the U.S. population was over the age of 65. By the year 2030, the number of Americans over age 65 will account for 20% of the population. This segment will include 76 million aging members of the baby boom generation, a group that already has relatively high rates of anxiety, depression, schizophrenia, and substance abuse (AoA, 2005). Life expectancy is also lengthening. By 2050, the number of Americans over age 85, known as the old-old, will increase fourfold or more, placing a significantly greater number of people at risk for mental disorders (National Institute on Aging [NIA], 2001). Box 43-1 provides an overview of the prevalence rates of selected psychiatric diagnoses in the current older population. The personal and economic consequences of mental disorders in this rapidly expanding cohort require heightened attention to the special mental health needs of older adults.

Box 43-1    **One-Year Prevalence Rates for Selected Psychiatric Diagnoses in Older Adults***

|  | Prevalence (%) |
|---|---|
| Any anxiety disorder | 11.4 |
| Simple phobia | 7.3 |
| Social phobia | 1 |
| Agoraphobia | 4.1 |
| Panic disorder | 0.5 |
| Obsessive-compulsive disorder | 1.5 |
| Any mood disorder | 4.4 |
| Major depressive episode | 3.8 |
| Unipolar major depression | 3.7 |
| Dysthymia | 1.6 |
| Bipolar I | 0.2 |
| Bipolar II | 0.1 |
| Schizophrenia | 0.6 |
| Somatization | 0.3 |

*Age 55 or older; based on data from epidemiologic catchment area.

Modified from U.S. Department of Health and Human Services: *Mental health: a report of the Surgeon General,* Rockville, MD, 1999, U.S. Department of Health and Human Services, Substance Abuse and Mental Health Services Administration, Center for Mental Health Services, National Institutes of Health, National Institute of Mental Health.

## CRITICAL THINKING QUESTION    1

Think of the last patient over the age of 65 for whom you cared during a medical-surgical clinical rotation. What factors could have placed the patient at risk for depression? If you noted any signs of depression, what actions were in the plan of care?

Modern American culture, which tends to celebrate youth, has placed little emphasis on understanding old age. This unfortunate bias has contributed to insufficient knowledge about mental health disorders in the older population, as well as public policies that adversely affect access to care. Recent research study results have increased the ability of health care providers to differentiate illness from normal aging and to identify differences between the clinical presentation and course of mental disorders in older adults and other age groups. Government agencies have joined together to investigate factors that influence older adults. A better understanding of the complex interplay of physical health, social factors, and emotional well-being in older adults is leading to mental health strategies tailored for the special needs of this group.

### Norm's Notes

*The geriatric population (those older than 65) is growing rapidly. There are more and more older people and thus more of their mental health problems for the health care system to deal with. Sometimes, those in need of mental health care have suffered during their younger years with the same problem(s) and have just grown older. Others, however, are growing older in a society in which work defines the person, and they no longer are working. Coupled with the mobility of our society, many older people find themselves without purpose (i.e., no job to do) and are alone. I get depressed just thinking about it.*

Nurses involved in the care of older adults should be familiar with prevention, detection, and treatment strategies for mental disorders throughout the continuum of care. This chapter presents an overview of mental health issues in older adults different from those of other age groups. Stressors, policy issues, barriers to mental health care, and common mental disorders occurring in older adults are discussed, along with assessment and psychotherapeutic management. Cognitive disorders, which account for some of the most frequently occurring mental disorders in older adults, are covered in Chapter 32.

## BARRIERS

Psychiatric disorders might lead to or exacerbate coexisting physical conditions by impairing older adults' physiologic function, independence, and ability to rally social support (USDHHS, 1999). Studies indicate that only half of older adults who acknowledge mental health problems receive any treatment, and only a fraction of those treated receive specialty mental health services (AoA, 2005). The unmet treatment needs result from patient barriers, provider barriers, and system-economic barriers.

### Patient Barriers

Attitudes of older adults themselves serve as a barrier to seeking mental health care. Patients and families who subscribe to stereotypes about normal aging might delay seeking care if they believe that conditions such as depression or memory loss are a normal part of aging. Additionally, older individuals might be reluctant to seek psychiatric care because admitting mental health problems is seen as a weakness and is more stigmatizing than it might be for a younger person. Seeking psychiatric care might also represent a loss of control and elicit fear of institutionalization. Furthermore, when outside help is required, people who grew up in an era that emphasized self-reliance are more likely to rely on family, friends, and other informal supports than on mental health professionals, who are often viewed with skepticism.

### Provider Barriers

Older adults are more likely to receive care from primary care physicians than from geriatric specialty providers. Despite the rapid growth in the over-65 population and recognition of their unique needs, geriatric specialists are scarce. Nurses and other health care providers who are not attuned to the complexities of geriatric care might miss opportunities to identify mental health disorders or predisposing factors.

Accurate assessment and diagnosis require familiarity with diagnostic tools, such as the Geriatric Depression Scale (see Evolve web site). Furthermore, individuals working with older adults must recognize that mental disorders might be expressed through somatic complaints and that symptoms of comorbid physical problems might compound the difficulty of diagnosing a mental disorder. An additional complication is physician reluctance to diagnose those mental disorders identified for fear of stigmatizing their geriatric patients (Tune, 2001).

Ageism, the negative stereotyping and devaluation of people solely because of their age, is also a significant barrier. Ageism is defined as the stereotypical view that mental health problems are part of the aging process. To serve older adults effectively, professionals must be attentive to their biases and stereotypes and increase their geriatric-specific knowledge.

### System-Economic Barriers

Diagnosis of psychiatric disorders in geriatric patients consumes time and resources not covered by medical insurance reimbursement. This and other funding issues, along with a lack of collabo-

ration and coordination among primary care, mental health, and aging services providers, thwart the provision and receipt of adequate mental health care for older adults (AoA, 2005). The cost of mental health care has been a major disincentive to providers and older adults who might otherwise seek psychiatric assistance. Historically, insurers, including federally funded Medicare and Medicaid, have placed severe limits on reimbursement for mental health care. Some insurers exclude mental health and substance abuse treatment altogether. Only in the last few years has legislative effort addressed parity in mental health coverage.

| CRITICAL THINKING QUESTION | 2 |
|---|---|

Many older adults have no insurance coverage to offset the high cost of prescription medications. How might this affect compliance?

## CONTINUUM OF CARE

Because of the prevalence and profound negative consequences of mental disorders in late life, nurses who encounter older adults in any setting should consider their physical, social, and emotional needs. Whenever possible, factors that place older adults at risk for mental disorders or problems stemming from mental illness should be identified and plans developed to meet the needs.

### PREVENTION

A balance of physical, social, and emotional functioning contributes to mental health. Many of the changes that accompany advancing age affect this balance, increasing older adults' vulnerability to mental disorders. A primary stressful event (e.g., broken hip [physical]) might lead to secondary stressors (e.g., emotional isolation). Health problems, acute and chronic, might lead to dependence, relocation, isolation, and financial hardship. A closer examination of these consequences might prove enlightening.

*Dependence:* Loss of independence, even temporarily, is terribly threatening in a person's later years because having to rely on others might signal a continued dependency.

Box 43-2    **Losses That Occur More Frequently Among Older Adults**

Loss of health
Loss of loved ones
Loss of hearing and vision
Loss of status
Loss of work
Loss of income
Loss of friends
Loss of cognitive skills
Loss of home and community
Loss of mobility

*Relocation:* Moving from familiar surroundings to a new environment is also threatening. To many older individuals, familiar surroundings represent a connection to all that is important in life. Additionally, the related changes can be overwhelming for some individuals with limited adaptive capacity.

*Isolation:* Most older individuals have fewer meaningful connections than they had earlier in life. Death, a mobile society, and estrangements are only a few reasons for this reality. Health care–related isolation can be particularly devastating for some older adults.

*Financial hardship:* Although many older individuals are financially secure, a significant number find unexpected medical expenses to be difficult or even impossible to meet on a fixed income. Most older adults have little, if any, ability to increase their income to meet additional unplanned expenses.

## Adaptive Mechanisms: Meaning, Control, Support

Losses common in the late years of life are listed in Box 43-2 and often precede the onset of mental disorders in older adults. Despite numerous inevitable changes, the majority of older adults adjust well and express a high degree of satisfaction with life (USDHHS, 1999). Exposure and adaptation to stressors vary with each older adult's economic and social resources, physical status, ethnicity, gender, and life experiences (AoA, 2005). Successful adaptation is enhanced by the ability to give *meaning* to experiences. Part of this process is comparing problems with what is experienced and expected by others who are the same age (Federal Interagency Forum on Aging [FIFA]–Related Statistics, 2000). This observation might account for 72% of older Americans reporting their health as good to excellent, despite multiple coexisting medical conditions and impairments (FIFA, 2000). As one sage older adult noted, at some point, simply being alive can be seen as a sign of good health. This coping skill is especially helpful when the stressor, such as a chronic health problem, is not easily modified.

Another adaptive mechanism that assists older adults to cope with stressful events is the use of mastery—the sense of ability to exercise *control* over circumstances. For this reason, unplanned stressors might be experienced as more negative than those that are planned. For example, adequate planning for the social and financial implications of retirement significantly affects adjustment to this major life change. Nurses can reinforce mastery by encouraging the older person's participation in care decisions.

*Support* systems (i.e., family, friends, private and government organizations) are valuable sources of emotional support and aid and are important predictors of physical and mental health and delayed institutionalization (FIFA, 2000). Measures that contribute to physical health and promote social functioning are important components of preventing mental disorders in older adults. Improved health care and programs developed to target older adults' needs have resulted in declines in the rates of disability and poverty, which are key indicators of well-being in older adults, reported by the AoA.

## Caregiver Training and Transportation

Specific legislation has led to funding programs to meet the special needs of an aging population. For example, the National Family Caregiver Support Program provides training, counseling, and respite for the caregivers of older adults, a group at risk for depression (AoA, 2005). Another example is the National Aging Network and Transportation Assistance program, established to address transportation needs (AoA, 2005). Lack of transportation has been cited as a factor in isolation and is a barrier to accessing health care. Nurses play a key role in illness prevention by providing information about mental health and available resources at sites where older adults are likely to visit.

### Local Area Agency on Aging

The government section of the telephone book contains the number for a local Area Agency on Aging (AAA). This organization is a valuable resource for older adults and their caregivers, who often have difficulty initiating a search for or negotiating access to care.

### CRITICAL THINKING QUESTION    3

If you have had the opportunity to meet the caregiver of an older person with a mental disorder, were both the patient and the caregiver participants in decision making? Did the caregiver treat the patient in the way that you would want to be treated in that situation? Describe both the positive and the negative aspects of nurse-patient-caregiver interactions.

## DETECTION

Measures that promote early detection of mental disorders in older adults include increasing public awareness of mental health issues, encouraging collaboration among service providers, and increased training of health professionals. Public education that emphasizes symptoms of mental disorders and treatment options does much to dispel the myths and stigma surrounding mental illness and empowers older adults to seek treatment. Some programs have been established to enhance community involvement. Public service workers such as grocery clerks, postal employees, and public utility workers are recruited and trained to identify and report vulnerable older adults. Nurses in all settings can contribute to early detection by assessing and reporting stressors and symptoms.

## TREATMENT SITES

Federal legislation has strongly influenced the care of older adults who have mental disorders. The Community Mental Health Act of 1963 initiated deinstitutionalization, resulting in a large number of individuals with severe and persistent mental disorders (SPMDs) being discharged from state and county mental hospitals to less restrictive settings. Many discharged older adults were placed in nursing homes, where inappropriate and inadequate care, including excessive use of physical

and chemical restraints, led to the passage of the Nursing Home Reform Act, known as the Omnibus Reconciliation Act of 1987 (OBRA). This legislation set stringent limits on the use of physical restraints and established guidelines for psychotropic drug use that regulate drug selection, dosing, and duration of treatment. In addition, to prevent nursing home placement for those who need psychiatric care in hospital or community programs, OBRA requires preadmission screening for all individuals with suspected mental disorders. Nursing home residents whose only need for nursing care stems from mental disorders were to be discharged. Nonetheless, many institutionalized older people with SPMDs continue to live in nursing homes. Most of these residents do not receive adequate psychiatric treatment because of a lack of mental health training for nursing home staff and inadequate Medicare and Medicaid funding to cover behavioral health care (AoA, 2005; Shea et al, 2000).

The majority of older adults with SPMDs live in the community. Currently, only a small percentage of community mental health centers have staff or services that target the needs of older adults, and primary care physicians are ill prepared and typically too rushed to treat mental disorders adequately (USDDHS, 1999). When care is provided, it is not uncommon for older adults to receive inappropriate psychotropic medication (USDHHS, 1999). Among the services needed to help community-based older adults with SPMD are the following:

1. Mental health outreach programs
2. Adult day services
3. Respite care and caregiver programs
4. Support groups
5. Self-help groups

## PSYCHOPATHOLOGY IN OLDER ADULTS

Unit V of this text provides an in-depth review of diagnostic classifications. This section is meant to supplement that information by detailing unique information on the presentation, course, and treatment of mental disorders in older adults. It is important for nurses in all practice areas to note that treating older adults with mental disorders benefits overall health by improving functional ability and compliance with health care instructions.

## DEPRESSION

As in other age groups, depression in older adults might result from psychosocial stress, biochemical changes, comorbid medical conditions, pharmaceutical agents, or a combination of factors. The effects of depression extend beyond well-known and emotionally distressing symptoms such as sadness, worthlessness, hopelessness, helplessness, fear, shame, and guilt. Less obvious effects include diminished social, cognitive, and physical functioning, along with increased mortality. This constellation of effects exacts an enormous personal and economic toll. Inadequate detection and treatment add to the burden.

Despite the fact that depression in older adults responds to the same interventions as those used in other age groups, nearly two thirds of older adults with depression do not get treatment, and treatment is thought to be adequate for only 11% of those who do receive care (NIMH, 2001). The cost of health care for depressed patients is about twice that for their elderly undepressed counterparts, the result of more medical hospitalizations, physician and emergency room visits, drug use, and often unnecessary tests and procedures (Campbell et al, 2000). In a global comparison of disease burden, depression ranked second only to ischemic heart disease in years of life lost to disability or death.

### INCIDENCE

The prevalence of late-life depression varies tremendously among reported studies. The rate of major depression diagnosed using the *Diagnostic and Statistical Manual of Mental Disorders,* Text Revision, Fourth Edition *(DSM-IV-TR)* criteria declines with age, but depressive symptoms increase (Forsell and Winblad, 1999). Table 43-1 demonstrates this trend and the increased risk for women over men. Rates for major depression increase in a linear fashion from 2% to 5% in community dwellers, to 5% to 10% in primary care settings, to 6% to 14% of medically ill older adults (Kayton, 2001). The co-occurrence of depression exacerbates the course of other diagnoses.

| Table 43-1 | Percentage of Noninstitutionalized Persons, Age 65 and Older, With Severe Depressive Symptoms (1998) | | |
|---|---|---|---|
| **Age (yr)** | **Total** | **Men** | **Women** |
| 65 to 69 | 15.4 | 12.1 | 18 |
| 70 to 74 | 14.3 | 10.3 | 17.2 |
| 75 to 79 | 14.6 | 10.4 | 17.4 |
| 80 to 84 | 20.5 | 17.1 | 22.4 |
| 85 or older | 22.8 | 22.5 | 23 |

From Federal Interagency Forum on Aging-Related Statistics: *Older Americans 2000: key indicators of well-being, Appendix A: detailed tables.* Federal Interagency Forum on Aging-Related Statistics, Washington, DC, 2000, U.S. Government Printing Office.
Also available at http://www.agingstats.gov/tables%202001/tables-healthstatus.html#Indicator%2016.

### PRESENTATION

Many factors complicate the detection of depression. Depression in older adults frequently does not align neatly with current *DSM-IV-TR* criteria, and many depressive symptoms can be attributed to physical causes in individuals with concurrent medical illnesses. Older adults are more likely to present with memory disturbance or somatic complaints than with the feelings associated with depression for which younger patients seek care. Older adults also might lack the range of vocabulary that younger individuals commonly possess to describe emotions. Rather than expressions of sadness, diminished self-esteem, irritability, or apathy, for example, older adults are more likely to complain of having the blues or feeling worthless. Cultural competence demands that professionals recognize differences in expression common to ethnic and cultural subgroups within the older population as well.

In addition to diagnostic barriers already discussed, the connection between medical conditions and depression complicates diagnosis. In fact, in a first episode of depression occurring after 60 years of age, the clinician should consider cerebrovascular disease (Sherman, 2005).

It is difficult to determine whether common physical indicators of depression in older adults, including weight loss, fatigue, insomnia, constipation, and multiple vague aches and pains, are the result of a mood disorder or symptoms of a medical problem. The *DSM-IV-TR* diagnosis of "mood disorder due to a general medical condition" can be given when mood symptoms are a direct physiologic consequence of medical conditions (American Psychiatric Association [APA], 2000). For example, depression coexists in 11% to 57% of patients with dementia and accounts for greater deficits than can be attributed to the primary diagnosis alone (Kales et al, 1999).

Although depression is caused by a medical illness in some cases, in other cases depression causes physiologic changes that enhance susceptibility to disease. Depression adversely affects endocrine, neurologic, and immune processes by increasing sympathetic tone, decreasing vagal tone, and causing immunosuppression (Penninx et al, 1999). People with depression are more likely to smoke, drink alcohol excessively, be physically inactive, and have poorer eating habits than those who are not depressed. These changes and health habits might be factors in depression as a predictor of coronary artery disease and diabetes and the increased risk of death following myocardial infarctions (Creed, 1999; Kayton, 2001).

### Depression or Dementia?

Because of the shared cognitive symptoms of depression and dementia, misdiagnosis of dementia occurs frequently. Depression that mimics dementia is termed pseudodementia. Shared symptoms include poor memory, disorientation, poor judgment, and agitation or psychomotor retardation. In addition to psychological tests, nursing observations can be critical to correcting misdiagnosis. Nurses should assess for higher functioning than would be expected in dementia and can also look for a downcast mood, which can help distinguish depression from the blander affect of true dementia. Differentiating these disorders is important for treatment because depression is highly treatable. Psychotic depression might also be confused with cognitive or other psychiatric disorders. When depression occurs for the first time after age 60, delusions are more common than with early-onset depression. Delusions of persecution or of having an incurable illness, as well as nihilistic delusions, are more frequent than delusions associated with guilt (Blazer and Koenig, 1996). Hallucinations, however, are an uncommon feature of psychotic depression. Many older adults with psychotic depression might ruminate, express suspiciousness, and voice multiple physical complaints. Psychotic depression is often resistant to traditional anti-

depressant medications and psychotherapy. As a result, electroconvulsive therapy (ECT) is frequently used in treatment.

## ELECTROCONVULSIVE THERAPY

ECT is often the treatment of choice for severe depression in older adults, especially those who are poor candidates for drug therapy or have failed to respond to other treatments. ECT offers a rapid response that is necessary when patients are suicidal or in danger of medical crisis. The safety and efficacy of ECT have been demonstrated for all age groups, including the old-old (Tew et al, 1999). Chapter 39 provides a thorough review of the topic.

## SUICIDE

Although suicide rates for the elderly are at the lowest point in 75 years, they are still 50% higher than for younger age groups (Jancin, 2005). As noted, older Americans are disproportionately more likely to commit suicide, the most serious and tragic consequence of missed or under-treated depression. Older adults comprise only 13% of the population but account for 19% of reported suicides. Table 43-2 demonstrates that the incidence of suicide increases with age and that Caucasian men over age 65 have the highest rate of all (Hoyert et al, 1999). However, when more finely tuned, data reveal that among non-Caucasian women in this age group, the rate is only 2.4 per 100,000, whereas for Caucasian men it is 34.2 per 100,000 (Jancin, 2005). Suicidal gestures and impulsiveness, common among young adults, are rare in older adults. In older adults, failed attempts

| Table 43-2 | Rate of Suicide Among Older Adults* |
|---|---|
| 55-64 years old | 13.5 |
| 65-74 years old | 14.4 |
| 75-84 years old | 19.3 |
| 85 years old and over | 20.8 |
| Caucasian men over 85 years old | 65 |
| Average rate across the life span | 10.6 |

*Rates per 100,000 population based on 1997 data.
From Hoyert DL, Kochanek KD, Murphey SL: Deaths: final data for 1997, In *National vital statistical report,* Hyattsville, MD, 1999, National Center for Health Statistics, USDHHS Publication No. 99-1120.

are usually not a cry for help; rather, they are a serious yet unsuccessful suicide bid. To underscore this point, older people tend to select highly lethal methods for suicide. For example, firearms are the most common method of suicide by both men and women 65 years and older, accounting for 78% of male and 34.8% of female suicides (NIMH, 1999b; Jancin, 2005).

The rate of suicide might be even higher than reported because statistics do not include what is known as *chronic suicide*. This term characterizes death caused by slower, less obvious means than the abrupt acts usually associated with suicide. Refusing to eat, noncompliance with medication, excessive alcohol intake, and physical risk taking might result in death but are not recorded as suicide (Butler and Lewis, 1995). Depression is a strong predictor of patients' decisions to support euthanasia or forego life-sustaining treatment (Blank et al, 2001). Suicide does not always arise from depression. For some individuals who face life-threatening illness, suicide is the ultimate means of exercising control over a situation. Rational or physician-assisted suicide is an area of great concern to society, practitioners, and legal decision makers.

Suicide prevention begins with the detection of risk (Box 43-3). It is important for nurses to listen to the themes of conversation and observe for signs that might signal suicidal risk or thoughts. Particular attention should be given to older individuals who are beginning to recover from depression: as energy returns, the risk of suicide increases. Intent might be signaled by a new preoccupation with religious issues, giving away possessions, changing a will, or other new behaviors. People might feel ashamed to plainly voice ideas of self-harm, so if negative statements or behaviors are detected, it is essential to ask directly about any intentions. The notion that these discussions can exacerbate suicidal thought is a myth.

## CLINICAL EXAMPLE

Mr. White is an 86-year-old Caucasian man who has outlived two wives. Mr. White has remained sexually active into his 80s but, within the last 2 years, he has had difficulty attaining an erection. Mr. White relates that a younger woman (mid-50s) recently asked about spending the night. She did, and Mr. White was unable to perform sexually. He said, "I'm just no good anymore." Mr. White said he was embarrassed by his sexual dysfunction. He states that he has had thoughts of suicide but would not act on them. He promises the nurse that he will call if he has an urge to harm himself.

## CLINICAL EXAMPLE

Mr. Timchuk is a 77-year-old Caucasian man with chronic obstructive pulmonary disease (COPD). He has great difficulty doing any physical activity. Mr. Timchuk is very despondent over his condition, and there is little hope that he will improve. Although he has not verbalized a desire to "end it all," he states that he would be better off dead. The nurse understands that he is at great risk for self-harm.

| Box 43-3 | **Predictors of Suicide Risk in Older Adults** |
|---|---|

Age older than 65 years
Male
White
Chronic or uncontrolled pain
Bereavement
Unmarried (widowed or divorced)
Social isolation
Retirement
Financial difficulty
Hopeless or helpless
Alcohol or drug abuse
History of previous attempt
Major depressive disorder, particularly psychotic depression or depression caused by a general medical condition

## MANIC EPISODES

Manic symptoms in older adults might be associated with bipolar disorder, medical and neurologic conditions, substance abuse, or medication. In older adults, bipolar disorder accounts for about 5% to 20% of mood disorders, most often as a recurrence of an existing disorder (Cassano et al, 2000). Late-onset bipolar disorder is defined as bipolar disorder in which symptoms first occur after age 40. Differences between early- and late-onset bipolar disorder suggest that they might be different types of manic-depressive illness (Schurhoff et al, 2000). For example, affective disorders are less common in first-degree relatives of those with late onset than in those with earlier onset (Cassano et al, 2000; Schurhoff et al, 2000). Late-onset bipolar disorder is generally less severe, with fewer and milder manic symptoms compared with early-onset bipolar disorder (Moon, 2005). Features might include grandiosity, disorientation, euphoria, or irritability. *Secondary mania* is the term used to describe manic symptoms associated with medical conditions or drugs. A substantial proportion of new-onset manic symptoms in older adults is associated with cerebral disorders or injuries and might run a bipolar course, with intervening periods of euthymia (Snowdon, 2000). Nursing interventions must address the negative impact of agitation and distractibility on self-care and self-protection in older adults.

## CLINICAL EXAMPLE

The local police department's community service officer brought Ms. Ellington, a 72-year-old Caucasian woman, to the hospital. She was found sitting outside a homeless shelter surrounded by boxes of personal belongings, drinking orange juice that had a strong odor of alcohol. She wore tight animal print leggings, a transparent blouse, and thigh-high white boots. A decorated wide-brimmed hat covered her sparse flame-red hair. On admission, Ms. Ellington was cursing loudly and threw her dentures at the first staff person who approached. Although she was well known to the staff, Ms. Ellington claimed that she was a Hollywood star who had been kicked out of her own mansion by friends, robbed of identification, and shipped to this city, where she would be unknown. In fact, according to police, she had been evicted from several shelters for disruptive behavior. An empty bottle of lithium and an unfilled prescription for more lithium were found in her purse.

## PSYCHOTIC DISORDERS

Psychotic disorders, characterized by delusions, hallucinations, disordered thoughts, bizarre behavior, or other evidence of impaired reality testing, are among the most severe psychiatric disorders. Symptoms often contribute to the institutionalization of older adults. Active psychosis is as disabling as quadriplegia on the disability component of the disability-adjusted life-years (DALYs) measure (NIMH, 2001). Nurses should be familiar with the numerous physical conditions and medications associated with psychosis in older adults (Box 43-4). A comprehensive assessment, including the nature and content of delusions and hallucinations, can facilitate identification of reversible causes and contribute to the accurate diagnosis necessary for determining the most effective course of treatment.

## SCHIZOPHRENIA

Although generally regarded as an illness with onset in late adolescence or early adulthood, symptoms first occur after age 40 in approximately 23.5% of all patients with schizophrenia, with a high female-to-male ratio (Howard et al, 2000). The most important characteristics for assessing a schizophrenic episode in an older person are hallucinations, delusions, and a history of a psychotic disorder (Alexopoulous et al, 2004).

Two classifications of schizophrenia in older adults are being investigated: late-onset schizophrenia (after age 40) and very late-onset (after age 60) (Howard et al, 2000). Late-onset and typical early-onset schizophrenia share some characteristics, including severe positive symptoms (delusions, hallucinations, bizarre or disorganized behavior, impaired communication) and a chronic course. Late-onset patients are more likely than their earlier-onset counterparts to present with bizarre, persecutory delusions; visual, tactile, and olfactory hallucinations; and accusatory or abusive auditory hallucinations (Howard et al, 2000; McClure et al, 1999). Disorganization and negative symptoms (withdrawal, apathy, and anhedonia) are less prominent than in early onset. A majority of individuals diagnosed with schizophrenia late in life have abnormal premorbid personality traits but, compared with persons with early-onset schizophrenia, are more likely to have better employment and marital histories. For many individuals, late-onset schizophrenia marks the beginning of a chronic disorder with periods of remission and symptom recurrence. The insidious deterioration of personality and social adjustment characteristic of early-onset schizophrenia also occurs; however, cognitive declines are no faster in older noninstitutionalized patients with schizophrenia than in normal comparison subjects (Eyler Zorrilla et al, 2000). In all age groups, antipsychotic medications are an effective treatment for

Box 43-4   **Disorders Associated With Psychosis in the Older Adult Population**

**Disorders**
Parkinson's disease
Alzheimer's disease
Pick's disease
Diffuse Lewy body disease
Vascular dementia
Seizure disorders
Hydrocephalus
Demyelinating diseases
Neoplasms
Encephalopathies
Neurosyphilis
Spinocerebellar degeneration

**Endocrinopathies**
Hyperthyroidism, hypothyroidism
Hyperparathyroidism, hypoparathyroidism
Addison's disease
Cushing's disease
Hypoglycemia

**Vitamin Deficiencies**
Thiamine
Niacin
Vitamin $B_{12}$
Folate

**Other Conditions**
Iatrogenic (secondary to drugs)
Lupus
Alcohol intake or withdrawal
Temporal arteritis
Hyponatremia
Delirium

**Differential Diagnosis**
Psychotic disorder caused by a general medical
   condition
Delirium
Dementia with delusions and hallucinations
Mood disorder with psychotic features
Delusional disorder
Psychosis secondary to substance abuse or
   dependence
Brief reactive psychosis
Psychosis not otherwise specified or schizophreniform
   disorder
Schizophrenia

From Jeste DV, Harris MJ, Paulsen JS: Psychosis. In Sadavoy J, Lazarus LW, Jarvik LF, et al, editors: *Comprehensive review of geriatric psychiatry-II,* ed 2 (pp. 593-614), Washington, DC, 1996, American Psychiatric Press; McClure FS, Gladsjo JA, Jeste DV: Late-onset psychosis: clinical, research, and ethical considerations, *Am J Psychiatry* 156:935, 1999.

many of the positive symptoms, especially when coupled with a structured environment (milieu), including social skills training and supportive nurse-patient interactions.

Research documenting the long-term course of schizophrenia is extremely limited; however, many chronic schizophrenic patients reach late life in spite of the high mortality associated with chronic early-onset schizophrenia. Mortality is associated with a high risk of suicide and medical problems, often related to comorbid substance abuse—especially nicotine dependence. Emphysema and other pulmonary and cardiac problems are common. The increase of movement disorders in older patients treated with traditional antipsychotics complicates medical management, increases the degree of disability associated with the disorder, and contributes to the high cost of services for older adult patients with schizophrenia.

Long-term institutionalization poses problems of learned dependence and decreases in problem-solving and coping skills. The negative symptoms of schizophrenia also contribute to impaired social functioning, which includes areas such as social appropriateness and grooming (Patterson et al, 2001). Nurses should note that older schizophrenic patients, especially those who are returned to the community after long-term institutionalization, might have significant deficits in daily living skills and lack the social networks important to successful adaptation. Thus, these individuals have a higher need for daily living services. Caregivers should emphasize problem-solving skills and interventions that promote social functioning.

## CLINICAL EXAMPLE

Ms. Auger is a 68-year-old Caucasian woman brought to the hospital by her sister, with whom she lives. She accuses her sister of forcing her into the hospital so that the sister can steal her money and car. The sister can recall no recent major stressor or signs of physical illness. She states that Ms. Auger has no history of psychiatric symptoms, but has always been a "loner." Despite obtaining a college degree, she had a stormy employment history because she was "unable to get along" with co-workers. She also was unable to sustain a long-term relationship with any man she dated. Ms. Auger's appearance is evidence of her inattention to dress and grooming. Although cooperative with

### CLINICAL EXAMPLE—cont'd

examination, her mood is dysphoric, and she has a flat affect. She admits to auditory hallucinations, particularly voices of people she knows, often conversing with each other. The voices tell her that they will steal from her, and they sometimes tell her to hurt herself.

A complete evaluation resulted in a diagnosis of schizophrenia. The geropsychiatrist ordered Zyprexa (olanzapine) 2.5 mg q hs.

## PARANOID THINKING

Paranoid symptoms are not uncommon in older adults. Delusions are generally chronic and well systematized and, unless associated with dementia or delirium, are not associated with memory loss, disorientation, or diminished cognitive function (Koenig et al, 1996). The content often involves persecution, jealousy (e.g., infidelity), or unusual situations that might conceivably occur in real life. It is important to investigate actual facts before labeling beliefs as delusional, because patients might relate bizarre tales that have a basis in reality. Because coping behaviors are compromised with age, paranoid thinking often emerges as a defense mechanism against a potentially hostile environment. Walking to the corner store in some neighborhoods might be perilous for older individuals because they are less able than younger people to fend off aggressors. A retreat into an environment that the fearful older adult can control results in increasing isolation. Although the threat might be based on reality, the resulting isolation and decrease in external stimuli, along with suspicious behaviors, can lead to paranoid thinking.

### CLINICAL EXAMPLE

Mrs. Justice is an 81-year-old African-American woman referred to the community mental health center by her primary care physician for treatment of psychosis. The neatly attired and spry woman tearfully relates that "haunts" have been breaking into her house at night, stealing money and other possessions. She sees the ghostly apparitions at least once a month, and when they appear, they speak to her, most often saying, "You stay out of the way, old woman, or we'll get you!" Before initiat-

ing pharmacologic intervention, a nurse practitioner conducted a home visit and found Mrs. Justice's home in disarray. Broken windows, gaps where kitchen appliances had been removed, and other findings led the nurse to request a police investigation. On the first night of their home surveillance, police arrested two young men dressed in white sheets who were hiding behind high shrubbery in front of the house. Interventions that were social rather than pharmacologic were instituted. (This actual case is an example of how cultural awareness and careful investigation prevented subsequent inappropriate diagnosis and treatment.)

## ANXIETY DISORDERS

The prevalence of anxiety disorders is the highest of all mental disorders in older adults. Little research has specifically addressed anxiety symptoms and syndromes in older adults, perhaps because epidemiologic data have revealed lower rates of anxiety disorders in community-dwelling older adults compared with younger groups (Lenze et al, 2000; USDHHS, 1999). As with other mental disorders, most anxiety disorders do not begin in later life but are a recurrence or worsening of a preexisting condition (Lang and Stein, 2001). Cognitive, behavioral, somatic, and physiologic symptoms are similar to those of other age groups (Box 43-5).

Many older adults have symptoms of anxiety that fail to meet diagnostic criteria for an anxiety disorder. As many as 23% to 38% of older adults with depression also experience anxiety, sometimes at a level that meets *DSM-IV-TR* criteria for generalized anxiety disorder, panic disorder, or a phobia (Lenze et al, 2000). Two anxiety disorders defined in the *DSM-IV-TR* might be overrepresented in older adults. "Anxiety due to a general medical condition" is a commonly used diagnosis resulting from the frequency of anxiety related to cardiovascular, endocrine, respiratory, and neurologic disorders in this age group (Keltner and Folks, 2005). "Substance-induced anxiety disorder" might be present in as many as 10% of community-dwelling older adults and 40% of nursing home residents, a consequence of substance abuse and dependence, as well as toxicity from prescription drugs (Folks and Fuller, 1997). Although anxiety is a normal emotion that alerts a person

## Box 43-5   Signs and Symptoms of Anxiety

**Gastrointestinal or Genitourinary Symptoms**
Abdominal pain
Anorexia
Butterflies
Dry mouth
Diarrhea
Nausea
Urinary frequency
Vomiting

**Cardiovascular Symptoms**
Chest discomfort
Diaphoresis
Dyspnea
Flushing
Hyperventilation
Pallor
Palpitations
Tachycardia

**Musculoskeletal Symptoms**
Backache
Fatigue
Muscle tension
Tremulous

**Neurologic Signs**
Dizziness or faintness
Paresthesia

**Psychological Manifestations**
Apprehensive
Compulsive
Fearful
Feelings of dread
Irritable
Intolerant
Panicky
Phobic
Preoccupied
Tense or worried

Modified from Keltner N, Folks D: *Psychotropic drugs,* ed 3, St. Louis, 2005, Mosby.

to impending danger or an unpleasant event, it can be considered maladaptive when it interferes with functioning (Sheikh, 1996).

## SUBSTANCE ABUSE

Substance abuse and dependence place older adults at tremendous risk of negative physical, psychological, and social consequences but often go undetected. Late-life alcohol and drug use and dependence are problems that have received little attention until recent years; thus a great deal is yet to be learned about geriatric-specific prevention, detection, and treatment options. Estimates of the current prevalence of alcohol abuse in older adults vary widely, from 1% to 15% (Blow, 2000; USDHHS, 1999). These numbers are expected to increase rapidly as a result of aging baby boomers, who have a greater history of alcohol abuse than the current older cohort. Similar expansion is expected with illicit drug use, currently a problem for only 0.1% of older adults (USDDH, 1999). A larger problem is the frequent misuse of prescription and over-the-counter (OTC) drugs, sometimes to the point that it can be characterized as drug abuse. It is important for nurses to understand factors that contribute to substance abuse and recognize presenting symptoms and potential consequences. Unless nurses and other health care providers recognize the serious problems that alcohol and prescription drugs pose for older adults and take measures to intervene, quality of life is diminished, independence compromised, and physical deterioration accelerated.

## ALCOHOL ABUSE AND DEPENDENCE

Alcohol abuse and dependence might occur for the first time in late life or might represent an unresolved problem from earlier life. More men than women approach late life with problem drinking, and although men represent the majority of older adults who abuse alcohol, late-onset alcohol abuse is more common in women than in men (Blow, 2000; Ludwick et al, 2000). A number of risk factors have been identified for late-onset problematic drinking. The presence of chronic medical disorders and sleep disturbances might lead some older adults to self-medicate with alcohol to control pain or induce sleep. Some isolated older adults or those with excessive free time use drinking to combat boredom or loneliness. Individuals who have lost a spouse are particularly at risk (Byrne et al, 1999). For some individuals, alcohol is seen as a means of decreasing or escaping the emotional distress of psychiatric disorders. When an alcohol use disorder is associated with another mental disorder, the term *dual diagnosis* is used.

Older adults' problematic alcohol use is often minimized or undetected by health care providers. Older adults often underreport alcohol consumption, the result of impaired recall, guilt, or shame. Social stigma is especially strong in older women, who are more likely than men to drink secretly at home and make efforts to conceal their drinking behavior (Ludwick et al, 2000). Along with assessment of the quantity of alcohol consumed, physiologic changes that occur with aging, medications, and certain conditions (e.g., cognitive disorders) that intensify alcohol's effects must be considered. Older adults show greater central nervous system sensitivity to alcohol than younger drinkers, so adverse effects on cognition and coordination will be more pronounced by comparison. Because of age-related changes, the same amount of alcohol will produce a blood alcohol level about 20% higher in a 65-year-old person than in a 30-year-old individual (Ganzin and Atkinson, 1996). Thus, even if older adults do not increase their level of alcohol consumption over that of earlier years, their bodies react as if they were drinking more.

*DSM-IV-TR* indicators for diagnosis of substance abuse are geared toward the impact of alcohol use on employment and driving, often irrelevant for older adults. Screening tools such as the CAGE test and the Geriatric Michigan Alcohol Screening Test (G-MAST) can assist identification of at-risk drinkers but are not routinely included in older adults' health assessments (Conigliaro et al, 2000). It is important to ask questions about alcohol consumption and its effects on life.

Nurses should also be attuned to the possibility of alcohol as a contributing factor in many problems seen in elderly medical and psychiatric patients. Box 43-6 lists some of the presenting features of older adult problem drinkers. Problem drinkers generally have more health-related complaints than their peers, and older women are particularly susceptible to alcohol's toxic effects (Ludwick et al, 2000). Unfortunately, withdrawal symptoms might be the first indication of alcohol dependence. Alcohol withdrawal includes a broad spectrum of symptoms and, although the severity of withdrawal symptoms is not appreciably different across age groups, physiologic changes and comorbid physical conditions place older adults at an increased risk (Wetterling et al, 2001). Nurses have a significant role in the management of alcohol withdrawal (Box 43-7).

A variety of interventions are available to support continued abstinence after withdrawal. For some late-onset drinkers, education and abstinence advice are effective (Blow, 2000). For other drinkers, including long-term alcohol abusers, formal structured programs are necessary. Greatest success is achieved when the program is geared specifically for older adults. Programs for older adults emphasize peer bonding and shared reminiscing in addition to cognitive-behavioral training that addresses themes such as self-efficacy, self-esteem, and relapse prevention strategies. Whenever possible, it is of paramount importance to address the factors that initially led to problem drinking.

---

**Box 43-6    Potential Alcohol-Related Problems in the Older Adult Population**

Fluctuations in activities of daily living and instrumental activities of daily living
Self-neglect
Trauma (e.g., falls, burns, accidents)
Weight loss
Dehydration
Gastrointestinal complaints (e.g., pain, bleeding, chronic diarrhea)
Incontinence
Increased medical complaints
Neuropathy
Jaundice
Ascites
Unexpected drug effects
Confusion or delirium
Dementia (Wernicke-Korsakoff syndrome)
Depression
Sleep disturbance
Family discord
Legal trouble (especially driving under the influence)

---

**Box 43-7    Nursing Care of Alcohol Withdrawal Syndrome in the Older Adult Population**

Assess withdrawal symptoms.
Assess vital signs.
Educate about withdrawal process.
Assist with activities of daily living.
Reduce environmental stimuli.
Supplement diet to meet nutritional needs.
Reorient patient.
Provide relaxation exercises.

---

## DRUG MISUSE AND ABUSE

Although older adults do not have a significant problem with illicit drug use, problems result from the overuse and misuse of prescription and OTC medications. Older adults use 25% to 30% of all prescription drugs and an even larger share of

## Box 43-8    Guidelines for Psychotropic Drug Use in Older Adults

**Initial Dose (Start Low—Go Slow)**
- Usually one third to one half of dose used for younger adults is effective.
- Start with a small dose and gradually increase until therapeutic effect or adverse side effects occur.

**Daily Dosage**
- Use the smallest dose that produces relief.
- Simplify dosing schedule.

**Individualization**
- Monitor blood levels when possible.
- Consider effect of other drugs and conditions.
- Partial symptom relief might be the most judicious and realistic goal.

**Discontinuation**
- Gradually taper off psychotropic drugs.
- If patients can manage without drug therapy, they should be allowed to do so.

without reliable information about medications that the others have prescribed. Confusion caused by generic and trade names can result in older adults taking the same medication under two names at the same time. Polypharmacy is common, so the nurse should be aware of potential complications and encourage patients to show the nurse all medications for cataloging. Drug regimens should be simplified and carefully explained.

### CRITICAL THINKING QUESTION    4

Do nurses at the facility where you have clinical rotations routinely include the same questions for alcohol and substance abuse in their assessments of geriatric patients as they do for younger adults? Do you feel comfortable asking your patients questions about the alcohol or drugs they ingest?

OTC agents (Substance Abuse and Mental Health Service Administration [SAMHSA], 2001). A large portion of prescriptions for this age group is for psychoactive, mood-changing drugs that have the potential for misuse, abuse, or dependency. Box 43-8 provides guidelines for the use of psychotropic drugs in older adults. Benzodiazepines, used for treatment of anxiety and insomnia, are of particular concern because they are frequently prescribed at inappropriately high doses and for excessive periods. This practice might lead to tolerance, physiologic dependence, and psychological dependence. Older women are more likely to receive and abuse psychoactive drugs than men (Blow, 2000; USDHHS, 1999).

Intentional and accidental misuse of drugs contributes to adverse health problems in older adults. An estimated 83% of adults over age 65 take at least one prescription drug, and 30% of adults take eight or more prescription drugs every day (SAMHSA, 2001). Compliance is a significant problem, exacerbated by poor vision and hearing, physical deficits, confusion, mental disorders, and inadequate instructions. Drug costs and packaging should also be considered as factors that promote noncompliance. Further complicating the situation, older adults might add several OTC agents, combine medications with alcohol, or take medication prescribed for others without notifying their physician. Many older adults see multiple physicians, each of whom might prescribe drugs

## ASSESSMENT OF OLDER ADULTS WITH MENTAL DISORDERS

Mental disorders are not isolated phenomena in older adults. Therefore, comprehensive psychosocial and physical assessments are required to determine factors that influence the older adult's level of function. Family members or other caregivers, who often play a pivotal role in the function of older adults, should be included in the assessment process whenever possible. The goals of the initial assessment and subsequent reassessments are to collect accurate information, identify problems and assets, plan interventions, predict outcomes, and measure changes over time. Because of the amount and depth of information needed, the nurse often works collaboratively with other disciplines to complete the assessment and contribute findings to an interdisciplinary team. Input from all disciplines, patient, and caregivers is used to develop goals and methods for care.

Nurses who are sensitive to the unique psychosocial and physical needs of older adults and adapt the assessment to accommodate these needs will increase the chances of obtaining data that accurately represent the patient. Interviews might produce anxiety because older adults are often reluctant to discuss problems with a stranger, especially a younger one. Older adult patients might be irritated by direct questions and view them as intrusive. Open-ended questions, which provide

| Box 43-9 | Enhancing Communication With Older Adults |
| --- | --- |

| *Considerations* | *Nursing Implications* |
| --- | --- |
| Slowed information processing | Do not rush; allow adequate time for questions to be answered. |
| | Avoid unnecessary interruptions. |
| Establishment of rapport | Offer a handshake. |
| | Make eye contact. |
| | Position at equal or lower level than patient. |
| | Address by title and last name unless asked to use another name. |
| Hearing deficits | Articulate words clearly. |
| | Face patient when speaking. |
| | Adjust volume of speech to patient's need; do not shout. |
| | Ensure use of hearing aid or amplifier. |
| | Use complementary nonverbal strategies (e.g., facial expressions, gestures). |
| Visual deficits | Provide adequate nonglare lighting. |
| | Ensure use of corrective lens. |
| Competing stimuli | Minimize background noise. |
| | Avoid times when patient is excessively tired, hurting, hungry, or has toileting needs. |
| | Provide privacy. |
| Education level | Match vocabulary to patient's level of use. |
| Decreased physical tolerance | Avoid overtiring. |

| Box 43-10 | Initial Assessment Information |
| --- | --- |

Demographics (age, marital status)
Spiritual and cultural values
Personal and family history
History of legal difficulties
Economic status and sources of income
Education and work history
Lifestyle and perception of current life situation
Current living arrangements
Interests, pleasures, and activities
Friendship and social interactions
Sexual functioning
Medical information and history
Prescription and over-the-counter drugs
Alcohol, tobacco, and other chemical use
Cognitive, behavioral, and emotional status
Goals and plans for the future

an opportunity for the patient to vent feelings and describe concerns and problems, often foster a healthy understanding of the patient's perspective of life and functioning. Strategies such as giving older people a measure of control, increasing self-esteem, using nonjudgmental wording, and providing positive reinforcement facilitate truthful information. Other strategies to enhance communication with older adults are listed in Box 43-9.

## PSYCHOSOCIAL ASSESSMENT

A wealth of clinical data can be obtained by listening to the stories that many older adults love to tell. Listening not only conveys a sense of appreciation for the individual's contributions across the life span, but also provides the patient a nonthreatening means of communicating pertinent information. The nurse should listen carefully during these conversations for persistent themes, such as a guilt, stress, grief, fear, or despair (Cully et al, 2001). By accepting expressed fears and concerns, the nurse assures the patient that these expressions will not result in rejection. Information about past experiences and coping strategies, along with personal strengths and weaknesses, might also be revealed. Formal assessment tools previously described might also be used to assess mental status, depression, and problem alcohol consumption. Box 43-10 lists information to obtain during the initial assessment.

Caregivers should be included in the assessment process. Not only can they provide information to clarify or expand on that given by the patient, their perspective of problems is also important for inclusion in a plan of care. Family members might be embarrassed to contradict information given by the patient in a joint interview. Because assessing family interaction is important, time should be spent interviewing the patient and family members, both separately and together. Nurses should use time with caregivers to assess their ability and willingness to provide care and support for the patient. Many caregivers, often spouses or children, fail to take care of their own needs and lack information about support services and respite care. Helping family members deal with the stressors of caregiving increases family and patient adjustment.

## PHYSICAL ASSESSMENT

Throughout this chapter, the connection between physical conditions and mental disorders has been stressed. Therefore, a complete physical examination is an essential component in the assessment of any older adult presenting with symptoms of mental disorders. The examination techniques for each subsystem do not differ substantially from the examination of younger adults. Numerous texts detail findings expected as a result of normal aging. Adaptations for decreased mobility and obvious impairments must be made. Careful attention to every subsystem is required because, in older adults, examination might reveal abnormalities in a system not suggested by the presenting symptoms. For example, subtle hearing loss can result in bizarre or incorrect responses, leading to erroneous assumptions about psychopathologic conditions. The nurse should use all senses during the examination, attending to the patient's visual presentation, odors, voice tone, and content. Blood tests, electroencephalography, and neuroimaging studies might be ordered to identify conditions that contribute to symptoms of mental disorders.

Special attention should be given to defining how physical problems interfere with the patient's functional ability. Older adults assign a great value to independence, and its loss can contribute to lower self-esteem and declines in mental health. The loss of key abilities might result in shame and frustration. Older adults who are dependent on others might resent the idea that others have to provide care and might believe that they have become a burden. The resulting anger can be directed internally and result in depression or withdrawal, or it might be directed at caregivers. Assessment of physical activities of daily living (PADLs) and instrumental activities of daily living (IADLs) provides a measure of the older adult's functional ability and guides the selection of interventions and services to meet identified needs. Box 43-11 identifies some of the variables for both PADLs and IADLs; Box 43-12 provides a sample question from the IADL scale. Patients, and sometimes their families, are often unable or unwilling to describe functional difficulties because of the threat to established patterns of lifestyle and interactions. According to the AoA (2000), 14% of older adults have difficulty carrying out PADLs and 21% report difficulties with IADLs. Observ-

---

### Box 43-11   Functional Assessment

| PADLs | IADLs |
| --- | --- |
| Bathing | Preparing meals |
| Dressing | Shopping |
| Eating | Managing money |
| Transferring | Using telephone |
| Walking | Using transportation |
| Toileting | Doing housework |

*IADLs,* Instrumental activities of daily living; *PADLs,* physical activities of daily living.

---

### Box 43-12   Sample Question: Instrumental Activities of Daily Living (IADLs) Scale

A. Ability to use telephone
  1. Operates telephone on own initiative—looks up and dials numbers, and so forth.
  2. Dials a few well-known numbers.
  3. Answers telephone but does not dial.
  4. Does not use telephone at all.

There are eight variables on this scale. The higher the score, the greater the disability. Other variables include shopping, food preparation, housekeeping, laundry, mode of transportation, responsibility for own medications, and ability to handle finances.

From Lawton MP, Moss M, Fulcomer M, Kleban MH: A research and service-oriented multilevel assessment instrument. *J Gerontol* 37:91, 1982.

---

ing task performance and carefully listening both to the patient and the collateral sources (e.g., family) as they describe daily activities might provide a more accurate picture of functional ability than direct questioning.

The physical examination should be used as an opportunity to assess for signs of abuse or neglect. Each state has laws that specify reporting requirements for intentional abuse, neglect, and exploitation of older adults. Laws also cover endangerment resulting from mental disorders. Chapter 5 discusses some legal issues that might stem from abuse or neglect.

## PSYCHOTHERAPEUTIC MANAGEMENT

### NURSE-PATIENT RELATIONSHIP

#### Attitude

Ageist attitudes, intergenerational differences, communication deficits, and the multiple problems of

Ms. Othelia Thatcher, a 78-year-old Caucasian woman with a 10-year history of severe depression, has been hospitalized twice in the last 2 years. She received a series of electroconvulsive therapy (ECT) treatments during each stay, with the last treatment given 11 months ago. Ms. Thatcher's cousin, a woman about 60 years old, brought the patient to the hospital emergency department this morning. The cousin described a gradual worsening of depressive symptoms over the past few months and says that Ms. Thatcher seems to need ECT approximately once a year. About 6 or 7 months after a course of ECT has been completed, the patient "goes bad again."

Ms. Thatcher complains of erratic sleep patterns and decreased appetite. She will not eat unless her cousin spoon-feeds her. The cousin reports that after a series of ECT, the patient is "easier to live with," plays with children, takes care of herself, helps with household tasks, and will "eat anything not nailed down."

The cousin estimates that the patient's depression began in the 1990s when "her only son, to whom she was very devoted," abandoned Ms. Thatcher to the welfare of the state and sold all her furniture. This occurred after the patient's extended hospitalization for treatment of pneumonia and a urinary tract infection. Since that time, Ms. Thatcher had reportedly lived in five different boarding homes before her cousin took her to the hospital 3 years ago.

The cousin states that Ms. Thatcher has never verbalized suicidal or homicidal thoughts, but she has a basically "paranoid view of life." The cousin cannot recall Ms. Thatcher ever having hallucinations.

older adults can pose significant obstacles to developing a therapeutic nurse-patient relationship. Nurses who are aware of their own feelings and reactions are able to focus on patients and their significant others in a therapeutic manner. By empathizing with the patient and caregivers and focusing on the patient's needs, the nurse can assist patients and their families manage the activities and demands of daily living and improve the overall quality of both physical and mental health.

## Understanding the Importance of Physical Health

Mental disorders have a significant effect on a patient's abilities to manage even the simplest of cognitive and physical tasks. Depression, psychosis, anxiety, and other disorders can result in inat-

tention or inability to perform routine ADLs. Therefore, it is essential for geropsychiatric nurses to ensure adequate fluid and nutritional intake, monitor elimination and hygiene, take protective measures in the face of impaired judgment, and remain vigilant for symptoms of physical illness and treatment complications. Some older adults have multiple physical complaints, the result of illness or psychological distress. The nurse should listen to complaints and evaluate potential causes. Summarizing and restating the patient's concerns out loud reinforce that the concerns have been heard. Interaction itself might be the real but unexpressed need of patients with persistent physical complaints (McCahill and Brunton, 1995).

## Communication

Communicating a sense of unconditional acceptance of the patient might be the most important intervention that the nurse can provide. Spending time with the patient outside that required for tasks such as medication administration and ADLs communicates an appreciation for the patient as a person of worth. Providing opportunities for the patient to participate in care decisions and control the sequence of events, such as allowing the patient to choose when to bathe, enhances self-esteem, self-worth, and decision-making skills. The nurse must be aware of problems and unspoken needs and incorporate them into the plan of care.

## Realistic Goals

Establishing both short- and long-term goals is important for nurses and patients. Discussions should be held with patients to stress the importance of goal setting. Often, ADLs can be a challenge, and developing a schedule of the day's activities with goals can help patients make decisions and cope with demands. Simple decisions might be difficult for older adults with mental disorders. Reducing the options available before allowing the patient choices can diminish frustration. For example, when it is time to dress, the nurse might restrict the choices of attire to two rather than offering an entire closet of options. The caregiver must be gentle and supportive, because additional time might be needed to achieve goals. Caregivers who base care decisions on the goal of restoring the patient to maximal

## Care Plan

Name: Ms. Othelia Thatcher                                    Admission Date: _____

*DSM-IV-TR* Diagnosis: Major depression

| | |
|---|---|
| Assessment | **Areas of strength:** Willingness to be treated; cooperative, good support system (cousin very concerned and wants patient back in home). |
| | **Problems:** Withdrawn, decreased interest in interactions and activities, decreased self-esteem, decreased energy, hopelessness, poor judgment. |
| Diagnoses | • Ineffective coping, disturbed sleep pattern, imbalanced nutrition; less than body requirements, impaired social interaction, self-care deficits |

| Outcomes | | Date met |
|---|---|---|
| | *Short-term goals:* | |
| | • Patient can maintain safety. | _____ |
| | • Patient can express feelings verbally. | _____ |
| | • Patient will have increased energy for self-care. | _____ |
| | *Long-term goals:* | |
| | • Patient will be able to talk about anger and disappointment related to son. | _____ |
| | • Patient will have an increase in self-concept. | _____ |
| | • Patient will maintain independence though living in cousin's home. | _____ |

| | |
|---|---|
| Planning/ Interventions | **Nurse-patient relationship:** Convey concern and acceptance without sympathy, encourage expression of feelings, interactions with others as tolerated, help patient explore anger with son. |
| | **Psychopharmacology:** Fluoxetine (Prozac) 20 mg q AM; risperidone (Risperdal) 0.5 mg q 12 hr; docusate sodium 100 mg bid. |
| | **Milieu management:** Provide adequate nutrition and hydration. Monitor patient for safety issues. Keep patient around others (not in room by self) as much as is reasonable. Keep naps short to facilitate sleep at night. |
| Evaluation | Patient expressed feelings of anger at being abandoned by son. Activity level increased. Minimal confusion post-ECT. Medication maintained. Will be discharged to return to cousin's home. |
| Referrals | Schedule visit with home health nurse for follow-up care. Schedule appointment with outpatient program coordinator within 7 days. |

independent function are likely to resist the urge to save time and energy by taking over tasks. Nurses should provide information on self-care and disease management at a pace that facilitates understanding. Patience, positive reinforcement, and consistency by the nurse benefit the patient.

## PSYCHOPHARMACOLOGY

Polypharmacy, physiologic changes, and comorbid physical disorders combine to increase the risk of unexpected drug effects in older adults. The negative impact of typical side effects is also exacerbated. Thus, the pharmacologic manage-

ment of psychiatric symptoms in older adults requires special consideration. Age-related changes that affect drug absorption, distribution, metabolism, and elimination are listed in Table 43-3 (Gareri et al, 2000). Co-administered drugs also affect *pharmacokinetics*. For example, antacids might delay absorption; proximal loop and potassium-sparing diuretics affect lithium excretion. *Pharmacodynamics* is the study of the actions and effects of drugs on organ tissue that bring about both intended effects and side effects. Knowledge of drugs' characteristics and their site and mechanism of action is important to understanding the sensitivity that older adults exhibit. For example, antipsychotic medications that act by blocking

| Table 43-3 | Age-related Changes: Effects on Pharmacokinetics |  |

| Physiologic Change | Effects | Special Considerations |
| --- | --- | --- |
| ↑ Gastric pH<br>↓ Absorptive surface<br>↓ Splanchnic blood flow<br>↓ Gastrointestinal motility<br>↓ Gastric emptying | Absorption | Delayed absorption of oral medication<br>Acid drugs more rapidly absorbed than base drugs |
| ↑ Body fat<br>↓ Lean body mass<br>↓ Total body water<br>↓ Serum albumin<br>↓ Cardiac output | Distribution | Extended half-life of lipid-soluble drugs, which accumulate in adipose tissue (e.g., barbiturates, phenothiazines, benzodiazepines, phenytoin, TCAs)<br>↓ Total plasma albumin = ↓ binding sites for protein-bound drugs, resulting in ↑ amount of free or active drug |
| ↓ Hepatic blood flow<br>↓ Hepatic mass<br>↓ Hepatic enzyme activity | Metabolism | Multiple drugs competing for same enzyme—might ↓ liver metabolism<br>High degree of genetic variability in available hepatic enzymes |
| ↓ Renal blood flow<br>↓ Glomerular filtration rate<br>↓ Tubular secretion<br>↓ Number of nephrons<br>↓ Creatinine production<br>↓ Creatinine clearance | Elimination | Creatinine clearance—can be reduced despite normal serum creatinine levels because of ↓ lean body weight and ↓ creatinine production<br>Reduction in renal clearance—might reduce dose requirements |

From Keltner N, Folks D: *Psychotropic drugs,* ed 3, St Louis, 2005, Mosby; Gareri P, Falconi U, De Fazio P, De Sarro G: Conventional and new antidepressant drugs in the elderly, *Prog Neurobiol* 61:353, 2000.

dopamine receptors have an increased likelihood of causing extrapyramidal side effects (EPSEs) in older adults who already have diminished dopamine concentrations. Nurses must observe and report both expected therapeutic and adverse medication reactions, as well as plan interventions to minimize the negative consequences of drug therapy. More extensive information is offered in the psychopharmacology unit of this text. Biologic changes affecting pharmacodynamics include increased receptor sensitivity, cholinergic degeneration, lower sedation threshold, nigrostriatal pathway changes, and the presence of other medical disorders.

## Antidepressants

Target symptoms of depression, side effect profiles, dose schedules, and cost are factors in antidepressant drug selection. The selective serotonin reuptake inhibitors (SSRIs), which are generally favored for older adults, are effective, have a favorable side effect profile and are not lethal in overdose. SSRIs are also used to treat primary anxiety disorders common to older adults (Compton and Nemeroff, 2001). Tricyclic antidepressants (TCAs) can be used in older adults, but their anticholinergic, antiadrenergic, and anti-

histaminic properties cause side effects that are particularly problematic for older adult patients. Hence, TCAs are not frequently prescribed.

Newer antidepressant agents, such as bupropion (Wellbutrin) and trazodone (Desyrel), have a better side effect profile than TCAs and are widely used. Bupropion causes little sedation, hypotension, anticholinergic response, or cardiotoxicity. Trazodone does not have anticholinergic effects but is sedating. The sedation distinction between antidepressants is important because depression is sometimes exhibited by agitation or sleep disturbance, and affected patients might benefit from the sedating properties of an antidepressant. When depression is exhibited by lethargy and excessive sleep, a more activating antidepressant is in order (e.g., bupropion, SSRIs). TCAs are not recommended for patients with known cardiac problems because of their association with changes in cardiac conduction, arrhythmias, and orthostatic hypotension. Patients should be carefully monitored for orthostatic changes, especially individuals who are also taking diuretics or vasodilators. Monoamine oxidase inhibitors (MAOIs) are rarely used in older adults, because these medications have potentially serious side effects and require dietary restrictions (Compton and Nemeroff, 2001). Similar to TCAs, MAOIs are lethal in overdose.

Full therapeutic response takes at least 2 to 4 weeks for most antidepressants. Many patients fail to respond to the first antidepressant prescribed. When this occurs, the nurse can reassure patients that this is not uncommon and that other drugs can be effective. Education about the importance of compliance and the need to continue antidepressant therapy, even when depressive symptoms resolve, is important. In most cases, antidepressants are continued for at least 6 months following symptom resolution to prevent relapse. Patients who are at high risk of relapse are maintained on antidepressants for longer periods (Whooley and Simon, 2000).

## Antipsychotics

Antipsychotic drugs are used in the treatment of schizophrenia, acute psychosis, aggressive behavior, and agitation. Atypical antipsychotics are regarded as the drugs of choice for treatment of older adults because of the favorable side effect profiles and efficacy of these drugs (Maixner et al, 1999). The term *atypical* was introduced to describe the low propensity of these agents to cause EPSEs and tardive dyskinesia (TD), a significant advantage for older adults who, because of neurodegenerative processes, are at risk for developing disabling and stigmatizing movement disorders. In fact, over a 1-year period taking conventional antipsychotics, older adults develop TD at a cumulative incidence rate of 28% compared with only 5% in younger patients (Jeste, 2004). With the atypical drugs, such as risperidone, this rate decreases significantly to 2.7%, (Jeste, 2004). As compared with traditional antipsychotics, atypical antipsychotics also show greater efficacy for both the positive and negative symptoms of schizophrenia and have fewer adverse cardiac effects and reduced sedative effects. Drugs in this class vary widely in their site of action and side effect profile. Table 43-4 presents guidelines for treating schizophrenia in older adult patients.

Traditional antipsychotic drugs are categorized as high potency or low potency. The high-potency drugs, such as haloperidol (Haldol) and fluphenazine (Prolixin), are associated with EPSEs. The low-potency antipsychotics, such as chlorpromazine (Thorazine) and thioridazine (Mellaril), cause sedative, anticholinergic, and antiadrenergic effects (particularly orthostatic hypotension) that make their use more problematic for older adults com-

| Table 43-4 | Expert Guidelines for Treating Schizophrenia in Older Patients | |
|---|---|---|
| **First-line Antipsychotic** | **Second-line Antipsychotics** | |
| Risperidone, 1.25-3.5 mg/day | Quetiapine, 100-300 mg/day | |
| | Olanzapine, 7.5-15 mg/day | |
| | Aripiprazole, 15-30 mg/day | |

From Alexopoulous G, Streim J, Carpenter D, Docherty JP: The expert consensus guidelines: using antipsychotic agents in older patients, *J Clin Psychiatry* 65(Suppl 2):1, 2004.

pared with high-potency agents. If one of the traditional drugs is used, it tends to be haloperidol. Antipsychotic drug dosages for older adults tend to be 50% or less those given to younger patients. Nurses must carefully monitor patients for side effects. Assessment tools—for example, the Abnormal Involuntary Movement Scale (AIMS)—can be used to identify EPSEs and TD.

## Antianxiety Agents

Anxiety is a common late-life problem, and its management often involves SSRIs, benzodiazepines, and buspirone (BuSpar) (Compton and Nemeroff, 2001; Keltner and Folks, 2005). A disproportionate share of prescriptions for benzodiazepines is written for older adults, despite the fact that this age group is particularly vulnerable to common side effects such as drowsiness, cognitive suppression, and ataxia (Heffern, 2000). An increased risk of falls, disinhibition characterized by violence or agitation, and retrograde amnesia are additional related concerns (Keltner and Folks, 2005). Federal guidelines, along with improved practice guidelines, for management of anxiety in older adults have encouraged the use of benzodiazepines such as lorazepam (Ativan) and oxazepam (Serax), which are metabolized by phase II mechanisms (i.e., nonoxidative). Benzodiazepines are recommended only for short-term management of anxiety. Because withdrawal syndrome (including withdrawal seizure) can occur when benzodiazepines are removed after 30 or more days of use, they should be withdrawn slowly over several weeks or longer. Benzodiazepines are relatively safe drugs when taken alone but can cause severe sedation and respiratory suppression when combined with alcohol or other sedatives. Buspirone

(BuSpar), a nonbenzodiazepine antianxiety agent, effectively manages anxiety without concerns for physical or psychological dependence. Furthermore, buspirone is not sedating and has no additive effect with alcohol. Its chief disadvantage is that its full therapeutic effects are delayed for 3 to 6 weeks (Keltner and Folks, 2005).

### Mood Stabilizers

Mood-stabilizing drugs used for treating bipolar disorders and mixed depressive episodes include lithium, valproates such as divalproex (Depakote), and the atypical antipsychotics. Lithium has long been the drug of choice for manic symptoms in patients of all ages; however, in recent years, the most commonly prescribed class of mood stabilizer appears to be the valproates (Sajatovic et al, 2005). As a group of drugs, atypical antipsychotics are prescribed about as often as the valproates and even more often in those with late-onset (i.e., older than age 60) bipolar disorder (Sajatovic et al, 2005).

With lithium, the serum levels are closely monitored in all patients and in older adults; both a therapeutic response (serum levels from 0.4 to 0.8 mEq/L) and a toxic response occur at lower levels. Older adults are also at a higher risk for toxic reactions related to altered fluid and electrolyte balance and co-administered medications, especially diuretics (Keltner and Folks, 2005; Snowdon, 2000). Because therapeutic effects of mood stabilizers take weeks to manifest, short-acting benzodiazepines are often considered as adjuncts to manage dangerous behaviors in the interval (Snowdon, 2000).

## MILIEU MANAGEMENT

Nurses responsible for older adults with mental disorders in inpatient or day care settings have a therapeutic responsibility to facilitate optimal function. Attention to all elements of the milieu can increase psychological functioning and prevent the deterioration resulting from withdrawal and disuse of skills that have been well documented in institutionalized older adults.

### Normalizing the Environment

Effective milieu management changes the quality of life in institutional environments by working with residents to normalize the environment as much as possible. The traditional associations of home involve control over people who come and go, as well as control of personal spaces, furnishings, and accessories (Katz, 1995). Furniture, at a height that facilitates independent mobility, can be placed in conversational groupings. Common rooms are best equipped with large-print books, games with large print and pieces, and stimulating pictures. Individual rooms can be deinstitutionalized by encouraging residents to use their own bedspreads, family pictures, favorite calendars, and other personal items. This same strategy, even in acute care settings, has the added benefit of providing orientation cues. Staff members often wear street clothes rather than traditional uniforms to encourage social interaction with residents and eliminate artificial barriers. It is important to remember privacy needs and respect personal space. Environmental adaptations that promote safety and independence for older adults are listed in Table 43-5.

| Selected Nursing Interventions for Assisting Older Adults With Depression |
| --- |
| Assess and meet physical needs. |
| Promote healthy behavior. |
| Maximize independence. |
| Promote sense of control. |
| Provide consistency. |
| Reinforce self-esteem. |
| Acknowledge individual's feelings. |
| Appreciate individual's uniqueness in context of entire life span and culture. |
| Reinforce genuine hope. |
| Identify available supports. |
| Consider family and caregivers. |

### Controlling Aggression

Controlling aggression is a major component of maintaining individual and environmental safety. Violent or agitated behavior might be the result of poor frustration tolerance, ineffective coping strategies, impulsivity, or real or imagined threats to personal space. Nurses must look at the environment and develop strategies to minimize precipitating factors. Careful attention should be paid to the potential for background stimuli such as constant music or television to cause distress. Physical and chemical restraints to control

| Table 43-5 | Environmental Adaptations |
|---|---|

| Considerations | Interventions |
|---|---|
| Decreased ability to distinguish colors | Use high-contrast colors in vivid hues. |
| Mobility impairments | Ensure nonslip floor surfaces. |
| | Provide adequate, nonglare lighting. |
| | Ensure well-fitting footwear. |
| | Provide chairs and toilets at comfortable height with armrests or handrails. |
| | Avoid placing rolling tables where patients might attempt to use them for stability. |
| | Provide shower stools, nonskid tub guards, and grab bars. |
| | Provide ambulation rails. |
| | Remove obstacles, clutter, and spills promptly. |
| Inability to read | Mark spaces with pictures or universal symbols. |
| Decreased thermoregulation | Ensure comfortable temperature. |
| | Observe for signs of hypothermia or hyperthermia. |
| | Provide sweaters, blankets. |
| | Ensure safe water temperature. |

behavior have numerous negative consequences, and alternative interventions should be attempted before use. Managing environmental stimuli, providing productive outlets for energy, and practicing redirection and diversion are important for reducing outbursts.

### Tailoring Activities

Therapeutic approaches should be based on the concept that all individuals have a need for human contact, social participation, and meaningful activity to maintain function. Individual and group interactions and activities should be planned to foster the greatest degree of independence and develop interpersonal and communication skills. A variety of activities can be tailored to match individual levels of physical and psychological function. Pet therapy helps fulfill patients' needs to give and receive affection through supervised sessions of holding, stroking, and playing with specially screened animals. Exercise therapy, tailored to all needs, even those with limited physical ability, provides outlets for the excess energy of anxiety and provides stimulation and socialization opportunities. Music is also an effective way to make contact with patients. Songbooks, hymnals, and records offer an array of music choices familiar to older adults, who often enjoy sing-alongs or simply listening to familiar and comfortable tunes. Nurturing and tending to plants can enhance physical function, relieve tension, and provide a sense of responsibility and accomplishment. These

therapeutic activities and others are important opportunities to provide patients with positive experiences and help them attain realistic goals.

### Valuing the Person Through Reminiscence and Life Review

Reminiscence is the process of recalling past experiences, which allows the listener insight into the patient's history and perspective. Patients can benefit from multiple dimensions of reminiscence, including clarifying their sense of self, connecting with others, providing instruction, restructuring recalled events, recalling previously used problem-solving strategies, and bringing closure and calmness in death preparation (Cully et al, 2001). Reminiscence groups can provide validation for each member and help participants establish new relationships while enhancing valuable communication and socialization skills.

Life review is a mechanism that uses reminiscence but is a different process. Evaluation of the entire life span through telling or writing a personal story is difficult work for the patient. During one-to-one interaction, the patient relates fears, conflicts, unresolved feelings, and unresolved losses, providing opportunities for therapeutic intervention.

### ▐ Study Notes

1. Despite the increase in the population of individuals 65 years of age and older, this group

experiences major barriers to obtaining quality mental health care because of issues such as ageism, their own attitudes, and cost of care.

2. Depression is a common mental disorder among older adults, but it is often overlooked, misdiagnosed, and inadequately treated.

3. Symptoms of other illnesses might mask depression because older adults might be preoccupied with physical rather than emotional symptoms.

4. Age-related life events, losses, changes, and physical decline are associated with the onset of depression.

5. The nurse-patient relationship focuses on helping patients achieve their highest level of function. Caregivers, when available, should be included in planning strategies to manage the activities and demands of daily living.

6. Adequate nutrition, socialization, and achievement of small realistic goals in daily living activities help reduce anxiety and maintain or restore psychological functioning.

7. Use of medications with older adults involves risks associated with polypharmacy, noncompliance, and altered pharmacokinetics.

8. SSRIs, bupropion, and trazodone are the recommended agents for treating depression in the older adult population.

9. When treating psychotic disorders, atypical antipsychotics are typically prescribed. If an older traditional agent is to be used, haloperidol is most often used because of its fewer antiadrenergic and anticholinergic effects.

10. Benzodiazepines using phase II metabolism, lorazepam and oxazepam, SSRIs, and the nonbenzodiazepine anxiety agents are prescribed most often for this age group.

11. ECT can be effective treatment for older adults suffering from depression.

## References

Administration on Aging: Factsheets. Available at http://www.aoa.gov/factsheets. Accessed November 22, 2005.

Alexopoulous G, Streim J, Carpenter D, Docherty JP: The expert consensus guidelines: using antipsychotic agents in older patients, *J Clin Psychiatry* 65(Suppl 2):1, 2004.

American Psychiatric Association [APA]: Mood disorders. In *Diagnostic and Statistical Manual of Mental Disorders, text revision*, ed 4 (pp. 345-428), Washington, DC, 2000, APA.

Blank K, Robison J, Doherty E, et al: Life-sustaining treatment and assisted death choices in depressed older patients, *J Am Geriatr Soc* 49:153, 2001.

Blazer DG, Koenig HG: Mood disorders. In Busse E, Blazer D, editors: *Textbook of geriatric psychiatry*, ed 2 (pp. 235-264), Washington, DC, 1996, American Psychiatric Press.

Blow F: Treatment of older women with alcohol problems: meeting the challenge for a special population, *Alcohol Clin Exp Res* 24:1257, 2000.

Butler RN, Lewis ML: Late-life depression: when and how to intervene, *Geriatrics* 50:44, 1995.

Byrne G, Raphael B, Arnold E: Alcohol consumption and psychological distress in recently widowed older men, *Aust N Z J Psychiatry* 33:740, 1999.

Campbell T, Franks P, Fiscella K, et al: Do physicians who diagnose more mental health disorders generate lower healthcare costs? *J Fam Pract* 49:305, 2000.

Cassano G, McElroy SL, Brady K, et al: Current issues in the identification and management of bipolar spectrum disorders in "special populations," *J Affect Disorders* 59:S69, 2000.

Compton M, Nemeroff C: The evaluation and treatment of depression in primary care, *Clin Cornerstone* 3:10, 2001.

Conigliaro J, Kraemer K, McNeil M: Screening and identification of older adults with alcohol problems in primary care, *J Geriatr Psychiatry Neurol* 13:106, 2000.

Creed F: The importance of depression following myocardial infarction, *Heart* 82:406, 1999.

Cully J, LaVoie D, Gfeller J: Reminiscence, personality, and psychological functioning in older adults, *Gerontologist* 41:89, 2001.

Eyler Zorrilla LT, Heaton RK, McAdams LA, et al: Cross-sectional study of older outpatients with schizophrenia and healthy comparison subjects: no differences in age-related cognitive declines, *Am J Psychiatry* 157:1324, 2000.

Federal Interagency Forum on Aging-Related Statistics: *Older Americans 2000: key indicators of well-being*, Federal Interagency Forum on Aging-Related Statistics, Washington, DC, 2000, U.S. Government Printing Office. Also available at http://www.agingstats.gov/chartbook2000.

Folks D, Fuller W: Anxiety disorders and insomnia in geriatric patients, *Psychiatr Clin North Am* 20:137, 1997.

Forsell Y, Winblad B: Incidence of major depression in a very elderly population, *Int J Geriatr Psychiatry* 14:368, 1999.

Ganzini L, Atkinson R: Substance abuse. In Sadavoy J, Lazarus LW, Jarvik LF, et al, editors: *Comprehensive review of geriatric psychiatry-II*, ed 2 (pp. 659-692), Washington, DC, 1996, American Psychiatric Press.

Gareri P, Falconi U, De Fazio P, De Sarro G: Conventional and new antidepressant drugs in the elderly, *Prog Neurobiol* 61:354, 2000.

Heffern W: Psychopharmacological and electroconvulsive treatment of anxiety and depression in the elderly, *J Psychiatr Ment Health Nurs* 7:199, 2000.

Howard R, Rabins PV, Seeman MV, Jeste DV: Late-onset schizophrenia and very-late-onset schizophrenia-like psychosis: an international consensus, *Am J Psychiatry* 157:172, 2000.

Hoyert DL, Kochanek KD, Murphey SL: Deaths: final data for 1997, *National vital statistics report*, Hyattsville MD, 1999, National Center for Health Statistics, DHHS Publication No. 99-1120.

Jancin B: New suicide data highlight toxicity of depression, *Clin Psychiatry News* 33:1, 6, 2005.

Jeste DV: Tardive dyskinesia rates with atypical antipsychotics in older adults, *J Clin Psychiatry* 65(Suppl 9):21, 2004.

Kales H, Blow FC, Copeland LA, et al: Health care utilization by older patients with coexisting dementia and depression, *Am J Psychiatry* 156:550, 1999.

Katz IR: Infrastructure requirements for research in late-life mental disorders. In Gatz M, editor: *Emerging issues in mental health and aging* (pp. 256-281), Washington, DC, 1995, American Psychiatric Press.

Kayton W: *The impact of major depression in patients with chronic medical illness,* Proceedings of the 154th Annual Meeting of the American Psychiatric Association, New Orleans, LA, 2001.

Keltner N, Folks D: *Psychotropic drugs,* ed 3, St. Louis, 2005, Mosby.

Koenig H, Christison C, Christison G, et al: Schizophrenia and paranoid disorders. In Busse E, Blazer D, editors: *Textbook of geriatric psychiatry,* ed 2 (pp. 265-278), Washington, DC, 1996, American Psychiatric Press.

Lang A, Stein M: Anxiety disorders. How to recognize and treat the medical symptoms of emotional illness, *Geriatrics* 56:24, 2001.

Lenze E, Mulsant BH, Shear MK, et al: Co-morbid anxiety disorders in depressed elderly patients, *Am J Psychiatry* 157:722, 2000.

Ludwick R, Sedlak CA, Doheny MO, Martsolf DS: Alcohol use in elderly women: nursing considerations in community settings, *J Gerontol Nurs* 26:44, 2000.

Maixner S, Mellow AM, Tandon R: The efficacy, safety and tolerability of anti-psychotics in the elderly, *J Clin Psychiatry* 60(Suppl 8):29, 1999.

McCahill M, Brunton S: The elderly patient with multiple complaints, *Hosp Pract* 30:49, 1995.

McClure FS, Gladsjo JA, Jeste DV: Late-onset psychosis: clinical, research, and ethical considerations, *Am J Psychiatry* 156:935, 1999.

Moon MA: Late-onset bipolar patients not as ill as counterparts, *Clin Psychiatry News* 33:48, 2005.

National Institute on Aging: *Strategic plan for fiscal years 2001-2005.* Available at http://www.nih.gov/AboutNIA/StrategicPlan/. Accessed May 30, 2006.

National Institute of Mental Health: *Crisis in geriatric mental health,* 1999a. Available at http://www.nimh.nih.gov/litalert/geriatriccrisis.cfm. Accessed August 18, 2001.

National Institute of Mental Health: *Suicide facts,* 1999b. Available at http://www.nimh.nih.gov/suicideprevention/suifact.cfm. Accessed May 30, 2006.

National Institute of Mental Health: *Older adults: depression and suicide facts,* NIMH Publication no. 01-4593, 2001. Available at http://www.nimh.nih.gov/healthinformation/elderlydepsuicide.cfm. Accessed May 30, 2006.

National Institutes of Health: *The impact of mental illness on society,* NIH Publication No. 01-4586, 2001. Available at http://www.nimh.nih.gov/publicat/burden.cfm. Accessed May 30, 2006.

Patterson T, Moscona S, McKibbin CL, et al: Social skills performance assessment among older patients with schizophrenia, *Schizophr Res* 48:351, 2001.

Penninx B, Geerlings SW, Deeg DJ, et al: Minor and major depression and the risk of death in older persons, *Arch Gen Psychiatry* 56:889, 1999.

Sajatovic M, Blow FC, Ignacio RV, Kales HC: New-onset bipolar disorder in later life, *Am J Geriatr Psychiatry* 13:282, 2005.

Schurhoff F, Bellivier F, Jouvent R, et al: Early and late onset bipolar disorders: two different forms of manic-depressive illness? *J Affect Disord* 58:215, 2000.

Shea D, Russo P, Smyer M: Use of mental health services by persons with a mental illness in nursing facilities: initial impacts of OBRA 87, *J Aging Health* 12:560, 2000.

Sheikh J: Anxiety disorders. In Sadavoy J, Lazarus LW, Jarvik LF, et al, editors: *Comprehensive review of geriatric psychiatry,* ed 2 (pp. 615-636), Washington DC, 1996, American Psychiatric Press.

Sherman C: Modify depression treatment for older patients, *Clin Psychiatry News* 33:54, 2005.

Snowdon J: The relevance of guidelines for treatment of mania in old age, *Int J Geriatr Psychiatry* 15:779, 2000.

Substance Abuse and Mental Health Service Administration (SAMHSA), The National Clearinghouse for Alcohol and Drug Information: *Use and abuse of psychoactive prescription drugs and over the counter medications,* 2001. Available at http://www.health.org/govpubs/BKD250/26f.htm. Accessed May 30, 2006.

Tew JD Jr, Mulsant BH, Haskett RF, et al: Acute efficacy of ECT in the treatment of major depression in the old-old, *Am J Psychiatry* 156:1865, 1999.

Tune L: Assessing psychiatric illness in geriatric patients, *Clin Cornerstone* 3:23, 2001.

U.S. Department of Health and Human Services: *Mental health: a report of the Surgeon General,* Rockville, MD, 1999, U.S. Department of Health and Human Services, Substance Abuse and Mental Health Services Administration, Center for Mental Health Services, National Institutes of Health, National Institute of Mental Health. Also available at http://:www.surgeongeneral.gov/library/mentalhealth/home.html. Accessed May 30, 2006.

Wetterling T, Driessen M, Kanitz RD, Junghanns K: The severity of alcohol withdrawal is not age dependent, *Alcohol Alcohol* 36:75, 2001.

Whooley M, Simon G: Managing depression in medical outpatients, *N Engl J Med* 343:1942, 2000.

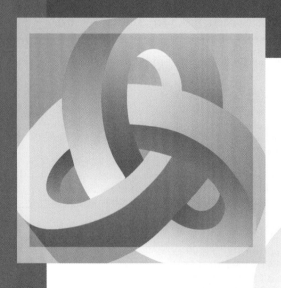

# Diagnostic Criteria for Mental Disorders, Text Revision (DSM-IV-TR)*

The following text represents the complete list of diagnoses found in the *DSM-IV-TR*. Many diagnoses have notations that increase specificity. These notations are not always included here. The following clarifications are made to assist you in understanding this material: *NOS* = not otherwise specified; *X* = a specific code number is required.

*Note to Students: This list represents all DSM-IV-TR diagnoses. It does not, however, reflect some of the subtleties of coding found in the DSM-IV-TR manual. The student is directed to the manual should finer discrimination be sought.*

## DISORDERS USUALLY FIRST DIAGNOSED IN INFANCY, CHILDHOOD, OR ADOLESCENCE

### MENTAL RETARDATION

*Note:* These are coded on Axis II.

| | |
|---|---|
| 317 | Mild Mental Retardation |
| 318.00 | Moderate Mental Retardation |
| 318.1 | Severe Mental Retardation |
| 318.2 | Profound Mental Retardation |
| 319 | Mental Retardation, Unspecified |

### LEARNING DISORDERS

| | |
|---|---|
| 315.00 | Reading Disorder |
| 315.1 | Mathematics Disorder |
| 315.2 | Disorder of Written Expression |
| 315.9 | Learning Disorder NOS |

### MOTOR SKILLS DISORDER

| | |
|---|---|
| 315.4 | Developmental Coordination Disorder |

### COMMUNICATION DISORDERS

| | |
|---|---|
| 315.31 | Expressive Language Disorder |
| 315.31 | Mixed Receptive–Expressive Language Disorder |
| 315.39 | Phonological Disorder |
| 307.0 | Stuttering |
| 307.9 | Communication Disorder NOS |

### PERVASIVE DEVELOPMENTAL DISORDERS

| | |
|---|---|
| 299.00 | Autistic Disorder |
| 299.80 | Rett's Disorder |

*Reprinted with permission from the American Psychiatric Association: *Diagnostic and statistical manual of mental disorders, text revision,* ed 4, Washington, DC, 2000, APA.

| | |
|---|---|
| 299.10 | Childhood Disintegrative Disorder |
| 299.80 | Asperger's Disorder |
| 299.80 | Pervasive Developmental Disorder NOS |

## ATTENTION-DEFICIT AND DISRUPTIVE BEHAVIOR DISORDERS

| | |
|---|---|
| 314.xx | Attention-Deficit/Hyperactivity Disorder |
| .01 | Combined Type |
| .00 | Predominantly Inattentive Type |
| .01 | Predominantly Hyperactive-Impulsive Type |
| 314.9 | Attention-Deficit/Hyperactivity Disorder NOS |
| 312.8 | Conduct Disorder |
| 313.81 | Oppositional Defiant Disorder |
| 312.9 | Disruptive Behavior Disorder NOS |

## FEEDING AND EATING DISORDERS OF INFANCY OR EARLY CHILDHOOD

| | |
|---|---|
| 307.52 | Pica |
| 307.53 | Rumination Disorder |
| 307.59 | Feeding Disorder of Infancy or Early Childhood |

## TIC DISORDERS

| | |
|---|---|
| 307.23 | Tourette's Disorder |
| 307.22 | Chronic Motor or Vocal Tic Disorder |
| 307.21 | Transient Tic Disorder |
| 307.20 | Tic Disorder NOS |

## ELIMINATION DISORDERS

| | |
|---|---|
| ___.__ | Encopresis |
| 787.6 | With Constipation and Overflow Incontinence |
| 307.7 | Without Constipation and Overflow Incontinence |
| 307.6 | Enuresis (Not Due to a General Medical Condition) |

## OTHER DISORDERS OF INFANCY, CHILDHOOD, OR ADOLESCENCE

| | |
|---|---|
| 309.21 | Separation Anxiety Disorder |
| 313.23 | Selective Mutism |
| 313.89 | Reactive Attachment Disorder of Infancy or Early Childhood |

| | |
|---|---|
| 307.3 | Stereotypic Movement Disorder |
| 313.9 | Disorder of Infancy, Childhood, or Adolescence NOS |

## DELIRIUM, DEMENTIA, AND AMNESTIC AND OTHER COGNITIVE DISORDERS

## DELIRIUM

| | |
|---|---|
| 293.0 | Delirium Due to . . . |
| ___.__ | Substance Intoxication Delirium |
| ___.__ | Substance Withdrawal Delirium |
| ___.__ | Delirium Due to Multiple Etiologies |
| 780.09 | Delirium NOS |

## DEMENTIA

| | |
|---|---|
| 290.xx | Dementia of the Alzheimer's Type, With Early Onset (also code 331.0 Alzheimer's disease on Axis III) |
| .10 | Without Behavioral Disturbances |
| .11 | With Behavioral Disturbances |
| 290.xx | Dementia of the Alzheimer's Type, With Late Onset (also code 331.0 Alzheimer's disease on Axis III) |
| .10 | Without behavioral disturbances |
| .11 | With behavioral disturbances |
| 290.xx | Vascular Dementia |
| .40 | Uncomplicated |
| .41 | With Delirium |
| .42 | With Delusions |
| .43 | With Depressed Mood |
| 294.1x | Dementia Due to HIV Disease |
| 294.1x | Dementia Due to Head Trauma |
| 294.1x | Dementia Due to Parkinson's Disease |
| 294.1x | Dementia Due to Huntington's Disease |
| 294.1x | Dementia Due to Pick's Disease |
| 294.1x | Dementia Due to Creutzfeldt-Jakob Disease |
| 294.1x | Dementia Due to . . . |
| ___.__ | Substance-Induced Persisting Dementia |
| ___.__ | Dementia Due to Multiple Etiologies |
| 294.8 | Dementia NOS |

## AMNESTIC DISORDERS

| | |
|---|---|
| 294.0 | Amnestic Disorder Due to . . . |
| ___.__ | Substance-Induced Persisting Amnestic Disorder |
| 294.8 | Amnestic Disorder NOS |

## OTHER COGNITIVE DISORDERS

294.9    Cognitive Disorder NOS

## MENTAL DISORDERS DUE TO A GENERAL MEDICAL CONDITION NOT ELSEWHERE CLASSIFIED

293.89    Catatonic Disorder Due to . . .
310.1     Personality Change Due to . . .
293.9     Mental Disorder NOS Due to . . .

## SUBSTANCE-RELATED DISORDERS

## ALCOHOL-RELATED DISORDERS

### Alcohol Use Disorders

303.90    Alcohol Dependence
305.00    Alcohol Abuse

### Alcohol-Induced Disorders

303.00    Alcohol Intoxication
291.81    Alcohol Withdrawal
291.0     Alcohol Intoxication Delirium
291.0     Alcohol Withdrawal Delirium
291.2     Alcohol-Induced Persisting Dementia
291.1     Alcohol-Induced Persisting Amnestic Dementia
291.x     Alcohol-Induced Psychotic Disorder
    .5    With Delusions
    .3    With Hallucinations
291.89    Alcohol-Induced Mood Disorder
291.89    Alcohol-Induced Anxiety Disorder
291.89    Alcohol-Induced Sexual Dysfunction
291.89    Alcohol-Induced Sleep Disorder
291.9     Alcohol-Related Disorder NOS

## AMPHETAMINE (OR AMPHETAMINE-LIKE)–RELATED DISORDERS

### Amphetamine Use Disorders

304.40    Amphetamine Dependence
305.70    Amphetamine Abuse

### Amphetamine-Induced Disorders

292.89    Amphetamine Intoxication
292.0     Amphetamine Withdrawal

292.81    Amphetamine Intoxication Delirium
292.xx    Amphetamine-Induced Psychotic Disorder
    .11   With Delusions
    .12   With Hallucinations
292.84    Amphetamine-Induced Mood Disorder
292.89    Amphetamine-Induced Anxiety Disorder
292.89    Amphetamine-Induced Sexual Dysfunction
292.89    Amphetamine-Induced Sleep Disorder
292.9     Amphetamine-Related Disorder NOS

## CAFFEINE-RELATED DISORDERS

### Caffeine-Induced Disorders

305.90    Caffeine Intoxication
292.89    Caffeine-Induced Anxiety Disorder
292.89    Caffeine-Induced Sleep Disorder
292.9     Caffeine-Related Disorder NOS

## CANNABIS-RELATED DISORDERS

### Cannabis Use Disorders

304.30    Cannabis Dependence
305.20    Cannabis Abuse

### Cannabis-Induced Disorders

292.89    Cannabis Intoxication
292.81    Cannabis Intoxication Delirium
292.xx    Cannabis-Induced Psychotic Disorder
    .11   With Delusions
    .12   With Hallucinations
292.89    Cannabis-Induced Anxiety Disorder
292.9     Cannabis-Related Disorder NOS

## COCAINE-RELATED DISORDERS

### Cocaine Use Disorders

304.20    Cocaine Dependence
305.60    Cocaine Abuse

### Cocaine-Induced Disorders

292.89    Cocaine Intoxication
292.0     Cocaine Withdrawal
292.81    Cocaine Intoxication Delirium
292.xx    Cocaine-Induced Psychotic Disorder

.11    With Delusions
.12    With Hallucinations
292.84    Cocaine-Induced Mood Disorder
292.89    Cocaine-Induced Anxiety Disorder
292.89    Cocaine-Induced Sexual Dysfunction
292.89    Cocaine-Induced Sleep Disorder
292.9    Cocaine-Related Disorder NOS

## HALLUCINOGEN-RELATED DISORDERS

### Hallucinogen Use Disorders

304.50    Hallucinogen Dependence
305.30    Hallucinogen Abuse

### Hallucinogen-Induced Disorders

292.89    Hallucinogen Intoxication
292.89    Hallucinogen Persisting Perception
          Disorder (Flashbacks)
292.81    Hallucinogen Intoxication Delirium
292.xx    Hallucinogen-Induced Psychotic
          Disorder
.11    With Delusions
.12    With Hallucinations
292.84    Hallucinogen-Induced Mood Disorder
292.89    Hallucinogen-Induced Anxiety
          Disorder
292.9    Hallucinogen-Related Disorder NOS

## INHALANT-RELATED DISORDERS

### Inhalant Use Disorders

304.60    Inhalant Dependence
305.90    Inhalant Abuse

### Inhalant-Induced Disorders

292.89    Inhalant Intoxication
292.81    Inhalant Intoxication Delirium
292.82    Inhalant-Induced Persisting Dementia
292.xx    Inhalant-Induced Psychotic Disorder
.11    With Delusions
.12    With Hallucinations
292.84    Inhalant-Induced Mood Disorder
292.89    Inhalant-Induced Anxiety Disorder
292.9    Inhalant-Related Disorder NOS

## NICOTINE-RELATED DISORDER

### Nicotine Use Disorder

305.10    Nicotine Dependence

### Nicotine-Induced Disorders

292.0    Nicotine Withdrawal
292.9    Nicotine-Related Disorder NOS

## OPIOID-RELATED DISORDERS

### Opioid Use Disorders

304.00    Opioid Dependence
305.50    Opioid Abuse

### Opioid-Induced Disorders

292.89    Opioid Intoxication
292.0    Opioid Withdrawal
292.81    Opioid Intoxication Delirium
292.xx    Opioid-Induced Psychotic Disorder
.11    With Delusions
.12    With Hallucinations
292.84    Opioid-Induced Mood Disorder
292.89    Opioid-Induced Sexual Dysfunction
292.89    Opioid-Induced Sleep Disorder
292.9    Opioid-Related Disorder NOS

## PHENCYCLIDINE (OR PHENCYCLIDINE-LIKE)–RELATED DISORDERS

### Phencyclidine Use Disorders

304.90    Phencyclidine Dependence
305.90    Phencyclidine Abuse

### Phencyclidine-Induced Disorders

292.89    Phencyclidine Intoxication
292.81    Phencyclidine Intoxication Delirium
292.xx    Phencyclidine-Induced Psychotic
          Disorder
.11    With Delusions
.12    With Hallucinations
292.84    Phencyclidine-Induced Mood Disorder
292.89    Phencyclidine-Induced Anxiety
          Disorder
292.9    Phencyclidine-Related Disorder NOS

## SEDATIVE-, HYPNOTIC-, OR ANXIOLYTIC-RELATED DISORDERS

### Sedative, Hypnotic, or Anxiolytic Use Disorders

304.10    Sedative, Hypnotic, or Anxiolytic
          Dependence

| | |
|---|---|
| 305.40 | Sedative, Hypnotic, or Anxiolytic Abuse |

### Sedative-, Hypnotic-, or Anxiolytic-Induced Disorders

| | |
|---|---|
| 292.89 | Sedative, Hypnotic, or Anxiolytic Intoxication |
| 292.0 | Sedative, Hypnotic, or Anxiolytic Withdrawal |
| 292.81 | Sedative, Hypnotic, or Anxiolytic Intoxication Delirium |
| 292.81 | Sedative, Hypnotic, or Anxiolytic Withdrawal Delirium |
| 292.82 | Sedative-, Hypnotic-, or Anxiolytic-Induced Persisting Dementia |
| 292.83 | Sedative-, Hypnotic-, or Anxiolytic-Induced Persisting Amnestic Disorder |
| 292.xx | Sedative-, Hypnotic-, or Anxiolytic-Induced Psychotic Disorder |
| .11 | With Delusions |
| .12 | With Hallucinations |
| 292.84 | Sedative-, Hypnotic-, or Anxiolytic-Induced Mood Disorder |
| 292.89 | Sedative-, Hypnotic-, or Anxiolytic-Induced Anxiety Disorder |
| 292.89 | Sedative-, Hypnotic-, or Anxiolytic-Induced Sexual Dysfunction |
| 292.89 | Sedative-, Hypnotic-, or Anxiolytic-Induced Sleep Disorder |
| 292.9 | Sedative-, Hypnotic-, or Anxiolytic-Related Disorder NOS |

## POLYSUBSTANCE-RELATED DISORDER

| | |
|---|---|
| 304.80 | Polysubstance Dependence |

## OTHER (OR UNKNOWN) SUBSTANCE-RELATED DISORDERS

### Other (or Unknown) Substance Use Disorders

| | |
|---|---|
| 304.90 | Other (or Unknown) Substance Dependence |
| 305.90 | Other (or Unknown) Substance Abuse |

### Other (or Unknown) Substance-Induced Disorders

| | |
|---|---|
| 292.89 | Other (or Unknown) Substance Intoxication |
| 292.0 | Other (or Unknown) Substance Withdrawal |
| 292.81 | Other (or Unknown) Substance-Induced Delirium |
| 292.82 | Other (or Unknown) Substance-Induced Persisting Dementia |
| 292.83 | Other (or Unknown) Substance-Induced Persisting Amnestic Disorder |
| 292.xx | Other (or Unknown) Substance-Induced Psychotic Disorder |
| .11 | With Delusions |
| .12 | With Hallucinations |
| 292.84 | Other (or Unknown) Substance-Induced Mood Disorder |
| 292.89 | Other (or Unknown) Substance-Induced Anxiety Disorder |
| 292.89 | Other (or Unknown) Substance-Induced Sexual Dysfunction |
| 292.89 | Other (or Unknown) Substance-Induced Sleep Disorder |
| 292.9 | Other (or Unknown) Substance-Related Disorder NOS |

## SCHIZOPHRENIA AND OTHER PSYCHOTIC DISORDERS

| | |
|---|---|
| 295.xx | Schizophrenia |
| .30 | Paranoid Type |
| .10 | Disorganized Type |
| .20 | Catatonic Type |
| .90 | Undifferentiated Type |
| .60 | Residual Type |
| 295.40 | Schizophreniform Disorder |
| 295.70 | Schizoaffective Disorder |
| 297.1 | Delusional Disorder |
| 298.8 | Brief Psychotic Disorder |
| 297.3 | Shared Psychotic Disorder |
| 293.xx | Psychotic Disorder Due to . . . |
| .81 | With Delusions |
| .82 | With Hallucinations |
| ___._ | Substance-Induced Psychotic Disorder |
| 298.9 | Psychotic Disorder NOS |

## MOOD DISORDERS

### DEPRESSIVE DISORDERS

| | |
|---|---|
| 296.xx | Major Depressive Disorder |
| .2x | Single Episode |
| .3x | Recurrent |

| 300.4 | Dysthymic Disorder |
|---|---|
| 311 | Depressive Disorder NOS |

## BIPOLAR DISORDERS

| 296.xx | Bipolar I Disorder |
|---|---|
| .0x | Single Manic Episode |
| .40 | Most Recent Episode Hypomanic |
| .4x | Most Recent Episode Manic |
| .6x | Most Recent Episode Mixed |
| .5x | Most Recent Episode Depressed |
| .7 | Most Recent Episode Unspecified |
| 296.89 | Bipolar II Disorder |
| 301.13 | Cyclothymic Disorder |
| 296.80 | Bipolar Disorder NOS |
| 293.83 | Mood Disorder Due to . . . |
| ___._ | Substance-Induced Mood Disorder |
| 296.90 | Mood Disorder NOS |

## ANXIETY DISORDERS

| 300.01 | Panic Disorder Without Agoraphobia |
|---|---|
| 300.21 | Panic Disorder With Agoraphobia |
| 300.22 | Agoraphobia Without History of Panic Disorder |
| 300.29 | Specific Phobia |
| 300.23 | Social Phobia |
| 300.3 | Obsessive-Compulsive Disorder |
| 309.81 | Posttraumatic Stress Disorder |
| 308.3 | Acute Stress Disorder |
| 300.02 | Generalized Anxiety Disorder |
| 293.89 | Anxiety Disorder Due to . . . |
| ___._ | Substance-Induced Anxiety Disorder |
| 300.00 | Anxiety Disorder NOS |

## SOMATOFORM DISORDERS

| 300.81 | Somatization Disorder |
|---|---|
| 300.81 | Undifferentiated Somatoform Disorder |
| 300.11 | Conversion Disorder |
| 307.xx | Pain Disorder |
| .80 | Associated With Psychological Factors |
| .89 | Associated With Both Psychological Factors and a General Medical Condition |
| 300.7 | Hypochondriasis |
| 300.7 | Body Dysmorphic Disorder |
| 300.81 | Somatoform Disorder NOS |

## FACTITIOUS DISORDERS

| 300.xx | Factitious Disorder |
|---|---|
| .16 | With Predominantly Psychological Signs and Symptoms |
| .19 | With Predominantly Physical Signs and Symptoms |
| .19 | With Combined Psychological and Physical Signs and Symptoms |
| 300.19 | Factitious Disorder NOS |

## DISSOCIATIVE DISORDERS

| 300.12 | Dissociative Amnesia |
|---|---|
| 300.13 | Dissociative Fugue |
| 300.14 | Dissociative Identity Disorder |
| 300.6 | Depersonalization Disorder |
| 300.15 | Dissociative Disorder NOS |

## SEXUAL AND GENDER IDENTITY DISORDERS

### SEXUAL DYSFUNCTIONS

#### Sexual Desire Disorders

| 302.71 | Hypoactive Sexual Desire Disorder |
|---|---|
| 302.79 | Sexual Aversion Disorder |

#### Sexual Arousal Disorders

| 302.72 | Female Sexual Arousal Disorder |
|---|---|
| 302.72 | Male Erectile Disorder |

#### Orgasmic Disorders

| 302.73 | Female Orgasmic Disorder |
|---|---|
| 302.74 | Male Orgasmic Disorder |
| 302.75 | Premature Ejaculation |

#### Sexual Pain Disorders

| 302.76 | Dyspareunia (Not Due to a General Medical Condition) |
|---|---|
| 306.51 | Vaginismus (Not Due to a General Medical Condition) |

### SEXUAL DYSFUNCTION DUE TO A GENERAL MEDICAL CONDITION

| 625.8 | Female Hypoactive Sexual Desire Disorder Due to . . . |
|---|---|

| 608.89 | Male Hypoactive Sexual Desire Disorder Due to . . . |
| 607.84 | Male Erectile Disorder Due to . . . |
| 625.0 | Female Dyspareunia Due to . . . |
| 608.89 | Male Dyspareunia Due to . . . |
| 625.8 | Other Female Sexual Dysfunction Due to . . . |
| 608.89 | Other Male Sexual Dysfunction Due to . . . |
| \_\_\_.\_ | Substance-Induced Sexual Dysfunction |
| 302.70 | Sexual Dysfunction NOS |

### *Paraphilias*

| 302.4 | Exhibitionism |
| 302.81 | Fetishism |
| 302.89 | Frotteurism |
| 302.2 | Pedophilia |
| 302.83 | Sexual Masochism |
| 302.84 | Sexual Sadism |
| 302.3 | Transvestic Fetishism |
| 302.82 | Voyeurism |
| 302.9 | Paraphilia NOS |

## GENDER IDENTITY DISORDERS

| 302.xx | Gender Identity Disorder |
| .6 | In Children |
| .85 | In Adolescents or Adults |
| 302.6 | Gender Identity Disorder NOS |
| 302.9 | Sexual Disorder NOS |

## EATING DISORDERS

| 307.1 | Anorexia Nervosa |
| 307.51 | Bulimia Nervosa |
| 307.50 | Eating Disorder NOS |

## SLEEP DISORDERS

## PRIMARY SLEEP DISORDERS

### *Dyssomnias*

| 307.42 | Primary Insomnia |
| 307.44 | Primary Hypersomnia |
| 347 | Narcolepsy |
| 780.59 | Breathing-Related Sleep Disorder |
| 307.45 | Circadian Rhythm Sleep Disorder |
| 307.47 | Dyssomnia NOS |

### *Parasomnias*

| 307.47 | Nightmare Disorder |
| 307.46 | Sleep Terror Disorder |
| 307.46 | Sleepwalking Disorder |
| 307.47 | Parasomnia NOS |

## SLEEP DISORDERS RELATED TO ANOTHER MENTAL DISORDER

| 307.42 | Insomnia Related to . . . |
| 307.44 | Hypersomnia Related to . . . |

## OTHER SLEEP DISORDERS

| 780.xx | Sleep Disorder Due to . . . |
| .52 | Insomnia Type |
| .54 | Hypersomnia Type |
| .59 | Parasomnia Type |
| .59 | Mixed Type |
| \_\_\_.\_ | Substance-Induced Sleep Disorder |

## IMPULSE-CONTROL DISORDERS NOT ELSEWHERE CLASSIFIED

| 312.34 | Intermittent Explosive Disorder |
| 312.32 | Kleptomania |
| 312.33 | Pyromania |
| 312.31 | Pathological Gambling |
| 312.39 | Trichotillomania |
| 312.30 | Impulse-Control Disorder NOS |

## ADJUSTMENT DISORDERS

| 309.xx | Adjustment Disorder |
| .0 | With Depressed Mood |
| .24 | With Anxiety |
| .28 | With Mixed Anxiety and Depressed Mood |
| .3 | With Disturbance of Conduct |
| .4 | With Mixed Disturbance of Emotions and Conduct |
| .9 | Unspecified |

## PERSONALITY DISORDERS

*Note:* These are coded on Axis II.

| 301.0 | Paranoid Personality Disorder |
| 301.20 | Schizoid Personality Disorder |

| | |
|---|---|
| 301.22 | Schizotypal Personality Disorder |
| 301.7 | Antisocial Personality Disorder |
| 301.83 | Borderline Personality Disorder |
| 301.50 | Histrionic Personality Disorder |
| 301.81 | Narcissistic Personality Disorder |
| 301.82 | Avoidant Personality Disorder |
| 301.6 | Dependent Personality Disorder |
| 301.4 | Obsessive-Compulsive Personality Disorder |
| 301.9 | Personality Disorder NOS |

## OTHER CONDITIONS THAT MAY BE A FOCUS OF CLINICAL ATTENTION

### PSYCHOLOGICAL FACTORS AFFECTING MEDICAL CONDITION

| | |
|---|---|
| 316 | ... [Specified Psychological Factor] Affecting ... [Indicate the General Medical Condition] |

Choose name based on nature of factors:

Mental Disorder Affecting Medical Condition

Psychological Symptoms Affecting Medical Condition

Personality Traits or Coping Style Affecting Medical Condition

Maladaptive Health Behaviors Affecting Medical Condition

Stress-Related Physiological Response Affecting Medical Condition

Other or Unspecified Psychological Factors Affecting Medical Condition

### MEDICATION-INDUCED MOVEMENT DISORDERS

| | |
|---|---|
| 332.1 | Neuroleptic-Induced Parkinsonism |
| 333.92 | Neuroleptic-Malignant Syndrome |
| 333.7 | Neuroleptic-Induced Acute Dystonia |
| 333.99 | Neuroleptic-Induced Acute Akathisia |
| 333.82 | Neuroleptic-Induced Tardive Dyskinesia |
| 333.1 | Medication-Induced Postural Tremor |
| 333.90 | Medication-Induced Movement Disorder NOS |

### OTHER MEDICATION-INDUCED DISORDER

| | |
|---|---|
| 995.2 | Adverse Effects of Medication NOS |

### RELATIONAL PROBLEMS

| | |
|---|---|
| V61.9 | Relational Problem Related to a Mental Disorder or General Medical Condition |
| V61.20 | Parent-Child Relational Problem |
| V61.1 | Partner Relational Problem |
| V61.8 | Sibling Relational Problem |
| V62.81 | Relational Problem NOS |

### PROBLEMS RELATED TO ABUSE OR NEGLECT

| | |
|---|---|
| V61.21 | Physical Abuse of Child |
| V61.21 | Sexual Abuse of Child |
| V61.21 | Neglect of Child |
| ___.__ | Physical Abuse of Adult |
| V61.12 | If by Partner |
| V62.83 | If by a Person Other Than Partner |
| ___.__ | Sexual Abuse of Adult |
| V61.12 | If by Partner |
| V62.83 | If by a Person Other Than Partner |

### ADDITIONAL CONDITIONS THAT MAY BE A FOCUS OF CLINICAL ATTENTION

| | |
|---|---|
| V15.81 | Noncompliance With Treatment |
| V65.2 | Malingering |
| V71.01 | Adult Antisocial Behavior |
| V71.02 | Child or Adolescent Antisocial Behavior |
| V62.89 | Borderline Intellectual Functioning |

*Note:* This is coded on Axis II.

| | |
|---|---|
| 780.9 | Age-Related Cognitive Decline |
| V62.82 | Bereavement |
| V62.3 | Academic Problem |
| V62.2 | Occupational Problem |
| 313.82 | Identity Problem |
| V62.89 | Religious or Spiritual Problem |
| V62.4 | Acculturation Problem |
| V62.89 | Phase of Life Problem |

## ADDITIONAL CODES

| | |
|---|---|
| 300.9 | Unspecified Mental Disorder (nonpsychotic) |
| V71.09 | No Diagnosis or Condition on Axis I |
| 799.9 | Diagnosis or Condition Deferred on Axis I |
| V71.09 | No Diagnosis on Axis II |
| 799.9 | Diagnosis Deferred on Axis II |

## MULTIAXIAL SYSTEM

Axis I   Clinical Disorders
         Other Conditions That May Be a
         Focus of Clinical Attention
Axis II  Personality Disorders (see above)
         Mental Retardation (see p. 680)
Axis III General Medical Conditions
Axis IV  Psychosocial and Environmental
         Problems
Axis V   Global Assessment of Functioning

## AXIS III: GENERAL MEDICAL CONDITIONS (WITH ICD-9-CM CODES)

Infectious and Parasitic Diseases (001-139)
Neoplasms (140-239)
Endocrine, Nutritional, and Metabolic Diseases and Immunity Disorders (240-279)
Diseases of the Blood and Blood-Forming Organs (280-289)
Diseases of the Nervous System and Sense Organs (320-389)
Diseases of the Circulatory System (390-459)
Diseases of the Respiratory System (460-519)
Diseases of the Digestive System (520-579)
Diseases of the Genitourinary System (580-629)
Complications of Pregnancy, Childbirth, and the Puerperium (630-676)
Diseases of the Skin and Subcutaneous Tissue (680-709)
Diseases of the Musculoskeletal System and Connective Tissue (710-739)
Congenital Anomalies (740-759)
Certain Conditions Originating in the Perinatal Period (760-779)
Symptoms, Signs, and Ill-Defined Conditions (780-799)
Injury and Poisoning (800-999)

## AXIS IV: PSYCHOSOCIAL AND ENVIRONMENTAL PROBLEMS

Problems with primary support group
Problems related to the social environment
Educational problems
Occupational problems
Housing problems
Economic problems
Problems with access to health care services
Problems related to interaction with the legal system/crime
Other psychosocial and environmental problems

## AXIS V: GLOBAL ASSESSMENT OF FUNCTIONING (GAF) SCALE

Consider psychological, social, and occupational functioning on a hypothetical continuum of mental health–illness. Do not include impairment in functioning due to physical (or environmental) limitations.

| Code | |
|---|---|
| | *Note:* Use intermediate codes when appropriate (e.g., 45, 68, 72). |
| 100<br><br>91 | Superior functioning in a wide range of activities, life's problems never seem to get out of hand, is sought out by others because of his or her many positive qualities. No symptoms. |
| 90<br><br><br><br><br><br>81 | Absent or minimal symptoms (e.g., mild anxiety before an exam), good functioning in all areas, interested and involved in a wide range of activities, socially effective, generally satisfied with life, no more than everyday problems or concerns (e.g., an occasional argument with family members). |
| 80<br><br><br><br><br>71 | If symptoms are present, they are transient and expectable reactions to psychosocial stressors (e.g., difficulty concentrating after family argument); no more than slight impairment in social, occupational, or school functioning (e.g., temporarily falling behind in schoolwork). |
| 70<br><br><br><br><br>61 | Some mild symptoms (e.g., depressed mood and mild insomnia) OR some difficulty in social, occupational, or school functioning (e.g., occasional truancy or theft within the household), but generally functioning pretty well, has some meaningful interpersonal relationships. |

60 | Moderate symptoms (e.g., flat affect and circumstantial speech, occasional panic attacks) OR moderate difficulty in social, occupational, or school functioning (e.g., few friends, conflicts with peers or

51 | co-workers).

50 | Serious symptoms (e.g., suicidal ideation, severe obsessional rituals, frequent shop-lifting) OR any serious impairment in social, occupational, or school function-ing (e.g., no friends, unable to keep a

41 | job).

40 | Some impairment in reality testing or communication (e.g., speech is at times illogical, obscure, or irrelevant) OR major impairment in several areas, such as work or school, family relations, judgment, thinking, or mood (e.g., depressed man avoids friends, neglects family, and is unable to work; child frequently beats up younger children, is defiant at home, and

31 | is failing at school).

30 | Behavior is considerably influenced by delusions or hallucinations OR serious impairment in communication or judg-ment (e.g., sometimes incoherent, acts grossly inappropriately, suicidal preoccu-pation) OR inability to function in almost all areas (e.g., stays in bed all day; no job,

21 | home, or friends).

20 | Some danger of hurting self or others (e.g., suicide attempts without clear expectation of death; frequently violent; manic excite-ment) OR occasionally fails to maintain minimal personal hygiene (e.g., smears feces) OR gross impairment in communi-

11 | cation (e.g., largely incoherent or mute).

10 | Persistent danger of severely hurting self or others (e.g., recurrent violence) OR persistent inability to maintain minimal personal hygiene OR serious suicidal act

1 | with clear expectation of death.

0 | Inadequate information.

# Glossary

**absence seizure** A type of generalized seizure in which there is an abrupt loss of consciousness (usually lasting less than 10 seconds); these seizures are nonconvulsive in nature and might not be noticed by others.

**abstinence syndrome** Physical signs and symptoms that occur when the addictive substance is reduced or withheld; also referred to as *withdrawal*.

**abstract thinking** The ability to find meaning in proverbs; the ability to conceptualize.

**abuse** Excessive use of a substance that differs from societal norms and causes clinically significant impairment.

**acceptance** The allowance of respect of individuality.

**acetylcholine (ACh)** A neurotransmitter synthesized by choline acetyltransferase from acetyl coenzyme A and choline. It is found in the peripheral nervous system at the myoneural junction, in the autonomic ganglia for parasympathetic or sympathetic systems, and in the parasympathetic postganglionic synapses, including cranial nerves (CNs) III, VII, IX, and X. Acetylcholine is found in the spinal cord, basal ganglia, and numerous sites within the cerebral cortex. Cortical acetylcholine is synthesized primarily in the nucleus basalis of Meynert and in the septal area near the hypothalamus.

**acrophobia** Dread of high places.

**active listening** Verbal and nonverbal skills used by the examiner to demonstrate interest and concern to the patient.

**acupressure** Use of pressure to restore balance by stimulating meridians.

**acupuncture** Ancient Chinese health practice that involves puncturing the skin with hair-thin needles at particular locations on the patient's body called *acupuncture points*. Acupuncture is believed to help reduce pain or change a body function. Sometimes, the needles are twirled, giving a slight electric charge.

**acute stress disorder** The development of characteristic anxiety, dissociative, and other symptoms that occur within 1 month after exposure to an extreme traumatic stressor.

**addiction** Psychological and physiologic symptoms indicating that an individual cannot control his or her use of psychoactive substances; termed *substance dependence* in the *DSM-IV-TR*.

**advocacy** Negotiating with others to develop, improve, and provide services for a patient.

**affect** Emotional range attached to ideas; outwardly demonstrated; feeling, mood, or emotional tone.

   **appropriate a.** Emotional tone in harmony with the accompanying idea, thought, or verbalization.

   **blunted a.** Disturbance manifested by a severe reduction in the intensity of affect.

   **flat a.** Absence or near-absence of any signs of affective expression.

   **inappropriate a.** Incongruence between the emotional feeling tone and the idea, thought, or speech accompanying it.

   **labile a.** Rapid changes in emotional feeling tone, unrelated to external stimuli.

**affective disorders** Group of psychiatric diagnoses characterized by mood disturbances on a continuum of depression to mania; termed *mood disorders* in the *DSM-IV-TR*.

**aggression** Forceful verbal or physical action—that is, the motor counterpart of the affect of anger, rage, or hostility.

**agitation** Anxiety associated with severe motor restlessness.

**agnosia** Difficulty in recognizing familiar objects; a symptom of organic brain disease.

**agnostic** One who is uncertain about whether there is a god (Greek *a,* no; *gnosis,* knowledge).

**agonist** In pharmacology, a substance that acts with, enhances, or potentiates a specific receptor type.

**agoraphobia** Fear of being in a place or situation in which escape might be difficult or embarrassing, or in which help might not be available in case of a panic attack.

**agranulocytosis** A significant drop in white blood cell count, which can have serious or lethal consequences. Clozapine can cause agranulocytosis.

**agraphia** Loss of the ability to write.

**AIDS dementia complex** A dementia attributed to HIV infection.

**akathisia** Motor restlessness, generally expressed as the inability to sit still, caused by the dopamine blockade by certain types of neuroleptic medications; an extrapyramidal side effect (EPSE).

**alcoholic** Individual whose compulsive use of alcohol causes problems at home, at work, or socially and who continues to use alcohol despite these adverse consequences.

**Alcoholics Anonymous (AA)** Self-help organization that uses a 12-step program to assist alcoholics to achieve and maintain sobriety; Al-Anon assists the spouses of alcoholics; Alateen assists the teenage children of alcoholics.

**alertness** Awareness and attentiveness to surroundings.

**alternative therapy** Broad range of healing philosophies and approaches that mainstream Western medicine does not commonly use, accept, study, understand, or make available.

**Alzheimer's disease** More correctly referred to as *dementia of the Alzheimer type* (DAT). DAT is the most common type of dementia. The characteristic symptoms are amnesia, aphasia, apraxia, and agnosia. It is a cognitive mental disorder resulting in dementia that is related to a progressive deterioration of brain tissue, described as plaques and neurofibrillary tangles.

**ambivalence** Opposing impulses or feelings directed toward the same person or object at the same time.

**amenorrhea** Absence of menstruation.

**amnesia** Partial or total inability to recall past information.

   **anterograde a.** Recent memory loss, as in the early stages of Alzheimer's disease.

   **global a.** Total memory loss, as in advanced stages of Alzheimer's disease.

   **retrograde a.** Remote memory loss, as in later stages of Alzheimer's disease.

   **short-term a.** Memory loss observed in alcoholic blackouts.

**amygdala** Cluster of nuclei in the medial temporal lobe involved with endocrine and behavioral functions and that plays a role in food and water intake, drive behavior, and emotions connected with those behaviors. In animal studies, electrical stimulation of the amygdala causes defensiveness, rage, and/or aggression.

**analytic worldview** Perception of the world that values detail to time, individuality, and possessions.

**anergia** Absence of energy caused by changes in brain chemistry, anatomy, or both.

**anger** Normal emotional response to the perception of a frustration of desires or threat to one's needs.

**anhedonia** Loss of pleasure in activities or interests previously enjoyed; a symptom noted in depression and schizophrenia.

**anorexia nervosa** Disorder characterized by a refusal to eat for a long period, resulting in emaciation, amenorrhea, disturbance in body image, and intense fear of becoming obese.

**Antabuse (disulfiram)** Drug given to alcoholics that blocks the breakdown of acetylaldehyde, producing nausea, vomiting, dizziness, flushing, and tachycardia if alcohol is consumed.

**antagonist** In pharmacology, a substance that blocks a receptor.

**anterior commissure** White matter tract that connects the olfactory structures bilaterally, as well as the temporal lobes and the amygdala.

**anticholinergic effect** Effect caused by drugs that block acetylcholine receptors. Common anticholinergic effects include dry mouth, blurred vision, constipation, and urinary hesitancy.

**antisocial personality** Personality disorder characterized by blatant disregard for social norms. Behavior is demonstrated on a continuum of mild to pathologic. Psychoanalytic theory attributes this disorder to an underdeveloped superego.

**anxiety** Nonspecific, unpleasant feeling of discomfort, with physiologic and psychological symptoms that generally result from a perception of a threat to safety and security.

**anxiety disorders** Patterns of symptoms and behaviors in which anxiety is either the primary disturbance or a secondary problem that is recognized when the primary symptoms are removed.

**anxiolytic** Antianxiety drug.

**apathy** Lack of feeling, interest, or emotion; indifference that is occasionally a mechanism for avoiding intense emotion.

**aphasia** Difficulty in searching for words.

**motor a.** Impaired speech as a result of an organic brain disorder in which understanding remains.

**nominal a.** Difficulty in finding the correct words in their appropriate sequence.

**sensory a.** Loss of ability to comprehend the meaning of words.

**appropriate** Suitable or fitting for a particular person, purpose, occasion, or situation, such as appropriate affect, response, or attire.

**apraxia** Inability to perform once known, purposeful, skilled activities in the absence of loss of motor function.

**assault** Legally, any behavior that physically or verbally presents an immediate threat of physical injury to another individual.

**assertiveness** Direct expression of feelings and needs in a way that respects the rights of others and self.

**asylum** (1) Place of safety or sanctuary; a refuge; (2) institution for the care of the mentally ill; often associated with mistreatment and callousness.

**atheist** One who believes that there is no deity (Greek *a*, no; *theos*, God)

**attention-deficit/hyperactivity disorder (ADHD)** Relatively common disorder of childhood onset characterized by inattention, impulsiveness, and overactivity.

**attitude** Pattern of mental views and feelings accumulated through past experiences and affected by present stimuli; a manner, disposition, tendency, or orientation with regard to a person or situation.

**atypical depression** Subtype of depression occurring more often in younger individuals; expressed by atypical symptoms—for example, increased appetite, weight gain, hypersomnia.

**autism** (1) Preoccupation with self without concern for external reality; a self-made private world of the individual with schizophrenia; (2) a disorder of markedly abnormal or impaired development in social interactions and communication occurring in early childhood.

**autistic thinking** Thoughts, ideas, or desires derived from internal, private stimuli or drives that are often incongruent with reality.

**autonomic nervous system** Division of the peripheral nervous system that is involuntary and innervates the viscera, heart, blood vessels, smooth muscle, and glands. It is divided into the parasympathetic (craniosacral) and sympathetic (thoracolumbar) systems.

**avolition** Lack of motivation.

**axon** Long process from the neuronal cell body that transmits impulses away from the cell.

**balance** Process by which patients are helped to achieve independence while conforming to norms.

**basal ganglia** Large nuclei, including the caudate nucleus, putamen, and globus pallidus, which are responsible for modulating voluntary movement.

**battery** Touching of the person of another, of his or her clothes, or anything else attached to his or her person without consent.

**behavior** Any observable, recordable, and measurable movement, response, or act of an individual (verbal and nonverbal).

**behavior therapy** Therapeutic approach that helps the patient modify behavior by modifying or changing old patterns of behavior.

**binge** Eating an unusually large amount of food in a relatively short period.

**binge eating** Disorder in which bingeing occurs without purging. Victims are generally overweight, because they do not purge.

**biofeedback** The use of a machine to communicate physical changes; used to train a person to reduce anxiety and modify behavioral responses.

**biologic variations** Physical differences between individuals or differences in body structure, skin color, other visible characteristics, enzymatic and genetic variations, electrocardiographic patterns, susceptibility to disease, nutritional preferences and deficiencies, and psychological characteristics.

**bipolar disorder** Affective or mood disorder characterized by at least one episode of mania, with or without a history of depression.

**biracial** Individual who crosses two racial and cultural groups.

**bizarre** Markedly unusual in appearance, thought, style, character, or behavior; absurd.

**blackout** Period in which the drinker functions socially but for which the drinker has no memory.

**blocking** Unconscious interruption in train of thought.

**blood-brain barrier** Guards the brain from fluctuations in body chemistry; regulates the amount and speed with which substances in the blood enter the brain.

**borderline personality disorder** Disorder with the essential feature of a pervasive pattern of unstable self-image, interpersonal relations, and mood.

**bradykinesia** Slow or retarded movement.

**brainstem** Vital structure that carries all information to and from the cerebral cortex and spinal cord. Because the brainstem is also responsible for respiration, its function is essential for life. It consists of the midbrain, pons, and medulla.

**bulimia** Compulsive binge eating accompanied by purging and an overconcern with body shape and weight. It is characterized by an insatiable craving for food, resulting in episodes of continuous eating and often followed by purging, depression, and self-deprivation.

**bulimia nervosa** Disorder characterized by binge eating, compensatory behavior, and over-concern with body shape and weight.

**bureaucracy** Excessive rules and structure that get in the way of efficient, responsive, and creative nursing care solutions.

**burnout** Spiraling process of decreased effectiveness.

**case management** Collaborative process for meeting health needs through the use of a variety of services in a cost-effective manner.

**catalepsy** State of unconsciousness in which immobility is constantly maintained.

**catatonia** Immobility as a result of psychological causes.

**catatonic behavior** Motor anomalies in nonorganic disorders, such as schizophrenia.

**catecholamines** Derived from the amino acid tyrosine, these substances include dopamine, norepinephrine, and epinephrine. Catecholamines are a subcategory of the monoamines, which also include serotonin and histamine. Catecholamines and their synthesis products are widely distributed in the central and peripheral nervous systems.

**caudate** Basal ganglia nucleus that protrudes into the anterior horn of the lateral ventricle.

**cerebral cortex** Narrow ribbon of gray matter that lies on the surface of the cerebrum. The gray matter lies on top of the white matter. The reverse is true in the spinal cord.

**child abuse** Harmful physical, emotional, sexual, and/or verbal behavior inflicted on a child.

**cholinergics** Substances that stimulate the cholinergic system. In the peripheral nervous system, cholinergic drugs constrict the pupil, increase the production of saliva and respiratory secretions, slow the heart, and increase gastrointestinal peristalsis and urinary output.

**chorea** Greek term for dance. The choreas are demonstrated as hyperkinetic disorders characterized by involuntary, unpredictable, and random movements of the trunk, head, face, and limbs.

**chromosome** The self-replicating genetic structure of cells containing the cellular DNA that bears in its nucleotide sequence the linear array of genes. Eukaryotic genomes (such as humans have) consist of a number of chromosomes whose DNA is associated with different types of proteins.

**circumstantiality** Digression of inappropriate thoughts into ideas, eventually reaching the desired goal.

**cirrhosis** Disease of the liver; characterized by the development of scar tissue in the liver. The person most likely to develop cirrhosis is a middle-aged man with chronic alcoholism.

**civil law** The part of the legal system concerned with the legal rights and duties of private persons. Civil lawsuits can recapture monetary loss from professionals who have been guilty of false imprisonment, defamation of character, assault and battery, or negligence.

**clang associations** Words similar in sound, but not in meaning, that conjure up new thoughts.

**clarification** Communication skill that helps define a patient's responses through the use of direct questions.

**claustrophobia** Dread of closed places.

**clinical depression** Another term for major depressive disorder that defines the disturbance of a person's mood according to *DSM-IV-TR* criteria.

**clinical supervision** Formal meeting among psychiatric nursing peers whose purpose is to provide a place for nurses caring for patients to examine attitudes, reactions, and conflicts with patients on the unit and to find new ways of approaching patient problems.

**clonic** State in which rigidity and relaxation succeed each other.

**closed-ended questions** Questions that generally elicit a "yes" or "no" response. Useful in gathering factual data.

**clouding of consciousness** Incomplete clarity of mind, with disturbance in perception and attitude (e.g., stupor).

**codependency** Stress-related preoccupation with an addicted person's life, leading to extreme dependence on that person.

**cognition** Act or process of knowing and perceiving.

**cognitive disorders** Those disorders that affect consciousness, memory, and other cognitive processes.

**cognitive dissonance** A state that arises when two posing beliefs exist at the same time.

**cognitive processes** Processes that pertain to perception, judgment, memory, and reasoning.

**coma** State of depressed consciousness wherein even extreme stimulation of the reticular activating system will not cause a response.

**command hallucinations** Hallucinations that tell the patient to take some specific action, such as to kill himself or herself or someone else.

**common law/case law** The term *common law* is applied to the body of principles that has evolved and continues to evolve and expand from judicial decisions that arise during the trial of actual court cases; law based on the outcome of cases.

**communication** Process that is the matrix for thought and relationships among all people, regardless of cultural heritage.

**community meeting** Meeting that is held in the therapeutic milieu and in which joint problem solving by community members is encouraged.

**community mental health** Application of the principles of psychiatric care to communities and groups of people. The goal of this effort is to maintain health, prevent mental illness when possible and, if treatment is indicated, treat the individual closer to his or her support systems.

**Community Mental Health Centers Act** 1963 legislation authorizing federal funds for the construction of comprehensive mental health centers.

**community worldview** Community needs and concerns are more important than individual ones. Quiet, respectful communication is valued, as well as meditation and reading as a learning style.

**comorbidity** Simultaneous existence of medical and psychiatric problems, each complicating the other.

**complementary therapy** Same as alternative therapy, but denotes therapy used as an adjunct to rather than as a replacement for conventional treatment.

**complex partial seizure** Formerly referred to as *temporal lobe* or *psychomotor seizure;* this seizure typically begins with a clouding of consciousness followed by some meaningless movement such as lip smacking or hand clapping; brief periods of forgetfulness are common.

**comprehension** Capacity to perceive and understand.

**compulsion** Uncontrollable impulse to perform an act or ritual repeatedly; might be in response to an obsession (unwilled, persistent thought), as in obsessive-compulsive disorder. The act or ritual serves to decrease anxiety. Examples of rituals include hand washing, cleaning, and checking (e.g., checking to see whether door is locked).

**concrete communication** Inability to think and communicate abstractly.

**concrete thinking** Use of literal meaning without ability to consider abstract meaning (e.g., "don't cry over spilt milk" might be interpreted as meaning, "Okay, I'll cry over the sink.")

**confabulation** Unconscious filling of gaps in memory with imagined or untrue experiences that the person believes but have no basis in reality.

**confidentiality** Treating the information about and from patients in a private manner; information about patients is confidential and requires patient approval before disclosure.

**conflict** Differing perspectives among staff or patients regarding various aspects of treatment.

**confused state** Bewildered, perplexed, or unclear. The type and degree of confusion should be specified.

**congruence** Accordant states. Example includes mood congruence, in which the person's visible emotional state correlates with his or her mood or feeling state.

**consciousness** State of awareness.

**conservator** Guardian; a legally appointed person who controls the affairs of a gravely disabled person, including the right to consent to or refuse psychiatric treatment.

**consultant-liaison nurse** Psychiatric mental health nurse who provides expert consultation for patients and staff in other parts of the hospital agency.

**consumer** Patient in treatment for psychiatric services.

**continuum of care** Levels of care through which an individual can move depending on his or her needs at a given point in time.

**contralateral** Opposite side of the body.

**conversion** Process by which a psychological event, an idea, a memory, or an impulse is represented by a bodily change or symptom, such as blindness or paralysis.

**coping mechanism** Any effort directed at stress management.

**corporate compliance** Health care provider's respon-sibility to comply with governmental laws and regulations.

**corpus callosum** Major connecting and communicating pathway between the hemispheres.

**cortisol** Glucocorticoid hormone found in the adrenal cortex that is involved in carbohydrate and protein metabolism. Cortisol hypersecretion occurs in many depressed individuals. Excretion of this hormone is not suppressed in many persons with major depression after an injection of dexamethasone.

**creed** Set formula that states the religious and spiritual beliefs of a community of faith (Latin, *credo,* I trust, believe).

**criminal law** Part of the legal system concerned with crime that is defined in state and federal statutes.

**crisis** A 4- to 6-week period of severe emotional disorganization following a major stressful event (e.g., divorce, job loss) as a result of the failure of coping mechanisms, lack of support, or both.

**cultural awareness** Process whereby the nurse acknowledges his or her cultural biases and recognizes that other individuals, groups, or communities have their unique cultural similarities and differences.

**cultural competence** Process whereby the nurse has developed cultural awareness, knowledge, and skills to promote effective and quality health care for patients.

**cultural diversity** Variety of cultural groupings; might include age, gender, socioeconomic status, religion, race, and ethnicity.

**cultural negotiation** Nurse's ability to work with a patient's cultural belief system to develop culturally appropriate interventions.

**cultural preservation** Nurse's ability to acknowledge, value, and accept a patient's cultural beliefs.

**cultural repatterning** Nurse's ability to incorporate cultural preservation and negotiation to identify patient needs, develop expected outcomes, and evaluate outcome plans.

**cultural values** Unique, individual expressions of beliefs related to culture that have been accepted as appropriate over time for persons in that culture.

**culturally diverse nursing care** Modification of nursing approaches to provide culturally competent care.

**culture** The internal and external manifestation of an individual's, group's, or community's beliefs, values, and norms that are used as premises for daily life and functioning.

**cupping** Alternative cultural or medical treatment that uses a small glass or cup to conduct the moxibustion treatment.

**custodial care** Process of caring for hygienic and nutritional needs in an institution, but not providing treatment for a mental disorder.

**cyclothymia** Chronic mood disturbance of at least 2 years' duration involving numerous hypomanic episodes and numerous periods of depression. It does not meet the criteria for a manic episode or major depression.

**deinstitutionalization** Shift in treatment location from large public hospitals to community settings.

**delirium** Disorder with alterations in consciousness and changes in cognition, usually caused by a general medical condition or is substance-induced. Typically, delirium develops over a short period and is treatable. It is (usually) a reversible bewildered state of clouded consciousness, generally accompanied by restlessness, disorientation, and fear. It might include periods of hallucinations.

**delusion** Fixed, false belief, not consistent with the person's intelligence and culture; unamenable to reason.

  **bizarre d.** Absurd belief.

  **nihilistic d.** False belief that the self, part of the self, or another object has ceased to exist.

  **paranoid d.** Oversuspiciousness leading to persecutory delusions.

  **persecution d.** False belief that one is being persecuted.

  **reference d.** False belief that the behavior of others in the environment refers to oneself; derived from ideas of reference in which one wrongly believes that he or she is being talked about.

  **somatic d.** False belief involving functioning of one's body.

**dementia** Disorder that causes pronounced memory and cognitive disturbances. Typically, dementias are gradual in onset and progressive in course.

**dendrites** Many projections from the neuron that transmit impulses to the cell body.

**denial** Avoidance of disagreeable realities or threats by ignoring or refusing to recognize them; an unconscious defense mechanism that might or might not be adaptive.

**deoxyribonucleic acid (DNA)** Molecule, primarily located in the nucleus of the cell, that encodes genetic information.

**dependence** State in which a drug user must take a usual or an increasing dose of a drug to prevent the onset of abstinence symptoms, withdrawal, or both.

**depersonalization** Feeling of unreality or strangeness related to one's self, body parts, bodily functions, or external environment.

**depression** Lowered or saddened mood state or major affective disorder, listed as a mood disorder in the *DSM-IV-TR.*

**derailment** Gradual or sudden deviation in train of thought, without blocking.

**derealization** Distortion of spatial relationships so that the environment becomes unfamiliar.

**devaluation** Criticism of others that defends against one's own feelings of inadequacy.

**dexamethasone suppression test (DST)** Diagnostic test for clinical depression that measures the function of the hypothalamic-pituitary axis (HPA).

**diencephalon** Posterior part of the forebrain; includes the thalamus, hypothalamus, epithalamus, and metathalamus.

**disinhibition** State in which a person is unable to suppress urges or statements that might be socially unacceptable (e.g., telling a dirty joke in an inappropriate situation).

**disoriented** Disturbance in orientation of time, place, or person.

**displacement** Shift of emotion from an object or a person who incites the emotion to a less threatening source; an unconscious defense mechanism that might or might not be adaptive.

**dissociation** (1) Removal from conscious awareness of painful feelings, memories, thoughts, or aspects of identity; (2) separation of mental or behavioral processes from the rest of the person's consciousness or identity; (3) splitting or separation of any group of mental or behavioral processes from the rest of the person's consciousness or identity.

**dissociative reaction** Process by which an individual blocks off part of his or her life from conscious recognition because of severe anxiety.

**distractibility** Inability to concentrate attention.

**dopamine** Brain neurotransmitter that influences muscle movement and emotions. The dopamine theory states that individuals with schizophrenia might have too much dopamine, which might account for their sensoriperceptual alterations. Research has refined this theory.

**double bind** Conflicting demands by significant individuals in a person's life. The person cannot meet both demands, so he or she is doomed to failure.

**dysarthria** Difficulty in articulating.

**dyskinesia** Disturbed coordination and motor activity, usually producing a jerky motion; an EPSE of neuroleptic medications related to their effect on dopamine receptors. (See also tardive dyskinesia.)

**dyslexia** Difficulty in reading.

**dysphagia** Difficulty in swallowing.

**dysphoria** Disorder of affect characterized by depression, malaise, and anguish; unpleasant mood state.

**dysthymia** Chronic mood disturbance involving a depressed mood for at least 2 years, more days than not.

**dystonia** Rigidity in muscles that control posture, gait, or ocular movement; an EPSE of neuroleptic medications that block dopamine.

**echolalia** Psychopathologic repeating of words of one person by another; noted in types of schizophrenia.

**echopraxia** Imitation of the body position of another.

**ecologic worldview** Perception of the world based on the belief that there is interconnectedness between a person and the earth, and that people have a responsibility to take care of the earth.

**ego** Personality process that focuses on reality, while striving to meet the needs of the id. The ego experiences anxiety and uses defense mechanisms for protection.

**electroconvulsive therapy (ECT)** Form of somatic therapy that uses electrically induced seizures to relieve a person's intractable depressive symptoms.

**emaciated** Made excessively thin by lack of nutrition.

**emotion** Complex feeling state with psychological, somatic, and behavioral components related to affect and mood.

**empathy** Objective understanding of how patients feel or how they see their situations.

**enkephalins** Widely distributed opioid-like neuropeptides that are part of the endorphin family. These substances mediate pain perception, taste, olfaction, arousal, emotional behavior, vision, hearing, neurohormone secretion, motor coordination, and water balance.

**environmental control** Ability of an individual to control nature by planning activities and tasks to assist in maintaining optimal balance in life.

**epidemiology** Study of the frequency and distribution of disease conditions in the population.

**epilepsy** Disorder of the central nervous system (CNS) in which the major symptom is a seizure. The seizure is caused by a temporary disturbance of brain impulses.

**ethnicity** Characteristic of a group whose members share a common social and cultural heritage passed on to each successive generation.

**ethnocentrism** Acknowledging and valuing only one's own culture.

**ethnopharmacology** Study of pharmacogenetic, pharmacodynamic, and pharmacokinetic influences based on different ethnic, racial, and cultural groups.

**etiology** Study of the causes of diseases, including both direct and predisposing causes.

**euphoria** False sense of elation or well-being; pathologic elevation of mood; complete lack of tension. It is most notable in the manic phase of bipolar disorder.

**euthymia** Normal, homeostatic mood state.

**excitement** Excited motor activity.

**existentialism** Philosophy that emphasizes the individual's ability and responsibility to make one's existence meaningful by making choices in the face of life's deep pain and uncertainty.

**expansive mood** Unrestrained expression of feelings.

**extrapyramidal side effects (EPSEs)** Involuntary muscle movements resulting from the effects of neuroleptic drugs on the extrapyramidal system. These drugs cause a dopamine blockade that creates a dopamine-acetylcholine (Ach) imbalance. EPSEs include akathisia, akinesia, dystonia, drug-induced parkinsonism, and neuroleptic malignant syndrome (NMS).

**extrapyramidal system** Outside the pyramidal (voluntary) tract; coordinates involuntary movements.

**eye contact** Occasional glancing into a person's eyes to demonstrate interest during an interaction.

**faith** Traditionally, the creed that one follows within one's religious community, but the term can be used more broadly to describe one's total life view, religiously based or not.

**family system** Field of influence exerted on one another by family members because of their complex interaction.

**fantasy** Imaginary sequence of events, common in childhood; appropriate as long as the person is aware of reality.

**fear** Anxiety as a result of consciously recognized and realistic danger.

**feedback** Articulation of one's perception of what another person has said or meant. This process requires at least two people.

**flashbacks** Cognitive, emotional, and physical reexperiencing of traumatic events.

**flight of ideas** Speech pattern demonstrated by a rapid transition from topic to topic, frequently without completing any of the preceding ideas; prominent in manic states.

**free association** In a therapeutic context, saying anything that comes to mind.

**fugue** Period of personality dissociation with memory loss.

**gait** Manner of progression in walking. For example, in an ataxic gait, the foot is raised high and the sole strikes down suddenly.

**gamma-aminobutyric acid (GABA)** Inhibitory amino acid neurotransmitter formed during the citric acid cycle from its precursor, glutamic acid. GABA receptors are widely distributed in the CNS and produce neuronal hyperpolarization through an influx of chloride ions. Drugs that increase the GABA level reduce anxiety and seizures.

**gender identity disorder** A profound discomfort with one's own gender and a strong and persistent identification with the opposite gender.

**genes** The fundamental physical and functional units of heredity. A gene is located in a sequence of nucleotides located in a particular position on a particular chromosome. There are about 30,000 different human genes.

**general leads** Interactive skills that facilitate the communication process by encouraging the patient to continue.

**generalized seizure** Involves both hemispheres of the brain at the onset of the seizure. Consciousness is usually impaired.

**genetic vulnerability** (1) Tendency to inherent traits, behaviors, and biologic characteristics of

one's ancestors; (2) inherited liability that increases the risk of exhibiting a psychiatric disorder.

**global memory loss** Total memory loss, as in advanced stages of Alzheimer's disease.

**globus pallidus** Gray matter structure located medial to the putamen. This portion of the basal ganglia is smaller and triangular in shape. It is subdivided into the globus pallidus externa and globus pallidus interna.

**glutamate** Major excitatory transmitter in the CNS with receptors throughout the brain. Glutamate stimulation of $N$-methyl-D-aspartate (NMDA)−activated channels permits excessive inflow of calcium ions and production of free radicals, which might cause neuronal death.

**grand mal seizure** Type of generalized seizure in which there is loss of consciousness and convulsions. This type of seizure is most frequently associated with epilepsy by laypersons.

**gravely disabled** Person who is unable to provide food, clothing, or shelter for himself or herself because of a mental illness.

**gray matter** Composed of the cell bodies and dendrites of neurons.

**grimacing** Contortion of facial muscles; might be an EPSE.

**gyri** Convolutions of gray matter on the cerebrum.

**half-life** The amount of time it takes the body to metabolize and excrete a drug. Half-lives can range from minutes to weeks.

**hallucination** False sensory perceptions not associated with real external stimuli; might involve any of the five senses: auditory, visual, olfactory, gustatory, or tactile.

> **auditory h.** Most prevalent in schizophrenia. The sounds might be perceived as thoughts or voices coming from any type of transmitter or from the patient's mind. The messages might be condemning or accusatory, or complimentary and encouraging. It is critical that the examiner be aware that the messages might be directing the patient toward harming self or others, so the message content cannot be ignored.

> **tactile h.** Common in alcohol withdrawal. Hallucinations might also be an effect of certain types of drugs, such as amphetamines, hallucinogens, and cannabis.

> **visual h.** Often associated with organic conditions.

**hebephrenia** Outdated schizophrenic subtype characterized by silliness, delusions, hallucinations, and regression.

**herbaceutical** Plant or plant part that produces and contains chemical substances that act on the body.

**here and now focus** Assisting patients to understand how their current behaviors influence daily living.

**highly active antiretroviral therapy (HAART)** Drug therapy in which three antiretroviral medications are used in combination to reduce the replication of HIV.

**HIV antibody** Antibody specific to HIV; usually appears within 6 weeks after HIV infection.

**holistic** Pertaining to totality or the whole (holistic care).

**homeless** Without a home. Homeless individuals, including whole families, might live on the street exclusively or might make use of community shelters, halfway houses, cheap hotels, or board-and-care homes.

**homeopathy** Unconventional Western medicine system based on the principle that "like cures like" (i.e., that the same substance in large doses produces the symptoms of an illness, and in very minute doses cures it). Homeopathic physicians believe that the more dilute the remedy, the greater its potency. Therefore, homeopathic practitioners use small doses of specially prepared plant extracts and minerals to stimulate the body's defense mechanisms and healing processes to treat illness.

**hostile** Feeling intense anger and resentment, exhibited by destructive behavior.

**hot or cold treatments** Cultural-medical approaches to maintaining or returning a person to a state of wellness. These approaches do not refer to the temperature of a treatment but to the fact that a specific, defined approach is appropriate for each state of wellness or illness.

**human immunodeficiency infection** Spectrum of illness caused by HIV that ranges from acutely or chronically HIV-infected adults to infants in the neonatal period.

**human immunodeficiency virus (HIV)** Virus that has been isolated and recognized as the causative agent of acquired immunodeficiency syndrome (AIDS). HIV is classified as a lentivirus in a subgroup of the retroviruses.

**human immunodeficiency virus, type 1 (HIV-1)** Retrovirus identified as the cause of AIDS.

**humanist** Individual who emphasizes people rather than other parts of the observable world or religion.

**Huntington's disease** Genetically transmitted disease that includes motor and cognitive changes.

**hydrotherapy** Use of water (wet sheet packs, 2- to 10-hour baths) for psychotherapeutic purposes.

**hyperactivity (hyperkinesis)** Restless, aggressive, often destructive activity; prominent in manic states.

**hypersomnia** Increased and prolonged sleeping.

**hypoactivity (hypokinesis)** Decreased activity or retardation (psychomotor retardation); slowing of psychological and physical functions.

**hypomania** Clinical syndrome similar to but less severe than that demonstrated in a full-blown manic episode.

**hypothalamus** Group of nuclei in the diencephalon that influences eating behavior, temperature regulation, emotional expression, and autonomic system. Dopaminergic neurons in the hypothalamus control lactation.

**id** Personality process that wants to experience only pleasure; is impulsive and without morals.

**idealization** Viewing others as perfect; exalting others.

**ideas of reference** Belief that some events have a special meaning (e.g., people laughing are perceived as laughing at the patient).

**idiopathic** Without known cause.

**illogical (thinking)** Contains erroneous conclusions or internal contradictions (irrational thoughts).

**illusion** Misinterpretation of a sensory input; observed in alcoholic withdrawal and delirious states.

**impaired parent** Parent whose nurturing capabilities are compromised or absent, related to psychiatric or substance abuse disorders.

**incidence** The rate at which a certain condition occurs, as the number of new cases of a specific mental disorder occurring during a certain period.

**independence** Taking actions for one's behalf, rather than asking others to do so.

**individual responsibility** Owning one's tasks, needs, feelings, and thoughts and taking action to address these responsibilities and needs.

**indoklon therapy** Convulsive therapy similar to electroconvulsive therapy (ECT); however, convulsions are induced by ether rather than by electrical stimulus.

**informed consent** Providing the patient with information about a specific treatment, including its benefits, side effects, and possible risks, that will enable him or her to make a competent and voluntary decision.

**insight** Recognition of motivational sources behind one's thoughts, actions, or behavior.

**insomnia** Inability to sleep or disrupted sleep patterns.

**intellectual functioning** Individual's general fund of knowledge, orientation, memory, mastery of simple mathematical equations, and capacity for abstract thinking.

**intellectualization** An (unconscious) defense mechanism; a process of thinking excessively about the philosophical or theoretical basis of a subject to the extent that anxiety-provoking issues are avoided.

**internal capsule** Broad band of myelinated fibers that separate the lentiform nuclei from the caudate nucleus and thalamus. Corticospinal (motor or pyramidal) tracts travel through the internal capsule, cerebral peduncles, and cerebral pyramids into the spinal cord, where they constitute the lateral corticospinal pathway. Damage to any of these structures can result in hemiparesis or hemiplegia.

**involuntary commitment** Commitment status in which a person who has the legal capacity to consent to mental health treatment refuses to do so and is involuntarily detained for treatment by the state.

**ipsilateral** Same side of body.

**irrational beliefs** Beliefs that are not logical but that influence feelings and behaviors.

**judgment and comprehension** Ability to understand, recall, mobilize, and constructively integrate previous learning in meeting new situations.

**kinesics** Study of body movements.

**Korsakoff's psychosis** Organic mental disorder with memory loss related to alcohol abuse.

**Kraepelin** German psychiatrist who initiated a classification system for psychiatry in 1896. He used the term *dementia praecox.*

**labile** Mood, affect, or behavior that is subject to frequent or unpredictable changes.

**least restrictive alternative** Environment that provides the necessary treatment requirements in the least restrictive setting possible. For example, a hospital setting is more restrictive than a board-and-care setting. If the board-and-care setting provides the necessary treatment requirements for a person, then that environment represents the least restrictive alternative.

**lentiform nuclei** Putamen and globus pallidus of the basal ganglia.

**lesion** Injury to tissue.

**Lewy bodies** Eosinophilic cytoplasmic inclusions seen in neuromelanin-containing neurons in Parkinson's disease.

**limit setting** Holding individuals to established norms with the intent of assisting them to function more constructively.

**limited or special power of attorney** Written document in which one person, the principal, authorizes another person, the attorney-in-fact, to act on the principal's behalf. In a limited power of attorney, the attorney-in-fact is granted only those powers specifically defined in the document.

**lipid solubility** Ability of a substance to dissolve in fat.

**lithium** Element or salt used in the treatment and prevention of manic episodes.

**locus ceruleus** Small nucleus ("blue spot") in the pontine tegmentum whose neurons are the major source of norepinephrine in the brain; present bilaterally.

**loose association** Pattern of speech in which a person's ideas slip off track onto another that

is completely unrelated or only slightly related.

**magical thinking** Belief that thoughts, words, or actions can cause or prevent an occurrence by some magical means.

**malingering** Deliberate feigning of an illness.

**malpractice** Negligence by a professional. Malpractice is a civil action that can be brought against a nurse if he or she has breached a standard of care that a reasonably prudent nurse would meet.

**managed care** Health care system that arranges the relationship among payers, providers, and consumers; monitors and influences the behavior of the mental health providers and the outcomes of care, and reimburses for services.

**mania** Disordered mental state of extreme excitement, hyperactivity, euphoria, and hyperverbal behavior.

**master-servant rule** As applied to the employer-employee relationship, this rule holds the employer responsible for the acts of employees as long as the employees are acting within the scope of their employment or authority.

**medially** Toward the midline.

**medulla** Approximately 3 cm long; the most caudal portion of the brainstem. It controls respiration and supplies innervation to the tongue and palate.

**melancholic depression** Subgroup generally seen in older individuals, often misdiagnosed as dementia; more often associated with dexamethasone nonsuppression. Depression usually worse in the morning, early morning awakening, psychomotor retardation or agitation, excessive or inappropriate guilt, and significant anorexia or weight loss are symptoms of melancholia.

**memory** Function by which information stored in the brain is later recalled to the conscious mind.

**meninges** Outer lining of the CNS composed of the dura mater, arachnoid, and pia mater.

**mental disorder** Disorder defined by the *DSM-IV-TR* as "A clinically significant behavioral or psychological syndrome or pattern . . . associated with present distress or disability."

**mental retardation** Lack of intelligence so great that it interferes with social and occupational performance.

**mental status examination (MSE)** Record of current findings that includes a description of a patient's appearance, behavior, motor activity, speech, alertness, mood, cognition, intelligence, reactions, views, and attitudes.

**meridian** Lines in a body that are representative of psychological or physical body functions. Cultural healers stimulate meridians and release harmful toxins or illness-producing spirits through the use of alternative treatment approaches such as moxibustion, cupping, coining, or skin scraping.

**mesocortical tract** Dopaminergic tract that projects from the ventral tegmental area near the substantia nigra to the neocortex, particularly the prefrontal cortex; involved in motivation, planning, behavior, attention, and social behavior.

**mesolimbic tract** Catecholaminergic neuronal tract (mostly dopaminergic) with cell bodies located in the ventral tegmental area of the midbrain and axons that project to the hippocampus, entorhinal cortex, amygdala, anterior cingulate gyrus, nucleus accumbens, and other limbic regions.

**metabolic tolerance** Process that occurs when the body is more efficient at metabolizing a substance.

**midbrain** Most rostral division of the brainstem. It contains important structures such as the cerebral aqueduct, superior and inferior colliculi, red nuclei, substantia nigra, cerebral peduncles, and oculomotor and trochlear cranial nerve nuclei.

**milieu** Environment or setting.

**milieu management** Purposeful manipulation of the environment to promote a therapeutic atmosphere.

**milieu therapy** Use of the environment to promote optimal functioning in a group or individual.

**minority** Social, religious, ethnic, occupational, or other group that constitutes less than a numeric majority of the population.

**model of care** Philosophy of causative and curative factors of mental illness that drives the nature of the care activities offered.

**monoamine oxidase** Enzyme that metabolizes monoamines such as dopamine, norepinephrine, and serotonin.

**monoamine(s)** Category of neurotransmitters that contain one amino group and are derived from amino acids. Subcategories of monoamines include the catecholamines (dopamine, norepinephrine, epinephrine), which are derived from tyrosine, and the indolamine serotonin, which is derived from tryptophan. Histamine is categorized as a monoamine but is biochemically different. Monoamine-synthesizing neurons are primarily found in the brainstem but have a wide net of influence because of the ubiquitous distribution of their axonal projections.

**monoamine oxidase inhibitors (MAOIs)** Antidepressant drugs that increase the bioavailability of certain neurotransmitters by interfering with their metabolism.

**mood** Individual's internal state of mind that is exhibited through feelings and emotions.

**mood disorder** Diagnostic category in the *DSM-IV-TR* that includes the affective disorders.

**mood disorder as a result of a general medical condition** Disorder resulting in a disturbance or alteration of a person's mood that is the result of a specific medical and/or physiologic condition.

**moxibustion** Alternative cultural medical treatment approach that uses moxa and heat to release illness-producing spirits from the body, mind, or spirit.

**mutism** Refusal to speak.

**NANDA** North American Nursing Diagnosis Association.

**narcissism** Extreme self-centeredness and self-absorption (narcissistic personality disorder).

**narcotherapy** Induction of a state of sedation by intravenous administration of sedatives (e.g., amobarbital) or stimulants (e.g., methylphenidate).

**National Institute of Mental Health** Government organization in the National Institutes of Health concerned with mental health issues in the United States.

**natural cause of illness** Belief that everyone and everything in the world is interrelated and that a disruption of this connectedness causes illness or disease.

**nature argument** This argument proposes that a specific mental disorder is caused by biological factors (e.g., neurotransmitter irregularities, pathoanatomy) rather than by psychodynamic factors (e.g., related to upbringing, life events, or other stressors).

**naturopathic physician** Alternative care practitioner who holds a doctor of naturopathy (ND) degree.

**naturopathy** Discipline that views disease as a manifestation of alterations in the processes by which the body naturally heals itself and emphasizes health restoration rather than disease treatment. Naturopathic physicians use an array of healing practices that include diet and clinical nutrition; homeopathy; acupuncture; herbal medicine; hydrotherapy (use of water in a range of temperatures and methods of applications); spinal and soft tissue manipulation; physical therapies involving electric currents; ultrasound and light therapies; therapeutic counseling; and pharmacology.

**negativism** Motiveless resistance to all instruction.

**negligence** Failure to do that which a reasonably prudent and careful person would do under the circumstances, or doing what a reasonable and prudent person would not do.

**neologism** New word created by the patient for psychological reasons; noted in some types of schizophrenia.

**neurofibrillary tangle** Mass of abnormal filamentous material located within the cell body of neurons. These tangles occur in several brain disorders, such as Alzheimer's disease, and are composed of cytoskeletal components.

**neuroleptic** Antipsychotic medication.

**neuron** Nerve cell.

**neurotransmitter** Chemical found in the nervous system (e.g., norepinephrine, serotonin, dopamine) that facilitates the transmission of nerve impulses across synapses between neurons.

**nihilistic ideas** Thoughts of nonexistence and hopelessness.

**noncompliance** Failure to take medication as prescribed.

**nonviolence** Solving conflictual situations by methods other than verbal or physical aggression.

**norepinephrine** Catecholamine neurotransmitter that is primarily synthesized in neurons of the locus ceruleus in the pons. Deficiencies of norepinephrine are linked to depression.

**norm** Expected behavior for a given therapeutic setting.

**nucleus accumbens** This nucleus is adjacent to the medial and ventral portions of the caudate and putamen. The neurons in this nucleus project to both the globus pallidus and the substantia nigra; a major component of the "reward pathway."

**nucleus basalis of Meynert** Located bilaterally, directly beneath the anterior commissure, it is the major brain site for the production of acetylcholine. Fibers from this nucleus project diffusely to the cerebral cortex.

**nurse-patient interaction** Purposeful use of the relationship between the patient and nurse for achieving patient treatment goals.

**nursing diagnosis** Statement that describes a patient's potential or actual problem or response to illness treatable by nurses.

**nurture argument** This argument proposes that a specific mental disorder is caused by psychodynamic factors (e.g., related to upbringing, life events, or other stressors) rather than by biological factors (e.g., neurotransmitter irregularities, pathoanatomy).

**obesity** Abnormal increase in the proportion of fat cells, mainly in the viscera and subcutaneous tissues of the body.

**objectivity** Process of remaining open, unbiased, and emotionally separate from a patient.

**obsession** Pathologic persistence of an unwilled thought, feeling, or impulse to the extent that it cannot be eliminated from consciousness by logical effort.

**obsessive-compulsive disorder** Disorder in which recurrent obsessions (thoughts) alternate with compulsions (behaviors). Both are unwilled.

**occupational therapy** Uses the activities of daily living to help people with mental disabilities achieve maximum functioning and independence at home and in the workplace.

**oculogyric crisis** Involuntary tonic muscle spasms of the eye. The eyes usually roll upward in a fixed stare. This very frightening dystonic reaction is caused by antipsychotic drugs.

**olfactory** Pertaining to the sense of smell.

**open posture** Relaxed yet attentive position with arms uncrossed; enhances patient's trust in the examiner.

**open-ended statement** Statement that elicits further exploration of the patient's problem by encouraging communication; can also be in the form of a question.

**openness** Atmosphere in which people are free to express their thoughts and feelings without fear of ridicule or censure.

**opportunistic illnesses** Illnesses that develop when the immune system is inactive or suppressed.

**organic mental disorders** Class of disorders of mental functioning caused by permanent brain damage or temporary brain dysfunction. The cause is known and might be primary (originating in the brain) or secondary to systemic disease. Cognition, emotions, and motivation are affected. The *DSM-IV-TR* uses the term *cognitive disorder*.

**orientation** Conscious awareness of person, place, and time.

**panic** State of extreme, acute, intense anxiety, accompanied by disorganization of personality and function.

**paranoia** Extreme suspiciousness of others and their actions.

**paranoid thinking** Oversuspicious thinking that might lead to persecutory delusions or projectile behavior patterns.

**parkinsonism** Cause (e.g., brain injury, antipsychotic drugs, carbon monoxide) of parkinsonism symptoms are known or suspected.

**parkinsonism symptoms** Masked facies, muscle rigidity, and shuffling gait. Symptoms are common in patients taking neuroleptic drugs; EPSEs are related to dopamine blockade.

**Parkinson's disease** Also known as *idiopathic parkinsonism*, where the cause is unknown. It pathologically presents as a loss of dopaminergic neurons in the substantia nigra and clinically exhibits a variety of motor and nonmotor signs and symptoms.

**partial seizure** Usually involves one hemisphere of the brain at the onset of the seizure.

**passive aggression** Anger expressed indirectly through subtle and evasive ways.

**pedophilia** Intense sexual arousal or desire and acts, fantasies, or other stimuli involving children.

**perception** Awareness of objects and relationships that follows stimulation of peripheral sense organs.

**perseveration** Psychopathologic repetition of the same word or idea in response to different questions.

**personal control** Exerting limits on one's own impulses to act in a manner that is contrary to one's best interests, treatment goals, or personal needs.

**personality disorder** Exaggerated, pathologic behavior patterns destructive to the individual and others.

**pervasive developmental disorder (PDD)** Any one of several conditions characterized by multiple social and cognitive delays.

**petit mal seizure** Variant of absence seizures characterized by three spikes per second and a wave electroencephalogram (EEG) pattern.

**pharmacodynamic tolerance** Tolerance seen when higher blood levels are required to produce a given effect.

**phobia** Exaggerated, pathologic dread or fear of some specific type of stimulus or situation.

**phobic disorder** Severe phobic behavior patterns that render the individual dysfunctional. Avoidance of the feared object or situation serves to assuage anxiety.

**physical or emotional security** Feeling safe from emotional, verbal, and physical assault.

**polymerase chain reaction (PCR)** Laboratory technique using molecular biology to identify the nucleic acid sequence of HIV in the cells of an infected individual; used in the early detection of perinatally exposed infants and in monitoring persons on clinical trials.

**postpartum depression** Subgroup of depression in the postpartum period occurring 30 days or less after childbirth.

**posttramantic stress disorder** development of characteristics symptoms (e.g., intense fear, helplessness, reexperiencing of events) following exposure to an extreme traumatic stressor.

**preconscious** Memories that can be recalled to consciousness with some effort.

**precursor** Something that precedes. Tyrosine is a precursor to dopamine in the synthesis of dopamine in the body.

**premorbid** State before onset of the disorder.

**prevalence** Estimate of the frequency of a disease condition in the population (e.g., ADHD affects 5% to 11% of school-age children).

**primary appraisal** Judgment an individual makes about an event.

**primary gain** Relief or expression of anxiety through impairment of disorder.

**privacy** Allowance of physical and emotional space for self and others.

**probable cause** Sufficient credible facts that would induce a reasonably intelligent and prudent person to believe that a cause of action exists.

**process recording** Written record of an encounter with a patient that is as nearly verbatim as possible, including both verbal and nonverbal behaviors of the nurse and the patient.

**professional chaplain** Also known as a spiritual care professional; one who has extensive postgraduate clinical training to offer spiritual care within a health care organization.

**projective identification** Placement of feelings on another to justify one's own expression of feelings.

**proxemics** Study of how people perceive and use environmental, social, and personal space in interactions with others.

**pseudodementia** A depressive condition of the elderly characterized by impaired cognitive function.

**psychiatric rehabilitation** Promotion of the patient's highest level of functioning in the least restrictive environment.

**psychoeducation** Strategy of teaching patients and families about disorders, treatments, coping techniques, and resources, based on the observation that people can be more effective participants in their own care if they have knowledge.

**psychomotor retardation** Markedly slowed speech and body movements.

**psychoneuroimmunology** Field of research focusing on the interactions of mind, environment, and bodily function, particularly immune system function.

**psychopathology** Study of underlying processes, both biological and psychosocial, that lead to mental disorders.

**psychosis** Inability to recognize reality, complicated by severe thought disorders and the inability to relate to others.

**psychosocial adversity** Environmental conditions such as poverty, unemployment, or overcrowded living conditions that do not support optimal development of a child.

**psychotherapeutic management** Model for nursing care that balances the three primary intervention models used by psychiatric nurses: therapeutic nurse-patient relationship, psychopharmacology, and milieu management.

**psychotic depression** Subtype of depression, in which a person experiences delusions and hallucinations; often misdiagnosed as schizophrenia or schizoaffective disorder.

**psychotropic drugs** Medications used in the treatment of mental illness.

**purge** Compensation for calories consumed by self-induced vomiting, laxative abuse, diuretics, or enemas.

**pyramidal system** Motor system for voluntary movement.

**race** Breeding population that primarily mates within itself.

**raphe nuclei** Nuclei located along the midline of the brainstem (*raphe,* seam). Serotonin is synthesized from these cells.

**reactive depression** Depressed mood related to some life event (e.g., divorce, losing one's job).

**reappraisal** Appraisal made after new or additional information has been received.

**receptor** A specialized area on a nerve membrane, blood vessel, or muscle that receives the chemical stimulation to activate or inhibit normal actions of nerves, blood vessels, or muscles.

**recreational therapist** Assists patients in finding leisure interests so that they can learn to balance work and play.

**relational worldview** Perception of the world grounded in the belief in spirituality and the significance of relationships and interactions among individuals.

**religion** Defined structures, rituals, beliefs, and values through which communities frequently address spiritual concerns.

**religiosity** Preoccupation with religious ideas or content.

**resiliency** Capability to withstand stressors without permanent dysfunction or developmental delay.

**respect for the individual** Acknowledgment and allowance of the rights of others to be unique.

**restraint** Physical control of a patient to prevent injury to the patient, staff, and other patients.

**reuptake** Physiologic process that occurs when a neurotransmitter is taken up into the presynaptic neuron after having been released into the synapse. Some psychotropic drugs are designed to prevent the reuptake of a specific neurotransmitter to increase the synaptic presence of that neurotransmitter.

**rigidity** Assumption of an inappropriate posture.

**satisfaction** Relaxation of the tension of physiologic needs.

**schizophrenia** Syndrome, illness, or mental health disorder heterogeneous in cause, pathogenesis, presenting picture, response to treatment, and prognosis. Symptoms generally reflect a progressive deterioration and disorganization of the individual's personality structure, affect, and cognition. The *DSM-IV-TR* lists the following types: paranoid, catatonic, disorganized, undifferentiated, and residual.

**scientific cause of illness** Belief that there are specific concrete explanations for every illness and disease. This explanation involves the entrance of pathogens such as viruses, bacteria, and germs into the body.

**seasonal affective disorder (SAD)** Subtype of depression occurring in late autumn or winter and lasting until spring.

**seclusion** Process of placing a patient alone in a specially designed room for protection and close observation.

**secondary appraisal** Evaluation an individual makes about potential actions to be taken.

**secondary gain** Attention and support received from others while ill.

**selective serotonin reuptake inhibitors (SSRIs)** Class of antidepressants; potent blockers of serotonin reuptake, thus increasing the level of serotonin in the synapse.

**serotonin (5-HT)** Monoamine neurotransmitter from the indolamine family. It is derived from the amino acid tryptophan. Deficiencies of serotonin are linked to depression.

**shuffling gait (parkinsonan gait)** Style of walking typically demonstrated by individuals whose dopamine stores have been blocked or depleted as a result of Parkinson's disease or antipsychotic medications.

**smudging** Common sacred rite of purification and cleansing practiced by many Native American nations. It includes the burning of cedar and sage for the purpose of fanning smoke with an eagle feather over or near the patient. It is seen as purifying the spirit and preparing the patient for a difficult spiritual journey such as illness or death, and is also used for other spiritual rituals.

**social organization** Culture around particular units, such as family, racial, or ethnic groups; religious groups; and community or social groups.

**social skills group** Group that helps psychiatric patients learn, practice, and develop skills for dealing with people in social situations.

**socialization skills** Skills necessary for negotiating daily interpersonal issues (e.g., acknowledging responsibility for one's behavior, using eye contact appropriately, interacting with others for purposes of sharing and support).

**somatic therapy** Therapeutic approach that uses physiologic or physical interventions to effect behavioral changes. For example, electroconvulsive therapy is a somatic treatment.

**somatization** Conversion of mental states or experiences into bodily symptoms; associated with anxiety.

**soul** Nonphysical, transcendent part of human beings involving their mind and will.

**space** Refers to distance and intimacy needs of culturally unique individuals in human interaction.

**spirituality** Awareness of relationships with all creation, an appreciation of presence and purpose that goes beyond the five senses and the physical world; includes a sense of meaning and belonging. It is often inclusive of religion.

**splitting** Inability to integrate good and bad aspects of self and others; person views self and others as all good or all bad.

**status epilepticus** Repetitive seizures; usually refers to repetitive grand mal seizures.

**statutory law** Statutory law is written law emanating from a legislative body. These laws are written by state and federal legislative authorities and passed in accordance with state and federal law.

**steady state** Desired state in anticonvulsant and other therapies, when the serum concentration of the drug is consistent and is maintained at a therapeutic level.

**step system** Process by which inpatients gain privileges and responsibilities based on their progress.

**stereotyping** Assumption that all people in similar cultural, racial, ethnic or other groups think and act alike.

**stereotypy** Continuous repetition of speech or physical activities.

**stressor** Stimulus perceived by the individual or the organism as challenging, threatening, or damaging.

**striatum** Basal ganglia that include the caudate and putamen.

**substance-induced mood disorder** Disorder that results from the disturbance or alteration of a person's mood caused by the ingestion of a prescribed or nonprescribed drug or medication or by exposure to a toxic substance.

substantia nigra Literally, black substance; a pigmented area of the midbrain where dopamine is synthesized.

suicidal ideation Individual's thinking about and inclination toward self-injury or self-destruction.

suicidal plan Specific method designed to inflict self-injury or self-destruction as verbalized by an individual.

suicide Self-inflicted death.

sulcus Groove separating gyri. Deep sulci are referred to as fissures.

superego Psychoanalytic structure of the mind equivalent to the conscience (sense of right and wrong). It develops in early childhood and provides the ego with an inner control to help cope with the id.

synapse Microscopic space between two neurons.

tangentiality Inability to have goal-directed associations of thought; never gets to desired goal from desired point.

tardive dyskinesia Extrapyramidal syndrome that usually emerges late in the course of long-term antipsychotic drug therapy; includes grimacing, buccolingual movements, and dystonia (impaired muscle tonus); might be irreversible.

teamwork Staff working together to achieve agreed-on goals for the unit and for patient care.

terror State of extreme tension.

theist One who believes in God, without necessarily conforming to a particular set of religious beliefs; from the Greek word for God, *theos*.

therapeutic In the psychotherapeutic management model, it is the communication of respect, a desire to help, and understanding to another person. Understanding includes knowledge of mental mechanisms, coping strategies, and stressors. Active listening is a crucial component of being therapeutic.

therapeutic communication Interactive verbal and nonverbal strategies that focus on the needs of the patient and facilitate a goal-directed, patient-oriented communication process.

therapeutic listening Listening that is focused on the patient and obtains therapeutically useful information about the patient.

therapeutic milieu Treatment environment managed in such a way that the environment itself is therapeutic.

therapy Means, usually with words, to cure or manage the course of another person's mental disorder. Nurses who practice psychotherapy are trained in a specific therapy model (e.g., psychoanalysis, cognitive therapy).

thinking Process of following a goal-directed flow of ideas, symbols, and associations to a logical conclusion in accordance with the person's developmental stage.

thought disorder Thinking characterized by loose associations, neologisms, and illogical constructs and conclusions.

time Either a physical quantity measured by a clock or patterns and orientations that relate to social processes.

time-out Disengaging the child from a specific situation (e.g., directing the child to sit in a chair facing away from other patients so that the child might regain self-control).

tolerance Need for increasing amounts of a substance to achieve the same effects.

tonic State of continuous tension.

transference Unconscious emotional reaction to a current situation that is actually based on previous experiences.

tricyclic antidepressants (TCAs) Drug classification of antidepressants that block the reuptake of norepinephrine and serotonin into the presynaptic neuron.

tuberoinfundibular tract Dopaminergic system with neurons in the arcuate nucleus of the hypothalamus that project to the pituitary stalk. This tract controls the secretion of prolactin.

tyramine Substance derived from the amino acid tyrosine and found in many common foods, such as aged cheeses, yogurt, and avocados. Tyramine-rich foods can cause a hypertensive crisis in a person being treated with MAOIs.

tyrosine Amino acid that is the precursor to dopamine.

unconscious Memories, conflicts, experiences, and materials that have been repressed and cannot be recalled at will.

undoing Defense mechanism by which a person symbolically acts out to reverse a previously committed act or thought; a common ritual in obsessive-compulsive disorder.

unit norm Expected behavior for a given therapeutic setting.

unnatural cause of illness Belief that outside forces such as a spell or a hex being cast on the sick person are the cause or the source of illness or disease.

validation Process of confirming an individual's intent by questioning the content of his or her message.

vascular dementia Results from the interruption of blood flow to the brain, which causes anoxia, ischemia, and subsequent infarction.

ventral tegmental area (VTA) Located in the midbrain, this region is dorsomedial to the substantia nigra and ventral to the red nuclei. The nuclei in this area produce dopamine. The efferent pathways from the VTA include the mesocortical and mesolimbic tracts.

ventricle System of connected brain cavities that are filled with cerebrospinal fluid, including the lateral ventricles (in the central portion of the telencephalon), the third ventricle (which runs between the thalami), the fourth ventricle (in the pons and medulla), and the connecting cerebral aqueduct (in the midbrain).

vesicle Storage sac at the synaptic terminal.

voluntary commitment Situation whereby the patient or his or her conservator or guardian requests psychiatric treatment and signs an application for that treatment. This person is also free to sign himself or herself out of the hospital.

Wernicke's area Sophisticated auditory association cortex located within the planum temporale that interprets spoken language.

Wernicke's encephalopathy Confusion and ophthalmoplegia caused by thiamine deficiency; most common in alcoholics. It results in necrosis and hemorrhage in the mammillary bodies and periventricular structures of the brainstem.

Western medicine Conventional clinicians use this term to describe the medicine practiced by the holders of Doctor of Medicine (MD) or Doctor of Osteopathy (DO) degrees, some of whom might also practice complementary and alternative medicines. Other terms for conventional medicine are allopathic medicine, regular medicine, mainstream medicine, and biomedicine.

white matter Substance in the brain composed of myelinated neuronal axons.

withdrawal (1) Act or process of turning inward to avoid a perceived environmental threat; (2) physiologic response to cessation of an addictive substance.

word salad Incoherent mixture of words or phrases.

# Index

Page references followed by "f" indicate figures, "t" indicate tables, and "b" indicate boxes.

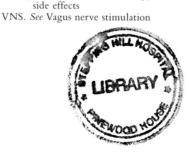
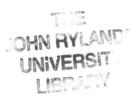

# NANDA-International Approved Nursing Diagnoses, 2005-2006

Activity intolerance
Activity intolerance, risk for
Airway clearance, ineffective
Allergy response, latex
Allergy response, latex, risk for
Anxiety
Anxiety, death
Aspiration, risk for
Attachment, impaired parent/infant/child, risk for
Autonomic dysreflexia
Autonomic dysreflexia, risk for

Body image, disturbed
Body temperature, imbalanced, risk for
Bowel incontinence
Breastfeeding, effective
Breastfeeding, ineffective
Breastfeeding, interrupted
Breathing pattern, ineffective

Cardiac output, decreased
Caregiver role strain
Caregiver role strain, risk for
Comfort, impaired
Communication, verbal, impaired
Communication, readiness for enhanced
Conflict, decisional (specify)
Conflict, parental role
Confusion, acute
Confusion, acute, risk for
Confusion, chronic
Constipation
Constipation, perceived
Constipation, risk for
Contamination
Contamination, risk for
Coping, community, ineffective
Coping, community, readiness for enhanced
Coping, defensive
Coping, family, compromised
Coping, family, disabled
Coping, family, readiness for enhanced
Coping, ineffective
Coping, readiness for enhanced

Death syndrome, sudden infant, risk for
Decision making, readiness for enhanced
Denial, ineffective
Dentition, impaired
Development, delayed, risk for
Diarrhea
Disuse syndrome, risk for
Diversional activity, deficient

Energy field, disturbed
Environmental intrpretation syndrome, impaired

Failure to thrive, adult
Falls, risk for
Family processes: alcoholism, dysfunctional
Family processes, interrupted
Family processes, readiness for enhanced
Fatigue
Fear
Feeding pattern, infant, ineffective
Fluid balance, readiness for enhanced
Fluid volume, deficient
Fluid volume, excess
Fluid volume, deficient, risk for
Fluid volume, imbalanced, risk for

Gas exchange, impaired
Glucose level, unstable, risk for
Grieving
Grieving, anticipatory
Grieving, complicated, risk for
Grieving, dysfunctional
Growth and development, delayed
Growth disproportionate, risk for

Health behavior, prone, risk for
Health maintenance, ineffective
Health-seeking behaviors
Home maintenance, impaired
Hopelessness
Human dignity, compromised, risk for
Hyperthermia
Hypothermia

Identity, personal, disturbed
Incontinence, urinary, functional
Incontinence, urinary, overflow
Incontinence, urinary, reflex
Incontinence, urinary, stress
Incontinence, urinary, total

From NANDA International: *NANDA nursing diagnoses: definitions and classifications, 2005-2006*, Philadelphia, 2005, NANDA International.